Contents

Colour plates in this volume

Figure 1.14 is reproduced with the permission of NeuroCom International Inc., 9570 SE Lawnfield Road, Clackamas, OR 97015-9611, USA

Contributors to this volume

Robert H. Ballagh MD, FRCS(C)
Consultant Otolaryngologist and Neurologist, Royal
Victoria Hospital, Barrie, Ontario, Canada; Formerly
Fellow in Neuro-otology and Skull Base Surgery,
Addenbrookes Hospital, Cambridge

John B. Booth MB, BS(Lond), FRCS, MRAeS, AKC
Consultant Otologist and Neuro-otologist,
St Bartholomew's Hospital and the Royal London
Hospital; Formerly Consultant, the Royal National
Throat, Nose and Ear Hospital, London; Civil
Consultant (Otology), Royal Air Force; Hunterian
Professor, Royal College of Surgeons of England;
Former Editor, *Journal of Laryngology and Otology*;
Honorary Member, American Otological Society

Gerald B. Brookes MB, ChB(Sheff), FRCS
Consultant ENT and Neuro-otological Surgeon, The
National Hospital for Neurology and Neurosurgery,
London and The Royal National Throat, Nose and
Ear Hospital; Honorary Senior Lecturer, Institute of
Neurology and Institute of Laryngology and
Otology, London

G. G. Browning MD, FRCS(Ed and Glas)
Professor of Otolaryngology, University of Glasgow;
Consultant in Administrative Charge, Department of
Otolaryngology, Royal Infirmary, Glasgow;
Consultant Otologist, Scottish Section, MRC
Institute of Hearing Research

J. E. T. Byrne MB, BCh, BAO(Dub), FRCSI
Consultant Ear, Nose and Throat Surgeon, Belfast
City Hospital

R. J. Canter MB, BS(Lond), FRCS(Eng), FRCS(Otol)
Consultant Otolaryngologist, Royal United Hospital,
Bath; Honorary Senior Lecturer, Postgraduate
School of Medicine, University of Bath

A. D. Cheesman BSc, MB, BS(Lond), FRCS
Consultant Otolaryngologist, Charing Cross Hospital
and the Royal National Throat, Nose and Ear
Hospital, London; Hunterian Professor, Royal
College of Surgeons of England

A. Forge BSc, MSc, PhD
Reader in Auditory Cell Biology, Institute of
Laryngology and Otology and University College,
London

I. Friedmann DSc, MD, FRCS, FRCPath
Emeritus Professor of Pathology, University of
London; Formerly Director, Department of
Pathology, Institute of Laryngology and Otology,
London; Honorary Consultant Pathologist, the
Royal National Throat, Nose and Ear Hospital and
Northwick Park Hospital and Clinical Centre;
Research Fellow, Imperial Cancer Research Fund
Laboratories, London; Visiting Professor of
Pathology, University of California, San Francisco,
Los Angeles and University of Colorado, Denver;
Consultant in Electron Microscopy, House Ear
Institute, University of Southern California, Los
Angeles, USA

Nicholas J. Frootko MB, ChB(Wits), MSc(Oxford), FRCS
Consultant Otolaryngologist, Whipps Cross Hospital,
London; Formerly Clinical Lecturer in
Otolaryngology, University of Oxford

R. R. Gacek MD, FACS
Professor and Chairman, Department of
Otolaryngology and Communication Sciences,
SUNY Health Sciences Center, USA

W. P. R. Gibson MD(Lond), FRCS, FRACS
Professor of Otolaryngology, The University of
Sydney, Australia; Formerly Consultant Neuro-
otologist, National Hospital for Nervous Diseases
and the Royal National Throat, Nose and Ear
Hospital, London

A. G. Kerr FRCS
Consultant Otolaryngologist, Royal Victoria
Hospital, Belfast and Belfast City Hospital; Formerly
Professor of Otorhinolaryngology, The Queen's
University, Belfast

B. Kotecha MB, BCh(Wales), FRCS, MPhil, DLO
Consultant ENT Surgeon, the Royal National
Throat, Nose and Ear Hospital, London

Harold Ludman MA(Camb), MB, FRCS
Consultant Otolaryngologist, King's College
Hospital, London; Consultant Surgeon in Neuro-
otology, National Hospital for Neurology and
Neurosurgery, London

Mark May MD, FACS
Clinical Professor, Department of Otolaryngology –
Head and Neck Surgery, University of Pittsburgh
School of Medicine; Director, Facial Paralysis Center,
Shadyside Hospital, Pittsburgh, Pennsylvania, USA

R. P. Mills MPhil, MS, FRCS
Consultant ENT Surgeon, Ninewells Hospital,
Dundee; Honorary Senior Lecturer, University of
Dundee

David A. Moffat BSc(Lond), MA(Camb), MB, BS(Lond), FRCS
Consultant Otoneurosurgeon, Addenbrookes
Hospital, Cambridge; Associate Lecturer, University
of Cambridge; Formerly Consultant ENT Surgeon,
Westminster Hospital, London; Honorary Member,
American Otological Society

A. Fitzgerald O'Connor MB, ChB(Birm), FRCS
Consultant Otolaryngologist, St Thomas' Hospital,
London

P. D. Phelps MD, FRCS, FFR, FRCR, DMRD
Consultant Radiologist, the Royal National Throat,
Nose and Ear Hospital, London

Richard T. Ramsden MB, ChB(StAnd), FRCS
Professor of Otolaryngology, Manchester Royal
Infirmary

Barry Schaitkin MD, FACS
Assistant Professor, Department of Otolaryngology –
Head and Neck Surgery, University of Pittsburgh
School of Medicine; Co-Director, Facial Paralysis
Center, Shadyside Hospital, Pittsburgh,
Pennsylvania, USA

O. H. Shaheen MS(Lond), FRCS
Consultant ENT Surgeon, The London Bridge
Hospital, London; formerly Consultant ENT
Surgeon, Guy's Hospital, London

Gordon D. L. Smyth DSc, MCh, MD(Belf), FRCS, DLO†
Formerly Consultant ENT Surgeon, Eye and Ear
Clinic, Royal Victoria Hospital, Belfast

J. G. Toner MB, BCh, BAO(Belf), FRCS
Consultant Otolaryngologist, Belfast City Hospital,
Belfast

H. Weerda MD, DMD
Director, Ear, Nose and Throat Clinic, University of
Lübeck, Germany

Carol Wengraf MB, BS(Lond), FRCS
Consultant Otolaryngologist, Royal Hull Hospitals
Trust, Hull

A. Wright MA, DM, FRCS, TechRMS, LLM
Professor of Otorhinolaryngology; Head of
Department, Institute of Laryngology and Otology,
London

David Wright MA(Camb), FRCS
Consultant Otolaryngologist, The Royal Surrey
County Hospital, Guildford; Honorary Consultant
Otolaryngologist to the Cambridge Military Hospital

Introduction

When I started work on this Sixth Edition I did so in the belief that my experience with the Fifth Edition would make it straightforward. I was wrong. The production of the Fifth Edition was hectic and the available time short. The contributors and volume editors were very productive and in under two and a half years we produced what we, and happily most reviewers, considered to be a worthwhile academic work. On this occasion, with a similar team, we allowed ourselves more time and yet have struggled to produce in four years. One is tempted to blame the health service reforms but that would be unfair. They may have contributed but the problems were certainly much wider than these.

The volume editors, already fully committed clinically, have again been outstanding both in their work and in their understanding of the difficulties we have encountered. Once again there was an excellent social spirit among the editors. They have been very tolerant of the innumerable telephone calls and it has always been a pleasure to work with them. The contributors have also been consistently pleasant to deal with, even those who kept us waiting.

There have been technical problems in the production of this work and I want to pay tribute to the patience of all those who suffered under these, not least the publishing staff at Butterworth-Heinemann. One of the solutions to the problems has been the use of a system of pagination that I consider to be ugly and inefficient for the user and I wish to apologize in advance for this. Unfortunately anything else would have resulted in undue delay in the publication date.

Medicine is a conservative profession and many of us dislike change. Some will feel that we have moved forward in that most Latin plurals have been replaced by English, for example we now have polyps rather than polypi. We have also buried acoustic neuromata, with an appropriate headstone, and now talk about vestibular schwannomas. It has taken about two decades for this to become established in otological circles and may take even longer again, to gain everyday usage in the world of general medicine.

I am pleased with what has been produced. Some chapters have altered very little because there have been few advances in those subjects and we have resisted the temptation of change for change's sake. There have been big strides forward in other areas and these have been reflected in the appropriate chapters.

Despite, and because of, the problems in the production of these volumes, the staff at Butterworth-Heinemann have worked hard and have always been pleasant to deal with. I wish to acknowledge the co-operation from Geoff Smaldon, Deena Burgess, Anne Powell, Mary Seager and Chris Jarvis.

It would be impossible to name all those others who have helped, especially my colleagues in Belfast, but I want to pay tribute to the forbearance of my wife Paddy who graciously accepted the long hours that were needed for this work.

As I stated in my introduction to the Fifth Edition, I was very impressed by the goodwill and generosity of spirit among my Otolaryngological colleagues and am pleased that there has been no evidence of any diminution of this during the nine years between the editions. I remain pleased and proud to be a British Otolaryngologist and to have been entrusted with the production of this latest edition of our standard textbook.

Alan G. Kerr

Preface

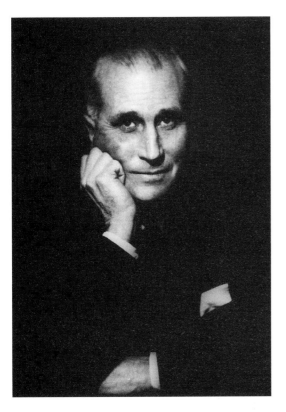

As one comes to write this Preface one is reminded that it is not only nine years since the last edition but also an exact period since Bill Scott-Brown died on 12th July 1987. Later that year in September was the memorial service to both Peggy and Bill held at the Priory Church of St Bartholomew immediately outside the hospital at which he had been a student some 70 years before. On a personal note I still miss his company, his kindness, his infectious enthusiasm and his encouragement though I still have the pleasure of seeing some of his old patients and seeing his familiar handwriting in the notes. He was a surgeon who always set himself the highest standards and every meeting we had is recalled with nostalgia. Quite apart from his surgery, he was dedicated to his wife and family, and was a consummate and passionate fisherman. When either of these left him free there was always his talent as a painter in oils or water colours but more usually pastels recalling either visits to Paris, France and elsewhere but above all his beloved Hampshire Avon and the beautiful surrounding countryside, particularly the river Test. As I now make my way to Bart's each week, I think of him frequently but always with gratitude and affection.

As for the authors of the various chapters, I have nothing but thanks and admiration for all the hard work they have put in. Their tolerance in accepting the suggestions and alterations from the Editor is much appreciated and their forbearance almost unbelievable when I am sure there must have been many occasions when they would curse under their breath. However, the ultimate objective has been to produce the very best of which we are all capable and this I hope we have gone some measure towards achieving. As previously I would like to thank the wives or partners and the families for the many hours which the contributors have put in and thereby denied themselves more humble pleasures! It is always a pleasure to thank Alan Kerr for his contribution but also for his unfailing tact when trying to apply the pressure.

Sadly, during the course of preparation, another colleague for whom I had the highest regard died. I hope that Gordon Smyth's chapter on otosclerosis will be read with lasting appreciation by all; it was written in the last year of his life, by an outstanding and truly dedicated otologist.

It is hoped that the reader will find the book both a source of information and reference and it will stand the test of time for a little while yet. Amazingly in the last edition HIV and AIDS were not even mentioned in my chapters; now their omission would be inconceivable!

John B. Booth

1

Examination of the ear

A. Fitzgerald O'Connor

The practice of medicine demands the taking of an accurate history and carrying out a careful clinical examination. This principle applies to otology as much as any other branch of medicine, and should not be forgotten in the rush for 'high technology' investigations which may be invasive and add little to the diagnostic process. The symptoms and signs associated with ear disease must be elicited, together with those which the patient may not recognize as being related to disorders of the ear.

History

Symptoms of ear disease include otalgia, discharge, disorders of auditory perception, mainly hearing loss, tinnitus, vertigo and headache.

Otalgia (see also Chapter 13)

Pain in the ear comes from pain receptors in the external or middle ear whose afferent fibres lie in the Vth, IXth and Xth cranial nerves and second and third cervical nerves.

As the skin is so closely applied to the meatal and auricular perichondrium, severe pain may be associated with an external otitis having minimal clinical signs. Senturia (1973) stated that severe otitis externa can be one of the most painful disorders known. Note must be taken of long-standing dermatitis, usually of the eczematous type. Trauma to the ear canal, when the patient attempts to remove wax, may predispose to infection but be forgotten in the history. Herpes zoster infections of the Vth and VIIth cranial nerves or the upper cervical nerves frequently begin with pain, the diagnosis only becoming apparent when the vesicular eruption on the pinna and meatus develops.

Other painful conditions of the external ear include polychondritis helicis (chondrodermatitis nodularis chronica helicis) and squamous carcinoma.

Myringitis bullosa haemorrhagica is a painful condition occurring spontaneously and resolving within several days. A vesicular eruption is seen on the tympanic membrane which may be associated with bleeding and serous discharge.

Otitis media, although a frequent cause of otalgia, is subject to overdiagnosis (Bluestone and Cantekin, 1979).

Children who have otitis media with effusion (glue ear) may have a history of previous upper respiratory tract infection and earache. Otalgia is said to occur in some children due to eustachian tube dysfunction when the middle ear pressure is markedly reduced leading to retraction of the tympanic membrane. The pain usually occurs at night when the child has been sleeping and may be due to venous congestion in the eustachian tube area with reduced frequency of swallowing and, consequently, failure of middle ear ventilation. On arising or sitting up the congestion clears, the eustachian tube opens and the pain disappears. Sometimes the child's crying, because of the pain, leads to hyperaemia of the tympanic membrane and the misdiagnosis of acute otitis media.

Sudden spontaneous resolution of pain in cases of true otitis media indicates perforation of the tympanic membrane. Pain is not a feature of chronic otitis media unless there is an associated otitis externa or more ominously dural inflammation. Less frequently, severe pain in a chronically discharging ear may reflect neoplastic change.

Pain may be referred to the ear from other areas supplied by the Vth, IXth and Xth cranial nerves and the upper cervical nerves. Thus, when otalgia is a presenting symptom and no local disease is found in the ear, a distant cause must be considered. Usual sources of referred otalgia are dental disease, lesions of the posterior tongue, pharynx and larynx.

Aural discharge (otorrhoea)

Otitis externa may present with itch and a watery odourless discharge. A clear fluid discharge from the ear after trauma may be indicative of a cerebrospinal fluid leak through a dural tear, often over the tegmen tympani and roof of the external auditory meatus.

When discharge contains mucus, it must have arisen from glands within the middle ear cleft, passing into the external auditory meatus either from an open mastoid cavity or through a tympanic membrane perforation.

A thick brown discharge of liquefied wax may occur in an otherwise healthy ear but often heralds an acute otitis media. In chronic otitis media, the discharge is often long-standing and characterized by a foul smell due to saprophytic organisms. Cholesteatomatous debris may be discharged, such patients frequently presenting because of the embarrassing nature of the smell. If it is a chronically discharging ear, the onset of bleeding may be an ominous sign, indicating the possibility of neoplastic change.

Bleeding from the ear usually follows trauma but, in rare cases, may occur from glomus tumours or vascular anomalies in the middle ear or external meatus.

Abnormalities of auditory perception

Deafness is the term most commonly used by patients to indicate an abnormality or change in their hearing acuity. Some idea of the level of hearing loss can be obtained from the history by asking about their difficulty in varying social situations. Conversation in a quiet environment is conducted around 40 dB hearing level, a doorbell output is, on average, 60 dB and conversation on the telephone between 40 and 70 dB within a limited frequency band of 200–1200 Hz. A person with a conductive loss appears to hear better in a noisy environment, usually because the speaker has raised the intensity of the voice and the masking effect of the background noise is reduced because of the hearing loss. This phenomenon is known as *paracusis Willisii* and is usually associated with otosclerosis. In sensorineural hearing loss, there is reduced discrimination of speech, particularly in background noise. The ability of a person with sensorineural deafness to discriminate speech is not necessarily helped when the speaker raises the intensity of the voice. Indeed the listener may say, 'Don't shout, I'm not deaf'.

Recruitment of loudness is characteristic of a cochlear hearing loss. A relatively small increase in the intensity of the auditory stimulus may cause frank discomfort to the listener. Poor speech discrimination without recruitment, especially if unilateral, suggests an auditory nerve lesion.

Tonal changes in auditory perception are usually expressed as 'one ear not sounding like the other' or 'tinny'. Diplacusis is the apparent difference in the pitch of a tone between the two ears and is associated with conditions causing endolymphatic hydrops.

Autophony is the abnormal perception of one's own breath and voice sounds and is often associated with a permanently open, or patulous, eustachian tube. The patient may also describe it as sounds echoing in the ear, or as if talking in a reverberating chamber.

Fluctuant hearing loss may result from disease causing either conductive or sensorineural pathology. The fluctuant nature of the hearing loss associated with upper respiratory tract infections, eustachian tube dysfunction and otitis media with effusion is well known. Menière's disease is characterized by a fluctuating sensorineural hearing loss, with the hearing deteriorating during each attack and partly recovering between attacks (Hood, 1980). In a variant of Menière's disease – Lermoyez's syndrome – the hearing drops before an attack, recovering as the vertigo begins.

Other features associated with the onset of the hearing loss should be noted. In the majority of cases of sudden deafness the cause is unknown, although many are assumed to be due to vascular disease. The deafness may be related to a recent viral infection, as seen in the classical unilateral mumps deafness. Severe infections such as meningitis and, abroad, malaria may pre-date the onset of hearing loss. Sudden deafness may be the presenting feature in up to 10% of patients with acoustic neuroma (Morrison and Booth, 1970) or be associated with a perilymph fistula resulting from an increased venous pressure due to straining or lifting.

Previous otological procedures should be noted, especially stapedectomy, which may have been performed many years previously.

It is important to enquire about a family history of hearing loss since this may reveal a hereditary cause, as in otosclerosis (Morrison and Bunday, 1970). There may be a history of noise trauma having occurred 20 or 30 years previously which has combined with the effect of ageing on the cochlea to produce a hearing disability. A clear history of occupational noise exposure and military service is required. In the UK, protection from industrial noise trauma has been supported by legislation for only a relatively short time so that many such cases still present to outpatient clinics. Social noise trauma includes pop music, rifle shooting and motor racing. Some people suffer irreversible hearing loss from relatively minor noise stimuli, whereas others are exposed to major noise trauma with little effect on their hearing.

The patient's past medical history is important since

the aminoglycoside antibiotics, used for life-threatening infections, and some of the 'loop' diuretics, are potentially ototoxic (Ballantyne and Ajodhia, 1984). It is generally considered that topical aminoglycoside antibiotics, as used in ear drops in discharging ears, do not cause hearing loss. More recently, the use of cytotoxic therapy has been implicated as cause of hearing loss. Salicylates bought 'over the counter' may be ototoxic to the susceptible user, as is quinine which used to be taken as an antimalarial drug.

In children, a history of poor speech development, lack of communication skills and education retardation may replace hearing loss as a symptom of ear disease.

Tinnitus

Tinnitus, like hearing loss, is a common presenting symptom of aural pathology. The nature of the tinnitus may be helpful in locating the lesion in the auditory pathway. A rhythmic beating or pounding tinnitus, synchronized with the pulse, is suggestive of a vascular lesion such as a glomus tumour. A dull, continuous tinnitus is sometimes found in association with a conductive hearing loss. This may represent normal noise levels in the temporal bone which have now become obvious to the patient because of the absence of the masking effect of environmental sound. Successful treatment of the conductive deafness, e.g. by stapedectomy, may alleviate this type of tinnitus. Body sounds transmitted via an abnormally patent (patulous) eustachian tube may be reported as tinnitus, and likewise the noise of a live insect in the ear canal.

Most cases are characterized by rushing, hissing or ringing sounds in the ear or head. The source of these may be in the cochlea, neural pathways or cerebral cortex.

Previous noise exposure and a history of having been given ototoxic drugs (aspirin, quinine, etc.) are important aetiological factors (Brown *et al.*, 1981; Meyerhoff *et al.*, 1983). Fluctuant tinnitus may be associated with Menière's disease and usually increases in intensity prior to a vertiginous attack, returning to its resting intensity in between.

Long-term tinnitus sufferers may well be unable to locate the offending noise in the ears and simply perceive head noise. Recognizable sounds such as voice, music and bells should not be considered to be evidence of ear disease, but more psychological, as in schizophrenia. Tinnitus, in general, may be caused by all of those agents which produce hearing loss and thus a similar history should always be taken.

Vertigo

The definition of vertigo is difficult. It may be defined as an 'hallucination of movement', i.e. the patients feel that they or their environment are moving. Elsewhere in this volume (Chapter 18), it is defined as a 'subjective sense of imbalance'.

The history is of paramount importance in making the diagnosis in cases of balance disorder. In many cases, the diagnosis can be made from the history alone. It is essential to elicit from the patient the exact sensation perceived, since the terms 'dizziness', 'vertigo' or 'light-headedness' mean different things to different people. The patient may have great difficulty describing the actual phenomenon (Hinchcliffe, 1973). This difficulty in description is a reflection of the small cortical representation of balance perception. The patient needs to rely on the mismatch of positional cues and the associated autonomic vegetative effects for their own description. It is important to identify symptoms not attributable to the vestibular system, such as the light-headedness, with blurring of consciousness, which accompanies cerebral anoxia. Anxiety states, in which the patient hyperventilates with resulting hypocarbia may also produce such symptoms (Evans and Trimm, 1966). The sensation of movement associated with vestibular lesions is most commonly rotatory, but can include swaying or tilting of either the patient or the surroundings. If nystagmus is present the environment is only perceived during the slow phase and since the images traverse the retina in the opposite direction, the environment appears to spin in the direction of the fast component. This may be useful on some occasions in trying to locate the offending labyrinth.

Peripheral lesions usually produce vertigo of sudden onset which may last for only seconds or up to a few days. In Menière's disease, the attacks are recurrent and usually associated with fluctuating hearing loss and tinnitus. Movement tends to make vertigo of peripheral origin worse. The best known example of this is the sudden onset of rotatory dizziness associated with certain head movements in patients with benign paroxysmal positional vertigo. Vertigo associated with coughing or sneezing suggests the presence of a perilymph fistula. Tullio's phenomenon is the vertigo caused by loud sounds and may be due to endolymphatic hydrops or a third labyrinthine window, as in a labyrinthine fistula (Kakkar and Hinchcliffe, 1970).

Central lesions tend to produce less intense vertigo. Positional changes have less effect, but the patient tends to have more disturbance of gait.

Vertebrobasilar ischaemia can cause sudden onset vertigo and drop attacks, without loss of consciousness, but is usually accompanied by other associated symptoms. A full medical history may reveal longstanding degenerative conditions such as diabetes mellitus or atherosclerosis. Life-threatening infections sometimes require potentially ototoxic antibiotics. Some of these, particularly gentamicin, may damage the vestibular system.

In summary, it is important to ask the patient if he

or she remembers the first attack and to describe it accurately. The onset, whether sudden or gradual, precipitating factors, duration of attack and associated symptoms are noted. The frequency and severity of attacks should be enquired about.

Oscillopsia

This descriptive term is used when the patient complains that the horizon rotates or jumps in a vertical plane when walking (Ramsden and Ackrill, 1982). Resulting spatial disorientation is corrected by the patient halting, holding on to a solid structure and focusing on a near image. It is due to an imbalance in the vestibulo-ocular reflex, which is necessary to stabilize the retinal image. Oscillopsia may follow loss of peripheral vestibular function, but it is also a feature of central lesions, especially when associated with an acquired pendular nystagmus (Rudge, 1984).

Clinical examination

The ear

Congenital absence of the auricle is termed 'anotia' and incomplete development 'microtia'. Anotia is associated with severe malformations of the ear canal, middle and inner ear; with microtia the auricular remnant is usually anteroinferior to the bony ear canal and the presence of a tragus is considered by some a good prognostic feature for middle ear reconstruction. Accessory auricles may be found and represent separate developments of the second branchial arch remnants. In all cases of congenital external ear dysplasia, a full examination should be made for other features which might allow the identification of a named syndrome.

Acquired lesions on the auricle include gouty tophi, squamous carcinoma, basal cell carcinoma and the painful nodules of chondrodermatitis helicis.

It is important to look behind the auricle for surgical scars. Postauricular incisions may be difficult to see deep in the retroauricular sulcus, and the more posteriorly placed incision associated with the formation of a Palva flap or excision of a vestibular schwannoma may be hidden in the hairline. Endaural incisions can usually be noted in the area between the tragus and helix, as indeed a preauricular incision can an undeclared rhytidoplasty. Examination behind the auricle may reveal evidence of acute inflammation in the form of erythema, tenderness or abscess formation. In children, a subperiosteal abscess tends to point posterosuperiorly to the external auditory meatus. In adults, the abscess points more posteriorly, reflecting the more extensive mastoid development. Pus from the mastoid may track anteroinferi-

orly along the sternomastoid muscle presenting as a mass in the neck (Bezold's abscess). Alternatively, it may track medially along the posterior belly of the digastric emerging in the submandibular triangle as Citelli's abscess (Shambaugh, 1967).

Lymphadenopathy, associated with ear infections, occurs occasionally in the preauricular node. Neoplastic infiltration of neck nodes in both anterior and posterior triangles occurs with aural carcinoma and is a grave prognostic feature.

The external auditory meatus is examined using either an auriscope or hand-held speculum and a headlight. In the adult, traction of the pinna upwards and backwards helps to straighten the canal and facilitate vision (Figures 1.1 and 1.2). If the view is obscured by wax this should be removed either by a wax probe or by syringing. Syringing is best avoided if there is a possibility that the tympanic membrane is perforated. It must not be forgotten that syringing can change the appearance of the tympanic membrane. It is often difficult to see the anterior sulcus of the canal because of a prominent anterior meatal wall. Canal stenosis may follow chronic otitis externa

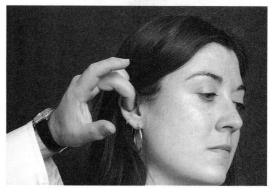

Figure 1.1 Use of Siegle speculum. Backward and upward retraction of the auricle with the middle finger

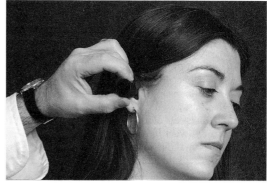

Figure 1.2 Use of Siegle speculum. Positioning and retention of the speculum in the meatus with the thumb and index finger

or surgery. Meatal osteomas, which are sometimes associated with cold water swimming, appear circumferential in the bony part of the meatus and may obstruct a clear view of the tympanic membrane.

Tympanic membrane

It is essential to identify the normal anatomical features of the tympanic membrane using either an auriscope or a speculum and headlight. The wide-angled lens of a Hopkins rod may be helpful and is useful for photography of the tympanic membrane. Some tympanic membranes are difficult to see and in these cases an operating microscope is useful.

If possible, the whole of the tympanic annulus should be seen, along with the handle and lateral process of the malleus. In most normal tympanic membranes there is the sharp reflection of the auriscope's light spreading anteroinferiorly in a cone shape. The mobility of the tympanic membrane is assessed by using a pneumatic bulb on the auriscope of a Siegle's speculum (Siegle, 1864) (Figure 1.3).

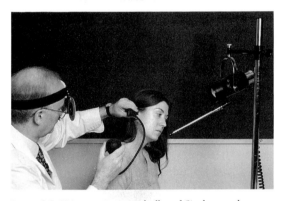

Figure 1.3 Using a pneumatic bulb and Siegle speculum with magnifying glass end

Alternating positive and negative pressures in the ear canal result in the normal tympanic membrane moving inwards and outwards. Where there is a perforation of the tympanic membrane or fluid in the middle ear, there is a loss of normal mobility.

The position of pathological features should be noted in relation to the normal anatomy, i.e. the pars tensa and pars flaccida. A perforation may be central, marginal or attic (in the pars flaccida). It is sometimes difficult to differentiate a retraction pocket from a perforation. In such cases pneumatic otoscopy with bacteriostatic powder blown on to the tympanic membrane helps to make the diagnosis. Assessment of the retraction pocket's adherence to middle ear structures (usually the incudostapedial joint) is important. If a perforation is present, the state of the middle ear mucosa should be assessed for inflammation, infection and oedema. When the stapes is visible through a perforation, its mobility can be assessed using the operating microscope by stimulating the other ear, if the hearing is normal, using a Barany noise box and looking for a crossed acoustic stapedius reflex. This technique may be helpful in the preoperative assessment of cases involving tympanosclerosis.

All preoperative cases should be viewed with the operating microscope in order to assess the meatal size, shape and to ascertain the surgical approach be it endural, postauricular or endomeatal. A lens with a focal length of 200 mm is needed.

Eustachian tube patency

The following manoeuvres indicate patency of the tube, although not necessarily normal function, as they are non-physiological.

Valsalva manoeuvre

The production of a high nasopharyngeal pressure by blowing out against closed lips and nose, normally results in an increase of middle ear pressure with the tympanic membrane bulging outwards. It is important to have the auriscope in place before the patient starts blowing as otherwise trauma to the external auditory meatus may occur with head movement.

Toynbee's manoeuvre

This occurs when a swallow is made with the lips and nose closed. A negative pressure in the nasopharynx and middle ear results in an indrawing of the tympanic membrane. This should return to its normal position with swallowing again with an open nose.

Frenzel manoeuvre (nasopharyngeal pressure test)

This manoeuvre was described, in 1938, by Hermann Frenzel, a prominent figure in German aviation medicine in World War II, and has been found to be more effective than the Valsalva or Toynbee test (Frenzel, 1950): 'with the nostrils and glottis closed, the air in the nasopharynx is compressed by the muscles of the floor of the mouth and tongue. The opening of the eustachian tube by this method is facilitated by the convexity of the tongue which places the soft palate and parts of the tube orifice to which it is connected into a more favourable position for opening the tube'.

Its advantage is that it can be performed in any phase of respiration and is independent of intrathoracic pressure. The disadvantage is that the procedure has to be learned, but once acquired it soon becomes unnecessary to hold the nostrils as these close automatically. This has an obvious advantage for those wearing a flying helmet, oxygen mask or both.

The subject has to acquire a feel for voluntary closing of the glottis and Frenzel suggested, 'the repeated production of a silent "ah" while expiring after a moderate inspiration'. Davison (1962) suggests: '. . . having the subject close the glottis after a moderate inspiration and then attempt to make an oral "ka" sound; if the subject partially compresses his nostrils while performing this manoeuvre, he can feel and hear the rush of air out of the anterior nares, thus demonstrating that the manoeuvre does diminish the volume of the nasopharyngeal space'.

Patulous eustachian tube

This is a not uncommon ear condition which frequently goes undiagnosed and is managed incorrectly (Bull, 1976). The patient complains of a sensation of blockage in the ear, but denies any hearing loss. The sensation of blockage disappears on lying down and may alter with certain positions of the head. Patients may also say that they hear the noise of themselves talking, eating or breathing.

The tympanic membrane is normal, but may in some cases be seen to move with respiration. If the patient is asked to breathe in and out through the nose with mouth open, air flow through a patulous tube is accentuated and the tympanic membrane movement is more easily visible (O'Connor and Shea, 1981).

The condition is often missed and treated as a eustachian tube obstruction with topical and systemic decongestants; these may make matters worse. The condition is common in people who have lost weight suddenly, usually from strict dieting but also in terminal malignancy, those on the contraceptive pill and in pregnancy. It may also be found in older patients given diuretics.

Treatment is usually unnecessary if the condition is explained to the patient and reassurance given that there is nothing seriously wrong. Some people obtain relief after insertion of a ventilation tube and, in rare instances, occlusion of the eustachian tube orifice in the nasopharynx by injection of Teflon paste around the eustachian cushion or electrocautery to the lumen using an intrinsic catheter may help (Hazel and Robinson, 1989). The instillation of mildly irritant nose drops may result in congestion of the eustachian tube orifice with relief of the symptoms (DiBartolomeo and Henry, 1992).

Fistula sign

If, following a pressure increase in the external auditory meatus, vertigo and nystagmus result, a positive fistula sign is said to be present. Such a pressure change can be achieved by simply compressing the tragus into the external auditory meatus. A similar effect can be obtained by using a pneumatic otoscope, Siegle's speculum or the air pump of a tympanometer. In cases of chronic suppurative otitis media, a positive fistula sign indicates the presence of a third window into the perilymphatic space enabling gross movement of the inner ear fluids and stimulation of the

vestibular end organs (Schuknecht, 1973). In ears with such disease, palpation of a fistula while probing the ear results in a violent vertiginous response.

Hennebert's sign

Hennebert's sign occurs when there is a positive fistula test with an intact tympanic membrane and no evidence of middle ear disease. The pathophysiology of this sign is unclear, but is thought to be due either to adhesions in the vestibule or to the presence of a third window somewhere in the labyrinth caused by osteitis (Schuknecht, 1993). It is seen most commonly in congenital or late tertiary syphilis, but is sometimes found in other conditions causing endolymphatic hydrops such as Menière's disease. Hennebert's sign is seen most clearly using the slow, sustained negative pressure change of the tympanometer.

The normal caloric response due to air currents that occurs during suction to the meatus or mastoid cavity should be recognized and not interpreted as a fistula sign.

Auscultation of the ear and temporal bone

This part of the examination is useful in some cases. The stethoscope is used, placing the bell over the ear canal and then lightly on the mastoid process; bruits from vascular anomalies or glomus tumours may be heard (Moffat and O'Connor, 1980). Recently, perception of cochlear emissions, which may or may not be associated with subjective tinnitus, have been reported (Harrison, 1986). In cases of patulous eustachian tube, a stethoscope end, or listening tube, inserted into the meatus will pick up the transmitted voice sounds from the nasopharynx.

Examination of the eyes

Inspection of the eyes may reveal features, such as hypertelorism or coloboma, associated with congenital hearing disorder syndromes. The presence of blue sclerae (osteogenesis imperfecta) (see Plate 3/15/I) and interstitial keratitis (congenital syphilis, Cogan's disease) should be noted.

Fundal examination

Examination of the fundus of the eye must be performed when there is a possibility of an intracranial lesion. Papilloedema may be seen with a space-occupying lesion, such as a cerebellopontine angle tumour or temporal lobe abscess, and also in otitic hydrocephalus where it is often chronic (O'Connor and Moffat, 1978). Optic nerve atrophy follows demyelinating conditions which may present with auditory and vestibular disturbances.

When looking at the fundus it is important to use optimum conditions, including a darkened room and mydriatic drops in order to see the fundus clearly. Remember, ophthalmologists regularly use these conditions: it would be wise for the infrequent 'ophthalmologist' to do the same.

Eye movements

Nystagmus is involuntary eye movement. Patients with nystagmus may describe an inability to focus on a still object or, when associated with rotational vertigo, movement of the visual field in the same direction as the nystagmus. Nystagmus is most easily seen in good light with the patient looking to the front (spectacles on, if usually worn!) and the observer viewing slightly from the side.

Visual fixation is obtained by placing a finger central to the eyes and at least 45 cm from the nose. The presence or absence of nystagmus is noted and the finger moved laterally in the same horizontal plane 30° to either side, asking the patient to follow the finger with his eyes (gaze).

Congenital nystagmus is characteristically pendular in type, when viewed in the 'neutral' central position and usually associated with visual defects.

Vestibular nystagmus may be horizontal or rotatory and has two components, a slow phase with a fast corrective phase in the opposite direction. The slow phase reflects an imbalance of input to the vestibular nuclei and the fast phase is a central righting response. The direction of the nystagmus is conventionally defined in terms of the direction of the fast phase. The intensity of the nystagmus is described in terms of the direction of gaze. Thus, a first degree nystagmus is visible only when the eyes are deviated to the side which is also the direction of the fast phase. A second degree nystagmus is visible in the above position and also with the eyes in the 'neutral', straight ahead position. A third degree nystagmus means that the nystagmus is present in all directions of gaze. If nystagmus changes direction with the gaze it is termed 'direction changing' and may be indicative of a central lesion.

The abolition of visual fixation accentuates a nystagmus associated with a peripheral lesion and may be viewed in the clinical setting using Frenzel's glasses – Frenzel's glasses or spectacles have + 15 to + 20 diopter lenses which almost completely suppress visual fixation. Within the superstructure of the frame there are battery run bulbs allowing the observer to observe eye movement without fixation and then the lenses may be swung superiorly and an assessment with fixation can be made (Figure 1.4).

It is also possible to abolish fixation by using a dark room where eye movements may be seen with an infrared viewer. In general, removal of visual fixation enhances the nystagmus due to a peripheral lesion but reduces that due to central lesions. These

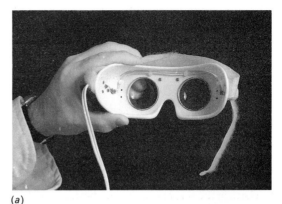

(a)

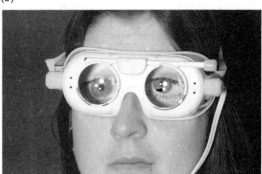

(b)

Figure 1.4 Frenzel's glasses; (a) showing illumination bulbs; (b) as worn during examination.

clinical techniques correlate well with the findings when electronystagmography is used.

If spontaneous nystagmus as described above is absent, nystagmus may be induced by positional changes, rotational or caloric stimulation. Nystagmus induced by changes in position may be associated with benign paroxysmal positional vertigo and is characterized by a brief delay in onset following the change in position (latent period), rotational or horizontal nystagmus directed towards the undermost ear, which lasts no longer than 20–30 seconds and is fatiguable. It is thought to be due to a 'benign' pathological process affecting the peripheral vestibular system (Schuknecht, 1969). A positionally induced nystagmus, that has no latent period, remains present while the patient is in the provocative position and is direction changing according to head position, is suggestive of a central lesion. If benign positional nystagmus has atypical features, the presence of a central lesion must be considered.

Corneal reflexes

The cornea is touched from the side with a fine wisp or cotton wool (NB: it is insufficient to touch the sclera). The normal response is a blink. The response of each cornea should be noted and compared. The loss of the corneal reflex is said to be the most sensitive indication of a lesion involving the trigeminal nerve, but is usually a late sign in vestibular schwannoma, indicating a large tumour which has expanded sufficiently so as to compress the nerve.

Facial nerve (VII)

Motor function

It is important to differentiate between an upper and lower motor neuron lesion. An upper motor neuron lesion paralyses only the lower part of the face, the forehead being spared as it has bilateral cortical representation. A lower motor neuron palsy involves all of that side of the face. The patient is asked to frown with the observer's thumb placed firmly in the midline to prevent muscle movement from the other side stimulating movement of the affected side. The patient is then asked to close and open the eyes, bearing in mind that the levator palpebrae muscle is partially innervated by the oculomotor nerve. The midface is examined by nose twitching and the lower face by showing the teeth. Various conventions have been suggested to quantify partial facial palsy, but all are open to observer differences. However, it should always be clearly stated whether the palsy is partial or complete.

Somatic sensory function

Touch sensation of the floor of the external auditory meatus has been noted to be absent in some cases of vestibular schwannoma (Hitselberger's sign).

Parasympathetic secretomotor function

Fibres passing in the nervus intermedius and then in the greater superficial petrosal nerve to the lacrimal gland may be tested by the tearing on a strip of filter paper placed over the lower lid (Schirmer's test). Only a gross difference between abnormal and normal sides is significant.

Special sensation

Taste from the anterior two-thirds of the tongue is examined, either by the use of test substances (salt, sugar and citric acid) or by electrogustometry. In this technique, a quantitative assessment may be obtained in terms of the electric current needed to elicit a metallic taste in the mouth; both methods are prone to false positives due to the hyposensitivity of many patients' taste buds.

Cranial nerves IX–XII

Glossopharyngeal (IX) nerve function is tested by touching the wall of the oropharynx or posterior third of the tongue. This is the afferent arm of the gag reflex whose efferent arm is mediated through the vagus, producing elevation of the palate and generalized movement of the oro-and hypopharynx. The palate should be examined in case of clicking tinnitus in order to exclude palatal myoclonus.

Indirect laryngoscopy will permit an assessment of vocal cord movement (vagus (X) nerve). To test accessory (XI) nerve function, the patient is asked to rotate the head against the observer's hand and the tension in the contralateral sternocleidomastoid muscle is felt. Shoulder shrugging is tested on each side.

Following hypoglossal (XII) nerve palsy, protrusion of the tongue from the mouth may lead to deviation towards the side of the lesion.

Examination of the nose and throat

A full examination of the nose and throat must always be carried out. Inspection of the nose may reveal rhinitis or sinusitis which is responsible for eustachian tube dysfunction. The postnasal space is examined using a mirror placed in the oropharynx. This necessitates the use of a tongue depressor and head mirror or head-lamp. The development of the fibreoptic rhinopharyngoscope permits the nasopharynx to be examined via the posterior choanae. Where there is evidence of a middle ear effusion, without an obvious explanation, the postnasal space must be examined, even if a general anaesthetic is required.

The rest of the upper air and food passages should be examined for the cause of a referred otalgia, e.g. carcinoma of the pyriform fossa.

Clinical tests of hearing

During the history taking and examination, the clinician should be making an assessment of the hearing threshold. The clinician should alter the voice level and avoid giving visual clues, and in this way gain an impression of how well the patient hears. This is of special importance in patients who are thought to have a non-organic hearing loss. An estimation of the hearing thresholds in each ear may be obtained with masking of the contralateral side by gently rubbing the orifice of the external auditory meatus with a finger.

Tuning fork tests

These tests are a most important part of any clinical examination of hearing and should be performed carefully. They are discussed in considerable detail in Volume 2. The tuning fork used most commonly has a frequency of 512 Hz. The note of the higher frequency forks tends to decay quickly, allowing insufficient time for the Rinne test to be performed. The lower frequency forks tend to enhance perception by vibration sensation.

Rinne test

Essentially this test consists of comparing the auditory acuity of each ear to bone and air conduction. The tuning fork is struck gently so as not to produce overtones and dysharmonics (usually by striking it on a bony prominence, belonging to the examiner not the patient!). The fork is placed firmly on the mastoid with the observer's hand steadying the head. Care is taken, especially in children, to have the fork placed firmly on bone and not on the sternomastoid muscle (Figure 1.5). The patient is asked to indicate when the sound disappears and the fork is then immediately placed erect and in line with the external auditory meatus about 2 cm from the orifice (Figures 1.6 and 1.7). If the patient still hears the note when the fork is placed in front of the ear the patient is termed 'Rinne positive' (air conduction being better than bone conduction). Alternatively, and more usually, in routine clinical practice, the patient is asked to compare the sound intensity of the fork in the mastoid position (bone conduction) with the meatal position (air conduction). If there is a significant sensorineural deafness, the fork will not be heard by bone conduction at all, but only by air conduction, and obviously in severe cases not by air conduction either. A conductive deafness of greater than 25 dB usually gives a negative Rinne test with a 512 Hz fork. However, with a 256 or 128 Hz fork, this may be reduced to 10–15 dB and, with the higher fre-

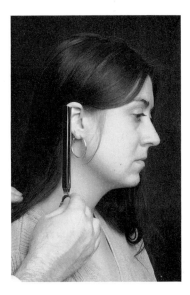

Figure 1.6 Rinne test. The tuning fork is placed erect 2 cm from the external auditory meatus

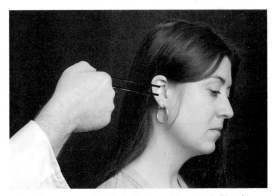

Figure 1.7 The tuning fork should *not* be dangled by the ear

quency forks (1028, 2048 and 4096 Hz), the conductive deafness needs to be greater than 25, 30 and 35 dB, respectively (Shambaugh, 1967; Girgis and Shambaugh, 1988).

False negative Rinne test

This is an important concept and its possibility should never be missed by the otologist. If the patient has no hearing in the test ear the bone conduction stimulus may be perceived by the contralateral (non-test) ear, although the patient often says that he hears it in the test ear. As there is no hearing by air conduction, the test result is labelled Rinne negative suggesting that the deafness is conductive in nature. This mistaken

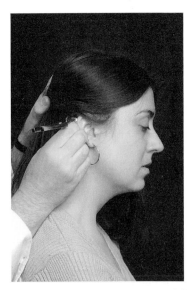

Figure 1.5 Rinne test. The tuning fork is pressed *firmly* on the mastoid bone

impression of function in a non-functioning ear is called a false negative Rinne test. In such cases the diagnosis is given by a combination of the Rinne and the Weber tests. In addition, the non-test ear can be masked by a Barany noise box (a clockwork-driven sound generator of about 90 dB) (Figure 1.8). This phenomenon occurs because the interaural attenuation for bone conduction is less than 5 dB, i.e. sound passes freely across the skull stimulating both ears equally, regardless of where the tuning fork is placed.

Weber test

The tuning fork is struck and the base placed on either the forehead, vertex or upper incisor teeth (Figure 1.9). The patient is asked where the sound is heard loudest. In a normal hearing person, the sound is related to the midline. In a patient with unilateral sensorineural deafness, it is referred to the good ear and in a patient with a conductive deafness to the affected ear. In cases of asymmetrical mixed (conduc-

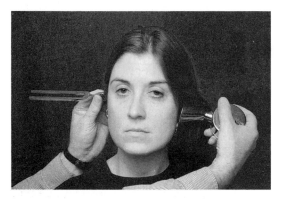

Figure 1.8 Masking the non-test ear with a Barany noise box during bone conduction testing

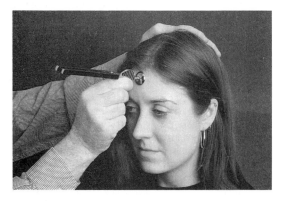

Figure 1.9 Weber test. The tuning fork is placed *firmly* on the forehead

tive plus sensorineural) deafness, no definite rules can be made, but the result interpreted in conjunction with the Rinne test. Obviously the Weber test is a great help in recognizing a false-negative Rinne test as it will be referred to the good ear. In long-standing cases of sensorineural deafness, the Weber test tends not to lateralize. A lateralized Weber in a conductive deafness may indicate a hearing loss of only 10–15 dB.

It should be understood that the abnormal test results in conductive deafness are not explained simply by lack of environmental masking, as they also occur in anechoic (soundless) chambers. Several theories have been put forward and it seems likely that the explanation differs in each type of conductive loss (Tonndorf, 1966).

The following tuning fork tests are of historical interest; with the wide availability of good audiometry they are rarely used.

Modified Schwabach test (absolute bone conduction test)

This compares the bone conduction of the patient with the bone conduction of a normal hearing person. The tuning fork is placed on the patient's mastoid with the meatus blocked and, when the patient no longer hears it, the fork is placed on the normal hearing person's mastoid (usually the examiner's), again with the meatus blocked. If the examiner hears the note, the patient's bone conduction is carried out in the same way but without occluding the meatus.

Several other tests are available which use the principle that, in a normal ear when the sound conducting mechanism of the external and/or middle ear is reduced, the bone conduction stimulus will be enhanced. If there is already a conductive deafness, there will be no change in the perception of the bone conduction stimulus.

Gelle test

The air pressure in the external auditory meatus is altered using a Siegle's speculum. In the normal individual, or those with a sensorineural loss, increasing the meatal pressure results in a decreased sensation of loudness from a bone conduction stimulus. No alteration of bone conduction thresholds indicates fixation of the stapes.

Bing test

Increased loudness for bone conduction stimuli less than 2 kHz, occurs in the normal patient or those with a sensorineural loss when the external meatus is occluded without altering meatal pressure. There is no change when a conductive deafness is present.

Tuning fork test in non-organic deafness

Stenger test

Principle: if sounds of identical frequency but different intensity are presented simultaneously to each ear, only the louder sound will be perceived. The test can be performed either with a pure-tone audiometer or tuning forks.

The examiner stands behind the patient. A tuning fork is struck and held 20 cm from the 'good ear'; the patient hears the sound. The fork is then removed and placed 5 cm from the 'bad ear'; the patient denies hearing the sound. Another fork is then held 15 cm from the good ear without the patient noticing.

If there is a genuine hearing loss the patient will hear the fork in the good ear, but if there is a non-organic hearing loss the patient will not be able to hear the fork in the good ear because the fork which is close, and therefore of louder intensity, is being heard in the bad ear.

Chimani–Moos test

This is a modification of the Weber test. When the tuning fork is placed on the vertex, the patient indicates that he hears it in the good ear and not in the deaf ear. The meatus of the good ear is then occluded. A genuinely deaf patient will still lateralize the sound to the good ear, the malingerer will usually deny hearing the sound at all.

Both of these tests should be used in conjunction with the clinical history (Is there a question of litigation? Was trauma involved?), and the clinical assessment of hearing during the examination.

Clinical tests of balance

Normal body position results from neural input into the cerebellum and brain stem from the receptors in the semicircular canals, the macula of the utricle, the proprioceptive and joint position sensors and the eyes along with reflex muscle activity.

During the clinical examination, each component of the system should be tested individually. If hypofunction of one input occurs, then compensation by the others usually takes place. However, when such compensation is removed, for example by closing the eyes, the resultant deficiency usually becomes obvious.

Romberg's test

The patient is asked to stand erect looking forwards with the feet together. If the patient is stable, he is asked to close the eyes. With a labyrinthine lesion the patient will sway often to the side of the lesion, a feature which is accentuated by closing the eyes. A

central lesion in the cerebellum results in symmetrical swaying that is less affected by eye closure. If the patient falls backwards in a rigid pose, but is able to regain balance before falling to the ground, there is a non-organic disturbance such as malingering or hysteria.

Unterberger's test

This test aims to reduce the input from the proprioceptive organs. The patient is asked to stand as for the Romberg test, but with the hands outstretched, and march on the spot with the eyes closed. The patient will rotate towards the side of a paralytic labyrinthine lesion. In the presence of an active irritative lesion, the balance disturbance is so significant that the patient cannot perform the test for more than a few seconds.

The gait test

The patient is asked to walk in a straight line between two points and then quickly turn to return on the same line. Patients with labyrinthine lesions deviate to the side of the lesion whereas marked imbalance on turning indicates a cerebellar lesion. The sensitivity of the test may be increased by asking the patient to walk on a bed of foam.

Caloric test

The classical Fitzgerald-Hallpike bithermal caloric test is the generally accepted method of evaluating vestibular function by caloric stimulation (Fitzgerald and Hallpike, 1942; Stahle, 1990).

The patient is placed supine on a couch with the head elevated to an angle of 30° to the horizontal. This brings the lateral semicircular canal into the vertical plane. Both ears are checked for wax or the presence of a perforation, as the latter would preclude caloric testing by this technique. Each ear is irrigated by water at 44°C and 30°C (7°C above and below normal body temperature) for 40 seconds. Warm water is used first and the tympanic membrane checked for a hyperaemic blush which indicates adequate irrigation. The eyes are observed for nystagmus with the patient focusing on a near object. The end point of the nystagmus is noted and its duration recorded. Frenzel's glasses are then used to reduce visual fixation and, if the nystagmus reappears, the new end point is noted. A normal caloric reaction results in nystagmus being visible between 90 and 140 seconds after the onset of irrigation, and prolongation by a further 60 seconds following the reduction of visual fixation (Figure 1.10). The affected ear is stimulated with warm water, then the contralateral ear is tested first with warm water, then with cold, and the test concluded by cold water irrigation of the affected ear. Between each irrigation a rest period of 7 minutes is allowed.

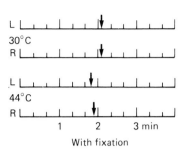

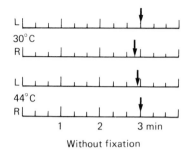

With fixation

Without fixation

Figure 1.10 Caloric test: normal reaction – with and without optic fixation

Cold water produces a nystagmus away from the stimulated ear (away cold = AC) and warm water towards the stimulated ear (towards hot = TH), thus the mnemonic ACTH.

Following bithermal caloric stimulation of a paretic labyrinth, nystagmus may be absent or decreased in amplitude and duration. Care should be taken to look for the end point prior to the reduction of visual fixation, which may prolong the nystagmus into the normal range (Figure 1.11).

When the nystagmus in one direction is significantly greater after bithermal testing, it is termed 'directional preponderance' (Figure 1.12). The significance of this is not fully understood.

Electronystagmography

Eye movements may be recorded electrically and expressed graphically using the technique of electronystagmography (electro-oculography).

There is a naturally occurring potential difference between the cornea and the pigmented layer of the retina. This corneoretinal potential, the cornea being positive in relation to the retina (300–1300 mV), is a function of the illumination of the eye. When electrodes are placed around the eye, movement of the globe results in different corneoretinal potentials relative to the fixed electrodes.

Pairs of electrodes are placed at the outer canthus for the horizontal plane and above and below the pupil distal to the eyelid for the vertical plane. A ground electrode is placed at the centre of the forehead. The signal picked up by the electrodes is enhanced by differential amplification and band pass filtering and then printed on moving paper. The impedance of the electrode–skin interface should be less than 5 kohms for a clear reading and there should be careful calibration at the outset of the test which needs to be repeated if the patient is tested in the dark because of the change in the intrinsic corneoretinal potential. The calibration is obtained by asking the patient to look straight ahead and then, with the head still, alternately to look between lights/spots positioned such that they are seen with a 30° eye movement to right and left (Figure 1.13a). The recorder is then adjusted so that a convenient pen movement can be expressed on degrees and the paper is run, usually at a speed of 1 cm/s.

The direction of eye movement in relation to the pen movement is noted (e.g. up, right and down, left) (Figure 1.13b).

The advantages of using electronystagmography for vestibular assessment are:

1 Total abolition of visual fixation is obtainable
2 Nystagmus may be quantified and qualified
3 A permanent record is available.

Other techniques include visualization of the eye movement using infrared detection and TV monitoring and these also have the advantage of assessing nystagmus without visual fixation, although neither can be used when the eyes are closed.

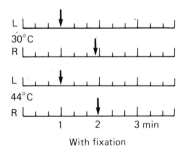

With fixation

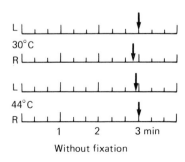

Without fixation

Figure 1.11 Caloric test: caloric left canal paresis

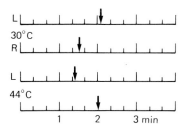

Figure 1.12 Caloric test: caloric right directional preponderance

Assessment of visual ocular control

There is discrete integration between the visual ocular pathways which allow fixation and pursuit of a subject across the visual field and the vestibular ocular pathways that enable assessment of labyrinthine function using caloric or motion stimuli (Hen, Young and Finley, 1974). When the efferent limb of the vestibulo-ocular reflex (VOR) is damaged, eye movement induced by visual stimuli is also abnormal. However, when the afferent limb of the reflex is damaged the visually controlled eye movement is usually normal. Lesion-producing abnormalities of the visual ocular pathway include brain stem and

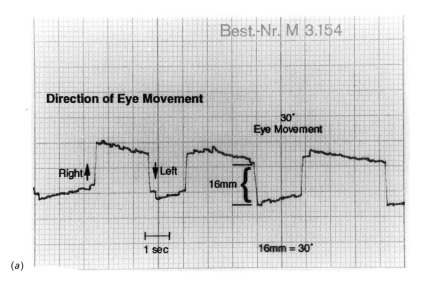

(a)

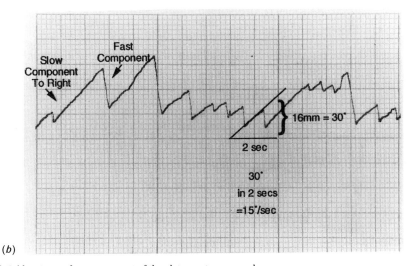

(b)

Figure 1.13a, b Calibrating and measurement of the elctronystagmograph

cerebello-pontine angle pathology and may be characterized by using the electronystagmogram (ENG).

The visual stimuli most commonly studied are *smooth pursuit*, *saccadic movement* and the so-called *optokinetic*.

Smooth pursuit stimuli are induced by asking the patient to follow a smoothly moving object, usually a pendulum. The resulting eye movement produces a sinusoidal graph on the ENG. Although abnormalities of the smooth pursuit occur with generalized CNS disorders, acute lesions of the peripheral labyrinth may transiently impair smooth pursuit movements on the contralateral side to the lesion as the eyes are moving against a tonic vestibular imbalance (Boloh, Honrubia and Sills, 1977). Interestingly, following a resolution of the vestibular abnormality, loss of the aberrant smooth pursuit movements occurs before spontaneous nystagmus in the dark disappears.

Saccadic eye movements occur when a patient looks sequentially at two objects across the visual field. Cerebellar disorders may result in dysmetria (eye movement extending beyond or reversing before the object) and if the changes are unilateral a cerebellopontine angle lesion should be considered.

Optokinetic nystagmus can be stimulated by either the patient being placed in a rotating cylinder which is marked by vertical white lines or asking the patient to carefully gaze at a rotating drum marked similarly on its surface. The electrophysiological basis for this phenomenon is complex and subject to different views by workers in the field; however abnormalities of optokinetic nystagmus give useful information to the clinician (Dix and Hood, 1971). The nystagmus is characterized by two components. The slow component reflecting the eye movement associated with fixation of the white line across the visual field and the fast component the reflex return of the eyes to the starting point. Unilateral disease of the brain stem and cerebellum may be associated with impaired optokinetic nystagmus when the stimulus moves towards the affected side. In cases of vestibular schwannoma, abnormalities of optokinetic nystagmus would indicate brain stem or cerebellar compression.

The addition of visual ocular control of assessment to the ENG following vestibular stimulation is quick, easy and cost-effective.

Computerized dynamic posturography

Computerized dynamic posturography aims objectively to measure the influence of each component involved in the balance process (visual, proprioceptive, vestibular, reflex muscle response) by assessing the patient's ability to stand in situations of increased difficulty (Lipp and Longridge, 1994). The examination is divided into two parts – a sensory organization test and a motor control test. The sensory organization test consists of the patient stand-ing on a dual forceplate that measures sway by integrating the patient's centre of gravity from pressure and sheer force. Various performance conditions are then undertaken and the amount of patient sway is compared to that of a normal population.

Condition 1 The patient stands looking at a fixed image of a horizon with blue sky at a distance of 1 m for 30 seconds

Condition 2 As for condition 1 with eyes closed

Condition 3 The patient stands looking at the image, as he sways naturally the image sways in tandem

Condition 4 As the patient naturally sways the forceplate moves with the feet (mobile forceplate)

Condition 5 As condition 4 with eyes closed

Condition 6 As condition 3 with mobile forceplate

	Vision	Proprioception	Vestibular
Condition 1	Present	Present	Present
Condition 2	Absent	Present	Present
Condition 3	Inaccurate	Present	Present
Condition 4	Visual	Inaccurate	Present
Condition 5	Absent	Inaccurate	Present
Condition 6	Inaccurate	Inaccurate	Present

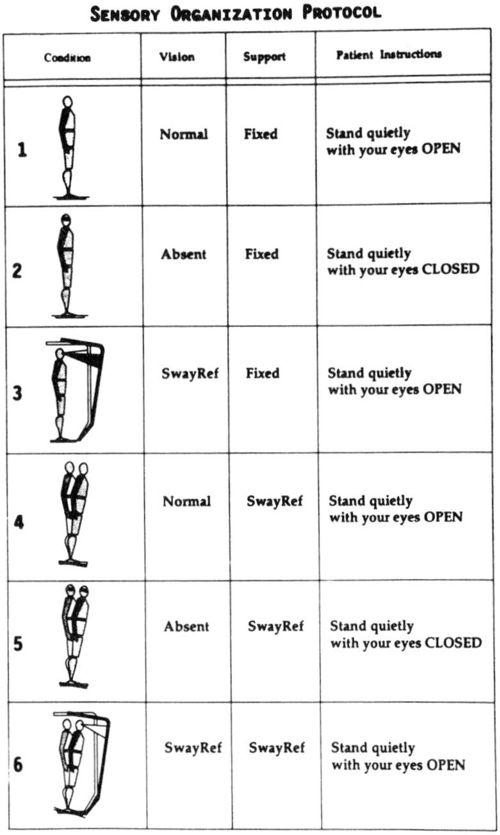

SENSORY ORGANIZATION PROTOCOL

Condition	Vision	Support	Patient Instructions
1	Normal	Fixed	Stand quietly with your eyes OPEN
2	Absent	Fixed	Stand quietly with your eyes CLOSED
3	SwayRef	Fixed	Stand quietly with your eyes OPEN
4	Normal	SwayRef	Stand quietly with your eyes OPEN
5	Absent	SwayRef	Stand quietly with your eyes CLOSED
6	SwayRef	SwayRef	Stand quietly with your eyes OPEN

Figure 1.14 Equitest Protocol.

Conditions 1 and 2 are analagous to eyes open and closed Romberg's tests. Condition 3 stresses balance and forces proprioception and vestibular response. Condition 4 forces visual and vestibular response and in conditions 5 and 6 the only normal input is vestibular (Figure 1.14).

In the motor control test the patient is given a brief impulsion by the forceplates and asked to maintain balance. The reflex response necessitates correct usage of the long loop latency reflex systems (Nashner and Grimm, 1977). The results are compared with normal patient data.

Tests for cerebellar dysfunction

Dysmetria and past pointing

The patient is asked to touch his nose and the examiner's finger alternately. The examiner's finger should be placed in front of the patient at a distance which necessitates very full extension of the patient's arms. The target finger is moved around. Failure by the patient to touch the examiner's finger or his own nose suggests the presence of a cerebellar lesion. If the test is performed satisfactorily the patient is asked to close the eyes and continue pointing. Straying from the targets now suggests a peripheral vestibular lesion (Marshall and Attia, 1983).

Asynergia

The patient is asked to tap the back of each hand in turn with the other hand. With the cerebellar lesions the accuracy of the tap and the discrete area of contact are lost.

Dysdiadochokinesis

In cerebellar lesions, asymmetry occurs when the patient is asked to pronate and supinate the hand on the side of the lesion.

Rebound

The patient's hands and arms are held out rigidly in front and the examiner pushes from above on one hand and from below on the other. The hands are then released. With a cerebellar lesion the patient's arms are unable to compensate for the change in resistance and move widely.

Audiometry

Modern audiometric techniques allow both quantitative and qualitative assessment of hearing. By utilizing different test techniques the anatomical site of the auditory dysfunction may be elicited (Table 1.1).

Table 1.1 Audiometric tests for characterizing hearing loss

Conductive hearing loss	Pure tone audiogram air-bone gap
	Tympanometry
	Absence of stapedial reflex
	Good speech discrimination score
	Auditory brain stem response: delayed wave III
	Bekesy type I
Sensorineural hearing loss	Pure tone audiogram threshold increase
	No air-bone gap
	Normal tympanogram
Cochlear hearing loss	Good speech discrimination score
	No tone decay
	Loudness discomfort
	Small stapedial reflex sensation level
	Bekesy type II
Retrocochlear hearing loss	Poor speech discrimination
	Tone decay
	Stapedial reflex decay
	Auditory brain stem response: wave V delay
	Bekesy type III/IV
Non-organic hearing loss	Pure tone audiogram threshold increase
	Air-bone gap may be present
	Auditory brain stem response: no delay
	Cortical evoked response audiometry threshold different to pure tone audiogram
	Bekesy type V

In general, audiometric analysis may be subjective (where the person being tested willingly responds to the stimulus) or objective where only passive cooperation of the subject is needed. Although objective audiometry tends to measure accurately one part of the auditory pathway, reasonable deduction may usually be made of the patient's ability to hear.

It is convenient to express hearing loss according to the site of the auditory dysfunction. Lesions of the external ear, ear canal, drums, ossicles including the oval window and middle ear result in a *conductive hearing loss*. If the lesion is in the cochlea or neural pathways, the term *sensorineural hearing loss* is used. A *mixed hearing loss* reflects pathology causing both conductive and sensorineural hearing losses.

A subdivision of sensorineural hearing loss may be made into cochlear and retrocochlear. The terms perceptive and neural hearing loss are now considered unhelpful. However, pathology in the cochlea may lead to neural degeneration (e.g. Menière's disease) and a retrocochlear loss may likewise be associated with cochlear degeneration (as in some patients with vestibular schwannoma); thus pure retrocochlear or cochlear hearing loss is uncommon.

A non-organic hearing loss is suggested when there is a disparity between the subjective and objective hearing thresholds and is seen in some psychiatric disorders or malingerers usually involved in litigation.

Procedure for pure tone audiometry

The air conduction tests using a pure tone audiometer are applicable to most adult patients and children over the age of 4 years depending on patient cooperation and the ability of the tester.

The patient should be visible to the tester and should respond by signalling (bell push or raising a finger). No visible or tactile clues should be available to the patient that may suggest the presentation of an auditory stimulus. The test should be conducted in a sound-proofed room.

Care should be taken not to present a sound stimulus during any change of the hearing level or frequency control. The duration of presentation should be 1–3 seconds (due to temporal integration, shorter duration bursts require greater sound pressure levels to be heard) (Yantis, 1985). Rhythmic presentation should be avoided which may lead to the patient anticipating near threshold levels and likewise regular automatic switching should not be used. Unduly long intervals between presentation may also lead to poor measured thresholds. It is important to familiarize the patient with the test procedure, this can be achieved by presenting a tone above the clinical hearing level and checking that the patient indicates the whole duration of the stimulus by changing the length of stimulus. If no response is obtained, the stimulus is increased by 20 dB and repeated until the response requirements are clearly understood by the patient.

The threshold of hearing for a pure tone is the minimum tone that can elicit a response from at least 50% of the individual presentations; in practice this is usually two out of three or four. The test starts with the better hearing ear (as related by the patient) in the following order: 1 kHz, 2 kHz, 4 kHz, 8 kHz, 0.5 kHz, 0.25 kHz.

For the first ear, a retest is performed at 1 kHz. If the retest value is more than 5 dB different from the earlier value then the next frequencies should be retested and so on. The better threshold is taken as the definitive value. In cases of high tone hearing loss and most importantly noise trauma compensation assessments, the frequencies 3 kHz and 6 kHz should also be tested.

The second ear is then tested in the same way with the retest beginning at 1 kHz. If there is a difference in the air conduction threshold exceeding 40 dB at any frequency, masking should be used or the threshold annotated on the audiogram as 'unmasked'.

Bone conduction threshold

Due to audiometer design and acoustic characteristics, bone conduction levels are measured between 0.5 kHz and 4 kHz. The position of the vibrator on the cranium is irrelevant as intra-aural attenuation for bone conduction is less than 5 dB. Bone conduction assessment is essential in all cases where a conductive hearing loss is clinically suspected. However, the limited accuracy in bone conduction audiometry due to audiometric measurement or inherent biological variability must be appreciated, especially in cases where assessment for compensation following noise trauma is being considered (Coles, Lutman and Robinson, 1991). Thus otoscopic, tympanometric and tuning fork information is of importance. The threshold estimation is performed as for air conduction testing, and masking is always used. The difference between the thresholds to air conduction and bone conduction is called the *air-bone gap*.

Masking

A sound stimulus presented to a test ear may be perceived by the non-test ear and the patient unable to judge clearly which ear is hearing the stimulus. Such a phenomenon can occur when the difference between the hearing thresholds of each ear to air conduction differs by 40 dB or more. Thus the inter-aural attenuation for air conduction is 40 dB. To be assured that the test ear is indeed being tested, a narrow band noise centred on the frequency of the tone being used on the test ear is presented to the non-test ear, thus preventing the non-test ear from perceiving the test stimulus. Care should be taken not to use too much masking noise as it may reduce the threshold of the test ear by cross masking (sound leakage around the head) or even by central masking.

Masking should be performed carefully and it is more important to mask properly at two or three frequencies than to fail to mask correctly at all frequencies on the audiogram.

Although there is no universal format for audiograms, most features required in routine clinical practice are found in the British Society of Audiology forms (British Society of Audiology, 1989).

Nomenclature on the pure tone audiogram

It should be noted there is no specific symbol for masked air conduction but the symbols ○ and X should be interpreted as having been masked if it was necessary.

○	Right air conduction
X	Left air conduction
△	Unmasked bone conduction
[	Masked right bone conduction
]	Masked left bone conduction
↓	Threshold beyond the output of the audiometer
L	Right uncomfortable loudness level
⌐	Left uncomfortable loudness level.

Although by definition a normal hearing threshold is 0 dB, hearing thresholds of − 10 dB to + 20 dB are considered 'within normal range'. However, in cases of medico-legal assessment any threshold depression may be considered relevant. No single audiometric pattern can be claimed to be pathognomonic. Various audiometric features are typical of otological pathology.

Conductive hearing loss

Otitis media with effusion (glue ear): a conductive loss maximal in the low frequencies with no sensorineural element (Figure 1.15).

Otosclerosis: a conductive hearing loss across the audiometric range with an increase in the bone conduction threshold (Carhart's notch) at 2 kHz in about 35% of affected people (Figure 1.16).

The Carhart notch, which may disappear after stapes surgery, reflects a loss in the inertial component of the stapes footplate (Gibb and Mal, 1973). It should be noted that the air conduction threshold does not parallel the Carhart notch (thus only the bone conduction is 'notched').

Sensorineural hearing loss

Low tone hearing loss: often seen in fluctuant sensorineural hearing loss commonly associated with Menière's disease (Figure 1.17).

High frequency loss: notched audiogram at 6 kHz (or 3 or 4 kHz) is typical of noise-induced hearing trauma (Figure 1.18).

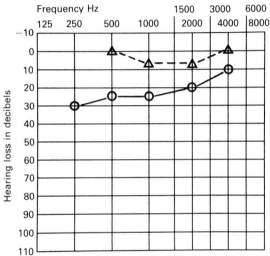

Figure 1.15 Conductive hearing loss, low tone (seromucinous otitis media/otitis media with effusion)

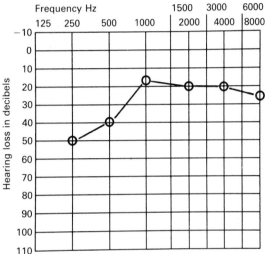

Figure 1.17 Sensorineural hearing loss, low tone (Menière's disease)

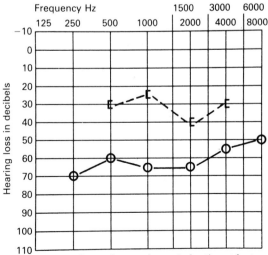

Figure 1.16 Conductive hearing loss – Carhart's notch at 2 kHz (otosclerosis)

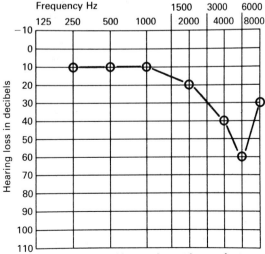

Figure 1.18 Sensorineural hearing loss with a notch at 6 kHz (noise-induced hearing loss)

Sloping high frequency: this occurs in presbyacusis (Figure 1.19).

Middle frequency loss: genetic recessive hearing loss (Figure 1.20).

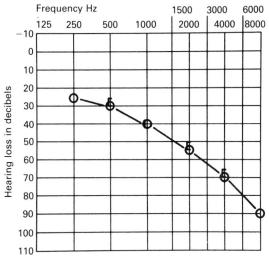

Figure 1.19 Sensorineural hearing loss high frequency sloping (presbyacusis)

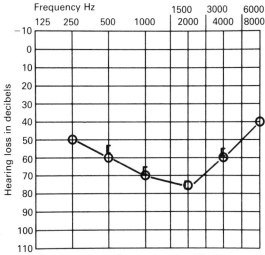

Figure 1.20 Sensorineural hearing loss – middle frequency (genetic recessive disorder)

Speech audiometry

The main function for human hearing is communication through language and therefore speech perception is of obvious importance. Assessment of speech perception may be made in many psychoacoustical forms, however speech audiometry is the simplest clinical tool.

The measure of speech discrimination is the percentage of phonetically-balanced monosyllabic words heard correctly when presented at different intensities. The intensities are obtained by simple biological calibration and expressed as relative speech levels (RSL) in dB. Various word lists are available and may be presented either through an audiometer or from a recorded tape. The Boothroyd word list is perhaps the most commonly used in the UK. The normal speech audiogram is a sigmoid-like curve with the maximum speech discrimination (100%) occurring at the 40 dB RSL and the 50% speech discrimination score half peak level (HPL) at 25 dB RSL.

A conductive hearing loss results in a shift of the curve to the right with 100% discrimination at a higher relative speech level (dB). In a sensorineural hearing loss, due to retrocochlear pathology, 100% discrimination is not attained and indeed at higher relative speech levels the discrimination may in fact be reduced due to desynchronization at a neural level. The half-peak level usually equates to the average pure tone loss in the speech frequencies; this observation may be useful when recognizing a non-organic hearing loss (Figure 1.21).

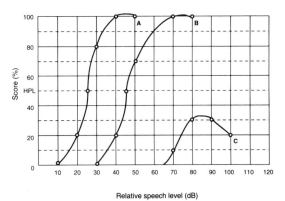

Figure 1.21 Speech audiogram. A. Normal curve; B. Conductive hearing loss; C. Sensorineural hearing loss – retrocochlear

A simplified speech discrimination test that can be used routinely consists of presenting the test ear with a list of 25 phonetically-balanced monosyllables at an intensity of 40–45 dB above the average air conduction thresholds of 0.5, 1 and 2 kHz. The number of words repeated correctly is expressed as a percentage (Kerr and Smyth, 1972).

Test of recruitment

Recruitment of hearing occurs with disorders of the cochlea and is characterized by an inappropriately increased perception of loudness with increasing sound intensity. The presence of auditory recruitment can be ascertained from several audiometric tests.

Fowler's test: alternate binaural loudness balance

The patient is presented with tones of the same frequency in each ear. After both thresholds have been obtained the normal ear is used as a reference (Priede and Coles, 1974). At each increment of 10 dB in the normal ear, the level of perceived equal loudness in the affected ear is obtained and plotted on a graph (Figure 1.22). The greater the slope of the graph the more recruitment is taking place and is indicative of cochlear pathology (Dix, Hallpike and Hood, 1948).

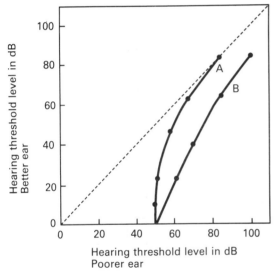

Figure 1.22 Loudness balance; A complete, B partial recruitment

Loudness discomfort level

This is a simple procedure which may be performed following pure tone threshold estimation. The test tone is increased above the threshold and the patient is asked to indicate when it becomes uncomfortable. The normal ear has a loudness discomfort (LDL) level of 90 dB HL. In patients with cochlear pathology, the loudness discomfort level can be as little as 10 dB above the pure tone level, indicating marked recruitment. This test is of special value when prescribing and managing hearing aids.

Tone decay

Tone decay or rather tonal decay, because it refers to the decay of a pure tone rather than a diminution in

frequency, remains a useful easy audiometric assessment of retrocochlear pathology. In physiological terms it is expressed as abnormal auditory adaptation. The simplest clinical test for tone decay uses the tuning fork. On testing bone conduction at the point when the tone is no longer heard, the fork is removed and then replaced (without restriking it); if it is heard then there is significant tone decay.

Audiometrically the Rosenberg (1971) modification of the Carhart test represents the easiest and most reliable technique (for technique see Volume 2, Chapter 12). Rosenberg classified tone decay as:

0–5 dB   normal
10–15 dB   mild
20–25 dB   moderate } Cochlear pathology
30–above   marked   Retrocochlear pathology.

Bekesy audiometry

In Bekesy audiometry the sound stimulus is presented automatically by the audiometer rather than by an audiometrician (Bekesy, 1947). However, careful explanation of the test is needed and an audiometrician's presence is usually necessary. The technique is used in occupational health examinations and health care screening programmes. Its accuracy compared with pure tone testing is extremely good.

The audiometer automatically produces a tone of continually changing frequencies starting at 125 Hz and sweeping to 8000 Hz. The patient keeps the intensity at a 'just audible level' by a switch which when pressed down decreases the intensity of the tone and when released increases the intensity of the tone. The frequency of the tone is plotted along the abscissa and the intensity along the ordinate of a Bekesy graph.

The stimulus is first presented as a pulse (2.5 interruptions/s) and then repeated with a continuous tone. Various features on the resulting graph give useful audiometric information and are expressed as Bekesy types I–V (Jerger 1960; Jerger and Herger, 1961).

Type I   overlapping of interrupted and continuous graph (normal or conductive hearing loss) (Figure 1.23)

Type II   overlapping to 1000 Hz and then dropping off of the continuous tone to no more than 20 dB of the interrupted tone (cochlear pathology). The width of the tracing usually decreases with a greater sensitivity to loudness difference limen (Figure 1.24)

Type III dropping off of the continuous below the interrupted from 125 Hz, with separation increasing across the range (retrocochlear pathology) (Figure 1.25)

Type IV   dropping off of the continuous tone graph, usually to 20 dB, then the continuous

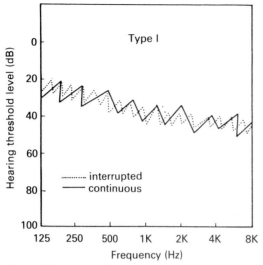

Figure 1.23 Bekesy audiogram: type I

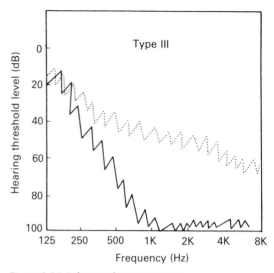

Figure 1.25 Bekesy audiogram: type III

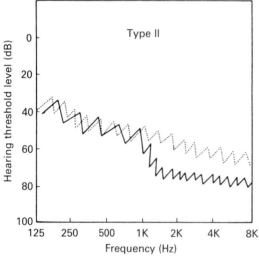

Figure 1.24 Bekesy audiogram: type II

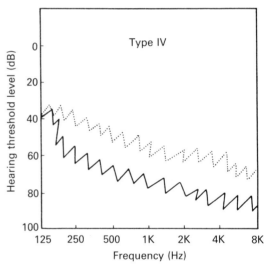

Figure 1.26 Bekesy audiogram: type IV

parallels interrupted across the range (retro-cochlear pathology) (Figure 1.26)

Type V dropping off of the interrupted trace, non-organic hearing loss (the malingerer is able to accentuate the hearing loss more easily with the interrupted tone) (Jerger and Herger 1961) (Figure 1.27).

Acoustic impedance measurements

As sound travels through the ear to the basilar membrane in the cochlea, it is impeded by the structures through which it passes in three separate ways. First, by their stiffness (mainly the tympanic membrane and ossicles); second, by their mass or inertial

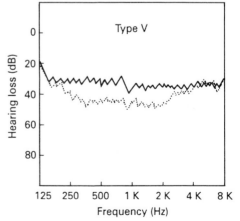

Figure 1.27 Bekesy audiogram: type V

effect (the ossicles); and third, by their frictional effect (cochlea). These effects cannot be calculated in a simple arithmetic fashion but need to be expressed in the form of a complex ratio of vector forces (Jerger and Northern, 1980). The development of the simple electroacoustic bridge by Terkildsen and Scott-Nielson (1960) has allowed this complicated, physical measurement to be utilized clinically in an extremely user-friendly way.

Although the term 'impedance' is used commonly it actually represents the resultant of the individual vectors, positive reactance (mass effect), negative reactance (stiffness effect) and acoustic resistance (resistance effect). Obviously for each impedance measurement (constraint of flow) there is a reciprocal (ease of flow). Thus:

For impedance, the reciprocal is admittance
For reactance, the reciprocal is susceptance
For resistance, the reciprocal is conductance.

Impedance and its vectors are expressed in acoustic ohms and admittance in acoustic mhos (ohms backwards). For routine clinical purposes the acoustic admittance is measured as an acoustic compliance (the acoustic analogue of electrical capacitance) in millilitres of air with *equivalent acoustic admittance* as, at low frequency, for practical purposes the middle ear behaves as a pure compliance. It is important to note that the volume measurement does not represent a real physical volume.

Design of an acoustic impedance meter

Essentially the impedance meter consists of four parts all connected to the ear canal by a soft airtight probe:

1 An oscillator producing a probe tone of fixed frequency (usually 220 Hz)
2 A microphone and meter registering the sound pressure level in the external auditory meatus
3 An air pump and manometer calibrated in millimetres of water from -600 mmH$_2$O to $+1200$ mmH$_2$O. A mechanism to alter and measure the air pressure in the external auditory meatus
4 An audiometer to produce pure tones varying in frequency and intensity for measurement of the stapedial reflex (ipsilateral through the probe and contralateral through a separate earphone).

Tympanometry

Altering the pressure in the external meatus results in changes in compliance because the drum is tensed and the ossicular chain stiffened. The point of maximum compliance occurs when the pressure in the meatus is equal to that in the middle ear. When the pressure exceeds or falls below the middle ear pressure the compliance will be reduced. Thus, indirectly,

the middle ear pressure can be calculated from the point of maximum compliance.

Normal ears

The maximum compliance range is from 0.39 ml to 1.30 ml in the normal population with normal middle ear pressures of between -100 mmH$_2$O and $+50$ mmH$_2$O. Such a tympanogram is often designated type A (Figure 1.28).

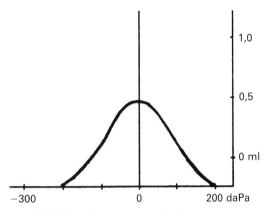

Figure 1.28 Normal tympanogram type A

Eustachian tube dysfunction

The point of maximum compliance occurs below -100 mmH$_2$O. This is designated type C (Figure 1.29).

Otitis media with effusion (seromucinous otitis media)

There is no change in the compliance (usually reduced at 0.06–0.81 ml) associated with external meatal air pressure change. The flat tympanogram, type B (Figure 1.30).

Ossicular discontinuity

The maximum compliance occurs at zero (atmospheric pressure) but is greatly increased and indeed the peak may be lost off the top of the graph (compliance greater than 3.5 ml) (Figure 1.31).

Stapedial and tensor tympani muscle reflex measurements

Contraction of both muscles leads to an increase in the stiffness of the ossicular chain and a reduction in the acoustic compliance. The tensor tympani contracts in response to tactile stimuli over the area subserved by the sensory supply of the trigeminal

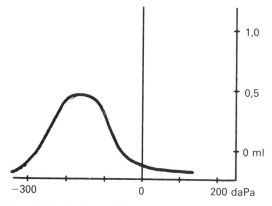

Figure 1.29 Negative middle ear pressure type C

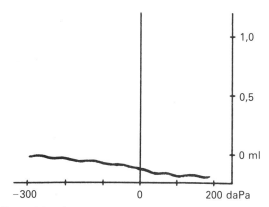

Figure 1.30 Flat tympanogram type B

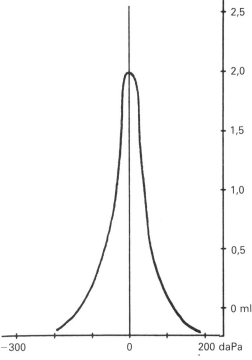

Figure 1.31 Hypercompliant tympanogram

nerve (Fee, 1981). Such testing is not used commonly in otological practice.

The acoustic (stapedial) reflex results from auditory stimulation of the ipsilateral or contralateral ear. The reflex arc is the VIIIth nerve, cochlear nucleus and complex brain stem internuclear connections to the ipsilateral and contralateral facial nuclei, facial nerve and the nerve to stapedius (Thompson, 1983). The minimal auditory stimulus that produces a contraction of the stapedius muscle is termed the acoustic reflex threshold and indicated on an audiogram by the letter Z. In a normal hearing ear the acoustic reflex threshold across the frequency range is 75–85 dB.

Uses of the acoustic reflex threshold measurement

Sensorineural hearing loss

In cases of a recruiting hearing loss the difference between the acoustic reflex threshold and the pure tone threshold is reduced, i.e. the acoustic reflex threshold sensation level decreases (Metz, 1952). An acoustic reflex threshold sensation level of 30 dB is not infrequently seen in Menière's disease. This objective assessment of recruitment can be of use in the management of hearing aids.

Where there is a retrocochlear pathology the acoustic reflex (if present) will decay inappropriately. A decay of 50% in the reflex within 10 s using an acoustic reflex stimulus of 10 dB above the acoustic reflex threshold is considered abnormal. Most significance is gained from the presence of reflex decays to wideband noise and pure tones of 1 kHz and less (Anderson, Barr and Wedenberg, 1970).

Objective threshold audiometry

In the diagnosis of non-organic hearing loss, the acoustic reflex may be of use. Although there is no direct relationship between the pure tone threshold and the acoustic reflex threshold, because of the possibility of recruitment several formulae have been devised utilizing both pure tone acoustic reflex threshold and the acoustic reflex threshold to broad band noise to predict the pure tone threshold. These methods are of most use when the true pure tone threshold is normal and in the paediatric population where there is no non-linear age effect. A normal hearing sensitivity is predicted when the broad band noise pure tone reflex threshold difference is greater than 20 dB and the acoustic reflex threshold at 1000 Hz is 95 dB SPL or less (Miller, Davies and Gibson, 1976; Jerger *et al.*, 1978).

Brain stem/cerebellopontine angle pathology

By recording the reflexes in each ear following ipsi- and contralateral acoustic stimulation, various patterns of response may indicate brain stem and associated pathology.

The presence of ipsilateral reflexes with absence of contralateral reflexes is suggestive of intra-axial *brain stem* lesions.

The absence of an ipsilateral reflex and the contralateral reflex along with the presence of both ipsi- and contralateral reflexes induced from the other ear is suggestive of unilateral afferent reflex arc abnormality (*VIIIth nerve lesion*). Subsequent loss of the remaining contralateral reflex with continual presence of the ipsilateral reflex may suggest a more progressive cerebellopontine angle lesion (*efferent reflex arc abnormality*).

A *facial nerve* lesion is characterized by an absent ipsilateral reflex and an absent contralateral reflex induced from the other ear.

Bell's palsy

The presence of an acoustic reflex in patients with an idiopathic facial palsy indicates an incomplete palsy and is a good prognostic sign for recovery of facial function as is the return of the acoustic reflex prior to any facial movement.

Neuromuscular disorders

Systemic diseases such as myaesthenia gravis, motor neuron disease, myotonic dystrophy and abnormalities of thyroid function may affect the efferent arm of the acoustic reflex. The reflex may be used in the diagnosis and the monitoring of the diseases in respect of both their natural history and response to therapy.

The acoustic reflex threshold is raised as compared with normal controls in patients with myaesthenia gravis and returns to normal after pyridostigmine (Laurian *et al.*, 1983). Reflex decay is a marked feature of both myaesthenia gravis and thyroid disorders.

Latency abnormalities are noted in all the above neurological conditions with increases in the initial reflex response, suggestive of abnormalities in neuromuscular transmission. In patients with myotonic dystrophy the rise time of the reflex is delayed, indicating a myopathic response which is confirmed by

failure in the growth of the reflex. In hypothyroidism the reflex growth is significantly abnormal and may be due to myxoedematous hypertrophy (Yamane and Normura, 1984).

Vascular abnormalities

Intratympanic vascular abnormalities produce cyclical changes in acoustic compliance at the tympanic membrane. These changes are synchronous with the heart rate. Glomus tumours, high uncovered jugular bulbs and arterial abnormalities (usually an internal carotid artery uncovered in the middle ear) are typical examples of this phenomenon. A vivid display of this phenomenon was described by Moffat and O'Connor (1980) where the impedance pattern associated with bilateral internal carotid aneurysms in the middle ear was displayed.

Patulous eustachian tube

Tinnitus, fullness and hearing loss may be the presenting symptoms of a patulous eustachian tube, with autophony becoming only evident on formal questioning. Vertigo may occur following Valsalva's manoeuvre when there is a sharp increase in nasopharyngeal pressure. The clinical signs associated with this condition include tympanic movement during nasal respiration which can be viewed otoscopically. The changes in middle ear pressure resulting in movement of the tympanic membrane may be seen as fluctuations in compliance on the tympanogram (O'Connor and Shea, 1981). Changing the head position from the erect to the supine may reduce the patulous nature of the eustachian tube due to venous congestion and reduction in the impedance fluctuations of the compliance.

Eustachian tube function

Eustachian tube dysfunction is characterized by a middle ear pressure of less than 100 mmH_2O. The pressure changes that result from a positive Toynbee's test (swallowing with the nose held closed) and Valsalva's manoeuvre (forced expiration against closed mouth and nose) can be seen graphically on the tympanogram. If the tympanic membrane is perforated or a ventilation tube is functioning, a flat tympanogram results usually close to zero (Holmquist, 1970). In this situation the measured volume is much higher than normal.

Non-acoustic intratympanic muscle reflexes

Both the stapedius and the tensor tympani muscle reflexes may be elicited by tactile stimuli to the skin subserved by branches of the trigeminal nerve. Their uses in clinical practice are limited and have been fully reviewed by Booth (1973).

Auditory evoked potentials

Electric response audiometry

The central nervous system generates random bioelectric activity which can be recorded using scalp electrodes (EEG). If specific sensory stimuli are introduced, the associated bioelectric event can be extracted from the continuous EEG by relating the event in time to the repetitive stimulus and averaging the responses. Following auditory stimulation the specific bioelectric events, *auditory evoked potentials*, occur at several levels in the auditory pathway and are measured to form the basis of electric response audiometry.

Electric response audiometry can be used in several areas of audiometry, namely threshold testing, site of lesion analysis and clinical diagnosis. In clinical practice, auditory brain stem responses, cortical evoked response audiometry and electrocochleography are the most commonly used auditory evoked potentials.

Auditory brain stem response

The auditory brain stem response is recorded from scalp electrodes (far field). The wave forms are remarkably standard and characterized by five major wave forms, the so-called Jewett waves labelled in Roman numerals I–V (Jewett and Williston, 1971). Their post-stimulatory latencies are extremely consistent in the general population and highly stable and reproducible in individuals. The neural potentials of each wave probably arise from discrete neural areas, namely wave I the VIIIth nerve, wave II the cochlear nucleus, wave III the superior olive, wave IV and wave V the inferior colliculus (Starr and Hamilton, 1976; Moeller, Janetta and Miller, 1982) (Figure 1.32).

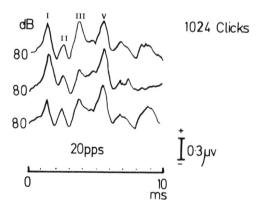

Figure 1.32 Jewett waves I–V

The stimuli used in auditory brain stem response testing are filtered clicks, producing a signal that represents sound in the 1–3 kHz band width, or tone pips. Auditory brain stem responses can be recorded in the presence of a general anaesthetic with relaxants or using sedation. Each wave is identified by the point of maximum potential that is followed by the maximum negative slope. The most prominent waves and the one most visible near to threshold is wave V (latency 5.3–6.3 ms at 80 dB HL) followed by wave III (3.6–3.9 ms) and wave I (1.7–1.9 ms).

Analysis of the auditory brain stem response is based mainly upon the latency measurement of waves I–V. The latency of wave I being abbreviated as T1, and wave II as T2 etc. The absolute latency of wave V (T5) has a wide range of normality (latency 5.3–6.3) and as a typical retrocochlear lesion (e.g. vestibular schwannoma) results in a delay of less than 1 ms, T5 delay is not a very sensitive test. However, in the individual, right and left auditory brain stem response latencies are equal (probably because they facilitate sound localization) and thus give a built in normal control for latency delay. The interaural latency delay for the wave V (IT5) in a normal population, is > 0.2 ms and any greater delay is considered abnormal. Using such criteria, an unacceptable false positive rate for the diagnosis of retrocochlear lesions remained. Formulae were devized to accomodate the degree of high frequency loss; Selters and Brackmann (1977) suggested that for every 10 dB hearing loss at 4 kHz above 50 dB, 0.1 ms could be subtracted from T5. Following this adjustment factor, if the T5 was still in excess of 2 ms then the false-positive rate for a retrocochlear lesion was only 8% and the false-negative rate 3%.

Not infrequently due to neural desynchronization, the auditory brain stem response is lost in cases of vestibular schwannoma (25% small tumours and 75% large tumours) and all absent responses should be further investigated.

The interpeak latencies can also be analysed and delays between waves III and V may indicate brain stem distortion.

Auditory brain stem response for threshold estimation is an extremely useful clinical tool, especially in children where an anaesthetic or sedation is required. Use of the rapid onset click stimulus leads to recognition of the auditory brain stem response (usually wave V) at stimulus levels very close to the subjective threshold (see Figure 1.32). The disadvantage of the click stimuli is in the frequency domains where only limited information is obtained, especially below 1 kHz. Moller and Blevgrad (1976) found the best correlation of the wave V threshold and the pure tone threshold at 2 and 4 kHz. Tone pip stimuli, although giving more frequency information, tend to correlate less accurately with pure tone thresholds (Mitchell and Clemis, 1977).

Auditory brain stem response testing may also be used in cases of suspected multiple sclerosis where patchy demyelination occurs within the brain stem, resulting in a distorted and aberrant wave pattern yet relatively normal hearing thresholds (Starr and Achor, 1975).

Electrocochleography

When information is required about the bioelectrical activity of the cochlea and VIIIth nerve specifically, electrocochleography is the investigation of choice. Although several recording techniques are available the near field transtympanic electrode that rests on the promontory gives the clearest and most reliable data (Ruth, 1990). Three major stimulus-related electrical potentials are commonly measured using electrocochleography: the cochlear microphonic, the summating potential and the compound action potential (Figure 1.33).

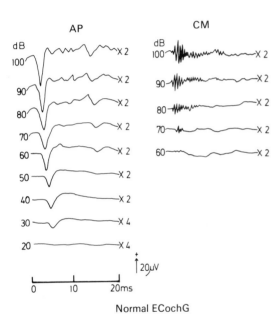

Figure 1.33 Normal electrocochleogram showing the action potential (AP) and cochlear microphonic (CM)

Cochlear microphonic

The cochlear microphonic is an alternating current response that is thought to reflect displacement-time patterns of the cochlear partition and seen to arise from the outer hair cells of the most basal turn of the cochlea (Gibson, 1978). The threshold and amplitude are of little clinical use as they are extremely dependent on specific electrode position. Waveform distortions are recognized with cochlear pathology, an example of which is 'after ringing' as seen in cases of Menière's disease. The presence of a cochlear micro-

phonic along with the absence of a compound action potential has been reported in patients with vestibular schwannoma (Gibson and Beagley, 1977).

Compound action potential

The compound action potential is derived from the first order neurons in the cochlear nerve (see Figure 1.33). The normal onset latency ranges from 1.2 ms at high intensity levels (110 dB HL) to 4.6 ms near threshold. The waveform is characteristically monophasic and very reproducible. It is an extremely accurate measure of auditory acuity across the frequency range of 1–4 kHz.

Summating potential

The second cochlear receptor potential is characterized by the same d.c. shift in the baseline of the response at the same latency as the compound action potential. In cases of Menière's disease, the summating potential is enhanced such that the ratio of the summating potential to the action potential is greater than 0.45 (Coats, 1986) (Figure 1.34).

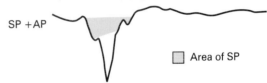

Figure 1.34 Summating potential (SP) and action potential (AP)

Cortical evoked response audiometry

The most significant advantage of cortical evoked response audiometry potentials is their close correlation at threshold with the psychoacoustical hearing thresholds. Pure tone stimuli can be used and the speech frequencies tested. The disadvantages are the relatively long test period (1–3 hours), the need for cognitive activity and the marked variability of responses in young children. The primary component, which can be traced to threshold is the P2 vertex positive peak (latency 150–200 ms). Further peaks occur at 50–75 ms vertex positive P1 and the vertex negative peaks, at 90–120 ms N1 and 260–300 ms N2 (Ruth and Lambert, 1991) (Figure 1.35). There is considerable intra- and inter-subject variability and the latencies tend to be more consistent than the amplitudes. Habituation tends to occur with responses being more prominent at the beginning of testing.

The test environment must be relaxed with good neck support as otherwise muscle activity will compromise the response. Masking of the contralateral

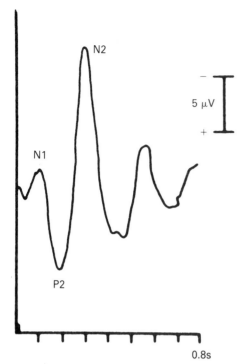

5 µV

N2

N1

P2

0.8s

Figure 1.35 Cortical evoked response audiogram

manoeuvres. Recent reports of electrocochleographic monitoring during endolymphatic sac surgery have displayed a reduction of the ratio of the summating potential: to the action potential following decompression. In a series of 97 patients with Menière's disease undergoing endolymphatic sac surgery, 45 had abnormal base summating potential:action potential ratios and 66% of these had significant reductions in the ratio following surgery. As the changes followed specifically decompression and drainage it has been suggested that intraoperative monitoring provides definitive identification of the sac and lumen.

Otoacoustic emissions

Otoacoustic emissions are acoustic signals produced in the cochlea that can be measured with a low noise microphone placed in the ear canal (Kemp, 1978) (Figure 1.36). They occur spontaneously in approximately 40% of the population and can be evoked by

ear is indicated as in conventional audiometry. Clinical uses of cortical evoked response audiometry relate to threshold testing especially in patients who by reasons of mental subnormality cannot comprehend routine testing and those with a non-organic hearing loss.

Intraoperative monitoring

Surgical procedures on the inner ear, VIIIth nerve and brain stem where hearing conservation is being considered require neurophysiological intraoperative monitoring of the cochlea, VIIIth nerve and brain stem function. Electrocochleography and auditory brain stem response monitoring are used in vestibular schwannoma surgery when the posterior fossa or middle fossa approaches are employed. Intraoperative changes in auditory function may be due to neural ischaemia, blood gas abnormalities and mechanical alteration of neural structures (Grundy *et al.*, 1983). Quick and continuous records are necessary in order to obtain near 'real time' responses. Although loss of the wave V or the electrocochleographic action potential is an extremely ominous sign, the prognosis of complete sensorineural hearing loss is not inevitable. Interest should not remain with the operative ear alone as contralateral testing may elicit (synchronous) brain stem dysfunction resulting from surgical

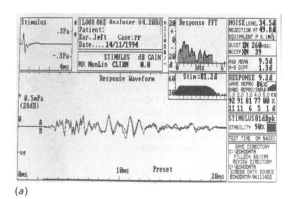

(a)

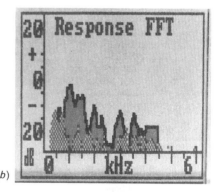

(b)

Figure 1.36 Otoacoustic emissions. (*a*) The response waveform of the acoustic response to the stimulus. In the standard IL088 mode, this shows the non-linear saturated component of the transient otoacoustic emission. (*b*) Frequency analysis shows response from 500 to 4.5 kHz indicating hearing better than 30 dB

various stimuli in 92–100% of a normal hearing population (Bray and Kemp, 1987). Both spontaneous and evoked otoacoustic emissions are thought to emanate from the outer hair cells. Evoked otoacoustic emissions are absent when the hearing loss is greater than 30 dB. The response under fixed test conditions is extremely stable and may be used to monitor transient changes in auditory function (Prieve, Gorga and Neely, 1991; Hall, *et al.*, 1994). Perhaps the most important use for otoacoustic emissions is the screening of newborn infants. Because the technique is quick, non-invasive, objective and gives specific information of cochlear function it is to be preferred to auditory brain stem response testing. However, it should be remembered that it gives no indication of the hearing threshold excepting that, when present, the hearing is near normal.

References

ANDERSON, H., BARR, B. and WEDENBERG, E. (1970) Early diagnosis of eight nerve tumours by acoustic reflex tests. *Acta Otolaryngologica*, Supplement 263, 232–237

BALLANTYNE, J. C. and AJODHIA, J. (1984) Iatrogenic deafness. In: *Vertigo*, edited by M. R. Dix and J. D. Hood. Chichester: John Wiley & Sons. pp. 217–247

BEKESY, G. V. (1947) A new audiometer. *Acta Otolaryngologica*, **35**, 411–422

BLUESTONE, C. D. and CANTEKIN, E. (1979) Otitis media and child development. *Annals of Otology, Rhinology and Laryngology*, **88**, (suppl. 60), 13–27

BOLOH, R. W., HONRUBIA, V. and SILLS, A. (1977) Eye tracking and optokinetic nystagmus results of quantitative testing in patients with well-defined nervous system lesions. *Annals of Otology, Rhinology and Laryngology*, **86**, 108–121

BOOTH, J. (1973) Tympanoplasty: factors in postoperative assessment. *Journal of Laryngology and Otology*, **87**, 27–67

BRAY, P. and KEMP, D. T. (1987) An advanced cochlear echo technique suitable for infant screening. *British Journal of Audiology*, **21**, 191–204

BRITISH SOCIETY OF AUDIOLOGY (1989) British Society of Audiology – recommended format for audiogram forms. *British Journal of Audiology*, **23**, 265–266

BROWN, R. D., PENNY, J., HENLEY, C., HODGES, K. G., KUPETZ, S. and GLENN, D. W. (1981) Ototoxic drugs and noise. In: *Tinnitus, CIBA Foundation Symposium 85*, edited by D. Evered and G. Lawrenson. London: Pitman. pp. 151–171

BULL, T. R. (1976) Abnormal patency of the eustachian tube. *British Medical Journal*, **283**, 1390

COATS, A. (1986) The normal summating potential recorded from the external ear. *Archives of Otolaryngology*, **112**, 759–768

COLES, R. R. A., LUTMAN, M. E. and ROBINSON, D. W. (1991) The limited accuracy of bone conduction audiometry: its significance in medico-legal assessments. *Journal of Laryngology and Otology*, **105**, 518–521

DAVISON, R. A. (1962) Ventilation of the normal and blocked middle ear. A review of mechanisms. *USAF School of Aerospace Medicine Review*, 7–62

DIBARTOLOMEO, J. R. and HENRY, D. F. (1992) A new medication to control patulous eustachian tube disorders. *American Journal of Otology*, **13**, 323

DIX M. R., HALLPIKE, C. S. and HOOD, J. D. (1948) Observations upon loudness recruitment phenomenon with special reference to the differential diagnosis of disorders of the internal ear and VIII nerve. *Proceedings of the Royal Society of Medicine*, **41**, 516–526

DIX, M. R. and HOOD, J. D. (1971) Further observations upon the neurological mechanisms of optokinetic nystagmus. *Acta Otolaryngologica*, **77**, 217–226

EVANS, J. H. and TRIMM, A. (1966) Dizziness. *Postgraduate Medical Journal*, **42**, 240–246

FEE, W. E. (1981) Clinical applications of new acoustic middle ear muscle stimulation. *Archives of Otolaryngology*, **107**, 224–226

FITZGERALD, E. and HALLPIKE, C. S. (1942) Studies in human vestibular function observations on the directional preponderance of caloric nystagmus resulting from cerebellar lesions. *Brain*, **65**, 1125–1137

FOWLER, E. (1937) The diagnosis of diseases of the neural mechanisms of hearing by the aid of sounds well above threshold. *Transactions of the American Otological Society*, **27**, 207–219

FRENZEL, H. (1950) Otorhinolaryngology. In: *German Aviation Medicine World War II*, vol. 2, Cap. 10-A. Washington DC: US Government Printing Office (translated into English). pp. 977–1004

GIBB, A. G. and MAL, K. R. (1973) Computer analysis of audiological aspects of otosclerosis. In *Disorders of Auditory Function*, edited by W. Taylor. New York: Academic Press. p. 229

GIBSON, W. P. R. (1978) Electrocochleography in essentials of clinical response. *Audiometry*. Edinburgh: Churchill Livingstone. p. 66

GIBSON, W. P. B. and BEAGLEY, H. A. (1977) Transtympanic electrocochleography in the revue in the investigation of retro-cochlear disease. *Revue de Laryngologie*, **97** (Supplement), 507–517

GIRGIS, T. F. and SHAMBAUGH, G. E. (1988) Turning forks: forgotten art. *American Journal of Otology*, **9**, 64–69

GRUNDY, B. L., JANETTA, P. J., PROCOPIO, D., LINA, A. and DOYLE, E. (1983) Intraoperative monitoring of brain stem auditory evoked potentials. *Journal of Neurosurgery*, **57**, 674–681

HALL, J. W., BAER, J. E., CHASE, P. A. and SCHWABER, M. K. (1994). Clinical application of otoacoustic emissions: What do we know about factors influencing measurement and analysis? *Otolaryngology – Head and Neck Surgery*, **110**, 22–38

HARRISON, R. V. (1986) Cochlear echoes, spontaneous emissions and some other recent advances in auditory science. *Journal of Otolaryngology*, **15**, 1–8

HAZEL, J. W. P. and ROBINSON, P. J. (1989) Patulous eustachian tube. The relationship with sensorineural hearing loss. Treatment by eustachian tube diathermy. *Journal of Laryngology and Otology*, **103**, 739–741

HEN, V. S., YOUNG, L. R. and FINLEY, C. (1974) Vestibular nucleus units in alert monkeys are also influenced by moving visual scenes. *Brain Research*, **71**, 144–149

HINCHCLIFFE, R. (1973) Investigation of vertigo. In: *Recent Advances in Otolaryngology*, edited by J. Ransome, H. Holden and T. R. Bull. Edinburgh: Churchill Livingston. pp. 103–126

HOLMQUIST, J. (1970) Size of mastoid air cell system in

relation to hearing after myringoplasty and eustachian tube function. *Acta Otolaryngologica*, **69**, 89–93

HOOD, J. D. (1980) Audiological considerations in Meniere's disease. *Journal for Oto-Rhino-Laryngology and its Borderlands*, **42**, 77–90

JERGER, J. (1960) Bekesy audiometry in analysis of auditory disorders. *Journal of Speech and Hearing Research*, **3**, 275–287

JERGER, J. and HERGER, G. (1961) Non organic hearing loss and Bekesy audiometry. *Journal of Speech and Hearing Research*, **26**, 390–392

JERGER, J. F. and NORTHERN, J. L. (1980) *Clinical Impedance Audiometry*, 2nd edn. Philadelphia: American Electromedics Corporation

JERGER, J. F., HAYES, D., ANTHONY, L. and MAUDLIN, L. (1978) Factors influencing prediction of hearing levels from the acoustic reflex. *Monographs in Contemporary Audiology*, **1**, 1–20

JEWETT, D. L. and WILLISTON, J. S. (1971) Auditory evoked far fields averaged from the scalp of humans. *Brain*, **94**, 681–696

KAKKAR, S. K. and HINCHCLIFFE, R. (1970) Unusual Tullio phenomena. *Journal of Laryngology and Otology*, **84**, 155–166

KEMP, D. T. (1978) Stimulated acoustic emissions from the human auditory system. *Journal of the Acoustical Society of America*, **64**, 1386–1391

KERR, A. G. and SMYTH, G. D. L. (1972) Routine speech discrimination tests. *Journal of Laryngology and Otology*, **86**, 33–41

LAURIAN, N., LAURIAN, L., SADOV, R., STRAUSS, M. and KALMANOVITZ, M. (1983) New clinical applications of the stapedial reflex. *Journal of Laryngology and Otology*, **97**, 1099–1103

LIPP, M. and LONGRIDGE, N. S. (1994) Computerised dynamic posturography. *Journal of Otolaryngology*, **23**, 177–183

MARSHALL, K. G. and ATTIA, E. L. (eds) (1983) Case 19. In: *Disorders of the Ear*. Bristol: John Wright. pp. 181–196

METZ, O. (1952) Threshold of reflex contractions of muscle of the middle ear and recruitment of loudness. *Archives of Otolaryngology*, **55**, 536–543

MEYERHOFF, W. L., MORIZON, O. T., SHADDOCK, L. C., WRIGHT, C. G., SHEA, D. A. and SIKORA, M. C. (1983) Tympanostomy tubes and otic drops. *Laryngoscope*, **93**, 1022–1027

MILLER, R., DAVIES, C. B. and GIBSON, W. P. R. (1976) Using the acoustic reflex to predict the pure tone threshold. *British Journal of Audiology*, **10**, 51–54

MITCHELL, C. and CLEMIS, J. D. (1977) Audiograms derived from brainstem responses. *Laryngoscope*, **8**, 1016–1022

MOELLER, A. R., JANETTA, P. and MILLER, M. B. (1982) Intracranially recorded auditory nerve responses in man. *Archives of Otolaryngology*, **108**, 77–82

MOFFAT, D. A. and O'CONNOR, A. F. (1980) Bilateral internal carotid aneurysms in the petrous bone. *Archives of Otolaryngology*, **106**, 172–178

MOLLER, K. and BLEVGRAD, B. (1976) Brainstem potentials in subjects with sensorineural hearing loss. *Scandinavian Audiology*, **5**, 115–127

MORRISON, A. W. and BOOTH, J. B. (1970) Sudden deafness – an otological emergency. *British Journal of Hospital Medicine*, **4**, 287–298

MORRISON, A. W. and BUNDAY, S. E. (1970) The inheritance of otosclerosis. *Journal of Laryngology and Otology*, **84**, 921–932

NASHNER, I. M. and GRIMM, R. J. (1977) Cerebral motor control in man longloop mechanism. In: *Progress in Clinical Neurophysiology*, vol. 4, edited J. E. Desmedt. Basel: Karger. pp. 804–103

O'CONNOR, A. F. and MOFFAT, D. A. (1978) Otogenic intracranial hypertension. *Journal of Laryngology and Otology*, **92**, 767–775

O'CONNOR, A. F. and SHEA, J. J. (1981) Autophony and the patulous eustachian tube. *Laryngoscope*, **91**, 1427–1434

PRIEDE, V. M. and COLES, R. R. A. (1974) Interpretation of loudness recruitment tests – some new concepts and criteria. *Journal of Laryngology and Otology*, **88**, 641–642

PRIEVE, B. A., GORGA, M. P. and NEELY, S. T. (1991) Otoacoustic emissions in adults with severe hearing loss. *Journal of Speech and Hearing Research*, **34**, 379–385

RAMSDEN, R. T. and ACKRILL, P. (1982) Bobbing oscillopsia from gentamicin toxicity. *British Journal of Audiology*, **16**, 147–150

ROSENBERG, P. E. (1971) Abnormal auditory adaption. *Acta Otolaryngologica*, **94**, 89

RUDGE, P. (1984) Central causes of vertigo. In: *Vertigo*, edited by M. R. Dix and J. P. Hood. Chichester: John Wiley & Sons. p. 456

RUTH, R. (1990) Trends in electro-cochleography. *Journal of the American Acadamy of Audiology*, **1**, 134–137

RUTH, R. A. and LAMBERT, P. R. (1991) Auditory evoked potentials. *Otolaryngologic Clinics of North America*, **24**, 349–370

SCHUKNECHT, H. (1969) Cupulolithiasis. *Archives of Otolaryngology*, **90**, 765–778

SCHUKNECHT, H. (ed.) (1993) Pathophysiology. In: *Pathology of the Ear*, 2nd edn. Malvern, Pennsylvania: Lea and Febiger. pp. 77–113

SELTERS, W. and BRACKMANN, D. E. (1977) Acoustic tumour detection with brain stem electrical responses audiometry. *Archives of Otolaryngology*, **103**, 181–187

SENTURIA, B. H. (1973) External otitis, acute diffuse evaluation of therapy. *Annals of Otology, Rhinology and Laryngology*, **82** (suppl. 8), 1–23

SHAMBAUGH, G. E. Jr (ed.) (1967) Diagnosis of ear disease. In: *Surgery of the Ear*, 2nd edn. London: W. B. Saunders. pp. 71–98

SIEGLE, E. (Deutch Klinik 1864) quoted by Polizer, A. (1909) *A Textbook of Disease of the Ear for Students and Practitioners*, 5th edn. Translated by M. J. Ballin and C. L. Heller. London: Balliere Tindall

STAHLE, J. (1990) Controversies on the caloric response. From Barany's Theory to Studies in Microgravity. *Acta Otolaryngologica*, **109**, 162–167

STARR, A. and ACHOR, J. (1975) Auditory brainstem responses in neurological disease. *Archives of Neurology*, **32**, 761–768

STARR, A. and HAMILTON, A. E. (1976) Correlation between confirmed sites of neurological lesions and abnormalities of far field brainstem responses. *Electroencephalography and Clinical Neurophysiology*, **41**, 595–608

TERKILDSEN, K. and SCOTT-NIELSON, S. (1960) An electroacoustic impedance measuring bridge for clinical use. *Archives of Otolaryngology*, **72**, 339–346

THOMPSON, G. (1983) Structure and function of the central auditory system. *Seminars in Hearing*, **4**, 1–13

TONNDORF, J. (1966) Bone conduction studies in experimental animals. *Acta Otolaryngologica Supplementum*, **213**, 1–132

YAMANE, M. and NOMURA, Y. (1984) Analysis of stapedial reflexes in neuromuscular disorders. *Otorhinolaryngology*, **46**, 84–96

YANTIS, P. A. (1985) Pure tone air conduction testing. In: *Handbook of Clinical Audiology*, 3rd edn, edited by J. Katz. Baltimore: Williams & Wilkins. pp.56–63

2

Radiology of the ear

P. D. Phelps

The petrous temporal bone is a complex structure containing important tiny bony objects such as the crura of the stapes and canals such as the vestibular aqueduct, which are less than 1 mm in diameter. These are close to the limits of resolution by imaging techniques. Good spatial resolution to allow adequate demonstration of these bony structures in the middle and inner ears has been an important requirement of radiographic equipment for many years. Spatial and density resolution are discussed in Volume 1, Chapter 17.

The major disadvantage of plain films is caused by overlapping of the structures which makes interpretation difficult. Historically, a great range of views has been described to try to overcome this problem. These specialized projections have now been almost entirely superseded by sectional imaging techniques.

Plain X-ray examination

Lateral view

Since the temporal bones are symmetrically placed, a true lateral view results in superimposition of the two sides; it is therefore necessary to angle the incident ray, or alternatively the skull, in order to prevent this. The greater the tilt, the more the attic (epitympanic recess) and antrum will be thrown clear of the mass of bone around the labyrinth, but this is offset by increased distortion. As shown in Figure 2.1a, the lateral projection of the petromastoid is obtained by placing the head in a true lateral position and angling the tube caudally 15°, thus preventing superimposition of the mastoid processes. The incident beam is centred 5 cm above the uppermost part of the external auditory meatus. The angled lateral view results in superimposition of the petrous bone on the mastoid

process and similarly of the internal and external auditory meatus (Figure 2.1b). The view allows assessment of the degree of pneumatization of the mastoid, the state of translucence of the air cells and the position of the sigmoid sinus and its relation to the tegmen tympani. The attic, aditus and mastoid antrum are also visible.

Oblique posteroanterior (Stenver's) view

In this view, the whole length of the petrous bone is demonstrated by placing it parallel to the X-ray film with the incident ray passing at right angles. When a 'skull table' is used, the patient sits erect, facing the film. With the radiographic baseline horizontal, the sagittal plane of the skull is rotated through 35° and tilted 15° away from the side to be examined. The incident ray is inclined at an angle of 12° cranially and is centred on a point 2 cm medial to the tip of the mastoid process. A radiograph in Stenver's position should demonstrate the petrous tip and internal auditory meatus, the semicircular canals (superior and lateral), the middle ear cleft, the mastoid antrum and the mastoid process (Figure 2.2).

Perorbital view

This is the best view of the internal auditory meatus if tomography is unavailable and should be carried out in the posteroanterior position to avoid radiation to the eyes. The orbitomeatal line is at right angles to the film. The tube is angled 5–10° caudally, centring between the orbits (Figure 2.3). The petrous pyramids and internal auditory meatus are thus projected through the orbits (Figure 2.4).

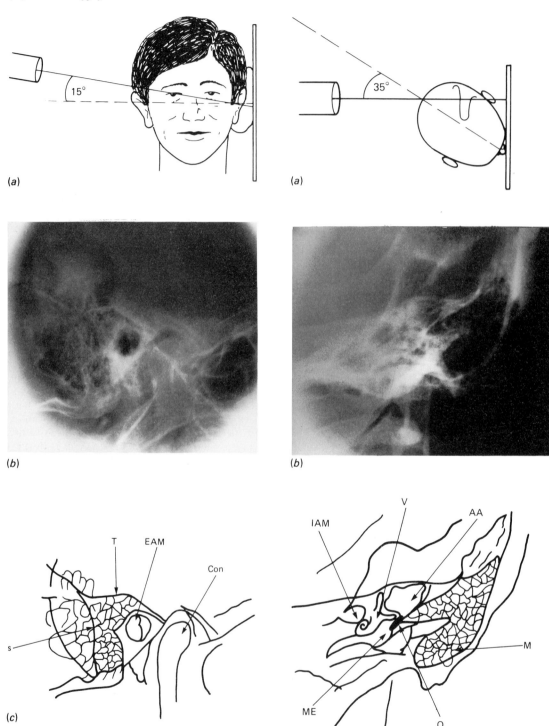

(a)

(b)

(c)

Figure 2.1 Lateral view showing mastoid air-cells. S = sigmoid sinus plate, T = tegmen, con = condyle of the mandible, EAM = external auditory meatus. (From *A Textbook of Radiological Diagnosis*, H. K. Lewis and Company Ltd, London and *Radiology of the Ear*, Blackwell Scientific Publications, Oxford)

Figure 2.2 Stenver's view showing mastoid process (M), attic and antrum (AA), as well as the vestibule (V) and semicircular canals. ME = middle ear, O = ossicles, IAM = internal auditory meatus

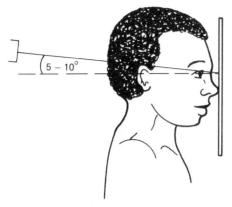

Figure 2.3 The position for the perorbital view

Computerized tomography (CT)

The ability of CT to show intracranial lesions was the first and most important contribution to diagnostic imaging and the premier role for the otologist is the demonstration of intracranial complications of suppurative ear disease, such as brain abscess, and the intracranial extension of tumours such as glomus and vestibular schwannoma. The introduction of thin section high resolution CT meant that very fine bone detail could be demonstrated in the petrous temporal bone. This is now the imaging investigation of choice, and has replaced conventional polytomography almost completely. However, the demonstration of soft tissue abnormalities in the middle ear has been disappointing. Virtually no tissue characterization is defined by CT and only the anatomical configuration and situation of a soft tissue mass gives a clue to the diagnosis, unless the mass contains abnormal calcification. Contrast enhancement of lesions in the petrous temporal bone has also been disappointing as an aid to diagnosis on a CT examination. A profound knowledge of the sectional anatomy is required, especially in the axial plane, which is the basis of the examination.

Radiation dose

Great care must be taken to limit radiation to the lens of the eye lens and cornea, especially if multiple sections are used in the axial plane. Despite the use of scout views with cursor lines and a machine with a tilting gantry, this can be difficult. We recommend a plane at 30° to the orbito-meatal baseline for most examinations of the ear. This is parallel to the roof of the orbit so that the globe is mostly below the sections (Figure 2.5).

Axial sections

Routine CT studies of the petromastoid use thin (1 or 2 mm) sections in the high resolution mode on 'bone algorithm'. These are viewed on a wide window setting of 3000 or 4000 HU. Contrast enhancement is almost never used for lesions of the petrous temporal bone. The lowest section shows the full length of the basal coil of the cochlea (arrow) (see Figure 2.6). The round window niche should be demonstrated in this section or in the next one up. The mid-modiolar is the next higher section; this shows all the coils of the cochlea and the stapes, oval window and vestibule. The next two important sections are at the level of the second part of the facial nerve (arrows) and the lateral

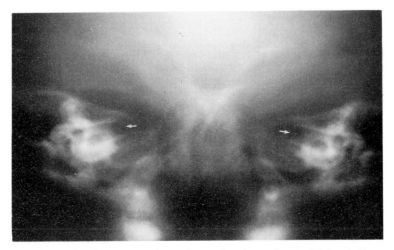

Figure 2.4 Zonogram of the internal auditory meatus (arrows); a similar view to the perorbital projection

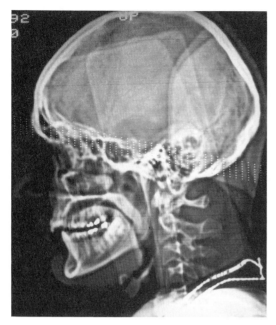

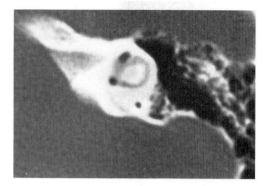

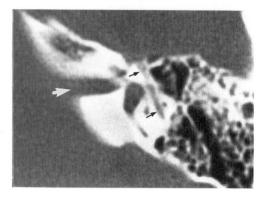

Figure 2.5 Lateral scout view showing the plane of a set of axial CT sections

semicircular canal respectively. The internal auditory meatus is seen in both these sections (white arrows). behind the middle ear cavity. Although the crura of the stapes may be seen, an adequate demonstration of the oval window is not obtained in the base plane. Four of the most important axial sections are shown in Figure 2.6.

Coronal sections

These are obtained in the head-hanging or chin-up position to supplement the axial views if required. Sections 1 or 2 mm thick are obtained as near as possible in the coronal plane aided by gantry tilt. The radiation dose to the eyes from coronal sections is very low as they are not in the X-ray beam. The sections are very similar to those for the standard study on the polytome which may have to be done if the patient cannot maintain the position for coronal CT.

The four most important coronal sections are shown in Figure 2.7. They begin at the level of the carotid canal (C) and curl of the central bony spiral of the cochlea. The malleus is well shown at this level. Further back the section at the level of the vestibule shows the internal auditory meatus (large arrow) as well as the stapes (small arrow) and oval window. Further back still, at the most prominent part of the lateral semicircular canal, the pyramidal eminence is shown between facial recess and sinus tympani and the round window niche (arrow). The descending facial canal and jugular fossa are assessed

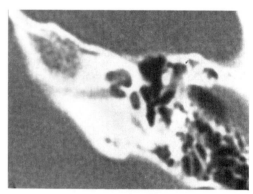

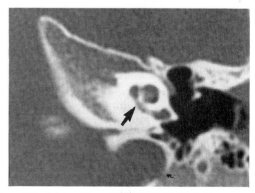

Figure 2.6 Axial sections of the petrous temporal bone

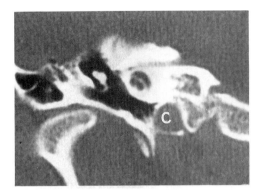

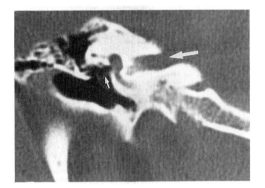

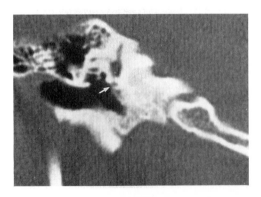

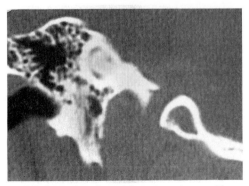

Figure 2.7 Coronal sections of the petrous temporal bone

and the examination finishes at the posterior semicircular canal, although further sections may be necessary to show the mastoid antrum and air cells.

CT examinations with intravenous contrast enhancement

These are now rarely performed since nuclear magnetic resonance became available. The standard procedure is to inject 50 ml of iodine-containing contrast medium, but for very vascular tumours such as glomus tumours, a rapid infusion of 250 ml is preferred, enabling the lesion to be enhanced in the vascular phase, i.e. with the contrast actually in the blood vessels rather than in the later extravasion phase with the contrast mainly in the extracellular spaces. This phase is more important for intracranial lesions.

Air meatography: the demonstration of the contents of the internal auditory meatus and cerebellopontine angle

Air CT meatography, otherwise known as gas cisternography, is no longer used as the definitive investigation to define a small intrameatal vestibular schwannoma unless contraindications or patient claustrophobia preclude MRI. The VIIth and VIIIth cranial nerves, as well as the loop of the anterior inferior cerebellar artery can usually be recognized (Figure 2.8). Air meatography needs to be performed with subsequent overnight hospital admission as, although it seems free of any serious complication, there is, nevertheless, a significant incidence of unpleasant side effects such as prolonged headache.

Other intrathecal contrast agents

These are rarely used in otoradiology. Large extra-axial masses in the posterior cranial fossa, if not clearly defined on the enhanced CT scan and MRI is not available, are best outlined by a positive intrathecal enhancing agent such as iopamidol (Niopam), which can show the relation of the tumour to the brain stem. An example of this is a cholesteatoma of congenital origin in the cerebellopontine angle (Figure 2.9).

Reformatted CT images

These can be obtained from multiple thin contiguous axial sections. Reformatted images can be made in any plane but the quality is always inferior to a direct examination and depends on two factors: (i) the number of sections and therefore the amount of raw data available for the reconstruction process; (ii)

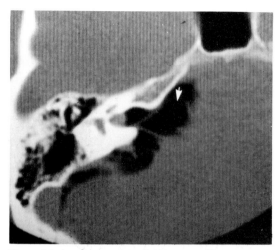

Figure 2.8 An air meatogram showing a small acoustic schwannoma in the fundus of the internal auditory meatus. Note besides the VIIth and VIIIth cranial nerves that the loop of the anterior inferior cerebellar artery has been demonstrated extending into the internal auditory meatus (arrow). These features would now be demonstrated by fast spin echo MRI

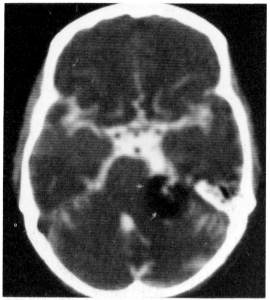

Figure 2.9 An iopamidol contrast study of the posterior cranial fossa. A well-defined area of low attenuation (arrows) is outlined. Congenital cholesteatoma of the cerebellopontine angle

absolute immobility of the patient while these sections are being obtained.

Sagittal reformatted views are useful for assessing a large vestibular aqueduct (Figure 2.10) and may also be used to show the descending facial canal and disruption between malleus and incus (Figure 2.11). MRI to demonstrate an enlarged endolymphatic sac and duct is probably more pertinent than using CT to show the bony outlines of the vestibular aqueduct

and this can now be achieved by thin section fast spin echo imaging.

Magnetic resonance imaging

The continuing development of new MR techniques means that the standard protocols for investigating

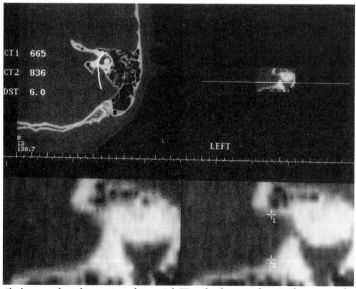

Figure 2.10 A large vestibular aqueduct demonstrated on axial CT and reformatted sagittal sections which are pretargetted slightly off the sagittal plane. The width of the descending limb of the vestibular aqueduct is measured in its mid portion at 6.0 mm

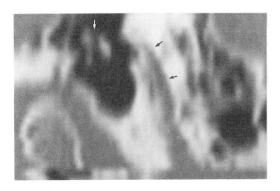

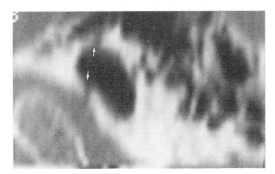

Figure 2.11 Sagittal reformatted views showing the descending facial nerve canal (black arrows) as well as disruption of the malleus and incus (white arrow). The lower section shows a fracture line through the bony external auditory meatus (white arrows)

deafness and lesions affecting the petrous temporal bone and posterior cranial fossa are subject to change. Clinical tests can usually give some idea of whether the abnormality is primarily in the petrous bone or the posterior cranial fossa. Audiometry, in particular the brain stem evoked responses, can help to decide whether sensorineural deafness is cochlear, i.e. end organ in type, or retrocochlear from lesions of the cranial nerves or their central connections. Magnetic resonance is the primary imaging investigation of choice for the retrocochlear type, but MR is secondary to CT for the assessment of the cochlear type of deafness. The protocols used for different pathologies will be described subsequently.

Bone produces a negligible signal on MR scans and so both the bone of the petromastoid and the air in the middle ear cleft and mastoid cell system appear as black areas on the scan, devoid of any of the bone detail so well demonstrated by tomography and high resolution CT. Thus, only soft tissue structures within the petrous temporal bone are imaged and this can be an advantage for the demonstration of the cranial nerves passing through the skull base, as the nerve itself will be shown, not the canal in which it lies. In contrast to the non-signal of compact bone, marrow spaces, which are very variable in extent but occur

mostly in the petrous apex, give an intense signal on T1-weighted images because of their large fat content (Figure 2.12).

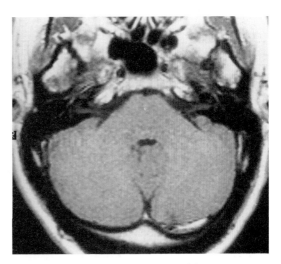

Figure 2.12 T1-weighted axial section of the posterior cranial fossa

The diagnostic protocol for MRI of the temporal bone and posterior fossa uses axial sections with long and short TR spin echo sequences after a short sagittal localizer. These repetition times are combined with long and short TEs to give T1- and T2-weighted images. The region of interest is portrayed in 4 mm thick slices. Recently a new technique of fast spin echo (FSE) has been introduced. This gives greatly improved spatial resolution and allows the individual nerves to be identified in the internal auditory meatus (Figure 2.13). Contrast enhancement using the paramagnetic agent gadolinium DTPA is used in most cases and has tended to replace the T2-weighted sequences. Most tumours show a significant degree of enhancement but studies with Gd are especially valuable for the demonstration of a vestibular schwannoma (see below).

Magnetic resonance angiography (MRA) can now be used as part of the MR examination, especially for vascular lesions such as glomus tumours or for vascular anomalies like a high jugular bulb if this is not differentiated convincingly by routine CT and MR protocols. Obstruction of the sigmoid sinus with demonstration of multiple venous collaterals can be usefully shown by MRA after arterial saturation (Figure 2.14). Occasionally, selective arterial MRA with elimination of venous flow may be useful for showing the blood supply to the tumour, usually from the posterior auricular or ascending pharyngeal arteries. Digital subtraction and catheter angiography are now only required for therapeutic embolization techniques preoperatively to reduce the blood supply to glomus tumours.

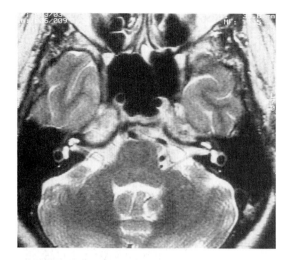

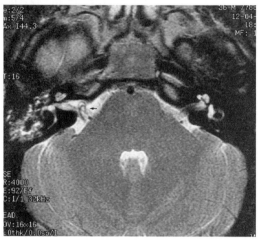

Figure 2.13 (*a*) T2-weighted fast spin echo of the posterior cranial fossa showing the VIIth and VIIIth nerves in the IAM; (*b*) a similar study from another case showing a vascular loop in the IAM (arrow). (Courtesy Dr M. Charlesworth and Mr J. B. Booth)

A major indication for arterial MRA is vessel displacement or compression. MRA is performed after conventional MRI but before gadolinium contrast is given. Evaluation of type and extent of vascular pathology can be severely hampered by alterations in the speed of blood flow. MRA can also be used to demonstrate the circulation in the vertebral arteries (see Volume 1, Chapter 17).

Demonstration of the facial nerve canal

The facial nerve runs a complicated course through the temporal bone. From the lateral end of the internal auditory meatus to the stylomastoid foramen, the facial canal is divided into three parts, corresponding to their directions. These are difficult to demonstrate

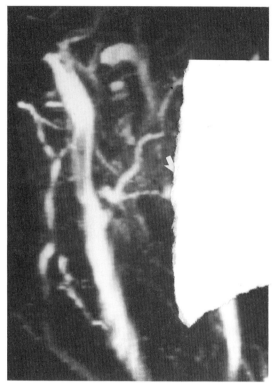

Figure 2.14 Venous MRA of the jugular veins showing normal perfusion of the right jugular vein and sigmoid sinus but occlusion of the left vein due to sigmoid sinus thrombosis (arrow). Note the venous collaterals. From *MRI of the Head and Neck*, Berlin: Springer Verlag, courtesy of Thomas J. Vogl)

with conventional radiography and the Stenver's view, which may show the descending part, is probably the only projection of value.

Labyrinthine part

Starting at the anterosuperior aspect of the lateral end of the internal auditory meatus, this short segment swings anteriorly above the cochlea to the pit for the geniculate ganglion, where the nerve turns sharply backwards to become the second part. This short length of canal may be shown by axial CT (Figure 2.15), but the sulcus for the geniculate ganglion is well demonstrated in coronal sections (see Figure 2.7).

Tympanic part

From the geniculate ganglion to the second bend, the nerve runs backwards above the oval window and below the lateral semicircular canal which overhangs it. It is surrounded by a thin bony sheath which may be dehiscent. Its course is somewhat oblique (Figure 2.16).

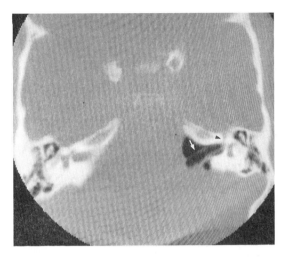

Figure 2.15 Facial nerve canal. Axial CT with air meatogram showing the facial nerve in the internal auditory meatus (white arrow) and the first part of the intratemporal canal (arrowhead)

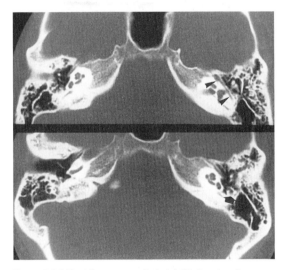

Figure 2.16 Facial nerve canal. Axial CT showing the tympanic part (arrowheads) and descending part (large arrow)

Mastoid or descending part

The third part of the nerve runs downwards from the second bend at the level of the pyramidal eminence to the stylomastoid foramen. Its length is partly dependent on the shape of the temporal bone and partly on the extent of pneumatization of the mastoid. Its width varies considerably. The bony canal is best demonstrated by coronal section and lateral CT (Figure 2.17). Recognition is easy where the nerve passes through solid bone, but may be difficult where

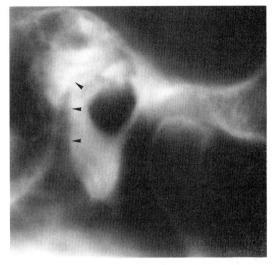

Figure 2.17 Facial nerve canal. Lateral view showing the descending part (arrowheads)

there is much pneumatization. In children with congenital ear lesions, it is important not to confuse the facial nerve canal with other dehiscences such as the tympanomastoid fissure.

Choice of investigation by imaging techniques

High resolution CT is now established as the most useful and versatile procedure for showing bony detail in the petrous pyramid, soft tissue abnormalities in the middle ear and extension of disease into the cranial cavity. It has supplanted conventional tomography and limited angiography. If the eyes are rigorously avoided, the good beam collimation of CT results in a corneal dose almost as low as polytomography with eyeshields. However, 20–25 slices, which included the orbits, were found to result in a considerable dose of radiation (12–25 cGy) using the most recent machine of a major manufacturer (see Volume 1, Chapter 17). Magnetic resonance is now the investigation of choice for showing soft tissue lesions in the petrous pyramid.

Otitis media is essentially a clinical diagnosis. Radiology shows only non-specific opacity of the middle ear cleft and is rarely required. It may, however, be useful for showing evidence of bone erosion in mastoiditis or alternatively for confirming that the air cells are indeed air containing. Similarly, the diagnosis of an acquired cholesteatoma with attic perforation is clinical, the treatment is surgical exploration, and radiology largely irrelevant, although it is now being claimed that a cholesteatoma as small as 3 mm in size can be diagnosed much earlier by the use of CT. For cholesteatoma behind an intact eardrum, imaging is as important as it is for vascular masses in the middle ear cavity (see below).

The demonstration of rarefaction of the labyrinthine capsule is sometimes useful to confirm the presence of otospongiosis.

A brief review of imaging techniques in some of these pathological processes is given below.

Congenital malformations

Congenital malformations of the inner, middle and external ear almost always present in childhood and are considered in Volume 6. This does not, however, apply to vascular anomalies which are usually discovered in late childhood or adulthood. The differential diagnosis of these vascular anomalies and their distinction from vascular neoplasms, especially glomus tumours, is almost entirely dependent upon radiology (Phelps and Lloyd, 1986).

Vascular anomalies

Angiography has been considered the definitive investigation and, in many cases, is mandatory when there appears to be a vascular mass behind the eardrum. Exceedingly rare abnormalities are a persistent stapedial artery or an aneurysm of the internal carotid artery (Glasscock *et al.*, 1980; Moffat and O'Connor, 1980). These can only be recognized by angiography. This discussion concerns aberrations in position of the internal carotid artery and jugular bulb.

The anatomy of the jugular bulb is variable, the right usually being larger than the left. Not infrequently, it extends above the inferior rim of the bony annulus, with or without a bony covering. The anatomy has been comprehensively reviewed by Graham (1974), who quoted dissections by other authors showing the jugular bulb extending above the inferior rim of the annulus in 6% of specimens, and a similar percentage showing dehiscence in the bony floor of the middle ear cavity.

When the jugular bulb is small, it is separated from the floor of the middle ear by a comparatively thick layer of bone, which is usually compact, but may contain air cells. Anteriorly the bulb is in relationship with the internal carotid artery. A spur or crest of bone separates the jugular fossa from the carotid canal at the skull base (Figure 2.18). When the jugular bulb is very large, it can extend up into the mesotympanum with a thin bony covering, which can easily be damaged at surgery (Figure 2.19). When there is dehiscence of this bony covering the exposed jugular bulb is at even greater risk. The soft tissue mass of a dehiscent jugular bulb cannot be adequately shown by conventional and tomographic imaging, but is well shown by CT, especially in the coronal plane, and by retrograde jugular venography (Figure 2.20).

Another aspect of the large jugular bulb is encroachment on inner ear structures. The internal auditory meatus, vestibular aqueduct and posterior semicircular canal may be affected, especially if there is an associated diverticulum from the bulb (Phelps and Lloyd, 1983).

Aberrations in the course of the internal carotid artery through the petrous temporal bone are extremely rare. Normally the artery ascends vertically, medial and anterior to the middle ear cavity before bending sharply anterior and medially below the eustachian tube and cochlea; it then passes through the foramen lacerum into the cranial cavity. A thin

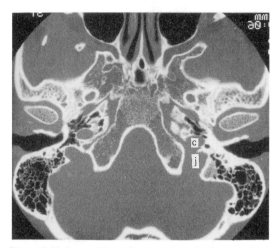

Figure 2.18 Lower CT axial section through the carotid canal (c) and jugular fossa (j). Note the condyle of the mandible and the anterior and posterior walls of the external auditory meatus are well demonstrated

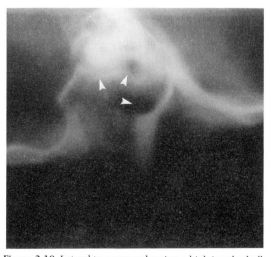

Figure 2.19 Lateral tomogram showing a high jugular bulb with thin bony covering forming the floor of the middle ear cavity (arrowheads)

between the carotid and the jugular bulb remains intact. In more severe aberrations, a soft tissue mass will be shown in the middle ear by CT (Figure 2.22), but the important differentiating feature on coronal CT is absence of the normal carotid canal and a laterally and more posteriorly placed vertical canal (Figure 2.23). These features need to be confirmed by angiography and no attempt at surgical interference should be made (Figure 2.24).

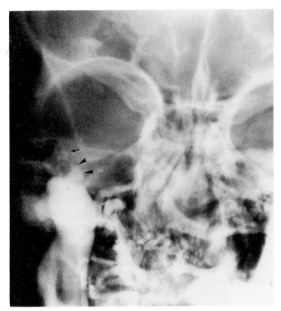

Figure 2.20 Retrograde jugular venogram showing a dehiscent jugular bulb in the middle ear cavity, but also a diverticulum extending medial to the labyrinth (arrowheads). The arrow indicates the crus commune. (From *Radiology of the Ear*, 1983, Blackwell Scientific Publications)

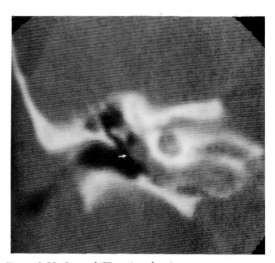

Figure 2.22 Coronal CT section showing a more severe aberration of the internal carotid artery which appears as a soft tissue mass in the middle ear cavity (arrow)

bony septum separates the artery from the hypotympanum (see Figure 2.7). There is said to be dehiscence in 1% of people (Glasscock *et al.* 1980), but the true incidence is probably much less than this. If the ascending part of the artery is more posteriorly placed than usual with a very acute bend, it is more likely to be dehiscent (Figure 2.21), although the spur

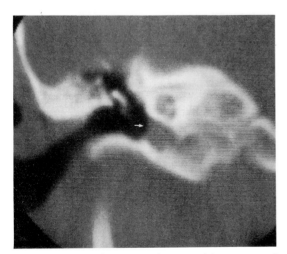

Figure 2.21 Coronal CT section showing a dehiscent carotid artery underneath the cochlea (arrow). The tympanogram showed characteristic pulsations

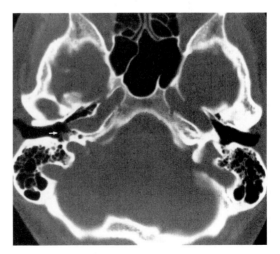

Figure 2.23 Dehiscent internal carotid artery in the middle ear cavity shown on this axial CT section. The arrow shows a separate stapedial artery. Compare with the other side

Differential diagnosis

Enlargement of the jugular fossa may be demonstrated on plain film X-ray by a transoral view or an undertilted submentovertical projection. However, the best method of demonstrating this anomaly is by high resolution CT scan when the jugular bulb can be seen

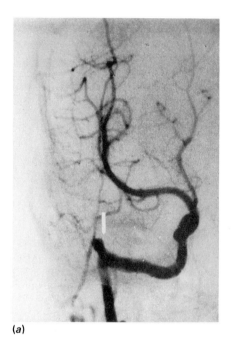

(a)

as a rounded or dome-shaped opacity encroaching upon the middle ear space (Figure 2.25). High resolution CT in the axial plane will also show both the enlargement of the jugular bulb and the integrity of the cortex at the margin of the jugular fossa. This allows a distinction to be made between a large jugular bulb and the enlargement that takes place in the presence of a glomus jugulare tumour.

In the anomaly of an aberrant carotid artery, it can be shown from angiographic studies that the vessel lies both more lateral than normal and more posteriorly. In this way, it may come to lie under the promontory in the middle ear, sometimes producing a small indentation. CT is again the definitive investigation, since it is possible to show both the soft tissue mass of the vessel in the middle ear and also the abnormal course of the carotid canal (Figure 2.26).

Trauma

The value of radiology for injuries involving the petrous temporal bone may be summarized:

1 To confirm the presence of a fracture line
2 To show the site of injury to the facial nerve
3 To demonstrate and confirm the pathway of a cerebrospinal fluid fistula
4 To show foreign bodies
5 In the late management of persistent conductive deafness, ossicular dislocations may be shown.

The radiological investigation should relate to and depend upon the clinical picture. To demonstrate a

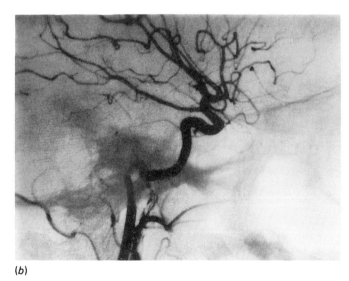

(b)

Figure 2.24 Angiographic confirmation of the aberrant carotid artery in the middle ear cavity. (*a*) Frontal view. The marker indicates the position of the medial wall of the middle ear cavity. The acute bend lies lateral to it. (*b*) The lateral view shows the posterior extension and acute bend in the artery. (Courtesy of Dr A. D. Lloyd, Walsgrave Hospital, Coventry)

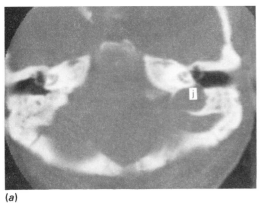
(a)

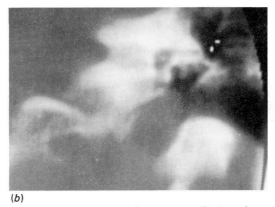
(b)

Figure 2.25 (*a*) Large jugular bulb (j) encroaches upon the middle ear cavity. Note the smooth bony margins. (*b*) Coronal CT section shows the soft tissue mass of the high jugular bulb in the middle ear cavity reaching to the level of the round window. Note the pyramidal eminence shown in this section

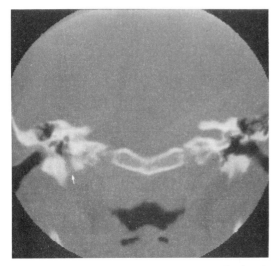

Figure 2.26 Coronal CT section showing a laterally placed carotid canal and artery in the middle ear cavity (arrow)

fracture, the X-ray beam must be in or close to the plane of the fracture line and several projections in different planes are necessary. Tomography or high resolution CT will show more fractures than will plain films and are valuable for demonstrating more precisely their path and extent. The examination needs to be performed in at least two planes.

Although fractures of the petrous temporal bone follow no set pattern, they are usually classified with reference to the long axis of the petrous pyramid as longitudinal or transverse.

The fracture line in the commoner longitudinal type is in the long axis of the petrous bone and, typically, it extends from the squama across the superior aspect of the bony external auditory meatus

and through the tegmen (Figure 2.27). The fracture line then passes in front of or behind the labyrinth.

Anterior longitudinal fractures usually involve the horizontal portion of the facial nerve canal in the region of the geniculate ganglion (Figure 2.28).

Posterior fractures involving the vertical portion of the canal or the posterior genu then proceed either along the roof of the eustachian tube or to one of the nearby foramina (the foramen lacerum, jugular foramen or internal auditory meatus). Longitudinal fractures are best shown by axial CT when the whole length of the fracture line can be shown, and by lateral tomography or reformatted lateral CT. The reformatting technique is particularly well suited to the demonstration of longitudinal fractures when the cross-sectional reconstruction can be made precisely

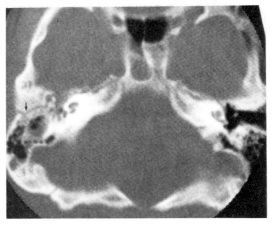

Figure 2.27 Axial CT scan showing longitudinal fracture through the roof of the external auditory meatus (arrows). Note the slight disruption of the joint between malleus and incus and fluid in the middle ear cavity

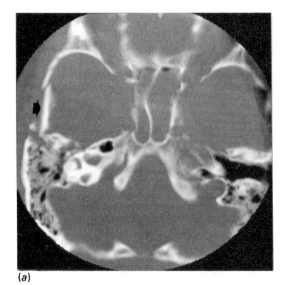

(a)

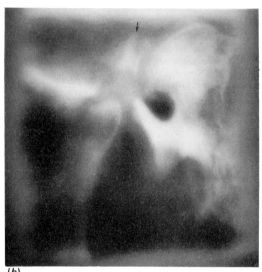

(b)

Figure 2.28 (*a*) Axial CT section showing a longitudinal fracture of the petrous temporal bone. There is a depressed fragment of the squamous temporal bone (arrow), fracture of the sphenoid sinuses with fluid levels. Although the ossicles are intact, there are small fragments of bone close to the geniculate ganglion. (*b*) Lateral tomogram showing disintegration of the articular fossa of the temporomandibular joint, and two fragments of bone (arrow) which were found to be impinging on the facial nerve at operation. (From *Tomography of the neurotological patient*, in *A Handbook of Neurotological Diagnosis*, edited by House and O'Connor, p. 238, by courtesy of Marcel Dekker Inc., New York, 1986)

in the plane of the fracture shown on the axial views.

Transverse fractures run at right angles to the long axis of the petrous bone. As classically described,

this type of fracture affects the pyramid, with the fracture line passing across the labyrinth or internal auditory meatus. It produces facial palsy and sensorineural deafness which may be complete and permanent. Some fractures, however, pass laterally to the pyramid, through the middle ear or external meatus and, because they are in the same plane, should strictly be classified as 'transverse', although the conductive deafness and other features make them very similar to the longitudinal type.

Transverse fractures are also best demonstrated by axial CT but they can usually be shown also by simple plain film views in the perorbital or Stenver's projections (Figure 2.29). Coronal CT sections will show the fluid level of a cerebrospinal fluid fistula.

Ossicular dislocations

When a head injury is followed by conductive deafness, it is most commonly the result of a simple haemotympanum or a traumatic rupture of the drum. However, if a hearing loss remains after the drumhead has healed, then disruption of the ossicular chain must be suspected.

Unfortunately, the commonest dislocation, namely that of the incudostapedial joint, cannot be satisfactorily demonstrated by tomographic methods. Displacement of the incus, rarely the malleus, and separation of the incudomalleolar joint can be demonstrated by axial and coronal tomograms or high resolution CT (Figure 2.30). Loss of the normal 'molar tooth' sign on the lateral views is another important sign of major ossicular displacement (see Figure 2.11).

Inflammatory disease

Acute otitis media and its complications are essentially diseases of childhood, and are considered in Volume 6. Chronic suppurative otitis media is usually described as:

1 Non-cholesteatomatous tubotympanic type in which radiology has a negligible role
2 Attico-antral type with cholesteatoma.

Adhesive otitis media involves the development of adhesions and tympanosclerosis, i.e. calcification in areas of hyaline degeneration. The only importance of tympanosclerosis, from an imaging point of view, is to be aware of its existence to avoid misinterpretation of plaques of calcification in the middle ear.

Radiology of complications of middle ear infection

These may follow any form of middle ear infection but, most commonly, acute mastoiditis and cholesteatomatous chronic suppurative otitis media.

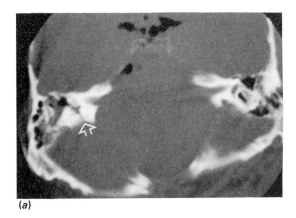

(a)

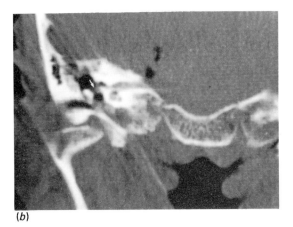

(b)

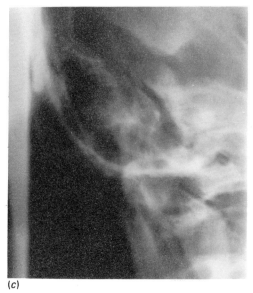

(c)

Figure 2.29 (*a*) Transverse fracture through the vestibule (open arrow) shown on this axial CT scan. Note the fluid level in the middle ear and the air in the cranial cavity. (*b*) Coronal CT section of the same case shows a traumatized but intact facial nerve (arrow) which was stretched across the fracture line. (*c*) Plain Stenver's view of the fracture. (From Tomography of the neurotological patient, in *A Handbook of Neurotological Diagnosis*, edited by House and O'Connor, p. 240, by courtesy of Marcel Dekker Inc., New York, 1986)

Labyrinthitis

The symptoms of vertigo in the presence of acute or chronic suppurative otitis media indicate the presence of labyrinthitis due to involvement of the labyrinthine fluids in the inflammatory process. Spread of the infection to the labyrinth may be via the intact oval window, the round window membrane or via an erosion in the labyrinthine capsule, the last usually being produced by a cholesteatoma. Radiology is likely to be informative only in cholesteatomatous disease, where the most common abnormality is an erosion of the bony capsule of the lateral semicircular canal, demonstrable on a Stenver's projection, coronal section tomography or CT. Suppurative labyrinthitis can also result from the spread of an infection from the blood stream or meninges. Following an episode of purulent labyrinthitis, which results in total destruction of the membranous labyrinth, the bony labyrinth may become filled with granulation tissue which often undergoes varying degrees of ossification. This so-called 'labyrinthitis obliterans' is, primarily, a histopathological diagnosis but the ossification is readily detectable by CT (Figure 2.31).

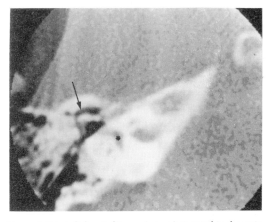

Figure 2.30 A dislocated incus (arrow) situated in the attic and no longer articulating with the malleus, which was shown on the section below this axial CT section. The asterisk indicates the vestibule

Partial obliteration of the bony labyrinth is probably a characteristic tomographic feature with a clear-cut margin seen between the parts obliterated

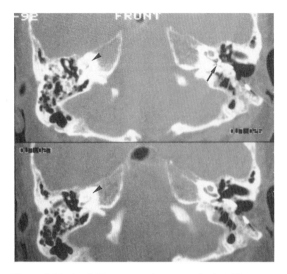

Figure 2.31 Axial CT sections of a patient deafened by meningitis. The coils of the cochlea on the right are partially obliterated (arrowheads) and there is a single channel implant in the round window niche on the left (arrow)

by bone and the portions seemingly unaffected. This appearance distinguishes post-suppurative labyrinthitis obliterans from advanced otosclerosis, in which the bone encroachment is much more diffuse.

Intracranial complications

These comprise one or more of the following: extradural abscess, subdural abscess, temporal lobe abscess, cerebellar abscess, meningitis and hydrocephalus. Suspicion of their presence is *par excellence* the indication for computerized tomography in acute or chronic suppurative otitis media.

The radiological diagnosis of brain abscess is based on the demonstration of a localized area of low attenuation and, after injection of contrast medium, a surrounding area of high attenuation. Distortion or displacement of the ventricles may be present if the lesion is large. Serial CT scans allow the development of a lesion to be monitored and give warning of incipient rupture into a ventricle, or they may be used to assess postoperative progress of the cavity. It is important to remember that up to 15% of brain abscesses of otitic origin are multiple. Occasionally, an abscess which is clinically silent may be demonstrated.

Extradural and subdural collections of pus will show a peripheral rim of low attenuation after contrast enhancement. Not infrequently, however, extradural abscesses are very shallow and not well demonstrated by computerized tomography, unless by chance a tomographic section passes through the centre of the pathological area.

Tuberculous otitis media in adults most commonly occurs in association with advanced pulmonary tuberculosis, but in children it may occur in isolation. Extensive ragged destruction in the mastoid and middle ear rather than sclerosis is the typical radiographic feature.

Malignant otitis externa

Malignant otitis externa is a rare condition in which an otitis externa, most often due to Pseudomonas infection and usually in a diabetic patient, spreads widely leading to osteomyelitis of the temporal bone; cranial nerve lesions may also occur according to the precise area of spread and occasionally death (Prasad, 1976).

Radiologically there is a typical appearance of rarefaction of the bone spreading symmetrically and centrifugally from the external auditory meatus. In an analysis of nine cases of diabetic malignant otitis externa, Mendez *et al.* (1979) found that when there was a unilateral facial paralysis or a jugular foramen syndrome, bone destruction was always demonstrable. Five cases had evidence of jugular fossa destruction, but only one had a jugular foramen syndrome. Retrograde jugular venography confirmed the presence of a high degree of venous obstruction at the jugular bulb.

A good demonstration of the extent of the disease is given by CT (Figure 2.32) but probably more important are isotope studies to show the degree of activity of the infective process (Mendez *et al.*, 1979). Nevertheless, early diagnosis is essential as prognosis seems to be related directly to the stage that the disease has reached at the onset of treatment (Mills, 1986).

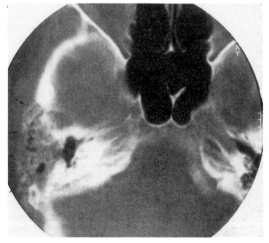

Figure 2.32 Malignant otitis externa. Axial CT scan at the level of the external auditory meatus, showing the infected bone on the side of the head

Cholesteatoma

The aetiology of this characteristic epidermoid cyst containing keratin is not fully understood. Two types are recognized, although they do not differ histologically.

1 Congenital cholesteatoma originating from ectodermal cell rests. This may arise in any of the cranial bones, the petrous temporal being the most commonly affected, or within the cranial cavity
2 Acquired cholesteatoma, in which there is ingrowth of the surface epithelium of the tympanic membrane.

In the vast majority the diagnosis is readily made on clinical grounds.

Congenital cholesteatoma

Congenital cholesteatoma may arise anywhere within the petrous temporal bone but may be conveniently classified into:

1 Cholesteatoma of the cerebellopontine angle
2 Cholesteatoma arising deep within the petrous pyramid
3 Cholesteatoma arising in the jugular fossa region
4 Congenital cholesteatoma of the middle ear cleft.

Classically, these lesions present in middle age with severe sensorineural deafness and facial spasm or weakness. This involvement of the facial nerve is a characteristic feature (Figure 2.33).

Cholesteatoma is the third most common tumour of the cerebellopontine angle, after vestibular schwannoma and meningioma. The CT brain scan shows an area of low attenuation (see Figure 2.9), but MR is the investigation of choice (Figure 2.34).

In the petrous pyramid

A large erosion is usually evident on plain films in a patient with cholesteatoma of the pyramid or petrous

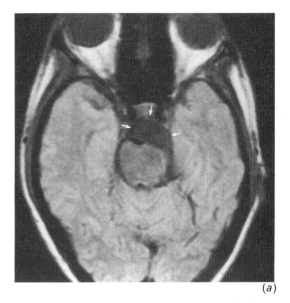

(a)

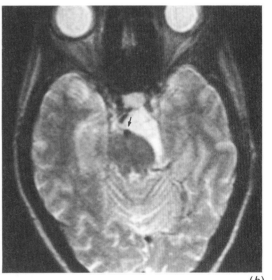

(b)

Figure 2.34 Two axial sections showing a cholesteatoma in the posterior cranial fossa impinging on the brain stem. (a) The T1-weighted protocol shows the mass with low signal (white arrow); (b) T2-weighted image shows high signal from the cholesteatoma. The black arrow indicates the vertebral artery

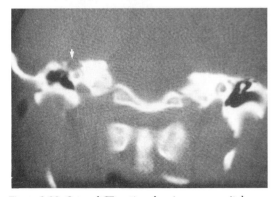

Figure 2.33 Coronal CT section showing a congenital cholesteatoma affecting the geniculate ganglion on the right (arrow)

apex. Tomograms show a clearly defined 'punched out' area of bone destruction. The clear-cut margins may be scalloped and the labyrinth is destroyed by a 'steam roller' effect, although individual coils of the cochlea and the modiolus may be identified after invasion of the cochlea has taken place. There may be thinning and elevation of the superior petrous ridge (Valvassori, 1974) (Figure 2.35). A CT scan

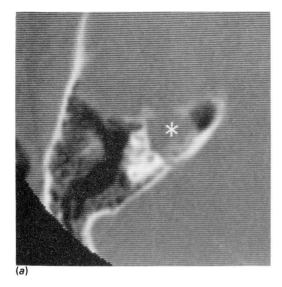

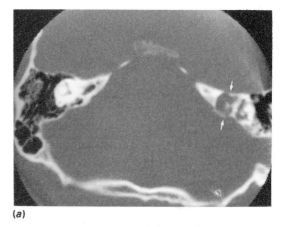

(a)

(a)

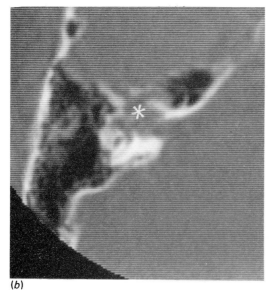

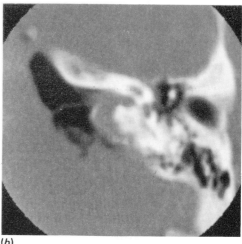

(b)

(b)

Figure 2.36 (*a*) Another congenital cholesteatoma of the petrous apex, which is causing expansion of the bony covering. (*b*) An air meatogram showing the VIIIth cranial nerve. The patient had normal VIIth and VIIIth nerve function in contrast to the previous case where there was complete loss of function of these nerves

Figure 2.35 Congenital cholesteatoma: two axial CT sections showing an expansile mass in a very well pneumatized petrous apex. The cholesteatoma (asterisk) is eroding into the top of the internal auditory meatus and medial aspect of the labyrinth

In the jugular fossa

A cholesteatoma arising in the region of the jugular fossa or skull base may mimic a glomus tumour, both radiologically and clinically. Although the destruction may be extensive, it is usually less ragged than that caused by a glomus tumour.

In the middle ear and mastoid

It is uncertain what proportion of the much more common cholesteatomas arising in the attico-antral region have a congenital origin but the percentage is probably small and they are, ultimately, indistinguishable from acquired cholesteatoma.

will demonstrate a non-enhancing mass of low attenuation, and high resolution CT demonstrates the characteristic expansile cyst-like lesion (Figure 2.36). The congenital cholesteatoma occurring in an extensively pneumatized pyramid can be difficult to diagnose radiologically.

There are two criteria which help to distinguish a cholesteatoma of the middle ear cleft which has a congenital rather than an acquired origin. These are:

1 An intact eardrum with no evidence of a previous perforation
2 An intact spur (scutum).

Acquired cholesteatoma

The vast majority of cholesteatomas arise from either the pars flaccida or the posterior segment of the tympanic membrane. From here they extend into any part of the tympanic cavity and backwards into the mastoid antrum and air cells. There is associated erosion of the walls of the middle ear cleft.

The most important single plain radiographic projection in the management of typical cholesteatoma is the lateral view, with the incident beam tilted 20° caudally. This will show the extent of pneumatization and erosion of the outer attic wall. The other mastoid projections will only demonstrate large erosions. Pneumatization is usually poor or absent and the mastoid sclerotic, but cholesteatoma may be encountered, with minimal bone destruction, in an extensive air-cell system.

Computed tomography in the coronal plane is the optimum method for demonstrating small cholesteatomas in the attic and antrum and is based mainly on the detection of bone erosion (Figure 2.37).

In the attic the following signs indicate the presence of a cholesteatoma:

1 Destruction of the lateral spur (scutum) of bone formed by the junction of the lateral boundary of the attic and the roof of the external auditory meatus
2 Bone destruction of the lateral attic wall
3 Destruction of the ossicles
4 Erosion of the medial attic wall. This is a less common sign, but may lead to involvement of the facial canal or a labyrinthine fistula. It should be noted that the presence of a fistula can only be confidently predicted if the lesion is present on two or more slices.

Similar erosive changes can be discerned on coronal CT, but its ability to depict precisely small soft tissue masses in the middle ear makes CT the best overall method of imaging cholesteatoma. Acquired cholesteatomas are diagnosed on CT by the presence of a non-dependent homogeneous soft tissue mass in an appropriate location (Swartz and Harnsberger, 1992). It is important to remember that CT imaging is unable to distinguish the soft tissues of a chole-

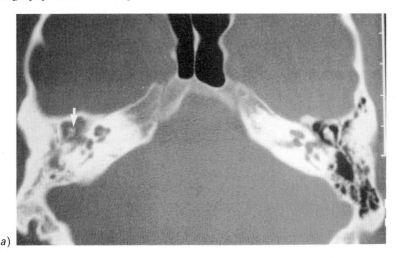

(a)

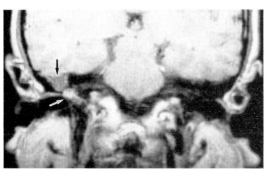

(b)

Figure 2.37 (a) Axial CT scan showing the soft tissue mass of a cholesteatoma with partial erosion of the ossicles (arrow); (b) coronal T1-weighted MR with gadolinium shows a granulomatous polyp as an enhancing mass in the lower middle ear cavity – such information is of little value to the surgeon. The black arrow shows the polyp, the white arrow the cholesteatoma

steatoma from polyps, granulation tissue mucosa, cholesterol cysts or fluid, by tissue characterization.

If a lesion is adequately assessed clinically, and a versatile surgical technique applied in the treatment, then radiological assessment is necessary only in those cases with unusual clinical features, e.g. suspicion of intracranial complications, facial palsy, positive fistula sign, and severe sensorineural deafness or disease in an only hearing ear.

A cholesteatoma may not, however, always be apparent on first inspection. House and Sheehy (1980) reported 41 cases of cholesteatoma with an intact eardrum (3.7% of their series). Cholesteatomas may also be associated with a central type of perforation. Such a true perforation is usually a feature of the safe tubotympanic type of disease, but it may also result from breakdown of a retraction pocket with the resultant isolation of squamous epithelium in the middle ear. Often polyps and granulation tissue obscure both types of disease. Invasion of the labyrinth by a cholesteatoma is not necessarily immediately associated with a dead ear, presumably due to a sealing off of the disease process. When there is a small fistula present in a semicircular canal, a piece of cholesteatoma matrix may be left over the defect in the hope of preserving the remaining cochlear function. In these circumstances, tomographic demonstration of the site of invasion of the labyrinthine capsule provides useful preoperative information (Figure 2.38).

Preservation of cochlear function in a labyrinth invaded by cholesteatoma, first described by Phelps in 1969, is now a well-recognized, though unusual phenomenon. Bagger-Sjobach and Phelps (1985) reviewed reported cases of this phenomenon and added three more (Figure 2.39).

Poor tissue characterization means therefore that CT is less than satisfactory for the demonstration of middle ear cholesteatoma which can only be suggested from the imaging by the morphology of the soft tissue mass and the character of the bone erosion. Can MRI improve this state of affairs? Cholesteatoma gives an intermediate signal on T1-weighted images and high signal on T2-weighted spin echo sequences. Thus it is possible to differentiate cholesteatoma from cholesterol granuloma, which is bright on T1 and T2 sequences (Figure 2.40). Granulation tissue is invariably present in association with an acquired cholesteatoma and being relatively vascular, unlike cholesteatoma, usually shows enhancement with gadolinium (see Figure 2.37). Other soft tissue contents of the middle ear and mastoid include fluid and yellow bone marrow which has a high fat content giving bright signal on the T1-weighted protocols.

In practice, such imaging assessments of an ear with an acquired cholesteatoma are difficult and have little practical application (Phelps and Wright, 1990). However, there are three situations where imaging can be very useful:

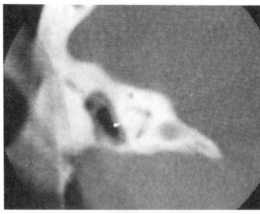

(a)

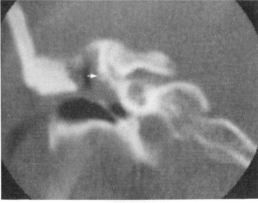

(b)

Figure 2.38 A patient with a positive fistula sign. A cholesteatoma is eroding into the lateral semicircular canal which can be seen to be eroded in these sections; (*a*) axial and (*b*) coronal

1 Encephalocoele in a mastoid cavity

Assessment of a mastoid cavity where it is uncertain whether a soft tissue mass is a recurrent cholesteatoma or an encephalocoele from descent of the brain through a deficient tegmen tympani. Brain tissue can be differentiated from cholesteatoma by MR (Figure 2.41) but, unfortunately, CSF has similar signal characteristics and therefore distinguishing cholesteatoma from a meningocoele is more difficult.

2 Lateral (sigmoid) sinus thrombosis

This is an important complication of suppurative ear disease and is difficult to diagnose. CT may demonstrate abnormal high density of the lumen of the sinus which does not enhance after intravenous contrast, although enhancement of the dura around the sinus may give the characteristic 'empty triangle' or 'delta sign'. However MR, and particularly MRA, is now the

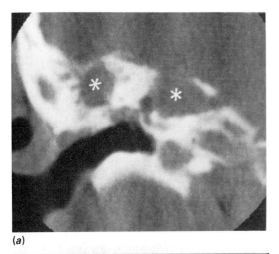

(a)

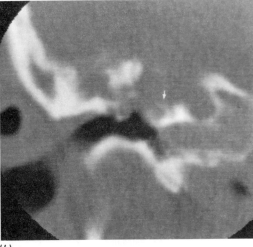

(b)

Figure 2.39 Two coronal CT sections showing a cholesteatoma (asterisk) (*a*) in the attic and extending to the medial side of the labyrinth, and (*b*) eroding into the back of the vestibule and top of the cochlea, leaving the central bony spiral exposed (arrow). Note the erosion of the spur and the intact malleus

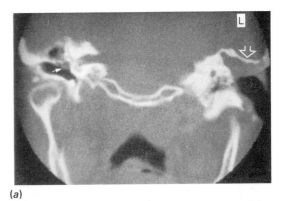

(a)

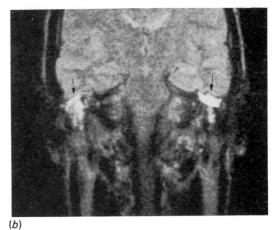

(b)

Figure 2.40 (*a*) Coronal section CT shows a small cholesteatoma in the right middle ear cavity (small arrow) confirmed by otoscopy. On the left there is a large radical cavity (open arrow) with a soft tissue mass in its roof; (*b*) T2-weighted coronal section MR shows intense signal (white) on both sides, although on the T1-weighted sections only the mass on the left gave a high signal. Surgery showed that the mass on the left was not in fact a cholesteatoma but a fluid filled cyst: a cholesterol granuloma

imaging investigation of choice. A fresh sinus thrombosis shows high signal intensity, but occlusion of the vein is best shown by venous MRA using a three-dimensional gradient echo sequence with flow compensation (Irving *et al.*, 1992). A dephasing radiofrequency (RF) pulse needs to be applied to the vessels in the neck to eliminate signal from inflowing (arterial) blood. Thus MRA demonstrates the thrombus as a total signal void of the sinus involved (see Figure 2.14).

3 Expansile lesion to the petrous apex

Both cholesteatoma and cholesterol granuloma occur in the petrous apex and both appear on CT as a clearly defined 'punched out' often expansile area of bone destruction. Magnetic resonance on the other hand can clearly distinguish the two types of pathology (Figure 2.42). Cholesterol granulomas have a high signal intensity on both T1- and T2-weighted protocols (Amedee, Marks and Lyons,

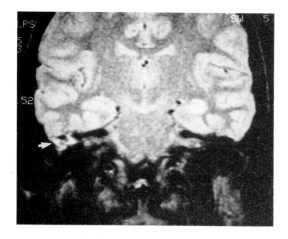

Figure 2.41 A soft tissue mass in a mastoid cavity which proved to be partly encephalocoele and partly recurrent cholesteatoma giving higher signal than brain on the T2-weighted coronal MR section (arrow)

1987) probably due to the presence of fluid in the cyst, rich in cholesterol crystals or to the presence of free methaemoglobin within the cyst, formed from the breakdown of red blood cells and acting as a paramagnetic contrast agent. The incidence of cholesterol granuloma in the petrous apex is thought to be more common than primary cholesteatoma or primary mucocoele (Lo *et al.*, 1984). The importance of the differentiation lies in the requirement for less radical surgery than if the lesion is a cholesteatoma (Lo *et al.*, 1984; Amedee, Marks, and Lyons, 1987).

Tumours of the middle ear and petrous temporal bone

Tumours may involve the middle ear, the mastoid and the petrous parts of the temporal bone, primarily, metastatically or by extension from adjacent sites such as the postnasal space, external auditory meatus, parotid gland or even from structures within the cranial cavity. Vestibular schwannoma is the most common tumour to erode the temporal bone. Primary neoplasms of the middle ear region are extremely rare, the most common being the glomus jugulare tumour (benign) and squamous cell carcinoma (malignant).

Benign neoplasms

A compact osteoma appears as a well-defined, usually single, although occasionally lobulated, bony mass of high density. Cancellous osteomas are more rare and present as a less dense, defined mass. They occur in the following situations:

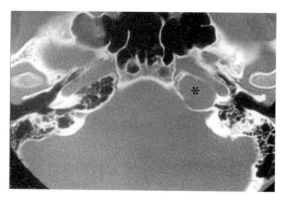

(a)

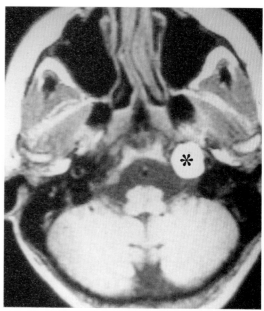

(b)

Figure 2.42 (a) Axial CT scan shows an expansile mass in the petrous apex after a head injury 3 months previously (asterisk); (b) axial MR T1-weighted section shows high signal suggesting cholesterol granuloma rather than cholesteatoma (asterisk)

1 External auditory meatus – where they are asymptomatic unless they become large enough to cause obstruction, with consequent hearing loss or retention of wax and skin debris
2 Squama of the temporal bone – where they cause a hard bulge above and behind the pinna
3 Mastoid – where they are asymptomatic unless encroaching upon the facial nerve canal, causing paralysis
4 Petrous pyramid – where they can occur in the region of the porus of the internal auditory meatus (Beale and Phelps, 1987)

5 Middle ear – where they may impinge upon the ossicular chain, causing a conductive hearing loss (Figure 2.43).

Glomus tumours

Sometimes called chemodectomas or paragangliomas, these arise from small structures called glomus bodies. The tumours are usually classified as glomus jugulare, vagale or tympanicum, depending on the site of origin. The glomus tympanicum may be entirely confined to the middle ear cavity but, usually, the tumour has reached such a size by the time of presentation that it is difficult to determine exactly where in the base of the skull or the upper part of the neck, it has arisen.

The glomus jugulare tumour located in the jugular bulb has ready access to various parts of the temporal bone and the foramina at the base of the skull since they spread along the lines of least resistance. Intracranial extension, therefore, can be along the carotid artery, through cranial nerve foramina, into the nasopharynx, intravascularly into the sigmoid sinus and inferior petrosal sinus, through the temporal bone air-cell systems to the petrous apex, or retrofacially into the mastoid process.

Classically, large tumours demonstrate ragged erosion of the base of the skull in the region of the jugular fossa and posteroinferior aspect of the petrous pyramid, with extension into the mastoid and adjacent occipital bone.

The first radiographic indication of a glomus jugulare tumour is an abnormality of the jugular foramen and fossa. The lateral (vascular) part of the fossa will be affected rather than the medial (nervous) part. The two fossae are rarely symmetrical and expansion may be difficult to asssess. It is most important, therefore, to look for evidence of bone erosion of the margins of the foramen (Figure 2.44). More extensive lesions show a ragged and irregular outline; this is more clearly defined than the erosion produced by an infiltrating lesion such as a carcinoma but not as smooth as the margins of a congenital cholesteatoma or neuroma.

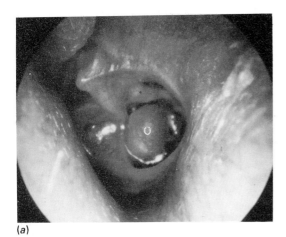

(a)

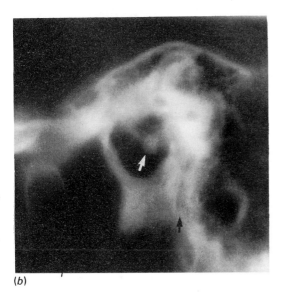

(b)

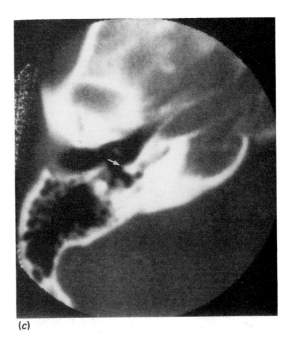

(c)

Figure 2.43 (a) The appearance of the ear drum, (b) lateral tomogram, (c) axial CT scan. A small osteoma (O) (white arrows) in the middle ear cavity. The black arrow points to the descending facial canal

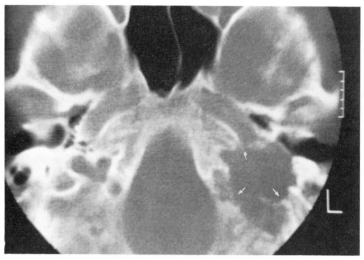

Figure 2.44 Axial section showing enlargement and erosion of the jugular fossa (arrows). Compare with the normal jugular foramen on the other side

Computerized tomography is superior to plain films, not only for assessment of the extent of bone destruction, but also for demonstrating the presence of a mass in the middle ear cavity. Minor erosion of the walls of the cavity and, especially, the promontory, by small glomus tympanicum tumours may also be shown.

We no longer use contrast enhanced CT to show the soft tissue extent of a glomus tumour as MRI before and after gadolinium enhancement is preferred for both jugulare and tympanicum tumours. Axial and coronal CT is used beforehand to assess the bony landmarks and any bone destruction. Sagittal MR views are particularly useful for large glomus jugulare tumours (Figure 2.45) and can show the down-ward extension into the internal jugular vein and neck, thereby replacing jugular venography in the initial assessment.

Glomus jugulare

If a glomus jugulare tumour extends anteriorly it may surround the internal carotid artery, and this is one of the major limitations to successful operative excision. Gadolinium-DTPA enhanced MRI in the axial plane will usually reveal the tumour surrounding the artery; axial CT of the base may confirm erosion of the carotid canal. Carotid angiography may also be useful. The use of gadolinium-DTPA enhanced MRI to demonstrate tumours surrounding the intrapetrous part of the internal carotid is complicated by the presence of bone marrow in the petrous apex, which gives a strong signal in T1-weighted images. A STIR (short tau inversion recovery) sequence may be useful to overcome this problem.

Fatty tissue also presents a diagnostic problem below the skull base; gadolinium-DTPA MRI will reveal glomus jugulare in the neck less distinctly from surrounding tissue planes containing fat, because both the tumour and the fatty tissue give strong signals in T1-weighted sequences (Figure 2.46). However, extension of the tumours down the lumen of the internal jugular vein is better shown by enhanced MRI than by retrograde jugulography which, at best, will reveal only the lower limit of the growth within the vein.

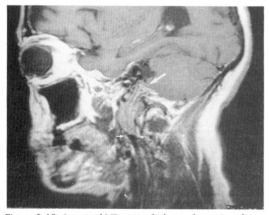

Figure 2.45 A sagittal MR view of a large glomus jugulare tumour. The arrows show the upper and lower extent of the mass

Glomus tympanicum

A small tumour on the promontory will be revealed

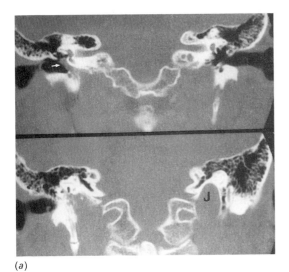

(a)

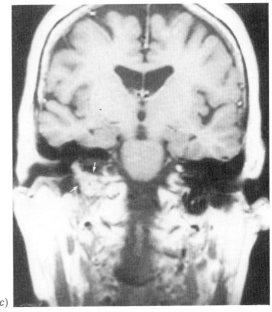

(c)

Figure 2.46 Three coronal sections showing a typical glomus jugulare tumour which has eroded up into the middle ear. (a) CT – arrow shows the mass in the middle ear. J = jugular fossa on the normal side; (b) unenhanced MR. The arrows show the tumour. (c) With gadolinium enhancement the tumour becomes more obvious in the middle ear but less clearly outlined against fat

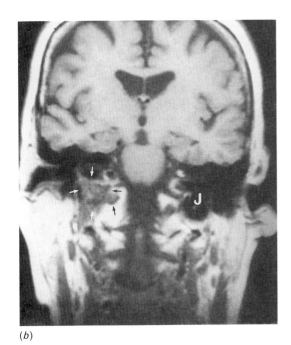

(b)

by CT as a soft tissue mass lying within an air-containing middle ear cavity (Figure 2.47). If this mass is surrounded by air, no further imaging is essential, although the intense enhancement of the tumour produced by gadolinium-DTPA enhanced MR helps to confirm the diagnosis.

As a glomus tympanicum tumour enlarges, two events occur which make confident diagnosis difficult:

1 The tumour reaches the floor of the middle ear cavity.
2 It occludes the eustachian tube, producing an obstructive serous otitis in the middle ear and mastoid. If a plate of thick bone separates the middle ear cavity from the jugular fossa, then no problem arises in differentiating a tympanicum from a jugulare tumour. However, this plate of bone may be very thin and also angulated, so that as a result of CT partial volume averaging, it may be impossible to be certain that it is intact. Gadolinium-DTPA enhanced MRI overcomes this problem by clearly distinguishing the very bright signal of the tumour from the signal void of the blood flowing through the jugular bulb (Figure 2.48). This technique will also distinguish the tumour from fluid in the mastoid air cells. The different appearances of a glomus tympanicum tumour, secondary serous otitis media and yellow marrow are well shown in Figure 2.48.

Angiography

Arteriography no longer has a role in the diagnosis of glomus tumours and is now only undertaken during a preoperative assessment when therapeutic

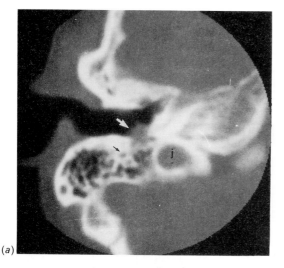

(a)

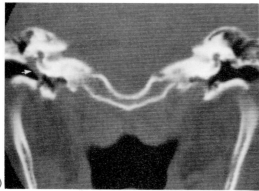

(b)

Figure 2.47 (*a*) Axial CT showing a small glomus tympanicum tumour (white arrow) in the posterior part of the middle ear cavity. This lies medial to the descending facial canal (black arrow) but is separate from the jugular fossa (j). (*b*) Coronal CT section at the level of the oval windows. A glomus tympanicum tumour in the mesotympanum. Note air above and below the tumour

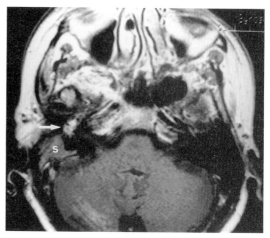

Figure 2.48 Axial MR section after gadolinium enhancement showing a small glomus tympanicum tumour in the middle ear (arrow), clearly distinguished from fluid in the mastoid air cells (s)

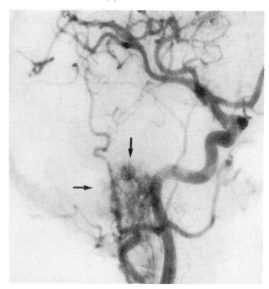

Figure 2.49 Typical angiographic appearance of a small glomus jugulare tumour showing the tumour blush and the supply from the ascending pharyngeal branch of the external carotid artery. (From *Diagnostic Imaging of the Ear*, 1990, edited by P. D. Phelps and G. A. S. Lloyd, Berlin: Springer Verlag, p. 146)

embolization can be used at the same time to reduce the vascularity of the tumour. The angiographic appearance is nearly always characteristic (Figure 2.49) with large vascular spaces, arteriovenous connections and dense homogeneous tumour staining. The blood supply is principally from the ascending pharyngeal artery which is the first branch of the external carotid. Other collaterals, from both external and internal systems, develop as the tumour enlarges and eventually there may be an additional supply from the vertebral system. The initial injection, therefore, should be into the common carotid artery, with subsequent selective catheterization and vertebral injection as required. Subtraction films are necessary.

The recent development of MRA means that this technique can supplement the MRI examination with a demonstration of the arterial supply and its relations to the tumour. For arterial MRA with fast blood flow a 3-D FISP (fast imaging with steady state precession) sequence is used. The venous flow is eliminated by one or two saturation pulses (Vogl, 1992) and post-processing displays the vessel without soft tissue. It is necessary, however, to perform the MRA after the plain MR examination and before contrast is given because of interference to the images from the enhanced mucosa in the nasal and oral cavities.

Recurrences of glomus jugulare tumours can be difficult to demonstrate after contrast enhancement, unless subtraction or fat suppression techniques are used (Figure 2.50).

Neuroma

Neuromas, more correctly called schwannomas, may arise from any of the cranial nerves but have a peculiar tendency to occur in the vestibular components of the VIIIth nerve within the internal auditory

meatus. They are the commonest tumour of the petrous temporal bone.

Neuromas of the facial nerve are slow-growing, rare tumours which may arise on any part of the facial nerve, and although they usually present with facial palsy, this is not always a feature.

Radiological diagnosis depends on the demonstration of localized erosion or expansion in the course of the facial nerve canal. The lesions are usually rounded or somewhat elongated (Figure 2.51). The region of the geniculate ganglion is often involved and so the pit for the geniculate ganglion above the cochlea should be carefully assessed on the coronal

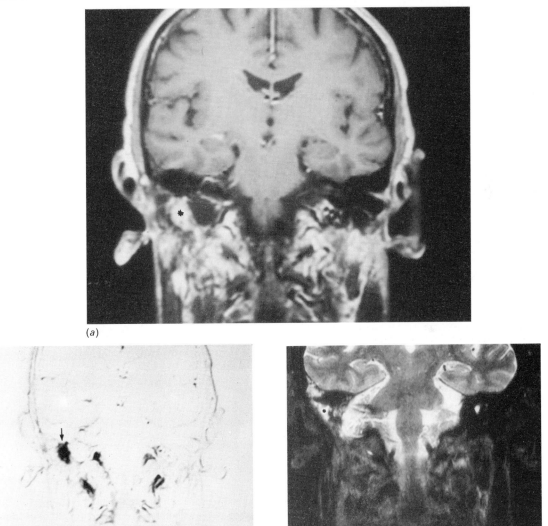

(a)

(b)　　　　　　　　　　　　　　　　　　(c)

Figure 2.50 (*a*) Coronal MR section with contrast enhancement showing a recurrent glomus jugulare tumour in the lower part of the right middle ear (*); (*b*) a photographic subtraction image from the pre-post gadolinium studies defines the tumour from the surrounding fat; (*c*) a study from the same patient at a later date using chemical shift fat suppression after gadolinium enhancement again shows the tumour (*) but does not distinguish it as well from the fat packed in the cavity

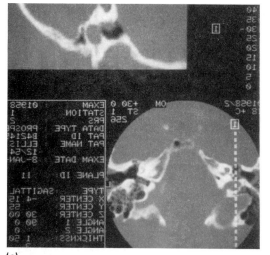

(a)

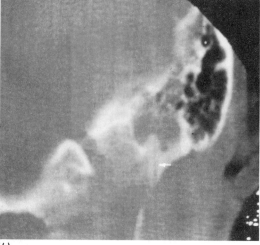

(b)

Figure 2.51 (*a*) Neuroma of the second and third parts of the facial nerve, axial and reformatted lateral section. (*b*) Coronal section. The arrow points to the unaffected part of the nerve above the stylomastoid foramen

CT cochlear cut for any erosion. Facial neuromas arising in the internal auditory meatus are virtually indistinguishable from acoustic tumours. The whole length of the facial nerve then needs to be shown by MR before and after gadolinium.

Vestibular schwannoma

Most vestibular schwannomas arise in the lateral one-third of the internal auditory meatus. Tumour growth takes place medially following the line of least resist-

ance and causes remodelling and expansion of the internal auditory meatus. Extension throughout the porus into the cerebellopontine angle then occurs.

A battery of clinical tests is available for the detection of a vestibular schwannoma but none is completely reliable nor indicates the size of the lesion. Radiological studies are therefore the definitive investigation for demonstrating or excluding the presence of a tumour on the VIIIth nerve. However, while most authorities agree with the desirability of demonstrating small tumours a few millimetres in size, the decision as to whether or not surgical removal is indicated becomes difficult, given the tumour's variable rate of growth. This decision will depend to a large extent on the age of the patient. Generally speaking, CT is now obsolete for the investigation of vestibular schwannoma (Figures 2.52 and 2.53).

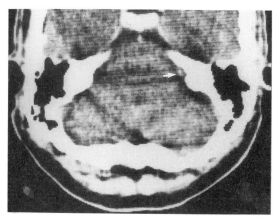

(a)

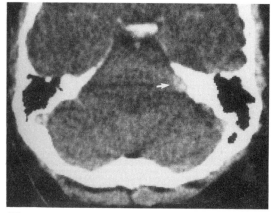

(b)

Figure 2.52 Contrast enhanced posterior fossa brain scan. The arrow shows a small vestibular schwannoma in the cerebellopontine angle. The two sections were taken 3 years apart and show the growth of the tumour. The patient refused operation

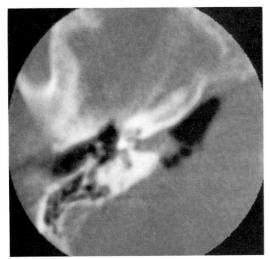

Figure 2.53 Air meatogram shows a small vestibular schwannoma protruding from the porus of the internal auditory meatus

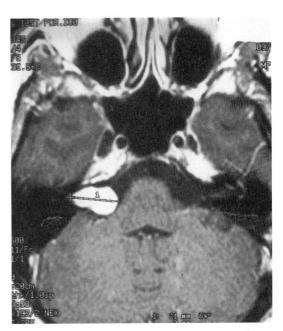

Figure 2.54 A typical medium-sized vestibular schwannoma measuring 30 × 20 mm shown on axial gadolinium enhanced MR scan

Initially magnetic resonance was little better than enhanced CT for identifying a vestibular schwannoma because of variable signal strengths from the tumours on T1 and T2-weighted images. It was the introduction of contrast enhancement with gadolinium DTPA that at last gave a definitive examination that is quick and easy and demonstrates reliably all vestibular schwannomas, large and small. Our policy has been to do only eight to 10 contiguous sections 4 mm thick through the posterior fossa in axial and coronal planes. For the smaller tumours where a policy of continuing assessment of rate of growth seems more satisfactory than surgery, measurements are made using the cursor on the MR machine for comparison with a repeat examination in 9–12 months (Figure 2.54). The recent introduction of fast spin echo (FSE) on our machine gives such good spatial resolution that we now do the initial MR examination without contrast (Figure 2.55). If the cranial nerves can be identified in the internal auditory meatus then a vestibular schwannoma has been excluded, but in doubtful cases gadolinium will have to be given to show that there is no enhancement of the nerve. Linear enhancement of the VIIth or VIIIth nerve in the internal auditory meatus may be due to inflammation. If no mass can be identified on the nerve then repeat examination in 9 months would seem more appropriate than exploratory surgery.

Other tumours within the cerebellopontine angle

Vestibular schwannomas account for 90% of tumours within the cerebellopontine angle. The differential diagnosis of large tumours is primarily the differentiation of masses in the posterior cranial fossa.

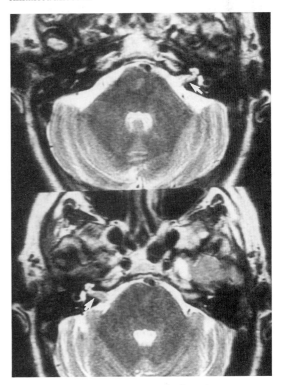

Figure 2.55 Fast spin echo T2-weighted axial sections showing the internal auditory meatus. The arrow points to normal cranial nerves in the upper section and a small vestibular schwannoma in the lower

Meningioma

Meningiomas are the next most common neoplasms that occur in the cerebellopontine angle. Several differentiating features have been described. Unlike vestibular schwannomas, meningiomas often calcify. They expand mainly posteriorly and medially and rarely have a broad attachment to the petrous bone.

Meningiomas may be oval, which is unusual with vestibular schwannomas acoustic tumours; surrounding oedema is said to occur more often with acoustic neuromas. Changes in the internal auditory meatus are rare with meningiomas and frequent with neuromas. Dense homogeneous enhancement, a smooth

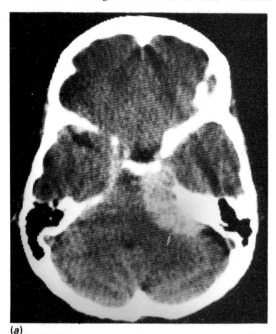

(a)

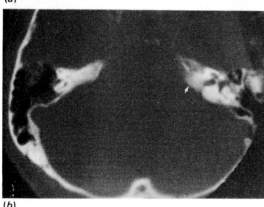

(b)

Figure 2.56 Enhanced axial CT scan showing a meningioma in the posterior cranial fossa attached to the petrous pyramid anteriorly. Section (*b*) shows that the hyperostosis is narrowing the internal auditory meatus

outline (Figure 2.56) and, sometimes, hyperostosis of the petrous ridge, are other features of a meningioma in the posterior fossa, although bony changes occur less often than when they arise in the region of the sphenoid ridge. Intense contrast enhancement occurs with GdMR (Figure 2.57).

Cholesteatoma

Cholesteatoma occurs in the angle or, more anteriorly, alongside the petrous apex. Non-enhancement of the lesion and low or even negative attenuation values are characteristic features (see above). Intermediate signal on T1 images and high signal on T2 are characteristic of the MR appearances.

Glioma

Gliomas, or large glomus jugulare tumours from below, may appear as enhancing masses in the region of the cerebellopontine angle. The pattern of bone erosion of the petrous pyramid will, however, suggest an extrinsic mass.

Neuroma

Neuromas arising from the trigeminal nerve or from the IXth, Xth and XIth nerves in the jugular fossa,

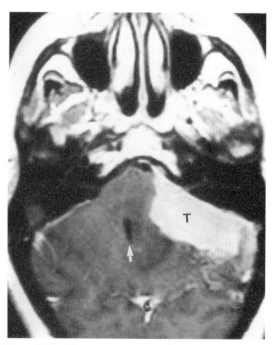

Figure 2.57 A large meningioma in the posterior cranial fossa (T) arising from the petrous ridge shown on enhanced axial MR scan. Note the displacement of the fourth ventricle (arrow)

may also extend up into the cerebellopontine angle. Neuromas of the last four cranial nerves involve the jugular foramen and cause expansion. It is usually impossible to determine the exact nerve of origin of these tumours at surgery, since the mass generally envelops them all. Radiologically, these tumours of the lower cranial nerves need to be differentiated from both a glomus jugulare tumour and from a vestibular schwannoma. They differ, radiologically, from glomus jugulare tumours in three respects: the contour of the bone is smooth and well defined with a neuroma (Figure 2.58) but poorly defined and irregular when the jugular fossa is expanded by a glomus tumour; a neuroma does not usually erode into the middle ear; and expansion of the hypoglossal canal is almost pathognomonic of a neuroma of the XIIth cranial nerve. As with all neuromas, the tumours are shown clearly by GdMR.

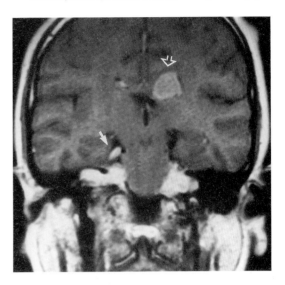

Figure 2.59 Neurofibromatosis type II; bilateral acoustic neuromas; a trigeminal neuroma (arrow) and a meningioma (open arrow) shown by coronal GdMR

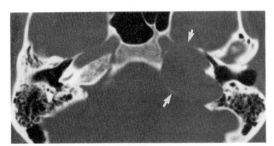

Figure 2.58 A neuroma of one of the lower three cranial nerves shown on an axial CT scan

Neurofibromatosis

There are two forms (NF1 and NF2) of the autosomal dominant disorder in which approximately 50% of the cases represent fresh mutations. The offending genes have been mapped to chromosome 17 for NF1 and chromosome 22 for NF2. Bilateral vestibular schwannomas and a high incidence of meningiomas are the characteristic features of NF2 (Figure 2.59). Gadolinium-enhanced MR of the whole brain and spinal cord is indicated.

Malignant neoplasms

Carcinoma arising in the cartilaginous part of the external auditory meatus tends to spread into the parotid gland and the postauricular sulcus, whereas a tumour arising from the deep bony meatus may perforate the eardrum at an early stage. It is, therefore, often impossible to assess the exact site of origin

of the tumour to decide whether it has arisen from the deep meatus or the middle ear cleft.

The diagnosis of carcinoma in the mastoid is usually made while performing a mastoidectomy in an effort to control presumed chronic mastoiditis, since preceding chronic ear infection is to be expected in at least 40% of patients. Sclerosis of the mastoid and clouding of the cells are therefore radiological signs of little value, but the presence of ragged erosion, usually extensive or in an unusual site, suggests neoplastic change (Figure 2.60). An important sign, on the lateral mastoid view, is erosion of the articular fossa of the temporomandibular joint. This was present on the initial radiographs in 30% of the author's cases.

The hard avascular bone of the labyrinthine capsule is relatively unaffected by carcinoma, and erosion of the capsule with direct invasion of the inner ear is a late radiological feature only present with extensive surrounding bone destruction. There are two important modes of spread of carcinoma of the middle ear (Figure 2.61). First, the tumour extends anteriorly and penetrates the bony septum separating the middle ear cavity from the carotid artery. It then spreads around the artery and extends down around the eustachian tube towards the postnasal space. Erosion of the carotid septum margins of the bony eustachian tube and soft-tissue extension of the tumour anteriorly can be demonstrated best by GdMR (Figure 2.62). Second, the tumour may spread upwards through the tegmen tympani and backwards

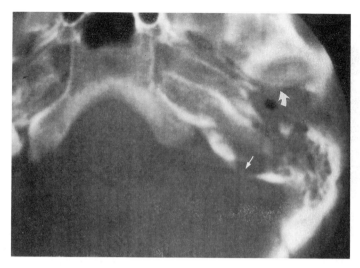

Figure 2.60 Extensive carcinoma of the ear eroding into the back of the temporomandibular joint (curved arrow), and posteriorly through the mastoid air cells (arrow)

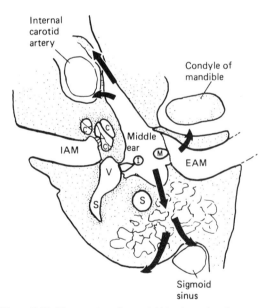

Figure 2.61 Diagram based on axial histological and tomographic sections of the petrous temporal bone. The arrows indicate the usual directions of spread of carcinoma in the middle ear and bony external auditory meatus. C = cochlea, V = vestibule, S = semicircular canal, I = incus, M = malleus. The top of the diagram is anterior. (From *British Journal of Radiology*, 1981)

through the mastoid air cells, then through the thin plate of bone forming the posterior wall of the petrous pyramid and underlying the lateral sinus.

Otosclerosis and bone dysplasias

The otic capsule forming the bony labyrinth of the inner ear is composed of hard, poorly vascularized, endochrondral bone which is metabolically inert and therefore relatively unaffected by systemic bone disease. Widespread bone disorders such as Paget's disease, hyperparathyroidism, rickets, osteogenesis imperfecta and fibrous dysplasia, may eventually affect the labyrinthine capsule causing sensorineural deafness, but the periosteal bone forming the remainder of the petrous temporal bone and base of skull is affected first in these diseases. The rare congenital dysplasias which are present at birth or appear during childhood are considered in Volume 6. Otosclerosis, the most common bone disorder causing deafness, affects only the labyrinthine capsule.

Otosclerosis (otospongiosis)

Otosclerosis is a localized disease of the bony labyrinth in which new bone, initially spongy and later denser, replaces the endochondral bone of the otic capsule and may cause ankylosis of the footplate of the stapes. The French term 'otospongiose' is more descriptive.

The immature woven bone of increased thickness, vascularity and cellularity has a lower radiographic density than that of the otic capsule. The focus becomes less active and more sclerotic with increasing maturity (and probably, also as a result of fluoride therapy).

Tomographic or CT demonstration of otosclerotic bone deposits depends mainly on the distortion of the

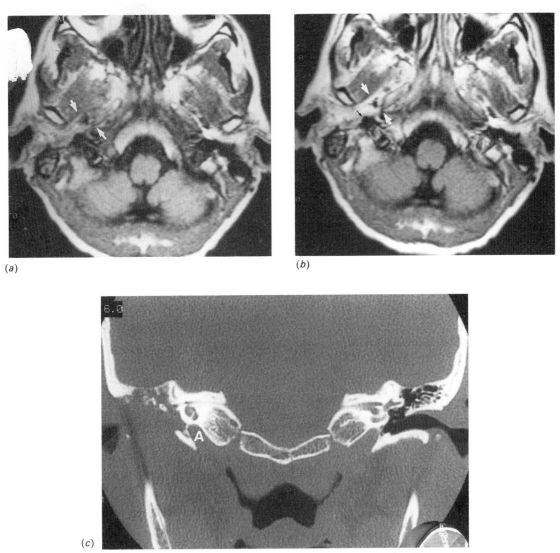

(a)

(b)

(c)

Figure 2.62 Axial MR scan before (a) and after (b) gadolinium enhancement showing high signal from a carcinoma of the external auditory meatus which is spreading forwards into the infratemporal fossa (white arrows). The black arrow points to the carotid artery. Coronal CT (c) shows the extensive bone destruction but unusually the carotid canal (A) does not seem to be involved. These findings were confirmed at surgery

normal clear-cut outline of the labyrinthine capsule. Otosclerotic foci must be large enough – 1 mm in diameter or more – to become radiographically visible. The normal labyrinthine capsule is the most dense bone in the body. It cannot become more radiopaque but, eventually, only thicker by apposition of otosclerotic bone.

Fenestral otosclerosis is essentially a clinical diagnosis based on the audiometric findings and only when severe will narrowing or obliteration of the oval window niche be shown. Follow up of patients after stapedectomy will be of more value to show displacement of a prosthesis (Figure 2.63). So-called cochlear otosclerosis, or rather otospongiosis, is much commoner than was considered previously and is well demonstrated by axial CT. Moreover, densitometry measurements at points in the cochlear capsule can help to confirm the rarefaction in a doubtful case and thereby assist the differential diagnosis of sensorineural deafness (Figure 2.64). Densitometry studies are important for two reasons: (i) as a relative contraindication to proposed surgery for a fixed

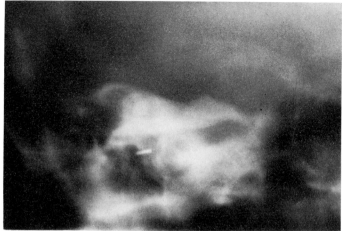

Figure 2.63 Coronal section tomogram showing a metallic prosthesis in the oval window. This would seem to extend too far medially

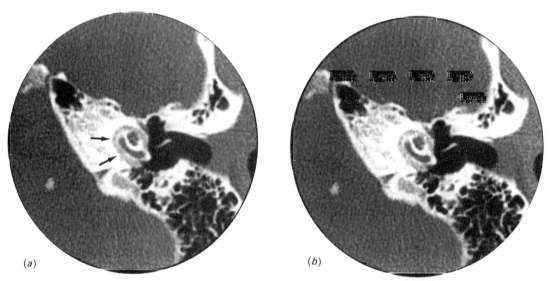

Figure 2.64 Otospongiosis. (*a*) A ring of rarefied bone surrounds the coils of the cochlea (arrows) on this axial CT scan; (*b*) with densitometry readings

stapes; (ii) if sodium fluoride therapy is proposed in an effort to arrest the deterioration of hearing. However, we have never observed recalcification as a result of NaF therapy.

Paget's disease (osteitis deformans)

The radiological appearance of the petrous pyramids is pathognomonic (Figure 2.65). The periosteal bone is affected first and the extensive demineralization that occurs makes the labyrinthine capsule stand out more clearly than normal in the initial stage, osteo-

porosis circumscripta. When the labyrinthine capsule becomes involved, the affected parts become almost impossible to identify, as they are replaced by amorphous bone. The remaining unaffected parts of the labyrinth may give the impression of floating in this grey, featureless, homogeneous, pagetoid bone. The medial ends of the petrous pyramids become tilted upwards due to bone softening and platybasia. Secondary degenerative changes in the cochlear duct seem to be the main cause of the deafness rather than narrowing of the internal auditory meatus. The margins of the meatus become difficult or impossible

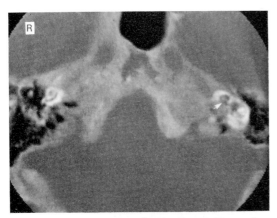

Figure 2.65 Axial CT section showing Paget's disease of the base of the skull. Note that the bony labyrinth on the right appears unaffected, but on the left the pagetoid bone is affecting the basal turn of the cochlea (arrow)

to define on the tomograms when surrounded by pagetoid bone. Finally, all recognizable features of the inner ear may be lost as progressive sclerosis occurs. The cause of the conductive component of the deafness seems to be involvement of the ossicles rather than stapedial ankylosis.

Fibrous dysplasia

Although monostotic fibrous dysplasia is not infrequently found affecting the facial bones, only a handful of cases have been reported in the petrous temporal region. These usually present with conductive deafness caused by a bony mass obstructing or occluding the external auditory meatus (Figure 2.66).

Although fibrous dysplasia, like Paget's disease, causes expansion of bone and affects the periosteal bone of the skull base rather than the labyrinthine capsule, the radiological differentiation is usually not difficult. Fibrous dysplasia occurs in a younger age group and the distinctive 'ground glass' appearance of fibrous dysplasia is unlike pagetoid bone.

Primary basilar impression (craniocervical dysplasia)

Primary basilar impression is the upward displacement of the skull base and upper cervical vertebrae into the cranial vault. It is a radiological diagnosis based upon Chamberlain's supposition that all parts of the axis and atlas lie caudad to the base of the skull. Elies and Plester (1980) suggested that such craniocervical dysplasia may result in a symptom-complex that in itself presents as a differential diagnosis from Menière's disease. They were able to display radiological evidence of primary basilar impression in 16% of patients presenting with non-specific dizziness and sensorineural deafness. Chamberlain's distance is the perpendicular length between the tip of the odontoid peg and a straight line (Chamberlain's line) drawn from the dorsal margin of the hard palate to the dorsal tip of the foramen magnum (Figure 2.67). Chamberlain's distance was considered positive if the odontoid peg was cephalad to Chamberlain's line, and negative if it was caudad. Kane, O'Connor and Morrison (1982) using this measurement showed a proclivity to basilar impression in patients with Menière's disease.

Secondary basilar impression may occur as a result of bone-softening pathologies, e.g. Paget's disease; the anterolateral impression is best measured by Bull's angle (Bull, Nixon and Pratt, 1955).

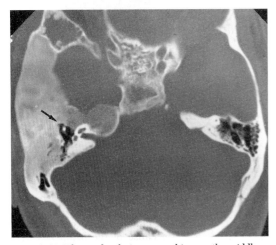

Figure 2.66 Fibrous dysplasia encroaching on the middle ear cavity (arrow) shown by axial CT scan

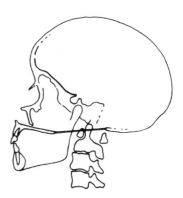

Figure 2.67 Chamberlain's line

Imaging for prospective cochlear implants

Radiology has a most important part to play particularly in the preoperative selection of suitable subjects for cochlear implants and, to a lesser extent, in the follow up. Implanting has proved most successful in post-lingual deafness, i.e. the small group of people who have become severely deaf after speech acquisition. Unfortunately, some of these disease processes not only damage the membranous labyrinth but also result in sclerosis and new bone formation in the sites of prospective implantation inhibiting or precluding insertion of the electrode.

Post-meningitic or otogenic labyrinthitis ossificans is the commonest condition that can be well demonstrated by thin section axial CT (Figure 2.68). The second commonest is severe otosclerosis/otospongiosis (Figure 2.69). The role of MRI in this assessment is uncertain at present but absence of the usual bright signal from the fluids in the coils of the cochlea on T2-weighted images suggests re-

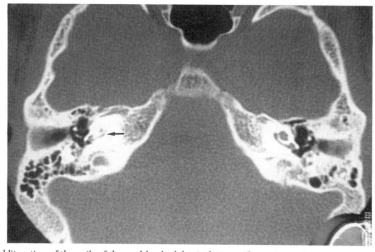

Figure 2.68 Partial obliteration of the coils of the cochlea by labyrinthitis ossificans (arrow). Compare with the normal side

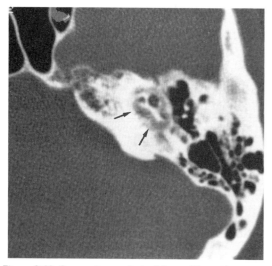

Figure 2.69 Severe otospongiosis of the cochlea with narrowing of the lumen of the coils (arrow). Axial CT scan

placement by fibrous tissue and is therefore a relative contraindication to an intracochlear implant (Figure 2.70).

Miscellaneous

Radionecrosis of the temporal bone

Radiation of bone may result in avascular necrosis and reparative fibrosis which is prone to secondary infection. This may be local or diffuse. The typical finding in the local form is dead bone in the external meatus (Figure 2.71) usually in the floor of the tympanic ring. Diffuse osteoradionecrosis is characterized by profuse pulsatile otorrhoea and deep boring pain. Computed tomography can demonstrate loss of bony architecture, sequestration and replacement of bone by fibrous tissue, and may mimic tumour formation.

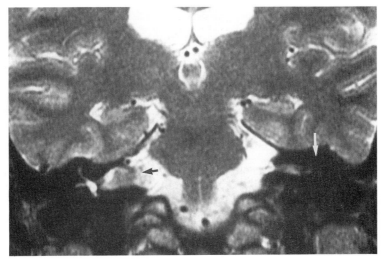

Figure 2.70 Coronal fast spin echo examination of a patient with a vestibular schwannoma in the right internal auditory meatus (black arrow) and post-meningitic labyrinthitis ossificans obliterating the left labyrinth (white arrow)

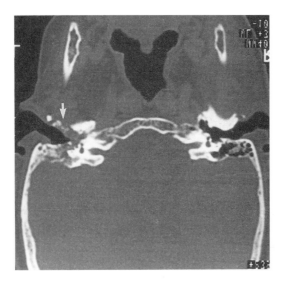

Figure 2.71 Osteoradionecrosis of the floor of the external auditory meatus (arrow). (Reproduced by kind courtesy of Mr J. B. Booth)

References

AMEDEE, R. G., MARKS, H. W. and LYONS, G. D. (1987) Cholesterol granuloma of the petrous apex. *American Journal of Otology*, **8**, 48–55

BAGGER-SJOBACH, D. and PHELPS, P. D. (1985) Cholesteatoma with extension to the cochlea. *American Journal of Otology*, **6**, 338–343

BEALE, D. and PHELPS, P. D. (1987) Osteomas of the petrous temporal bone, a report of 3 cases. *Clinical Radiology*, **38**, 67–69

BULL, J. W. D., NIXON, W. L. B. and PRATT, R. T. C. (1955) The radiological criteria and familial occurrence of primary basilar impression. *Brain*, **78**, 229–247

ELIES, W. and PLESTER, D. (1980) Basilar impression: a differential diagnosis of Menière's disease. *Archives of Otolaryngology*, **106**, 232–233

GLASSCOCK, M. E., DICKINS, J. R. E., JACKSON, C. G. and WIET, R. J. (1980) Vascular anomalies of the middle ear. *Laryngoscope*, **90**, 77–88

GRAHAM, M. D. (1974) The jugular bulb: its anatomic and clinical consideration in contemporary otology. *Laryngoscope*, **84**, 105–124

HOUSE, J. W. and SHEEHY, J. L. (1980) Cholesteatoma with intact tympanic membrane: a report of 41 cases. *Laryngoscope*, **90**, 70–76

IRVING, R. M., JONES, N. S., HALL-CRAGGS, M. A. and KENDALL, B. (1991) CT and MR imaging in lateral sinus thrombosis. *Journal of Laryngology and Otology*, **105**, 693–695

KANE, R. J., O'CONNOR, A. F. and MORRISON, A. W. (1982) Primary basilar impression: an aetiological factor in Menière's disease. *Journal of Laryngology and Otology*, **96**, 931–936

LO, W.M., SOLTI-BOHMAN, A. G., BRACKMANN, D. E. and GUSKIN, P. (1984) Cholesterol granuloma of the petrous apex: CT diagnosis. *Head and Neck Radiology*, **153**, 705–711

MENDEZ, G. JR, QUENCER, R. M., DONOVAN POST, M. J. and STOKES, N. A. (1979) Malignant otitis externa: a radiologic clinical correlation. *American Journal of Roentgenology*, **132**, 957–961

MILLS, R. (1986) Malignant otitis externa. *British Medical Journal*, **292**, 429–430

MOFFAT, D. A. and O'CONNOR, A. F. F. (1980) Bilateral internal carotid aneurysms in the petrous temporal bone. *Archives of Otolaryngology*, **106**, 172–175

PHELPS, P. D. (1969) Preservation of hearing in the labyrinth invaded by cholesteatoma. *Journal of Laryngology and Otology*, **83**, 1111–1114

PHELPS, P. D. and LLOYD, G. A. S. (1983) *Radiology of the Ear*. Oxford: Blackwell Scientific Publications

PHELPS, P. D. and LLOYD, G. A. S. (1986) Vascular masses in the middle ear. *Clinical Radiology*, **37**, 359–364

PHELPS, P. D. and WRIGHT, A. (1990) Imaging cholesteatoma. *Clinical Radiology*, **41**, 156–162

PRASAD, U. (1976) Malignant external otitis. *Journal of Laryngology and Otology*, **90**, 963–965

SWARTZ, J. D. and HARNSBERGER, H. R. (1992) *Imaging of the Temporal Bone*. New York: Thieme Medical Publishers. p. 84

VALVASSORI, G. E. (1974) Benign tumours of the temporal bone. *Radiologic Clinics of North America*, **12**, 533–542

VOGL, T.J. (1992) *MRI of the Head and Neck*. Berlin: Springer Verlag. p. 233

3

Aetiopathology of inflammatory conditions of the external and middle ear

G. G. Browning

Anatomy and pathology of the squamous epithelium of the external ear

The pinna and external auditory meatus are lined with keratinized squamous epithelium which is identical to the skin that covers the rest of the body (Figure 3.1). The deeper or basal cells are cuboidal in shape and rest upon a basement membrane. This layer is constantly undergoing cell division and the progeny of the original cells gradually move towards the surface becoming flatter in the process. As they reach the top layer the cells shrink, lose their nucleus, and die. When dry the surface cells contain a tough protein called keratin, hence the name keratinized squamous epithelium. Finally the surface cells are shed.

In the external auditory meatus, the epithelium varies in thickness, being thickest in the cartilaginous portion where there are rete pegs, thinner in the bony portion where there are no pegs and thinnest of all on the tympanic membrane where the number of layers of cells is considerably reduced.

As squamous epithelium, the skin of the meatus obeys the well recognized laws of repair. If a break occurs in the basal layer due either to trauma or inflammation the cells migrate until they meet another epithelial surface; this may be either epithelium of the same or of a different type. Hence, if a tympanic membrane defect occurs, the squamous epithelium will advance and one of three things may happen: the gap may be bridged resulting in a healed tympanic membrane; the epithelium may fail to bridge the defect and join at some position with the middle ear mucosa, although this need not necessarily be at the edge of the defect; and finally, it may not meet up with middle ear mucosa in the region of the tympanic membrane, perhaps because the mucosa has been destroyed, but grows into the middle ear until it finally does so. Why the ear should heal in one way rather than another is uncertain, but it is probably related to how much epithelium is lost and over which structures the epithelium has to migrate. These may be normal anatomical structures such as the middle ear mucosal folds, pathological tissue, such as granulations, secretions or pus, or perhaps a surgically inserted graft.

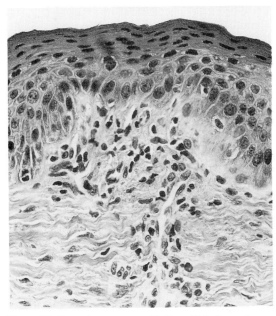

Figure 3.1 Normal squamous epithelium. This shows the progressive maturation of the cuboidal basal cells to become flattened and eventually keratinized squamous epithelial cells

Anatomy and pathology of the mucosa of the middle ear and mastoid

The ciliated, pseudostratified columnar epithelium of the respiratory tract extends up the eustachian tube as far as the anterior part of the middle ear cavity (Figure 3.2). These cells are capable of producing mucus. In addition there are goblet cells and mucus-secreting glands. More posteriorly, the mucosa changes patchily into a simple cuboidal or stratified epithelium with no secretory elements. The medial aspect of the tympanic membrane and the mastoid air cells are lined by a single layer of cells ranging in shape from cuboidal to flat.

In the early stages of inflammation, whatever its cause, there is vasodilatation of the submucosal tissues. Glandular secretion is stimulated with the production of a thin mucoid fluid. Some of the epithelial cells die and the bacteria that are normally in the area multiply in the denuded areas and aggravate the condition. A polymorphonuclear reaction occurs from the neutrophils in the blood and a mucopurulent discharge results. This may remain stagnant within the middle ear and mastoid air cell system because of immobility or loss of the cilia including those of the eustachian tube.

Most frequently, resolution will occur but if the condition is prolonged for some reason, such as the inability of the secretions to drain down the eustachian tube, the number of glands and goblet cells will increase and the areas formerly covered by cuboidal or flat epithelium will change into a similar but perhaps less well differentiated pseudostratified columnar epithelium (Figure 3.3). Differentiation into squa-

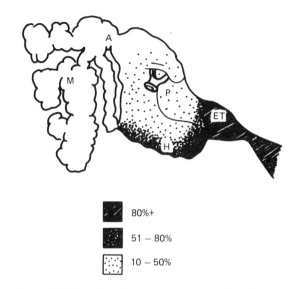

	80%+
	51 – 80%
	10 – 50%

Figure 3.2 Extent of respiratory type mucosa within the middle ear represented by the percentage of ciliated mucus secreting cells per unit area (after Shimada and Lim, 1972). A, antrum; ET, eustachian tube; H, hypotympanum; M, mastoid; P, promontory

mous epithelium, most frequently non-keratinized, can also occur.

Granulation tissue is an end result of non-resolution of an inflammatory process. Localized areas of the mucosa become hyperplastic with invasion of fibroblasts, capillaries and macrophages, plasma cells

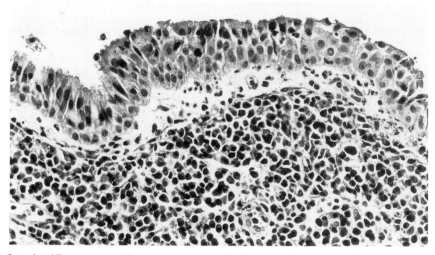

Figure 3.3 Inflamed middle ear mucosa. There is an increase in the thickness of the mucosa which shows several different cell types, secretory on the left and early metaplasia to squamous epithelium on the right. There is an intense inflammatory reaction, mainly of plasma cells in the subepithelial tissues

and lymphocytes. Granulation tissue can be covered by all the variations in mucosal types described above but is also frequently ulcerated so that it does not have a mucosal covering.

A variety of chemical mediators of inflammation have been described which have been categorized into the following groups: histamine, lipid mediators, plasma enzyme systems, kinins, cytotoxins and neurogenic subtances (Turner, 1992). Of particular importance in otitis media are the mediators of the cytokine group which include the various interleukins. An example of the work that has been going on in this field recently is the discovery that the bone resorbing activity of cholesteatoma with chronic otitis media may be attributed to interleukin-1α (Kurihara *et al.*, 1991).

Bacteriology of the external and middle ear

Like skin elsewhere, that of the external auditory meatus has a normal commensal flora such as *Staphylococcus epidermidis (albus)*, and *Corynebacterium* spp. (diphtheroids). In addition *Staph. aureus* and *Streptococcus viridans* can frequently be present without causing any ill effects (Sipila *et al.*, 1981). When the skin's natural defence mechanism breaks down, such as in otitis externa, the resident bacteria multiply because of the more favourable environment and other organisms such as *Proteus* and *Pseudomonas* spp., which are normal commensals of other parts of the body, may then flourish. The fact that these bacteria can be isolated is more likely to imply that they are secondary invaders rather than the cause of the condition. Naturally their local multiplication will increase the degree of the inflammatory response, but what is less certain is whether their elimination, say by antibiotic therapy, will be of material, clinical benefit.

In normal individuals with an intact tympanic membrane, the culture of swabs taken from the middle ear mucosa will not usually grow any bacteria. In some, however, an upper respiratory tract flora such as *Streptococcus* and *Pneumococcus* spp. may be isolated and this should not be considered surprising because of the continuity of the middle ear with the nasopharynx. If, however, skin commensals such as *Staph. epidermidis* or *Corynebacterium* spp. are isolated then they are most likely to be contaminants picked up during the sampling of the middle ear.

When a tympanic membrane defect is present the normal flora of the external auditory meatus has easy access to the middle ear. In most instances, the mucosa should be no less able than that of the nose or throat to deal with such contamination. In some, however, if the mucosa is more susceptible or already inflamed for some other reason, bacterial colonization is likely to occur, both with the normal skin commensals and the bowel-type flora normally found around the body. When this occurs, the question has to be asked: what part do the bacteria have in the condition? The fact that an average of two different species of bacteria can be isolated from active ears (Sweeney, Picozzi and Browning, 1982) would suggest that secondary colonization rather than primary infection is a strong possibility.

The role of antibiotic therapy in inflammatory conditions of the external auditory meatus is controversial, but the needless prescribing of them should be condemned on bacteriological grounds because of the likelihood of the development of resistant strains particularly those that produce β-lactamase. The penicillins (including ampicillin) and the cephalosporins are only effective because they have a β-lactam ring to which various chemical radicals can be added to make different antibiotics. Bacteria can develop resistance to these antibiotics by producing β-lactamase (previously called penicillinase) and what is of concern is that the genetic ability to do so can be passed relatively easily from one bacterial species to another. The indiscriminate prescribing of the penicillins and the cephalosporins will increase the number of resistant strains within the population. This might be of little consequence in the management of ear disease but is of considerable importance for infections elsewhere in the body.

Otitis externa

Definition

The term 'otitis externa' covers any inflammatory condition of the skin of the external auditory meatus, but when used in an unqualified manner it implies diffuse dermatitis/eczema of the canal skin. (In dermatological terms there is no difference between dermatitis and eczema.)

Classification

Several different classifications have been used (Mawson, 1963; Peterkin, 1973) which are based on fine clinical distinctions concerning the appearance of the lesion and the likely aetiological factors. Unfortunately, there is no histological or other quantifiable distinction in these classification systems. An alternative is to classify otitis externa as to the extent of the lesion (Table 3.1).

Incidence

Few data apart from anecdote appear to be available concerning the incidence of the various forms of otitis externa but perhaps the commonest type in both general and hospital practice is diffuse otitis externa. Furunculosis is also fairly common but invasive otitis externa and keratosis obturans are rare.

Table 3.1 Classification of otitis externa

Classification	Subclassification
Localized (furunculosis)	
Diffuse otitis externa	Idiopathic
	Traumatic
	Irritant
	Allergic
	Bacterial/ fungal
	Climatic/ environmental
Part of generalized skin conditions	Seborrhoeic dermatitis
	Allergic dermatitis
	Atopic dermatitis
	Psoriasis
Invasive (granulomatous/necrotizing/ malignant)	
Other (keratosis obturans)	

Localized otitis externa

The most common form is a boil (furunculosis) of one of the sebaceous glands of the outer third of the canal where the skin is hair bearing. Pathologically, there is no difference between boils in this site and anywhere else in the skin.

Diffuse otitis externa

Here the pathological process is initially limited to the skin of the cartilaginous portion of the external auditory meatus and perhaps the concha. With more extensive involvement, the bony canal and tympanic membrane become affected.

Aetiology

Idiopathic

In most instances, there will be no obvious reason why diffuse otitis externa has developed and it must therefore be considered idiopathic. In most instances, it is likely to be due to a combination of factors superimposed upon a breakdown, for some as yet unknown reason, in the skin's natural defence mechanism and in particular of the sebaceous and ceruminous glands whose lipid secretions coat the squamous epithelium of the meatus. It then requires only the addition of another minor factor, such as trauma, for the condition to commence.

Traumatic

It is a natural reaction to poke or scratch an itchy ear with whatever is available (fingernail, matchstick, paper or hair clip). Though this might give patient satisfaction, it could break the skin and allow, for example, secondary infection to occur. In addition, the poking instrument itself might cause an irritant or allergic reaction (see below).

Irritant

Many chemicals when applied to the skin will cause an irritant rather than an allergic reaction. The difference between the two reactions is that the former will occur in everyone if the application of the irritant is sufficiently prolonged and its concentration is high enough. Irritant reactions are more severe if the skin surface is moist and its natural defence mechanism is compromised. Allergic reactions only occur in some individuals who develop a type IV hypersensitivity after a period of sensitization to the allergen.

Irritants are frequently instilled into the ear in the form of solvents (e.g. propylene glycol, triethanolamine oleyl polypeptide) in wax softeners and in some medicinal ear drops. Sixty per cent of hospital patients with otitis externa will have an irritant reaction to such agents when they are applied in the same concentration as in the proprietary preparation (Holmes *et al.*, 1982).

Allergic

In most instances where an allergy is present, it is to topical medications which have been instilled into the meatus and under these circumstances they must be considered potentiators rather than initiators of the condition. The commonest allergens are antibiotics (e.g. neomycin, framycetin, gentamicin, polymyxin), antibacterials (e.g. clioquinol) (Holmes *et al.*, 1982) and antihistamines. Other potent sensitizers are metals and in particular nickel which is often present in paper and hair clips which may be used to scratch the ear. In addition, some of the constituents in fingernail varnish, cosmetics and hair preparations can cause allergic reactions. It has been estimated that in one to two-thirds of patients attending a hospital clinic with otitis externa, there will be an allergic component, mainly to topical medications (Rasmussen, 1974; Smith, Keay and Buxton, 1990).

Bacterial/fungal

The role of bacteria in uncomplicated otitis externa is controversial. Normally only diphtheroids and *Staph. epidermidis* can be cultured from the canal skin, but in otitis externa, potentially pathogenic organisms can be cultured from at least 75% of ears (Leventon *et al.*, 1967). The identity of the most common organism varies between published series but the most prevalent would appear to be *Pseudomonas* spp., coliforms, *Proteus* spp. and *Staphylococcus aureus* in that order (Singer *et al.*, 1952; Leventon *et al.*, 1967).

When anaerobes are looked for they can be isolated from 20% of ears (Brook, Frazier and Thompson, 1992). However, the fact these organisms are isolated does *not* mean that they are responsible. In unilateral otitis externa, approximately 40% of the non-affected ears will grow similar, potentially pathogenic bacteria; this is significantly more common than the figure of approximately 3% in normal ears (Leventon *et al.*, 1967). Bacteria frequently colonize any inflamed skin surface, e.g. burns, and once the otitis externa has resolved clinically, approximately 40% will still have the same type of flora (Leventon *et al.*, 1967). Though the bacteria most commonly isolated are bowel commensals, it is unlikely that they colonize the skin of the ear because of poor personal hygiene and the non-washing of hands. Bowel-type flora can be isolated from anywhere on body skin after a night in bed and the fact that they persist in the external auditory meatus is more likely to be due to a loss of the normal skin protective mechanisms allowing secondary colonization.

Otitis externa is often found in association with active chronic otitis media and some have postulated that this is due to an allergic reaction to the bacteria in the mucopus rather than a direct irritant reaction to the moist discharge. There is no evidence to support this concept and the organisms isolated grow elsewhere in the body, as commensals, without causing allergic problems.

Fungi, though not infrequently seen growing in the debris of the meatus, in non-tropical countries are secondary invaders usually following the use of antibiotic–steroid ear drops. This is confirmed by the ease with which they can be eliminated by removing the debris and ceasing medication.

Climatic/environmental

Those who have worked in hot and humid climates will state that otitis externa is much more frequent there than in cold climates. There are many potential reasons for this, one being that more individuals go swimming in hot weather and, if the skin defence mechanism is already compromised, the combination of getting their ears wet and perhaps irritated by the chemicals in the pool water causes the condition to erupt. This is confirmed in swimmers; the incidence of otitis externa is related to the time spent swimming (Calderon and Mood, 1982). Whether the ears become infected with the swimming water is doubtful as the water is usually not contaminated with bacteria when patients develop otitis externa (Calderon and Mood, 1982) and the bacteria isolated are the same in swimmers and non-swimmers alike (Feinmesser *et al.*, 1982). If, however, a patient develops otitis externa while swimming in a pool that is contaminated with, for example, *Pseudomonas* spp., then the ear will understandably become colonized with that organism (Seyfried and Fraser, 1978).

Pathology

The basic pathology of diffuse otitis externa (Figure 3.4) is that of dermatitis (eczema) anywhere in the

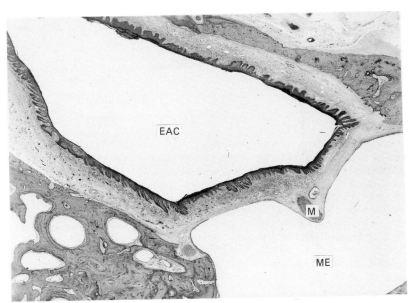

Figure 3.4 Otitis externa. In comparison to the normal external auditory meatus (see Figure 3.15), in otitis externa the eithelium and subepithelial spaces are thickened including that over the tympanic membrane. Note the rete pegs which are normally absent in the inner two-thirds of the external auditory canal (EAC). M, malleus; ME, middle ear. (Collection MEEI)

skin and it is impossible to distinguish on histological grounds between one clinical type or aetiology and another.

There are several stages through which the lesions can pass. First, there is an acute stage with hyperaemia and intercellular oedema (spongiosis). As the oedema increases small vesicles develop which contain serous fluid within which are some inflammatory cells. In the next stage, the vesicles rupture and serous fluid exudes onto the skin surface. The distinction between the stratum granulosum and corneum is lost with the production of nucleated keratotic cells (parakeratosis) which scale off. Though the condition is usually reversible it can pass into a chronic fibrotic and indurated phase.

Though secondary damage to the ceruminous glands with loss of their protective secretions is postulated as one reason for failure of resolution of the condition in some patients, no histological evidence has been presented to support this (Figure 3.5). In other inflammatory dermatological conditions there is no loss of pilosebaceous cell function; indeed it is often the reverse and there may be hyperplasia.

Generalized skin conditions

In every patient with otitis externa, it is important to look for evidence of more extensive skin involvement particularly behind the ear, on the scalp or face and neck. Dermatologists, on the basis of their own experience, may attribute other disease labels, but the aetiological factors are just the same as for diffuse otitis externa, that is they are most commonly unknown.

Seborrhoeic dermatitis

This is a non-specific term used to describe any dermatitis that is neither irritant nor allergic in origin which affects the sebum-producing areas such as the scalp, face, and the back of the neck; dandruff is a mild form. The condition is often made worse when it affects a moist area between two areas of skin that are in contact, e.g. in the postauricular sulcus. Intertrigo is a more specific name to attach to this and is obviously akin to diffuse otitis externa. There is some evidence from specific antifungal therapy that yeasts of *Pityrosporum* spp. may be an important factor in seborrhoeic dermatitis (Ford *et al.*, 1984), but their role in otitis externa would not appear to have been studied.

Allergic dermatitis

There is no pathological difference between irritant and allergic reactions that are confined to the ear and those that are part of a more general reaction. The reaction need not always be confined to the area with which the allergen is in contact; satellite lesions can occur, e.g. on the neck.

Atopic dermatitis

In atopic children with the triad of dermatitis, allergic rhinitis and bronchitis, the external auditory meatus can be involved, but the distinction from classical otitis externa should be easy to make. Topical medications are more likely to cause irritant (but not allergic) reactions in atopic as opposed to other children.

Psoriasis

Psoriasis affects in the region of 2% of Caucasians, and a lesser proportion of other ethnic groups, at some time in their life. Histologically, it is distinguishable from dermatitis by the presence of nucleated keratinized squames (parakeratosis) and elongation of

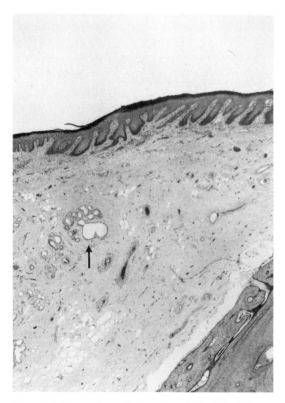

Figure 3.5 Otitis externa. Section through the skin of the outer third of the meatus showing the presence of ceruminous glands (arrowed) in otitis externa. (Collection MEEI)

the rete pegs. The lesions are white and scaly because the transit time of cells from the basal layer to the surface is about 3 days compared with the normal 28 days. Rubbing the lesion with a spatula will cause the skin to produce scales leaving some fine bleeding points. When the ear is affected the lesion is primarily of the concha and the adjacent cartilaginous meatus. The differential diagnosis is not difficult because of the almost invariable presence of other psoriatic lesions.

Invasive (granulomatous/necrotizing/malignant) otitis externa

Many different names have been ascribed to this condition which almost invariably presents with granulation tissue in the external auditory meatus initially at the junction of the cartilaginous and bony parts.

Pathology

Invasive otitis externa is considered to be due to an opportunistic infection with *Pseudomonas aeruginosa* though there are often multiple bacteria. It usually affects those over 50 years of age and most patients have evidence of microvascular disease. Most, though by no means all, have diabetes mellitus which may or may not be insulin dependent and well or poorly controlled (*Lancet*, 1982). Immunosuppression such as AIDS should also be considered.

The term 'necrotizing' is used because in many there is necrosis of the adjacent cartilage or bone of the meatus. The granulomatous condition may then spread through the soft tissues to the base of the skull where it can involve the lower cranial nerves. Alternatively, *Pseudomonas aeruginosa* may spread via the mastoid bone to affect the facial nerve or go on to give rise to intracranial complications. How the pathology spreads is often confused by the fact that a high proportion of patients have had some form of earlier mastoid surgery, commonly resulting in an open cavity.

The term 'malignant' is used because there is a high mortality if the disease process spreads outside the external auditory meatus (Chandler, 1977).

The condition is assumed by many to originate in the external auditory meatus, but in some reports the condition appears to have arisen from acute otitis media (six out of 15 patients reported by Meyerhoff, Gates and Montalbo, 1977) or is associated with active chronic otitis media (four out of 11 patients where the tympanic membrane was described by Doroghazi *et al.*, 1981).

Hyperkeratosis of canal skin (keratosis obturans)

Hyperkeratosis of canal skin is an extremely rare condition and can either be focal or generalized. In both, lack of the normal migratory pattern of exfoliation of canal skin is considered to be the problem (Soucek and Michaels, 1993). When focal, it gives rise to a localized collection of epithelial squamous and debris either on the tympanic membrane or deep in the meatus. This can expand and locally corrode the meatus bone, at which stage it might be called a canal cholesteatoma (Pierpergerdes, Kramer and Behnke, 1980; Naiberg, Berger and Hawke, 1984; Holt, 1992). When the hyperkeratosis is generalized it leads to retention of a hyperkeratotic plug deep in the canal, frequently called keratosis obturans. Clinically, this has to be distinguished from retention behind a canal narrowing or a wax plug (Black and Chaytor, 1958; Naiberg, Berger and Hawke, 1984). In one report from an English suburban town, an association with bronchiectasis in children with keratosis obturans was noted (Morrison, 1956).

Middle ear
Acute otitis media
Definition

Classically the term 'acute otitis media' is taken to imply a bacterial or viral infection which affects the mucosal lining of the middle ear and mastoid air cell system. This leads to clinical signs of infection with a bulging inflamed tympanic membrane. More recently, acute otitis media is also considered to be one end of a continuous spectrum of the otitis medias that affect young children, the other end being otitis media with effusion (Giebink, 1992).

Incidence

Acute otitis media is reported to be the commonest otological condition in childhood, with an incidence of nearly 50% in the first year of life (Figure 3.6). The incidence remains high in the first 5 years of life, but thereafter tails off to become relatively infrequent in teenagers. There appears to be a marginally higher incidence in boys. Such figures are reported from the community by non-specialists and as such have to be treated with caution as they are likely to include many children who have otalgia for other reasons, less than half of those with otalgia being considered to have acute otitis media when seen by specialists (Ingvarsson, 1982).

Acute otitis media is more frequent in the colder months of the year when upper respiratory tract infections are also more frequent and in children from urban as opposed to rural homes (Pukander, Sipila and Karma, 1984). The relative risks of an infant having recurrent episodes of acute otitis media are shown in Table 3.2 (after Alho *et al.*, 1993). The greatest risk is if they attend a nursery school when they are 3.2 times more likely to have recurrent

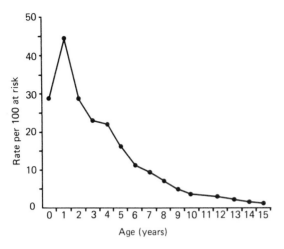

Figure 3.6 Incidence of acute otitis media (after Ingvarsson *et al.*, 1983)

Table 3.2 Relative risks for recurrent acute otitis media in children up to 2 years. (Modified from Alho *et al.*, 1993)

Atopy	1.8
Breast-fed (months)	
0–3 versus 4–6	1.0
0–3 versus 7–12	1.1
0–3 versus > 12	1.3
Daycare	
Family	1.8
Nursery	3.2
High no. of sibs	1.9
Parental smoking	1.4
Sex (boys)	1.8

episodes than a child who is looked after at home. Thereafter, boys, multiple sibs, atopy and family day care are the most important factors.

Whether the incidence of acute otitis media is changing over the years is uncertain mainly because of the inadequate ways there are of assessing this. Although the number of antibiotic prescriptions given for acute otitis media is increasing, this could solely reflect a change in prescribing practice. If Table 3.2 is looked at, the decline of breast-feeding and the increase in day-care nursery attendance in recent decades, might suggest a likely increase in the incidence but this has to be balanced against a smaller family size and less parental smoking. What is certain is that in developed countries complications are now rare. For example, the risk of clinically developing

acute mastoiditis currently is about 0.04% (van Buchem, Peeters and Van't Hof, 1985).

Aetiology

Relationship with otitis media with effusion

In attempting to identify the aetiological factors that might be responsible for acute otitis media, it is often difficult to do so because many authors fail to distinguish between acute otitis media and otitis media with effusion. While accepting that they may be the two ends of a continuous spectrum, there is no doubt that they are two clinically distinct conditions that affect two different age spectra.

Viral and bacterial infections

Most children have a history of a preceding upper respiratory tract infection, which initially will be viral and will affect not only the mucosa of the respiratory passages but also that of the eustachian tube and middle ear. Second, bacterial infection can then occur and, if the eustachian tube is functionally blocked by oedema, a middle ear abscess will result. The bacteria involved are almost invariably those normally resident in the upper respiratory tract and in one-third of patients more than one organism will be cultured. *Streptococcus pneumoniae* and *Haemophilus influenzae* are the commonest organisms, making up about 80% of the isolates. Thereafter, *Moraxella (Branhamella) catarrhalis*, *Staphylococcus aureus* and *Pseudomonas aeruginosa* are isolated in that order (Chonmaitree *et al.*, 1992). Interestingly, in about 20% of ears no bacteria or virus can be isolated and viruses alone are isolated from 16% of ears (Chonmaitree *et al.*, 1992). Antibiotic therapy for recurrent episodes increases the number of isolates from individual ears and makes *Haemophilus influenzae* the predominant organism (Harrison, Marks and Welch, 1985).

Eustachian tube

The eustachian tube has two main functions: to maintain the middle ear pressure at atmospheric pressure and to allow the normal secretions of the respiratory type mucosa, with which it and part of the middle ear are lined, to pass on into the nasopharynx. It achieves this during swallowing by the muscular contraction of the levator palati dilating the pharyngeal opening and the tensor palati opening the cartilaginous tube (Honjo, Okazaki and Kumazawa, 1980). It seems reasonable to postulate that the adynamic bony part could be physically blocked by the mucosal oedema associated with an upper respiratory tract infection and be an aetiological factor in acute otitis media.

It is known that normal 3-year-old children are less able than adults to equalize an artificially induced negative middle ear pressure. This inability gradually disappears, until by about the age of 12 an adult ability has developed (Bylander, 1980). The reason for this is unknown, as it is difficult to conjecture why the relative shortness and horizontal position of the eustachian tube in childhood should affect its function. However, the more horizontal position of the tube might allow easier access of bacteria from the nasopharynx to the middle ear. This could be combined with poor tubal function which allows children to create a high negative middle ear pressure by sniffing (Magnuson, 1981a) so sucking a bolus of infected mucus into the middle ear. The fact that acute otitis media is more frequent in children with Down's syndrome and those with cleft palates would support some role for eustachian tube dysfunction.

Allergy

As stated earlier, from some studies atopic children appear to be more at risk though the majority of children with acute otitis media are not atopic.

Pathology

The earliest stage is hyperaemia of the middle ear and eustachian tube mucosa which is followed by a serous exudate with polymorphonuclear leucocytes (neutrophils). The lining mucosa of the middle ear

hypertrophies and there is metaplasia with conversion from simple cuboidal epithelium to one with mucus-producing cells (Figure 3.7). The metaplastic process can extend to the mastoid air cells. The air in the middle ear and mastoid spaces is absorbed and replaced by an inflammatory exudate, under increasing tension, of mucus, serum, leucocytes and bacteria. The tympanic membrane bulges and, in about 30% of untreated cases, will rupture spontaneously through a small hole in the pars tensa (Ingvarsson, 1982). This perforation may be difficult to see because of the associated oedema.

In the majority of children, acute otitis media resolves spontaneously and this is independent of whether the tympanic membrane ruptures or antibiotic therapy is given (van Buchem, Dunk and Van't Hof, 1981). In up to one-third of ears there will still be sufficient middle ear fluid 4 weeks later to give a 20 dB conductive hearing impairment but this again would appear to be independent of whether a myringotomy has been performed or antibiotics have been given. It is often said that the incidence of residual fluid is higher if courses of antibiotics have not been completed but this remains to be proven and indeed the evidence is against it, the incidence being no different whether 3 or 10 days of antibiotics are prescribed (Chaput de Saintonge *et al.*, 1982; Bain, Murphy and Ross, 1985). The incidence of long-term middle ear fluid is very low, 95% of children having no otoscopic evidence of fluid and a normal tympano-

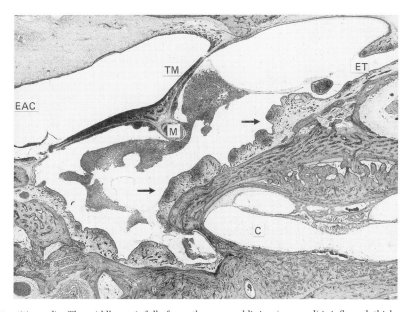

Figure 3.7 Acute otitis media. The middle ear is full of pus, the mucosal lining (arrowed) is inflamed, thickened and metaplastic. The tympanic membrane (TM) though still intact is hyperaemic. C, cochlea; EAC, external auditory canal (meatus); ET, eustachian tube; M, malleus; TM, tympanic membrane. (Collection MEEI)

gram 11 weeks later (Wheeler, 1986). In the majority, the tympanic membrane will heal without any sequelae but, in some, tympanosclerosis will develop (see below). The middle ear and mastoid spaces will return to normal but, in some, cholesterol granulomas will form and fibrous sclerosis of the air cells occurs (see below).

In a few children, for some as yet unknown reason, the process can take a more destructive course with the development of acute mastoiditis. Though the mastoid mucosa will almost invariably be affected in acute otitis media, it is only when the infected material is prevented from draining from the mastoid air cells, most probably because of oedema around the ossicular chain, that clinical symptoms related to the mastoid develop. In some, this will progress to what, in effect, is osteomyelitis with bone resorption and remodelling by osteoclasts. The mastoid abscess will probably either rupture externally through the cortex or intracranially if it is not drained surgically. The infection can spread to the venous sinuses (thrombophlebitis) or to the inner ear (labyrinthitis). Though inner ear damage might seem likely in some, to date in well controlled human studies there does not appear to be an increased risk of developing a sensorineural hearing impairment (Rahko, Karma and Sipila, 1989). A facial nerve palsy may develop because of pressure.

Bullous myringitis

Definition

Bullous myringitis (myringitis bullosa haemorrhagica) is a clinical diagnosis based on finding serous fluid containing vesicles (blebs) in the superficial layer of the tympanic membrane.

Incidence

Vesicles on the tympanic membrane are not uncommon in children and young adults presenting with symptoms suggestive of acute otitis media.

Aetiology

It has long been assumed that the blebs on the tympanic membrane are due to a viral infection, but, in the majority, a virus cannot be isolated (Roberts, 1980). The sole evidence then for a viral aetiology rests upon the commonly reported association with an upper respiratory tract infection and the occasional association with a cranial nerve palsy. The alternative is that the blebs are a manifestation of acute otitis media since bacteria can be isolated from middle ear aspirates as frequently and of a similar type to those isolated in acute otitis media (Coffey, 1966). Contrary to some suggestions the mycoplasmas do not appear to be isolated more frequently.

Pathology

The histological appearances do not appear to have been described.

Granular myringitis

Definition

In granular myringitis, there are areas of granulation tissue on the tympanic membrane sometimes, but not invariably, in association with middle ear pathology.

Pathology

The pathological findings (Figure 3.8) are of non-specific granulation tissue affecting the superficial epithelial layers of the tympanic membrane to a variable extent (Khalifa *et al.*, 1982). In some, the process gradually extends to the skin of the meatus and a fibrotic stenosis results. In some, the granulation tissue is a manifestation of acute or chronic otitis media with a small tympanic membrane defect which cannot be seen because of the granulations (Hoshino *et al.*, 1982).

Otitis media with effusion

Definition

Many different terms have been used for the chronic condition where there is an accumulation of non-purulent fluid in the middle ear. None of them has achieved universal recognition mainly because each can be criticized etymologically. Chronic otitis media with effusion is a clumsy term and can be confused with the standard usage of chronic otitis media. The term 'effusion' does not differentiate between purulent and non-purulent effusions. Otitis media with effusion is slightly better but still clumsy. Secretory otitis media assumes that the middle ear fluid is a secretion which it may not be. Serous otitis media is incorrect because the fluid is not serum. Glue ear is a good lay description but the fluid is not an adhesive. Non-purulent otitis media is considered incorrect by some because bacteria can sometimes be isolated. Of them all, otitis media with effusion is perhaps the best and for consistency this term will be used.

The time that the fluid has to be present in the middle ear for the condition to be considered chronic is usually taken as 12 weeks (Bluestone, 1984).

Incidence

Many sequential studies have reported that between 20% and 50% of children will have an episode of otitis media with effusion at some time between the ages of 3 and 10 years. For example, of 404, 3-year-

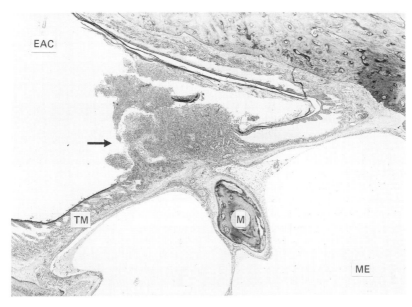

Figure 3.8 Granular myringitis. There is an area of non-specific granulation tissue (arrowed) on the tympanic membrane (TM) in the region of the handle of the malleus (M). The middle ear (ME) in this case is normal. EAC, external auditory canal (meatus). (Collection MEEI)

old children followed up over a winter 6-month period and using strict tympanometric and acoustic reflex criteria for diagnosis, 42% had the problem (Fiellau–Nikolajsen, 1983). In 94% of these children, the condition had resolved within 3 months, but in the 6% in whom it persisted, spontaneous resolution over the following 3 months was unlikely.

Aetiology in children

The factors responsible in a specific child are likely to be multifactorial and a combination, in varying degrees, of the following:

Environmental

The most important determinant as to whether a child has persistent or recurrent otitis media with effusion is the amount of contact they have with other children. Thus, those in large families and those attending for group care or education in day nurseries, creches, playgroups, and school are significantly more likely to have problems. This is the same as for acute otitis media and the natural conclusion is that both are related to recurrent upper respiratory tract infections. This would appear indeed to be the case, but the evidence is that depending on a child's predisposition, some will develop recurrent otitis media with effusion, some acute otitis media and others tonsillitis (Schilder *et al.*, 1992). Because of the association with upper respiratory tract infection there is obviously a higher seasonal incidence in the

winter months (Fiellau–Nikolajsen, 1983; Zielhuis *et al.*, 1989). Passive smoking has also been blamed but care has to be exercised to ensure that other environmental factors have been controlled for.

Sex

Though girls and boys, once other factors have been controlled for, appear to be equally likely to develop otitis media with effusion, boys have episodes that are likely to be more persistent (Teele *et al.*, 1990).

An age-old question is whether a sclerotic mastoid predisposes a child to having recurrent episodes because the lesser air reservoir is unable to compensate for changes in middle ear pressure. Children who have had otitis media with effusion have smaller mastoids than children who have not, but there is a considerable overlap in size (Tos and Stangerup, 1984). Over a 5-year period, the mastoid air cell system will increase in size in only 40% of ears that have been affected by the condition (Hussl and Welzl–Mueller, 1980). What is required is a longitudinal study in children from birth correlating episodes of otitis media with effusion with the radiological size of the mastoid.

Eustachian tube malfunction

As was discussed under acute otitis media, children have poorer eustachian tube function than adults, but there is some evidence that it is even poorer in those with otitis media with effusion. However, it could just be that the eustachian tube malfunction is a result of the frequently associated mucosal oedema rather than because of poor muscle function (see below). There is considerable evidence that once the otitis media settles the eustachian tube function improves markedly (Poulsen and Tos, 1977; Virtanen, 1983) which would argue for its being a secondary phenomenon.

It is known that children with a cleft palate have a higher incidence than normal of otitis media with effusion but this does not mean that their poor eustachian tube function need be the reason. Not all children with a cleft palate have the problem (Bess, Schwartz and Redfield, 1976), so even in those who do there must be a combination of factors which makes them more susceptible to otitis media with effusion.

It has been argued that the problem with the eustachian tube is not that it does not open, but that it opens too easily. If air does not get up the tube, the air within the middle ear will be absorbed but this alone does not create a negative middle ear pressure of the magnitude seen in established cases. Many children are habitual sniffers and this itself will cause negative middle ear pressure (Magnuson, 1981a). The ability to create a negative middle ear pressure is partly related to good eustachian tube function (Bylander, 1980) and unfortunately in children with unilateral otitis media with effusion, sniff-positive ears (that is those in whom the pressure could be changed by sniffing) were as common in the normal as in the pathological ears (Magnuson, 1981b).

Perhaps the main reason why it has not been possible to prove that eustachian tube function has a role is that the tests are often unrepeatable; they assess the ear in artificial situations and only when the child has the condition.

The consensus, but by no means all the evidence, is that children with otitis media with effusion have poorer muscular function than normal but they can still maintain an adequate middle ear pressure under normal conditions (Bylander, Tjerstrom and Ivarsson, *et al.*, 1983). It just makes them a population at risk for some additional aetiological factor(s).

Adenoid hypertrophy

The role of adenoid hypertrophy has been much debated, the most commonly suggested mechanism being displacement of the eustachian tube orifice rather than its obstruction. In addition, some consider that, together with the tonsils, the adenoids constitute a reservoir of infection. In children, the adenoids are almost invariably enlarged and there is little evidence to suggest that large adenoids are more frequently associated with otitis media with effusion than with normal ears (Hibbert, 1982; Maw, Jeans and Cable, 1983). If there were unequivocal evidence that surgical removal of the adenoids had an effect then their

role would have been proven. Unfortunately, there is disagreement about the role of adenoidectomy though there is increasing evidence from randomized controlled trials that it is beneficial (Maw, 1983; Gates *et al.*, 1987; Dempster, Browning and Gatehouse, 1993). Interestingly it is likely to do this by mechanisms other than changing eustachian tube function (Dempster and Browning, 1989).

Unresolved acute otitis media

There is no doubt that fluid can remain in the middle ear following an episode of acute otitis media, but prospective studies would suggest that only about 5% will have middle ear fluid after 12 weeks and none will have any 8 months later (Wheeler, 1986). It appears to make little difference to the incidence of retained fluid 4 weeks later whether antibiotics were prescribed or not (van Buchem, Dunk and Van't Hof, 1981) and, when they were, whether it is for short (3-day) or long (10-day) periods (Chaput de Saintonge *et al.*, 1982; Bain, Murphy and Ross, 1985).

Many children with otitis media with effusion do not have a past history of acute otitis media but it is suggested that in them there may have been a subclinical infection. If bacteria that are likely to be contaminants from the external auditory meatus are excluded, culture of middle ear fluid will isolate an upper respiratory tract flora in 10–20% of ears (e.g. Pelton *et al.*, 1980). The types of flora are similar to those isolated in young children with acute otitis media, predominantly β-haemolytic streptococcus and *Haemophilus influenzae*, but their isolation does not mean that there is a cause–effect relationship. Similar bacteria have been isolated from ears with otosclerosis (Sipila *et al.*, 1981). Antibodies to bacteria within the middle ear fluid have been looked for and do not always correspond to the bacteria which are isolated at the same time (Bernstein *et al.*, 1980). If a factor, the bacteria probably produce endotoxins (de Maria *et al.*, 1984) which can either have a direct effect on the middle ear mucosa or affect the cilia in the eustachian tube.

Allergy

The question as to whether allergy is an important factor is controversial, but the balance of scientific evidence is that it is not.

Atopic allergy in the form of asthma, rhinitis and dermatitis has been calculated to affect about one-third of children at some time in the first 10 years of life when otitis media with effusion is also common. It is vital then that, when the incidence of allergy is being investigated in children with this condition, a comparison be made with a well-matched control group. There is some evidence which suggests that the incidence of otitis media with effusion is marginally higher in children with an allergic diathesis, but even this does not mean that in these children the problem is an allergic one. It could just be that they are more prone to develop otitis media with effusion, e.g. because of the eustachian tube oedema associated with their rhinitis.

If otitis media with effusion were to have an allergic basis it would be expected that the levels of IgE in the middle ear fluid would be higher than in the serum. This does not appear to be the case in children with no allergic diathesis (Lim, 1979) and raised levels are found in only approximately 15% of children with allergic rhinitis (Bernstein *et al.*, 1983).

Aetiology in adults

Idiopathic

In adults it is important to consider a postnasal space tumour but fortunately this is not a common cause of otitis media with effusion except in the Chinese. They have a genetic predisposition to such tumours; the actual incidence depending on where in the world they reside. The problem has been studied considerably less in adults than in children and, in most, no cause can be found. Even a history of an upper respiratory tract infection may be irrelevant because of its prevalence in the community.

Barotrauma

On descent in an aeroplane, it can sometimes be difficult to equalize the negative middle ear pressure by autoinflation and, if the negative pressure is prolonged, a mild serous transudate may result.

Nasopharyngeal carcinoma

Two-thirds of patients with a nasopharyngeal tumour will have otitis media with effusion but it is incorrect to think that this is the sole presenting symptom. Symptoms and signs are most frequently multiple (Table 3.3).

Table 3.3 The most frequent clinical signs of nasopharyngeal tumours

Sign(s)	Percentage incidence
Cervical adenopathy	86
Auditory	67
Nasal obstruction	67
Epistaxis	64
Neurological	28

From Cammoun, Vogt Hoerner and Mourali, 1974

Radiotherapy

Radiotherapy can cause fibrosis around the eustachian tube resulting in its malfunction. As the most frequent reason to give radiotherapy in this area is for a nasopharyngeal tumour, separating the two aetiologies can be difficult.

Acquired immunodeficiency syndrome (AIDS)

Individuals with AIDS have a higher incidence of otitis media with effusion (Lalwani and Sooy, 1992). This is presumably due to an increased incidence of upper respiratory tract infections, lymphoid hypertrophy of the adenoids and more rarely nasopharyngeal tumours. Otitis media with effusion is also a frequent terminal event in patients with AIDS (Michaels, Soucek and Liang, 1994).

Pathology

The changes (Figure 3.9) that occur in the middle ear, mastoid and eustachian tube mucosa in otitis media with effusion have been well described in biopsy specimens from the middle ear (Lim and Birck, 1971; Bremond and Coquin, 1972; Gunderson and Gluck, 1972; Tos, 1980; Palva, Makinen and Rinne, 1981) and temporal bone sections (Ishii, Toriyama and Suzuki, 1980; Tos, 1980). Once otitis media with effusion has become established the normal flat cuboidal middle ear and mastoid mucosa is patchily replaced by thickened pseudostratified mucus-secreting epithelium with varying degrees of specialization, such as the development of cilia. Goblet cells are frequently present and sometimes mucus-secreting glands are formed. The ciliary lining would appear to be less efficient at moving the secretions into the nasopharynx than normal, but whether this is a primary or secondary phenomenon is unknown (Karja, Nuutinen and Karjalainen, 1983). Certainly, children with a primary abnormality of the cilia, such as that in Kartagener's syndrome, frequently develop otitis media with effusion (*Lancet*, 1980), but in general, ciliary dysfunction is more likely to be secondary. The submucosa is oedematous and inflamed with dilated blood vessels and an increased number of macrophages, plasma cells and lymphocytes. The same histological findings pertain to otitis media with effusion in cleft palate children, in animals when it is produced experimentally and in adults with nasopharyngeal tumours.

What is frequently debated is the origin of the fluid within the middle ear and mastoid air cell system. In surgical practice, this is usually categorized by its consistency as being either serous or mucoid. This is obviously a gross simplification of the situation as there will be a full spectrum of fluid types made up of a mixture of the secretions of the epithelial cells, the goblet cells and the mucous glands along with the inflammatory exudate/transudate which comes through the intercellular spaces from the inflamed submucosa.

The cells which are often present in the middle ear fluid have been analysed in the hope that this

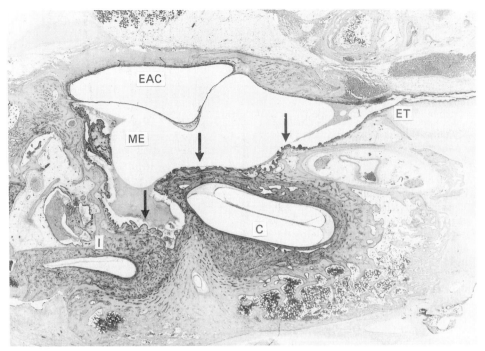

Figure 3.9 Otitis media with effusion. Minimal effusion remains post-mortem but the mucosa (arrowed) of the middle ear over the promontory and in the facial recess is hypertrophied, hyperaemic and slightly polypoid. The bony eustachian tube (ET) is patent. C, cochlea; EAC, external auditory canal (meatus); ME, middle ear. (Collection MEEI)

may give some indication of the aetiology. Bacteria are sometimes isolated (see above) as are all types of inflammatory cells (neutrophils, lymphocytes and monocytes). The types of cell isolated vary considerably between patients and there would appear to be no correlation with the aetiology. For example, atopic individuals and those with cleft palate have similar proportions of cells (Sipila and Karma, 1982).

The biochemical constituents of the middle ear fluid have also been analysed in an attempt to determine whether it is a transudate or a secretion and if it is part of an immunological reaction. In general, the total protein concentration is higher than in serum in both serous and mucoid effusions (Juhn, 1984). This is primarily because of the local production of enzymes and antibodies, but there is nothing unexpected in this because this will occur in an inflammatory reaction irrespective of the aetiology. The only aspect that biochemical studies appear to have answered is that an IgE (allergic) response is not a major cause of the fluid (Lim, 1979).

An age-old question is whether a sclerotic mastoid predisposes to recurrent episodes or is a result thereof. The latter is now considered more likely. There is no doubt that children with otitis media with effusion have smaller mastoids than normal (Tos and Stangerup, 1984). Recent longitudinal studies support the concept that progressive pneumatization is least

in those with recurrent episodes (Nakano and Sato, 1990).

In the majority of children, the condition resolves and the middle ear mucosa returns to normal. In some, the sequelae of any type of inflammation in the middle ear cleft, such as tympanosclerosis and cholesterol granuloma can occur. What perhaps is more relevant is the formation of permanent retraction (atelectatic) pockets which may or may not be adherent to the middle ear structures. However, it is doubted whether these can occur in the absence of associated episodes of acute otitis media (Sadé and Berco, 1976).

Congenital cholesteatoma

Definition

Congenital (primary) cholesteatomas are squamous epithelial cysts that can arise anywhere within the temporal bone. Aetiologically they have no relationship to acquired cholesteatoma.

Incidence

The incidence of congenital cholesteatoma is unrecorded but in clinical practice they are rare. It might be expected that because they are congenital in origin, they would present in the neonatal period.

This is not the case as it takes time for them to grow to a sufficient size to cause symptoms. There are two common ages and modes of presentation. If they arise within the middle ear cleft, they present with a hearing loss in childhood when it affects the ossicular chain. Alternatively, if their origin is within the petrous apex of the temporal bone, they present in adulthood when they press on the facial nerve or brain stem.

Aetiology

Fairly convincing histological evidence has now been presented from serially sectioned temporal bones that squamous epithelial cell rests are a frequent finding in the mucosa in the fetal mastoid antrum (Michaels, 1986) (Figure 3.10). It is as-

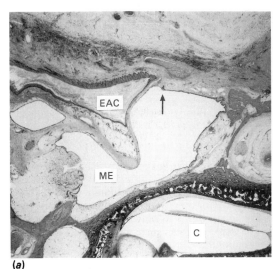

(a)

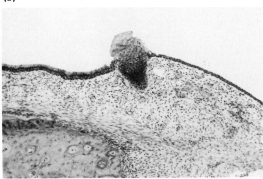

(b)

Figure 3.10 (*a*) Congenital cholesteatoma. Arrow indicates an epidermoid formation in the superior anterolateral part of the middle ear of a 20-week fetus which it is suggested in some ears may progress to a congenital cholesteatoma. (*b*) High power view of arrowed area. C, cochlea; EAC, external auditory canal (meatus); ME, middle ear. (Figures from Michaels, 1986)

sumed that, in the majority, these rests disappear but occasionally they may persist to form a congenital cholesteatoma.

Pathology

Histologically, a congenital cholesteatoma is identical to an epithelial retention cyst (see Figure 3.30) and is not usually associated with active mucosal disease (Friedberg, 1994).

Chronic suppurative otitis media

Definitions

Over the years many different terms have been used for the different clinical types of chronic suppurative otitis media. Inevitably this has led to confusion and has made it difficult for the trainee to understand. In the early days of otology, when the tympanic membrane could only be seen by using reflected sunlight, the main distinction that could be made was whether the disease affected the pars tensa or the pars flaccida. This anatomical distinction led to the use of the terms 'tubotympanic' and 'atticoantral', respectively. Another anatomical distinction that was relatively easy to make was whether the tympanic membrane defect was central or extended to the margin of the meatus, especially in the posterosuperior quadrant. Today, these anatomical terms are less frequently used for diagnostic purposes mainly because of increased ability to assess the ear, especially with an operating microscope, and to determine not only where the pathology is, but what type of disease is present. Thus, when the disease affects the attic, it is usually possible to decide whether or not a cholesteatoma is present. Therefore, pathological definitions are increasingly being used in preference to anatomical ones and are those which are used in this chapter.

Healed otitis media

Here the pars tensa and pars flaccida are intact and in a normal position but abnormal in appearance. This may be due to various degrees of scarring, thickening, chalk patches, tympanosclerotic plaques or healed perforations. These are all signs that at some time in the past there was inflammation in the middle ear cleft, most likely otitis media but also possibly surgical trauma due to a ventilation tube. Such an ear is burnt out with regard to activity and, the disability, if any, will be a hearing impairment due to ossicular chain fixation or disruption. In addition, there are many ears that if looked at histologically will have evidence of old otitis media but the tympanic membrane is normal (da Costa *et al.*, 1992).

Inactive (mucosal) chronic otitis media

Here there is a permanent defect of the pars tensa but there is currently no evidence of inflammation either of the middle ear mucosa or tympanic membrane. The ossicular chain may be eroded or fixed. The natural history of such an ear is to become active or remain inactive.

Active (mucosal) chronic otitis media

In addition to the tympanic membrane defect the middle ear mucosa is inflamed and oedematous with the production of excess mucus or mucopus. Such activity may be intermittent or continuous. In some ears, granulation tissue or polyps can develop.

Active squamous epithelial chronic otitis media: cholesteatoma

Here, in addition to active mucosal chronic otitis media as defined above, there is a squamous epithelially lined pocket full of squamous epithelial and inflammatory debris. This most frequently arises in the pars flaccida but can occur from a pars tensa retraction pocket. A cholesteatoma is the most common clinical term used but keratoma, cholesteoid, epidermoid cholesteatoma, epidermoidosis have all been used. The adjective 'acquired' is sometimes used to distinguish such a cholesteatoma from a congenital one.

Inactive squamous epithelial chronic otitis media: retraction pocket

Various degrees of retraction of the pars flaccida must be considered normal but when part of the retraction is out of vision for the otoscopist this is considered abnormal because of its potential to retain squamous epithelial debris which might lead to active squamous epithelial disease, i.e. a cholesteatoma. The various stages of pars flaccida retraction have been well described by Tos, Stangerup and Larsen (1987) (Figure 3.11).

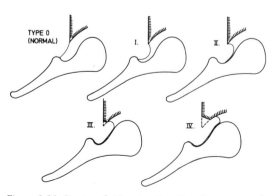

Figure 3.11 Staging of attic retraction (Tos, Stangerup and Larsen, 1987)

Table 3.4 Population prevalence (%) of adult otitis media (Browning and Gatehouse, 1992). The 95% confidence intervals are in parentheses

	Healed otitis media	Inactive chronic otitis media	Active chronic otitis media
Overall	11.9 (10.2–13.6)	2.6 (1.8–3.4)	1.5 (1.1–1.9)
Age (years)			
18–40	10.1 (8.6–14.4)	2.5 (1.0–4.0)	0.9 (0.2–1.6)
41–60	11.5 (9.3–13.7)	2.1 (1.2–3.0)	2.1 (1.3–2.9)
61–80	16.2 (12.8–19.6)	2.7 (1.6–3.8)	2.1 (1.3–2.9)
Sex			
Women	11.3 (9.3–13.3)	2.4 (1.7–3.1)	1.2 (0.8–1.6)
Men	12.6 (9.8–15.4)	2.8 (1.4–4.2)	1.9 (1.1–2.7)
Occupation			
Non-manual	10.1 (7.7–12.5)	1.9 (0.8–3.0)	0.8 (0.4–1.2)
Manual	13.5 (11.0–16.0)	3.3 (2.3–4.3)	2.2 (1.5–2.9)

Retraction of the pars tensa can also occur and again, if part is out of vision, this could give rise to active disease, i.e. a cholesteatoma. Unfortunately, some surgeons because of the suggested propensity of retraction pockets to become active, describe their surgery of inactive retraction pockets as cholesteatoma surgery.

Prevalence

The majority of reports of the incidence of chronic otitis media are from clinic data. These tend to reflect the referral pattern to that clinic rather than the prevalence in the general population. The British Medical Research Council National Study of Hearing looked at adults randomly selected from the general population (Table 3.4). The overall incidence of healed, inactive and active otitis media is 12, 2.6 and 1.5% respectively; it unfortunately has not been possible to subdivide the inactive and active ears into mucosal and squamous epithelial disease. However, in clinical practice, up to 50% of active ears will be associated with a cholesteatoma (Smyth, 1976). Interestingly, there is no obvious lessening of the incidence in recent years, those in the 18–40-year age group being just as likely to have chronic otitis media as the 40–60-year group. As might be expected, those in manual occupations are more likely to have chronic otitis media, but there was no difference in the incidence between men and women.

Aetiology: general

Environmental

As with many medical conditions, there is a close correlation between patients with chronic otitis media and socioeconomic group, the lower groups having a higher incidence. It is not known why this is the case, but almost certainly it relates to general health, diet, and overcrowding in the home. When investigating such factors it is difficult to allow for others such as genetics, climate, method of screening and previous management of the condition (Hinchcliffe, 1977). What is known is that in disadvantaged populations such as Maori children (Giles and Asher, 1991) and Innuits (Pedersen and Zachau–Christiansen, 1988) the incidence is higher than in Britain.

Genetic

The question as to whether one race is more predisposed to chronic otitis media remains unanswered, mainly because of the inability to control for many of the factors mentioned above. It is, for example, suggested that American Negroes are less likely to have the condition than White Americans (Harell, Pennington and Morrison, 1982) but this could simply be due to different patterns of attendance for medical treatment.

The importance of genetic factors was much debated earlier this century, in particular whether the incidence was related to the size of the mastoid air cell system which was considered to be genetically determined (Diamant, 1982). The mastoid air cell system is smaller in individuals with otitis media, but it is not known whether this is a primary or secondary event. Histologically, there is no doubt that with repeated inflammation, the mastoid air cell system becomes progressively more sclerotic (see above). The degree of initial mastoid aeration may be a predisposing factor, but once the condition has developed the cell system will decrease in size.

Previous otitis media

It appears to be generally held that chronic otitis media is a sequela of acute otitis media and/or otitis media with effusion, but it is not known what factors make one ear, and not another, progress to the chronic condition. It has been suggested that with the chronic retraction of the tympanic membrane which is associated with otitis media with effusion, there is a loss of the fibrous tissue layer (Smyth, 1980) which will not heal if there is a subsequent acute perforation. Though this theory might initially appear attractive, there is little evidence to support it and destruction of fibrous tissue by unspecified enzymes in the middle ear fluid is pathologically unlikely.

Unfortunately, there is little evidence that surgical or medical management of these childhood conditions makes any difference to the incidence of chronic otitis media. It could even be that surgery makes the matter worse, particularly by the creation of tympanosclerotic patches in the tympanic membrane (Ambegaokar, Brown and Richards, 1978).

Infective

Bacteria can almost invariably be isolated from the mucopus or from the mucosa of the middle ear in active chronic otitis media provided that the correct culture methods are used (Figure 3.12). The proportion of the different organisms varies between series but they are mainly Gram-negative, bowel-type flora and often several different organisms will be cultured from the one ear. Contrary to an opinion that is often expressed, the types of flora are no different if a cholesteatoma is present (Sweeney, Picozzi and Browning, 1982).

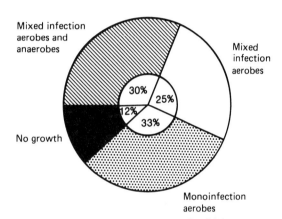

Figure 3.12 Percentage of organisms isolated from ears with active mucosal otitis media. A total of 55% of ears will grow several organisms. (After Sweeney, Picozzi and Browning, 1982)

The fact that organisms can be isolated so frequently is usually taken to imply that bacterial infection of the mucosa is the main reason for the continued activity. However, the role of bacteria can be questioned for several reasons. When the tympanic membrane is intact, bacteriological cultures taken from the middle ear can, on occasion, isolate organisms which are unlikely to be contaminants from the external auditory meatus (Sipila *et al.*, 1981). In addition, in nearly 50% of ears with inactive chronic otitis media, an identical flora to that isolated from active ears can be cultured (Picozzi *et al.*, 1982). Another finding is that although anaerobic organisms can be isolated from at least 40% of ears, their elimination by metronidazole therapy does not cause the ear to become inactive (Browning *et al.*, 1983).

Thus, it could be argued that the bacteria in ears with chronic otitis media are secondary invaders of a mucosa which is inflamed because of other factors, rather than that they are the primary cause of the disease. This does not mean that they do no damage. There is considerable evidence that bacteria can produce substances that affect ciliary function (Wilson and Cole, 1988) and hence would encourage stasis of secretions in the middle ear. There is also evidence that polymicrobial colonization is more damaging than monomicrobial (Brook, 1987).

Tuberculosis is much less common than formerly but should be considered when active disease does not respond to medical or surgical management. The route of infection can be haematogenous from another focus such as the lungs or via the eustachian tube, e.g. from the ingestion of infected milk.

Upper respiratory tract infections

Though it has not been studied scientifically, many patients will state that their ear starts to discharge after an upper respiratory tract infection. The postulate, here, would be that the viral infection would also affect the mucosa of the middle ear making it less resistant to the organisms that are normally present in the middle ear, allowing bacterial overgrowth.

Tradition would also suggest that patients with chronic otitis media frequently have chronic disease of the respiratory tract, such as sinusitis. The frequency with which this occurs has not been reported, but clinical experience in the 1980s would suggest that it is uncommon. It remains a reasonable postulate that, if one area of the respiratory tract mucosa is affected, there is an increased likelihood that another part will also be affected, but it does not mean that management of one condition is necessary before the other can be successful.

Autoimmunity

It seems likely that individuals with established autoimmune disease will have a higher incidence of chronic otitis media, but to date rheumatoid arthritis is the only condition to have been studied and in this condition this appears the case (Camilleri *et al.*, 1992).

Allergic

Though postulated by some as an important factor, it remains to be proven that allergic individuals have a higher incidence of chronic otitis media than non-allergic subjects. In some, allergy to the antibiotics in ear drops or to the bacteria or their toxins is an interesting but as yet unproven possibility.

Eustachian tube malfunction

In active chronic otitis media, the eustachian tube is frequently blocked by oedema but whether this is a primary or secondary phenomenon is unknown. Certainly reconstructive surgery is frequently successful in such ears which would suggest that, in these ears at least, it was a secondary event. In inactive ears, various methods have been used to evaluate eustachian tube function and most would suggest that the tube is unable to return a negative pressure to normal.

Aetiology: acquired cholesteatoma

There has been considerable debate about the aetiology of cholesteatoma and the question still remains unanswered as it was 80 years ago. The protagonists of each of the three main theories (Figure 3.13) are vociferous in support of their own cause, but the answer is almost certainly that they are all relevant, some applying more to a specific patient than others. The way to answer the debate is to follow up several thousand children over many years and, if this were to be combined with an assessment of the effect of surgery, many important questions could be answered. Until then, opinions as to the aetiology are based on clinical impressions as animal models and studies *in vitro*, though innovative and interesting, are of questionable relevance to the human situation.

Negative middle ear pressure

It is suggested that continued negative middle ear pressure, which is often associated with childhood otitis media with effusion, will cause the pars flaccida to retract resulting in a squamous epithelial-lined pocket. The question is why pars flaccida rather than pars tensa retraction occurs. The fibrous layer is less organized, there are mucosal folds and perhaps a bony plate between the supratubal recess and the epitympanum (Morimitsu *et al.*, 1989) which might cause differential negative pressures. Once a retraction occurs, it is suggested that because of its narrow isthmus epithelial debris will be retained which subsequently becomes infected and expands under tension. The antrum will then become blocked producing an inflammatory reaction with osseous sclerosis of the mastoid akin to that seen in chickens when the ostium of their pneumatized humerus is occluded (Beaumont, 1966).

Evidence to support this concept comes from the high rate of recurrent retraction pockets in individuals who have been operated upon for cholesteatoma and in whom the defect has been grafted. This would suggest that these patients do indeed have poorly functioning eustachian tubes but the majority of these retractions do not progress to form a cholesteatoma. When a cholesteatoma occurs after surgery, it is most likely to be due to residual squamous

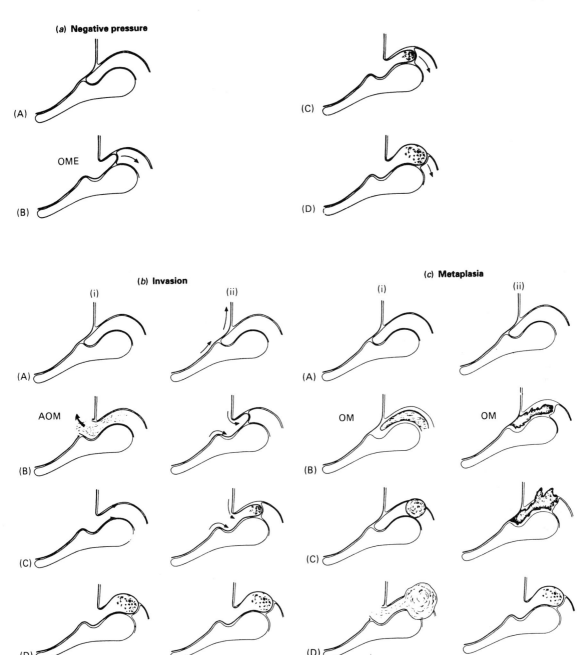

Figure 3.13 Alternative theories of development of cholesteatoma. (*a*) *Negative pressure*: continued negative pressure associated with otitis media with effusion (B) causes a progressive retraction pocket in the attic (C) which because of its narrow neck becomes a cholesteatoma (D). (*b*) *Invasion: mechanism i.* Acute otitis media causes an attic perforation (B) following which the squamous epithelium grows in from the external auditory meatus (C), to cause a cholesteatoma (D). *Invasion: mechanism ii.* The normal direction of migration of the squamous epithelium is outward (A). With continued migration (B) a retraction pocket (C) and eventually a cholesteatoma is formed (D). (*c*) *Metaplasia: mechanism i.* Subsequent to otitis media the mucosa undergoes metaplasia to a squamous epithelium (B) which forms into a cyst (C) which, because it cannot drain, enlarges and subsequently bursts externally as a cholesteatoma (D). *Metaplasia: mechanism ii.* Otitis media irritates the squamous epithelium overlying the attic causing it to hypertrophy (B). This hypertrophy continues (C) and a cholesteatoma is eventually formed (D)

epithelium being left behind the graft. Several other arguments would suggest that negative pressure is unlikely to be the sole aetiology. One is that the pressure is unlikely ever to be great enough to cause indrawing of the normal pars flaccida and the otoscopic progression of an attic retraction to a cholesteatoma does not appear to have been documented. In addition, the surgical management of retraction pockets with ventilation tubes does not appear to influence their long-term position. Some will return to a normal position without and others will remain retracted with management (Sade, Avraham and Brown, 1982). However, part of the reason for this could be adhesions rather than eustachian tube function being irrelevant.

Invasion

Two main ways have been postulated as to how an abnormal growth of the squamous epithelium of the skin of the external auditory meatus or tympanic membrane may cause a cholesteatoma. The more widely held concept is that the epithelium takes advantage of a temporary defect in the pars flaccida, caused by an episode of acute otitis media, to grow into the attic. For some as yet undiscovered reason, the epithelium is thought not to obey the normal reparative laws of contact inhibition so that when it meets the middle ear mucosa it continues to invade.

The evidence to support this concept is tenuous. It is easy to see how a temporary defect in the pars flaccida could allow a retraction pocket to occur but the evidence is lacking for an invasive quality for the epithelium. The histology of the epithelium within a cholesteatoma is identical to that of the meatus and shows no evidence of increased mitoses or early neoplasia. Tissue culture techniques may show slightly different patterns of epithelial (Proops, Hawke and Parkinson, 1984) or fibroblast growth (Parisier *et al.*, 1993) from cholesteatoma tissue but the culture methods are so artificial that their relevance has been doubted (*Lancet*, 1986).

Some will attempt to draw a parallel with inclusion dermoids which can occur when squamous epithelium is left behind a tympanomeatal skin flap or a tympanic membrane graft. These, like residual parts of a cholesteatoma which may form a 'pearl' (see Figure 3.30), are histologically distinct from cholesteatoma (see Figures 3.18 and 3.25) and are more akin to inclusion epithelial dermoids which can occur anywhere in the body subsequent to implantation.

The alternative concept of invasion is that the epithelium itself is normal but its direction of migration, instead of being out, is inwards which causes a retraction pocket to continue to expand. The normal pattern of migration of the epithelium from the centre of the tympanic membrane towards the external

auditory meatus was initially described by Litton (1963) and Alberti (1964) but expanded upon by Michaels (1989). Migration from the pars tensa appears to be distinct from the pars flaccida (Figure 3.14). What could be postulated is that once a retraction pocket forms, the normal direction of outward growth is lost and is replaced by an inward growth pattern which would cause the retraction pocket to expand. If this were to be the case, it is unnecessary to invoke a pathological nature for the epithelium.

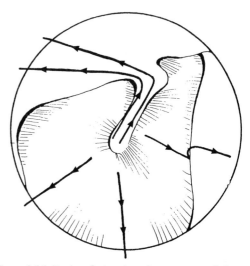

Figure 3.14 Routes of migration of squamous epithelium. (Adapted from Michaels, 1989)

Metaplasia

It is postulated that secondary to episodes of inflammation, areas of metaplasia to squamous epithelium occur in the middle ear mucosa and these expand to create cysts, as is known to occur with surgically implanted squamous epithelium. These cysts, it is postulated, enlarge and then burst through the pars flaccida, or less frequently the pars tensa, to create a cholesteatoma. Metaplasia of mucosa into a squamous epithelium, which is sometimes keratinized, is not uncommon in the lower respiratory tract secondary to irritation and the fact that this also occurs in the ear is shown by the frequent finding of squamous epithelium in granulation tissue and aural polyps (see Figure 3.24b), even when there is no evidence of a cholesteatoma (Palva and Makinen, 1983).

Though metaplasia may be the mechanism in congenital cholesteatoma, the evidence to support it as a cause in acquired cholesteatoma is less persuasive.

Animal experiments have shown that artificially induced inflammation in the middle ear will be associated with metaplasia into squamous epithelium, but the finding of epithelial cysts in chronic mucosal otitis media has not been recorded, unless there has been previous surgery when implantation may have occurred. It is also difficult to conjecture why these metaplastic areas should preferentially produce cysts in the attic. Animal experiments that occlude the external auditory meatus or irritate the lateral aspect of the tympanic membrane produce 'cholesteatomas' in the pars flaccida (Steinbach, Pusalkar and Heumann, 1988).

Non-specific pathology: potentially present in all types of chronic otitis media

Tympanosclerosis

Tympanosclerosis is a result of continued inflammation in the middle ear cleft and is present histologically in one-quarter of ears with chronic otitis media, irrespective of type (Meyerhoff, Kim and Paparella, 1977). Pathologically, tympanosclerosis is the end point of a healing process in which the collagen in fibrous tissue hyalinizes, loses its structure and becomes fused into a homogeneous mass (Schuknecht, 1974). Thereafter calcification and perhaps ossification may occur to a variable extent. Tympanosclerosis most frequently affects the tympanic membrane (Figure 3.15), but the ossicular ligaments, interosseous joints (Figures 3.16 and 3.17), muscle tendons and submucosal space can also be affected causing varying degrees of immobility of the ossicular chain (Igarashi *et al.*, 1970). Clinical reports of surgical findings suggest that tympanosclerosis is rare in active ears (Gristwood and Venables, 1982) and particularly in ears with a cholesteatoma (Plester, 1971), but pathological studies of temporal bones would not support this distinction (Meyerhoff, Kim and Paparella, 1977). Though clinical intuition might suggest that tympanosclerosis is irreversible, series that have followed up ears with tympanosclerosis of the tympanic membrane secondary to childhood otitis media for many years have shown it to disappear in a proportion (Ambegaoker, Brown and Richards, 1978; Tos, Bonding and Poulsen, 1983).

Ossicular erosion

Ossicular chain erosion occurs in ears both with and without cholesteatoma and, because in most ears with a cholesteatoma there is also active mucosal disease, the question arises as to whether there are one or two mechanisms by which erosion may occur. The consensus is that in most instances the erosion is a non-specific result of the hyperaemia associated with mucosal inflammation. In any condition in which there is an area of inflammation in contact with bone, resorption and remodelling will occur. Granulation tissue is found more frequently around the ossicular chain than anywhere else in the middle

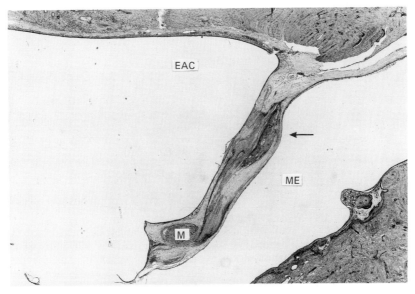

Figure 3.15 Tympanosclerosis. Within the fibrous tissue layer of the tympanic membrane there is a large tympanosclerotic plaque which is partly ossified (arrow). EAC, external auditory canal (meatus); M, malleus; ME, middle ear. (Collection MEEI)

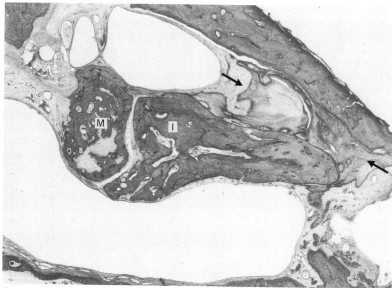

Figure 3.16 High power view showing fixation of the incus in the fossa incudis by tympanosclerosis (arrow). I, incus; M, malleus. (Collection MEEI)

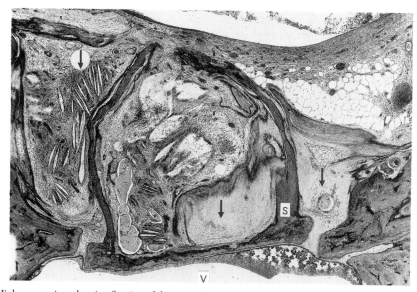

Figure 3.17 High power view showing fixation of the stapes (arrows on right hand side of the figure) by tympanosclerosis. Note cholesterol crystals in the inflammatory tissue (arrowed) on the left hand side of the figure. S, stapes; V, vestibule. (Collection MEEI)

ear cleft. This could be a result of the mucosal folds directing the spread of inflammation (Proctor, 1964) as well as their position in the antrum, where even a mild degree of oedema will block secretions within the mastoid air cells. The reason that the long process of the incus and the stapes superstructure are the parts of the chain which are most frequently affected

is likely to be due to their delicate structure, rather than their tenuous blood supply (Thomsen *et al.*, 1974).

With increasing knowledge and the development of immunohistological and chemical methods, attention is increasingly being turned to looking at the various cytokines that are involved in inflammatory reactions and neoplasia. As might be expected, cholesteatoma tissue has been investigated to see if it is different from the epithelium of a normal tympanic membrane or if the inflammatory reaction associated with it is different from that in active mucosal disease. Thus the various epidermal growth factors (EGF), transforming growth factors (TGF), tumour necrosing factors (TNF), interleukins and prostaglandins have been identified singly and in combination in cholesteatoma tissue. However, as they are also found in any inflammatory reaction and as the normal interplay of these cytokines is complex, it will be difficult to show that cholesteatoma tissue is any different.

Histologically, when there is a cholesteatoma associated with bone erosion there is invariably underlying hyperaemic inflamed tissue associated with it (Figure 3.18a,b) (Thomsen *et al.*, 1974; Tos, 1979; Sade *et al.*, 1981). Although the ossicular chain is perhaps more frequently eroded when there is cholesteatoma in association with active mucosal chronic otitis media, it is probably a function of where it is located rather than the pathology itself. It is unlikely that the squamous epithelial lining of a cholesteatoma secretes any noxious substance or enzyme which destroys bone, though this is contested (Abramson, Moriyama and Huang, 1984). The clinical evidence cited for this is the erosion of the long process of the incus by a retraction pocket which can occur over the years without any obvious clinical activity.

Numerous papers have been published as to how bone destruction occurs. To date there is no substantive evidence that it is a different process from elsewhere in the body where osteoclasts are responsible for bone absorption in association with various enzymes (Ohsaki *et al.*, 1988; Lannigan, O'Higgins and McPhie, 1993).

Fibrous sclerosis

During the reparative phase of any inflammation, fibrous tissue is laid down by fibroblasts and, in the middle ear and mastoid air cells, this can result in adhesions between the tympanic membrane, ossicles and the middle ear mucosa.

Mastoid sclerosis

Subsequent to fibrous sclerosis, there is remodelling and deposition of new bone mainly by the action of osteoblasts which results in a sclerotic mastoid (Figure 3.18a). Interestingly, if the external opening of the pneumatized humerus in a chicken is blocked off, fibrocystic sclerosis and new bone formation, which is histologically similar to mastoid sclerosis, will result (Ojala, 1957; Beaumont, 1966).

Cholesterol granuloma

This is primarily a histological rather than a clinical term for a pathological process which can occur anywhere in the middle ear cleft and is independent of whether the ear is active or inactive and whether or not a cholesteatoma is present. Histologically, there is a giant cell reaction around cholesterol crystals (see Figure 3.17) indicating an inflammatory reaction of the middle ear mucosa to them. The origin of the cholesterol crystals is debated, but it has been suggested that they are due to the breakdown of extravasated blood cells as iron deposits are often found in association (Friedmann, 1959). On the other hand, it is argued that middle ear secretions, in particular those associated with otitis media with effusion, contain cholesterol and gross haemorrhage is not a common feature of otitis media (Sade and Teitz, 1982).

Otologists often use the term 'cholesterol granuloma' when they find thick yellow fluid in the mastoid or middle ear space at surgery. The latter can often be suspected otoscopically by the presence of a blue drum (Ranger, 1949). This yellow fluid will indeed contain cholesterol, but it is wrong to call it a cholesterol granuloma because this is a mucosal pathology. In such ears, there will be cholesterol granulomas in the mucosa, but they will also be found in inactive ears where the otologist would never think of applying the term. The better clinical term to use would be 'cholesteatosis'.

Labyrinthitis

Clinically vestibular problems are not uncommon in active chronic otitis media with or without cholesteatoma. In most instances it is likely to be an irritative labyrinthitis because of inflammation in the round window area. As a result the round window membrane thickens (Sahni *et al.*, 1987) but this obviously does not eliminate the problem. Alternatively, in ears with a cholesteatoma a lateral semicircular canal 'fistula' can result (Figure 3.19).

Endolymphatic hydrops is a not infrequent secondary occurrence in bones with chronic otitis media (Plantenga and Browning, 1979; Paparella, Schachern and Goycoolea, 1988) and this possibility should be borne in mind clinically if there are vestibular problems.

Sensorineural hearing impairment

There are many potential reasons why an individual with chronic otitis media may have a mixed rather than a purely conductive impairment: the disease process may itself affect the cochlea; potentially ototoxic ear drops are often given; surgery itself can cause damage; the patient might have an unrelated sensorineural hearing impairment; and the artificial elevation of the bone conduction thresholds due to the Carhart effect have to be corrected for. Histologically the evidence for the disease itself causing a sensorineural hearing impairment is scant (Walby, Barrera and Schuknecht, 1983). Clinically also the evidence is weak once all the other possible factors

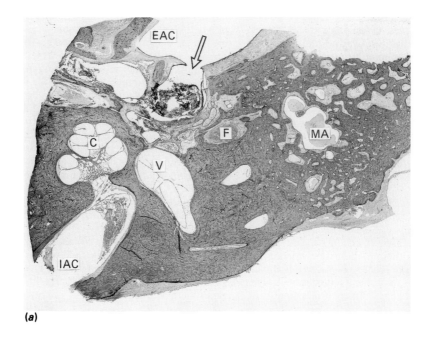

(a)

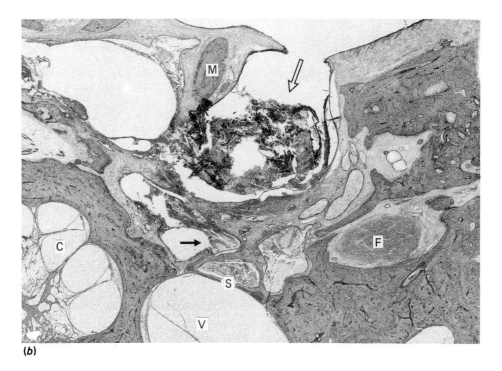

(b)

Figure 3.18 Cholesteatoma. (*a*) Transverse section at the level of the stapes showing a cholesteatoma (clear arrow) in the middle ear. Note the fibrosclerosis of the mastoid air cell system. (*b*) High power view showing the squamous epithelial debris in a narrow necked retraction pocket associated with inflammatory tissues (black arrow) which has eroded the stapes superstructure. C, cochlea; EAC, external auditory canal (meatus); F, facial nerve; IAC, internal auditory canal (meatus); M, malleus; MA, mastoid air cells; S, stapes: V, vestibule. (Collection MEEI)

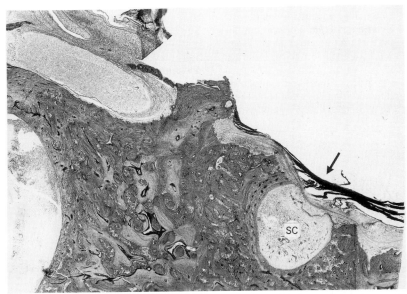

Figure 3.19 Fistula of semicircular canal. The bone over the semicircular canal (SC) is eroded and covered by squamous epithelium (arrow). In this instance the meatus is obliterated with fibrous tissue. (Collection MEEI)

are controlled for (Dumich, Harner and Rochester, 1983; Browning and Gatehouse, 1989).

Specific pathology

Inactive chronic otitis media

By definition, the tympanic membrane is abnormal in inactive chronic otitis media and the clinical appearance depends on the method of healing, but in all instances there is a loss of the fibrous tissue layer of the tympanic membrane. Thus, in the replacement, there is a membrane bridging the defect composed only of an outer layer of squamous epithelium and an inner mucosal one (Figure 3.20). When a perforation is present, the squamous epithelium of the outer tympanic membrane meets the middle ear mucosa at

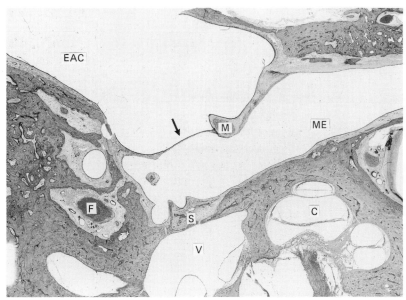

Figure 3.20 Replacement tympanic membrane. The replacement tympanic membrane (arrowed), unlike the remainder of the tympanic membrane anteriorly, does not have a fibrous tissue layer. Note the tympanosclerotic plaque in the anterior tympanic membrane. C. cochlea; EAC, external auditory canal (meatus); M, malleus; ME, middle ear; S. stapes; V, vestibule; F. facial nerve. (Collection MEEI)

a variable position, frequently within the middle ear (Figures 3.21a,b). This has practical implications for myringoplasty. If there is any residual drum, there may be a tympanosclerotic plaque in the fibrous layer.

Clinically what constitutes a marginal as opposed to a central perforation is confusing, some equating a marginal perforation with one that extends to the bony meatus. Others (Figure 3.22, from Diamant, 1982) would equate it with disease which is primarily located in the posterosuperior quadrant and therefore more likely to be associated with a cholesteatoma. Pathologically, the difference has not been clearly defined but some would suggest that it depends on whether or not the annulus is destroyed.

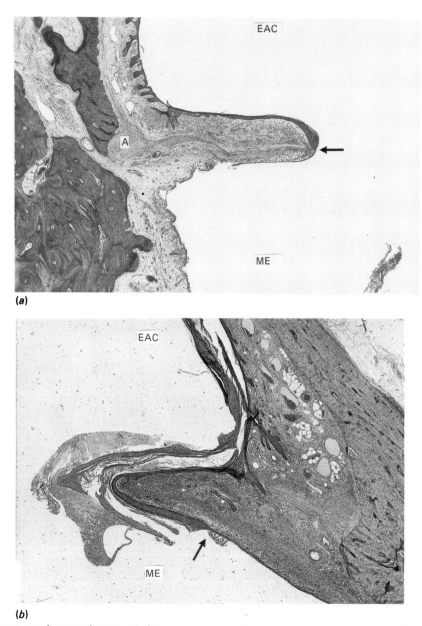

(a)

(b)

Figure 3.21 Tympanic membrane perforation. (a) Chronic tympanic membrane perforation showing (arrowed) the junction of the squamous epithelium and the ear mucosa at the edge of the defect. Note the mild otitis externa, secondary to middle ear activity. (b) Chronic tympanic membrane perforation showing (arrowed) the junction of the squamous epithelium of the external auditory meatus (EAC) with the middle ear mucosa to be within the middle ear (ME). A, annulus. (Collection MEEI)

Central perforations

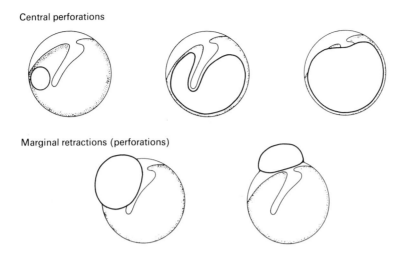

Marginal retractions (perforations)

Figure 3.22 Diagrammatic distinction between perforations of the tympanic membrane that are classified as central as opposed to marginal (after Diamant, 1982)

Active mucosal disease (including polyps)

The extent to which the lining of the middle ear and mastoid air cells are affected varies. In the middle ear the usually non-secretory mucosa is replaced by a respiratory type, mucus-secreting mucosa with goblet cells. The mucosa is generally hyperaemic with an underlying inflammatory response (Figure 3.23). Areas of granulation tissue may form especially in non-draining areas, such as around the ossicles.

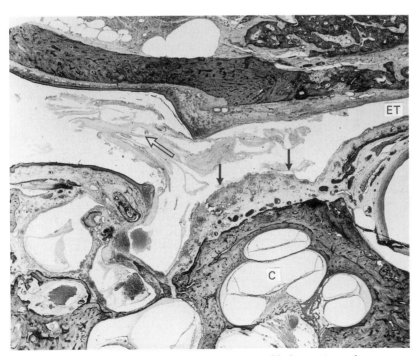

Figure 3.23 Active mucosal chronic otitis media. The middle ear mucosa (black arrow) over the promontory and eustachian tube (ET) is hypertrophied and inflamed with the production of a mucopurulent discharge (clear arrow) which is draining via a chronic tympanic membrane perforation. C, cochlea. (Collection MEEI)

Depending on its severity, there can be active resorption and bone remodelling, irrespective of whether a cholesteatoma is present, which can lead to dehiscence of the fallopian canal. Surprisingly the mastoid mucosa seldom undergoes metaplasia to a secretory lining, granulation tissue being more common (Schachern *et al.*, 1991).

For some as yet unknown reason polyps can sometimes arise from this hyperaemic inflamed mucosa (Figure 3.24*a*) and progressively enlarge so that they block off drainage via the external auditory meatus. Their surface can be ulcerated, covered in a hyperaemic respiratory type mucosa or have areas of squamous metaplasia (Figure 3.24*b*).

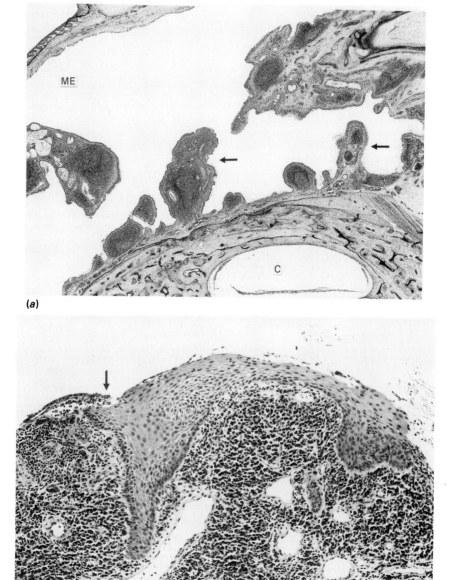

Figure 3.24 Polyps on promontory. (*a*) Early polyposis (arrows) of the middle ear mucosa. These polyps are covered by a respiratory type mucosa and the stalk shows an intense inflammatory reaction, mainly of plasma cells. C, cochlea; ME middle ear. (*b*) This high power view of a different polyp shows an area of squamous metaplasia, the junction with the respiratory type mucosa being indicated with an arrow. (Collection MEEI)

Active chronic otitis media with cholesteatoma

A cholesteatoma has nothing whatsoever to do with cholesterol. It is a keratinized, squamous epithelial-lined pocket containing keratinous debris (Figures 3.18*a,b* and 3.25*a,b*) which it would be histologically more correct to call a keratoma (Schuknecht, 1974). A cholesteatoma is distinguished from a re-

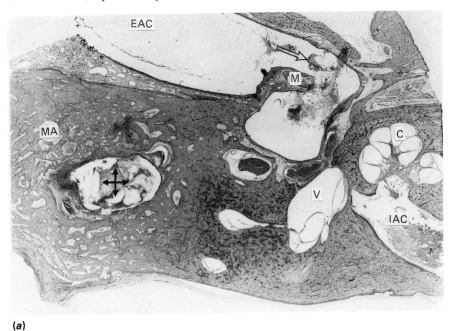

(a)

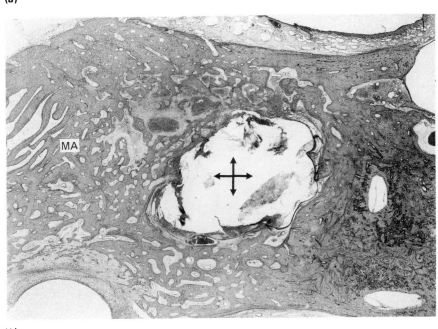

(b)

Figure 3.25 Cholesteatoma. (*a*) Squamous epithelial lined retraction pocket (clear arrow) which is full of debris and which lines the middle ear cavity and extends via the antrum (seen in associated sections) to the mastoid (black arrow) which is sclerotic. The cholesteatoma is surrounded by an inflammatory reaction. C, cochlea; EAC, external auditory canal (meatus); IAC, internal auditory canal (meatus); M, malleus; MA, mastoid air cells; V, vestibule. (*b*) High powered view showing the cholesteatoma within the mastoid air cells (MA). (Collection MEEI)

traction pocket (Figure 3.26) or areas of squamous metaplasia (see below) by its retention of keratinous debris.

Histologically, there would appear to be little difference between the squamous epithelium of a cholesteatoma and that of skin, all the recognized layers being present. The number of Langerhans' cells may be increased but this is taken to be a result of the underlying inflammation rather than a finding which is specific to a cholesteatoma (Lim and Saunders, 1972). Almost invariably when keratinous debris is retained, there will be an associated inflammatory response in the subepithelial connective tissue (see Figure 3.18*b*), but whether the two are connected is uncertain. Granulation tissue will often develop in association with a cholesteatoma and this may present at its margins and even develop into an aural polyp.

Pathology following surgery

Homo/autograft ossicles: prostheses

The method whereby repositioned ossicles become integrated into the ear appears to be independent of how they have been preserved, if at all, or whether they are homografts or autografts. They become covered by a layer of mucosa and most commonly the general structure of the ossicle remains, but as dead bone with few, if any, osteocytes. Usually there is a slight degree of inflammation and vascularization of the haversian canals along with some erosion or new bone growth on the surface (Figure 3.27*a*). Ceramics are incorporated in the same manner.

Implants that have a lattice structure, such as porous polyethylene (Plastipore), allow the ingrowth of fibrous tissue but often this is associated with a chronic giant cell inflammatory reaction which encourages their extrusion (Figure 3.27*b*).

Mastoid cavity

An open mastoid cavity that has healed and is inactive is usually lined by keratinized squamous epithelium on a layer of fibrous sclerosis that extends into any residual mastoid air cells (Figure 3.28). If an area remains active, it is because of superficial granulation tissue which may take on a polypoidal

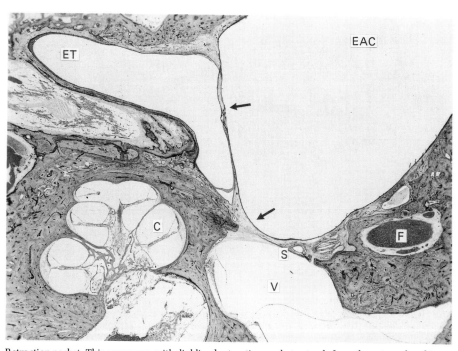

Figure 3.26 Retraction pocket. This squamous epithelial lined retraction pocket extends from the external auditory meatus (EAC) into the middle ear, over the eustachian tube (ET) and over the stapes footplate (S) whose superstructure has been previously eroded. Note the cholesterol crystals in the fibrous tissue posterior to the stapes footplate. C, cochlea; V, vestibule; F, facial nerve. (Collection MEEI)

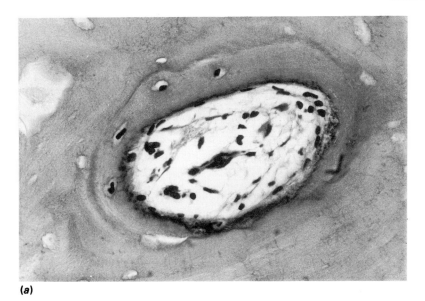

(a)

(b)

Figure 3.27 (*a*) Autograft ossicle. New bone deposition on dead transplanted bone in a haversian canal in an autologous incus after 9 years in the middle ear. (Reproduced by kind permission of Mr A. G. Kerr and the Editor of the *Journal of Laryngology and Otology*). (*b*) A Plastipore prosthesis after 18 months in the middle ear. There is a good fibrous tissue capsule but, deep in it, a multinucleated foreign body giant cell is seen engulfing polythene (arrow). (Reproduced by kind permission of Mr A. G. Kerr and the Editor of *Clinical Otolaryngology*)

character (Figure 3.29) rather than because of continued discharge from respiratory type epithelium or osteitis in the underlying bone (Pettigrew, 1980; Youngs, 1992).

If part of a cholesteatoma is left within a closed middle ear cleft, one of two things may happen. The first, and perhaps the more likely, is that the squamous epithelium undergoes metaplasia to middle ear-type mucosa. The evidence for this comes from surgical operations where part of the cholesteatoma matrix has been left over a semicircular canal fistula and, when the ear has been re-explored many months later, there has been no evidence of squamous epithelium (Smyth, 1980). The alternative is

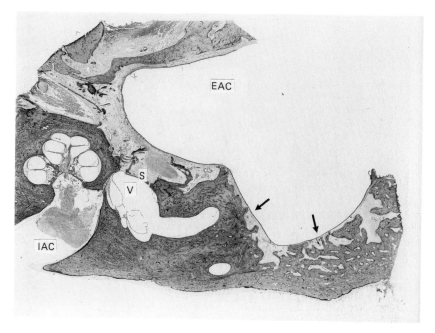

Figure 3.28 Inactive mastoid cavity. There is a squamous epithelial lined mastoid cavity which is in continuity with a squamous epithelial lined, but obliterated, middle ear space. The remaining air cells are obliterated with fibrous tissue. EAC, external auditory canal (meatus); IAC, internal auditory canal (meatus); S, stapes; V, vestibule. (Collection MEEI)

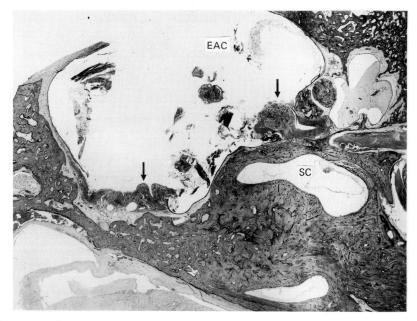

Figure 3.29 Active mastoid cavity. There is granulation tissue in the mastoid bowl and on the promontory (arrowed). The mastoid air cells underlying this granulation tissue are sclerotic and not the source of the inflammation. The remainder of the cavity and middle ear space is covered by squamous epithelium. EAC, external auditory canal (meatus); SC, semicircular canal. (Collection MEEI)

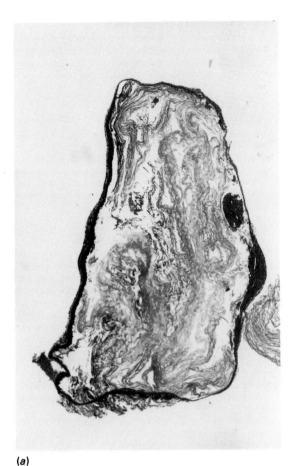

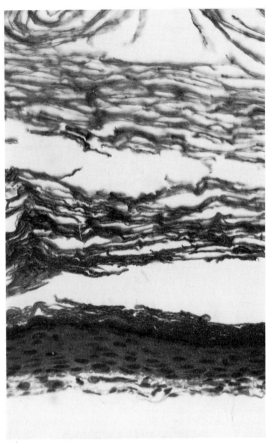

(a) **(b)**

Figure 3.30 Cholesteatomatous pearl. (*a*) The cyst is lined by squamous epithelium and is full of keratinous debris. (*b*) High power view showing epithelium identical to normal skin (see Figure 3.1)

that a 'cholesteatoma pearl' will develop (Figure 3.30*a,b*). Histologically, the main difference between such squamous epithelial retention cysts and an acquired cholesteatoma is that there is no external opening and the associated inflammation is considerably less. As such they more closely resemble congenital rather than acquired cholesteatomas. The natural history of these cysts is unknown, but they can disappear spontaneously. However, some fear that if they are not removed surgically they may become a cholesteatoma.

Acknowledgements

We are deeply indebted to Professor H. F. Schuknecht for the generous way in which he put at our disposal the temporal bone material in his collection at the Massachusetts Eye and Ear Infirmary. These sections are identified as 'Collection MEEI'.

References

ABRAMSON, M., MORIYAMA, H. and HUANG, C. C. (1984) Pathogenic factors in bone resorption in cholesteatoma. *Acta Otolaryngologica*, **97**, 437–442

ALBERTI, P. W. R. M. (1964) Epithelial migration of the tympanic membrane. *Journal of Laryngology and Otology*,, **78**, 808–830

ALHO, O. P., KILKKU, O., OJA, H., KOIVU, M. and SORRI, M. (1993) Control of the temporal aspect when considering risk factors for acute otitis media. *Archives of Otolaryngology – Head Neck Surgery*, **119**, 444–449

AMBEGAOKAR, A. G., BROWN, M. J. K. M. and RICHARDS. S. H. (1978) Grommets and glue ear: a five-year follow up of a controlled trial. *Journal of the Royal Society of Medicine*, **71**, 353–356

BAIN, J., MURPHY, E. and ROSS, F. (1985) Acute otitis media: clinical course among children who received a short course of antibiotic. *British Medical Journal*, **291**, 1243–1246

BEAUMONT, G. D. (1966) The effects of exclusion of air from pneumatised bones. *Journal of Laryngology and Otology*, **80**, 236–249

BERNSTEIN, J. M., KOSINSKI, D., MYERS, D., NISENGARD, R. and WICHER, K. (1980) Antibody coated bacteria in otitis media with effusions. *Annals of Otology, Rhinology and Laryngology*, **89**, Suppl. 68

BERNSTEIN, J. M., LEE, J., CONBOY, K., ELLIS, I and LI, P. (1983) The role of IgE mediated hypersensitivity in recurrent otitis media with effusion. *American Journal of Otology*, **5**, 66–69

BESS, F. H., SCHWARTZ, D. M. and REDFIELD, N. P. (1976) Audiometric, impedance, and otoscopic findings in children with cleft palates *Archives of Otolaryngology*, **102**, 465–469

BLACK, J. I. M. and CHAYTOR, R. G. (1958) Wax keratosis in childrens ears. *British Medical Journal*, **2**, 673–675

BLUESTONE, C. D. (1984) State of the art: definitions and classifications. In: *Recent Advances in Otitis Media with Effusion. Proceedings of the IIIrd International Conference*, edited by D. J. Liu, C. D. Bluestone, J. O. Klein and J. D. Nelson. Ontario: Decker and Mosby

BREMOND, G. and COQUIN, A. (1972) Ultrastructure of normal and pathological middle ear mucosa. *Journal of Laryngology and Otology*, **86**, 457–472

BROOK, I. (1987) The role of anaerobic bacteria in otitis media: microbiology, pathogenesis, and implications on therapy. *American Journal of Otolaryngology*, **8**, 109–117

BROOK, I., FRAZIER, E. H. and THOMPSON, D. H. (1992) Aerobic and anaerobic microbiology of external otitis. *Clinical Infectious Diseases*, **15**, 955–958

BROWNING, G. G. and GATEHOUSE, S. (1989) Hearing in chronic suppurative otitis media. *Annals of Otology, Rhinology and Laryngology*, **98**, 245–250

BROWNING, G. G. and GATEHOUSE, S. (1992) The prevalence of middle ear disease in the adult British population. *Clinical Otolaryngology*, **17**, 317–321

BROWNING, G. G., PICOZZI, G. L., SWEENEY, G. and CALDER, I. T. (1983) Role of anaerobes in chronic otitis media. *Clinical Otolaryngology*, **8**, 47–51

BYLANDER, A. (1980) Comparison of eustachian tube function in children and adults with normal ears. *Annals of Otology, Rhinology and Laryngology*, **89**, (suppl. 68), 20–24

BYLANDER, A., TJERSTROM, O. and IVARSSON, A. (1983) Pressure opening and closing functions of the eustachian tube in children and adults with normal ears. *Acta Otolaryngologica*, **95**, 55–62

CALDERON, R. and MOOD, E. W. (1982) An epidemiological assessment of water quality and 'swimmer's ear'. *Archives of Environmental Health*, **37**, 300–305

CAMILLERI, A. E., SWAN, I. R. C., MURPHY. E. and STURROCK, R. D. (1992) Chronic otitis media: a new extra articular manifestation in ankylosing spondylitis. *Annals of Rheumatic Diseases*, **51**, 655–657

CAMMOUN, M., VOGT HOERNER, G. and MOURALI, N. (1974) Tumors of the nasopharynx in Tunisia. An anatomic and clinical study based on 143 cases. *Cancer*, **33**, 184–192

CHANDLER, J. R. (1977) Malignant external otitis: further considerations. *Annals of Otology, Rhinology and Laryngology*, **86**, 417–428

CHAPUT DE SAINTONGE, D. M., LEVINE, D. F., TEMPLE SAVAGE, I., BURGESS. G. W. S., SHARP, J., MAYHEW, S.. R. *et al.* (1982) Trial of three-day and ten-day courses of amoxycillin in otitis media. *British Medical Journal*, **284**, 1078–1081

CHONMAITREE, T., OWEN, M. J., PATEL, J. A., HEDGPETH, D., HORLICK, D. and HOWIE, V. M. (1992) *Journal of Pediatrics*, **120**, 856–862

COFFEY, J. D. (1966) Otitis media in the practice of pediatrics. *Pediatrics*, **38**, 25–32

DA COSTA, S. S., PAPARELLA, M. M., SHACHERN, P. A., YOON, T. H. and KIMBERLEY, B. P. (1992) Temporal bone histopathology in chronically infected ears with intact and perforated tympanic membranes. *Lanryngoscope*, **102**, 1229–1236

DE MARIA, T. F., PRIOR, R. B., BRIGGS, B, R., LIM, D. J. and BIRCK, H. G. (1984) Endotoxin in middle-ear effusions from patients with chronic otitis media with effusion. *Journal of Clinical Microbiology*, **20**, 15–17

DEMPSTER, J. H. and BROWNING, G. G. (1989) Eustachian tube function following adenoidectomy: an evaluation by sniffing. *Clinical Otolaryngology*, **14**, 411–414

DEMPSTER, J. H., BROWNING, G. G. and GATEHOUSE, S. (1993) A randomized study of the surgical management of children with persistent otitis media with effusion associated with a hearing impairment. *Journal of Laryngology and Otology*, **107**, 284–289

DIAMANT, M. (1982) Mastoid pneumatization and cholesteatoma – the genetic question. In: *Cholesteatoma and Mastoid Surgery. Proceedings of the IInd International Conference*, edited by J. Sade. Amsterdam: Kugler. pp. 105–110

DOROGHAZI, R. M., NADOL, J. B., HYSLOP, N. E., BAKER, A. S. and AXELROD, L. (1981) Invasive external Otitis. Report of 21 cases and review of the literature, *American Journal of Medicine*, **71**, 603–614

DUMICH, P. S., HARNER, S. G. and ROCHESTER, M. N. (1983) Cochlear function in chronic otitis media. *Laryngoscope*, **93**, 583–586

FEINMESSER, R., WIESEL. Y. M., ARGAMAN, M. and GAY, I. (1982) Otitis externa – bacteriological survey. *Journal for Oto-rhino-laryngology and its Borderlands*, **44**, 121–125

FIELLAU-NIKOLAJSEN, M. (1983) Epidemiology of secretory otitis media. *Annals of Otology, Rhinology and Laryngology*, **92**, 172–177

FORD, G. P., PARR, P. M., IVE. F. A. and SHUSTER, S. (1984) The response of seborrhoeic dermatitis to ketoconazole. *British Journal of Dermatology*, **111**, 603–607

FRIEDBERG, J. (1994) Congenital cholesteatoma. *Laryngoscope*, **104** (Suppl. 62), 1–24

FRIEDMANN, I. (1959) Epidermoid cholesteatoma and cholesterol granuloma experimental and human. *Annals of Otology, Rhinology and Laryngology*, **68**, 57–59

GATES, G. A., AVERY, C. A., PRIHODA, T. J. and COOPER, J. C. (1987) Effectiveness of adenoidectomy and tympanostomy tubes in the treatment of chronic otitis media with effusion. *New England Journal of Medicine*, **317**, 1444–1451

GIEBINK, G. S. (1992) Otitis media update: pathogenesis and treatment. *Annals of Otology, Rhinology and Laryngology*, **101**, 21–23

GILES, M. and ASHER, I. (1991) Prevalence and natural history of otitis media with perforation in Maori school children. *Journal of Laryngology and Otology*, **105**, 257–260

GRISTWOOD, R. E. and VENABLES, W. N. (1982) Cholesteatoma and tympanosclerosis. In: *Cholesteatoma and Mastoid Surgery. Proceedings of the IInd International Conference*, edited by J. Sade. Amsterdam: Kugler. pp. 133–137

GUNDERSEN, T. and GLUCK, E. (1972) The middle ear mucosa in serous otitis media *Archives of Otolaryngology*, **96**, 40–44

HARELL, M., PENNINGTON, F. R. and MORRISON, W. V. (1982) Prevalence of cholesteatoma in black Americans. In: *Cholesteatoma and Mastoid Surgery. Proceedings of the IInd International Conference*, edited by J. Sade. Amsterdam: Kugler. pp. 97–104

HARRISON, C. J., MARKS, M. I. and WELCH, D. F. (1985)

Microbiology of recently treated acute otitis media compared with previously untreated acute otitis media. *Pediatric Infectious Disease*, **4**, 641–646

HIBBERT, J. (1982) The role of enlarged adenoids in the aetiology of serous otitis media. *Clinical Otolaryngology*, **7**, 253–256

HINCHCLIFFE, R. (1977) Cholesteatoma: epidemiological and quantitative aspects. In: *Cholesteatoma. Proceedings of the First International Conference*, edited by B. F. McCabe, J. Sade and M. Abramson. Alabama: Aesculapius. pp. 277–286

HOLMES, R. C., JOHNS, A. N., WILKINSON, J. D., BLACK, M. M. and RYCROFT, R. J. G. (1982) Medicament contact dermatitis in patients with chronic inflammatory ear disease. *Journal of the Royal Society of Medicine*, **75**, 27–30

HOLT, J. J. (1992) Ear canal cholesteatoma. *Laryngoscope*, **102**, 608–613

HONJO, I., OKAZAKI, N. and KUMAZAWA, T. (1980) Opening mechanism of the eustachian tube. A clinical and experimental study. *Annals of Otology, Rhinology and Laryngology*, **89**, (suppl. 68), 25–27

HOSHINO, T., YANO, J., ICHIMURA, K., HASHIMOTO, H. and NOZUE, M. (1982) Chronic myringitis and chronic suppurative otitis media. *Archives of Otorhinolaryngology*, **234**, 219–223

HUSSL, B. and WELZL-MUELLER, K. (1980) Secretory otitis media and mastoid pneumatization. *Annals of Otology, Rhinology and Laryngology*, **89**, (Supplement 68), 79–82

IGARASHI, M., KONISHI, S., ALFORD, B. R. and GUILDFORD, F. R. (1970) The pathology of tympanosclerosis. *Laryngoscope*, **80**, 233–243

INGVARSSON, L. (1982) Acute otalgia in children – findings and diagnosis. *Acta Paediatrica Sandinavica*, **71**, 705–710

INGVARSSON, L., LUNDGREN, K., OLFSSON, B. and WALL, S. (1983) Epidemiology of acute otitis media in children. *Acta Otolaryngologica Supplementum*, **388**

ISHII, T., TORIYAMA, M. and SUZUKI, J-I. (1980) Histopathological study of otitis media with effusion. *Annals of Otology, Rhinology and Laryngology*, **89**, (Supplement 68). 83–86

JUHN, S. (1984) Biochemistry of middle ear effusion; state of the art. In: *Recent Advances in Otitis Media with Effusion. Proceedings of the IIIrd International Conference*, edited by D. J. Lim, C. D. Bluestone, J. O. Klein and J. D. Nelson. Ontario: Decker and Mosby

KARJA, J., NUUTINEN, J. and KARJALAINEN, P. (1983) Mucociliary function in children with secretory otitis media. *Acta Otolaryngologica*, **95**, 544–546

KERR, A. G. (1981) Proplast and Plastipore. *Clinical Otolaryngology*, **6**, 187–191

KHALIFA, M. C., EL FOULY, S., BASSIOUNY, A. and KAMEL, M. (1982) Granular myringitis. *Journal of Laryngology and Otology*, **96**, 1099–1101

KURIHARA, A., TOSHIMA, M., YUASA, R. and TAKASAKA, T. (1991) Bone destruction mechanisms in chronic otitis media with cholesteatoma: specific production by cholesteatoma tissue in culture of bone-resorbing activity attributable to interleukin-1 alpha. *Annals of Otology, Rhinology and Lanryngology*, **100**, 989–998

LALWANI, A. K. and SOOY, C. D. (1992) Otologic and neurotologic manifestations of acquired immunodeficiency syndrome. *Otolaryngologic Clinics of North America*, **25**, 1183–1197

LANCET (1980) Flagellating cilia. i, 346–347

LANCET (1982) Necrotising otitis externa. i. 207

LANCET (1986) Culture crafts of keratinocytes: a growth industry. ii, 183

LANG, J., KERR, A. G. and SMYTH, G. D. L. (1986) Long term viability of transplanted ossicles. *Journal of Laryngology and Otology*, **100**, 741–747

LANNIGAN, F. J., O'HIGGINS. P. and MCPHIE. P. (1993) The cellular mechanism of ossicular erosion in chronic suppurative otitis media. *Journal of Laryngology and Otology*, **107**, 12–16

LEVENTON, G., MAN, A., KRAUS, P. and ALTMANN, G. (1967) External otitis: study of recurrences. *Journal of Laryngology and Otology*, **81**,413–418

LIM, D. J. (1979) Normal and pathological mucosa of the middle ear and eustachian tube. *Clinical Otolaryngology*, **4**, 213–234

LIM, D. J. and BIRCK, H. (1971) Ultrastructural pathology of the middle ear mucosa in serous otitis media. *Annals of Otology, Rhinology and Laryngology*, **80**, 838–853

LIM, D. J. and SAUNDERS, W. H. (1972) Acquired cholesteatoma: light and electron microscopic observations. *Annals of Otology, Rhinology and Laryngology*, **81** 2–12

LITTON, W. B. (1963) Epithelial migration over the tympanic membrane and external canal. *Archives of Otolaryngology*, **77**, 254–257

MAGNUSON, B. (1981a) On the origin of the high negative pressure in the middle ear space. *American Journal of Otolaryngology*, **2**, 1–12

MAGNUSON, B. (1981b) Tubal opening and closing ability in unilateral middle ear disease. *American Journal of Otolaryngology*, **2**, 199–209

MAW, A. R. (1983) Chronic otitis media with effusion (glue ear) and adenotonsillectomy: prospective randomised controlled study. *British Medical Journal*, **287**, 1586–1588

MAW, A. R., JEANS, W. D. and CABLE, H. R. (1983) Adenoidectomy: a prospective study to show clinical and radiological changes two years after operation. *Journal of Laryngology and Otology*, **97**, 511–518

MAWSON, S. R. (1963) *Diseases of the Ear*, London: Arnold Ltd.

MEYERHOFF, W. L., GATES, G. A. and MONTALBO, P. J. (1977) Pseudomonas mastoiditis. *Laryngoscope*, **87**, 483–492

MEYERHOFF, W. L., KIM, C. S. and PAPARELLA, M. M. (1977) Pathology of chronic otitis media. *Annals of Otology, Rhinology and Laryngology*, **87**, 749–760

MICHAELS, L. (1986) The epidermoid formation in the developing middle ear; possible source of cholesteatoma. *Journal of Otolaryngology*, **15**, 169–174

MICHAELS, L. (1989) Biology of cholesteatoma. *Otolaryngologic Clinics of North America*, **22**, 869–881

MICHAELS, L., SOUCEK, S and LIANG, J. (1994) The ear in the acquired immunodeficiency syndrome: 1. Temporal bone histopathologic study. *American Journal of Otology*, **15**, 515–522

MORIMITSU, T., NAGAI, T., NAGAI, M., IDE, M., MAKINO, K., TONO, T. *et al.* (1989) Pathogenesis of cholesteatoma based on clinical results of anterior tympanotomy. *Auris Nasus larynx (Tokyo)*, **16** (Supplement 1), S9–S14

MORRISON, A. W. (1956) Keratosis obturans. *Journal of Laryngology and Otology*, **70**, 317–321

NAIBERG, J., BERGER. G., and HAWKE, M. (1984) The pathologic features of keratosis obturans and cholesteatoma of the external auditory canal, *Archives of Otolaryngology*, **110**, 690–693

NAKANO, Y. and SATO, Y. (1990) Prognosis of otitis media with effusion in children and size of the mastoid air cell system. *Acta Otolaryngologica Supplementum*, **471**, 56–61

OHSAKI, K., YAMASHITA, S., FUJITA, A., MASUDA, Y., UEDA, S., SUGIURA, T. *et al.* (1988) Mechanism of bone destruction due to middle ear cholesteatoma as revealed by laser-raman spectrometry. *American Journal of Otolaryngology*, 9, 117–126

OJALA, L. (1957) Pneumatisation of the bone and environmental factors; experimental studies on chick humerus. *Acta Otolaryngologica Supplementum*, 133

PALVA, T. and MAKINEN, J. (1983) Why does middle ear cholesteatoma recur? Histological observations. *Archives of Otolaryngology*, 109, 513–518

PALVA, T., MAKINEN, J. and RINNE, J. (1981) Middle ear mucosa in chronic effusions. *Otorhinolaryngology*, 43, 241–247

PAPARELLA, M. M., SHACHERN, P. A. and GOYCOOLEA, M. V. (1988) Multiple otopathologic disorders. *Annals of Otology, Rhinology and Laryngology*, 97, 14–18

PARISIER, S. C., AGRESTI, C. J., SCHWARTZ, G. K., HAN, J. C. and ALBINO, A. P. (1993) Alteration in cholesteatoma fibroblasts: induction of neoplastic-like phenotype. *American Journal of Otology*, 14, 126–130

PEDERSEN, C. B. and ZACHAU-CHRISTIANSEN, B. (1988) Chronic otitis media and sequelae in the population of Greenland. *Scandinavian Journal of Social Medicine*, 16, 15–19

PELTON, S. I., TEELE, D. W., SHURIN, P. A. and KLEIN, J. O. (1980) Disparate cultures of middle ear fluids. *American Journal of Diseases of Children*, 134, 951–953

PETERKIN, G. A. G. (1973) Otitis externa. *Journal of Laryngology and Otology*, 88, 15–21

PETTIGREW, A. M. (1980) Histopathology of the temporal bone after open mastoid surgery. *Clinical Otolaryngology*, 5, 227–234

PICOZZI, G. L., SWEENEY, G., BROWNING, G. G. and CALDER, I. T. (1982) Bacteriology of different activity states of chronic otitis media. *Clinical Otolaryngology*, 7, 137

PIERPERGERDES, J. C., KRAMER, B. M. and BEHNKE, E. E. (1980) Keratosis obturans and external auditory canal cholesteatoma. *Laryngoscope*, 90, 383–391

PLANTENGA, K. R. and BROWNING, G. G. (1979) The vestibular aqueduct and endolymphatic sac and duct in endolymphatic hydrops. *Archives of Otolaryngology*, 105, 546–552

PLESTER, D. (1971) Tympanosclerosis. *Journal of the Otolaryngological Society of Australia*, 3, 325–326

POULSEN, G. and TOS, M. (1977) Tubal function in chronic secretory otitis media in children. *Otorhinolaryngology*, 39, 57–67

PROCTOR, B. (1964) The development of the middle ear spaces and their surgical significance. *Journal of Laryngology and Otology*, 78, 631–648

PROOPS, D. W., HAWKE, W. M. and PARKINSON, E. K. (1984) Tissue culture of migratory skin of the external ear and cholesteatoma: a new research tool. *Journal of Otolaryngology*, 13, 63–69

PUKANDER, J., SIPILA, M. and KARMA, P. (1984) Occurrence of and risk factors in acute otitis media. In: *Recent Advances in Otitis Media with Effusion, Proceedings of the IIIrd International Conference*, edited by D. J. Lim, D. Bluestone, J. O. Klein and J. D. Nelson. Ontario: Decker and Mosby. pp. 9–13

RAHKO, T., KARMA, P. and SIPILA, M. (1989) Sensorineural hearing loss and acute otitis media in children. *Acta Otolaryngologica*, 108, 107–112

RANGER, D. (1949) Idiopathic haemotympanum. *Journal of Laryngology and Otology*, 63, 672–681

RASMUSSEN, P. A. (1974) Otitis externa and allergic contact dermatitis. *Acta Otolaryngologica*, 77, 344–347

ROBERTS, D. B. (1980) The etiology of bullous myringitis and the role of mycoplasmas in ear disease: a review. *Pediatrics*, 65, 761–766

SADÉ, J., AVRAHAM, S. and BROWN, M. (1982) Dynamics of atelectasis and retraction pockets. In: *Cholesteatoma and Mastoid Surgery. Proceedings of the IInd International Conference*, edited by J. Sade. Amsterdam: Kugler. pp. 267–282

SADÉ, J. and BERCO, E. (1976) Atelectasis and secretory otitis media. *American Journal of Otolaryngology*, 85, (Supplement 25), 66–72

SADÉ, J., BERCO, E., BUYANOVER, D. and BROWN, M. (1981) Ossicular damage in chronic middle ear inflammation. *Acta Otolaryngologica*, 92, 273–283

SADÉ, J. and TEITZ, A. (1982) Cholesterol in cholesteatoma and in the otitis media Syndrome. In: *Cholesteatoma and Mastoid Surgery. Proceedings of the IInd International Conference*, edited by J. Sadé. Amsterdam: Kugler. pp. 125–132

SAHNI, R. S., PAPARELLA, M. M., SCHACHERN, P. A., GOYCOOLEA, M. V. and LE, C. T. (1987) Thickness of the human round window membrane in different forms of otitis media. *Archives of Otolaryngology – Head Neck Surgery*, 113, 630–634

SCHACHERN, P., PAPARELLA, M. M., SANO, S., LAMEY, S. and GUO, Y. (1991) A histopathological study of the relationship between otitis media and mastoiditis. *Laryngoscope*, 101, 105–1055

SCHILDER, A. G. M., ZIELHUIS, G. A., STRAATMAN, H. S. and VAN DEN BROEK, P. (1992) An epidemiological approach to the etiology of middle ear disease in the Netherlands. *European Archives of Oto-Rhino-Laryngology*, 249, 370–373

SCHUKNECHT, H. F. (1974) *Pathology of the Ear*. Boston: Harvard University Press

SEYFRIED, P. L. and FRASER, D. J. (1978) *Pseudomonas aeruginosa* in swimming pools related to the incidence of otitis externa infection. *Health, Laboratory Science*, 15, 50–57

SHIMADA, T. and LIM, D. J. (1972) Distribution of ciliated cells in the human middle ear. Electron and light microscopic observations. *Annals of Otology, Rhinology and Laryngology*, 81, 203–211

SINGER, D. E., FREEMAN, E., HOFFERT, W. R., KEYS, R. J., MITCHELL, R. B. and HARDY, A. V. (1952) Otitis externa. Bacteriological and mycological studies. *Annals of Otology, Rhinology and Laryngology*, 61, 317–333

SIPILA, P., JOKIPII, A. M. M., JOKIPII, L. and KARMA, P. (1981) Bacteria in the middle ear and ear canal of patients with secretory otitis media and with non-inflamed ears. *Acta Otolaryngologica*, 92, 123–130

SIPILA, P. and KARMA, P. (1982) Inflammatory cells in mucoid effusion of secretory otitis media. *Acta Otolaryngologica*, 94, 467–472

SMITH, I. M., KEAY, D. G. and BUXTON, P. K. (1990) Contact hypersensitivity in patients with chronic otitis externa. *Clinical Otolaryngology*, 15, 155–158

SMYTH, G. D. L. (1976) Tympanic reconstruction. *Journal of Laryngology and Otology*, 90, 713–741

SMYTH, G. D. L. (1980) Aetiology of chronic suppurative otitis media. In: *Chronic Ear Disease*. New York: Churchill Livingstone. pp. 3–20

SOUCEK, S. and MICHAELS, L. (1993) Kerotosis of the tympanic membrane and deep external auditory canal. *European Archives of Otorhinolaryngology*, 250, 140–142

STEINBACH, E., PUSALKAR, A. and HEUMANN, H. (1988) Cholesteatoma – pathology and treatment. *Advances in Oto-Rhino-Laryngology*, 39, 94–106

SWEENEY, G., PICOZZI, G. L. and BROWNING, G. G. (1982) A quantitative study of aerobic and anaerobic bacteria in chronic suppurative otitis media. *Journal of Infection*, **5**, 47–55

TEELE, D. W., KLEIM. J. O., CHASE, C., MENYUK, P. and ROSNER. B. A. (1990) Otitis media in infancy and intellectual ability, school achievement, speech, and language at age 7 years. *Journal of Infectious Diseases*, **162**, 685–694

THOMSEN, J., JORGENSEN, M. B., BRETLAW, P. and KIRSTENSEN, H. K. (1974) Bone resorption in chronic otitis media. *Journal of Laryngology and Otology*, **88**, 975–992

TOS, M. (1979) Pathology of the ossicular chain in various chronic middle ear diseases. *Journal of Laryngology and Otology*, **93**, 969–980

TOS, M. (1980) Middle ear epithelia in chronic secretory otitis. *Archives of Otolaryngology*, **106**, 593–597

TOS, M. and STANGERUP, S. E. (1984) Mastoid pneumatization in secretory otitis. *Acta Otolaryngologica*, **98**, 110–118

TOS, M., BONDING, P. and POULSEN, G. (1983) Tympanosclerosis of the drum in secretory otitis after insertion of grommets. A prospective, comparative study. *Journal of Laryngology and Otology*, **97**, 489–496

TOS, M., STANGERUP, S. E. and LARSEN, P. (1987) Dynamics of eardrum changes following secretory otitis. *Archives of Otolaryngology – Head Neck Surgery*, **113**, 380–385

TURNER, N. C. (1992) The response to injury. Acute inflammation. In: *Oxford Textbook of Pathology*, edited by O'D McGee, P. Isaacson and N. A. Wright, Oxford: Oxford University Press. pp. 351–365

VAN BUCHEM, F. L., DUNK, J. H. M. and VAN'T HOF, M. A. (1981) Therapy of acute otitis media: myringotomy, antibiotics, or neither? *Lancet, ii*, 883–887

VAN BUCHEM, F. L., PEETERS, M. F., and VAN'T HOF, M. A. (1985) Acute otitis media: a new treatment strategy. *British Medical Journal*, **290**, 1033–1037

VIRTANEN, H. (1983) Eustachian tube function in children with secretory otitis media. *International Journal of Pediatric Otorhinolaryngology*, **5**, 11–17

WALBY, A. P., BARRERA, A. and SCHUKNECHT, H. F. (1983) Cochlear pathology in chronic suppurative otitis media. *Annals of Otology, Rhinology and Laryngology*, **92** (Supplement 103), 3–19

WHEELER, T. K. (1986) Tympanometry in children with treated acute otitis media. *Lancet, i*, 529–531

WILSON. R. and COLE, P. J. (1988) The effect of bacterial products on ciliary function. *American Review of Respiratory Diseases*, **138**, S49–S53

YOUNGS, R. (1992) The histopathology of mastoidectomy cavities, with particular reference to persistent disease leading to chronic otorrhoea. *Clinical Otolaryngology*, **17**, 505–510

ZIELHUIS, G. A., HEUVALMANS-HEINEN, I W., RACH, G. H. and BROEK, P. V. D. (1989) Environmental risk factors for otitis media with effusion in preschool children. *Scandinavian Journal of Primary Health Care*, **7**, 33–38

4

Pathology of the cochlea

I. Friedmann

The delicate structures of the ear are housed in a comparatively inaccessible part of the skull as Du Verney, a French pioneer in this field, has so aptly described in a postscript to his great thesis *Traité De L'Organe De L'Ouie* (1683): 'Of all the Organs assign'd to the Use of Animals, we have the least knowledge of those of the Senses: but there is none more obscure than that of Hearing; the Minuteness and Delicacy of the Parts which compose it, being inclos'd by other Parts render Enquiries into them more difficult, and their Structure so intricate, that there is much trouble in explaining as there was in discovering them' (Asherson, 1979).

The sensory organ of hearing was described by Alfonso Corti (Figure 4.1) who was born at Gambarana, near Pavia in Lombardy, Italy, on 15 June, 1822 and died in 1876 at his villa in Mazzolino. He was 19 when he entered medical school at the University of Pavia, but did not complete his course because, at the age of 23, he was attracted by the growing fame of Vienna University where he later received his medical degree. There he attended the Institute of Anatomy and, guided by the great anatomist Joseph Hyrtl, Corti concentrated on the research of the anatomy of the inner ear; subsequently working with Albert von Kölliker at the University of Würzberg, he was the first to describe the sensory epithelium of the inner ear.

In his experiments, Corti used material as fresh as possible and placed tissue specimens with a diameter of a few millimetres between two slides, bonding them with a mastic material. He then allowed a fixative to run between the slides and, after fixation, he stained his preparations with a carmine solution. Thus, he was the first to use carmine in histology. In his studies, Corti used a light microscope allowing magnification of 20–500 times.

Applying this procedure, Corti was not only the first to recognize the bipolar cells of the spiral ganglion, but was able to describe in some detail the basilar membrane, the inner spiral sulcus cells, the pillar cells, as well as the foramina nervosa. Further-

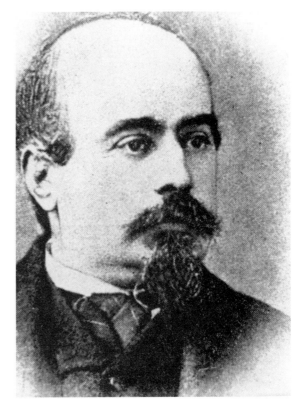

Figure 4.1 Portrait of Alfonso Corti who, in 1851 described the organ bearing his name

more, he detected the three rows of the outer hair cells and he was the first to describe the tectorial membrane and the stria vascularis in his paper *Recherches sur l'organe de l'ouie des mammiféres* in 1851. In spite of the great advances in our knowledge of the organ of Corti, much of the outline given by Corti has remained valid and the organ justly bears his name (Kley, 1986).

Remarkably little has been written about Ernst Reissner (1824–1878) who discovered the vestibular membrane in the cochlear duct. His thesis, published in 1851 under the title *De Auris Internae Formatione*, was based on a meticulous study of the fowl embryo ear at different stages of development (Nsamba, 1979).

It is interesting to note that recent intensive research on the fowl and mammalian embryo otocyst mainly in tissue culture, essentially reflects Reissner's method (Fell, 1929; Friedmann, 1956; Orr, 1965; Van de Water and Ruben, 1971; Sobkowicz, Berman and Rose, 1975; Sobkowicz, Loftus and Slapnick, 1993).

Development of the labyrinth

From the medial aspect of the otocyst (Figure 4.2), a hollow diverticulum appears which becomes elongated to form the endolymphatic canal. The otocyst itself divides into the pars superior or vestibular (utricular) pouch and the pars inferior or cochleosaccular pouch. From the vestibular pouch three semicircular canals develop: first, the superior semicircular canal, followed by the posterior and lateral or horizontal canals. The cochlear duct appears around the fifth week as a diverticulum of the cochlear pouch and the saccule develops from its upper portion. This rapid development of the inner ear takes place between the twenty-sixth and the forty-second day; a comparatively short period of time which seems to suffice to transform the simple otocyst into the complicated structures of the membranous labyrinth. After this period, the speed of growth slows down considerably. At this vital period the embryo is most susceptible to teratogenic damage.

The structural differentiation of the cochlea is completed by the third month (length of embryo 25–70 mm). The cochlear nerve fibres induce the sensory epithelium on the inner wall to proliferate, whereas the outer wall continues its longitudinal growth; as a result of this uneven growth the cochlea develops into a spiral organ of two and a half coils.

The complete cytological differentiation of the cochlea and the ossification of the otic capsule may be completed between the fourth to the sixth month (embryo length approximately 70–200 mm). It reaches completion with the formation of the three rows of outer hair cells and the single row of inner hair cells with their supporting cells. An area of resorption between the internal and external hair

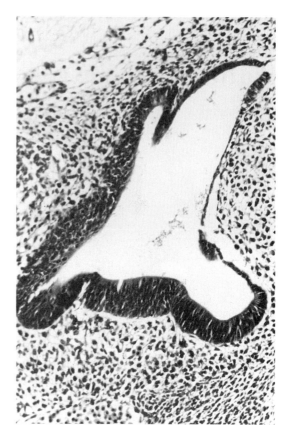

Figure 4.2 Fowl embryo otocyst – 3½ days old

cells leads to the formation of the tunnel of Corti (Figure 4.3).

Gross anatomy (Figure 4.4)

The inner ear is located in the petrous portion of the temporal bone and is protected by the toughest part of the skull, the otic capsule. The labyrinth, an essential part of the auditory organ, is a complex structure. It consists of a membranous tube lined by epithelium (membranous labyrinth) filled with endolymph and is contained within a bony tube, the osseous labyrinth, which is of corresponding complexity of shape and contains the perilymph. The membranous labyrinth is supplied by branches of the auditory nerve and its cochlear branch passes to the organ of Corti (Figure 4.4).

The cytoskeleton

The investigation of the pathology of the cochlea requires the application of a wide range of scientific methods. Histochemical and immunological studies

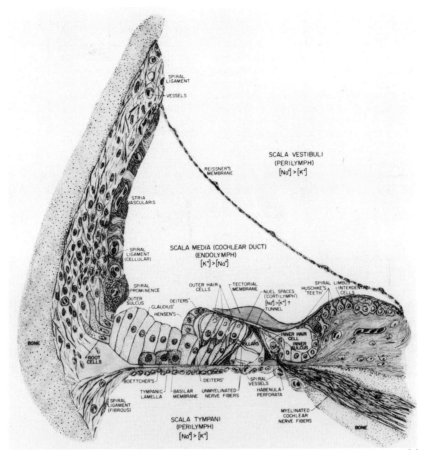

Figure 4.3 Diagram of the human organ of Corti (after Hawkins). The diagram shows the intricate structure of the organ of hearing located in the scala media or cochlear duct filled with the endolymph

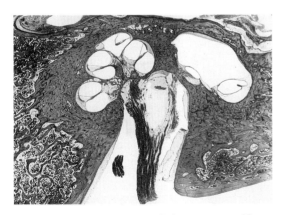

Figure 4.4 Midmodiolar section of a human temporal bone showing the labyrinth. Note the cochlea, the vestibule and the branching auditory nerve (in the internal auditory meatus)

as well as both transmission and scanning electron microscopy have provided an increasing amount of in-

formation on the morphology of the inner ear in health and disease (Friedmann, 1963; Lim and Lane, 1969; Engstrom and Ades, 1973; Hunter-Duvar, 1978).

The cytoplasm of most of the higher eukaryotic cells contains a filamentous network which forms the cytoskeleton. Its characteristic structure differs from the actins, myosins, tubulins and some of the other microtubular proteins. They are the so-called intermediate filaments (IF), proteins forming the basic elements of some of the mammalian cells in the body and in tissue culture. They measure 7–14 nm in diameter and fall between the larger microtubules of 22 nm, the myosin filaments of 15 nm and the microfilaments, including the actins, of 6 nm in diameter.

There are five classes of intermediate filaments:

1 The cytokeratins (praekeratins) with a molecular weight of 45 kd and 60 kd. They are characteristic for epithelial cells with desmosomes.
2 Desmin filaments with molecular weight of 53 kd. They occur in the striated and smooth muscle cells, in cardiac cells and in the muscle coat of vessels.
3 Glial filaments have a molecular weight of 55 kd.

They occur exclusively in astrocytes and in the Bermann-type glial cells.

4 Neurofilaments form three subgroups with molecular weights of 68 kd, 145 kd and 220 kd respectively. Present in most neurons of cervical and peripheral nerves.

5 Vimentin filaments with a molecular weight of 45 kd are characteristic for mesenchymatous cells.

The cytoskeleton of the organ of Corti was investigated by immunohistochemical methods and the neuronal structures of the inner ear and the innervation of the organ of Corti identified (Friedmann and Arnold, 1993). (Table 4.1; Figure 4.5).

Cytokeratin was expressed by all the supporting elements of the human organ of Corti, including cytokeratin 5, 8, 18 and 19. It is interesting to note

Table 4.1 Expression of intermediate filament proteins in the fetal and adult human inner ear (from Friedmann and Arnold, 1993)

Structural/cell type	Cytokeratins		Vimentin		Neurofilaments	
	Fetal	Adult	Fetal	Adult	Fetal	Adult
Inner ear ganglia						
Spiral ganglion cells	+	+	+ or −	−	+ or −	+ or −
Vestibular ganglion cells	+	+	+	−	+ or −	+ or −
Schwann cells	−	−	+	+	−	−
Organ of Corti						
IHC	+	−	+	−	−	−
OHC-1	+	−	+	−	−	−
OHC-2	+	−	+	−	−	−
OHC-3	+	−	+	−	−	−
Border cell	+	+	+	−		
Inner pillar cell	+	+	+	+	−	−
Outer pillar cell	+	+	+	+	−	−
Deiters' cell	+	(+)	+	−	−	−
Hensen's cell	+	+	−	−	−	−
Claudius' cell	+	+	−	−	−	−
Boettcher's cell	+	− ?	−	−	−	−
Vestibular organs						
Hair cells (types I and II)						
Crista	+	−	+	−	−	−
Utricle	+	−	+	−	−	−
Saccule	+	−	+	−	−	−
Non-sensory cells						
Crista	+	+	+	−	−	−
Utricle	+	+	+	−	−	−
Saccule	+	+	+	−	−	−
Epithelia involved in inner ear fluid homeostasis						
Stria vascularis						
Marginal cells	+	+	−	−	−	−
Intermediate cells	−	−	+	+	−	−
Basal cells	−	−	+	+	−	−
Reissner's membrane						
Epithelial cells	+	+	+	+	−	−
Mesenchymal cells	−	−	+	+	−	−
Dark cells	+	+	−	−	−	−
Endolymphatic duct	− or +	− or +	− or +	− or +	−	−
Endolymphatic sac	− or +	− or +	− or +	− or +	−	−
Spiral prominence cells	+	+	(+)	+	−	−
Root cells	+	+	+	+	−	−
Epithelial lining of the membranous labyrinth						
Inner sulcus cells	+	+	+	−	−	−
Outer sulcus cells	+	+	+	+	−	−
Spiral limbus cells	+	(+)?	−	−	−	−
SCC	− or +	− or +	− or +	−	−	−

IHC: inner hair cells; OHC: outer hair cells; SCC: semicircular canal

that these were expressed strongly by the inner and outer pillar cells, by the phalangeal processes and by their apical processes (reticular lamina). There was no reaction by the hair cells or by the bodies of the Deiters' cells. There exists a gradient of increasing cytokeratin expression from the cochlear base to the apex. In the stria vascularis only the marginal (epithelial) cells expressed cytokeratin and the reaction was uniform in all the coils of the cochlea (Figure 4.5).

Histopathology of the organ of Corti

The pathological changes of the different constituents of the inner ear can be assessed in familiar, general pathological terms (Table 4.2).

Changes of the sensory epithelium may be complex (Friedmann, 1974). The neuroepithelium of the organ of Corti may be totally absent, as in various congenital syndromes, or there may be partial degeneration or absence of the hair cells and supporting cells. Basophilic deposits form in the stria vascularis, the nature of which remains obscure. The tectorial membrane may be deformed and the ultrastructural changes of the sensory epithelium of the inner ear can be extensive (Figure 4.6). The cytoplasm of hair cells may show protrusions or ballooning followed by rupture of the outer cell membrane, distension of the rough endoplasmic reticulum with multiple Hensen bodies and marked reduction of the number of the ribosomes. Dense bodies and phagosomes may be present (Table 4.3).

Table 4.2 Histopathological findings in sensorineural deafness

Site	Lesion	Aetiology of deafness
Sensory epithelium	Total absence or loss	Congenital; ageing
	Partial absence or degeneration	Noise
		Drugs
	Inclusions	Chromosome abberations
Tectorial membrane	Shrinkage; retraction adhesions	Congenital; anencephaly
		Viral (rubella, measles and mumps)
Reissner's membrane	Distension	Menière's syndrome
	Adhesions	Anencephaly
	Collapse	Meningitis
	Rupture	Trisomy 22
		Otosclerosis
Stria vascularis	Atrophy	Ageing, presbyacusis
	Congestion and hyalinization	Diabetes mellitus
	PAS-positive deposits	Lange-Jervell syndrome
		Toxoplasmosis
	Basophilic concrements	Budd-Chiari syndrome
		Alport's syndrome
	Vacuolation	Ototoxic agents
	Granulations	Noise
		Viruses (rubella, measles)
Spiral limbus	Vacuolation	Cytotoxic agents
	Granulations	Viral (rubella, measles)
Otic capsule and scalae	Ossification and remodelling of bone	Meningococcal or pneumococcal meningitis
		Pendred's syndrome
		Cogan's syndrome
		Chronic otitis
		Labyrinthitis ossificans
		Systemic bone disease; Paget's disease
		Vascular obstruction
		Syphilis, congenital
		Otosclerosis
		Leukaemia
Perilymph and endolymph	Increase of protein content	Syphilis
		Viral disease
		Infective disease
		Neoplastic, e.g. schwannoma of auditory nerve
VIIIth nerve	Demyelination	Rickettsiosis
	Nodular infiltrates	Rickettsiosis

Table 4.3 Ultrastructural changes

Cytoplasm of hair cells	Protrusion-rupture of outer cell membrane (see Figure 4.6)
	Distension of rough endoplasmic reticulum
	Hyperplasia of smooth endoplasmic reticulum
	Multiple Hensen bodies
	Dense bodies + + +
	Phagosomes + + +
	Golgi apparatus – concentration of ototoxic secretory and toxic substances
Ototoxic antibiotics	
Mitochondria	Damage and rupture of cristae
	Vacuolation and vesiculation
Nucleus	Aggregation of chromatin
Ribosomes	Reduction
Nerves	Bulging and rupture – myelin inclusions, atrophy
Neurons	Lipofuscin
	Lysosomes
	Vacuolation
	Nissl substance-reduced
	Protein crystalline inclusions (Figure 4.7)
Basal lamina	Multiplication and production of long-spaced collagen (Figure 4.8)

The mitochondria are often damaged and contain ruptured cristae. Peripheral aggregations of chromatin and intranuclear viral inclusions may be present. Crystalline, laminated or striated inclusions may be seen in the hair cells (Friedmann, Cawthorne and Bird, 1965a; Slepecky, Hamernik and Henderson, 1980, 1981) (Figure 4.7).

The stria vascularis forming the lateral wall of the cochlear duct is the site of various well-defined pathological lesions associated with several syndromes and diseases: atrophy in ageing and presbyacusis (Kimura and Schuknecht, 1970 a,b; Schuknecht, 1974); congestion and hyalinization in diabetes; periodic acid-Schiff (PAS) positive deposits in the Jervell-Lange-Nielsen syndrome; calcification and adhesions in the Budd-Chiari syndrome, toxoplasmosis and Alport's syndrome; vacuolation caused by ototoxic substances and by noise and inflammatory granulations in viral diseases (rubella, measles).

Basophilic deposits in the stria vascularis were studied by Zaytoun (1983). In 42 temporal bones from 22 patients with hearing loss, atrophy of the stria was seen in 12 cases and substrial fibrosis in three; cystic structures were noted in four and the stria appeared to be normal in seven cases. In 18 cases, bilateral deposits were noted and there were deposits in two or all three coils of the cochlea; the middle coil was the most common site. The deposits presented in the marginal zone of the stria vascularis and protruded into the endolymphatic space. The

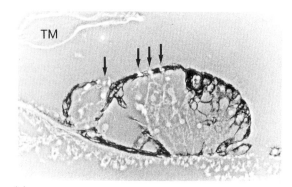

(*a*)

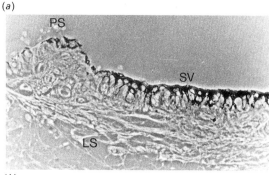

(*b*)

Figure 4.5 (*a*) Strong expression of cytokeratin in the organ of Corti (apical coil). Arrows pointing at perforations in the reticular membrane represent the negative reaction of the cuticular plates of the hair cells. Monoclonal antibody used; TPA-7. TM-Tectorial membrane. (*b*) Note that in the stria vascularis (SV) cytokeratin is only expressed by the marginal cells. PS-Spiral prominence. LS-spiral ligament. (From Friedmann and Arnold (1993) *Pathology of the Ear.*)

organ of Corti often showed mild to severe loss of the hair cells and/or total degeneration.

Microscopically, the deposits showed a striking variation in size and shape. Some were elongated or crescent-shaped, others were rounded or polygonal with a concentric lamellar pattern. Still others exhibited a fibrillar pattern. Occasionally, the deposits caused the stria vascularis to be detached from the spiral ligament. In some, the deposits showed a crystalline pattern with sharp edges and fine spicules as described in a case of long-standing profound sensorineural deafness (Nadol and Burgess, 1982) and in Jervell-Lange-Nielsen syndrome (Friedmann, Fraser and Froggatt, 1966; Friedmann, Froggatt and Fraser, 1968).

Classification of hearing loss

The classification of hearing loss has remained complicated and the simple division into conductive, sensorineural and mixed types contrasts sharply with the elaborate schemes developed by various authors.

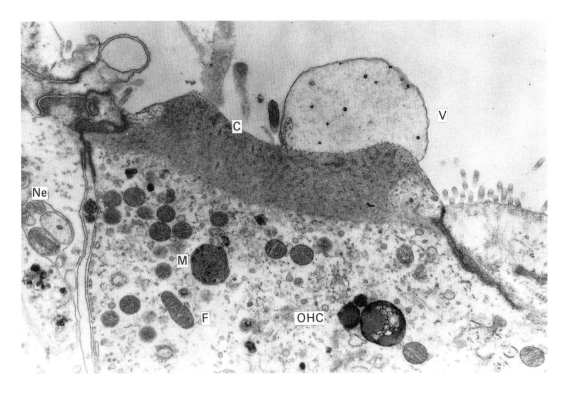

Figure 4.6 Transmission electron micrograph showing the surface of an outer hair cell (OHC) of the organ of Corti of a guinea-pig treated with neomycin. Note the large vesicular structure protruding from the softened cuticular plate (C). There are numerous dense bodies and mitochondria (M) present and there is a layer of cisternae alongside the outer cell membrane. Also desmosomes and gap junctions linking the hair cell with the neighbouring cells. Ne = nerve. F = filaments ($\times$ 21 000)

In trying to distinguish between congenital and acquired deafness, the progress made in recent years has to be considered. The isolation of the rubella virus by Weller and Neva (1962) marked a turning point in the laboratory diagnosis of this condition. This and other advances in virology have thrown some light on the causes of deafness. Furthermore, the rapid progress of genetic and chromosome studies has contributed to a better understanding of the genetic influence playing such an important role in the causation of hearing loss. It is interesting to mention that William Wilde was the first otologist to recognize that heredity played a role and might be the cause of hearing loss in man (Ruben, 1991). However, Toynbee in his book, published in 1860, does not mention Wilde and is silent about the hereditary aspect of deafness. It was Politzer who accepted heredity as a cause of deafness (Politzer, 1902). In a recent review of the history of the genetics of hearing impairment, Ruben noted the significance of animal genetics and animal research which has greatly enhanced our knowledge of the biological mechanisms controlling 'the processes of the inner ear which result in normal and abnormal function' (Ruben, 1991; Friedmann and Arnold, 1993).

Pathogenesis

Hearing loss in the newborn may be caused by failure to develop one or more parts of the auditory system or to an interruption at any stage in the process of development. It may also be the result of some factor which disturbs or causes the degeneration of the already wholly or partly developed hearing mechanism. Ormerod (1960) tabulated the pathology of congenital deafness as follows:

1 Failure to develop or interruption of development as the result of genetic factors, or toxic influence caused by certain forms of maternal illness during the first 3 months of pregnancy (aplasia)
2 Interruption of development
3 Degeneration of parts of the auditory apparatus which have already developed in some degree or have reached maturity (abiotrophy):

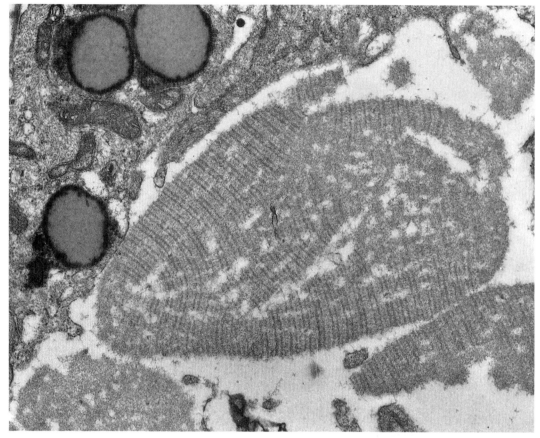

Figure 4.7 A crystalline-type inclusion of lipoid and proteinaceous material found in the hair cells under normal or disease conditions

a of the cochlear duct or scala media
b of the sensory end organs
c of the nerve elements.

The pathology of deafness may be conveniently classified according to the following scheme. No new categories are proposed, all have been selected from previous writings on the subject (Friedmann, 1974), although there may be differences of opinion about the interpretation of some of the syndromes.

1 Pathology of deafness of genetic origin
   lesions of the conductive apparatus
   lesions of the sensorineural apparatus
   aplasia
   abiotrophy (heredodegenerative lesions)
   chromosome aberrations
2 Embryopathies
   antenatal: rubella, syphilis, toxoplasmosis; other infections – viral and bacterial; hormonal
   perinatal: infections; asphyxia; kernicterus; toxic; hormonal; metabolic

postnatal: infection – viral and bacterial; neoplasms; hormonal; environmental – exposure to noise; ageing; toxic.

Aplasia

These are hereditary lesions of a degenerative nature, not apparent at birth but revealed at a later period of life, of a progressive nature and associated with deafness. Several classical types are recognized (Schuknecht, 1967a):

1 Michel type (complete failure of development of the inner ear)
2 Mondini type (Illum, 1972) (incomplete development of the bony and membranous labyrinth). (Figure 4.8)
3 Scheibe type (cochleosaccular aplasia)
4 Alexander type (membranous cochlear aplasia).

Membranous cochleosaccular aplasia as described by Scheibe (1892) is the most common pathological

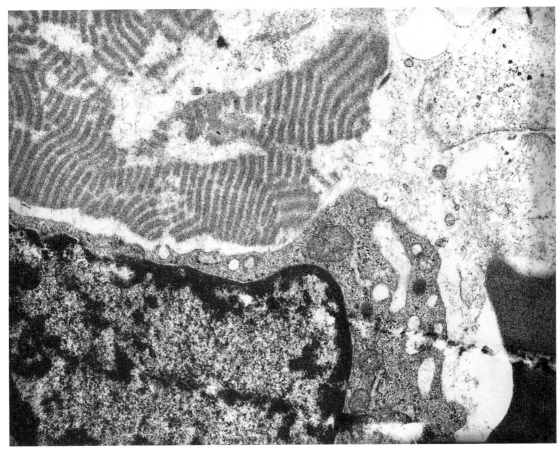

Figure 4.8 Long-spaced collagen bands (also called Luse bodies) occur in schwannomas; Menière's disease and some neoplasms

lesion in congenital sensorineural deafness of any cause.

Suehiro and Sando (1979) developed a new elaborate classification of labyrinthine anomalies which, however, has not been widely applied and may prove complicated to otologists.

Anencephaly

Anencephaly may be accompanied by major structural deformities of the labyrinth and a Mondini-type malformation of the cochlea was described in most cases (Illum, 1972; Kelemen and Etschenbacher, 1978; Friedmann, Wright and Phelps, 1980) (Figure 4.9a,b).

Heredodegeneration (abiotrophy)

These conditions are of considerable general interest. Heredodegenerative deafness occurs alone or in com-

bination with other abnormalities in which case they are known as 'syndromes'. There are about 70 phenotypically-distinct types of syndrome which may be classified as mesodermal, ectodermal and neuroectodermal, according to the combination of anomalies which are present:

1 Occurring alone: in infants or in adults
2 Associated with other abnormalities
   a essentially ectodermal, e.g. Waardenburg's syndrome; Usher's syndrome; Cogan's syndrome
   b essentially mesodermal, e.g. Alport's syndrome; Jervell-Lange-Nielsen (cardioauditory) syndrome; Pendred's syndrome; Hurler's syndrome (gargoylism); Marfan's syndrome
   c essentially neuroectodermal, e.g. von Recklinghausen's disease; Refsum's syndrome; Jamaican neuropathy.

Chromosomal aberrations are responsible for a number of severe anomalies. The presence of an extra chromosome (trisomy) may lead to anomalies associated with deafness.

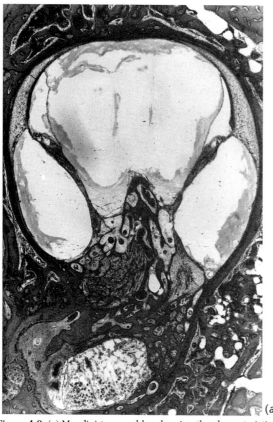

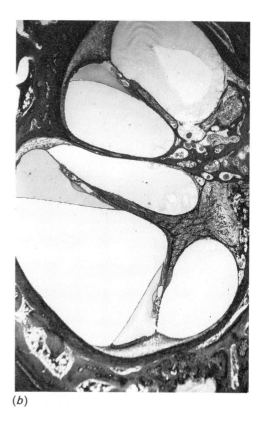

(b)

(a)

Figure 4.9 (*a*) Mondini-type cochlea showing the characteristic absence of the interscalar septum in the upper part of the cochlea with the formation of a scala communis. There is much inspissated perilymph present in the perilymphatic spaces and Reissner's membrane appears to be collapsed onto the organ of Corti. Note the presence of nerves and neurons (skull of an anencephalic fetus). (*b*) Mondini-type cochlea from another anencephalic fetus (Hallpike collection)

Neuroectodermal syndromes

Waardenburg's syndrome

In 1951, P. J. Waardenburg, a Dutch ophthalmologist, described a genetically determined (autosomal dominant) syndrome of which unilateral deafness is a feature. The partial albinism of the hair scalp has given the condition one of its names – white forelock syndrome. The commonest and most important feature is sensorineural deafness with eyelid deformity and heterochromia or deep blue eyes.

The histopathology (Figure 4.10) of the temporal bones of a child with Waardenburg's syndrome studied by the present author, showed total absence of the organ of Corti, atrophy of the stria vascularis and absence of the neurons of the spiral ganglion (Friedmann, 1974).

Since the original description, over 1200 cases of the syndrome have been reported, not only in patients of Dutch extraction but also in English, American, African, Indian, Oriental and Black persons (Hageman, 1977; Wang, Karmody and Pa-

shayan, 1981; Galich, 1985). Waardenburg's syndrome seems to consist of two genetically distinct entities which can be differentiated clinically into Waardenburg's syndrome with or without dystopia canthorum (type 1 and type 2 respectively). Congenital deafness in both ears may occur in about 25% of the patients with Waardenburg's syndrome type 1 and in about 50% of those with type 2 (Liu, Newton and Read, 1995).

Oto-retinal abiotrophies

Cockayne's syndrome

This consists of sensorineural deafness associated with retinal atrophy and dwarfism. There are additional features such as kyphoscoliosis, prognathism, cataracts, premature senile appearance and mental deficiency (Cockayne, 1936).

The post-mortem findings were described by Paddison, Moossy and Derbes (1963) who found extensive

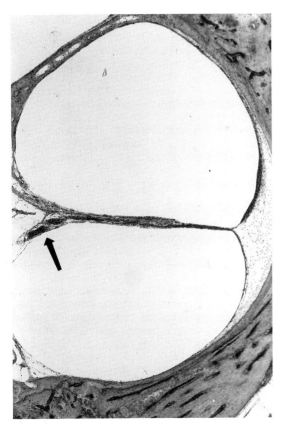

Figure 4.10 Waardenburg's syndrome. The temporal bones of a 3½-year-old girl with profound deafness, partial heterochromia of the irides and the typical eyelid deformities of Waardenburg's syndrome were obtained soon after death (Dr L. Fish). Microscopy shows total absence of the organ of Corti. There was atrophy of the stria vascularis and loss of the cochlear neurons. Reissner's membrane appeared to be missing. Note the bundle of surviving spiral nerves fibres (arrow)

corticosubcentral atrophy with secondary hydrocephalus. There was widespread loss of neurons of the cerebral cortex and fibrosis of the leptomeninges. Calcareous deposits (probably sidero-calcific) were found in numerous capillaries. There were no chromosome abnormalities.

Usher's syndrome

This consists of retinitis pigmentosa and sensorineural deafness. The histopathological findings include malformation of the cochlea, cochleosaccular dysplasia and degeneration of the spiral ganglion (Usher, 1914).

Two types of Usher's syndrome have been identified but other genotypic forms might be discovered in the future. Progressive pigmentary retinopathy is the es-

sential diagnostic feature of both types. A set of clinical criteria is recommended for the diagnosis of the two genetically distinct types I and II which have been adopted by the Usher Consortium (Smith *et al.*, 1994).

A more recent report has presented evidence that a defective myosin VIIA gene was responsible for Usher's syndrome type IB. The mutations identified might be responsible for the absence of a functional protein so that this type might be defined as a 'primary cytoskeletal protein defect' (Well *et al.*, 1995).

Cogan's syndrome

Non-syphilitic interstitial keratitis associated with vestibuloauditory dysfunction was first described by Cogan in 1945. Twenty-seven cases were reviewed by Cody and Williams (1960) and two cases were added by Bellucci, Grobeisen and Sah (1974). Fifty-three cases have been reviewed by Cheson, Bluming and Alroy (1976) (including one of their own). In 72% of the affected patients there was an underlying systemic, often vascular, process. Ten per cent had fatal or near fatal aortic valvular disease, which proved to be amenable to surgical intervention. Other systemic manifestations have included congestive heart failure, gastrointestinal haemorrhage, adenopathy, splenomegaly, hypertension, musculoskeletal involvement and eosinophilia.

Morgan, Hochman and Weider (1984) described two patients, a 26-year-old woman and a 61-year-old man. The younger woman responded promptly to corticosteroid treatment in the form of prednisolone 80 mg daily. While the condition of the older man improved, his hearing loss remained unchanged, in spite of high doses of prednisolone and cyclophosphamide.

The clinical course of Cogan's syndrome is as variable as its modes of presentation. Some patients have died within months of onset; others have lived up to 15 years after diagnosis. Most patients regain and retain good vision, but permanent severe hearing loss is the rule (Wolff *et al.*, 1965).

Histopathology

Necrotizing vasculitis may be present, affecting the heart, aorta, kidneys and gastrointestinal system. The inner ear shows degeneration of the organ of Corti and of the spiral ganglion. Endolymphatic hydrops and ossification of the labyrinth may occur.

The aetiology and pathology of the syndrome remain obscure. It has been suggested that the syndrome is a manifestation of polyarteritis nodosa (Cheson, Bluming and Alroy, 1976). The pattern of multisystem involvement can be almost identical in these entities and, in fact, sudden nerve deafness may occur in polyarteritis nodosa.

Wildervanck's syndrome

Wildervanck's syndrome consists of the triad of Klippel-Fell deformity of the cervical spine, the ocular motility syndrome and congenital hearing loss: it is also called the cervico-oculo-acoustic syndrome. West, Ghelkar and Ramsden (1989) described a patient with this syndrome with unilateral Mondini-type deformity of the inner ear identified by CT, an important diagnostic tool in the assessment of congenital hearing loss.

The ear and the kidneys – mesodermal syndromes

There exists a close relationship between the kidneys and the inner ear, which appears to be immunological, as well as biochemical and functional (Quick, Fish and Brown, 1973; Arnold, 1980). Evidence of a shared antigenicity between the two organs has been recognized: antibodies against the glomerular basement membrane act against the basement membrane of the strial capillaries. Furthermore, animal experiments have provided evidence of an antigenic similarity of the epithelial components of the kidney and of the stria vascularis (Quick, Fish and Brown, 1973; Arnold and Weidauer 1975; Arnold, Weidauer and Seelig, 1976; Weidauer, Arnold and Seelig, 1977). The ultrastructural organization of both organs shows considerable similarities of functional importance (Schuknecht, 1974; Arnold, 1980). It is, therefore, not surprising that renal diseases and their treatment may be accompanied by hearing disorders (Arnold, 1984).

Familial thin basement membrane

Nephropathy

There is a broad spectrum of hereditary nephropathies, often accompanied by sensorineural hearing loss, ranging from the relatively less severe 'familial thin basement membrane nephropathy' (FTBMN) to the more severe Alport's syndrome (Dische, Weston and Parsons, 1985; Gauthier *et al.*, 1989; Friedmann and Arnold, 1993).

Alport's syndrome

This can be defined as familial nephropathy, usually accompanied by sensorineural deafness. Alport (1927) described a 14-year-old boy suffering with nephritis and severe bilateral nerve deafness and discovered that he belonged to the fourth generation of a family with hereditary nephritis, first described by Guthrie in 1902. Alport's investigations revealed that 11 of the 24 members of the family examined had a hearing loss: five were described as being 'stone deaf'.

In 1965, Dubach and Nager reported the first case of Alport's syndrome in Switzerland. Arnold (1984) described the histopathology of four temporal bones from two patients with Alport's syndrome. Celis-Blaubach *et al.* (1974) studied the vestibular disorders in two patients with Alport's syndrome. More recently the genetics of 41 families with Alport's syndrome were studied by Flinter *et al.* (1988) and the genetics of renal tract disorders by Crawford (1988). Molecular genetics began to unravel Alport's syndrome, but early hopes were dashed (Lancet, 1991).

Clinical features

Alport's syndrome can be defined as familial nephropathy, usually accompanied by sensorineural deafness (Alport, 1927). It is inherited as an autosomal dominant trait and is more severe in men than women. The disease begins in childhood, usually with haematuria following an acute upper respiratory infection. Hearing loss is slowly progressive, and different in both ears. The discrimination score remains normal until severe hearing loss ensues (Arnold, 1984).

Development of high—tone sensorineural deafness is one of the most useful signs in a patient with haematuria, and will suggest the diagnosis of Alport's syndrome, even in the absence of renal bipopsy or a family history of renal disease (Bergstrom *et al.*, 1973). An audiogram should be obtained in any patient presenting with unexplained haematuria as subclinical hearing impairment might otherwise be missed (Flinter *et al.*, 1988).

Histophathology

The changes in the stria vascularis range from mild perivascular oedema with thickening of the capillary walls and fragmentation or splitting of the basement membrane, to complete degeneration and atrophy. The spiral prominence is less affected, although severe perivascular oedema may be present. In cases of severe deafness there is a loss of inner and outer hair cells and of ganglion cells, particularly in the basal turn. Non-specific basophilic deposits may occur (Gregg and Becker, 1963; Crawford and Toghill, 1968; Bergstrom and Thompson, 1983; Nadol and Arnold, 1987).

However, according to Fujita and Hayden (1969) consistent inner ear pathology is conspicuous by the absence of any characteristic histological findings. A normal organ of Corti with a normal spiral ganglion and acoustic nerve was found in some cases (Wood and Knight, 1966). It has been suggested that many of the degenerative changes noted in the hair cells of the organ of Corti could be attributed to autolysis (Miller *et al.*, 1970).

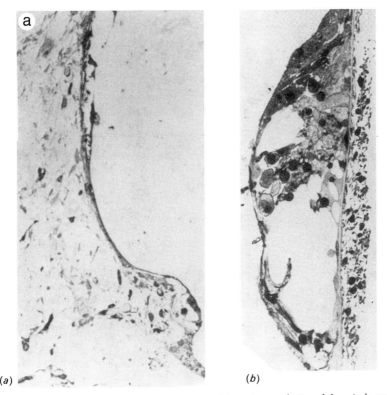

Figure 4.11 (*a*) Alport's syndrome. There is complete degeneration of the stria vascularis and the spiral prominence was oedematous in every coil of the cochlea. (*b*) Alport's syndrome. Showing the degenerated organ of Corti. (By courtesy of Professor W. Arnold)

Arnold (1984) studied four temporal bones from two patients with Alport's styndrome, diagnosed by their family history and electron microscopically, by fine needle bipopsy of the kidney. There was marked degeneration of the stria vascularis (Figure 4.11). The hair cells and the cells of the spiral ganglion were degenerated where the stria vascularis was atrophied (Figure 4.10). Electron microscopic studies of the ear revealed a multilayered basement membrane of the vas spirale, consistent with the abnormalities found in the glomerular basement membrane and lens capsule. Characteristic ultrastructural changes of the glomerular basal lamina have been described in hereditary nephritis showing an extensive 'basket-weave' pattern, as confirmed by Yoshikawa, Cameron and White (1981).

The renal changes combine various features of chronic glomerulonephritis, pyelonephritis and interstitial nephritis. Lipid-laden foam cells are present in the tissue forming long rows and clusters in the renal cortex. This is considered a characteristic feature of hereditary nephritis (Krickstein, Gloor and Balogh, 1966).

Concretions in the basement membrane in Bowman's capsule of the renal glomeruli and in the proximal convoluted tubules of the kidney were described by Magori *et al.* (1983). Crystalline deposits in the glomerular basement membrane were noted in patients with renal failure (Sanfillippo *et al.*, 1981).

Pathogenesis

The pathogenesis of the sensorineural hearing loss is not understood. It is not clear whether it has resulted from a special type of glomerulonephritis as suggested by Arnold (1984) or whether this congenital disorder was based on a primary degeneration of the inner ear.

There can be no doubt that the syndrome is of genetic origin (Arnold, 1980; Hasstedt, Atkin and San Juan, 1986; Crawfurd, 1988; Barker *et al.*, 1990). The sensorineural hearing loss may be a genetically determined autoimmune lesion triggered by the diseased kidneys. Flinter *et al.* (1988) described 41 families with the classical Alport's syndrome, all of whose pedigrees were compatible with an X-linked inheritance. According to these authors, Alport's syndrome includes two different diseases: an X-linked hereditary nephritis with sensorineural deafness and an autosomal dominant hereditary nephritis without deafness (Flinter *et al.*, 1988).

Since deafness has been reversed by renal transplantation, the mechanism causing hearing loss might be considered secondary to renal disease. McDonald, Anderson and Ott (1978) described eight patients with Alport's syndrome who had undergone successful renal transplantation. One of these patients showed substantial hearing improvement, while the hearing of the others became stabilized.

Oda *et al.* (1974) reported that 43 of 290 renal transplant patients suffered some hearing loss, directly attributable to the treatment of the kidney disease. Bergstrom *et al.* (1980; Bergstrom and Thompson, 1983) found that 40% of all patients on long-term dialysis and 47% of the children studied had lost their hearing. Microscopy of the examined temporal bones showed the stria vascularis to contain heavy basophilic deposits but there was no correlation between the degree of the hearing loss and the presence of the strial deposits. Moreover, many patients who have undergone long-term dialysis and/or have received renal transplants have retained their normal hearing.

Potter's syndrome

First described in 1946 (Potter, 1946) the syndrome is characterized by complete renal agenesis, pulmonary hypoplasia and a peculiar facial expression. It affects approximately one in 3000 babies.

Saito *et al.* (1982) described the histopathological findings in a newborn infant with Potter's syndrome. The principal feature was the Mondini-type cochlea. There were also extensive deformities of the external and of the middle ear with absence of the ossicles, atresia of the oval window and an abnormal course of the facial nerve. In addition, there was renal aplasia and pulmonary hypoplasia.

Marfan's syndrome

Marfan's syndrome (Marfan, 1896) is caused by a generalized defect of the connective tissue, affecting collagen and bone formation almost equally. It is usually hereditary in origin and it is characterized by multiple abnormalities, in particular of the skeleton (arachnodactyly), of the eyes (ectopia lentis); the external ears lacking in cartilaginous support show hypertrophy of the helix and occasionally of the stapes. The cardiovascular system is frequently involved (aneurysms).

The syndrome is usually recognized by the orthopaedic surgeon and the otologist may only rarely be confronted by a deaf child with deformities of the external ears and other signs of Marfan's syndrome (McKusick, 1972). The hearing loss can be of conductive type (Everberg, 1959), or sensorineural in character (Schilling, 1936).

Kelemen (1966) studied the histopathological findings in the right temporal bone of an 11-month-old girl with arachnodactyly and other signs of Marfan's syndrome. There was no deformity of the external ear. In the inner ear an abnormal bony lip caused narrowing of the vestibular aqueduct.

Jervell–Lange-Nielsen syndrome

The Jervell–Lange-Nielsen, or cardioauditory syndrome, consists of congenital deafness with an abnormal electrocardiogram and fainting attacks, frequently causing the sudden death of a child so affected. This rare syndrome was first described in 1957, by Jervell and Lange-Nielsen in four of six siblings of a Norwegian family (Jervell, Thingstad and Thor-Osten, 1966). The fainting attacks had originated in childhood and three of the children had died at the ages of 4, 5 and 9 years respectively. The deaf children showed striking abnormalities of the electrocardiogram, previously undescribed, and characterized mainly by a gross prolongation of the Q–T interval. Levine and Woodworth (1958) during the

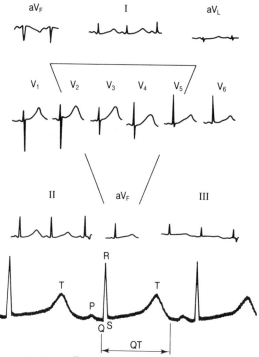

Figure 4.12 Jervell–Lange-Nielsen syndrome. The electrocardiogram shows the characteristic prolongation of the Q–T interval

screening of several thousand deaf persons, described the syndrome in a boy of Finnish ancestry who died suddenly at the age of 13. Nine further cases in Britain and Ireland were ascertained (Friedmann, Fraser and Frogatt, 1966; Friedmann, Frogatt and Fraser, 1968). The attacks are considered to be syncopal as a result of cardiac insufficiency secondary to cardiac arrest or some transient arrhythmia and the syndrome is inherited in an autosomal recessive manner (Figure 4.12).

Histopathology

The most constant finding is a widespread degeneration of the sensory end organs of the cochlea and the vestibular apparatus; Reissner's membrane is collapsed and adheres to the stria vascularis, to the tectorial membrane and/or the remnants of the organ of Corti. The stria vascularis contains unusual spherical inclusions of some eosinophilic hyaline matter in every coil which seem to be most abundant in the apical coil. The deposits filling distended vessels protrude into the cochlear duct. The ragged surface of the stria vascularis appears to have been ruptured by the underlying fibrillar or crystalline material forming the deposit or inclusion. The deposited material is PAS-positive; this suggests that it contains mucopolysaccharides or allied substances (Figures 4.13, 4.14, 4.15a,b). Special investigation of the conducting system of the heart revealed considerable narrowing of the sinuatrial artery with intimal hyperplasia. The gradual narrowing of this artery and its intraneural

branches may result in arrhythmia; should this become uncontrollable, death may ensue during a fainting attack.

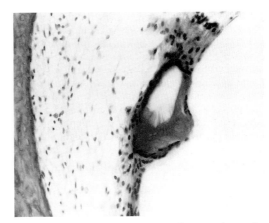

Figure 4.14 As Figure 4.13. The protruding vessel is partly filled by the PAS-positive material displaying a delicate border of crystalline needles

Pendred's syndrome

Pendred's syndrome usually consists of bilateral profound childhood deafness and the development in childhood of diffuse or nodular colloid goitre. The mental and physical development of the child is otherwise normal.

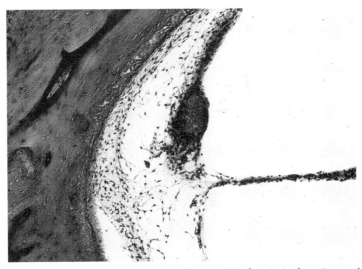

Figure 4.13 Jervell–Lange-Nielsen syndrome. The characteristic PAS-positive deposits in the stria vascularis protrude into the scala media; probably within a distended vessel. The patient was a 12-year old girl who suffered with the cardioauditory syndrome of Jervell–Lange-Nielsen

Histopathology of the ear shows malformed cochlear structures and degenerative changes in the inner ear. Hvidberg-Hansen and Jorgensen (1968) described the temporal bone findings from a 60-year-old man who had been born deaf and from about the age of 25 had developed a goitre which was first removed at the age of 49. The histological diagnosis was of a colloid nodular goitre. At the age of 60, the recurrent goitre had to be removed after unsuccessful thyroid hormone replacement therapy.

The bilateral developmental arrest of the labyrinth was of the Mondini type. Apart from this malformation, however, there were also signs of atrophy of the organ of Corti and of the tectorial membrane, endolymphatic hydrops, connective tissue formation in the saccule and utricle, and an increased amount of periotic connective tissue with endosteal ossification of the cochlea.

A recent study by Johnsen, Jorgensen and Johnsen (1986) of five temporal bones from four patients with Pendred's syndrome has confirmed an earlier finding that the malformed cochlea in Pendred's syndrome resembles that of the Mondini-type (Illum, 1972; Illum *et al.*, 1972).

Mucopolysaccharidoses

These form a group of lysosomal storage diseases caused by inherited deficiency of an enzyme capable of degrading glycosaminoglycans (Table 4.4). Hurler's disease (mucopolysaccharidosis (MPS I)) is an autosomal recessively inherited lysosomal storage disease caused by α-L-iduronidase deficiency. Therefore, in Hurler's disease, glycosaminoglycans (mucopolysaccharides) accumulate in the tissues and are excreted in the urine. Hurler's disease is distinct from the X-linked recessively inherited Hurler's disease (MPS II), the severe variants of which superficially resemble the former clinically.

Deafness is a well-recognized component of the clinical phenotype in both Hurler's and Hunter's diseases (Hurler, 1919; Kittel, 1963). Although both these diseases are invariably fatal, deafness often makes an appreciable contribution to the overall morbidity in the earlier stages of their evolution. Hearing loss is also an important practical problem in the clinically milder syndromes associated with α-L-iduronidase deficiency, Scheie disease (MPS IS) and Hurler Scheie disease (MPS IH/S), and in the mild variants of Hunter's disease. Briedenkamp *et al.* (1992) in a comprehensive review of 45 children with mucopolysaccharidoses have determined the frequency of complications related to the head and neck. Recurrent respiratory infections occurred in 3% and chronic recurrent middle ear infections with effusions occurred in 73% of the patients. The significance of these complications lies in the fact that their continuing care is often 'the primary management issue of these patients' (Briedenkamp *et al.*, 1992). All cases of otitis media but one responded to antibiotic treatment and dry ear precautions. One patient required mastoidectomy and there was a great deal of granulation tissue present filling the middle ear. Histological examination of this tissue showed the typical foamy histiocytes with deposits of intracellular mucopolysaccharides as described in our cases of Hurler's disease (Friedmann *et al.*, 1985). Sensorineural hearing loss was observed in four patients.

Histopathology

Characteristic vacuolated Hurler or gargoyle cells were noted disrupting the fascicles of the vestibulo-cochlear nerve within the temporal bone in two cases of Hurler's disease (Schachern, Shea and Paparella, 1984; Friedmann *et al.*, 1985), the perivascular spaces of the mastoid process contained many vacuolated cells, and large areas of the mastoid process were replaced by accumulated Hurler cells (Figure 4.16). The neuroradiological features in these cases were described by Watts *et al.* (1981) and post-mortem biochemical and general pathological studies were reported by Crow *et al.* (1983).

Deafness associated with chromosomal aberrations

The presence of an extra chromosome (trisomy) may lead to anomalies associated with deafness (Beighton, 1990).

Table 4.4 The mucopolysaccharidoses

Eponym	Organs mainly affected
Hurler	Central nervous system
	Skeleton
	Viscera
Scheie	Skeleton (mild relative to Hurler)
	Viscera (mild relative to Hurler)
Hurler/Scheie	Phenotype intermediate
	between Hurler and Scheie
Hunter	Central nervous system
	Skeleton
	Viscera
Sanfilippo-A	Central nervous system
Sanfilippo-B	Central nervous system
Sanfilippo-C	Central nervous system
Sanfilippo-D	Central nervous system
Morquio A	Skeleton
Morquio B	Skeleton
Maroteaux-Lamy	Skeleton
Sly	Central nervous system

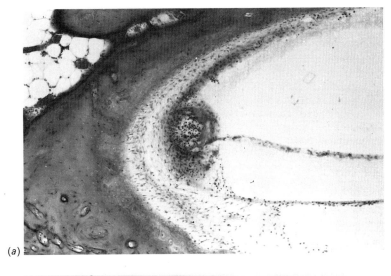

(a)

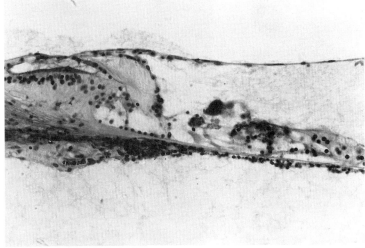

(b)

Figure 4.15 (a) Jervell–Lange-Nielsen syndrome. From the collection of the Temporal Bone Laboratory of the Institute of Laryngology and Otology: no. 1537. In some contrast with the previous case the distended (aneurysmatic) vessel protruding from the stria vascularis contains large numbers of mononuclear cells. Note the sagging Reissner's membrane. (b) This shows the degenerated organ of Corti. Note globular deposits of PAS-positive material attached to the remnants of outer hair cells. The dislodged tectorial membrane is adherent to the sagging Reissner's membrane

Trisomy 13–15 or D

Patau *et al.*, in 1960, described multiple anomalies associated with the presence of an additional chromosome in trisomy 13–15. The principal features include deafness, anophthalmia, absence of the olfactory bulb and tracts, cleft palate, hare-lip, low-set ears, polydactyly and cardiac disorders.

Cochlear changes may include absence of apical and middle coils, missing hook portion, shortened and underdeveloped cochlea. The organ of Corti may be degenerated and the tectorial membrane rolled up. A Mondini-type scala communis may be present between the middle and basal coils (Kos, Schuknecht and Singer, 1966; Kahn and Adour, 1978). However normal conditions were noted by Kelemen, Hooft and Kluyskens (1968) in the temporal bone from a patient with trisomy 13–15.

Kos, Schuknecht and Singer (1966) described multiple cochlear lesions in two cases of trisomy 13–15. The organ of Corti was replaced by fibrous tissue in the basal coil. Reissner's membrane was absent and the stria vascularis was atrophic. Collapse of Reissner's membrane was noted in other parts of the

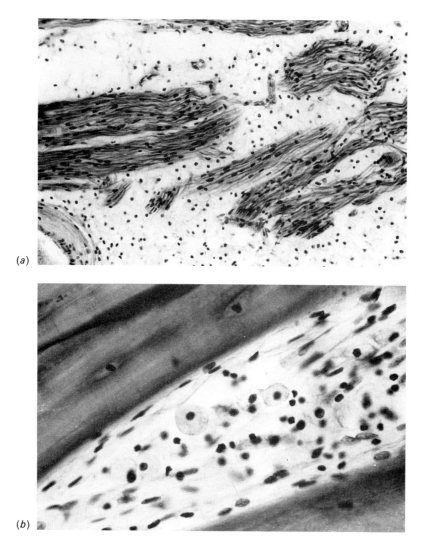

Figure 4.16 (*a*) Hurler's disease. The cochleovestibular nerve is infiltrated by clear Hurler cells splitting the nerve tissue into short fragments. (*b*) Note several large clear Hurler cells among the mainly mononuclear cells in and around a small vessel in the bone of the mastoid process. The patient was a 6-year old girl with Hurler's disease who had also suffered from otitis media with effusion or 'glue ear'

cochlea covering the remnants of the organ of Corti and of the atrophic stria vascularis. Other cases were studied by Sando *et al.* (Sando and Wood, 1971; Sando *et al.*, 1975). In addition to cochlear malformations, there were multiple middle ear anomalies and persistence of the stapedial artery.

Trisomy 17–18 or E (Edward's syndrome)

Trisomy of chromosomes 17–18 was described by Edwards *et al.* (1960). Further cases were reported by Patau *et al.* (1961) and Crawfurd in 1961. Kos,

Schuknecht and Singer (1966) described the histopathological findings of the ears in a case of trisomy 18. There were grossly malformed ossicles and the modiolus of the cochlea was underdeveloped (right ear). The organ of Corti and the maculae were normal. The left cochlea appeared to be flattened and displayed a Mondini-type scala communis. Sando and Wood (1971) noted middle ear anomalies associated with malformations of the external and of the inner ear.

Trisomy 21–22 or G (Down's syndrome)

This was first described by Down in 1866. Subsequently, in 1959, Lejeune, Gauthier and Torpin discovered trisomy for the chromosome 21 as the cause of Down's syndrome. It might result from a trisomy interchange or translocation (Polani *et al.*, 1965). About 90% of males afflicted with trisomy 21 have 47 instead of the normal 46 chromosomes at birth.

The temporal bone findings are less well documented (Friedmann and Arnold, 1993). Igarashi *et al.* (1977) described a 'slightly shortened' cochlea in four pairs of temporal bones from patients with this syndrome. This was confirmed by Bilgen *et al.* (1996).

Viral diseases

The ear is potentially open to infection by any of the respiratory viruses and it is a widely accepted assumption that bacterial otitis is often preceded by viral otitis. Although some respiratory viruses have on occasions been isolated from the middle ear, there is no evidence that any of them could invade the middle ear and cause a pure viral otitis media.

Various viruses can cause fetal damage and congenital malformations affecting the ear, and the role of certain specific viruses is well established; for example rubella, cytomegalovirus (Davis, 1979), herpes simplex, varicella-zoster, influenza, mumps and measles (Table 4.5).

Table 4.5 Causes of postnatal deafness

Infections
  May cause loss of hearing and subsequent deafness:
bacterial purulent labyrinthitis in otitis media
Cerebrospinal meningitis
  Meningococcal or pneumococcal:
  osification of the cochlea
Typhoid
  Toxic effect
TB meningitis
  Endolymphatic hydrops
Rickettsial infection
Treponemal infection
  Ossification of cochlea

Parasitic
  Malaria
  Toxoplasmosis

Virus
  Mumps
  Cytomegalovirus and rubella
  Varicella zoster virus
  Hepatitis virus/Australia antigen
  Epstein-Barr virus (infectious mononucleosis or glandular fever)

The ear in maternal rubella

The special vulnerability of the eye, ear and heart of the developing fetus in maternal rubella during the first trimester of pregnancy is well recognized and, although the period of greatest danger to the fetus from rubella is in the first trimester, infection in the second and third trimesters can cause deafness.

Histopathology

By contrast with the rapid progress of the epidemiology and virology new knowledge of the histopathology of rubella deafness has remained fragmentary, because of the relatively small number of temporal bone specimens available (Friedmann, and Wright, 1966; Lindsay, 1973b). Microscopy of the cochlea showed partial collapse of Reissner's membrane with adherence of the membrane to the stria vascularis and organ of Corti. Small granulomas may be present between the stria vascularis and Reissner's membrane (Figure 4.17). The tectorial membrane was found to be rolled up lying in the internal sulcus. Collapse of the saccule was observed, and the membrane was found to be collapsed and adherent to the macula sacculi suggestive of a recent acute inflammatory process. There were only minor changes in the organ of Corti. The hair cells were plentiful, as were the pillar cells, and appeared to be normal. There were some areas of cystic dilatation at the junction of Reissner's membrane and the spiral ligament.

The granulomatous lesions described by several authors appear to have occurred when the organ of Corti had reached morphological maturation (Friedmann and Wright, 1966; Bordley and Hardy, 1969; Brookhauser and Bordley, 1973; Lindsay, 1973a). This could be interpreted as consistent with the degeneration of the preformed neuroepithelial structures, reflecting continued virus cell interaction, as suggested by other stigmata of the rubella syndrome. Unusually large granulomas have been noted in the stria vascularis of the cochlea from an 8-year-old deaf boy (Figures 4.17, 4.18 and 4.19). His mother had suffered from an unrecognized, viral infection, probably rubella in the fourth month of her pregnancy. The boy suffered from deafness and renal disease. At post mortem (Dr A. C. Cameron, consultant pathologist, The Children's Hospital, Birmingham), various features of the rubella syndrome were identified: there was absence of the falx cerebri and the ductus arteriosus was patent. The serum antibody titre for rubella was higher than 1:512.

Prenatal rubella is recognized as a cause of congenital deafness, but its importance may not be fully appreciated (Brookhauser and Bordley, 1973). One reason is that a woman may have a silent rubella infection during pregnancy and pass the virus to the fetus without any clinical evidence of her own infection (Alford, Neva and Weller, 1964; Menser, Dods and Harley, 1967). Of 84 pregnant women infected with the rubella virus, but without clinical disease, 10 gave birth to children from whom the virus was isolated (Bordley *et al.*, 1968).

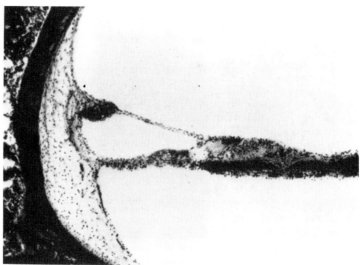

Figure 4.17 Rubella. The stria vascularis is infiltrated by inflammatory cells forming small non-specific granulomas in other cochlear coils. Reissner's membrane is attached to the inflamed stria vascularis and the organ of Corti had been damaged although the pillar cells are still recognizable as are some of the outer hair cells. The patient was a 5-day-old baby whose mother had rubella in the fifth week of pregnancy

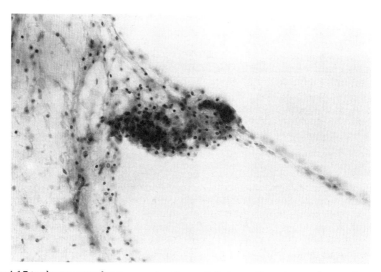

Figure 4.18 As Figure 4.17 to show a granuloma occupying the angle between the stria vascularis and Reissner's membrane. There is marked degeneration of the organ of Corti and there is widespread cellular infiltration

A study of the effect of rubella on the frequency of congenital deafness for 5 years after an epidemic in 1960, in an island population, revealed that of 87 congenitally deaf children born the year after the epidemic, all but one had suffered deafness as the only demonstrable congenital abnormality. Only 20 gave a history of first trimester rubella, so by the usual classification the remaining 67 cases would be labelled as idiopathic, all known causes having been ruled out. However, serological tests for rubella anti-

bodies on 30 of the 'idiopathic' deaf children were positive in 74% compared with 30% in a control group born within the same year (Karmody, 1968).

In the investigation of congenital deafness in a child, a test for rubella antibodies should be performed. With increasing age a positive result becomes less significant, but the absence of rubella antibodies would exclude the virus as a cause and focus attention on other factors.

The affinity of certain viruses, in particular, the

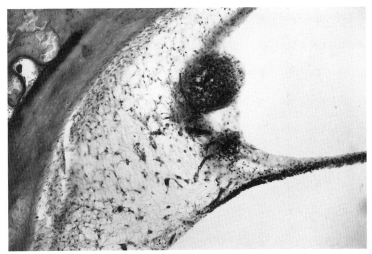

Figure 4.19 Rubella. From the collection of the Temporal Bone Laboratory of the Institute of Laryngology and Otology. no. M1515. There is a large and a smaller non-specific granuloma in the inflamed stria vascularis. Note the congested vessels and the oedematous spiral ligament

paramyxoviruses and tocoviruses, for the cochleo-vestibular system has been recognized. There is mounting evidence of a viral infection in otosclerosis. The application of immunohistochemical methods has revealed the expression of antigens of rubella, mumps and measles in the otosclerotic footplates examined (Arnold and Friedmann, 1988). The viral antigens are more strongly expressed by the cells of the perivascular tissue in otospongiosis and by various inflammatory cells and also osteoclasts in the resorption lacunae of otosclerosis (Friedmann and Arnold, 1993).

Herpes zoster oticus

The classical syndrome, described by Ramsay Hunt in 1907, is uncommon, and it is a more complicated disease than the original conception of 'geniculate ganglionitis' would indicate. Multiple cranial nerves may be affected, but the facial nerve and its ganglion is perhaps the most commonly involved.

The case described by Blackley, Friedmann and Wright (1967) involved the VIIth and VIIIth cranial nerves. The patient, a 69-year-old woman who complained of sudden deafness and right facial palsy, died of carbon monoxide poisoning some 214 days from the onset of herpes zoster of the ear.

Histopathology

The most striking feature of the histopathology was the presence 7 months after the herpetic eruption, of intense perivascular, perineural and intraneural round cell aggregations in the facial nerve, the auditory nerve, the cochlea (Figure 4.19) and in the mastoid process. The organ of Corti was damaged

and, with the atrophic stria vascularis, was covered by the collapsed Reissner's membrane.

A notable feature was a capillary in the midmodiolar angle of the basal coil packed with red blood corpuscles and surrounded by a dense lymphocytic infiltrate, shown in detail in Figure 4.20. Sections of the temporal bone of the clinically affected side contained extensive lymphocytic or round cell infiltration of the nerve throughout its length and also of the auditory nerve. There was considerable perivascular 'cuffing' by lymphocytes in the modiolus, in the perineural tissue of the facial nerve, the chorda tympani and the skin of the external auditory meatus. The vestibular, spiral and geniculate ganglia contained numerous apparently normal neurons, although there was scattered lymphocytic infiltration of the surrounding nerve tissue.

These findings were in complete accordance with the main histopathological findings of the four cases previously described: that is profuse and widespread lymphocytic infiltration in the facial nerve which is in striking contrast to the microscopical findings in Bell's palsy (Friedmann, 1974).

Acyclovir, a virostatic drug, has been given intravenously to a patient with herpes zoster resulting in restored facial motion and rapid resolution of hearing loss and dizziness at the end of the 7-day regimen (Dickins, Smith and Graham, 1988).

Mumps

Mumps appears to be the virus infection most commonly associated with sudden deafness. It may be a more frequent cause of deafness since mumps infec-

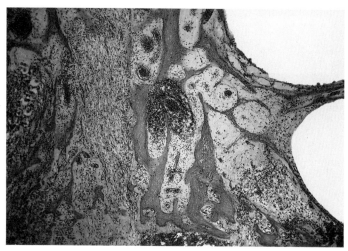

Figure 4.20 (*a*) Herpes zoster. The midmodiolar area of the cochlea showing dense diffuse and perivascular infiltration. Note perivascular 'cuffing' of several vessels and the loss of neurons

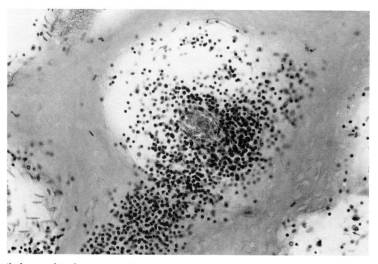

Figure 4.20 (*b*) Detail of a vessel in the otic capsule enveloped by a dense aggregation of mononuclear cells and lymphocytes

tion without parotitis is not uncommon and can remain undiagnosed.

Unilateral deafness as a complication of vaccination against mumps, measles and rubella has been reported by Nabe-Nielsen and Walter (1988).

Measles

Endolymphatic labyrinthitis caused by infections with measles virus is well recognized. The virus may reach the endolymphatic system from the blood stream and cause destruction of the neuroepithelium.

Lindsay and Hemenway (1954) described the histopathological findings in the temporal bones of a 7-month-old deaf child, following measles infection (Figure 4.21). Giant cells were present in the endolymph, and the tectorial membrane was rolled up (Figure 4.22). Nager (1907) described the pathology in a 3-year-old patient, and Beal, Davey and Lindsay (1967) in an infant of 16 months. On the whole, our knowledge of pathological details is scanty (Bordley and Kapur, 1977).

Experimental evidence suggests a specific trophism for structures of the inner ear by viral infections (Spector, 1976). This hypothesis has been based on

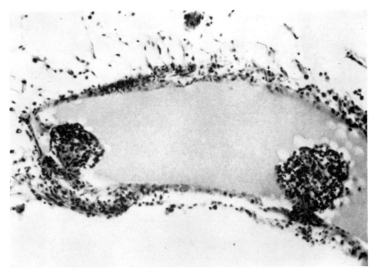

Figure 4.21 (*a*) Granulomatous proliferation in the membranous labyrinth in measles. (By courtesy of the late Dr J. R. Lindsay, University of Chicago)

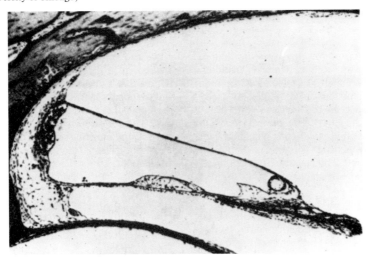

Figure 4.21 (*b*) The cochlea of a 7-month-old deaf baby after measles

the relevant studies of Davis (1981). Davis inoculated the inner ear of hamsters with hampster-adapted strains of influenza, mumps and rubella viruses which resulted in characteristic histopathological features: mumps virus affecting the organ of Corti, stria vascularis and Reissner's membrane; the influenza virus spreading in the perilymphatic spaces. The rubella virus appeared to infect the crista and semicircular canals in contrast to the findings in the human cochlea (Friedmann and Arnold, 1993).

Viral encephalopathy

Viral labyrinthitis may be associated with viral encephalitis. The temporal bones of three children with viral encephalopathy studied by Karmody (1983) included a

4½-year-old child who died of chicken pox and a 12-month-old girl with congenital encephalopathy. Herpes zoster infection was suspected in the latter but the characteristic perivascular cellular infiltrations appeared to be lacking. The third case, a 2-year-old boy, is of additional interest because he died of Reye's syndrome complicated by an upper respiratory tract infection. The inner ear was extensively damaged. The organ of Corti was degenerated and there were granulations in the degenerated stria vascularis and the spiral ligament appeared to be separated from the otic capsule.

Reye's syndrome

This syndrome was described by Reye, Morgan and Baral (1963) as encephalopathy with fatty degen-

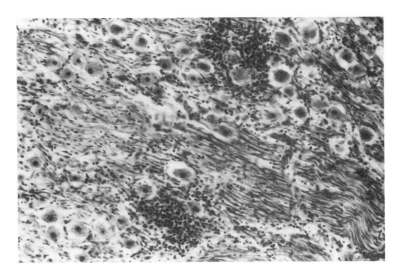

Figure 4.22 Scrub typhus fever. Auditory nerve showing two typhus nodules within the fibres of the vestibular branch surrounded by the ganglion cells of Scarpa's ganglion. Note the mononuclear cells forming the nodules. × 150. The clinical diagnosis of epidemic typhus has been revised as 'scrub typhus' caused by *R. tsutsugamushi*. I am indebted to Dr Frank W. Kiel for his expert advice

eration of the viscera, mainly the liver and kidney, in children 1–12 years of age. There is usually a preceding viral illness such as chicken pox or influenza B. The syndrome has been related to aspirin administration (Rarey *et al.*, 1983, 1984; Rarey, Davis and Deshmukh, 1984). The clinical symptoms may include progressive, frequently haemorrhagic vomiting, convulsions and coma. Some patients present with a characteristic posture. The aetiology is obscure but some patients may recover (Deshmukh, Massab and Mason, 1982).

Hinojosa and Lindsay (1977) described the histopathology of the temporal bone from a 9-year-old girl with Reye's syndrome who died in a coma 10 days after admission to hospital. The fundus of the internal auditory meatus showed vascular haemorrhagic congestion of the nerves. All structures within the endolymphatic system showed advanced degeneration, with the exception of the tectorial membrane and cupulae. There was vascular congestion in one ear with the formation of thrombi and free haemorrhage within the modiolus and the spiral ganglion. The type and extent of the degeneration in the inner ears in this case resembled those noted in a series of experiments on the guinea-pig in which the blood supply was surgically interrupted (Perlman and Kimura, 1957; Lindsay, 1973b), rather than the fatty change predominating in Reye's syndrome.

Refsum's disease – hereditary neuropathy

The syndrome first described by Refsum in 1946 is an inherited autosomal recessive disorder belonging to a group of diffuse peripheral polyneuropathies caused by a defect in myelin metabolism (Refsum, 1946, 1981; Rake and Saunders, 1966; Campbell and Williams, 1967). The syndrome consists of peripheral neuropathy, cerebellar ataxia, retinitis pigmentosa, cardiac abnormalities, deafness. Cataracts, ichthyosis and anosmia are other characteristic features. A raised plasma phytanic acid level is diagnostic (Alexander, 1966). Early diagnosis is essential (Goldman *et al.*, 1985), because the plasma phytanic acid level can be lowered by long-term adherence to special diets (Gibberd *et al.*, 1985; Britton and Gibberd, 1988; Dickson *et al.*, 1989).

Histopathology

There is diffuse thickening of the peripheral nerves in the form of concentric lamellae formed by hyperplastic connective tissue around individual axons (onionskin formation). Hallpike described the histopathology of the inner ear in a patient with Refsum's disease (Hallpike, 1967). His findings resembled the hereditary cochleosaccular degeneration as described by Scheibe (1891). A similar case was described by Rake and Saunders (1966) showing the facial nerve and geniculate ganglion thickened by collagen. There was an excess of phytanic acid in both serum and the sural nerve which showed complete loss of myelin sheaths but not of the axons. The kidneys may be affected (Pabico *et al.*, 1981).

Hypokalaemia was noted in a 24-year-old woman with acute Refsum's disease (Dick *et al.*, 1993). There was retinitis pigmentosa and sensorineural hearing loss in this patient and the phytanic acid level was high. The polyneuropathy of this patient had responded to treatment but the hearing loss persisted.

Rickettsial infection

Epidemic typhus fever caused by *Rickettsia prowazekii* and 'scrub typhus' caused by *Rickettsia tsutsugamushi* has been a curse of armies (Stephenson, 1944) and civilians at war or living in insanitary or overcrowded conditions such as in prisons, prisoner of war camps and, in particular, in concentration camps (Richet, 1945; Davis, 1947; Friedmann, Frolich and Wright, 1993). Vaccination and insecticidal measures, such as spraying with DDT, have reduced the incidence of typhus fever but there were many reports of outbreaks of typhus during World War II (1939–1945) by medical officers serving with both the Allied and the German armies (Friedmann, Frolich and Wright, 1993).

Hearing loss is a frequent and comparatively early complication of the disease as well documented by Seiferth (1944), a German ENT-specialist. Daggett (1946), in a review of the cause of hearing loss in British servicemen, referred to hearing loss among soldiers who suffered from scrub typhus during the Burma campaign.

Friedmann, Frolich and Wright (1993) have described the microscopical findings in the inner ear from five British servicemen who died of scrub typhus during the South Asia campaign in 1944 and who suffered hearing loss described as deafness by the attending RAMC Officer. The latter excised the temporal bones which reached Dr Hallpike's Ferens Laboratory in perfect condition in 1945. The sections (by S. Bishop), now in the Hallpike collection at the Institute of Laryngology and Otology, offered a unique opportunity, augmenting the experience of the present author in the histopathological lesions caused by *Rickettsia*, which had been obtained during a fatal outbreak of typhus among civilian prisoners in a town in Slovakia in 1945.

Histopathology

Microscopy of the inner ear revealed the characteristic 'typhus nodules' first described by Fraenkel in 1921 after the Great War (1914–1918). The VIIIth nerve, in particular its vestibular branch, and Scarpa's ganglion contained nodular aggregations of mononuclear cells (Figure 4.22) scattered widely in the cochlea. There were similar aggregations of mononuclear cells attached to the organ of Corti and in the macula of the saccule and elsewhere. There was extensive interstitial neuritis of the VIIIth nerve and of the facial nerve and patchy demyelination within the nerves (Figures 4.23 and 4.24). Thus the cause of hearing loss and of the vestibular symptoms lies in the inner ear and VIIIth nerve infected by the organism (*Rickettsia prowazekii*).

Syphilis

Invasion of the central nervous system by *Treponema pallidum* occurs during the early stages of infection.

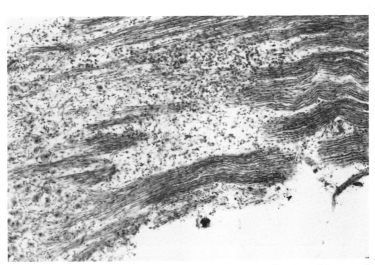

Figure 4.23 As Figure 4.22. Interstitial neuritis of the VIIIth nerve. Note diffuse infiltration of the nerve by mononuclear cells separating and disrupting the nerve fibres. × 150

Deafness may occur in both acquired and congenital syphilis.

Acquired syphilis

The pathology of the deafness is obscure. The principal lesions are those of the tertiary stage of the disease, which may become manifest within a few or many years after infection. The skin and cartilage of the external ear may be infected. The middle ear and temporal bone may be the sites of destructive gummatous processes of tertiary syphilis (Figure 4.25).

Congenital syphilis

The stillborn or young infant may exhibit syphilitic changes in the middle ear and cochlea which may become ossified. Severe endolymphatic hydrops and degeneration of the organ of Corti and spiral ganglion have also been described (Karmody and Schuknecht, 1966) (Figures 4.26).

Neuropathology in AIDS

The nervous system is often involved in the acquired immunodeficiency syndrome (AIDS) by infections and infestations, by neoplasms and by several diseases of uncertain pathogenesis (Gonzales and Davis, 1988).

The most common pathological changes are caused by the HIV agent itself, e.g. 'HIV-associated subacute encephalitis'. Cytomegalovirus (CMV) is the commonest secondary virus and toxoplasmosis a frequent

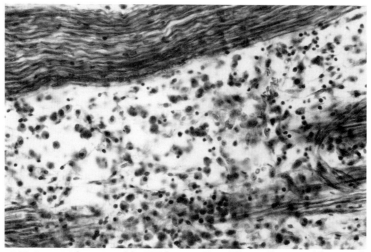

Figure 4.24 As Figure 4.23. Interstitial neuritis of the VIIIth nerve. Note diffuse infiltration of the nerve by mononuclear cells separating and disrupting the nerve fibres. × 400

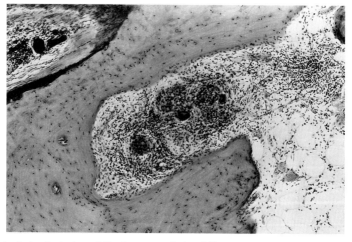

Figure 4.25 Giant cellular lesion in the bone following congenital syphilis

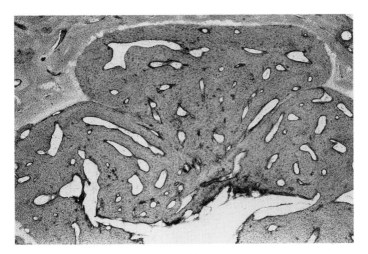

Figure 4.26 Ossification of the cochlea following congenital syphilis

cause of abscess formation. Fungeal infections by *Cryptococcus* are often the cause of meningitis. Michaels *et al.* (1994) have studied 49 temporal bones from 24 patients with AIDS and found severe otitis media in five patients, low-grade otitis media in 15 patients, labyrinthine cryptococcosis in 2 patients, cytomegalovirus inclusion-bearing cells in the inner ear and middle ear in 6 patients and deposits of Kaposi's sarcoma in the VIIIth nerve of one patient. These almost heroic investigations confirm that the ear is as susceptible to AIDS-associated diseases as any other organ and particularly prone to cytomegalovirus infection. Davis *et al.* (1995) have pointed out that histopathological changes of the inner ear were rare and that some viral inner ear infections may be both asymptomatic and nonpathogenic in AIDS patients.

Primary CNS B-cell lymphoma, often multiple, accounts for a major percentage of the lymphomas seen in AIDS. Various peripheral neurophathies may also occur.

Toxoplasmosis

Toxoplasmosis, one of the most widespread protozoal infections in humans, presents in two forms: the congenital and the acquired form. The congenital form presents at birth as a generalized disease. In the acquired form generalized lymphadenopathy is the prominent clinical finding. Chloroidoretinitis and various cerebral lesions may ensue. However, many infants infected *in utero* may appear healthy at birth but after a long interval may develop choroidoretinitis and other symptoms and signs of cerebral damage (Stern *et al.*, 1969).

Although the inner ear may be a site of the parasite or suffer when the brain damage involves the higher centres it has been suggested that it is not a signifi-

cant cause of congenital or infantile deafness (Ristow, 1966; Wright, 1971).

Idiopathic sudden sensorineural hearing loss

The condition can be defined as spontaneous sudden hearing loss in patients with no previous apparent otological problems. Its pathogenesis has remained speculative despite some, mainly empirical, improvement of its clinical management.

The cause of so-called idiopathic sudden deafness is often obscure. Morrison and Booth (1970) have compiled a long list of causes of sudden deafness (Table 4.6). Progressive or sudden hearing loss can be caused by localized or systemic vascular disease. A recent study by Gates *et al.* (1993) has revealed a statistically significant association of cardiovascular disease and hearing loss in a cohort of 1662 elderly men and has confirmed that low-frequency presbyacusis was associated with microvascular disease leading to atrophy of the stria vascularis. The vessels of the stria vascularis and of the internal auditory artery and its branches, which are terminal arteries, play a significant role also in diabetes mellitus and in various congenital syndromes associated with deafness.

Histopathology

The pathological changes resemble those occurring in labyrinthitis of known viral aetiology.

The principal histopathological changes involve the organ of Corti and the tectorial membrane with less frequent and less severe lesions of the stria vascularis and of the vestibular labyrinth. In two of the 12 cases studied by Schuknecht and Donovan (1986), the severe-hearing loss was attributed to the atrophy

Table 4.6 Causes of sudden deafness (Morrison and Booth, 1970)

Central
Diffuse cortical encephalitis
Sudden psychogenic deafness

Retrocochlear lesions
Multiple sclerosis
Penicillin hypersensitivity
Brain-stem encephalitis
Herpes zoster oticus
Vestibular schwannoma
Idiopathic sudden deafness

Cochlear lesions
Post-meningitis
Post-measles
Post-mumps
Suppurative labyrinthitis
Profound anaemia
Congenital syphilis
Rickettsial infection
Menière's disease
Following spinal anaesthesia
Vascular lesions
Sludging from sickle-cell trait
Idiopathic
Ototoxic agents

Traumatic lesions
Head injury – dislocation or fracture of the stapes with perilymph fistula

of the tectorial membrane and one of the cases showed atrophy of the cochlear neurons as the probable cause (Figure 4.27).

A histological study of sudden deafness resulting from rupture of cochlear membranes first in the left ear, and then 3 years later in the right ear, in a patient with vertebrobasilar arteriosclerosis was reported by Gussen (1983). Two healed ruptures were shown on the right side, one in the hook portion of the cochlea and one in the area of the promontory; the latter was adherent to the saccule, distorting it inferiorly. In the left temporal bone, a healed rupture was shown. Although the patient's vertebrobasilar artery disease and her sudden deafness are considered separate entities, one must at least consider whether such long-standing vascular insufficiency might predispose to more readily ruptured membranes with sudden pressure changes in the inner ear.

Hearing loss due to noise

The effect of noise or any acoustic trauma (Table 4.7) is of considerable industrial and public health importance. Repeated exposure to high levels of noise is a major cause of deafness, particularly in certain industrial occupations and in places of public or private entertainment where there is over amplification of sound. Proximity to explosions or to gunfire is also liable to result in deafness. Noise-induced degenerative patterns in the human ear exhibit a characteristic 'knife-sharp' demarcation line between the damaged and undamaged areas (Lim and Dunn, 1979).

In nature sound seldom exceeds 100 dB (Cudennec *et al.*, 1986). Industrial noise pollution produces louder noise which tends to last much longer. These

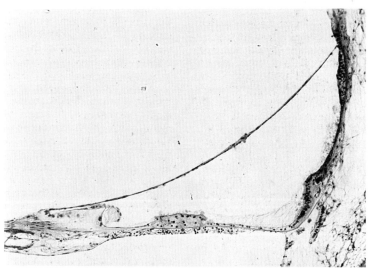

Figure 4.27 Sudden deafness. Scala media in the middle coil of the cochlea (left) showing that the pillar cells and the Deiters's cells were missing but not the hair cells. About 60% of the stria vascularis was atrophic and the tectorial membrane was displaced into the inner sulcus covered by a layer of endothelial cells. (By courtesy of Professor H. F. Schuknecht)

Table 4.7 Hearing loss due to physical agents

Mechanoacoustical causes
Direct trauma to the ears and/or head; blast; pressure-
  dysbarisms; noise, vibration

Electromagnetic causes
Electric shock; ionizing radiations

Thermal causes
Cold – cryosurgery; heat – ultrasound

Hearing loss following head injury
(Hinchcliffe, 1970)

Conductive
1 Haemorrhagic
      blood clot in external auditory meatus
      haemotympanum
2 Scarring: across external auditory meatus or middle ear
3 CSF in middle ear
4 Ossicular damage
      Malleus
        dislocation
        fracture
      Incus
        incudostapedial joint separation
        dislocation
      Stapes:
        avulsion
        fractured crura

Sensorineural
1 Receptor organ
      Stimulation hearing loss
      Labyrinthine capsule fracture (longitudinal fracture of
        petrous part of temporal bone)
2 Neuronal
      Transverse fracture of petrous part of temporal bone
3 Brain damage

include aircraft noise, noise caused by construction equipment and rivetting tools, etc., and from 50 to 60% of all industrial workers are exposed to 85 or more decibels for 8 hours a day – i.e. about 25% of their working life (Falk, 1977). Noise from dental drills and music from personal cassette players tends to be much overrated (Coles, 1986). However, an investigation of 505 students found significant hearing losses in those who admitted frequent attendance at pop music entertainment, in contrast to a control group with a different taste (Hanson and Fearn, 1975).

There has been a good deal of controversy about the deleterious effect of loud rock music delivered, either by the instruments themselves or by amplifiers and by personal head phones (Buffe *et al.*, 1986). Drake-Lee (1992) has tested four members of a heavy metal band before and within half an hour following their concert. One member had an ear protector but the other three members, with unprotected ears, 'showed a temporary threshold shift in the lower frequencies'. The author concluded that there was a small, but definite risk to rock musicians developing sensorineural hearing loss and tinnitus. Members of an audience attending such concerts are less at risk than has been claimed but tinnitus might ensue with its inherent discomfort to the individual (Drake-Lee, 1992).

Acoustic trauma may cause sensory cell damage by direct mechanical action, by metabolic disturbances resulting from impaired blood circulation, or as a result of the altered permeability of the cell membrane. The inner hair cells are more resistant to acoustic trauma regardless of their site (Bohne, 1976), but greater hearing loss is caused by the loss of the inner than the outer hair cells. By contrast, the outer hair cells display a varied susceptibility in different coils of the cochlea. The morphological changes include proliferation and vacuolation of the endoplasmic reticulum, swelling of the mitochondria, and degeneration of the cuticular plate. The swollen sensory cell may rupture and perish (Hawkins and Johnsson, 1976).

The sensory cells are joined by attachment zones and gap junctions as first described in tissue cultures of the otocyst (Friedmann and Bird, 1961a). Subsequently, it has been shown that the cell junctions of the organ of Corti are disrupted by noise (Beagley, 1965).

The hair cells and the cochlear nerve endings can degenerate within days following excessive exposure to sound. In the cochlear nucleus, the small cochlear nerve endings are especially susceptible to acoustic trauma. It is noteworthy that there is evidence for both a differential sensitivity of inner and outer hair cells and of a selective susceptibility of different auditory pathways in the central nervous system to acoustic overstimulation (Kent and Bohne, 1983).

Spoendlin (1985) emphasized the great variability of cochlear damage caused by sound or noise; in particular, the metabolic delayed type damage to hearing varies greatly and is the predominant type in the present noisy environment. There are critical intensity levels determining the type and extent of the damage. Intensive noise leads to total destruction of the organ of Corti, especially in the upper basal turn.

In regions where the organ of Corti is completely destroyed, the cochlear neurons undergo a slow progressive retrograde degeneration over a period of months, resulting in an almost 90% loss of cochlear neurons including their ganglion cells within the spiral ganglion. This event is influenced only by the loss of the inner hair cells but does not follow when only the outer hair cells are missing (Spoendlin, 1975).

High intensity sound (noise) produces considerable changes in the cilia, which may be converted into large complex 'giant' structures affecting the function of the sensory cells. Lim (1986), in a comprehensive review, has drawn renewed attention to the important role of the ciliary apparatus in the normal transduction of sound and any damage may considerably impair its function. Various stereociliary changes may be caused by acoustic trauma (also by ototoxic agents). These have been described as floppy, fanned-out, fractured, fused, giant and dissolved cilia. Following mechanical overstimulation or acoustic trauma, the stereocilia show a reduction in stiffness, as measured directly in isolated organs of Corti. They may return to their pre-exposure stiffness in about 15 minutes, following mechanical stimulation (Miller, Canlon and Flock, 1985; Saunders and Flock, 1985).

Splayed (fanned-out) stereocilia may be caused by the tightening of the contractile proteins that are attached to the rootlets in the cuticular plate (Friedmann, Cawthorne and Bird, 1965a; Slepecky, Hamernik and Henderson, 1980, 1981). Another mechanism could be the result of the altered consistency of the cuticular plate because of depolymerization, leading to an exaggerated pivoting of the rootlets. Seemingly minor changes of the stereocilia–cuticular plate complex have a profound effect on the auditory and/or vestibular function (Friedmann, Cawthorne and Bird, 1965b; Lim, 1986).

'Extra-auditory effects', other than hearing reactions, can be caused by noise or loud sounds resulting from the interaction of sounds with other sensory functions, e.g. vision.

Experimentally produced endolymphatic hydrops in guinea-pigs by obliteration of the endolymphatic sac was treated by exposure of the animals to noise. There was marked sludging of red corpuscles in the arterioles of the stria vascularis and scattered loss of outer hair cells on the hydropic side, confirmed by electron microscopy. Hydropic ears appear to be highly vulnerable to noise (Nakai *et al.*, 1991). Asymptomatic patients may display clinical signs when exposed to external insults, e.g. noise. Noise affects the stereocilia of the hair cells causing marked disarray (Cho *et al.*, 1991).

An increased risk of noise-induced hearing loss was noted in persons taking moderate doses of aspirin or salicylates (McFadden, Plattsmier and Pasanen, 1984).

Symphonic musicians suffer from hearing loss caused by symphonic music (Ostri *et al.*, 1989). Violinists have a poorer hearing of higher frequencies in the left ear.

The response to mechanical injury for the afferent nerve endings was studied in tissue culture by Sobkowicz and Slapnick (1992). Electron microscopy showed vigorous sprouting of nerve endings with synaptic formation between hair cells and growth cones of nerves.

Fractures of the temporal bone

More young adults are now killed and injured in automobile accidents than from any other cause. More than 75% of these injuries are to the head, and the ear is the most frequently injured sensory organ in the body (Hough and Stuart, 1968). Temporal bone or basilar skull fractures are extremely common in any injury to the head (Murakami *et al.*, 1990).

Injuries to the temporal bone may be considered in three groups: those affecting the external auditory meatus (extralabyrinthine fractures), those largely affecting the middle ear cleft (tympanolabyrinthine), and those affecting the internal ear (labyrinthine fractures). Many injuries, however, involve all these structures. Ballantyne (1962) first drew attention to the effect of skull trauma on the middle ear.

Ototoxic drugs

There is a wide range of drugs which are capable of causing deafness and/or dizziness, either by producing toxic degeneration of the inner ear, or of the higher centres of hearing and equilibrium. The peculiar sensitivity of the VIIIth nerve has not yet been satisfactorily explained. Many ototoxic drugs have no apparent chemical similarity (for instance thalidomide, ethacrynic acid and the arsenical compound atoxyl), but most ototoxic antibiotics belong to the 'useful but unruly' family of basic streptomyces antibiotics (Hawkins, 1976), or aminoglycoside antibiotics and to the so-called 'loop diuretics'.

Histopathology

It has been shown that the effect of some ototoxic antibiotics differed from that of acoustic trauma which usually started at the base of the cochlea extending to its apex. This applies equally to neomycin, gentamicin and kanamycin. Neomycin seemed to act initially upon the hook area and apical coil, whereas gentamicin and kanamycin would initially cause simultaneous destruction of the outer hair cells in the upper basal coil and in the hook area. Neomycin may also act on the apical inner hair cells which are only seldom damaged by gentamicin or kanamycin (Figure 4.29) (Hawkins, 1959; Friedmann and Bird, 1961b; Friedmann, Dadswell and Bird, 1966). The lesions caused by atoxyl usually start at the apex (Anniko, 1976a,b).

There exist great variations among individual animals (and humans) in their reaction to the ototoxic antibiotics necessitating individual evaluation of the hair cell damage.

The mechanism of action of the aminoglycosides has been studied by means of an improved fixation method using gentamicin with particular reference to its ultrastructural effects (De Groot, 1989). It was noted that gentamicin accumulated in the hair cells mainly in lysosomes and in multivesicular structures suggesting an endocytotic pathway for the uptake of these drugs. Release into the endoplasmic reticulum and Golgi complex may ensue as previously recognized (Friedmann and Bird, 1961b; Friedmann, 1974; Friedmann and Arnold, 1993). Anniko (1976b) believes that the primary changes occurred in the stria vascularis altering the ionic composition of the endolymph with consequent vesicular degeneration of the inner and outer hair cells.

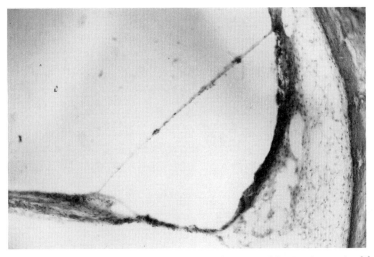

Figure 4.28 Patient treated with kanamycin. There is total absence of the organ of Corti and necrosis of the stria vascularis. Reissner's membrane shows nodular thickening, a characteristic lesion of ototoxicity

Transmission electron microscopy

As has been shown in animals, and in tissue culture, ototoxic antibiotics are ribosomal and mitochondrial poisons (Friedmann and Bird, 1961b).

The earliest ultrastructural signs of degeneration of the organ of Corti, regardless of the antibiotic administered, occur in the outer hair cells (see Figure 4.6). The cisternae along the outer cell membrane become distended and dense bodies accumulate in the subcuticular cytoplasm of the hair cells. Subsequently the distended cisternae become vacuolated and eventually the outer cytoplasmic membrane will rupture. The intracellular organelles are expelled into Nuel's space leading to their complete disintegration.

Sensorineural deafness may be caused by the 'loop diuretics', frusemide (furosemide) and ethacrynic acid, which inhibit cellular metabolism and the enzymes participating in electrolyte transport. Ethacrynic acid causes oedema and cystic degeneration of the stria vascularis. Studies of the combined effect of kanamycin and ethacrynic acid show that the concurrent administration of two or more ototoxic drugs has an enhanced toxic effect on the inner ear. On the other hand, the selective ototoxicity of atoxyl can be employed as a model system for comparative studies of various ototoxic agents (Anniko, 1976a; Anniko and Wersall, 1976).

The effect of prussic acid on neurons has been demonstrated on tissue cultures of the isolated fowl embryo otocyst exposed to sodium cyanide (Friedmann and Bird, 1972). The degenerative changes observed were comparable to those observed in patients with the kassava syndrome. Kassava root is a widely consumed food in Africa, which contains a cyanogenic compound linamarin; and it has been recognized that multiple neuropathy associated with deafness might ensue in persons consuming this otherwise simple food.

Scanning electron microscopy (Figure 4.29)

The effect of gentamicin has been studied by scanning electron microscopy on guinea-pigs (Forge, 1985; Lim, 1986). A variety of lesions has been noted at the hair cell apex. The stereocilia were fused or foreshortened, apparently disintegrating. The surfaces of the outer hair cells where stereocilia were almost completely destroyed appeared to be roughened. The cuticular surfaces were bulging and became detached from the reticular lamina. 'Crooked' rootlets with bent stereocilia, floppy cilia, fusion of stereocilia and giant cilia have been observed on cochlear hair cells exposed to ototoxic agents (Figures 4.29, 4.30 and 4.31).

The detached hair cell remnant could be seen beneath the surfaces of the expanded or swollen supporting cell possessing microvilli and occluding the space beneath the vanishing hair cell debris (Forge, 1985; Lim, 1986). This process is probably electrochemical in nature and acts through the gap junctions linking the two cell groups. This type of necrosis of the cell has been likened by Forge (1985) to the 'apoptosis' occurring in developing organs which require a programmed regularly timed cell death (Willie, 1981).

A partial or total loss of outer hair cells alone, in a given segment of the cochlea, was not associated with any corresponding rarefaction or loss of neurons. When the inner hair cells had also degenerated, the number of neurons in the spiral ganglion and spiral osseous lamina was markedly reduced, provided the survival time was long enough for degeneration to have run its course. The secondary

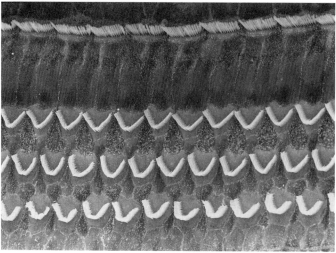

Figure 4.29 Scanning electron micrograph of the normal organ of Corti. (By courtesy of Dr A. Forge)

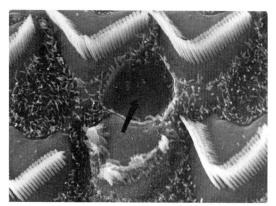

Figure 4.30 A pit (arrow) in place of an outer hair cell in the first row. The surface of the pit floor is covered with microvilli. (By courtesy of Dr A. Forge)

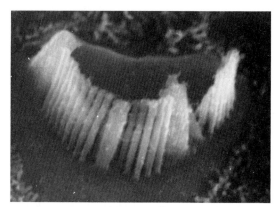

Figure 4.31 Various alterations of the stereocilia as viewed by scanning electron microscopy. Fusion of some stereocilia may be seen. Other stereocilia were foreshortened and apparently disintegrating. (By courtesy of Dr A. Forge)

degeneration of first order neurons following any damage to the organ of Corti, appeared to be a delayed phenomenon; its full development was not apparent until at least 4 weeks after the cessation of treatment with gentamicin.

Aminoglycosides can cross the placenta and damage the developing embryo. Sprague-Dawley rat embryos exposed to retinoids prenatally developed craniofacial malformations. Pregnant rats were treated with 40 mg/kg retinoic acid or 10 mg/kg etretinate (Granstrom and Kulaa-Mikkonen, 1990). Similar lesions were noted on the fetuses of hamsters treated with retinoic acid (Shenefelt, 1990).

Fermin and Igarashi (1983) have raised the question 'why aminoglycosides were preferentially attracted to the epithelia of the inner ear and kidneys.' These authors employed the chick which is considered to provide a satisfactory developmental model

for the study of ototoxic drugs *in vivo* as we have shown in tissue cultures of the isolated chick embryo otocyst (Friedmann, 1956; 1974).

Tissue culture studies

Tissue culture studies (Friedmann and Bird, 1961b) on isolated chick embryo otocysts exposed to various antibiotics confirmed that ototoxic antibiotics act as mitochondrial poisons causing far-reaching morphological changes in the mitochondria of the sensory cells affected. Other organelles and cells may also suffer. There were widespread mitochondrial changes in the neurons and the nerve fibres in otocyst cultures exposed to dimycin or neomycin (Friedmann and Bird, 1961b). In cultures treated with neomycin, the initial zone of degeneration was localized around the

Golgi apparatus of the sensory cells, causing degeneration of the mitochondria of the perinuclear region. Subsequently, the process extended to the numerous mitochondria aggregated in the intermediate zone – 'the power house' of the cell. The breakdown of this vital part of the cell can lead to the loss of function of the sensory cells.

Parallel histochemical investigations of otocyst cultures exposed to dimycin or neomycin (McAlpine and Friedmann, 1963) have shown that some enzyme systems remain active. This paradox might be explained by the fact that even small fragments of mitochondrial membrane may contain relatively intact enzyme systems, including the enzymes necessary for coupling phosphorylation to electron transport (Lehninger *et al.*, 1958).

It is interesting to note that rudimentary kinocilia appear to survive the higher doses of gentamicin, e.g. $600 - 1200$ μg, which may arrest the differentiation of the sensory epithelium. The general pattern of the damage caused by different ototoxic antibiotics follows a similar course in the experimental animal and in tissue culture (Friedmann and Bird, 1961a,b; Friedmann, Dadswell and Bird, 1966).

Osteoradionecrosis

Osteoradionecrosis of the temporal bone is a well recognized complication of radiotherapy of neoplasms of the head and neck. Characteristically the development of osteoradionecrosis may be long delayed after the time of radiotherapy. Hariri and Small (1990) have described an interesting case of osteoradionecrosis of the temporal bone presenting 40 years after radiotherapy to the ipsilateral mandible, with symptoms and signs of a cerebellopontine angle lesion. Severe radionecrosis of the temporal bone as a potentially lethal condition has been discussed in a study of a series of seven such cases by Birzgalis *et al.* (1993).

Delayed effects of ionizing radiation on the ear

Patients with carcinoma of the brain, nasopharynx, tonsil and parotid gland have been treated with doses of radiation which range from 5000 to 7000 cGy over a period of 5–7 weeks. Depending on the size and site of the tumour, one or both temporal bones may receive a nearly equivalent dose of radiation. Several studies have shown that some patients so treated developed hearing difficulties during therapy (Bohne, Marks and Glasgow, 1985).

The question of damage to the ear from exposure to ionizing radiation was studied by exposing groups of chinchillas to fractional doses of radiation (200 cGy/day) for total doses ranging from 4000 to 9000

cGy. In order to allow any delayed effects of radiation to become manifest, the animals were sacrificed 2 years after completion of treatment and their temporal bones were examined. The most pronounced effect of treatment was degeneration of the sensory and supporting cells and the loss of VIIIth nerve fibres in the organ of Corti. The degree of damage found in many of these ears proved to be the cause of permanent sensorineural hearing loss.

Ageing and hearing loss

Hearing loss and degeneration of balance control in the aged is of gradual onset and forms part of the progressive deterioration of the physiological functions associated with the ageing process. These are of a general nature, affecting any cell of any tissue or organ, although different cell systems may become vulnerable in particular ways.

The true nature of the pathogenesis of hearing loss of the aged (presbyacusis) has remained obscure. The principal lesions to be recognized are a loss of hair cells in the basal and apical areas of the cochlea, a loss of neurons and nerve fibres of the spiral ganglion and spiral nerve, and vascular changes and atrophy affecting the stria vascularis (Schuknecht, 1974; Suga and Lindsay, 1976a, b; Nadol and Arnold, 1987).

Four distinct clinical patterns have been recognized in the ageing population with typical histopathological correlates:

1 Degeneration and loss of neural elements or 'neural presbyacusis'
2 Degeneration and loss of hair cells or 'sensory presbyacusis'
3 Inner ear biochemical defect or 'metabolic presbyacusis'
4 Degeneration or inefficiency of inner ear supportive elements or 'mechanical presbyacusis'.

Neural presbyacusis

The loss of cochlear neurons is the most consistent pathological change in the ageing ear, commencing at an early age and continuing throughout life. A loss of neurons of the cochlea in the presence of a functional end organ produces a distinctive pattern of auditory malfunction characterized by a progressive loss of word discrimination in the presence of stable pure tone thresholds (Schuknecht and Gacek, 1993). For neuronal presbyacusis the criterion is a loss of 50% or more of cochlear neurons compared with the mean.

Early degeneration affects the dendritic processes of the osseous spiral lamina. In areas of severe degeneration there may be marked loss of spiral ganglion cells and afferent axons (Figure 4.32).

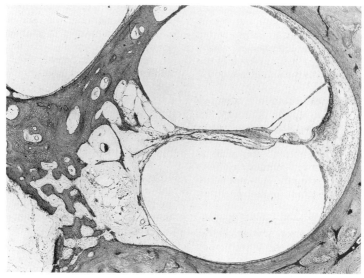

Figure 4.32 Neural presbyacusis showing total absence of spiral neurons. The patient experienced bilateral progressive hearing loss, worse in the left ear, during the later years of his life and died at the age of 75 years. (By courtesy of Professor H. F. Schuknecht)

Sensory presbyacusis

Sensory hair cell losses at the extreme basal end of the cochlea are common in the ageing cochlea. An important collaborative study by Wright *et al.* (1987) has provided reliable data on the distribution of sensory hair cells in the normal human cochlea, coupled with the evaluation of age-related changes in the hair cell density. The material consisted of 53 cochleae (including nine from fetuses) preserved by perilymphatic perfusion with fixation taking place shortly after death and the material allocated to one of six age bands. For each age band, average cytocochleograms have been drawn for both inner and outer hair cells.

The average cytocochleograms showed a progressive age-related loss of the outer hair cells, mainly at the apical and basal ends of the cochlea. The loss of the inner hair cells, though less marked than that of the outer hair cells, occurred also at the base but not at the apex of the cochlea. A simple linear equation is suggested allowing the quantitative assessment of hair cell loss in individual cases exposed in life to cochleotoxic agents (Wright *et al.*, 1987).

Many aged cochleae show an island of hair cell loss in the 8–12 mm region of the 4 kHz frequency. This loss is probably caused by acoustic trauma. The earliest ultrastructural changes, such as loss of the stereocilia are followed by a slight distortion and flattening of the organ of Corti and loss of the supporting cells. Eventually only an undifferentiated epithelial mound is left resting on the basilar membrane. There is a concomitant loss of dendrites and, to a lesser extent, of neuronal bodies (Schuknecht and Gacek, 1993).

The criterion established by the authors for sensory presbyacusis is the presence of any total loss of hair cells beginning at the basal end of the cochlea, that is at least 10 mm in length, encroaching on the speech frequency area of the cochlea.

Metabolic or strial presbyacusis

Schuknecht (1964a,b) described a common type of sensorineural hearing loss which has its onset in middle age, is slowly progressive, and is characterized by a flat audiometric pattern. It is associated with degenerative changes of the stria vascularis of the middle and apical turns of the cochlea (Figures 4.33 and 4.34).

Atrophy of the stria vascularis is an important cause of sensorineural hearing loss of ageing. The pathological changes consist of degeneration of all three layers of the stria vascularis, most prominently in the apical region of the cochlea, affecting most severely the marginal cells, then the intermediate and least severely, the basal cells. Schuknecht and Igarashi (1964), Pauler, Schuknecht and White (1988), Schuknecht and Gacek (1993) and Masutani, Takahashi and Sando (1992) have noted that hearing loss occurred when there were strial losses of about 30% or greater. The organ of Corti and the spiral ganglion appear to be normal. This is clinically associated with a comparatively flat audiogram but excellent speech discrimination.

The cells and vessels of the stria vascularis may be totally absent but small remnants may survive around a small vessel near the attachment of Reis-

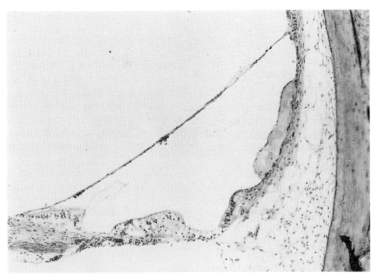

Figure 4.33 Strial metabolic presbyacusis. There is a homogeneous encapsulated deposit replacing the atrophied stria vascularis. The other structures are normal. (By courtesy of Professor H. F. Schuknecht)

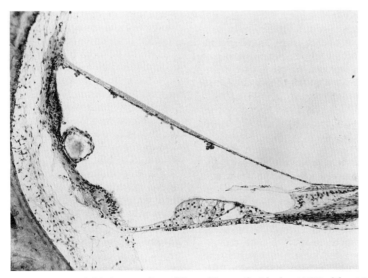

Figure 4.34 Same patient as in Figure 4.33 showing the middle cochlear coil with about 50% of the stria vascularis atrophied and replaced by an encapsulated cystic structure containing some basophilic matter. Figures 4.33 and 4.34 are from a 68-year-old woman who suffered with bilateral symmetrical hearing loss exhibiting flat threshold patterns with relatively good speech discriminating scores. (By courtesy of Professor H. F. Schuknecht)

sner's membrane. There may be basophilic granules and occasionally cysts present. Atrophy of the stria vascularis may alter the biochemical composition and the bioelectrical properties of the endolymph and is associated with a nearly uniform threshold loss for all frequencies (Schuknecht and Ishii, 1966; Pauler, Schuknecht and White, 1988). It appears to be the

Achilles heel of the inner ear (Johnsson and Hawkins, 1972).

The stria vascularis possesses important functional roles including secretory functions and the production of the endolymph. Any morphological change might adversely affect its functioning and lead to the formation of an abnormal endolymph disturbing the proper function of the auditory and vestibular sensory organs.

Cochlear conductive presbyacusis
(Ramadan and Schuknecht, 1989)

This is characterized by a linear descending audiogram which occurs not only as a manifestation of ageing but may be associated with otosclerosis and Paget's disease of the temporal bone. It has been suggested that this hearing loss might be caused by the resonance characteristics of the cochlear duct that determine frequency distribution.

There are other cellular and subcellular processes participating in various degenerative syndromes which find expression in extreme old age. The hair cell population decreases with age in parallel with atrophy of the spiral nerves (Wright *et al.*, 1987). The vestibular end organs may also be affected and there is an age-related progressive reduction of the number of vestibular sensory cells and nerve fibres over the age of 40 years. The cells contain a great deal of lipofuscin, yet the physiological ability of such persons may not be substantially impaired, probably as a result of compensation by the surviving cells.

The basilar membrane becomes progressively narrower and thicker from apex to base. Ageing may lead to an atrophy of both the spiral ligament and of the basilar membrane. Lipidosis of the basilar membrane occurring in the aged could also be the cause of hearing loss (Nomura, 1970).

Mixed presbyacusis

Although 'the basic tenet of four pathological types of presbyacusis has remained valid', Schuknecht and Gacek (1993) in a recent paper have emphasized that 'many aging ears show combinations of pathological types'. A particular type may predominate but 'its occurrence in total isolation from the others is the exception rather than the rule'.

The loss of sensory cells, usually located in the basal part of the cochlea, appears to be the least important cause of hearing loss in the elderly. Impaired cell function rather than cell attrition may be the cause of cochlear dysfunction, in particular, in a group defined by Schuknecht and Gacek as 'intermediate presbyacusis', forming a large proportion of ill-defined types of presbyacusis.

Neuronal losses are a constant finding as well as atrophy of the stria vascularis in the middle and apical coils associated with a flat audiometric pattern. However, there are about 25% of flat audiograms in the aged 'which cannot be explained by light microscope studies' (Schuknecht and Gacek, 1993). There is no medical treatment for the degenerative changes of the ageing cochlea at present.

Vascular diseases causing hearing loss

Progressive or sudden hearing loss can be caused by localized or systemic vascular disease. In the first category, the vessels of the stria vascularis and the internal auditory artery and its branches, which are terminal arteries, play a significant role, for example in diabetes mellitus and in various congenital syndromes associated with deafness. The vestibular end organs appear to be more resistant than the organ of Corti to the effects of surgical severance of the labyrinthine artery.

The cause of so-called idiopathic sudden deafness varies. Vascular disorders such as spasm, oedema or arteritis, or a combination of several vascular factors, have been incriminated. Polyarteritis nodosa and Wegener's granulomatosis involving the ear may cause deafness (Friedmann and Bauer, 1973; Rowe-Jones, Macallan and Soroshan, 1990).

Wegener's granuloma of the ear

In Wegener's granulomatosis, the ear is frequently affected so that pain in the ear, aural discharge, aural polyp, loss of hearing or total deafness of mixed conductive and sensory type may first bring the patient to medical attention (Figure 4.35). This may subsequently be followed by deterioration of the patient's general condition, pulmonary signs such as haemoptysis, or haematuria with subsequent renal failure leading to death from uraemia (Friedmann and Arnold, 1993).

McGaffrey, McDonald and Pacer (1980) reviewed 112 patients with Wegener's granulomatosis, seen at the Mayo Clinic between 1970 and 1978. Conductive deafness was present in 21 patients, as noted by others (Kornblut, Wolfe and Fauci, 1982). This common condition is caused by serous otitis. Sensorineural hearing loss occurs and may respond to treatment with prednisone and cyclophosphamide (McGaffrey and McDonald, 1979).

Limited Wegener's granuloma

There is a growing recognition of the fact that some of the features of Wegener's granulomatosis which are regarded as classic are not always present (Friedmann and Arnold, 1993). It is important to recognize the disease in its earlier limited form also in the upper respiratory tract.

Systemic bone diseases affecting the temporal bone

The temporal bone may be affected by any systemic bone disease but it may also be the solitary site of the disease. Hearing loss may ensue. The diseases include fibrous dysplasia, Paget's disease, osteogenesis imperfecta, osteopetrosis, histiocytosis X, eosinophilic granuloma, and giant cell reparative granuloma.

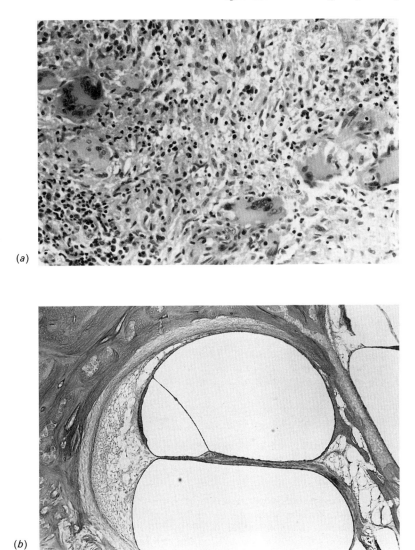

(a)

(b)

Figure 4.35 (a) Wegener's granulomatosis. There was an extensive giant cellular granulomatous lesion in the temporal bone. (b) The organ of Corti was deranged: note the missing inner hair cells and the inflammatory infiltration of the basilar membrane and of the stria vascularis. There is extensive oedema of the spiral ligament

Brookes and Booth (1987) presented a broader view having included genetic hyperostoses and genetic dysplasias of the skull affecting the temporal bone, e.g. genetic craniotabular hyperostoses and genetic craniotabular dysplasia of various kinds.

There are considerable characteristic biochemical, radiological and other features in these bone diseases (see Brookes and Booth, 1987), which will be included under the various headings.

A unique morphological feature of the human temporal bone are the 'globuli interossei' formed by embryonic cartilage remnants. They appear to be implicated in various bone diseases affecting solely the critical area in otosclerosis or wider areas affected by systemic bone diseases, e.g. osteogenesis imperfecta and, in particular, osteopetrosis.

Mechanism of mineralization

Katchburian's working hypothesis of mineralization (Katchburian, 1973) has universal appeal and can be confirmed on the basis of our observations on tympanosclerosis and otosclerosis. Early stages of mineralization are characterized by the appearance of matrix vescicles from cells in the collagenous

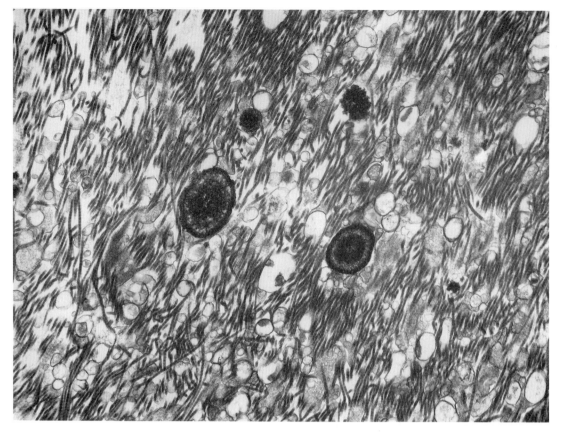

Figure 4.36 Note the large number of matrix vesicles and several calcospherules in collagenous tissue (from a specimen of tympanosclerosis)

matrix (fibroblasts, inflammatory cells, epithelial cells). The membrane of matrix vesicles, which contains calcium and phosphate ions, may become altered due to lack of renewal, followed by loss of water and supersaturation inside the matrix vesicles (Anderson, 1969; Friedmann, Hodges and Graham, 1980).

Supersaturation leads to incipient calcification and crystal formation, and will proceed spontaneously, resulting in the production of calcospherules in the collagenous tissue (Figure 4.36). Progressive mineralization follows with a gradual increase in the number of inclusions, frequently accompanied by mineralization beyond the matrix vesicles. Eventually confluent mineralized masses or plaques are formed. This applies to any bony dysplasia. The matrix vesicles may only be responsible for the mineralization of the non-fibrillar phase of the matrix (Katchburian, 1973). Mineral deposits in the inter-fibrillar region could lead to the creation of ionic conditions in the matrix, thus facilitating the initial precipitation of calcium phosphate within the collagen fibres and causing dystrophic calcification.

Osteogenesis imperfecta (*Van der Hoeve and de Kleyn syndrome*)

Osteogenesis imperfecta is a rare condition characterized by fragility of the bones, leading to multiple fractures. Malebranche (1694) first described the disease in a 20-year-old man. Lobstein (1935) named it 'osteopathyrosis idiopathica'. Vrolik (1849) describing the condition for the first time in a new-born infant with numerous intrauterine fractures of the long bones and a poorly ossified calvarium, called it osteogenesis imperfecta.

The lesions may present in two forms: as osteogenesis imperfecta congenita at birth, and as osteogenesis imperfecta tarda, when the changes become evident during childhood or adolescence (Looser, 1906; Seedorff, 1949). The incidence of the disease is estimated as from 1 in 15 000 births to 1 in 60 000. Taitz (1987) warns against implicating osteogenesis imperfecta as a cause of unexplained fractures in otherwise healthy babies and that may apply also to fractures of the base of the skull.

Osteogenesis imperfecta is a complex disease of the

bone. There are four subtypes resulting from genetically determined abnormalities of connective tissue especially type 1 pro-collagen (Smith, 1984). The temporal bone may be affected by this generalized skeletal abnormality, which may result from a specific dominant gene abnormality. Nager (1922) and Altmann (1962) were among the first to describe the temporal bone findings and Altmann noted the thin stapedial crura as a characteristic feature of the stapes in osteogenesis imperfecta (Zajtchuk and Lindsay, 1975).

Histopathology (Figures 4.37 and 4.38)

In the congenital form the lamellar bone is replaced by a spongy network of non-lamellar bone, which permeates the entire temporal bone or the otic capsule, and may involve the oval window region and stapes, when it can be difficult to distinguish from otosclerosis. Periosteal and endosteal bone appear sponge-like and their ossified matrix less compact than normal. The endochondral bone is relatively normal.

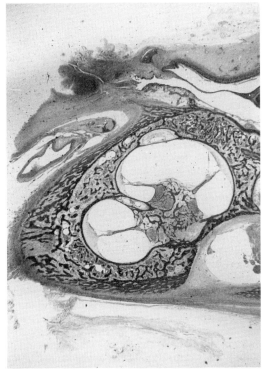

Figure 4.37 Congenital osteogenesis imperfecta. A spongy network of non-lamellar bone permeated the entire otic capsule (no. C 289–Temporal Bone Collection Institute of Laryngology and Otology)

The basic defect appears to lie in the maturation of collagen that does not mature beyond the reticulin stage. Therefore, during ossification the hydroxyapatite crystals are laid down on a faulty framework. This and the reduced hydroxyapatite content greatly reduces the stress resistance of the bone resulting in pathological fractures.

In older individuals the bones are brittle ('fragilitas ossium'). The histological features display no characteristic pattern that might be of differential diagnostic significance. The changes may be regarded as the result of a functional abnormality of osteoblasts.

As regards the underlying mechanism, a cross-linking defect in the collagen has been recognized (Bauze, Smith and Francis, 1975) in severe cases of osteogenesis imperfecta. It has been noted in tissue cultures of fibroblasts from patients with osteogenesis imperfecta that the production of collagen was defective, incriminating the cells (Brown, 1973).

When collagen molecules have been synthesized intermolecular cross-links are formed between adjacent molecules. Defective cross-linking would have extensive effects in any collagen-containing tissue (Byers, Barsh and Holbrook, 1982).

Conductive hearing loss, common in osteogenesis imperfecta has been attributed to coincidental otosclerosis. It is more likely that it is caused by fixation of the footplate or fibrous replacement of the suprastructure of the stapes. Zajtchuk and Lindsay (1975) described the temporal bone changes in a 66-year-old woman operated on repeatedly to alleviate her progressive hearing loss caused by the effect of osteogenesis imperfecta on the stapes. There was a family history of the triad of blue sclerae, deafness and fractures in her mother, her only nephew and herself.

Stapes and stapes fragments from 14 stapedectomies were studied by Brosnan *et al.* (1977). The footplates appeared to be softer than in otosclerosis due to the faulty reticulin framework and the reduced hydroxyapatite content greatly reducing the stress resistance of bone. The histopathology of osteogenesis imperfecta was compared with that of otosclerosis. There was a greater degree of structural disorganization and a greater area occupied by resorption spaces present, distinguishing the new bone formed in osteogenesis imperfecta from otosclerosis. This has been confirmed (Igarashi *et al.* 1980; Sando *et al.*, 1981; Pedersen *et al.*, 1985; Milroy and Michaels 1990, and others).

The genetics of osteogenesis imperfecta have remained obscure, but the most frequent form, accounting for about 80% of cases, is an autosomal disorder type I usually associated with blue sclerae (Schoenfeld, Fried and Ehrenfeld, 1975; Smith, 1984; British Medical Journal, 1987). Type II is a very severe form of osteogenesis imperfecta causing multiple fractures at birth, and death.

A common aetiology for otosclerosis and osteogenesis imperfecta as favoured by earlier authors (Wullstein *et al.*, 1960; Ogilvie and Hall, 1962, and others) has received some support; immunohistochemical studies have furnished some evidence of a possible role of paramyxoviruses in both bony dyscrasias (Arnold and Friedmann, 1988).

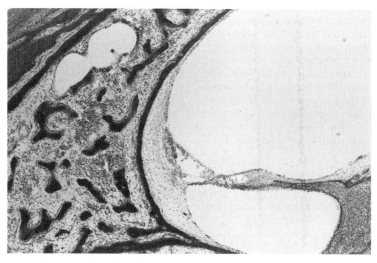

Figure 4.38 As Figure 4.37 showing in detail the affected otic capsule in the upper coil of the cochlea. Reissner's membrane appears to be adherent to the atrophic stria vascularis. (By courtesy of Milroy and Michaels)

Paget's disease

Paget's disease is a heritable abiotrophy of the collagen matrix of the bone (McKusick, 1972; Nager, 1975) affecting mainly the skeleton and progressively also the skull and the temporal bones. This causes enlargement of the bone and extensive alteration of the architecture of the petrous pyramid, the middle ear, the otic capsule and the external auditory meatus. Subsequently, hearing loss and vestibular disturbances may ensue.

Paget's disease affecting the skull may cause obstruction of the external auditory meatus, giving rise to conductive deafness; obliteration of the labyrinth and sensorineural deafness are less common symptoms. Some of the features which distinguish it from otosclerosis include the later age of onset, lack of family history, sensorineural deafness showing rapid deterioration, tinnitus, radiological evidence of Paget's disease of the skull.

Patients with extensive disease of the skull may have no complaints at all until ear trouble develops, e.g. tinnitus or unilateral hearing loss (Perlman, 1967). Hearing loss occurs in about 30–50%. Smaller localized lesions may remain undetected (Collins and Winn, 1955). Serum alkaline phosphatase activity is raised. Acid phosphatase, an index of osteoclastic activity, and urine hydroxyproline which indicates the breakdown of bone collagen, are also elevated but of little diagnostic value (Brookes and Booth, 1987). The disease affects mainly men over 40 years of age but women can also be affected causing substantial disability (Kanis, 1991).

Histopathology

Histologically there is evidence of disordered and very active reconstruction of the bone (Friedmann, 1974). There are, in the active phase, numerous multinucleated osteoclasts lying in the perivascular fibrous tissue or in the deep lacunae they have produced. Elsewhere, chains of osteoblasts are prominent lining newly formed bony trabeculae. Alternating resorption and apposition of bone culminates in the classical mosaic of irregular cement lines. In the inactive lesion remodelled bone, displaying the characteristic mosaic pattern of cement lines, has been formed. This must not be confused with the similar pattern observed in the sclerotic mastoid bone following chronic infective diseases. The author has studied the temporal bones of a woman who died at the age of 81; the petrous temporal bones were almost totally affected by the process. Her deafness was, in fact, only moderate and it had been easy to communicate with her. The process obstructed the external auditory meatus and obliterated the tympanic cavity but not the cochlea; the organ of Corti was present (Figure 4.39). There is a similarity with otosclerosis, in that there is a sharp zone of demarcation between the diseased and the normal bone (Figure 4.40). A woven pattern is displayed under polarized light (Figure 4.41a). The histopathological changes commence with osteoclastic resorption of bone followed by osteoblastic regeneration and the formation of primitive osteoid bone resulting in the characteristic 'mosaic' pattern of the reconstructed bone. (Figure 4.41b). Vascular hypertrophy and extensive arteriovenous shunting may occur.

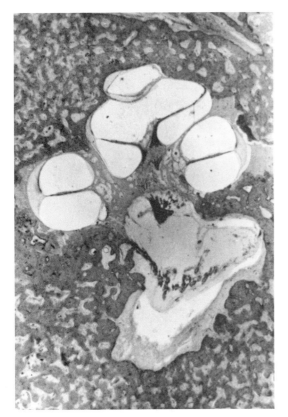

Figure 4.39 Paget's disease of bone surrounding the apparently normal cochlea and the internal auditory meatus

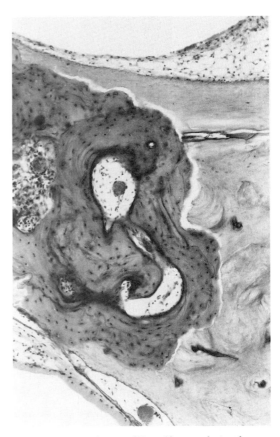

Figure 4.40 Large plaques of 'Paget' bone replacing the lamellar bone of the otic capsule

Paget's disease of the temporal bone affects the entire temporal bone, although the cochlea seems, in most cases, to escape total obliteration (Lindsay and Lehman, 1969). The otic capsule, in particular the periosteal layer, may be replaced or eroded by diseased bony tissue (Nager, 1975; Milroy and Michaels, 1990). The endosteal layer may also be affected. Milroy and Michaels studied three cases by the micro-slicing technique (Michaels, Wells and Frohlich, 1983), and noted, in two grossly affected patients, that the otic capsule was eroded in places by diseased bone. Remodelling and the enhanced stromal and osteogenic activity may account for the development of various benign and malignant neoplasms. In about 10% of cases with Paget's disease sarcomatous changes developed in the skull, including the facial bones (McKenna *et al.*, 1964; Friedmann and Osborn, 1982).

There exist various osteoclast-activating factors (Chambers, 1988). Jandinski (1988) has confirmed that the osteoclast activating factor is interleukin-1 beta. Horowitz *et al.* (1984) have shown that a bone resorbing factor was produced by the interaction of T cells with macrophages; B cells alone, or with macrophages, produced no detectable bone resorbing factor.

Treatment with calcitonin and the biphosphonate etidronate were shown swiftly to reduce osteoclast mediated bone resorption (Bickerstaff *et al.*, 1990). The effect of injected calcitonin was striking but temporary. There was both biochemical and clinical improvement; bone pain was relieved; bone resorption slowed; paraparesis and leontiasis from maxillary Paget's disease could be halted and possibly reversed (Smith, 1992).

There are strong clues about its cause; that Paget's disease of the bone is a slow viral infection of the paramyxoviridiae family (Mills *et al.*, 1984). Using modern methods of molecular biology, however, Nuovo *et al.* (1992) have failed to confirm the role of the measles virus in the causation of Paget's disease of the bone.

Fibrous dysplasia of bone

The term fibrous dysplasia was introduced by Lichtenstein in 1936 replacing no less than 33 different

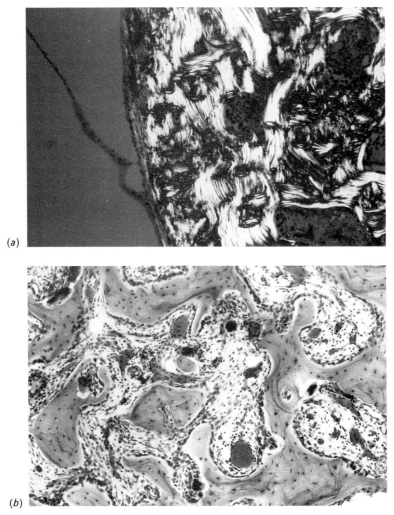

(a)

(b)

Figure 4.41 (*a*) Paget's disease of bone under polarized light to show its woven pattern. (*b*) Microscopical features of Paget's disease of the bone showing the disorganized bone of the mastoid process of a patient (T29 250 Institute of Laryngology and Otology collection). There are large numbers of osteoclasts present but also osteoblasts lining the abnormal bone

names used by various authors to describe this disease (Lichtenstein, 1938; Lichtenstein and Jaffe, 1942; Reed, 1963). Fibrous dysplasia produces circumscribed lesions usually in the long bones; but it is not uncommon in the skull, particularly in the maxilla. The temporal bone may be affected alone (Figure 4.42). Monostotic or polyostotic fibrous dysplasia is, therefore, distinguished. The aetiology is obscure. The histological features may vary and there is a wide spectrum of fibrosseous lesions of the bone representing variants of fibrous dysplasia. These lesions are distinguished according to their predominant histological features and clinical correlates (Fu and Perzin, 1974).

The primary histological component consists of connective tissue with metaplastic new bone formation;

this is of woven pattern and a lamellar organization may be lacking. There are comparatively slender bony trabeculae present forming a network surrounded by fibrous connective tissue. Immature osteoblasts staining unevenly may be present. Osteoclasts can be seen tunnelling into the mineralized interior of the trabeculae scalloping and fragmenting them. The resorbed areas become filled with cellular fibrous tissue (Figure 4.42).

The *temporal bone* may be the site of monostotic, less frequently, of polyostotic fibrous dysplasia. The patient complains of a progressive hearing loss caused by increasing narrowing of the external auditory meatus. Less commonly, the size of the temporal bone may be increased by a painless flat or spherical postauricular swelling, or by an intracranial space-

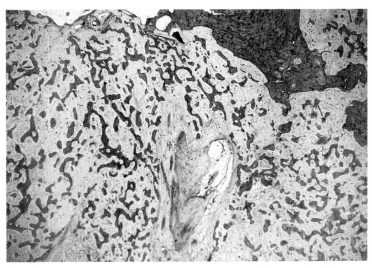

Figure 4.42 Fibrous dysplasia of the mastoid process (Hallpike collection H 236) diagnosed as fibrosarcoma. Microscopy shows a dense network of newly formed bony trabeculae within dense fibrous tissue. Presented clinically as massive tumour-like enlargement of the mastoid process

occupying mass (Nager, Kennedy and Kopstein, 1982). Stenosis of the external auditory meatus may reform after surgical treatment.

A patient with massive fibrous dysplasia of the temporal bone mistaken for an osteoma was described by Chatterji (1974). Fibrous dysplasia of the mastoid process was described by Friedmann and Arnold (1993). The patient was a young woman whose principal complaint was unusually severe pain in and around the ear. On examination, the cortex of the mastoid process and the attic were found to consist of soft bone displaying, microscopically, a dense network of newly formed bony trabeculae in dense fibrous tissue (see Figure 4.42).

Fibrous dysplasia is a benign process. The fibroblasts of the fibrous component appear to be comparatively uniform in size and shape and there are only scant mitoses to be seen. The ratio of fibrous tissue to bone varies from case to case and from site to site in the same lesion (Fu and Perzin, 1974). Occasional cases of malignant transformation have been reported; usually after radiotherapy (Schwartz and Alpert, 1964). Another type of fibrous dysplasia is characterized by disseminated and extraskeletal manifestations; the McCune-Albright syndrome (McCune, 1936; Albright *et al.*, 1937). Clinically skin pigmentation and various endocrine disorders such as pubertas praecoz and hyperthyroidism may be associated with the lesions.

Osteopetrosis (*marble bone disease or Albers-Schonberg disease*)

Osteopetrosis as described by Jaffe (1972) is a rare heritable disorder of the bony skeleton characterized by enhanced bone density and brittleness while the medullary spaces are obliterated by osteocartilaginous trabeculae.

There are two types of osteopetrosis: osteopetrosis fetalis leading to early death (malignant type) and osteopetrosis tarda adult-type osteopetrosis (Milroy and Michaels, 1990).

Histopathology

The abnormality is caused by a failure of adult bone formation and the failure of resorption or replacement of primitive bone. Myers and Stool (1969) examined the temporal bones of a $2\frac{1}{2}$-year-old Negro girl who died of the sequelae of osteopetrosis (anaemia and pulmonary haemorrhage). Sections of the temporal bones showed that the enchondral layer was most severely affected and there was bony obliteration of the mastoid air cell system. There were no inner ear changes attributable directly to the abnormal bone.

Recurrent progressive facial palsy and deafness are frequently encountered (Hamersma, 1970; Hawke, Jahn and Bailey, 1981). Acute recurrent attacks of facial palsy identical with Bell's palsy usually start in childhood. The disease is probably the result of a congenital metabolic disorder of bone resulting in a failure of resorption of cartilage and mature bone. Milroy and Michaels (1990) described a 62-year-old woman with benign adult-type osteopetrosis. She died of chronic renal failure. At autopsy, her bones were found to be densely sclerotic. The skull was greatly thickened and the sclerotic vertebrae contained only small foci of bone marrow.

Microscopy showed an increased number of calcified

globuli interossei in the otic capsule (Figures 4.43 and 4.44). The ossicles were thickened and fixation of the stapes contributed to the patient's hearing loss – the prominent clinical feature in this patient's history. There was bone deposition in the narrowed mastoid air cells and the eustachian tube was narrowed on both sides. The narrowing of the internal auditory meatus on both sides may have accounted for a degree of sensorineural hearing loss. The aetiology has remained obscure and it is debatable whether there is overproduction of bone or reduced absorption of the bone tissue.

Bonucci, Sartori and Spina (1975) reported the results of an electron microscopic and biochemical study of costochondral biopsies from a male baby with osteopetrosis fetalis. There was an increased zone of degenerated chondrocytes filled with large vacuoles formed by degenerated mitochondria. The structure of the osteoclasts was abnormal and their brush border either absent or excessively developed. The intracellular acid phosphatase activity was enhanced, a characteristic function of osteoclasts in osteopetrosis.

Bonucci, Sartori and Spina (1975) suggested that osteopetrosis is the result of the combined effect of degenerated chondrocytes, delayed calcification of the matrix and the reduced rate of absorption of the bone tissue by abnormal osteoclasts.

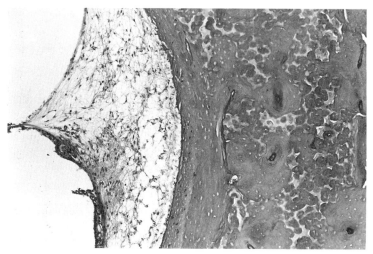

Figure 4.43 Osteopetrosis of the temporal bone. Note the calcified globuli interossei in the enchondral layer of the otic capsule. The endosteal layer is normal. (By courtesy of Dr C. H. Milroy)

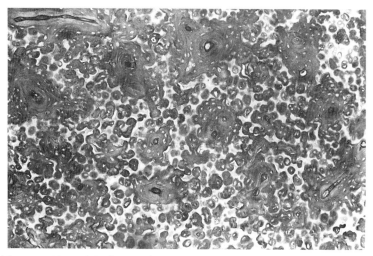

Figure 4.44 Detail of the case in Figure 4.43 showing the vast number of calcified globuli

Idiopathic histiocytosis (also called non-lipoid histiocytosis, histiocytosis X or, more recently, Langerhans histiocytosis)

This non-committal title describes a triad of diseases: Letterer-Siwe disease, Hand-Schuller-Christian disease and eosinophilic granuloma of bone. All have in common focal accumulations or large macrophages in various organs. These diseases have attracted a great deal of attention among otolaryngologists, in particular eosinophilic granuloma.

Eosinophilic granuloma of the temporal bone

Extensive surveys have been published by Druss (1936), Goodhill (1950), Kelemen (1960) and Tos (1966). More recent reports include a review of 22 cases from the Mayo Clinic (McGaffrey and McDonald, 1979).

Incidence

Toohill, Kidder and Eby (1973) reviewed the literature between 1952 and 1972, and found 13 reported cases; to these they added three of their own – among that total, five had bilateral temporal bone involvement. Levy, Sarfaty and Schindel (1980) reported five more cases with bilateral bone involvement. McGaffrey and McDonald (1979) reviewed 22 patients seen at the Mayo Clinic between 1926 and 1978. Fradis, Podoshin and Ben-David (1989) described four children of Bedouin and Druz ethnic origin with eosinophilic granuloma.

Eighteen of 62 children diagnosed with Langerhans' cell histiocytosis at the Children's Hospital of Pittsburgh between 1970 and 1986 demonstrated ear and temporal bone involvement. In six children, such otological disease was their sole presenting manifestation (Cunningham *et al.*, 1989).

Clinical features

Solitary eosinophilic granuloma presents with symptoms and signs which may be interpreted as chronic otitis media. There is discharge from the ear, and polypoid granulations may be found in the external auditory meatus. In other cases, the granuloma presents as a painful, bony swelling infiltrating the postauricular area when it has to be distinguished from a malignant neoplasm. Radiologically, an area of destruction may be noted. To the naked eye, the lesion is usually a circumscribed soft, yellowish brown mass, thus accounting for the punched out appearance on X-ray.

Histopathology

The microscopical picture shows characteristic features in varying proportions. Eosinophils are always present either as a diffuse infiltrate or as more localized mases and noteworthy is the relative maturity of these cells. Interspersed are larger cells with large pale-staining, ovoid or indented nuclei, while cytoplasmic boundaries show variable definition, some cells being sharply delineated while others present a syncytial appearance (Friedmann and Osborn, 1982).

Aetiology and pathogenesis

The cause of the condition is completely unknown and attempts to link it with Schuller-Christian syndrome and Letterer-Siwe disease has confused rather than elucidated the problem. The common feature of histiocytic infiltration hardly justifies the concept of a unified pathology. Eosinophilic infiltration is a more prominent feature in the granuloma, but it also represents a reaction to a variety of aetiological agents and is, therefore, somewhat lacking in specificity.

Most cases of eosinophilic granuloma remain solitary but may cause local bone destruction giving rise to a clinical and radiological impression of a malignant tumour. Eosinophilic granuloma is radiosensitive and has a good prognosis.

Sensorineural deafness and otosclerosis

Large otosclerotic foci may reach the cochlea and damage the spiral ligament. Kelemen and Linthicum (1969) suggested a correlation between the atrophy of the spiral ligament and the extent of the sensorineural hearing loss, subsequently confirmed by others. Schuknecht and Barber (1985) have cast doubt on the significance of the involvement of the cochlear endosteum on inner ear function. However, they reported one case where they accept that otosclerosis has resulted in sensorineural deafness without stapes fixation. The otosclerotic inner ear syndrome, as described by McCabe (1966) consists of vertigo and unilateral conductive deafness. It is probably caused by the biochemical alteration of the perilymph by an otosclerotic lesion reaching the endosteal layer at a site in the pars superior of the labyrinth as confirmed by Ghorayer and Linthicum (1978).

The venous shunts first described by Ruedi in 1968 are abnormal vascular connections between the veins of the membranous labyrinth and the vascular spaces in active otosclerotic foci and in Paget's disease. The resultant venous congestion may damage the inner ear.

The pathogenesis of otosclerosis has remained unresolved but modern immunohistochemical methods have shown that otosclerotic bone may contain the antigens of the paramyxoviruses measles and mumps and also of the rubella virus (Table 4.8). This raises the question whether infections with these viruses in childhood may predispose the individual to otosclerosis later in life (Friedmann and Arnold, 1993).

Immunology

Immunological mechanisms play an aetiological role in ear diseases, many of which have been considered to be of idiopathic nature (Veldman, 1987; Arnold, Altermatt and Gebbers, 1984). Various cellular constituents of the immune system, as well as immunoglobulins, have been identified within the inner ear, suggesting that it may possess an active immune system. While it is possible that many of the idiopathic diseases will eventually prove not to be immunologically mediated, the result of the intensive investigation carried out will assist in a better understanding of some of the basic mechanisms of host immunity involved in ear disease (Gloddeck and Harris, 1989; Veldman, Harada and Meeliwsen, 1993).

Pathology of the ear in autoimmune disease

Organ-specific autoimmune disease of the inner ear is difficult to diagnose. McCabe in 1979 reported the first series of patients with progressive bilateral sensorineural hearing loss that have responded well to immunosuppressive treatment. The diagnosis of autoimmune disease of the inner ear has been based on a correlation of clinical findings, laboratory tests and the response to steroid or immunosuppressive treatment.

The external and middle ear may be involved in relapsing polychondritis, Wegener's granuloma, polyarteritis nodosa. The inner ear may be severely affected in polyarteritis nodosa associated with Cogan's syndrome. Other autoimmune diseases affecting the inner ear are: relapsing polychondritis, giant cell arteritis, sarcoidosis, lupus erythematosus.

Schuknecht (1991) described the histopathological findings in the temporal bones of a man of 55 who had suffered with periods of vertigo and progressive hearing loss for several years. He had been treated with steroids because an underlying immunological process had been suspected, but died in his sixty-third year. The temporal bones showed extensive destruction of the tissues of the inner ear, including the sensory elements, their supporting structures and of the membranous labyrinth (Figure 4.45). Scattered perivascular mononuclear infiltrates (Figure 4.46) and free-floating aggregations of these cells were noted. The diagnosis of autoimmune disease was based on the exclusion of viral labyrinthitis, Ménière's disease, sudden deafness and other known causes.

Polyarteritis nodosa

Polyarteritis nodosa is a systemic vasculitis affecting the small and medium-sized muscular arteries at their sites of bifurcation, causing segmental necrosis and inflammatory changes in all the layers of the arterial wall. Sensorineural hearing loss may be, though rarely, the presenting condition (Friedmann and Arnold, 1993). The temporal bone findings were first described by Druss and Maybaum in 1934 as early vascular lesions in the smaller arterioles of the bone marrow of the petrous pyramid; other vessels displayed subendothelial proliferation and fibrinoid necrosis occasionally with aneurysmal dilatation.

The second description of the histopathological findings in the temporal bone has been credited to Rossle (1937) who described characteristic polyarteritis nodosa-like changes in the mucosa of the middle ear. Gussen in 1977 described the histopathological findings in the temporal bone of a 66-year-old woman who became deaf 7 months before her death caused by polyarteritis nodosa. The left internal auditory artery showed polyarteritis nodosa lesions and there was fibrosis and ossification in the labyrinth. Another case of polyarteritis nodosa was described by Jenkins, Pollack and Fisch (1981) in a 48-year-old man who developed sudden deafness.

An interesting combination of pathological lesions was described by Adkins and Ward (1986) in a 60-

Table 4.8 Immunohistochemistry of footplate otosclerosis *versus* osteogenesis imperfecta, postinflammatory footplate sclerosis and normal footplate

Stapes footplate	IgG	IgM	IgA	IgD	Measles	Rubella	Mumps
Otosclerosis							
Resorptive stage	+ + +	+ +	+ +	−	+ + +	+ + +	+ + +
Sclerotic stage	+ +	−	(+)	−	+ (+)	+ (+)	+ (+)
Osteogenesis imperfecta	+ + +	+ +	+ +	−	+ + +	+ + +	+ + +
Postinflammatory sclerosis	+ +	−	−	−	−	−	−
Normal	−	−	−	−	−	−	−

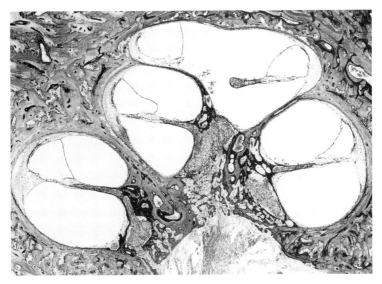

Figure 4.45 Autoimmune disease causing hearing loss. There was extensive degeneration of the inner ear including the sensory elements and their supporting structures

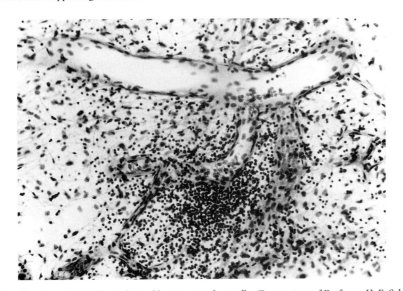

Figure 4.46 Scattered perivascular infiltrate formed by mononuclear cells. (By courtesy of Professor H. F. Schuknecht)

year-old man with well-documented hearing loss, who had classical polyarteritis nodosa, rheumatoid arthritis and bilateral otosclerosis. Autopsy revealed an occult schwannoma of the VIIIth nerve. There was extensive polyarteritis nodosa of the arteries of the facial canal and in the geniculate ganglion.

Wegener's granuloma of the ear

The ear is frequently affected by Wegener's granu-loma in particular of the 'limited' type (Friedmann

and Bauer, 1973; Friedmann and Arnold, 1993). Hearing loss, of a mixed conductive and sensory type, may bring the patient to medical attention. There have been many reports about patients whose otological symptoms and signs appeared to be the first manifestation of Wegener's granulomatosis (Friedmann and Bauer, 1973; Calonius and Chris-tensen, 1980; McGaffrey, McDonald and Pacer, 1980; Friedmann and Arnold, 1993). A valuable serological test employing an antineutrophil cytoplasmic antigen (ANCA) has proved less specific but should be carried out on all suspected cases (Rasmussen and Wilk, 1955; Kempf, 1989; Wackym, Mamas and McCabe. 1993; Carrie, Hughes and Watson, 1994).

Experimental autoimmune labyrinthitis

The time course of hearing impairment and cellular infiltration into the inner ear was studied by Yamanobe and Harris (1992) after systemic sensitization of guinea-pigs with a single intradermal injection of bovine inner ear antigen (IEAg) in complete Freund's adjuvant (CFA). Lymphocytes and polymorphonucleo-cytes appeared mainly in the scala tympani on days 7–14, and in addition there was thickening and cellular infiltration of the round window membrane at day 14. These cellular infiltrations resolved after day 28. Some sensitized animals ($n = 5$) had spontaneous remissions after day 28; however, the hearing thresholds did not completely recover. The authors noted that 'clearance of the cochlear cellular infiltration and improved hearing thresholds can occur spontaneously'.

There is some evidence for a passage of antibodies from the middle ear into the perilymph. Harris and Ryan (1984) have suggested that the perilymph communicating with the cerebrospinal fluid is 'a lymphatic of sorts' and have referred to the endolymphatic sac as a possible source of antibody producing cells, as shown by Rask-Anderson and Stahle (1980) and of immunoglobulins (Arnold, Altermatt and Gebbers, 1984).

The perilymph contains IgG and Harris *et al.* believe that the inner ear has immunological functions including autoimmunity, as confirmed experimentally by Gloddek and Harris (1993).

Ulcerative colitis and hearing loss

The association of inflammatory bowel disease and autoimmune disorders including autoimmune sensorineural deafness is well documented (Summers and Harker, 1982; Weber, Jenkins and Coker, 1984; Dowd and Rees, 1987; Jacob *et al.*, 1990).

The precise aetiology of sensorineural deafness in ulcerative colitis remains unclear, though in some patients there is evidence of an immune complex vasculitis (Kanzaki and Oguchi, 1983).

Hirschsprung's disease and hearing loss

Congenital deafness has been described in a small number of patients with Hirschsprung's disease. In none of these patients has this association been familial (McKusick, 1973; Lowry, 1975). However, Weinberg, Currarino and Besserman (1977) described a family with deafness associated with Hirschsprung's disease in three consecutive generations. Enhanced susceptibility to ototoxic drugs has been incriminated in some patients as the cause of deafness (Lowry, 1975).

Miscellaneous infectious and neoplastic causes of hearing loss

Purulent labyrinthitis complicating acute or chronic otitis media and purulent meningitis can cause partial or total ossification of the cochlea (Figures 4.47, 4.48 and 4.49).

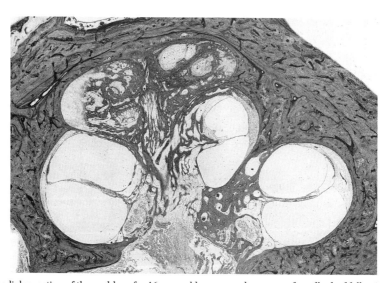

Figure 4.47 Midmodiolar section of the cochlea of a 46-year-old woman who was profoundly deaf following meningitis at the age of 3 years. There is severe atrophy of the auditory sense organ and the apical region of the cochlea is obliterated by fibrous tissue and bone. (By courtesy of Professor H. F. Shuknecht and Professor L. Ruedi)

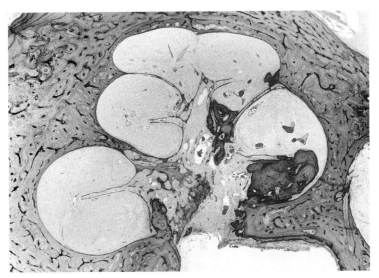

Figure 4.48 The cochlea of a 22-year-old woman suffering with systemic lupus erythematosus and chronic serous otitis media. Microscopy shows the membranous structures to be missing. There is a great deal of patchy ossification present. There is a total loss of ganglion cells. (By courtesy of Dr M. M. Paparella)

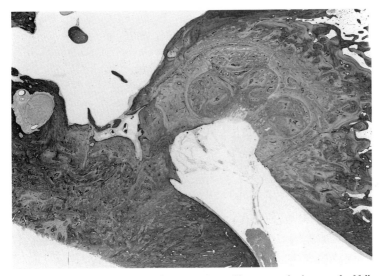

Figure 4.49 Midmodiolar section of the temporal bone from a 74-year-old woman who became deaf following meningitis. Microscopy shows a normal intact otic capsule surrounding the completely ossified cochlea. Labyrinthitis ossificans following meningitis. (By courtesy of Dr M. M. Paparella)

Schwannoma of the VIIIth nerve may form satellite tumours in the cochlea (Figure 4.50). It may cause degeneration of the inner ear by obstruction of the vascular circulation in the internal auditory meatus (Schuknecht, 1974; Suga and Lindsay, 1976b).

Various malignant neoplasms can spread to the cochlea, e.g. rhabdomyosarcoma, paraganglioma, malignant melanoma or lymphoma. Leukaemic deposits may occur.

The so-called acoustic neuroma is a misnomer.

The precise histopathological term is vestibular schwannoma as it most commonly arises from the Schwann cells of the vestibular branch of the VIIIth cranial nerve. Strictly speaking a 'neuroma' is a non-neoplastic overgrowth of perineural fibres, Schwann cells and scar tissue.

The temporal bone and the ear may be the site of secondary neoplasms (Figure 4.51) and may be directly invaded along the facial nerve or the eustachian tube by a growth in the pyriform fossa or in

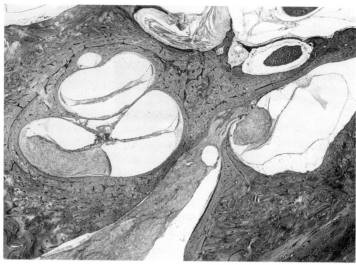

Figure 4.50 Schwannoma in the cochlea and vestibule

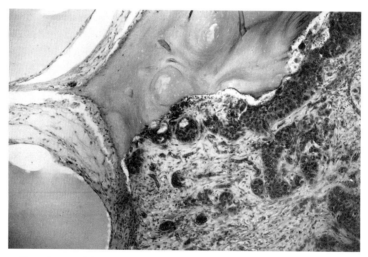

Figure 4.51 Squamous cell carcinoma of the middle ear invading the otic capsule. Note osteoclasts forming the advance guard – characteristic Carter-phenomenon in neoplastic invasion of bone

the nasopharyngeal region. Secondary neoplasms of the ear are more common than the number of published cases would indicate, partly because of the pathologists' lack of interest in the apparently barren regions of the temporal bone.

Intracochlear implants

Cochlear implants have been widely used in the treatment of acquired or congenital hearing loss.

However, careful selection of suitable patients is essential so as to avoid disappointment. Gray *et al.* (1991) reported three patients in whom ultra high resolution CT was of great assistance in the pre- and postoperative management of these patients. Imaging of the petrous temporal bones as developed at the Royal National Throat and Nose Hospital by Phelps and Lloyd (1990) has been mandatory for any patient who is being considered for an intracochlear implant (Phelps, 1992).

Structural deformities of the inner ear are often

associated with profound and progressive hearing loss. Bony irregularities of the cochlear duct such as partial or complete bony obliteration make full insertion of a multichannel electrode impossible. There were 14% such cases in a series by Balkany, Gantz and Nadol (1988), and 28% of selected patients in the series of Harnsberger *et al.* (1987).

Cochlear implants in children may face some anatomical difficulties. Although the cochlea is of adult size at birth, the mastoid in contrast is small, soft and still growing, making it difficult to anchor the implanted electronics (O'Donoghue, 1992).

Histopathology

Johnsson, House and Linthicum (1979) and Larsen *et al.* (1982) have described cochlear lesions in a patient implanted for several years (Johnsson, House and Linthicum, 1979).

The potential histopathological changes resulting from intracochlear implants have been studied on various experimental animal models. Perforation of the round window membrane can cause endothelial lesions in the scala membrane, followed by fibrosis and ossification. The osseous spiral lamina and the basal lamina may be damaged (Schindler and Bjorkroth, 1979; Miller and Sutton, 1980; Pfingst *et al.*, 1981; Sutton *et al.*, 1983).

Simmons, Schuknecht and Smith (1986) have examined the temporal bones from a 57-year-old man deafened 6 years before by neomycin and implanted with four electrodes 5 years before his death. Only the right temporal bone was available and microscopy showed the empty tract of the electrodes lined by fibrous tissue containing a small number of foreign-body giant cells. Two of the electrodes had reached the internal auditory meatus. There was some fibrous tissue and new bone formation in the scala tympani of the basal coil.

The potential histopathological changes have been studied on experimental animal models (Simmons, 1979). It was noted that electrical stimulation may cause degenerative changes not only in the surrounding connective tissue but also in the nerves and affect eventually the central nervous system of experimental animals.

Most of the potential lesions have been minimized in human patients by the application of modern surgical methods and improved electrodes.

Acknowledgements

The excellent secretarial work of Mrs Jeanette Suckling (formerly at the Clinical Research Centre) is gratefully acknowledged. The late Tony Frolich contributed many of the best illustrations enhancing the quality of the chapter.

References

ADKINS, W. Y. and WARD, P. H. (1986) Temporal bone showing polyarteritis nodosa, otosclerosis and occult neurinoma. *Laryngoscope*, **96**, 645–653

ALBRIGHT, F., BUTLER, A. M., HAMPTON, A. C. and SMITH, P. (1937) Syndrome characterized by osteitis fibrosa disseminata, areas of pigmentation and endocrine dysfunction with precocious puberty in females. Report of 5 cases. *New England Journal of Medicine*, **216**, 727–746

ALEXANDER, W. S. (1966) Phytanic acid in Refsum's syndrome. *Journal of Neurology, Neurosurgery and Psychiatry*, **29**, 412–416

ALFORD, C. A. JR, NEVA, F. A. and WELLER, T. H. (1964) Virologic and serologic studies on human products of conception after maternal rubella. *New England Journal of Medicine*, **271**, 1275–1281

ALPORT, A. C. (1927) Hereditary familial congenital haemorrhagic nephritis. *British Medical Journal*, **1**, 504–505

ALTMANN, F. (1962) The temporal bone in osteogenesis imperfecta congenita. *Archives of Otolaryngology*, **75**, 486–497

ANDERSON, H. C. (1969) Vesicles associated with calcification in the matrix of epiphyseal cartilage. *Journal of Cell Biology*, **41**, 59–72

ANNIKO, M. (1976a) Atoxyl-induced damage to the sensory cells in the organ of Corti in the guinea-pig cochlea. *Virchows Archiv B. Cell Pathology*, **21**, 267–277

ANNIKO, M. (1976b) Surface structure of the vascular stria in the guinea-pig cochlea. Normal morphology and atoxyl-induced pathological changes. *Acta Otolaryngologica*, **82**, 343–353

ANNIKO, M. and WERSALL, J. (1976) Afferent and efferent nerve terminal degeneration in the guinea-pig cochlea following atoxyl administration. *Acta Otolaryngologica*, **82**, 325–336

ARNOLD, W. (1980) Uberlegungen zur Pathogenese der cochleorenalen Syndrome. *Acta Otolaryngologica*, **89**, 330–341

ARNOLD, W. (1984) Inner ear and renal disease. *Annals of Otology, Rhinology and Laryngology*, **93**, 119–123

ARNOLD, W. and FRIEDMANN, I. (1988) Otosclerosis – an inflammatory disease of the otic capsule of viral aetiology. *Journal of Laryngology and Otology*, **102**, 865–871

ARNOLD, W. and WEIDAUER, W. (1975) Experimental studies on the pathogenesis of inner ear disturbances in renal disease. *Archiv für Oto-Rhino-Laryngologie*, **211**, 217–221

ARNOLD, W. ALTERMATT, N. I. and GEBBERS, J. O. (1984) Qualitativer Nachweis von Immunoglobulinen im menschliche Saccus endolymphaticus. *Laryngologie, Rhinologie and Otologie*, **63**, 464–467

ARNOLD, W. and WEIDAUER, W. and SEELIG, H. P. (1976) Experimenteller Beweis einer gemeinsamen Antigenizitat zwischen Innenohr und Niere. *Archives of Otorhinolaryngology*, **212**, 99–117

ASHERSON, N. (1979) Du Verney's 'Traité de l'organe de l'ouie'. *Journal of Laryngology and Otology*, **93**, Supplement 2, 1–110

BALKANY, T., GANTZ, B. and NADOL, J. B. (1988) Multichannel cochlear implants in partially ossified cochleas. *Annals of Otology, Rhinology and Laryngology*, **97**, 3–7

BALLANTYNE, J. C. (1971) *Deafness*, 2nd edn. London: Churchill

BARKER, D., HOSTIKKA, S. L., ZHOU, J., CHOW, L., OLIPHANT, A. R., GERKIN, S. L. *et al.*, (1990) Identification of mutations in the Col 4A5 collagen gene in Alport's syndrome. *Science*, **248**, 1224–1227

BAUZE, R. J., SMITH, R. and FRANCIS, M. J. O. (1975) A new look at osteogenesis imperfecta. *Journal of Bone and Joint Surgery*, **59B**, 2–12

BEAGLEY, H. A. (1965) Acoustic trauma in the guinea pig. II. Electron microscopy including the morphology of cell junctions in the organ of Corti. *Acta Otolaryngologica*, **60**, 479–495

BEAL, D. D., DAVEY, P. R. and LINDSAY, J. R. (1967) Inner ear pathology of congenital deafness. *Archives of Otolaryngology*, **55**, 134–142

BEIGHTON, P. (1990) Hereditary deafness In: *Principles and Practice of Medical Genetics*, edited by A. E. H. Emery and D. L. Rimoin. Vol. 1. London: Churchill Livingstone. pp. 733–748

BELLUCCI, R. J. GROBEISEN, B. and SAH, B. C. (1974) Bilateral suden deafness in Cogan's syndrome. *Bulletin of the New York Academy of Medicine*, **50**, 672–681

BERGSTROM, L. and THOMPSPON, P. (1983) Hearing loss in pediatric renal patients. *International Journal of Pediatric Otorhinolaryngology*, **5**, 227–234

BERGSTROM, L., JENKINS, R., SANDO, I. and ENGLISH, G. M. (1973) Hearing loss in renal disease: clinical and pathological studies. *Annals of Otology, Rhinology and Laryngology*, **82**, 555–574

BERGSTROM, L., THOMPSON, P., SANDO, I. and WOOD, R. (1980) Renal disease – its pathology, treatment and effects on the ear. *Archives of Otolaryngology*, **106**, 567–572

BICKERSTAFF, D. R., DOUGLAS, D. L., BURKE, P. H., O'DOHERTY, D. P. and KANIS, J. A. (1990) Improvement in deformity of the face in Paget's disease treated with diphosphonates. *Journal of Bone and Joint Surgery*, **72B**, 132–136

BILGIN, H., KASEMSHWAN, L., SCHACHERN, P. A., PAPARECMA, H. M. and LE CHAP, T. (1996) Temporal bone study of Down's syndrome. *Archives of Otolaryngology – Head and Neck Surgery*, **122**, 271–275

BIRZGALIS, A. R., RAMSDEN R. T., FARRINGTON W. T. and SMALL M. (1993) Severe radionecrosis of the temporal bone. *Journal of Laryngology and Otology*, **107**, 185–187

BLACKLEY, J. B., FRIEDMANN, I. and WRIGHT, I. M. (1967) Herpes zoster oticus with facialis nerve palsy and auditory nerve symptoms. *Acta Otolaryngologica*, **63**, 533–550

BOHNE, B. A. (1976) Mechanisms of noise damage in the inner ear. In: *Effects of Noise on Hearing*, edited by D. Henderson, R. P. Hamernik, D. S. Dosanjh and J. H. Mills. New York: Raven Press. pp. 41–68

BOHNE, B. A., MARKS, J. E. and GLASGOW, G. P. (1985) Delayed effects of ionizing radiation on the ear. *Laryngoscope*, **95**, 818–828

BONUCCI, E., SARTORI, E and SPINA, M. (1975) Osteopetrosis fetalis. Report on a case with special reference to ultrastructure. *Virchow's Archiv A Pathologische Anatomie*, **368**, 109–121

BORDLEY, J. E. and HARDY, J. M. B. (1969) Laboratory and clinical observations on prenatal rubella. *Annals of Otology, Rhinology and Laryngology*, **78**, 917–928

BORDLEY, J. E. and KAPUR, Y. P. (1977) Histopathologic changes in the temporal bone resulting from measles infection. *Archives of Otolaryngology*, **103**, 162–168

BORDLEY, J. E., BROOKHAUSER, P. E., HARDY, J. and HARDY, W. G. (1968) Prenatal rubella. *Acta Otolaryngologica*, **66**, 1–9

BREDBERG, G. (1967) The human cochlea during development and ageing. *Journal of Laryngology and Otology*, **81**, 739–758

BRIEDENKAMP, J. K., SMITH, M. E., DUDLEY, J. P., WILLIAMS, J. D., GRUNLEY, H. L. and CROCKETT, D. M. (1992) Otolaryngologic manifestations of the mucopolysaccharidoses. *Annals of Otology, Rhinology and Laryngology*, **101**, 472–478

BRITISH MEDICAL JOURNAL (1987) Child abuse and osteogenesis imperfecta. **295**, 1082–1087

BRITTON, T. C. and GIBBERD, F. B. (1988) A family with heredopathia atactica polyneuritiformis (Refsum's disease). *Journal of the Royal Society of Medicine*, **81**, 602–603

BRONSON, E. (1917) Fragilitas osseum and its association with blue sclera and otosclerosis. *Edinburgh Medical Journal*, **16**, 240–281

BROOKES, G. B. and BOOTH, J. B. (1987) Diseases of the temporal bone. In: *Scott-Brown's Otolaryngology*, 5th edn., edited by A. G. Kerr, Vol. 3 Otology, edited by J. B. Booth. London: Butterworths. pp. 360–380

BROOKHAUSER, P. E. and BORDLEY, J. F. (1973) Congenital rubella deafness: pathology and pathogenesis. *Archives of Otolaryngology*, **98**, 252–257

BROSNAN, M., BURNS, H., JAHN, A. F. and HAWKE, M. (1977) Surgery and histopathology of the stapes in osteogenesis imperfecta tarda. *Archives of Otolaryngology*, **103**, 294–298

BROWN, D. M. (1973) Collagen metabolism in fibroblasts from patients with osteogenesis imperfecta. In:*Clinical Aspects of Metabolic Bone Diseases*. edited by B. Frame. Amsterdam: Excerpta Medica. pp. 303–307

BUFFE, P., CUDENNEC, I. F., BEN AZZOUZ, M. B., BASSOUMI, T. and FEMENON, J. J. (1986) Enquete sur la nuisance de l'ecoute de la musique au casque. *Annales d'Oto-laryngologie (Paris)*, **103**, 351–355

BYERS, P. H., BARSH, G. S. and HOLBROOK, K. A. (1982) Molecular pathology in inherited disorders of collagen metabolism. *Human Pathology*, **13**, 89–95

CALONIUS, I. H. and CHRISTENSEN, C. K. (1980) Hearing impairment and facial palsy as initial signs of Wegener's granulomatosis. *Journal of Laryngology and Otology*, **94**, 649–657

CAMPBELL, A. M. C. and WILLIAMS, E. R. (1967) Natural history of Refsum's syndrome in a Gloucestershire family. *British Medical Journal*, **3**, 777–779

CARRIE, S., HUGHES, K. B. and WATSON, M. G. (1994) Negative ANCA in Wegener's granulomatosis. *Journal of Laryngology and Otology*, **108**, 420–422

CELIS-BLAUBACH, A., GARCIA-ZOZAYA, J. L., PEREZ-REQUEJO, J. L. and BRESSE, K. (1974) Vestibular disorders in Alport's syndrome. *Journal of Laryngology and Otology*, **88**, 663–674

CHAMBERS, T. J. (1988) *The Regulation of Osteoclastic Development and Function in Cell and Molecular Biology of Vertebrate Hard Tissues*. Chichester: Wiley, (Ciba Foundation Symposium 136) pp. 92–107

CHATTERJI, P. (1974) Massive fibrous dysplasia of the temporal bone. *Journal of Laryngology and Otology*, **88**, 179–183

CHESON, B. D., BLUMING, A. Z. and ALROY, J. (1976) Cogan's syndrome: a systemic vasculitis. *American Journal of Medicine*, **60**, 549–555

CHO, H., SAKAMOTO, H., HACHIKAWA, K. and NAKAI, Y. (1991) Electron microscope observations on the communication between inner ear stereocilia under normal and noise-stimulated conditions. *Acta Otolaryngologica*, Supplement 486, 13–18

COCKAYNE, E. A. (1936) Gargoylism (Chondro-osteodystrophy, Hepatosplenomegaly, Deafness) in Two Brothers. *Proceedings of the Royal Society of Medicine*, **30**, 104–107

CODY, D. T. R. and WILLIAMS, H. L. (1960) Cogan's syndrome. *Laryngoscope*, **70**, 447–478

COGAN, D. G. (1945) Syndrome of nonsyphilitic interstitial keratitis and vestibulo-auditory symptoms. *Archives of Ophthalmology*, **33**, 144–149

COLES, R. R. A. (1986) Development, characteristics and effects of noise-induced hearing loss (NIHL.). In a lecture to the Section of Otology of the Royal Society of Medicine

COLLINS, D. H. and WINN, J. M. (1955) Focal Paget's disease of the skull (osteoporosis circumscripta). *Journal of Pathology and Bacteriology*, **69**, 1–9

CORTI, A. (1851) Recherches sur l'organe de l'ouie. *Zeitschrift für Wissenschaftliche Zoologie*, **3**, 109–169 (reproduced by H. I. Wullstein)

CRAWFURD, D'A. (1961) Multiple congenital anomalies associated with an extra chromosome. *Lancet*, ii, 22–24

CRAWFURD, M. D'A. (1988) Nephritis with deafness (Alport's syndrome). In: *The Genetics of Renal Tract Disorders*. Oxford Monographs on Medical Genetics. No. 14. Oxford: Oxford University Press

CROW, J., GIBBS, D. A., COZENS, W., SPELLACY, E. and WATTS, R. W. E. (1983) Biochemical and histopathological studies on patients with mucopolysaccharidoses, two of whom have been treated with fibroblast transplantation. *Journal of Clinical Pathology*, **36**, 415–430

CUDENNEC, Y. F., DE ROTALIER, P., AUBERT, C., COHAT, J. P., BEN AZZOUZ, M. and BUFFE, P. (1986) Fulguration d'oreille, *Annales d'Oto-laryngologie (Paris)* **103**, 343–349

CUNNINGHAM, M. J., CURTIN, H. D., JAFFE, R. and STOOL, S. E. (1989) Otologic manifestations of Langerhans' cell histiocytosis. *Archives of Otolaryngology Head and Neck Surgery*, **115**, 807–813

DAGGETT, W. I. (1946) Discussion on war deafness and the care of deafened ex-servicemen. *Proceedings of the Royal Society of Medicine*, February, 508–516

DAVIS, G. L. (1979) Congenital cytomegalovirus infection and hearing loss: clinical and experimental observations. *Laryngoscope*, **89**, 1681–1688

DAVIS, G. L. (1981) In vitro models of virus-induced congenital deafness. *American Journal of Otology*, **3**, 156–160

DAVIS, G. L. and STRAUSS, M. (1973) Viral disease of the labyrinth II. An experimental model using the mouse cytomegalovirus. *Annals of Otology, Rhinology and Laryngology*, **82**, 584–593

DAVIS, L. E., RAREY, K. E. and MCLAREN, L. C. (1995) Clinical viral infections and histologic temporal bone studies of patients with AIDS. *Otolaryngology – Head and Neck Surgery*, **113**, 695–701

DAVIS, W. A. (1947) Typhus at Belsen, control of the typhus epidemic. *American Journal of Hygiene*, **46**, 66–83

DE GROOT, J. C. M. J. (1989) Cell biological aspects of gentamicin cochleootoxicity. MD-Thesis. University of Utrecht, OMI Utrecht

DEKABAN, A. S. (1968) Abnormalities in children exposed to X-ray irradiation during various stages of gestation: tentative timetable of radiation injury to the human fetus. Part I. *Journal of Nuclear Medicine*, **9**, 422–477

DESHMUKH, D. R., MASSAB, H. F. and MASON, M. (1982) Interaction of aspirin and other potential etiologic factors in an animal model for Rye's syndrome. *Proceedings of the National Academy of Science*, **79**, 7557–7660

DICK, J. F. R., GIBBERD, F. B., MEERAN, K. and ROSE, C. F. (1993) Hyperkalaemia in acute Refsum's disease. *Journal of the Royal Society of Medicine*, **86**, 171–172

DICKINS, J. R. S., SMITH, T. J. and GRAHAM, S. S. (1988) Herpes zoster oticus. Treatment with intravenous Acyclovir. *Laryngoscope*, **98**, 776–779

DICKSON, N., MORTIMER, J. G., FAED, J. M., POLLARD, A. C., STYLES, M., PEART, M.D. et al. (1989) A child with Refsum's disease: successful treatment with diet and plasma exchange. *Developmental Medicine and Child Neurology*, **31**, 81–97

DISCHE, F. E., WESTON, M. J. and PARSONS, V. (1985) Abnormally thin glomerular basement membranes associated with haematuria and proteinuria or renal failure in adults. *Journal of Nephrology*, **5**, 103–109

DOWD, A. and REES, W. D. W. (1987) Treatment of sensorineural deafness associated with ulcerative colitis. *British Medical Journal*, **295**, 26

DOWN, J. L. H. (1866) Clinical description of mongolian imbeciles. *Reports of London Hospital*, **3**, 259–263

DRAKE-LEE, A. B. (1992) Beyond music: auditory temporary threshold shift in rock musicians after a heavy metal concert. *Journal of the Royal Society of Medicine*, **85**, 617–619

DRUSS, J. G. (1936) Aural manifestations of lipoid granulomatosis (Hand-Schuller-Christian disease). *Annals of Otology, Rhinology and Laryngology*, **45**, 693–703

DRUSS, J. G. and MAYBAUM, D. L. (1934) Periarteritis nodosa of the temporal bone. *Archives of Otolaryngology*, **19**, 502–507

DUBACH, U. C. and NAGER, G. T. (1965) Familial nephropathy and deafness First observation in a family in Switzerland. *Helvetica Medica Acta*, **12**, 36–43

DU VERNEY, J. G. (1683) Traité de l'organe de l'ouie, contenant la structure, les usages et les maladies de toutes les parties de l'oreille, Paris: E. Michallet. See also Stewart F. F. (1965) J. G. Du Verney (1684–1730) Author of the first scientific account of the ear. *Proceedings of the Royal Society of Medicine*, **58**, 753–755

EDWARDS, J. H., HARNDEN, D. G., CAMERON, A. H., CROSS, V. M. and WOLFF, V. H. (1960) A new trisomic syndrome. *Lancet*, i, 787–790

EKMAN, O. J. (1788) *Descriptio et Casus Aliquot Osteomalaciae Upsaliae*. cf. Bauze, R. J. Edman J. F.

ELWOOD, J. H. (1976) Anencephaly and spina bifida in the British Isles. In: *Birth Defects. Risks and Consequences*, edited by S. Kelly, E. B. Hook, D. T. Janerich and I. H. Porter. New York: Academic Press. pp. 21–39

ENGSTROM, H. D. and ADES, H. W. (1973) Ultrastructure of the cochlea. In: *The Ultrastructure of Animal Tissues and Organs*, Part 2, edited by I. Friedman. Amsterdam: Elsevier. pp. 85–151

EVERBERG, G. (1959) Marfan's syndrome associated with hearing defects. Report of a case in one of a pair of twins. *Acta Paediatrica*, **481**, 70–76

FALK, S. A. (1977) Pathophysiological responses of the auditory system to excessive sound. In: *Handbook of Physiology*, edited by D. H. K. Lee. Chapter 2. Section 9. Reactions to environmental agents. Bethesda, Maryland: American Physiological Society. pp. 17–30

FELL, H. B. (1929) The development in vitro of the isolated otocyst of the embryonic fowl. *Archives für experimentelle Zellforschung*, **7**, 69

FERMIN, C. D. and IGARASHI, M. (1983) Aminoglycoside ototoxicity in the chick inner ear: 1. The effects of kanamycin and netilmicin on the basilar papilla. *American Journal of Otolaryngology*, **4**, 174–183

FLINTER, F. A. CAMERSON, J. S., CHANTLER, C., HOUSTON, I. and BOBROW, M.. (1988) Genetics of classic Alport's syndrome. *Lancet*, ii, 1005–1007

FORGE, A. (1985) Outer hair cell loss and supporting cell expansion following chronic gentamicin treatment. *Hearing Research*, **19**, 171–182

FRADIS, M., PODOSHIN, L. and BEN-DAVID, J. (1989) Eosinophilic granuloma of the temporal bone. *Journal of Laryngology and Otology*, **103**, 435–437

FRAENKEL, E. (1921) Die Haut bei der Fleckfiebererkrankung. In: *Hanbuch der erztlichen Erfahrungen im Weltkriege* **8**, 117–126

FRIEDMANN, I. (1945) Epidemic typhus fever in Eastern Slovakia, Unpublished observations

FRIEDMANN, I. (1956) In vitro culture of the isolated otocyst of the embryonic fowl. *Annals of Otology, Rhinology and Laryngology*, **65**, 98–107

FRIEDMANN, I. (1963) Electron microscopy in the pathology of the ear, nose and throat: experimental and human. In: *The Scientific Basis of Medicine*, British Postgraduate Medical Federation, Annual Reviews. London: Athlone Press. pp. 302–318

FRIEDMANN, I. (1974) *Pathology of the Ear*. Oxford: Blackwell

FRIEDMANN, I. and ARNOLD, W. (1993) *The Pathology of the Ear*, (revised edition). Edinburgh: Churchill Livingstone

FRIEDMANN, I. and BAUER, F. (1973) Wegener's granulomatosis causing deafness. *Journal of Laryngology and Otology*, **87**, 449–464

FRIEDMANN, I. and BIRD, E. S. (1961a) Attachment zones of cells in organ cultures of the isolated fowl embryo otocyst. *Journal of Ultrastructure Research*, **5**, 44–50

FRIEDMANN, I. and BIRD, E. S. (1961b) The effect of ototoxic antibiotics and of penicillin on the sensory areas of the isolated fowl embryo otocyst in organ cultures. *Journal of Pathology and Bacteriology*, **81**, 81–90

FRIEDMANN, I. and BIRD, E. S. (1972) The effect of sodium-cyanide on the chick embryo otocyst in vitro. *Acta Otolaryngologica*, **72**, 280–289

FRIEDMANN, I. and OSBORN, D. A. (1982) *Granulomas and Neoplasms of the Nose and Paranasal Sinuses*. Edinburgh: Churchill Livingstone

FRIEDMANN, I. and WRIGHT, I. M. (1966) Histopathological changes in the foetal and infantile inner ear by maternal rubella. *British Medical Journal*, **2**, 20–23

FRIEDMANN, I., CAWTHORNE, T. and BIRD, E. S. (1965a) Broad-banded striated bodies in the sensory epithelium of the human macula and in neurinoma. *Nature*, **207**, 171–174

FRIEDMANN, I., CAWTHORNE, T. and BIRD, E. S. (1965b) The laminated cytoplasmic inclusions in the sensory epithelium of the human macula. *Ultrastructure Research*, **12**, 92–103

FRIEDMANN, I. DADSWELL, J. V. and BIRD, E. S. (1966) Electron microscope studies of the neuroepithelium of the inner ear in guinea-pigs treated with neomycin. *Journal of Pathology and Bacteriology*, **92**, 415–422

FRIEDMANN, I., FRASER, G. R. and FROGGATT, P. (1966) Pathology of the ear in the cardio-auditory syndrome of Jervell and Lange-Nielsen (recessive deafness with electrocardiographic abnormalities). *Journal of Laryngology and Otology*, **80**, 451–470

FRIEDMANN, I., FROGATT, P. and FRASER, G. R. (1968) Pathology of the ear in the cardio-auditory syndrome Lange-Nielsen and Jervell. *Journal of Laryngology and Otology*, **82**, 883–896

FRIEDMANN, I., FROLICH, A. and WRIGHT, A. (1993) Epidemic typhus fever and hearing loss: a histologic study. *Journal of Laryngology and Otology*, **107**, 275–283

FRIEDMANN, I., HODGES, M. and GRAHAM, M. M. (1980) Tympanosclerosis – an electron microscope study of matrix vesicles. *Annals of Otology, Rhinology and Laryngology*, **89**, 241–245

FRIEDMANN, I., SPELLACY, E., CROW, J. and WATTS, R. W. R. (1985) Histopathological study of the temporal bones in Hurler's disease. *Journal of Laryngology and Otology*, **99**, 29–41

FRIEDMANN, I., WRIGHT, J. W. and PHELPS, P. D. (1980) Temporal bone studies in anencephaly (2). *Journal of Laryngology and Otology*, **94**, 929–944

FU, Y. S. and PERZIN, K. H. (1974) Non-epithelial tumours of the nasal cavity paranasal sinuses and nasopharynx: a clinico-pathological study. II. Osseous and fibroosseous lesions including osteoma, fibrous dysplasia, ossifying fibroma, osteoblastoma, giant cell tumour and osteosarcoma. *Cancer*, **33**, 1289–1305

FUJITA, S. and HAYDEN, R. C. (1969) Alport's syndrome. *Archives of Otolaryngology*, **90**, 453–466

GALICH, R. (1985) Temporal bone involvement in Waardenburg's syndrome. *Ear, Nose and Throat Journal*, **64**, 441–445

GATES, G. A., COBB, J. I. D., D'AGOSTINO, R. B. and WOLF, P. H. A. (1993) The relation of hearing in the elderly to the presence of cardiovascular disease and cardiovascular risk factors. *Archives of Otolaryngology Head and Neck Surgery*, **119**, 156–161

GAUTHIER, B., TRACHTMAN, H., FRANK, R. and WALDERRAMA, L. (1989) Familial thin basement membrane nephropathy in children with asymptomatic microhematuria. *Nephron*, **51**, 502–508

GHORAYER, R. Y. and LINTHICUM, F. H. JR (1978) Otosclerotic inner ear syndrome. *Annals of Otology, Rhinology and Laryngology*, **87**, 85–90

GIBBERD, F. B., BILLIMORIA, J. D., GOLDMAN, J. M. and CLEMENTS, M. E. (1985) Heredopathia atactica polyneuritiformis. *Acta Neurologica Scandinavica*, **72**, 1–17

GLODDEK, B. and HARRIS, J. P. (1989) The role of lymphokines in the immune response of the inner ear. *Acta Otolaryngologica*, **108**, 68–75

GOLDMAN, J. M., CLEMENS, M. E., GIBBERD, F. B. and GILLIMORIA, J. B. (1985) Screening of patients with retinitis pigmentosa for heredopathia atactica polyneuritiformis. *British Medical Journal*, **290**, 1109–1110

GONZALES, M. F. and DAVIS, R. L. (1988) Neuropathology of acquired immunodeficiency syndrome. *Journal of Neuropathology and Applied Neurobiology*, **14**, 345–363

GOODHILL, V. (1950) Histiocytic granuloma of skull (a triphasic clinicopathologic syndrome previously termed Letterer-Siwe's disease, Hand-Schuller-Christian's disease and eosinophilic granuloma): Report of 18 cases. *Laryngoscope*, **60**, 1–54

GRANSTROM, G. and KULAA-MIKKONEN, A. (1990) Experimental craniofacial malformations induced by retinoids and resembling branchial arch syndromes. *Scandinavian Journal of Plastic and Reconstructive Surgery*, **24**, 3–12

GRAY, R. E., EVANS, R. A., FREE, C. E. L. SZUTOWICZ, H. L. and MASKELL, J. F. (1991) Radiology for cochlear implants. *Journal of Laryngology and Otology*, **105**, 85–88

GREGG, J. B. and BECKER, S. F. (1963) Concomitant progressive deafness, chronic nephritis and ocular lens disease. *Archives of Ophthalmology*, **69**, 293–299

GUSSEN, R. (1977) Polyarteritis nodosa and deafness. A

human temporal bone study. *Archives of Otolaryngology*, **217**, 263–271

GUSSEN, R. (1983) Sudden deafness associated with bilateral Reissner's membrane ruptures. *American Journal of Otolaryngology*, **4**, 27–32

GUTHRIE, L. G. (1902) 'Idiopathic' or congenital hereditary and familial haematuria. *Lancet*, i, 1243–1246

HAGEMAN, M. J. (1977) Audiometric findings in 34 patients with Waardenburg's syndrome. *Journal of Laryngology and Otology*, **91**, 575–584

HALLPIKE, C. S. (1967) Observations on the structural basis of two rare varieties of hereditary deafness. In: *Myotatic Kinesthetic and Vestibular Mechanisms*. CIBA-Foundation symposium, edited by A. V. S. de Reuck, and J. Knight. London: Churchill. p. 285

HAMERSMA, H. (1970) Osteopetrosis (marble bone disease) of the temporal bone. *Laryngoscope*, **80**, 1518–1539

HANSON, D. R. and FEARN, R. W. (1975) Hearing acuity in young people exposed to pop music and other noise. *Lancet*, ii, 283

HARNSBERGER, H. R., DART, D. J., PARKIN, J. L., STOKER, W. K. and OSBORN, A. G. (1987) Cochlear implant candidates: assessment with CT and MNR imaging. *Radiology*, **164**, 53–57

HARIRI, M. A. and SMALL, M. (1990) Radionecrosis of the temporal bone, presenting as a cerebello-pontine lesion. *Journal of Laryngology and Otology*, **104**, 423–425

HARRIS, J. P. and RYAN, A. F. (1984) Immunobiology of the inner ear. *American Journal of Otolaryngology*, **5**, 418–425

HASSTEDT, S. J., ATKIN, C. L. and SAN JUAN, A. C. (1986) Genetic heterogeneity among kindreds with Alport's syndrome. *American Journal of Human Genetics*, **38**, 940–953

HAWKE, M., JAHN, A. F. and BAILEY, D. (1981) Osteopetrosis of the temporal bone. *Archives of Otolaryngology*, **107**, 278–282

HAWKINS, J. E. JR (1959) Antibiotics and the inner ear. *Transactions of the American Academy of Ophthalmology and Otology*, **63**, 206–216

HAWKINS, J. E. JR (1976) Drug ototoxicity. In: *Handbook of Sensory Physiology*, edited by W. D. Keidel and M. D. Neff. vol. 5. Auditory system, part 3; clinical and special topics. Berlin: Springer. pp. 707–748

HAWKINS, J. E. JR and JOHNSSON, L.-G. (1976) Patterns of sensorineural degeneration in human ears exposed to noise. In: *The Effects of Noise on Hearing – Critical Issues*, edited by D. Henderson and R. P. Hamernik. New York: Raven Press. pp. 91–110

HINCHCLIFFE, R. (1971–1972) Hearing loss due to physical agents. *Reports of the Institute of Laryngology and Otology*, **20**, 58–77

HINOJOSA, R. and LINDSAY, J. R. (1977) Inner ear degeneration in Reye's syndrome. *Archives of Otolaryngology*, **103**, 634–640

HOROWITZ, M., VIGNERY, A., GERSHON, R. R. and BARRER, R. (1984) Thymus derived lymphocytes and their interactions with macrophages are required for the production of osteoclast-activating factor in the mouse. *Proceedings of the National Academy of Science*, **81**, 2181–2185

HOUGH, J. V. D. and STUART, W. D. (1968) Middle ear injuries in skull trauma. *Laryngoscope*, **78**, 899–937

HOUSE, W. F. (1976) Cochlear implants. *Annals of Otology, Rhinology and Laryngology*, **85**, Supplement 27, 3–6

HUNT, J. R. (1907) Herpetic inflammation of the geniculate ganglion. *Journal of Laryngology and Otology*, **25**, 405–411

HUNTER-DUVAR, I. M. (1978) Electron microscopic assessment of the cochlea. *Acta Otolaryngologica*, Supplement 381, 1–44

HURLER, G. (1919) Uber einen typ multipler abartungen vorwiegend im skelett-system. *Zeitschrift für Kinderheilkunde*, **24**, 220–234

HVIDBERG-HANSEN, J. and JORGENSEN, S. M. (1968) The inner ear in Pendred's syndrome. *Acta Otolaryngologica*, **66**, 129–143

IGARASHI, M., TAKAHASHI, M., ALFORD, B. R. and JOHNSON, P. E. (1977) Inner ear morphology in Down's syndrome. *Acta Otolaryngologica*, **83**, 175–181

IGARASHI, M., KING, A. I., SCHWENZIELER, C. W., WATANABE, T. and ALFORD, B. R. (1980) Inner ear pathology in osteogenesis imperfecta. *Journal of Laryngology and Otology*, **94**, 697–705

ILLUM, P. (1972) The Mondini type of cochlear malformation: a survey of the literature. *Archives of Otolaryngology*, **96**, 305–311

ILLUM, P., KIAER, H. W., HINDBERG-HANGE, J., and SONDERGAARD, C. (1972) Fifteen cases of Pendred's syndrome. Congenital deafness and sporadic goitre. *Archives of Otolaryngology*, **96**, 297–304

JACKLER, R. K., LUXFORD, M. M., SCHINDLER, R. A. and MCKERROW, W. S. (1987) Cochlear patency problems in cochlear implantation. *Laryngoscope*, **97**, 801–805

JACOB, A., LEDINGHAM, J. G., KERR, A. I. G. and FORD, M. J. (1990) Ulcerative colitis and giant cell arteritis associated with sensorineural deafness. *Journal of Laryngology and Otology*, **104**, 889–890

JAFFE, H. L. (1972) *Metabolic Degeneration and Inflammatory Diseases of Bone and Joints*. Philadelphia: Lea and Fiebiger

JANDINSKI, J. J. (1988) Osteoclast-activating factor is now interleukin-1 beta: historical perspective and biological implications. *Journal of Oral Pathology*, **17**, 145–152

JENKINS, H. A., POLLACK, A. M. and FISCH, U. (1981) Polyarteritis nodosa as a cause of sudden deafness. *American Journal of Otolaryngology*, **2**, 99–107

JERVELL, A. and LANGE-NIELSEN, F. (1957) Congenital deafmutism, functional heart disease with prolongation of the QT interval and sudden death. *American Heart Journal*, **54**, 59–68

JERVELL, A., THINGSTAD, R. and THOR-OSTEN, E. (1966) The surdocardiac syndrome. Three new cases of congenital deaths with syncopal attacks and Q-T prolongation in the electrocardiogram. *American Heart Journal*, **72**, 582–593

JOHNSEN, T., JORGENSEN, M. B. and JOHNSEN, S. (1986) Mondini cochlea in Pendred's syndrome. A histological study. *Acta Otolaryngologica*, **102**, 239–247

JOHNSSON, L.-G. and HAWKINS, J. E. JR (1972) Sensory and neural degeneration with aging, as seen in microdissections of the human inner ear. *Annals of Otology, Rhinology and Laryngology*, **1**, 179–193

JOHNSSON, L.-G. and HAWKINS, J. E. JR (1976) Degeneration patterns in human ears exposed to noise. *Annals of Otology*, **85**, 725–739

JOHNSSON, L.-G., HOUSE, W. F. and LINTHICUM, F. H. (1979) Bilateral cochlear implants: histological findings in a pair of temporal bones. *Laryngoscope*, **89**, 759–762

KAHN, Z. M. and ADOUR, K. K. (1978) Histologic findings in the temporal bone in trisomy D (D/D translocation). *Archives of Otolaryngology*, **104**, 22–25

KANIS, J. A. (1991) *Pathophysiology and Treatment of Paget's Disease of Bone*. London: Martin Dunitz

KANZAKI, J. and OGUCHI, T. (1983) Circulating immune complexes in steroid-responsive hearing loss. Long term observation. *Acta Otolaryngologica*, Supplement 393, 77–84

KARMODY, C. S. (1968) Subclinical maternal rubella and congenital deafness. *New England Journal of Medicine*, **278**, 809–814

KARMODY, C. S. (1983) Viral labyrinthitis: early pathology in the human. *Laryngoscope*, **93**, 152–1533

KARMODY, C. S. and SCHUKNECHT, H. F. (1966) Deafness in congenital syphilis. *Archives of Otolaryngology*, **83**, 18–27

KATCHBURIAN, E. (1973) Membrane-bound bodies as indicators of mineralization. *Journal of Anatomy*, **116**, 285–302

KELEMEN, G. (1960) Histiocytosis involving the temporal bone (Letterer-Siwe, Hand-Schuller-Christian). *Laryngoscope*, **70**, 1284–1304

KELEMEN, G. (1966) Marfan's syndrome and the hearing organ. *Acta Otolaryngologica*, **59**, 23–32

KELEMEN, G. and ETSCHENBACHER, E. (1978) Das gehororgan bei einem Falle von anencephalie. *Archives of Otorhinolaryngology*, **218**, 221–227

KELEMEN, G. and LINTHICUM, F. H. JR (1969) Labyrinthine otosclerosis. *Acta Otolaryngologica*, Supplement 253, 1–68

KELEMEN, G., HOOFT, C. and KLUYSKENS, P. (1968) The inner ear in autosomal trisomy. *Practica Oto-Rhino-Laryngologica*, **30**, 251–258

KEMPF, H. G. (1989) Ear involvement in Wegener's granulomatosis. *Clinical Otolaryngology*, **14**, 451–456

KENT, M. D. and BOHNE, B. A. (1983) Noise-induced degeneration in the brain and representation of inner and outer hair cells. *Hearing Research*, **9**, 145–151

KIMURA, R. S. and SCHUKNECHT, H. F. (1970a) The ultrastructure of the human stria vascularis. Part I. *Acta Otolaryngologica*, **69**, 415

KIMURA, R. S. and SCHUKNECHT, H. F. (1970b) The ultrastructure of the human stria vascularis. Part II. *Acta Otolaryngologica*, **70**, 301–318

KITTEL, G. (1963) Pfaundler Hurler disease or gargoylism from the otorhinolaryngological aspects. *Zeitschrift für Laryngologie, Rhinologie und Otologie*, **42**, 206–217

KLEY, W. (1986) Alfonso Corti (1822–1876) – discoverer of the sensory end-organ of hearing in Wurzburg. *Oto-Rhino-Laryngologie*, **48**, 61–67

KORNBLUT, A. D., WOLFE, S. M. and FAUCI, A. S. (1982) Ear disease in patients with Wegener's granulomatosis. *Laryngoscope*, **92**, 713–717

KOS, A. O., SCHUKNECHT, H. F. and SINGER, J. B. (1966) Temporal bone studies in 13–15 and 16 trisomy syndromes. *Archives of Otolaryngology*, **83**, 439–445

KRICKSTEIN, H. L., GLOOR, F. G. and BALOGH, K. (1966) Renal pathology in hereditary nephritis with nerve deafness. *Archives of Pathology*, **82**, 506–517

LANCET (1989) Herpes simplex latency (Editorial), 194–195

LANCET (1991) Congenital rubella – 50 years on. Noticeboard. i, 668

LANCET (1991) Alport's syndrome (Editorial), 338, 1201

LARSEN, S. A., ASHER, D. I., BALKANY, T. H. J. and RUCKNER, N. C. (1983) Histopathology of the auditory nerve and cochlear nucleus following intracochlear stimulation. *Otolaryngologic Clinics of North America*, **16**, 233–248

LEHNINGER, A. L., WASKINS, C. H. L., COOPER, C., DEVLIN, T. M. and JAMBLE, J. L. JR (1958) Ototoxic antibiotics. *Science*, **128**, 450–456

LEJEUNE, J., GAUTHIER, M. and TORPIN, R. (1959) Etudes des chromosomes somatiques de 9 enfants mongoliennes. *Comptes rendus de l'Academie des Sciences (Paris)*, **248**, 1721–1722

LEVINE, S. A. and WOODWORTH, C. R. (1958) Congenital deafmutism, prolonged QT-interval, syncopal attacks and sudden death. *New England Journal of Medicine*, **259**, 412–417

LEVY, R., SARFATY, S. M. and SCHINDEL, I. (1980) Eosinophilic granuloma of the temporal bone. *Archives of Otolaryngology*, **106**, 167–171

LICHTENSTEIN, L. (1938) Polyostotic fibrous dysplasia. *Archives of Surgery*, **36**, 874–898

LICHTENSTEIN, L. and JAFFE, H. L. (1942) Fibrous dysplasia of bone. *Archives of Pathology*, **33**, 777–816

LIM, D. J. (1986) Effects of noise and ototoxic drugs at the cellular level in the cochlea: a review. *American Journal of Otolaryngology*, **7**, 73–99

LIM, D. J. and DUNN, D. E. (1979) Anatomic correlates of noise-induced hearing loss. *Otolaryngologic Clinics of North America*, **12**, 493–511

LIM, D. J. and LANE, W. C. (1969) Cochlear sensory epithelium. A scanning electron microscopic observation. *Annals of Otology, Rhinology and Laryngology*, **78**, 827–841

LINDSAY, J. (1973a) Histopathology of deafness due to postnatal viral disease. *Archives of Otolaryngology*, **98**, 258–264

LINDSAY, J. R. (1973b) Profound childhood deafness: inner ear pathology. *Annals of Otology, Rhinology and Laryngology*, **82**, 98–99

LINDSAY, J. R. and HEMENWAY, W. G. (1954) Inner ear pathology due to measles. *Annals of Otology, Rhinology and Laryngology*, **63**, 754–771

LINDSAY, J. R. and LEHMAN, R. H. (1969) Histopathology of the temporal bone in advanced Paget's disease. *Laryngoscope*, **79**, 213–227

LINTHICUM, F. H. JR and ANDERSON, W. (1991) Cochlear implantation of totally deaf ears. *Acta Otolaryngologica*, **111**, 327–331

LIU, X., NEWTON, V. and READ, A. (1995) Hearing loss and pigmentary disturbances in Waardenburg syndrome with reference to WS type II. *Journal of Laryngology and Otology*, **109**, 96–100

LOBSTEIN, J. F. (1935) *Lehrbuch der pathologischen Anatomie* Stuttgart: Thieme. Vol 2 p. 179 (published also in French in 1933)

LOOSER, E. (1906) Zur Kenntniss der Osteogenesis imperfecta congenita et tarda. *Mitteilungencien der Grenzebeite Medizin und Chirurgie*. **15**, 161. (also in Proceedings of the German Pathology Society 1904)

LOWRY, R. B. (1975) Hirschsprung's disease and congenital deafness. *Journal of Medical Genetics*, **12**, 114–115

LUBS, H. A., ULMAN KENIG, E. and BRANDT, J. K. (1961) Trisomy 13–15: a clinical syndrome. *Lancet*, ii, 1001–1002

MCALPINE, J. C. and FRIEDMANN, I. (1963) A histochemical study of the effects of ototoxic antibiotics on the isolated embryonic otocyst of the fowl (Gallus domesticus). *Journal of Pathology and Bacteriology*, **86**, 477–486

MCCABE, B. F. (1966) Otosclerosis and vertigo. *Proceedings of the TransPacific Oto-Ophthalmologic Society*, **47**, 37

MCCABE, B. F. (1979) Autoimmune sensorineural hearing loss. *Annals of Otology, Rhinology and Laryngology*, **88**, 585–589

MCCAFFREY, T. V., MCDONALD, T. J. C., FACER, G. W. and DEREMEER, A. (1980) Otologic manifestations of Wegener's granulomatosis. *Otolaryngology – Head and Neck Surgery*, **88**, 586–593

MCCAFFREY, T. V. and MCDONALD, D. J. (1979) Histiocytosis X of the ear and temporal bone. A study of 28 cases. *Journal of Bone and Joint Surgery*, **89**, 1735–1742

MCCUNE, D. J. (1936) Osteitis fibrosa cystica: the case of a 9-year old girl who also exhibits precocious puberty, multiple pigmentation of the skin and hyperthyroidism. *American Journal of Diseases of Childhood*, **52**, 745–748

MCDONALD, TH. J., ANDERSON, C. F. and OTT, N. T. (1978) Reversal of deafness after renal transplantation in Alport's syndrome. *Laryngoscope*, **88**, 38–42

MCFADDEN, D., PLATTSMIER, H. S. and PASANEN, E. G. (1984) Temporary hearing loss induced by combinations of intense sounds and non-steroidal anti-inflammatory drugs. *American Journal of Otolaryngology*, **5**, 235–241

MCKENNA, R. J., SCHWINN, C. P., SOONG, K. and HIGGINBOTHAM, N. L. (1964) Osteogenic sarcoma in Paget's disease. *Cancer*, **17**, 42–66

MCKUSICK, V. A. (1972) *Heritable Disorders of Connective Tissue*. St Louis: Mosby. pp. 718–723

MCKUSICK, V. A. (1973) Congenital deafness and Hirschprung's disease. *New England Journal of Medicine*, **228**, 690

MCNEIL, N. F., BERKE, M. and REINGOLD, I. M. (1952) Polyarteritis nodosa causing deafness in an adult. *Annals of Internal Medicine*, **37**, 1253

MAGORI, A., ORMOS, J., FAZEKAS, M., SOMKODI, S., RUDAS, L. and TURI, S. (1983) Concretions of the renal basement membranes. *Diagnostic Histopathology*, **6**, 195–200

MAINS, B. (1989) Wegener's granulomatosis. False positive antineutrophil cytoplasmic antibody test. *Journal of Laryngology and Otology*, **103**, 324–325

MALEBRANCHE (1678) (cf. Seedorff, 1949) *Traite de la recherche et de la verite*. Paris

MARFAN, A. B. (1896) Un cas de deformation des quatre membres plus prononcée aux extremites caracterisée par l'alongement des os avec un certain degree d' amincissement. *Bulletin Societé Medicale Paris*, **15**, 3 seri 220

MASUTANI, H., TAKAHASHI, H. and SANDO, I. (1992) Stria vascularis in Meniere's disease: a quantitative histopathological study. *Auris-Nasus-Larynx*, **19**, 145–152

MAYER, O. (1919–1920) Das anatomische Substrat der Amterschwerhorigkeit. *Archiv fur Ohren, Nasen Kehlkopfheilkunde*, **105**, 1–13

MENSER, M. A., DODS, I. L. and HARLEY, J. D. (1967) A twenty-five year follow-up of congenital rubella. Special article. *Lancet*, ii, 1347–1350

MICHAELS, L., WELLS, M. and FROHLICH, A. (1983) A new technique for the study of temporal bone pathology. *Clinical Otolaryngology*, **8**, 77–85

MICHAELS, L., SOUCEK, S. and LIANG, J. (1994) The ear in AIDS – a temporal bone histologic study. *American Journal of Otology*, **15**, 515–522

MILLER, G. W., JOSEPH, D. I., COZAD, R. L. and MCCABE, B. F. (1970) Alport's syndrome. *Archives of Otolaryngology*, **92**, 419–432

MILLER, J., CANLON, B. and FLOCK, A. (1985) High intensity noise effects on stereocilia mechanics. *Abstracts of the Eighth Midwinter Research Meeting*, Association for Research in Otolaryngology. p. 50

MILLER, J. M. and SUTTON, D. (1980) Cochlear prosthesis: morphological considerations. *Journal of Laryngology and Otology*, **94**, 359–366

MILLS, B. G., SINGER, F. R., WEINER, I. P., SUFFIN, S. C., STABILE, E. and HOLST, P. (1984) Evidence for both respiratory syncytial virus and measles virus antigens in the osteoclasts of patients with Paget's disease of bone. *Clinical Orthopaedics and Related Research*, **183**, 303–311

MILROY, C. M. and MICHAELS, L. (1990) Pathology of the otic capsule. *Journal of Laryngology and Otology*, **104**, 83–90

MONDINI, C. (1791) Anatomica surdi nati secto. Bononiensi

Scientarium et artium instituto atque academia commentarii. *Bonaniae*, VII, 419–428

MORGAN, J. C., HOCHMAN, R. and WEIDER, D. J. (1984) Cogan's syndrome: acute vestibular and auditory dysfunction with interstitial keratitis. *American Journal of Otolaryngology*, **5**, 258–261

MORRISON, A. W. and BOOTH, J. B. (1970) Sudden deafness, an otological emergency. *British Journal of Hospital Medicine*, **4**, 287–298

MURAKAMI, M., OHTANI, I., AIKAWA, T. and ANZAI, T. (1990) Temporal bone findings in two cases of head injury. *Journal of Laryngology and Otology*, **104**, 986–989

MYERS, E. N. and STOOL, S. (1969) The temporal bone in osteopetrosis. *Archives of Otolaryngology*, **89**, 460–469

NABE-NIELSEN, J. and WALTER, B. (1988) Unilateral deafness as a complication of the mumps measles and rubella vaccination. *British Medical Journal*, **297**, 489

NADOL, J. B. JR (1979) Electronmicroscopic findings in presbycusis degeneration of the basal turn of the human cochlea. *Otolaryngology – Head and Neck Surgery*, **87**, 818–836

NADOL, J. B. and ARNOLD, W. J. (1987) The ear. In: *Atlas of Histopathology of Diseases of the Ear, Nose and Throat*, edited by J. Laissue, W. Arnold, I. Friedmann and H. Naumann. Stuttgart: Thieme. pp.1–54

NADOL, J. B. and BURGESS, B. (1982) Cochleosaccular degeneration of the inner ear and progressive cataracts inherited as an autosomal dominant trait. *Laryngoscope*, **92**, 1028–1037

NAGER, F. R. (1907) Beitrage zur histologies der erworbenen taubstummheit. *Zeitschrift der Ohrenheilkunde*, **54**, 217–244

NAGER, F. R. (1922) Die Labyrinkapsel bei angeborenen Knochenerkrankungen. *Archiv für Ohren Nasen Kehlkopfheilkunde*, **109**, 81–103

NAGER, G. T. (1975) Paget's disease of the temporal bone. *Annals of Otology, Rhinology and Laryngology*, **84**, (Supplement 22), 32

NAGER, G. T., KENNEDY, D. W. and KOPSTEIN, E. (1982) Fibrous dysplasia. A review of the disease and its manifestations in the temporal bone. *Annals of Otology, Rhinology and Laryngology*, **91** (Supplement 92), 5–52

NAKAI, Y., MASUTANI, H., MORIGUCHI, M., MATSUNAGA, K. and SUGITA, M. (1991) The influence of noise exposure on endolymphatic hydrops. *Acta Otolaryngologica*, Supplement 486, 7–10

NOMURA, Y. (1970) Lipidosis of the basilar membrane. *Acta Otolaryngologica*, **69**, 352–357

NSAMBA, C. (1979) Ernst Reissner. Historical vignette. *Archives of Otolaryngology*, **105**, 434–435

NUOVO, N. A., NUOVO, J., MACCONNELL, PH., FORDE, A. and STEINER, G. O. (1992) In situ analysis of Paget's disease of bone for measles-specific PCR-amplified cDNA. *Diagnostic Molecular Biology*, **1**, 256–265

ODA, M., PRECIADO, M. C., QUICK, C. A. and PAPARELLA, M. M. (1974) Labyrinthine pathology of chronic renal failure in patients treated with hemodyalisis and kidney transplantation. *Laryngoscope*, **84**, 1489–1506

O'DONOGHUE, G. M. (1992) Cochlear implants in children. *Journal of the Royal Society of Medicine*, **85**, 635–637

OGILVIE, R. F. and HALL, I. S. (1962) On the aetiology of otosclerosis. *Journal of Laryngology and Otology*, **76**, 84

ORMEROD, F. C. (1960) The pathology of congenital deafness. *Journal of Laryngology and Otology*, **74**, 919–950

ORR, M. F. (1965) Development of acoustic ganglia in tissue

culture of embryonic chick otocysts. *Experimental Cell Research*, **40**, 68–77

OSTRI, B., ELLER, N., DAHLIN, E. and SKYEU, G. (1989) Hearing impairment of orchestral musicians. *Scandinavian Audiology*, **18**, 243–249

OTTE, J., SCHUKNECHT, H. F. and KERR, A. G. (1978) Ganglion cell population in normal and pathological human cochleae. Implication for cochlear implantation. *Laryngoscope*, **88**, 1231–1246

PABICO, K. C., GRUEBEL, B. J., MCKENNA, B. A., HOLLANDER, J. WEISSBACHER, J. and PANNER. B. J. (1981) Renal involvement in Refsum's disease. *American Journal of Medicine*, **79**, 1136–1143

PADDISON, R. M., MOOSSY, J. and DERBES, V. J. (1963) Cockrayne's syndrome. *Dermalogica Tropica*, **2**, 195–203

PATAU, K., SMITH, D. W., THERMAN, E., INHORN, S. L. and WAGNER, H. P. (1960) Multiple congenital anatomy caused by an extra chromosome. *Lancet*, i, 790–792

PATAU, K., THERMAN, E., SMITH, D. W. and DEMARS, R. I. (1961) Trisomy chromosome 18 in man. *Chromosoma*, **12**, 280–285

PAULER, M., SCHUKNECHT, H. and THORNTON, A. R. (1986) Correlative studies of cochlear neuronal loss with speech discrimination and pure-tone thresholds. *Otorhinolaryngology*, **243**, 200–206

PAULER, M., SCHUKNECHT, H. F. and WHITE, J. A. (1988) Atrophy of the stria vascularis as cause of sensorineural hearing loss. *Laryngoscope*, **98**, 754–759

PEDERSEN, U., MELSEN, F., ELBROND, O. and CHARLES, P. (1985) Histopathology of the stapes in osteogenesis imperfecta. *Journal of Laryngology and Otology*, **99**, 451–458

PERLMAN, H. B. (1967) Some labyrinth capsule diseases and inner ear deafness. In: *Sensorineural Hearing Processes and Disorders*, edited by B. Graham. Boston: Little, Brown and Co. pp. 465–479

PERLMAN, H. B. and KIMURA, R. (1957) Experimental obstruction of venous drainage and arterial supply of the inner ear. *Annals of Otology Rhinology and Laryngology*, **66**, 537–547

PFINGST, B. E., SUTTON, D., MILLER, J. M. and BOHNE, B. A. (1981) Relation of psycho-physical data to histopathology in monkeys with cochlear implants. *Acta Otolaryngologica*, **69**, 1–13

PHELPS, P. D. (1992) Cochlear implants for congenital deformities. *Journal of Laryngology and Otology*, **106**, 967–970

PHELPS, P. D. and LLOYD, G. A. S. (1990) *Diagnostic Imaging of the Ear*. Berlin; Springer, p. 43

PHELPS, P. D., ANNIS, J. A. D. and ROBINSON, P. J. (1990) Imaging for cochlear implants. *British Journal of Radiology*, **63**, 512–516

POLANI, P. E., HAMARTON, J. L., GIANELLI, F. and CARTER, C. O. (1965) Cytogenetics of Down's syndrome (mongolism) III. Trisomies and mutation rates of chromosome interchanges. *Cytogenetic Cell Genetics*, **4**, 193–206

POLITZER, A. (1902) *Diseases of the Ear*. London: Bailliere Tindall Co

POPE, F. M., MARTIN, G. R., LICHTENSTEIN, J. R., PENTINNEN, R., GERSON, B., ROWE, D. R. *et al.* (1975) Patients with Ehlers-Danlos syndrome type IV lack type 111 collagen. *Proceedings of the National Academy of Sciences, USA*, **72**, 1314–1316

POTTER, E. L. (1946) Bilateral renal agenesis. *Journal of Pediatrics*, **29**, 68–76

PRITCHARD, J. L. (1956) General anatomy and histology of bone In: *Biochemistry and Physiology of Bone*, edited by G. H. Bourne. London: Academic Press. pp. 1938–1959

QUICK, C. A., FISH, A. and BROWN, C. (1973) The relationship between cochlea and kidney. *Laryngoscope*, **83**, 1469–1482

RAKE, M. and SAUNDERS, M. (1966) Refsum's disease: a disorder of lipid metabolism. *Journal of Neurology, Neurosurgery and Psychiatry*, **29**, 417–422

RAMADAN, H. H. and SCHUKNECHT, H. F. (1989) Is there a conductive type of presbycusis. *Otolaryngology – Head and Neck Surgery*, **100**, 30–34

RAREY, K. E., DAVIS, J. A., DAVIS, L. E. and HAWKINS, J. E. (1983) Inner ear pathology associated with Reye's syndrome. *International Journal of Pediatric Otorhinolaryngology*, **6**, 255–263

RAREY, K. E., DAVIS, J. A. and DESHMUKH, J. R. (1984) Inner ear changes in the ferret model for Reye's syndrome. *American Journal of Otolaryngology*, **5**, 191–192

RAREY, K. E., DAVIS, J. A., PUSH, N. L. and DESHMUKH, J. R. (1984) Effects of influenza infection, aspirin and an arginin-deficient diet on the inner ear in Rey's syndrome. *Annals of Otology, Rhinology and Laryngology*, **93**, 551–557

RASK-ANDERSON, H. and STAHLE, J. (1980) Immunodefence of the inner ear. *Acta Otolaryngologica*, **106**, 409–416

RASMUSSEN, N. and WILK, A. (1955) Autoimmunity in Wegener's granulomatosis. In: *Immunology, Autoimmunity and Transplantation in Otolaryngology*, edited by J. E. Veldman, B. F. McCabe and E. M. Huizing. Amsterdam: Kugler. pp. 231–236

REED, R. J. (1963) Fibrous dysplasia of bone – a review of 25 cases. *Archives of Pathology*, **75**, 480–495

REFSUM, S. (1946) Heredopathia atacticapoly neuritiformis: a familial syndrome not hitherto described. A contribution to the clinical study of hereditary disorders of the nervous system. *Acta Psychiatrica Scandinavica*, Supplement 38, 1–303

REFSUM, S. (1981) Refsum's disease – phytanic acid storage disease, a biochemically well defined disease with a specific dietary treatment. *Archives of Neurology*, **38**, 605–606

REISSNER, E. (1851) De auris internae formatione. Thesis. Cf. Nsamba, C. (1979)

REYE, R. D. K., MORGAN, G. and BARAL, J. (1963) Encephalopathy and fatty degeneration of the viscera. A disease entity in childhood. *Lancet*, ii, 749–752

RICHET, C. (1945) Notes sur le typhus exanthematique observé à Buchenwald. *Bulletin Société Medicale des Hôpitaux de Paris*, **61**, 183–187

RISTOW, W. (1966) Zur Frage der aetiologischen Bedeutung der Toxoplasmose für Hörschadigung und Taubstummheit. *Zeitschrift für Laryngologie, Rhinologie and Otologie*, **45**, 251–264

ROSSLE, R. (1937) Die Veranderungen der Schleimhaute der Nebenhohlen des Kopfes durch rheumatische Gefassentzundurgen. *Archiv für Ohren-Nasen-Kehlkopfheilkunde*, **142**, 193–204

ROWE-JONES, J. M., MACALLAN, D. C. and SOROOSHAN, M. (1990) Polyarteritis nodosa presenting as bilateral sudden onset cochleovestibular failure in a young woman. *Journal of Laryngology and Otology*, **104**, 562–564

RUBEN, R. J. (1991) The history of the genetics of hearing impairment. Genetics of Hearing Impairment. *Annals of the New York Academy of Sciences*, **630**, 6–14

RUEDI, L. (1968) Are there cochlear shunts in Paget's disease and Von Recklinghausen's disease? *Acta Otolaryngologica*, **65**, 13–24

SAITO, R., TAKATA, N., MASUMOTO, M., KOIDE, I., FUJITA, A.,

OGURA, Y. *et al.* (1982) Anomalies of the auditory organ in Potter's syndrome. Histopathologic findings in the temporal bone. *Archives of Otolaryngology,* **108,** 484–489

SANDO, I., LEIBERMANN A., BERGSTROM, L., IZUMI, S. and WOOD, R. (1975) Temporal bone histopathological findings in trisomy 13 syndrome. *Annals of Otology, Rhinology and Laryngology,* **84** (Supplement 21)

SANDO, I., HINOJOSA, R. MYERS, D. and HARADA, T. (1981) Osteogenesis imperfecta tarda and otosclerosis. A temporal bone histopathology report. *Annals of Otology, Rhinology and Laryngology,* **90,** 199–203

SANFILLIPPO, F., WISEMAN, C. H., INGRAM, P. and SHENBURNE, J. (1981) Crystalline deposits of calcium and phosphorus. Their appearance in glomerular basement membranes of a patient with renal failure. *Archives of Pathology and Laboratory Medicine,* **105,** 594–598

SAUNDERS, J. C. and FLOCK, A. (1985) Changes in cochlear hair-cell stereocilia stiffness following overstimulation. *Abstracts of the Eight Midwinter Research Meeting.* Association for Research in Otolaryngology. p. 51

SCHACHERN, P. A., SHEA, D. A. and PAPARELLA, M. M. (1984) Mucopolysaccharidosis I-H (Hurler's syndrome) and human temporal bone histopathology. *Annals of Otology Rhinology Laryngology,* **93,** 65–69

SCHEIBE, A. (1891–92) Ein Fall von Taubstummheit mit Acusticusatrophie u. Bildungsanomalien im Heutigen Labyrinth beiderseits. *Zeitschrift für Hals, Nasen und Ohrenheilkunde,* **22,** 11–33

SCHILLING, V. (1936) Striae Distensae Als Hypophysares Symptom Beim Basophilen Vorderlappen-Adenom und Arachno Daktylie mit Hypophysen-Tumor. *Medizinische Welt,* **10,** 724–729

SCHINDLER, R. A. and BJORKROTH, B. (1979) Traumatic intracochlear electrode implantation. *Laryngoscope,* **89,** 752–758

SCHINDLER, R. A. and MERZENICH, M. M. (1974) Chronic intracochlear implantation: cochlear pathology and acoustic nerve survival. *Annals of Otology, Rhinology and Laryngology,* **83,** 202–214

SCHOENFELD, Y. and ESENBERG, D. A. (1981) The mosaic of autoimmunity. *Immunology Today,* **10,** 123–126

SCHOENFELD, Y., FRIED, A. and EHRENFELD, N. E. (1975) Osteogenesis imperfecta. *American Journal of Diseases of Children,* **129,** 679–687

SCHUKNECHT, H. F. (1964a) Presbycusis. *Laryngoscope,* **65,** 402–419

SCHUKNECHT, H. F. (1964b) Further observations on the pathology of presbycusis. *Archives of Otolaryngology,* **80,** 369–382

SCHUKNECHT, H. F. (1967a) Pathology of sensorineural deafness of genetic origin. In: *Deafness in Childhood,* edited by F. McConnell and P. H. Ward. Nashville: Vanderbilt University Press. pp. 69–90

SCHUKNECHT, H. F. (1967b) The effect of aging on the cochlea. In: *Sensorineural Hearing Processes and Disorders,* edited by A. B. Graham. Boston: Little Brown & Co. pp. 393–401

SCHUKNECHT, H. F. (1974) *Pathology of the Ear.* Cambridge, Mass: Harvard University Press

SCHUKNECHT, H. F. (1991) Ear pathology in autoimmune disease. In: *Advances in Oto-Rhino-Laryngology,* edited by C. R. Pfaltz. Basel: Karger. **46,** 50–70

SCHUKNECHT, H. F. (1993) *Pathology of the Ear,* 2nd edn. Philadelphia: Lee and Feibiger

SCHUKNECHT, H. F. and BARBER, W. (1985) Histologic variants of otosclerosis. *Laryngoscope,* **95,** 1307–1317

SCHUKNECHT, H. F. and DONOVAN, E. D. (1986) The pathology of idiopathic sudden sensorineural hearing loss. *Archives of Otolaryngology,* **243,** 1–15

SCHUKNECHT, H. F. and GACEK, M. R. (1993) Cochlear pathology in presbycusis. *Annals of Otology, Rhinology and Laryngology,* **102** (suppl. 158), 1–16

SCHUKNECHT, H. F. and IGARASHI, M. (1964) Pathology of slowly progressing sensorineural deafness. *Transactions of the American Academy of Ophthalmology and Otolaryngology,* **68,** 222–242

SCHUKNECHT, H. F. and ISHII, T. (1966) Hearing loss caused by atrophy of the vascular stria. *Japanese Journal of Otology,* **69,** 1825–1833

SCHUKNECHT, H. F., GACEK, R. R. and IGARASHI, M. (1965) The pathological types of cochleosaccular degeneration. *Acta Otolaryngologica,* **59,** 154–167

SCHUKNECHT, H. F., WATANUKI, K., TAKAHASHI, T., BELAL, A. A., KIMURA, R. S., JONES, D. D. *et al.* (1974) Atrophy of the stria vascularis; a common cause of hearing loss. *Laryngoscope,* **84,** 1777–1821

SCHWARTZ, D. T. and ALPERT, M. (1964) The malignant transformation of fibrous dysplasia. *American Journal of Medical Sciences,* **247,** 35–54

SEEDORFF, K. S. (1949) Osteogenesis imperfecta. A study of clinical features and heredity based on 55 Danish families (180 members). University of Arhus. Thesis. (See also for a long list of references up to 1948)

SEIFERTH, L. B. (1944) Uber die Storungendes Hor-und Gleichgewichtapparates und uber entzundliche Ohrenerkrankungen beim Fleckfieber. *Deutsche Medizinische Wochenschrift,* **70,** 23–24

SHENEFELT, R. E. (1990) Morphogenesis of malformations in hamsters caused by retinoic acid. *Teratology,* **5,** 103–118

SIMMONS, F. B. (1979) Electrical stimulation of the auditory nerve in cats. Long term electrophysiological and histological results. *Annals of Otology, Rhinology and Laryngology,* **88,** 533–539

SIMMONS, F. B., SCHUKNECHT, H. F. and SMITH, L. (1986) Histopathology of an ear after 5 years of electrical stimulation. *Annals of Otology, Rhinology and Laryngology,* **95,** 132–134

SLEPECKY, N., HAMERNIK, R. P. and HENDERSON, D. (1980) The sensory hair cell. A reexamination of a hair cell organelle in the cuticular plate region and its possible relation to active processes in the cochlea. *Hearing Research,* **2,** 413–421

SLEPECKY, N. HAMERNIK, R. and HENDERSON, D. (1981) The consistent occurrence of a striated organelle (Friedmann body) in the inner hair cells of the normal chinchilla. *Acta Otolaryngologica,* **191,** 189–190

SMITH, R. (1984) Osteogenesis imperfecta. *British Medical Journal,* **189,** 194–195

SMITH, R. (1992) Paget's disease of bone. Advance, and controversy. (Editorial). *British Medical Journal,* **305,** 1379–1380

SMITH R. J. H., BERLIN, C. I., HEJTMANCIK, J. F., KEATS, B. J. B., KIMBERLING, W. J., LEWIS, R. A. *et al.,* (1994) Clinical diagnosis of the Usher syndrome. *American Journal of Medical Genetics,* **50,** 32–38

SOBKOWIC, Z. H. M. and SLAPNICK, S. M. (1992) Neuronal sprouting and synapse formation in response to injury in the mouse organ of Corti in culture. *International Journal of Developmental Neuroscience,* **10,** 545–566

SOBKOWICZ, H. M., BERMAN, B. and ROSE, J. E. (1975) Organotypic development of the organ of Corti in tissue culture. *Journal of Neurocytology,* **4,** 543–572

SOBKOWICZ, H. M., LOFTUS, J. M. and SLAPNICK, S. M. (1993) Tissue culture of the organ of Corti. *Acta Otolaryngologica*, Supplement 502, 3–36

SPECTOR, G. J. (1976) Histopathologic and experimental models of sensory and neural deafness. *Annals of Otology, Rhinology and Laryngology*, 85, 802–813

SPOENDLIN, H. (1975) Retrograde degeneration of the cochlear nerve. *Acta Otolaryngologica*, 79, 266–275

SPOENDLIN, H. (1985) Histopathology of noise-deafness. *Journal of Otolaryngology*, 14, 282–286

STEPHENSON, C. S. (1944) Epidemic typhus and other rickettsial diseases of military importance. *New England Journal of Medicine*, 213, 407–413

STERN, H., BOOTH, J. C., ELEK, S. D. and FLECK, D. G. (1969) Microbial causes of mental retardation: the role of prenatal infections with cytomegalovirus, rubella virus and toxoplasmosis. *Lancet*, ii, 443–445

SUEHIRO, S. and SANDO, I. (1979) Congenital anomalies of the inner ear. Introducing a new classification of labyrinthine anomalies. *Annals of Otology, Rhinology and Laryngology*, 88, 1–24

SUGA, F. and LINDSAY, J. R. (1976a) Temporal bone histopathology in osteopetrosis. *Annals of Otology, Rhinology and Laryngology*, 85, 15–25

SUGA, F. and LINDSAY, J. R. (1976b) Inner ear degeneration in acoustic neurinoma. *Annals of Otology, Rhinology and Laryngology*, 85, 343–349

SUMMERS, R. and HARKER, L. (1982) Ulcerative colitis and sensorineural hearing loss. Is there a relationship? *Journal of Clinical Gastroenterology*, 4, 251–252

TAITZ, L. S. (1987) Child abuse and osteogenesis imperfecta. *Britsh Medical Journal*, 295, 1082–1083

TOOHILL, R. J., KIDDER, T. M. and EBY, L. G. (1973) Eosinophilic granuloma of the temporal bone. *Laryngoscope*, 83, 877–889

TOS, M. (1966) A survey of Hand-Schuller-Christian's disease in otolaryngology. *Acta Otolaryngologica*, 62, 217–228

TOYNBEE, J. (1860) *The Diseases of the Ear. Their Nature, Diagnosis and Treatment*. London: John Churchill

USHER, C. (1914) On the inheritance of retinitis pigmentosa with notes of cases. *Reports of the Royal London Ophthalmic Hospital*, 191, 130–236

VAN DE WATER, T. R. and RUBEN, R. J. (1971) Organ culture of the mammalian inner ear. *Acta Otolaryngologica*, 71, 303–312

VELDMAN, J. E. (1987) *Immunobiology, Histophysiology, Tumor Immunology in Otorhinolaryngology*. Amsterdam: Kugler

VELDMAN, J. E., HARADA, T. and MEELIWSEN, F. (1993) Diagnostic and therapeutic dilemmas in rapidly progressive sensorineural hearing loss and sudden deafness. A reappraisal of immune reactivity in inner ear disorders. *Acta Otolaryngologica*, 113, 303–306

VELDMAN, J. E., MEELIWSEN, F. and HUIZING, E. H. (1987) Advances in oto-immunology: new trends in functional pathology of the temporal bone. *Laryngoscope*, 97, 413–421

VELDMAN, J. E., ROORD, J. J., O'CONNOR, A. F. and SHEA, J. J. (1984) Autoimmunity and inner ear disorders: an immune-complex mediated sensorineural hearing loss. *Laryngoscope*, 94, 501–507

VROLIK, W. (1849) Tabulae ad illustrandum embryogenesis hominis et mammalium, tam naturalem quam abnormem. Amsterdam, London: G. M. P. (c.f. Jaffe, H. L. (1972) *Metabolic Degenerative and Inflammatory Diseases of Bones and Joints*. Philadelphia: Lea and Feibiger, p. 162.)

WAARDENBURG, P. J. (1951) A new syndrome combining developmental anomalies of the eyelids, eyebrows and nose roof with pigmentary defects of the iris and head hair with congenital deafness. *American Journal of Human Genetics*, 3, 195–253

WACKYM, PH. A., MAMAS, J. D. and MCCABE, B. F. (1993) Early diagnosis of otologic Wegener's granulomatosis using the serologic marker c-ANCA. *Annals of Otology, Rhinology and Laryngology*, 102, 337–341

WANG, I., KARMODY, C. S. and PASHAYAN, H. (1981) Waardenburg's syndrome: variations in expressivity. *Otolaryngology – Head and Neck Surgery*, 80, 666–670

WATTS, R. W., SPELLACY, E., KENDALL, B., DU BOULAY, G. and GIBBS, D. A. (1981) Computerized tomography studies on patients with mucopolysaccharidoses. *Neuroradiology*, 21, 9–23

WEBER, R. S., JENKINS, H. A. and COKER, N. J. (1984) Sensorineural hearing loss associated with ulcerative colitis. *Archives of Otolaryngology*, 110, 810–812

WEIDAUER, H., ARNOLD, W. and SEELIG, H. P. (1977) Nachweis von Basal-membranantikorpern im Innenohr bei experiemnteller Masuginephritis. *Zeitschrift für Laryngologie, Rhinologie und Otologie*, 56, 850–857

WEINBERG, A. G., CURRARINO, G. and BESSERNAN, A. M. (1977) Hirschsprung's disease and congenital deafness. Familial association. *Human Genetics*, 38, 157–161

WELL, D., BLANCHARD, S., KAPLAN, J., GUILFORD, P., GIBSON, F., WALSH, J. *et al.* (1945) Defective myosin VII gene responsible for Usher syndrome type IB. *Nature*, 374, 60–61

WELLER, T. H. and NEVA, F. A. (1962) Propagation in tissue culture of cytopathic agents from patients with rubella-like illness. *Proceedings of the Society of Experimental Biology and Medicine*, 111, 215–225

WEST, F. D. B., GHELKAR, A. and RAMSDEN, R. T. (1989) Wildervanck's syndrome – unilateral Mondini dysplasia identified by computed tomography. *Journal of Laryngology and Otology*, 103, 408–411

WILDE, W. (1853) *Practical Observations on Aural Surgery*. Philadelphia: Blanchard and Lee.

WILLIE, A. H. (1981) Cell death: a new classification separating apoptosis from necrosis. In: *Cell Death in Biology and Pathology*, edited by I. D. Bowen and R. A. Lockshin. London: Chapman and Hall. pp. 9–34

WOLFF, D., BERNHARD, W. G., TSUTSUMI, S., ROSS, I. S. and NUSSBAUM, H. E. (1965) The pathology of Cogan's syndrome causing profound deafness. *Annals of Otology, Rhinology and Laryngology*, 74, 507–520

WOOD, T. J. and KNIGHT, L. W. (1966) A family with Alport's syndrome of hereditary nephritis and deafness. *Australian Annals of Medicine*, 15, 227–235

WRIGHT, A., DAVIS, A., BREDBERG, G., ULEBRI, L. and SPENCER, H. (1987) Hair cell distributions in the normal human cochlea. A report of a European working group. *Acta Otolaryngologica*, Supplement 436, 15–24

WRIGHT, J. L. W., PHELPS, P. D. and FRIEDMANN, I. (1976) Temporal bone studies in anencephaly. *Journal of Laryngology and Otology*, 90, 919–927

WRIGHT, M. I. (1971) *The Pathology of Deafness (an introduction)*. Manchester: Manchester University Press

WULLSTEIN, H. I., KLEY, W., RAUCH, S. and KOZTLIN, R. (1960) Zur biochemie der perilymphe operierten otosklerosen. *Zentralblatt für Laryngologie und Rhinologie*, 39, 665–672

YAMANOBE, S. and HARRIS, J. P. (1992) Spontaneous remission in experimental autoimmune labyrinthitis. *Annals of Otology, Rhinology and Laryngology*, 101, 1007–1014

YANAGITA, N., YOKOI, S., KOIDE, J., TORIYAMA, M. and ISHII, T. (1987) Acute bilateral deafness with nephritis: a human temporal bone study. *Laryngoscope*, **97**, 345–352

YOSHIKAWA, W. N., CAMERON, A. H. and WHITE, R. H. R. (1981) The glomerular basal lamina in hereditary nephritis. *Journal of Pathology*, **135**, 199–209

ZAJTCHUK, J. T. and LINDSAY, J. R. (1975) Osteogenesis imperfecta congenita and tarda: a temporal bone report. *Annals of Otology, Rhinology and Laryngology*, **84**, 350–359

ZAYTOUN, G. M. (1983) Basophilic deposits in the vascular stria; a clinicopathological update. *Annals of Otology, Rhinology and Laryngology*, **92**, 242–248

Further reading

ALEXANDER, G. (1904) Zur Kentniss der Missbildungen des Gehorganges besonders des Labyrinths. *Zeitschrift der Ohrenheilkunde*, **46**, 245–253

ALTMANN, F. (1950) Histologic picture of inherited nerve deafness in man and animals. *Archives of Otolaryngology*, **51**, 852–890

BALLANTYNE, J. C. (1962) Injuries of the ear. *Journal of Laryngology and Otology*, **76**, 661–664

BURNS, H. and ROBINSON, D. W. (1970) *Hearing and Noise in Industry*. London: HMSO

COHEN, A. (1977) Extraauditory effects of acoustic stimulation. In: *Handbook of Physiology*, edited by D. H. K. Lee. Chapter 3. Section 9. Reactions to environmental agents. Bethesda, Maryland: American Physiological Association. pp. 31–34

CRAWFURD, M. D'A. and TOGHILL, P. J. (1968) Alport's syndrome of hereditary nephritis and deafness. *Quarterly Journal of Medicine*, **37**, 563–576

FISCH, U. (1974) Facial paralysis in fractures of the petrous bone. *Laryngoscope*, **84**, 2141–2154

FISHER, E. R. and HELLSTROM, H. R. (1961) Cogan's syndrome and systemic vascular disease. *Archives of Pathology*, **72**, 96

FRIEDMANN, I. (1969) The innervation of the developing fowl embryo otocyst in vitro and in vivo. *Acta Otolaryngologica*, **67**, 224–238

GUSSEN, R. (1968) Mondini type genetically determined deafness. *Journal of Laryngology and Otology*, **82**, 41–55

ISHII, T. (1977) The fine structure of lipofuscin in the human ear. *Archives of Otorhinolaryngology*, **215**, 213–221

ISHII, T., MURAKAMI, Y., KIMURA, R. S. and BALOGH, K. Jr (1967) Electron microscopic and histochemical identification of lipofuscin in the human inner ear. *Acta Otolaryngologica*, **64**, 17–29

JAFFE, H. L. (1958) *Tumours and Tumorous Condition of the Bones and Joints*. Philadelphia: Lea and Febiger

JOHNSSON, L.-G., FELIX, H., GLEESON, F. H., and POLLAK, A. (1990) Observations on the pattern of sensorineural degeneration in the human cochlea. *Acta Otolaryngologica*, Supplement 470, 88–96

LAXDAL, O. E., SINHA, R. P., MERIDA, J. *et al.* (1969) Reye's syndrome. Encephalopathy in children associated with fatty change in the viscera. *American Journal of Disease of Children*, **117**, 717–721

LECK, J. (1966) Incidence and endemicity of Down's syndrome. *Lancet*, ii, 457–460

LIM, D. J. (1976) Ultrastructural changes in the cochlea following acoustic hyperstimulation and ototoxicity. *Annals of Otology, Rhinology and Laryngology*, **85**, 741–742

MOODY, D. B., STEBBINS, W. C., JOHNSSON, L.-G. and HAWKINS, J. E. Jr (1976) Noise-induced hearing loss in non-human primates. In: *The Effects of Noise on Hearing – Critical Issues*, edited by D. Henderson, R. P. Hamernick, D. S. Dogandh and J. H. Mills. New York: Raven Press

MOODY, D. B., STEBBINS, W. C., HAWKINS, J. E. Jr and JOHNSSON, L. (1978) Hearing loss and cochlear pathology in the monkey (Macaca) following exposure to high levels of noise. *Archives of Otorhinolaryngology*, **220**, 47–72

MORTON, E. W. D. and COGAN, D. G. (1959) Syndrome of nonsyphilitic interstitial keratitis and vestibuloaudtitory symptoms. A long-term follow-up. *Archives of Ophthalmology*, 695

NYLEN, B. (1949) Histpathological investigations of the localization number activity and extent of otosclerotic foci. *Journal of Laryngology and Otology*, **63**, 321–327

ORNVOLD, K., and NIELSEN, M. H. (1985) Disseminated histiocytosis; a clinical and immunohistochemical retrospective study. *Acta Pathologica, Microbiologica et Immunologica Scandinavica*, **93**, 311–316

PAPARELLA, M. M., SCHACHERN, P. A. and GOYCOLEA, M. V. (1988) Multiple otopathologic disorders. *Annals of Otology, Rhinology and Laryngology*, **97**, 14–18

PENROSE, L. S. (1961) Familial examples of mongolism. *British Medical Bulletin*, **17**, 184–189

PERKOFF, G. T., STEPHENS, F. F., DOLOWITZ, D. A. and TYLER, F. H. (1951) A clinical study of hereditary interstitial pyelonephritis. *Archives of Internal Medicine*, **88**, 191–200

PHELPS, P. D. (1986) Congenital cerebrospinal fluid fistulae of the petrous temporal bone. *Clinical Otolaryngology*, **11**, 79–92

PHELPS, P. D., REARDON, W., PERBREY, M. E., BELLMAN, S. and LUXON, L. (1991) X-linked deafness, stapes gushers and a distinctive defect of the inner ear. *Neuroradiology*, **33**, 326–330

REVESZ, T., EARL, C. J. and BARNARD, R. O. (1988) Superficial siderosis of the central nervous system presenting with longstanding deafness. *Journal of the Royal Society of Medicine*, **81**, 479–481

SANDO, I. and WOOD, P. R. (1971) Congenital middle ear anomalies. *Otolaryngologic Clinics of North America*, **4**, 291–318

SMITH, D. W., PATAU, K., THERMAN, E. and INHORN, S. L. (1963) The D-trisomy syndrome. *Journal of Pediatrics*, **62**, 326–332

5

Pathology of the vestibular system

R. R. Gacek

Knowledge of the pathophysiology of vestibular disorders is essential for a logical, accurate evaluation and management of the vertiginous patient. The diagnosis of vestibular system disease, particularly peripheral disorders, depends primarily on a carefully obtained history with some assistance from tests of hearing function and vestibular sensitivity (caloric, positional tests). Radiological tests (CT, MRI) are helpful in the evaluation of neoplastic and inflammatory disorders which affect the labyrinth, VIIIth cranial nerve and central nervous system (posterior fossa). A reliable body of information necessary to derive an accurate diagnosis of vestibular systems disease comes from our study of temporal bones from patients with vestibular disorders.

Vertigo or dysequilibrium is a result of an asymmetry in the peripheral or central portions of the vestibular system. The severity of dysequilibrium depends on the magnitude and speed of onset of the asymmetry. Compensatory mechanisms usually correct for small asymmetries, thus rendering the patient almost asymptomatic. However, recurrent and progressive asymmetries produce troublesome vestibular symptoms. Since other sensory modalities also participate in spatial orientation, pathologies involving the visual, proprioceptive systems, cerebellum and reticular formation may also be responsible for dysequilibrium. However, the present discussion will be limited to pathologies involving the input from vestibular labyrinthine sense organs which project to the brain stem forming important motor reflex connections. The asymmetries in the vestibular pathway may be located in the sense organ, the first order vestibular neuron, the vestibular nuclei and their connections to the extraocular muscles, contralateral vestibular nuclei, the vestibulocerebellum and the vestibulospinal tracts. It is appropriate to discuss these pathologies at the peripheral and central levels. A number of

reports have emphasized that the majority of clinical disorders producing vertigo are located peripherally, that is in the sense organ or the first order vestibular neuron. Central vestibular pathways are less frequently responsible for dysequilibrium.

Peripheral vestibular system

Significantly more information is available about the pathology affecting vestibular sense organs and their nerve supply than any other segment of the vestibular pathway. The vulnerability of the peripheral vestibular system to various intrinsic and extrinsic pathologies along with a more complete histopathological documentation of these disorders are responsible for our present level of knowledge of vestibular pathologies. Pathology in the peripheral vestibular system produces clinical symptoms by significant alteration of the action potentials directed through the vestibular nerve into the brain stem. It may be useful therefore to subdivide further the peripheral pathologies into those that affect the sense organ and those that affect the first order neuron. A helpful approach for discussing these pathologies for diagnostic and therapeutic reasons is from the viewpoint of the pathophysiological mechanism responsible for vestibular asymmetry.

End organ pathology
Mechanical stimulation

Several pathological situations may be responsible for recurrent or chronic dysequilibrium by mechanical stimulation of the vestibular sense organs in an unphysiological fashion. Essentially this mechanism produces an unphysiological change in the action potentials leading from a specific end organ by such mechanical stimulation. There are several well known clinical examples of this form of pathology.

Erosion of the bony labyrinth

Erosion of the bony labyrinth capsule by cholesteatoma may occur as a result of pressure from the enlarging cholesteatoma sac and/or a chemical process of bone erosion probably mediated through collagenolytic enzymes (Abramson, 1969; Abramson and Gross, 1971). When fenestration of the bony labyrinth capsule has occurred, an opportunity for the transmission of pressure from the ear canal to the membranous labyrinth is present (Figure 5.1). True fistulization of the perilymphatic space and the middle ear space through such bony fistulae is extremely rare. Of course the transmission of positive or negative pressure in the ear canal by displacing the cupula of the fenestrated bony canal will activate the vestibulo-ocular reflex accompanied by the symptoms of rotatory vertigo. The lateral, superior and posterior semicircular canals may be involved by this pathology in decreasing order of frequency (Ritter, 1970; Gacek, 1974). The bony wall of the cochlea may also be eroded or fistulized by cholesteatoma or chronic osteitis (Figure 5.2). Such erosion is usually in association with fistulization of the bony vestibular labyrinth and is manifested by a sensorineural hearing loss which may assume a descending or flat threshold pattern. The most frequent location of erosion of the cochlear wall is over the basal end (promontory) (Gacek, 1974). Since fistulization of the cochlear wall is not indicated by a specific diagnostic test, the condition is usually recognized during surgery for

cholesteatoma. It should be suspected in all cases undergoing surgery for extensive cholesteatoma. It should be mentioned that along with the bony fistulization of the labyrinth capsule, varying degrees of a localized inflammatory process occur along the endosteal membrane and perilymphatic space adjacent to the fistula. Undoubtedly such inflammatory reactions are also responsible for dysequilibrium in addition to the vertigo produced by activating the fistula mechanically. Therefore this pathological circumstance has an inflammatory as well as a mechanical mechanism for dysequilibrium. Since the cholesteatoma membrane is pathological tissue, surgical removal is a desirable goal. A general rule suggests that the cholesteatoma matrix can usually be removed safely from a small fistula (< 2 mm) without tearing the underlying endosteal membrane (Gacek, 1974). However, safe removal of the cholesteatoma is usually not possible over a large fistula because of the greater duration of the pathological erosion with a greater degree of adherence by fibrous tissue to the membranous labyrinth. However, this is not an inviolate rule.

Hennebert's sign

A positive vestibulo-ocular response with clinical symptoms may also occur in the presence of a normal tympanic membrane and middle ear space when positive or negative pressure is applied to the tympanic membrane. Dysequilibrium and ocular deviation in the absence of clinical middle ear disease is referred to as Hennebert's sign and can be explained on the basis of mechanical stimulation of vestibular sense organs by depression and withdrawal of the

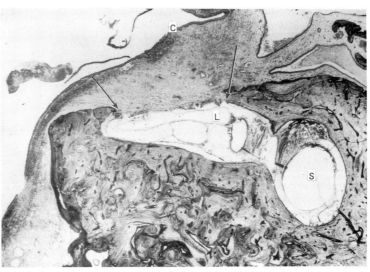

Figure 5.1 Photomicrograph demonstrating fistulization of the bony labyrinth (arrows) over the lateral semicircular canal (L) by cholesteatoma membrane (C). S = superior semicircular canal ampulla

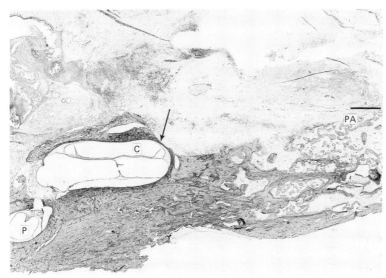

Figure 5.2 Osteitis and abscess formation in the petrous apex (PA) produce near fistulization (arrow) of the cochlear wall (C). P = posterior semicircular canal ampulla

stapes footplate in the oval window (Nadol, 1977). The mechanical stimulation depends on distension of the membranous wall of vestibular sense organs especially the saccular wall which may contact the undersurface of the stapes footplate (Figure 5.3). A pushing or pulling effect on the membranous walls by the footplate initiates the mechanical displacement of vestibular sense organs. Contact with other vestibular sense organs (cristae ampullaris) may then allow transmission of pressure introduced through the ossicular chain producing vestibular stimulation and ocular deviation.

Prosthetic stimulation of the vestibular sense organs

Mechanical stimulation of the vestibular sense organs may occur as a result of a stapedectomy procedure used to correct the hearing loss due to otosclerosis.

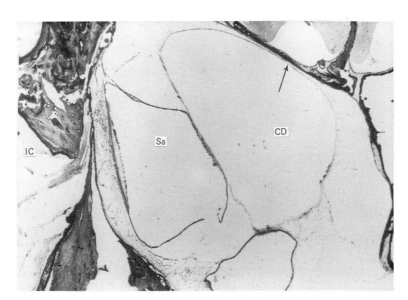

Figure 5.3 Progressive endolymphatic hydrops may result in a dilated cochlear duct (CD) which establishes contact between the stapes footplate (arrow) and the saccule (Sa) or other vestibular end organs. IC = internal auditory canal

Because the utricular macula lies close to the oval window in the vestibule, it may be contacted by a prosthesis which extends excessively beyond the level of the window into the vestibule. Particularly in the case of the piston type prosthesis which must be inserted beyond the level of the window to prevent refixation by bony and fibrous tissue, an excessively long prosthesis may make contact with the utricular macula (Figure 5.4). Depression of the incus during surgery while the patient is under local anaesthesia can be used to determine the proper length of the prosthesis. The long prosthesis syndrome is usually manifested by ataxia exacerbated by the Valsalva manoeuvre, heavy lifting or bending over, and usually taking the form of dysequilibrium or ataxia rather than rotatory vertigo. Unrelieved mechanical stimulation by a stapes prosthesis in this manner may result ultimately in a sensorineural hearing loss because of the traumatic labyrinthitis which is produced.

Cupulolithiasis

Cupulolithiasis is a well known form of pathology responsible for paroxysmal positional vertigo (type III Aschan). The accumulated histopathological evidence indicates that the posterior semicircular canal is responsible for the vertigo and nystagmus produced in the head-down position with the Hallpike manoeuvre (Gacek, 1985). The nystagmus provoked in the head extended and ear-down position (Hallpike manoeuvre) is a rotatory nystagmus directed toward the downmost ear (clockwise with left ear down, counter-clockwise with right ear down) which is visible with the unaided eye 1–3 seconds after the provocative position is assumed. The duration of nystagmus is short (20–25 s), reappears briefly in reversed direction when the sitting position is resumed and fatigues on repeated provocation. The neural pathways from the posterior canal sense organ which input to the brain stem and extraocular muscles explain the direction of nystagmus provoked in this position by a gravity-sensitive cupula and also the nystagmus resulting from selective ablation of the innervation of the posterior canal crista. Histopathological observations (Schuknecht, 1969; Schuknecht and Ruby, 1973) of the posterior canal crista in patients with benign paroxysmal positional vertigo revealed basophilic deposits embedded into the cupula of the posterior semicircular canal of the undermost ear in the provocative position (Figure 5.5). Presumably these deposits are derived from the otoconial blanket located over the utricular macula, the probable source for otoconia in the pars superior of the labyrinth. These otoconia are thought to be dislodged from the utricular macula as a result of head trauma, acute and chronic inflammatory conditions, ageing, or surgical insult to the labyrinth. The otoconia gravitating into the most dependent portion of the labyrinth (i.e. posterior canal ampulla) are most likely to become embedded into the cupula of the posterior canal rendering it gravity sensitive during the positional test. Clinical proof that the posterior canal crista is responsible for the symptomatology in this syndrome is available in the form of the complete relief afforded by selective denervation of the posterior canal in the undermost ear (Gacek, 1985). Experimental evidence that increasing the specific gravity of the cupula allows it to respond to gravity has been pro-

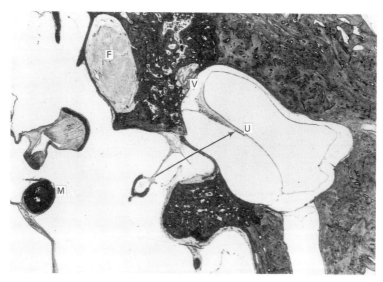

Figure 5.4 A vertical section through the oval window region demonstrates the opportunity for contact with the utricular macula (U) by a long stapedectomy prosthesis (arrow). F = facial nerve, V = superior division of vestibular nerve surrounded by otosclerotic bone, M = manubrium of malleus

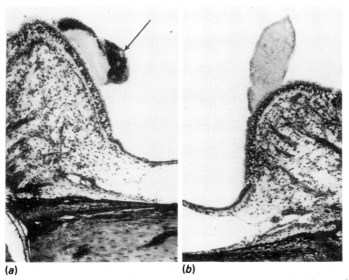

(a)   **(b)**

Figure 5.5 (*a*) The arrow indicates basophilic deposit in cupula of posterior canal crista of undermost labyrinth from a patient with benign paroxysmal positional vertigo. (*b*) Note absence of deposit in contralateral posterior canal cupula

duced by using deuterium oxide to increase the specific gravity of the cupula (Money and Myles, 1974). In both the experimental animal and human subjects this results in positional nystagmus of the peripheral type.

Vestibular atelectasis

Merchant and Schuknecht (1988) have described a condition which they have called vestibular atelectasis. A group of temporal bones in the Massachusetts Eye and Ear Infirmary Collection from patients with vestibular symptoms were separated out from the known vestibular disorders such as Menière's disease, vestibular schwannoma, labyrinthitis and brain stem and cerebellar neoplasms. In a significant number of these temporal bones the pathological findings consisted of a collapse of the membranous labyrinth including the walls of the ampullae, the utricle and the saccule. They used the term vestibular atelectasis since no other pathological correlate could be identified to explain the disturbance of the vestibular system. Strict histological criteria were used to rule out post-mortem artefact as a cause of the collapse. The principal clinical symptom in these patients was chronic unsteadiness, particularly noted on head movement. Short episodes of a rotatory vertigo were also noted in some patients. Because of the absence of other histological findings, sufficient to explain the vestibular system disorder, they attributed the patient's symptoms to the collapse of the membranous labyrinth which in some way disturbs the motion mechanics of the cupulae (Figure 5.6a) and the otolithic membranes (Figure 5.6b). The collapse of the

membranous labyrinth may be caused by a traumatic insult (viral, ageing, vascular, head trauma) which destroys the tethering support of the perilymphatic trabeculae and weakens the rigidity of the membranous walls. The collapsed ampullary, utricular or saccular walls interfere with vestibular function by entrapment or compression of the cupulae and otolithic membranes.

The condition is subdivided into primary and secondary vestibular atelectasis. *Primary vestibular atelectasis* is characterized by an initial vestibular symptom of paroxysmal type in the absence of auditory or central nervous system signs. These symptoms have a duration of several days and following resolution are followed by a period of dysequilibrium characterized by persistent unsteadiness aggravated by head movement. In some patients, the symptoms become less pronounced with time and in others they may be insidious and have a prolonged duration.

Secondary vestibular atelectasis refers to collapse of the membranous labyrinthine walls in association with other underlying pathology of the peripheral vestibular system. Some of these pathologies are the degeneration of ageing, endolymphatic hydrops and temporal bone fracture. In some instances, such as in the degeneration of ageing where sufficient degeneration of the sensory structures is present, the vestibular symptoms may be minimal or not present. The primary alternative diagnosis which may simulate primary vestibular atelectasis is acute vestibular neuritis. The main differentiation would be that vestibular neuritis has characteristic paroxysms of vertigo lasting one to several days while the clinical symptoms in vestibular atelectasis are chronic

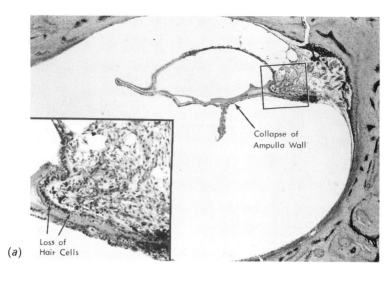

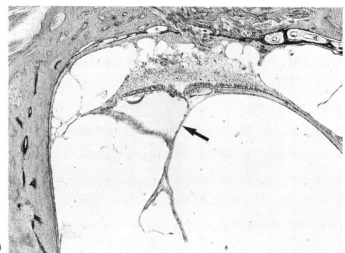

Figure 5.6 (*a*) Vestibular atelectasis represented by collapse of the ampullary wall onto the cupula and crista ampullaris. Inset demonstrates a partial loss of hair cells. (*b*) The utricular wall (arrow) is collapsed on to the macula which has a partial loss of supporting and hair cells

dysequilibrium precipitated or aggravated by head movement. Similarly, the chronic dysequilibrium precipitated by head movement seen occasionally in Ménière's disease, vestibular schwannoma or other vestibular disorders may be on the basis of secondary or associated vestibular atelectasis. The mechanism of interference with motion mechanics by collapse of the vestibular labyrinth seems a reasonable hypothesis to explain vestibular symptoms in those patients where other histological correlates such as degeneration of sense organs or the vestibular nerve, or endolymphatic hydrops are absent.

Inflammation

Inflammation of the labyrinth is termed labyrinthitis and may be classified as either bacterial or viral. Bacterial labyrinthitis may occur as an extension of infection from the middle ear space or the intracranial cavity. Acute or chronic bacterial otitis media may extend into the labyrinth either through a bony labyrinthine fistula associated with cholesteatoma or by way of the round window membrane (Figure 5.7) or the oval window (Figure 5.8). Suppurative labyrinthitis may also occur as an extension of bacterial meningitis along the fluid pathways that

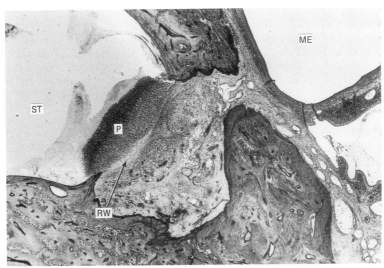

Figure 5.7 Purulent exudate (P) in suppurative labyrinthitis as a result of extension by suppurative middle ear disease through the round window membrane (RW). ME = Middle ear space, ST = scala tympani

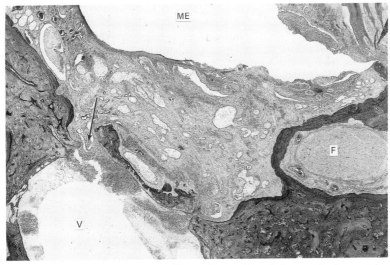

Figure 5.8 Demonstration of extension by suppurative middle ear disease through the annular ligament (arrow) into the vestibule (V). F = Facial nerve, ME = middle ear space

communicate the subarachnoid space with the perilymphatic space of the cochlea. These are the cochlear aqueduct or the cribrose area in the base of the modiolus of the cochlea.

Bacterial labyrinthitis can be classified into four stages (Schuknecht, 1974a):

1 acute or toxic (serous)
2 acute suppurative
3 chronic suppurative
4 fibrosseous.

The acute toxic or serous form of labyrinthitis will occur as a result of chemical changes in the perilymphatic space caused by a toxic or suppurative process which impinges on a membrane barrier of the labyrinth, such as the round window membrane, or the membrane covering a bony fistula. During this stage chemical changes in the perilymphatic space may occur without the invasion of bacterial organisms and the inflammatory cell component which accompanies bacterial invasion. Although vertigo with nystagmus may be present at this stage, the disturbance in vestibular physiology is reversible if the toxic (inflammatory) process adjoining the vestibular labyrinth is controlled medically or surgically. The second stage of acute suppurative labyrinthitis occurs when invasion of the perilymphatic space by bacterial organisms has occurred with an accompanying response from the host organism in the form of inflammatory cells and fibrocytes (Figure 5.9). At this stage irreversible destruction of auditory and vestibular function has occurred and the goal of treatment is to control the extension of infection so that invasion of the subarachnoid space is prevented. Adequate treatment with chemotherapeutic agents may suffice to control acute suppurative disease, but surgical drainage may also be necessary. The third stage in suppurative labyrinthitis is the chronic stage where involvement of the labyrinth by bacterial organisms with an inflammatory tissue response has occurred over a long period of time usually as an extension of chronic inflammatory middle ear and mastoid disease. Complete irreversible loss of vestibular and auditory function invariably occurs and the primary goal is to eradicate the inflammatory process in order to prevent intracranial extension. The final or healed stage of suppurative labyrinthitis is the fibrosseous response that is generated by the host organism as the inflammatory process has been successfully controlled (Figure 5.10). At first, a dense fibrous tissue response occurs to obliterate the labyrinthine spaces with a resultant complete loss of auditory and vestibular function and then, ultimately, calcification and osteoneogenesis may occur to obliterate some or all of the labyrinthine spaces (labyrinthitis ossificans) (Figure 5.11).

The most common bacterial organisms responsible for acute serous or suppurative labyrinthitis are pneumococci, streptococci and *Haemophilus influenzae*, while the chronic form is caused by a mixture of Gram-negative bacilli (*Pseudomonas, Proteus, Escherichia coli*).

A more common form of labyrinthitis is that which is seen as a result of invasion by viral agents (Bordley, Brookhauser, and Worthington, 1972). Viruses such as the mumps virus, the influenza viruses, adenoviruses and other viral agents have been associated with an acute disturbance of auditory and vestibular function manifested as sustained vertigo and nystagmus lasting 3–5 days with a gradual lessening of the spontaneous nystagmus and vagal symptoms. As these symptoms abate and the patient recovers balance by use of the compensatory mechanisms, varying degrees of residual permanent loss of auditory and vestibular function may be seen. The viraemia reaches the fluid pathways of the labyrinth either directly from the blood stream or by way of the subarachnoid space. The viral agents probably affect the structures located within the scala media and the sense organs of the vestibular labyrinth (Karmody, 1983). Hair cells of the organ of Corti, as well as the stria vascularis and spiral ganglion may be affected by the viral infection (Figure 5.12). Cystic degeneration, hair cell loss, and round cell infiltrates are the characteristic findings in the end organs of both the auditory (Figure 5.13) and vestibular labyrinth

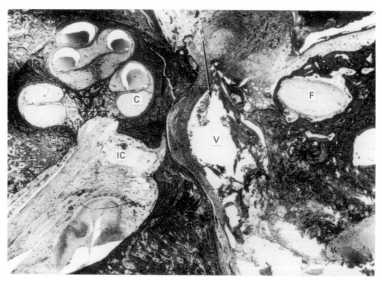

Figure 5.9 Extensive suppurative labyrinthitis in vestibular (V) and cochlear (C) portions of the labyrinth with associated involvement of meninges of internal auditory canal (IC) as a result of invasion through the oval window (arrow). F = Facial nerve

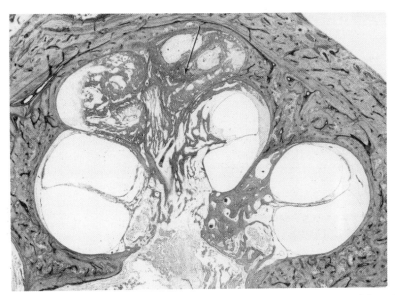

Figure 5.10 Arrow indicates the osseous reparative response in the cochlea following suppurative labyrinthitis

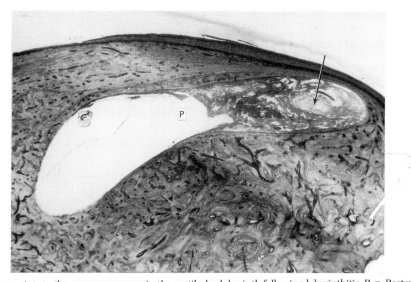

Figure 5.11 Arrow points to the osseous response in the vestibular labyrinth following labyrinthitis. P = Posterior semicircular canal

(Figure 5.14). Of course, viral labyrinthitis is beyond the presently available therapeutic management programme. However, steroids have been shown to be of some benefit to hearing recovery in those patients where hearing loss is not greater than 90 dB (Wilson, Byl and Laird, 1980). Recovery from vestibular symptoms after viral labyrinthitis is gradual and depends primarily on compensatory mechanisms involving the visual, proprioceptive and cerebellar pathways. Fortunately, viral labyrinthitis is usually unilateral and

therefore function of the contralateral ear is sufficient to enable a patient to function reasonably well.

Degeneration

Degeneration of the sensory cells of the vestibular sense organs is associated with vestibular symptoms and eventually may lead to a loss of vestibular sensitivity. Since the hair cell is the transducer by which

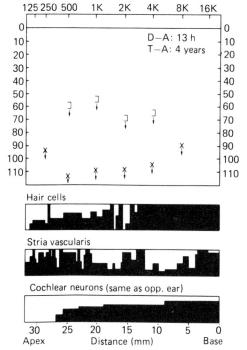

Figure 5.12 Audiogram and assessment of sensory, neural and secretory structures in the cochlea as a result of viral labyrinthitis. D-A = Death to autopsy interval, T-A = test to autopsy interval

the mechanical stimulation of the sense organ is transformed into an electrical impulse (action potential) in the vestibular nerve fibres, deterioration of these sensory cells is important in the normal func-

tion of the vestibular apparatus. Two well-known causes of vestibular sensory cell degeneration are ototoxic drugs, and the ageing process.

Ototoxicity

Most therapeutic agents, particularly the aminoglycosides, that are harmful to the labyrinth will cause degeneration of the vestibular sensory cells as well as severe toxic effects on the organ of Corti. Streptomycin (McGee and Olszewski, 1962; Wersall and Hawkins, 1962) and gentamicin (Lundquist and Wersall, 1967) are unique because of their ability to affect the vestibular hair cells before affecting the hair cells of the organ of Corti. Therefore, these drugs are potent vestibulotoxic agents. Since the hair cells are surrounded in a perilymph fluid environment, blood-borne chemicals will reach the sensory cells of the vestibular and auditory neuroepithelium by way of perilymph which is a derivative of blood. A large number of animal experiments supported by clinical trials in patients treated for vestibular disorders (Schuknecht, 1957) have demonstrated that streptomycin sulphate administered parenterally will cause degeneration of the hair cells of the cristae and the maculae of the labyrinth. This effect will be manifested clinically by ataxia after approximately 20–25 g streptomycin and will usually result in a loss of vestibular function as measured by absence of a vestibulo-ocular reflex at 30–40 g total dosage. If the streptomycin is discontinued at the point where the vestibulo-ocular reflex is absent following a strong ice-water stimulus, no auditory deficit will occur. Therefore this method of destroying vestibular hair cells is useful in the management of patients with disabling bilateral Menière's disease or in patients

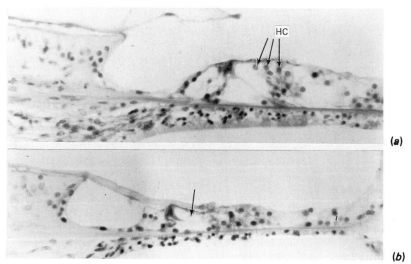

Figure 5.13 (*a*) Organ of Corti from uninvolved ear of patient with hearing loss shown in Figure 5.12. HC = Outer hair cells. (*b*) Arrow indicates missing hair cells in organ of Corti of ear with severe hearing loss

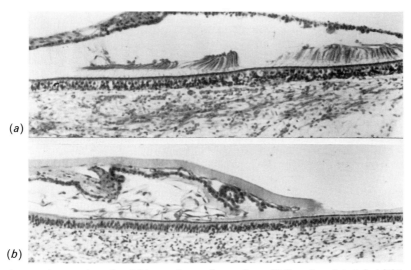

Figure 5.14 (*a*) The saccular macula and otolithic membrane of normal ear. (*b*) Shrunken distorted otolithic membrane with loss of hair cells in the saccular macula of ear following viral labyrinthitis

who have Menière's disease in an only hearing ear. The temporal bones of patients treated with streptomycin sulphate have demonstrated almost complete loss of vestibular hair cells in the cristae with a partial loss in the maculae (Figure 5.15). The vestibulotoxic effect therefore appears to be more severe on the sense organs of the semicircular canals. Patients who have been treated with streptomycin sulphate and have bilateral vestibular hair cell ablation compensate well, not only because of other equilibrium systems, but also because residual hair cell function in the maculae serves as an important vestibular input.

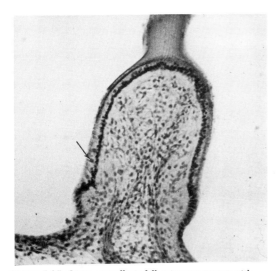

Figure 5.15 Crista ampullaris following treatment with streptomycin sulphate. Arrow points to remaining hair cell nuclei in the neuroepithelial layer

Ageing

Although vertigo and dysequilibrium are common complaints in the elderly, (Sheldon, 1948; Droller and Pemberton, 1953) being estimated at 38–60%, the usual vestibular tests show variable responses with ageing. Vestibular function as measured by the caloric method may be decreased (Arslan, 1957) or normal (Forgacs, 1957), but rotational tests which are more physiological, show a more consistent decrease with ageing (Wall, Black and Hunt, 1984). Vestibulospinal reflex measurements with the posture platform method, rather consistently demonstrate decreased function with increased age.

Along with these tests of function in the ageing population, various studies have shown morphological changes in both the sense organ and the first order vestibular neuron. Loss of hair cells in the crista ampullares, the maculae of the saccule and the utricle has been demonstrated with a greater loss of sensory cells in the cristae (Rosenhall, 1973). The saccular macula appears to have a higher incidence of sensory cell loss than the utricular macula (Johnsson, 1971). Other morphological changes in the sensory epithelium such as cyst formation and the accumulation of lipofuscin are also increased in greater age groups (Ishii *et al.*, 1967). Changes in the first order vestibular neurons, both in terms of decreased number (Richter, 1980) and in decreased myelination (Bergstrom, 1973) have also been described in the ageing individual. Finally, degenerative changes of the otolithic membrane and macula of the saccule and utricle as well as collapse of the vestibular membranous walls have been documented in the ageing individual (Merchant and Schuknecht, 1988).

A useful classification of the various clinical syndromes of dysequilibrium in the ageing population correlated with the morphologies of the sensory and neural components as well as the architecture of the vestibular labyrinth has been proposed by Nadol and Schuknecht (1990). Their classification basically divides the forms of dysequilibrium into those that are inducible and transient, and a form which is non-inducible or chronic and unremitting. The inducible transient forms of vertigo are related to, or initiated by, change in body or head position. The first of these is cupulolithiasis which is caused by a change in the specific gravity of the cupula of the posterior semicircular canal usually from degenerated otoconia from the utricular macula in the pars superior as a result of ageing. This form of cupulolithiasis presents a rather typical form of severe paroxysmal positional vertigo manifested by rotatory nystagmus in the provocative head-down position. This syndrome is de-

scribed in a previous section of this chapter. It should be mentioned that this form of cupulolithiasis in the ageing individual may be most severe and is frequently chronic and not intermittent. In selected individuals ablation by singular neurectomy has proven to be a very useful therapeutic approach.

The other two forms of inducible transient vertigo are characterized by a concept of vertigo initiated or aggravated by change in either body axis or by angular rotation of the head. The type induced by change in body axis is relative to gravity such as changing from coming from a recumbent to an erect position has been called the macular dysequilibrium of ageing and is thought to be produced by morphological changes in the membranous walls of the utricular and saccular maculae with or without sensory and supporting cell pathology (Figure 5.16a). It

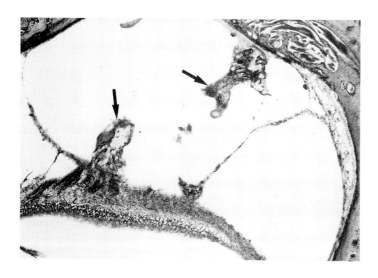

Figure 5.16 (*a*)

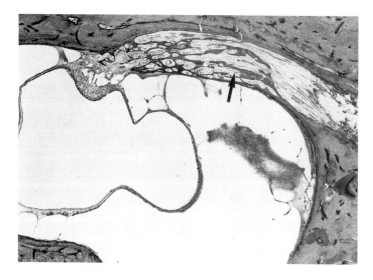

Figure 5.16 (*b*)

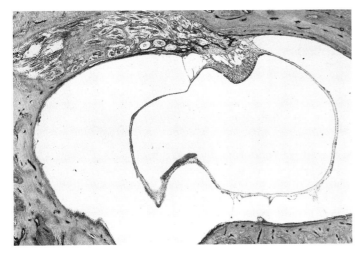

Figure 5.16 (*c*)

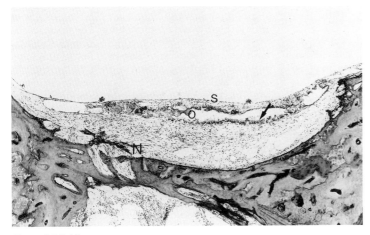

Figure 5.16 (*d*)

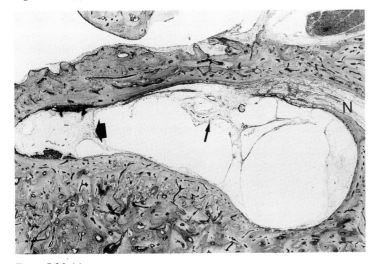

Figure 5.16 (*e*)

Figure 5.16 (*a*) The abnormal proliferation of tissue (arrows) near the utricular macula may be responsible for macular dysequilibrium of ageing. (*b*) Degenerated vestibular neurons (arrow) and normal crista ampullaris in a 73-year-old woman who experienced sudden onset of vertigo for several days and constant dysequilibrium thereafter. (*c*) The contralateral ear in this patient revealed normal neural and sensory units. (*d*) Collapse of thickened saccular wall (S) onto a degenerated otolithic membrane (O) and degenerated sensory epithelial structures (arrow) in autoimmune inner ear disease. The vestibular nerve fibres are also degenerated (N). (*e*) Similar changes in the pars superior where there is thickening and collapse of the ampullary wall (arrow), degenerated sense organ (C) and vestibular nerve (N). A fibrosseous response is seen in the perilymphatic space (large arrow)

has been described by Merchant and Schuknecht (1988) as vestibular atelectasis, and may be a result of either vascular or ageing structural changes in the membranous walls of the utricle or saccule which collapse onto the otolithic membrane causing a disturbance in the motion mechanics of the sense organ.

The final form of inducible transient vertigo is that formerly described as the ampullary dysequilibrium of ageing which is induced by angular rotation of the head. It is typically induced by turning the head from side to side and is thought to be related to collapse of the membranous ampullary wall onto the cupula and cristae of the semicircular canals. Sensory and supporting cell pathology may or may not be associated with this form of vestibular atelectasis. The chronic or unremitting form of dysequilibrium in ageing frequently takes the form of a constant sense of motion or dysequilibrium but may be aggravated by body and head movements. The aetiology of this degeneration may be vascular, infectious, neoplastic, or idiopathic. Degeneration of the sensory cells and neural units (Figure 5.16b, c) down to a level which is incapable of receiving the numerous physiological stimuli which impact on these physical activities may be the histological correlate of this chronic form of dysequilibrium.

Ageing in the central vestibular pathway undoubtedly also occurs in the ageing individual. However, post-mortem morphological material documenting such age-related changes or decreases in neuronal complement is not available.

Autoimmune inner ear disease

During the past decade the recognition and pathology of autoimmune inner ear disorders have been abundantly documented. Auditory and vestibular symptoms as a manifestation of an immune process directed at the inner ear structures has been well documented both clinically and histopathologically. The labyrinth may be involved in an autoimmune process as part of a systemic or non-organ specific disease or as an isolated instance of organ specific autoimmunity.

The pathological correlates have been described in a number of temporal bones in non-organ specific autoimmunity conditions such as polyarteritis nodosa (Gussen, 1977; Jenkins, Pollak and Fisch, 1981) and Cogan's syndrome (Wolff *et al.*, 1965; Rarey, Bicknell, and Davis, 1986). In addition to the symptoms caused by multisystem involvement (kidneys, skeletal system, cardiovascular system, nervous system), patients with polyarteritis nodosa may experience sensorineural hearing loss prior to the onset of other system complaints or after the full development of polyarteritis nodosa. The hearing loss is usually sudden in onset

and rapidly progressive; it may affect one or both ears and may be associated with vestibular symptoms. Vestibular, like the auditory, symptoms are usually abrupt in onset and may be either mild or severe. The histopathological changes in the vestibular labyrinth and the cochlea reflect the result of occlusive vasculitis of the labyrinthine artery with resulting ischaemic changes in the sense organs of the labyrinth. These changes primarily involve the cochlea but may involve the vestibular labyrinth as well. The typical changes are a fibrosseous reaction in the cochlea with subsequent degeneration of hair cells in the organ of Corti and cochlear neurons. The vestibular system will also exhibit a fibrosseous reaction in both the perilymphatic and endolymphatic compartments with degeneration of the sense organs of the otolith and semicircular canal structures. The vestibular nerve may also show evidence of degeneration.

Cogan's syndrome consisting of audiovestibular symptoms as well as an interstitial keratitis may also be associated with iritis, vasculitis of the retinal artery, scleritis and exophthalmus. The audiovestibular symptoms are often suggestive of endolymphatic hydrops or Menière's disease. Fluctuating sensorineural hearing loss and episodic rather than the sudden audiovestibular vertigo caused by ischaemia are the rule. If untreated, the hearing loss may progress to severe deafness. These audiovestibular symptoms are different from those in polyarteritis nodosa in that the symptoms are more recurrent, are not as rapidly progressive as in polyarteritis nodosa, but the vertigo is episodic and severe. Nevertheless, the inner ear pathology consists of a fibrosseous reaction in the vestibular and auditory labyrinth with degeneration of sensory and neural structures similar to that seen in polyarteritis nodosa. The involvement of the vestibular system is more severe in Cogan's syndrome than in polyarteritis nodosa. It has been suggested that the changes in Cogan's syndrome are more consistent with an autoimmune response to proteins of the membranous labyrinth rather than an occlusive vasculitis (Schuknecht, 1991).

Audiovestibular symptoms have also been described in relapsing polychondritis, a third condition where multisystem involvement by the autoimmune process is thought to occur. This syndrome consists of inflammatory reaction in multiple cartilages of the head and neck (auricle, nose), iritis, fever, malaise, and fatigue. Chondrocytes lose their cytoplasm and are replaced by fibrous tissue. Plasma cells and lymphocytes occur at the interface of cartilage and fibrous tissue.

The hearing loss can be bilateral or unilateral and may be sudden and profound, or slowly progressive. Vertigo may also occur with the hearing loss. Histological documentation of degenerated sense organs of the auditory and vestibular labyrinth with fibrous and osseous reaction in the scala tympani and lateral canal suggest that the pathology is secondary to occlusive vasculitis of the labyrinthine artery and its branches (Hoshino *et al.*, 1980).

The description of organ specific autoimmune inner ear disease by McCabe (1979) initiated a new interest and heightened index of suspicion to the clinical recognition of this entity. The typical clinical presentation is that of a bilateral sensorineural hearing loss which is progressive and usually somewhat fluctuant along with vestibular symptoms that are severe and episodic. Differentiation from Ménière's disease may be difficult. A number of clinical tests attempting to identify the immunological response have been described and implemented in diagnosis of this entity but have not demonstrated a high specificity. These are C-reactive protein, screening for rheumatoid factors and antinuclear antibodies. The identification of non-specific sedimentation elevation has been used in the identification of autoimmune inner ear disease. The diagnosis is primarily based on a positive clinical response to the use of steroids or immunosuppressant agents (McCabe, 1979).

Very few temporal bones have been studied in organ-specific autoimmune inner ear disease. Schuknecht (1991) has described one case of a patient with a bilateral progressive, primarily high frequency sensorineural hearing loss with falling speech discrimination which, over a period of 3 years, reached a level of profound deafness. This patient experienced episodic vertigo and ataxia over the period of time and demonstrated only a slightly elevated sedimentation rate with a normal antinuclear antibody (ANA) titre and immunoglobulins A, G and M; however, the IgE fraction was significantly elevated. The temporal bones revealed advanced degeneration of the organ of Corti but with normal cochlear neurons. Fibrous tissue and new bone formation were present in the scala tympani and focal collections of lymphocytes and plasma cells were noted in various areas such as the spiral ligament, tympanic lamella and Rosenthal's canal. Similar changes were noted in the vestibular labyrinth where degeneration of the sense organs including the ampullary ridge, the saccular macula and the utricle were described. There was collapse of the membranous labyrinth into the saccular and utricular maculae (see Figure 5.16d). The ampullae were collapsed onto the cristae. The histological findings, therefore, in organ specific autoimmune inner ear disease are degeneration of inner ear structures, such as the sense organs, and collapse of the membranous labyrinth. Focal infiltrates of lymphocytes, plasma cells and macrophages are noted throughout the membranous labyrinth and associated structures and a proliferation of bone and fibrous tissue were noted in the perilymphatic spaces (see Figure 5.16e).

Trauma

Trauma to the temporal bone and the vestibular sense organs may occur in several forms. Usually the injury results from a fracture through the bony labyrinthine capsule or disruption of the fibrous and bony barriers in the oval or round windows of the labyrinth. Before discussing these categories of direct and indirect trauma to the vestibular labyrinth, it should be noted that injury to the vestibular labyrinth with clinical symptoms may occur in the absence of any disruption of the bony vestibular labyrinth. Labyrinthine concussion as a result of head injury is a well known clinical phenomenon resulting in dysequilibrium, vertigo and positional vertigo (Bárány, 1921; Dix and Hallpike, 1952). The histopathology of this injury is not well documented because of the absence of temporal bone material procured at the time of such injury. However, experimental evidence indicates that injury to the otoconial blanket of the macular sense organs with disruption of the otoconia is one effect that follows concussion (Schuknecht, 1962). A release of a significant number of otoconia which then become embedded into the posterior canal cupula may produce the condition known as cupulolithiasis. Furthermore, bleeding into the perilymphatic space is known to occur following head blows in the experimental animal (Schuknecht and Davison, 1956). The chemical change in the perilymphatic fluid resulting from blood causing a chemical labyrinthitis is also a possible explanation for dysequilibrium.

Temporal bone fractures

Temporal bone fractures are divided into longitudinal and transverse fractures. Although the more common, longitudinal fracture (80%) frequently involves the middle ear, ossicular chain, and facial nerve canal; it does not usually directly involve the vestibular labyrinth. However, transverse fracture of the petrous portion of the temporal bone as a result of severe injury to the base of the skull frequently produces a fracture line through the bony labyrinth and/or the internal auditory meatus (Stenger, 1909). This occurs because it is the weakest point in the petrous segment of the temporal bone. The fracture through the vestibular labyrinth will produce the clinical signs of severe labyrinthine injury with vertigo and a sustained spontaneous nystagmus which gradually resolves over the period of several days to a week. The injury to the blood supply and the membranous structures of the labyrinth results in degeneration of the vestibular sense organs and ultimately in fibrosseous obliteration of the vestibular labyrinth (Figure 5.17). Vestibular symptoms gradually subside as the loss of vestibular and auditory function becomes complete. If residual vestibular function is present, it may be responsible for persistent dysequilibrium. Complete

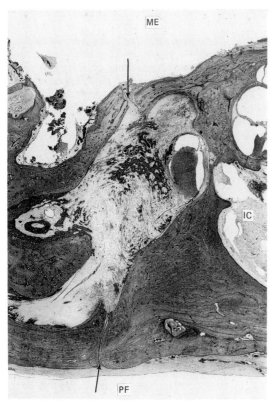

Figure 5.17 The fibrosseous response in the vestibular labyrinth following transverse temporal bone fracture (arrows) may obliterate the bony labyrinth and isolate vestibular sense organs. IC = Internal auditory canal, ME = middle ear space, PF = posterior cranial fossa

ablation in the form of labyrinthectomy or vestibular nerve section may be required to relieve symptoms.

An unusual, but potentially significant long-term complication of temporal bone fracture which extends through the external auditory meatus is cholesteatoma which develops from entrapped stratified squamous epithelium in the fracture line. Such cholesteatomas may reach considerable size eventually destroying both labyrinthine and facial nerve function.

Surgical fistulization

Surgical fistulization of the vestibular labyrinth usually involves the lateral semicircular canal prominence. Such surgical fistulization is caused by inadequate awareness of landmarks in a temporal bone obscured not only by pathology, but also by a poorly developed air cell system. Should surgical fistulization of the bony vestibular labyrinth occur, a serous and serofibrinous labyrinthitis with ultimate degeneration of the vestibular and auditory sense

organs will follow if preventive measures are not taken (Altmann, 1946). These preventive measures may be a form of firm sealing of the surgical bony fistula, using bone wax or tissue, to prevent a persistent communication between the fluid spaces of the labyrinth and the middle ear.

Direct penetrating injury

Direct penetrating injury to the oval window may occur from a slender instrument introduced into the ear canal and through the tympanic membrane. Such accidental introduction of a penetrating instrument may sublux or fracture the stapes footplate producing an oval window to middle ear fistula (Figure 5.18). The perilymphatic fistula results in a serous and serofibrinous labyrinthitis with various degrees of dysequilibrium and vertigo. The dysequilibrium gradually subsides even if there is degeneration of the vestibular system. However, auditory function will eventually be lost if the fistula is not repaired as soon as possible after the injury (Arragg and Paparella, 1964).

Perilymph fistula

Perilymphatic to middle ear fistula may occur through either the oval or round windows as a result of indirect injury to the window membranes. Such indirect injury occurs as a result of abrupt severe changes in the middle ear or subarachnoid space (CSF) pressure (Goodhill, 1971; Pullen, 1972). Injuries such as these are associated with severe barotrauma, extreme physical exertion or impact noise. Symptoms associated with perilymph fistula may include a variety of vestibular and auditory symptoms and findings. The fistula test is often negative and therefore not always helpful in identifying a fistula. The persistence of vertigo and nystagmus with or without auditory deficit over a prolonged period of time (1–2 weeks) following an injury associated with sudden pressure changes should raise the suspicion of a perilymph fistula. Repair of the fistula is essential to achieve reversal of the serous labyrinthitis before progression to fibrinous or degenerative labyrinthitis has occurred. However, clear identification of a membrane defect by adequate surgical exposure is a prerequisite to accurate diagnosis and successful repair with an appropriately placed tissue graft (Figure 5.19).

Vascular injury

Vascular injury to the vestibular and auditory labyrinth can be divided into those that result from occlusion of the blood supply to the labyrinth and those that occur as a result of excessive bleeding into the labyrinth.

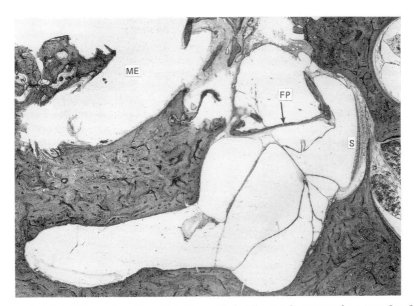

Figure 5.18 The stapes footplate (FP) may be subluxed into the vestibule following direct ossicular injury. S = Saccular macula, ME = middle ear space

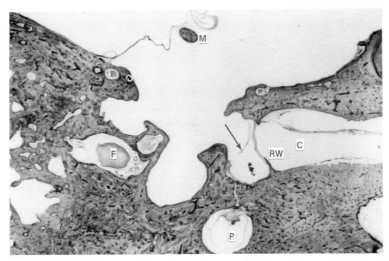

Figure 5.19 A mucous membrane fold (arrow) with ventilatory fenestra often covers the round window niche and must be differentiated from the round window membrane (RW) in order to identify surgically a perilymphatic fistula of the RW. C = Cochlea, P = posterior canal ampulla, F = facial nerve, M = manubrium of malleus

Occlusion of vascular supply

Occlusion of arterial vessels to the vestibular labyrinth can produce degeneration of both the neural and sensory components of the vestibular labyrinth. The best known example of this is occlusion of the anterior vestibular artery (Lindsay and Hemenway, 1956). The clinical manifestations of this event are the acute onset of vertigo which is sustained over several days with spontaneous resolution. Loss of function of the sense organs supplied by the superior division of the vestibular nerve occurs while hearing remains unaffected if cochlear branches are not occluded. The histopathology of this condition shows degeneration of the superior division of the vestibular nerve and its branches along with the sense organs supplied by the superior vestibular division (Figure 5.20). Although complete compensation of this partial vestibular deficit usually occurs, persistent vestibular symptoms in the form of paroxysmal positional vertigo may result if the otoconial loss from the utricular macula is large and becomes embedded into the cupula of the posterior canal.

Excessive bleeding into the labyrinth

Excessive bleeding into the vestibular labyrinth has been documented as a result of subarachnoid haemor-rhage or spontaneous intralabyrinthine bleeding secondary to a major blood dyscrasia. Massive bleeding into the perilymphatic space along with increased subarachnoid pressure may force significant amounts of blood elements into the perilymphatic spaces of both the vestibular (Figure 5.21) and auditory (Figure 5.22) labyrinth along the communicating channels between perilymph and cerebrospinal fluid (Perlman and Lindsay, 1939; Holden and Schuknecht, 1968). These channels are the cochlear aqueduct, the cribrose area of the cochlea and other channels that surround the vestibular nerve fibres as they penetrate

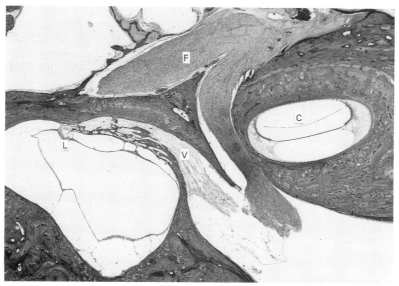

Figure 5.20 Degeneration of the superior division of the vestibular nerve (V) and sense organs (L = lateral canal crista) is observed following occlusion of the anterior vestibular artery. C = Cochlea, F = facial nerve

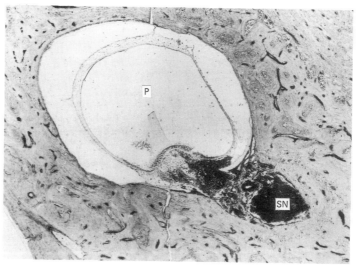

Figure 5.21 In subarachnoid haemorrhage elements of blood are forced into the channels carrying vestibular nerve fibres. SN = singular canal and nerve, P = posterior canal ampulla

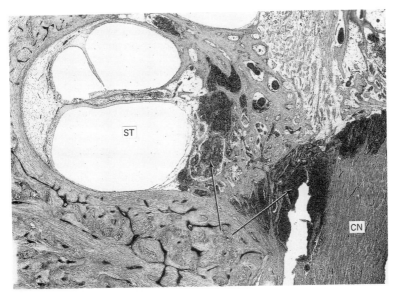

Figure 5.22 Massive degree of extravasated blood from subarachnoid space along the cochlear nerve (CN) fibres (arrows) into the cochlea. ST = Scala tympani

the otic capsule. Massive bleeding into the perilymphatic space is responsible for sustained dysequilibrium and hearing loss probably as a result of a chemical alteration in the perilymphatic environment surrounding the vestibular and auditory nerve fibres. Bleeding into the perilymphatic space may also occur as a result of spontaneous haemorrhage associated with a blood dyscrasia (Figure 5.23). A well known example of such haematological disorder is leukaemia, where extensive bleeding into the perilymphatic spaces of the vestibular and auditory labyrinth was responsible for the sustained vertigo and nystagmus with loss of auditory function (Schuknecht, Igarashi and Chasin, 1965). The ultimate loss of labyrinthine function resulted from the chemical labyrinthitis caused by the massive infusion of blood elements in the perilymphatic compartments.

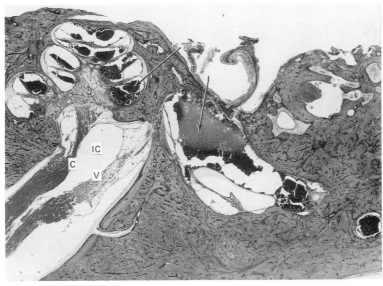

Figure 5.23 Spontaneous haemorrhage (arrows) into the perilymphatic spaces of the labyrinth may occur with haematological disorders such as leukaemia. IC = Internal auditory canal, C = cochlear nerve, V = vestibular nerve

Neoplasia

Neoplasia originating in the vestibular labyrinth has been reported in the form of neural tumours or schwannomas arising from the peripheral branches of the vestibular nerve or the cochlear nerve within the bony labyrinth. Intralabyrinthine schwannomas have been described by several authors (Wanamaker, 1972; Stewart, Liland and Schuknecht, 1975; DeLozier, Gacek and Dana, 1979). Unlike the intracanalicular form of schwannoma, intralabyrinthine vestibular schwannomas produce significant vestibular symptoms resembling those seen in Menière's disease. Recurrent episodic vertigo and fluctuating sensorineural hearing loss have been the usual clinical symptoms associated with this entity. The preoperative clinical diagnosis of surgically subsequently proven intralabyrinthine schwannomas, has been Menière's disease or atypical Menière's disease. The histopathological picture consists of a schwannoma arising from the myelinated labyrinthine segments of the vestibular and auditory nerves which then expands to occupy the perilymphatic compartment of the vestibule. The tumours which arise from the cochlear nerve proliferate into the scala tympani but are also associated with episodic vertigo and sensorineural hearing loss (Figures 5.24 and 5.25). The episodic vertigo may be the result of chemical changes produced by the tumour which then affect the vestibular nerve fibres. It is also possible that the episodic vertigo is a result of progressive endolymphatic hydrops caused by tumour obstruction of the drainage system (ductus reuniens). Endolymphatic

hydrops has also been observed in temporal bones containing an intralabyrinthine schwannoma. Since the vestibular ganglion is remotely located in the internal auditory meatus and therefore not affected by the enlarging tumour, the vestibular nerve input to the brain stem remains capable of transmitting pathological input, thereby accounting for the severity of vestibular symptoms with this form of schwannoma. Other forms of neoplasia which may involve the labyrinth include malignancies such as squamous cell carcinoma or adenocarcinoma which may destroy the bony otic capsule and eventually affect the vestibular labyrinth. However, the otic capsule is generally resistant to neoplastic invasion from an extrinsic source and is violated only late in the course of such metastatic disease.

Metabolic alteration

This category includes vestibular pathologies which result in labyrinthine symptoms because of chemical or ionic changes in the fluid environment of the labyrinth, namely the perilymphatic and endolymphatic compartments. Normal function of the labyrinth depends on the maintenance of normal ionic and chemical composition of endolymph and perilymph. The vastly different ionic composition of endolymph and perilymph (endolymph – high in potassium, low in sodium; perilymph – low in potassium, high in sodium) permits a standing potential differential of approximately 120 mV to exist between endolymph and the compartment surrounding

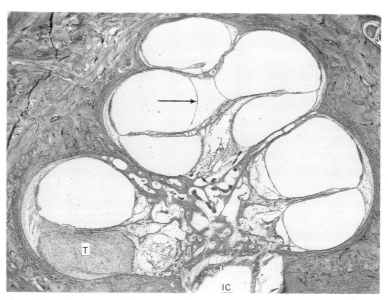

Figure 5.24 This intracochlear schwannoma (T) is associated with endolymphatic hydrops evidenced by a distended Reissner's membrane (arrow). IC = Internal auditory canal

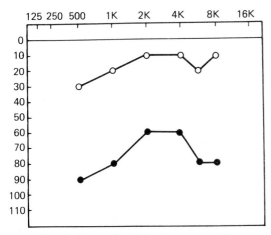

Figure 5.25 The hearing loss (left ear) in a surgically proven case of intracochlear neuroma resembles the threshold pattern associated with endolymphatic hydrops

the hair cells and nerve fibres (perilymph). An alteration in this chemical composition will lead to dysfunction and dysequilibrium because of a change in the action potentials of the vestibular nerve. Such changes are more likely to occur in the perilymphatic fluid since it is the compartment most easily affected by various inflammatory or traumatic insults to the otic capsule or its natural fenestrae (oval and round windows). Furthermore, this is the fluid environment which is critical for normal hair cell and vestibular nerve function. Common examples of an alteration in perilymph composition affecting vestibular physiology are:

1 the serous labyrinthitis which occurs following oval window surgery (Hohmann, 1962)
2 sensorineural hearing loss with vertigo associated with chronic inflammatory disease in the round window niche (Figure 5.26).

Following stapedectomy, dysequilibrium (especially positional) and sensorineural hearing loss are common for several days. Gradual resolution of symptoms with return of cochlear function parallels the readjustment in clinical changes produced by the surgery. A similar resolution of labyrinthine symptoms occurs when chronic inflammatory middle ear disease is surgically controlled. The term serous labyrinthitis is used to describe such reversible forms of labyrinthine irritation.

A second example of labyrinthine physiology distributed by chemical alteration in the fluid compartments is that responsible for the clinical symptoms of Menière's disease. It is now established that the pathological correlate of Menière's disease is progressive endolymphatic hydrops as a result of endolymphatic sac dysfunction (Figure 5.27). This pathology has been demonstrated in human temporal bone material (Hallpike and Cairns, 1938; Lindsay, 1942; Schuknecht, Benitez and Beekhuis, 1962) as well as in the experimental animal (Kimura, 1967; Schuknecht, Northrop and Igarashi, 1968). The progressive endolymphatic hydrops may require various time intervals in different species to develop following sac dysfunction (destruction). Eventually progressive distension of the endolymph compartment leads to disruption of the membranous walls of either the pars inferior or the pars superior of the labyrinth (Figure 5.28). Theoretical (Lawrence

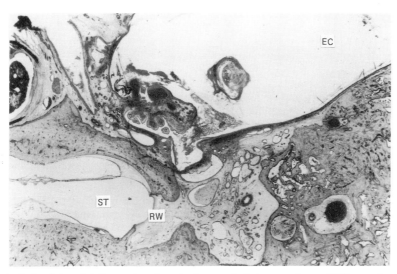

Figure 5.26 The proximity of chronic inflammatory tissue to the round window membrane (RW) may allow chemical changes in the scala tympani (ST) to affect labyrinthine neural function (serous labyrinthitis). EC = External auditory canal

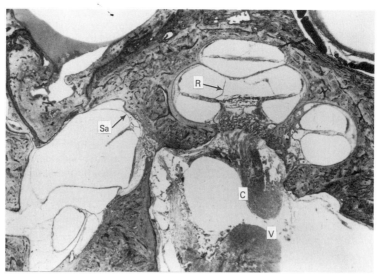

Figure 5.27 The histopathological correlate of Menière's disease is progressive endolymphatic hydrops demonstrated here by distended Reissner's membrane (R) and saccular wall (Sa). C = Cochlear nerve, V = vestibular nerve

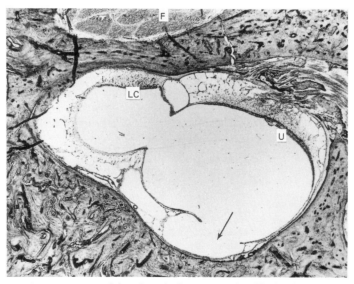

Figure 5.28 In the pars superior progressive endolymphatic hydrops is manifested by breaks in the wall of the membranous labyrinth (arrow) with sealing off (herniation) by fibrous tissue. LC = Lateral canal crista, U = utricular macula, F = facial nerve

and McCabe 1959; Dohlman, 1965) as well as experimental evidence (Silverstein, 1970) indicates that these events permit release of high potassium endolymph which drastically alters the ionic composition of perilymph by raising the potassium level. High potassium levels in the perilymph diminish the standing action potentials in the vestibular nerve resulting in a sudden asymmetry of input to the vestibular nuclei. Clinically these changes are manifested by dysequilibrium and nystagmus. After the membrane breaks heal, ion composition in perilymph gradually returns to a normal level. Nerve action potentials also recover to a normal pattern resulting in symmetry of input to the brain stem. The resolution of vestibular symptoms follows.

The sensorineural hearing loss which occurs in Menière's disease can be accounted for by a similar pathophysiological mechanism. Early in the development of endolymphatic hydrops when hearing loss is the earliest presenting symptom, a low frequency sensory pattern of loss is seen. The accumulation of endolymph in the scala media with the gradient being greatest at the apical turn and less in the basal turn is consistent with the ascending threshold elevation pattern. Furthermore, changes in endolymph volume are consistent with the fluctuations in threshold sensitivity which are characteristic of Menière's disease. Long durations of endolymphatic hydrops with episodic vertigo are commonly associated with increased sensorineural hearing loss frequently with loss of speech discrimination. Although light microscopic evaluation of the organ of Corti fails to reveal corresponding sensory lesions to account for the sensory and neural deficits (Figure 5.29), degeneration of apical spiral ganglion cells has been observed in Menière's disease (Lindsay, Kohut and Sciarra, 1962). It seems possible that ultrastructural degenerative

changes in auditory nerve terminals within the organ of Corti may also help to explain some of the permanent neural auditory deficits (speech discrimination loss) seen in later stages of the disease. Such nerve terminal injury could result from repeated potassium intoxication following membrane ruptures of the pars inferior.

In a similar way, morphological changes in terminal portions of vestibular neurons may occur following repeated insults from potassium contamination of the surrounding perilymph. Degeneration of vestibular ganglion cells has not been observed in temporal bones from patients with Menière's disease. However, it is well known that vestibular ganglion cells do not degenerate readily following injury to their axonal processes while cochlear ganglion cells are very susceptible to such injury. Therefore, the decreased vestibular sensitivity often seen later in the course of Menière's disease may be explained by ultrastructural morphological changes in peripheral terminal portions of vestibular neurons.

Neural (first order vestibular neuron) pathology

Inflammation

The vestibular ganglion located in the internal auditory meatus may be affected by various viral agents resulting in the condition called vestibular neuritis (neuronitis). Vestibular neuritis is manifested clinically by a sudden onset of sustained vertigo and dysequilibrium accompanied by a spontaneous nystagmus lasting from 3 to 7 days followed by gradual resolution. These vestibular signs and symptoms usually occur in the absence of involvement of the auditory system, thus supporting the supposition that the selective involvement of the vestibular system is extra-labyrinthine, i.e. at the vestibular nerve level. Clinical supporting evidence that viral agents are responsible for this condition is based on epidemiological evidence of an increased incidence of this vestibular syndrome during an epidemic of viral infections and clinical evidence that an upper respiratory viral disorder frequently precedes the vestibular syndrome (Stahle, 1966; Coats, 1969). Vestibular neuritis may take one of two clinical forms, acute or chronic. The acute form is manifested by a single prolonged vestibular disorder which does not recur after resolution. The chronic form includes those patients who have recurrent vestibular attacks without hearing loss following the initial episode (Dix and Hallpike, 1952). These recurring attacks of episodic vertigo may be of varying durations. Although the vestibular attacks usually last one or more days, they may occasionally resemble the original episode. Nevertheless, the episodes are longer in duration than the attacks which are observed in Menière's disease. The clinical diagnosis is

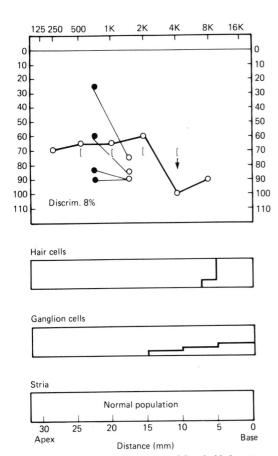

Figure 5.29 The audiometric pattern of threshold elevation in Menière's disease is not compatible with the loss of sensory and neural elements

based upon a history of a preceding viral episode, the length of the attacks, the exclusion of auditory symptoms and a reduced vestibular sensitivity in one ear in the presence of normal hearing. Although vestibular neuritis is usually unilateral, bilateral involvement may occur in a small number of cases.

The histopathological observations in this disorder demonstrate degeneration of the vestibular ganglion and its processes in the presence of a normal auditory end organ and nerve (Figure 5.30). In addition to the reduced number of vestibular ganglion cells and nerve fibres, a round cell infiltrate is frequently observed surrounding the vestibular nerve fibres in the internal auditory meatus. Treatment of vestibular neuritis may be necessary only for the chronic form. A progressive degeneration of the vestibular nerve in the chronic form will usually permit episodes of diminishing severity which may be managed non-surgically. However, occasionally severity of symptoms and the magnitude of disability may justify selective vestibular ablation in a particular patient.

Degeneration

Degeneration of the vestibular nerve may be caused by non-inflammatory agents. Demyelination and degeneration of vestibular neurons has been observed in carcinomatous encephalopathy (Schuknecht, 1974b) and diabetes mellitus (Naufal and Schuknecht, 1972). The degeneration of the first order vestibular neuron is responsible for varying severities and forms of dysequilibrium ranging from episodic vertigo to ataxia. A persistent or recurring dysequilibrium frequently having a duration of days or weeks is usually seen with these forms of degenerative neuropathy. The degenerative process may also involve the auditory nerve or may involve primarily the vestibular nerve. Histopathological documentation exists in the form of degeneration of the vestibular nerve and its ganglion in the presence of normal sense organs (Figure 5.31). Of course, decreased vestibular sensitivity determined by the caloric test is the clinical correlate of this degenerative process. Demyelination of the vestibular nerve has not been documented in demyelinating disorders such as multibular sensitivity determined by the caloric test is the clinical correlate of this degenerative process. Demyelination of the vestibular nerve has not been documented in demyelinating disorders such as multiple sclerosis and amyotrophic lateral sclerosis where dysequilibrium and ataxia are common clinical features. It is presumed that the vestibular system and other equilibrium modalities are affected centrally in these neurological disorders. Degeneration of the vestibular nerve may also occur as a result of the ageing process on neural and vascular structures of the labyrinth. Patients with degenerative ageing processes affecting the vestibular nerve usually also have sensorineural hearing loss as a result of degeneration of the auditory nerve.

Trauma

Although transverse fractures of the temporal bone usually involve the vestibular labyrinth and the internal auditory meatus when vestibular symptoms are

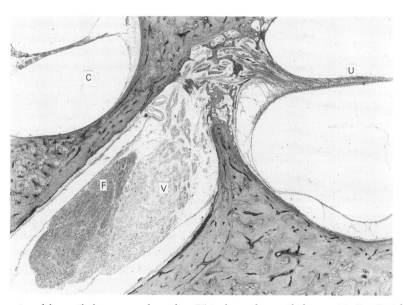

Figure 5.30 Degeneration of the vestibular nerve and ganglion (V) is observed in vestibular neuritis. F = Facial nerve, C = cochlea, U = utricular macula and nerve

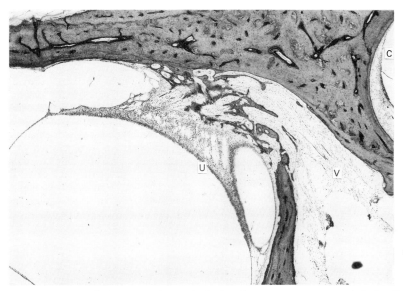

Figure 5.31 Degeneration of the vestibular nerve (V) may also be found in carcinomatous encephalophy. U = Utricular macula. C = cochlea

present, occasionally the fracture line will skirt the vestibular labyrinth and sense organs and extend into the bony channels through which the vestibular nerve branches reach the sense organs. Fractures which injure vestibular nerve fibres in this way produce a self-limiting form of vertigo, because of the adjustment to partial vestibular ablation that is made by the host. Auditory function will be preserved provided that the fracture has spared the cochlea. No treatment is required for such an injury which is identified clinically by demonstration of a decrease in vestibular function, but the presence of normal auditory function.

Postlabyrinthectomy neuroma

An unusual complication of labyrinthectomy is the amputation neuroma arising from transected vestibular dendrites producing episodic vertigo. At least four cases have been reported in the literature of episodic vertigo following transtympanic labyrinthectomy for disabling vertigo from progressive endolymphatic hydrops (Pulec, 1974; Linthicum, Alonso and Denia, 1979) or surgical (stapedectomy) traumatic labyrinthitis (Hilding and House, 1965). These case reports described a fibrous tissue mass filling the vestibule excision of which provided relief of the patient's vertiginous symptoms. Histological examination of these masses revealed proliferating nerve fibres in bundles surrounded by varying amounts of fibrous tissue. There was no evidence of a neoplasm in these specimens. The following case illustrates this sequela of labyrinthectomy.

A 28-year-old woman who had lost hearing in the right ear early in childhood and with a normal

hearing left ear presented with severe episodic vertigo, 1–2 hours in duration for 2–3 years. The diagnosis of delayed endolymphatic hydrops was made and a transcanal labyrinthectomy performed. The patient experienced complete relief of her episodic vertigo for a period of one year. She then began to experience episodic vertigo of similar duration to her pre-labyrinthectomy symptoms. An enhanced MRI revealed a mass in the region of the right vestibule with a normal internal auditory meatus (Figure 5.32a). A transmastoid exposure of the vestibule was carried out and a firm tissue mass was excised from the vestibule. Histological examination of this mass revealed regenerating, myelinated and unmyelinated nerve fibres in various fascicles and bundles surrounded by varying amounts of fibrous tissue and round cells (plasma cells and lymphocytes) (Figure 5.32b, c). The patient has experienced complete relief following excision of this mass.

A traumatic neuroma following labyrinthectomy consists of regenerating nerve fibres presumably from the dendritic processes of remaining Scarpa's ganglion cells. However, animal studies suggest that vestibular neurons and ganglion cells undergo retrograde degeneration following amputation of sense organs and distal dendrites (Schuknecht, 1982; Gacek, unpublished observation). These findings would argue against the regeneration of afferent neuron processes as responsible for the neuroma. It is possible that these regenerating nerve fibres may represent regenerating axons of the efferent vestibular component which would also have been transected in the labyrinthectomy procedure. However, since the efferent nerve cell bodies do not have direct connections with the vestibular reflex pathways

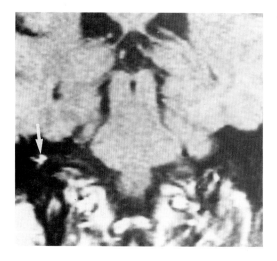

Figure 5.32 (*a*)

(vestibulo-ocular, vestibulospinal), it is more likely that Scarpa's ganglion neurons are responsible for the abnormal neural input initiated in the traumatic neuroma. The nature of the inciting stimulus for this input is unknown.

The traumatic neuroma is differentiated from the neoplasm of Schwann cells (schwannoma) which is often referred to in the literature as an acoustic neuroma. The regeneration neuroma following amputation of nerve processes is not a neoplastic process but an abnormal regeneration of nerve fibres and their myelin sheaths. Should an excised postlabyrinthectomy neuroma recur, excision of Scarpa's ganglion by a transmastoid approach would be indicated.

Compression

Compression of the VIIth and VIIIth cranial nerves

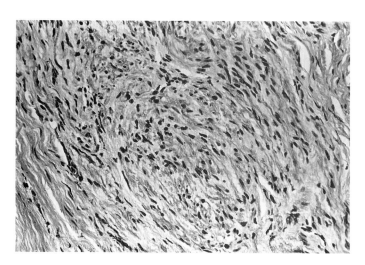

Figure 5.32 (*b*)

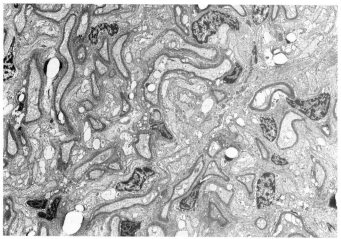

Figure 5.32 (*c*)

Figure 5.32 (*a*) This MRI revealed an enhanced mass (arrow) in the vestibule of a patient who experienced recurrent vertigo 8 months after a successful labyrinthectomy. (*b*) Light and (*c*) electron microscopic evidence of regenerating myelinated and unmyelinated nerve fibres are observed in the excised mass

may occur in the internal auditory meatus from vascular, neoplastic and osseous disorders.

Vascular

Although it is possible that a large vessel such as the anterior inferior cerebellar artery or a tortuous basilar artery may significantly compress the VIIth or VIIIth nerves in or near the internal auditory meatus, this condition probably exists less frequently than it has been clinically reported. A loop of the anterior inferior cerebellar artery resting against the facial and vestibular nerves within the internal auditory meatus is a common finding in normal temporal bone specimens (Figure 5.33). Yet dysfunction of these nerves was not a clinical finding in patients from whom the temporal bones were acquired. Reisser and Schuknecht (1991) studied the incidence of anterior inferior cerebellar artery loops in the internal auditory meatus in the Massachusetts Eye and Ear Infirmary temporal bone collection and found that the incidence of a loop in cases with unexplained vertigo was no different from that in the collection as a whole. They presented convincing morphological evidence supporting the contention that the vessel loop in the internal auditory meatus is a normal anatomical occurrence and there is no statistical evidence that it is a significant cause of auditory or vestibular dysfunction. Nevertheless, a number of clinical reports (Janetta, 1980) have indicated that a loop of vessel resting on the vestibular or VIIth nerves in the internal auditory meatus is responsible for various vestibular and facial nerve symptoms. Relief of these symptoms is purported to follow when the vessel has been dissected away from the nerve structures and cushioned with an intervening sponge implant. Pressure against the nerves in the internal auditory meatus by a pulsating vessel which may become more tortuous with age is a possible mechanism by which vestibular symptoms may occur at the neuronal level. Since this neural-vascular arrangement is often not associated with clinical symptoms, convincing documentation that such vascular compression is responsible for the clinical disorder must be made carefully with an unbiased approach.

Neoplasm

The VIIth and VIIIth nerves may be compressed in the internal auditory meatus or cerebellopontine angle as a result of extrinsic compression by a neoplasm from an adjacent part of the temporal bone. Benign expanding tumours arising from the petrous apex (Gacek, 1975; DeLozier, Parkins and Gacek, 1979) (epidermoid, mucocoele, abscess, cholesterol granuloma, neurofibroma, chondroma, meningioma) or the jugular foramen (Gacek, 1983) (neurofibroma, paraganglioma, meningioma, chondroma) may compress the nerves in the internal auditory meatus (Figures 5.34 and 5.35). The auditory deficit produced is a retrocochlear pattern of sensorineural hearing loss. The pathological correlate is degeneration of cochlear neurons with an intact organ of Corti (Figure 5.36). Vestibular symptoms vary from intermittent dysequilibrium, episodic vertigo to positional vertigo. Although the vestibular ganglion does not degenerate as readily as the cochlear ganglion cells, atrophy of the vestibular ganglion cells will occur eventually (years) after compression of their axons (Figure 5.37).

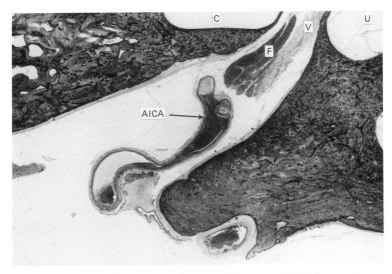

Figure 5.33 This prominent vascular loop of the anterior inferior cerebellar artery (AICA) has an intimate relationship with the facial (F) and vestibular (V) nerves in the internal auditory meatus but was not associated with facial or vestibular nerve signs. C = Cochlea, U = utricle

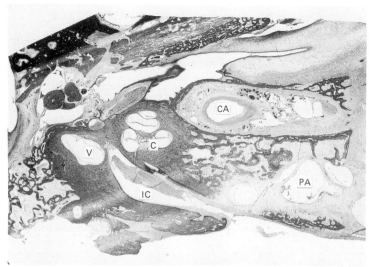

Figure 5.34 A petrous apex (PA) abscess may compress the nerves of the internal auditory meatus (IC). V = Vestibule, C = cochlea, CA = internal carotid artery

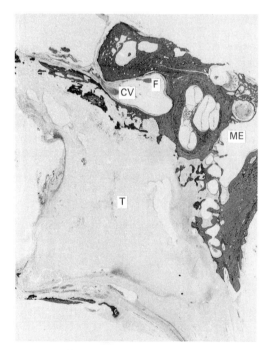

Figure 5.35 This neurofibroma (T) of the jugular foramen compressed the cochleovestibular nerve (CV) complex and the facial nerve (F) in the internal auditory meatus. ME = Middle ear space

Osseous compression

Compression of the nerves in the internal auditory meatus may be produced by disorders of bone metabolism. Sclerosteosis is a rare inherited bone disorder where periosteal bone growth continues and obliterates the bony channels of the temporal bone which carry neural and vascular structures (Nager and Hammersma, 1986). Vestibular and auditory symptoms of VIIIth nerve compression are similar to those described from neoplastic compression. Decompression of venous drainage channels has been successful in prolonging life in these patients.

It is conceivable that other disorders of bone metabolism (fibrous dysplasia, osteopetrosis) may also be responsible for VIIth and VIIIth nerve symptoms as a result of compression in the internal auditory meatus.

A more common association of dysequilibrium and a disorder of the otic capsule is seen in otosclerosis. Vestibular symptoms are frequently present in patients with otosclerosis. The exact pathophysiological mechanism responsible for vestibular symptoms, ranging from episodic vertigo to dysequilibrium, in this condition which is primarily manifested by a conductive auditory deficit is not known. However, compression of vestibular nerve fibres by the otosclerotic focus as they pass through the optic capsule is a plausible explanation (see Figure 5.4).

Compression by hereditary conditions

Pressure atrophy of the vestibular and auditory neurons may occur within the bony channels of the cribrose portion of the innervation pathway to the labyrinth. Khetarpal *et al.* (1991) have described in five temporal bones from three subjects of two kindreds with an inherited form of sensorineural hearing loss (autosomal dominant), the accumulation of an acid mucopolysaccharide within the bony channels of the dendrites of the VIIIth nerve causing

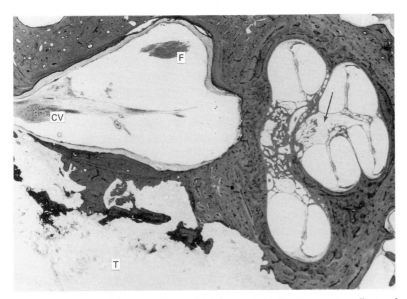

Figure 5.36 This higher magnification of the case in Figure 5.35 demonstrates the degenerative effect on the spiral ganglion (arrow) of the compression by tumour (T). CV = Cochleovestibular nerve, F = facial nerve

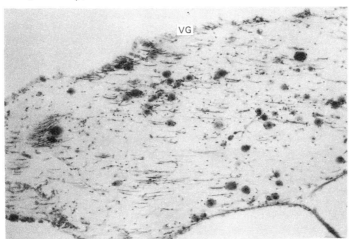

Figure 5.37 The vestibular ganglion (VG) also shows marked degeneration from nerve compression in the internal auditory meatus

degeneration of neural and sensory structures. All of these patients demonstrated a progressive high frequency sensorineural hearing loss since early adulthood but only one had a history of recurrent vertigo. However, all the temporal bones showed consistent pathological findings of the mucopolysaccharide material obliterating the bony channels of the vestibular (Figure 5.38a, b) and cochlear innervation pathway. Based on this series as well as previous reported temporal bones of this form of sensorineural hearing loss, the authors proposed two phenotypes of autosomal dominant sensorineural hearing loss:

1 The progressive sensorineural hearing loss with an onset in the third to the fifth decades having the appropriate pathological correlates of sensory and neural degeneration in the organ of Corti but with a normal vestibular labyrinth. Vestibular symptoms are absent in this phenotype.

2 The sensory and neural degeneration is present in both the auditory and vestibular labyrinth with the mucopolysaccharide material obliterating the bony channels in the cribrose areas of the labyrinth producing retrograde degeneration of both the vestibular and auditory neurons. This accumulation of mucopolysaccharide is also responsible for degeneration of hair cells and supporting cells of end organs by infiltration of the stroma of the sense organs. The proposed mechanisms by which the mucopolysaccharide material may cause neural

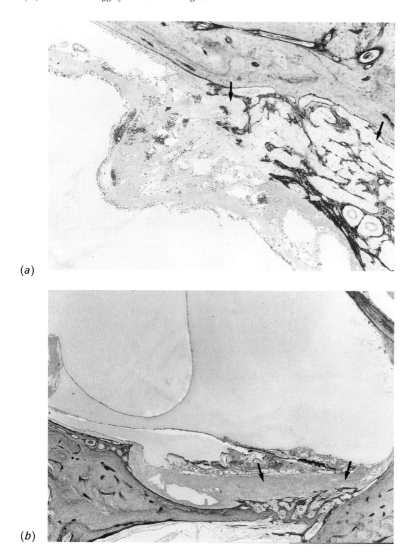

(*a*)

(*b*)

Figure 5.38 A homogeneous acidophilic deposit (arrow) fills the bony channels and stromal regions of the sense organs of (*a*) the cristae and (*b*) maculae causing degeneration of the vestibular neurons. There is degeneration of the sense organs possibly secondary to ischaemic compromise by the mucopolysaccharide filling of the bony channels in the cribrose areas

and sensory degeneration is by compression of the dendritic processes of the neurons, alteration of the fluid environment of the neurons or compromise of the blood supply to the neurons and sense organs. It is quite possible that a combination of all three mechanisms may be present in this particular form of hereditary degeneration of the labyrinth.

Neoplasia

The vestibular nerve may be affected by either benign or malignant neoplasms. The most common benign tumour to involve the nerves contained within the internal auditory meatus is the VIIIth nerve schwan-noma which usually arises from the myelinated segment of the vestibular division (Figure 5.39). Since the Schwann cell (myelinated) portion of the VIIIth nerve is located lateral (distal) to the glial–Schwann cell junction, these tumours arise within the internal auditory meatus and extend into the cerebellopontine angle when they have filled the meatus. Most of the vestibular schwannomas (60–70%) arise from the superior division of the nerve which makes up a majority of the vestibular nerve fibre population. Rarely a schwannoma may arise from the cochlear division of the VIIIth nerve.

These Schwann cell tumours are divided into two histological types: Antoni A and B. The Antoni A variety is formed of tightly packed flattened Schwann

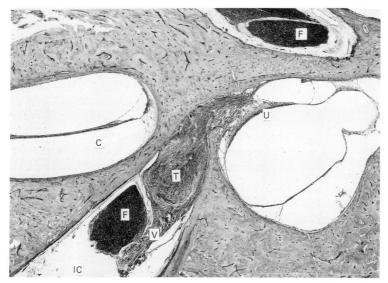

Figure 5.39 The small asymptomatic canalicular schwannoma (T) arises from distal portions of the vestibular nerve (V) in the internal auditory canal (IC). F = Facial nerve, C = cochlea, U = utricular macula

cells whose nuclei are frequently stacked in layers (palisading) with dense cytoplasm forming the substance of the tumour. Surgically these tumours are firm, relatively avascular and well encapsulated. The Antoni B form of schwannoma is made up of plump cells with foamy cytoplasm, loosely arranged and mixed with areas undergoing fatty and cystic degeneration. These tumours surgically appear soft, cystic, somewhat vascular and with a thin capsule.

It is not surprising that the vestibular sensitivity test (ENG) is the most frequently abnormal study in the diagnosis of VIIIth nerve schwannoma (Erickson, Sorenson and McGavran, 1965). This is often the case even though vestibular symptoms (vertigo, ataxia, positional vertigo) are usually mild or absent. The relatively mild vestibular symptoms are probably explained by the slow destruction of vestibular neuronal units, thus allowing for compensation by the host. This relationship is emphasized by the observation of small occult vestibular schwannomas in temporal bones from patients without balance symptoms during life.

The vestibular schwannoma usually presents clinically as a result of the effects produced on adjacent nerve structures in the bony internal auditory meatus (Figure 5.40). Of the two nerves in the internal

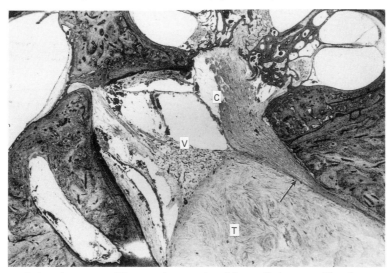

Figure 5.40 Larger vestibular schwannoma (T) causes degeneration of the vestibular nerve (V) and compression of the cochlear nerve (arrow). C = Cochlear nerve

auditory meatus, the cochlear nerve is more susceptible to compression. Therefore, the most common
clinical effects are hearing loss and tinnitus (Erickson,
Sorenson and McGavran, 1965). The typical hearing
deficit produced by nerve compression (retrocochlear
lesion) with subsequent degeneration of cochlear neurons is a severe loss in speech (word) discrimination
out of proportion to the pure tone threshold elevation
(Figure 5.41). An additional common pattern is a
high frequency pure tone loss which is related to
compression of the neurons innervating the basal
turn of the cochlea since they are located near the
periphery of the cochlear nerve trunk in the internal
auditory meatus. However, many variations in the
audiometric picture of hearing loss may be demonstrated as a result of cochlear nerve compression by a
vestibular schwannoma. Therefore additional pathophysiological mechanisms of sensorineural hearing
loss may be responsible. Ischaemia of various segments
of the end organ secondary to vascular compression in
the internal auditory meatus by the tumour and
changes in the perilymph surrounding the cochlear
nerve fibres (Figure 5.42) and hair cells are two
additional abnormalities which may account for sensorineural hearing deficits. Although slow compression of the facial nerve in the internal auditory meatus
by the schwannoma slowly results in flattening of the
nerve trunk with an ostensible loss of axons, motor
paralysis of the facial muscles is not a common clinical
finding even with large VIIIth nerve tumours. This
paradox is best explained by the fact that surviving
motor axon terminals sprout to re-innervate adjacent
denervated facial muscle fibres over time and provide
adequate motor function. Although the schwannoma
is the most common benign neoplasm to involve the
VIIth and VIIIth nerves in the internal auditory
meatus, other tumours which may also simulate this
picture are meningioma, epidermoid, haemangioma,
arachnoid cyst, lipoma, and granuloma.

Malignant neoplasms may metastasize to the temporal bone in two ways: haematogenous spread to the
marrow space of the petrous apex, and to the internal
auditory meatus by way of the subarachnoid space.
Neoplastic replacement of the marrow in the petrous
apex causes deficits of the Vth and VIth cranial
nerves early in development and affect the VIIth and
VIIIth nerves in the internal auditory meatus when
they attain large size. However, when malignant
tumours spread to the subarachnoid space of the
internal auditory meatus, facial nerve paralysis and
VIIIth nerve symptoms are frequent and prominent
(Figure 5.43).

The clinical picture produced by involvement of
the nerves in the internal auditory meatus by malignant neoplasm differs greatly from the clinical presentation of a slow growing benign tumour such as the
schwannoma. Vestibular symptoms are prominent
and sustained because of the rapid onset of a significant asymmetry produced when neoplasm destroys

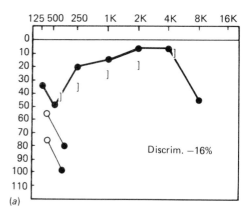

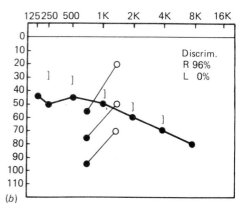

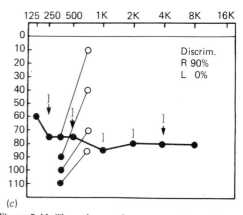

Figure 5.41 These three audiograms emphasize the
variation in pure tone threshold sensitivity with a marked
loss in speech discrimination score which is associated with
a retrocochlear lesion

significant numbers of vestibular neurons. Of course,
sensorineural hearing loss, usually of the typical retrocochlear pattern, accompanies the vestibular deficit.
Infiltration and destruction of the facial nerve motor

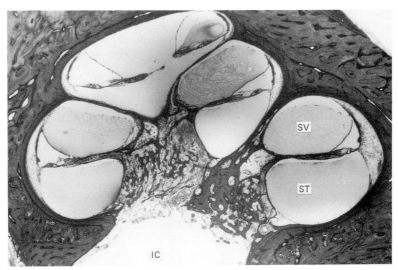

Figure 5.42 Abnormally high perilymph protein levels are characteristically seen with vestibular neuroma. The alteration in chemistry may also explain auditory and vestibular deficits. SV = Scala vestibuli, ST = scala tympani, IC = internal auditory canal

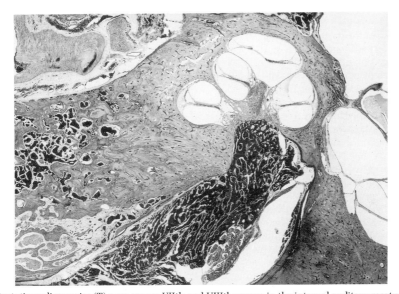

Figure 5.43 Metastatic malignancies (T) may encase VIIth and VIIIth nerves in the internal auditory meatus manifesting as marked hearing loss, dysequilibrium and facial palsy

axons caused by the malignant tumour cells is manifested by paralysis of the facial musculature. The most common primary malignancies that metastasize to the internal auditory meatus are carcinoma of the breast, lung, kidney and prostate gland (Schuknecht, Allam and Murakami, 1968). Carcinoma of the middle ear or nearby nasopharynx may extend into the labyrinth resulting in sensorineural hearing loss and vertigo from a serofibrinous labyrinthitis. Of course, such extension from the middle ear space across the bony labyrinth capsule does not occur

readily because of the resistant nature of otic capsular bone. This barrier may be crossed by tumour cells either through the oval or round windows, or through a fenestration of the otic capsule.

Central vestibular system

Since a small percentage (less than 10%) of patients presenting with vertigo represent central nervous system pathology (Barber, 1984), the recognition of these disorders is dependent on a strong index of suspicion. The major portion of the central vestibular pathways are located in the brain stem and cerebellum so that most central vestibular pathology is located in the posterior cranial fossa (infratentorial). As indicated in the discussion of the peripheral vestibular disorders, pathology affecting the central nervous system may also be of inflammatory, neoplastic, vascular, congenital or degenerative type.

Central vestibular disorders of neoplastic, degenerative or vascular causes usually demonstrate multiple neurological deficits in addition to vestibular symptoms and signs. These additional neurological deficits should be documented by a full neurological examination. Intrinsic lesions of the posterior fossa (vascular, neoplastic) involve significant portions of the brain stem and frequently affect the nearby nuclei such as the abducens nucleus, the facial nucleus, nucleus ambiguus and the trigeminal nucleus and tracts producing neurological signs which permit a relatively obvious diagnosis. Two vascular occlusive disorders which affect the portion of the brain stem containing the vestibular nuclei are lateral brain stem medullary syndrome and thrombosis of the anterior inferior cerebellar artery. The lateral medullary syndrome results from occlusion of the posterior inferior cerebellar or vertebral artery (Fisher, Karnes and Kubik, 1961). The symptom complex may come on slowly or rapidly. It consists of pain in the side of the face, vertigo with vomiting, dyslexia, dysphasia and dysphonia without loss of consciousness. The typical findings result from involvement of the descending trigeminal tract, the sympathetic autonomic system in the reticular formation and ipsilateral paralysis of the soft palate, larynx and pharynx as well as VIth, VIIth and VIIIth nerve involvement. Thrombosis of the anterior inferior cerebellar artery is more uncommon, and is characterized by nausea and vomiting as well as facial paralysis, sensory disturbances and cerebellar symptoms. The vertigo and hearing loss may be caused by involvement of the vestibular and auditory nuclei in the brain stem and/or the membranous labyrinth because of occlusion of the labyrinthine artery. Hinojosa and Kohut (1990) described a case of anterior inferior cerebellar artery thrombosis with resulting ischaemic defects in the brain stem, vestibular and auditory nuclei with relatively little ischaemic change in the labyrinth. In this case the VIIIth nerve symptoms can be explained on the basis of brain stem involvement. However, early neoplasms of the cerebellum, particularly the cerebellar vermis may initially produce only positional vertigo and nystagmus of the non-fatiguing variety (type I or type II) (Gregorius, Crandall and Baloh, 1976). Hearing and vestibular (ENG) tests are usually normal at this early stage. Extrinsic lesions (cerebellar tumours and cysts, the Arnold Chiari malformation) may compress the brain stem and interrupt vestibulo-ocular pathways within the brain stem or near the surface of the IVth ventricle. Interruption of these pathways may be manifested by unique signs such as downbeat nystagmus, upbeat nystagmus, positional nystagmus, or perverted induced nystagmus. An understanding of the involvement of these pathways is helpful to diagnosis of central vestibular disorders.

Positional nystagmus

Positional nystagmus of central origin is usually of the non-fatiguing variety (type I and type II), but occasionally the fatiguing variety (type III) may be associated with central pathology (Harrison and Ozsahinoglu, 1975; Watson *et al.*, 1981). However, usually types I and II are central in origin, whereas type III is usually peripheral in origin. Positional nystagmus is frequently seen in cerebellar lesions particularly when the vestibulocerebellum (flocculonodular lobe) is involved primarily or secondarily by neoplasm. This clinical sign is probably caused by a loss of the inhibitory effect of the cerebellum on the vestibular nuclei where vestibulo-ocular neurons are located.

Downbeat spontaneous nystagmus

This form of spontaneous nystagmus may reflect lesions which interrupt the excitatory pathways to the inferior rectus muscle (Baloh and Spooner, 1981). This excitatory pathway which relays the input from the posterior semicircular canal originates from the medial vestibular nucleus in the caudal brain stem, crosses the mid-line to send its fibre projection in the contralateral medial longitudinal fasciculus and terminates in the trochlear nucleus and the inferior rectus subnucleus of the oculomotor complex. Brain stem lesions such vascular infarcts, demyelinating disorders and the Arnold Chiari malformation have been identified as causes for spontaneous downbeat nystagmus. The mechanism of the downbeat nystagmus is based on an interruption of the excitatory pathway to the inferior rectus muscle. The unopposed contraction of the superior rectus which receives it excitatory input from the anterior semicircular canal by way of the brachium conjunctivum is responsible for the upward drift of the globe while the fast phase in a downward direction represents the compensatory movement. Downbeat spontaneous nystagmus may also be associated with lesions of the cerebellar flocculus due to loss of the inhibitory input to the superior rectus at the level of the superior vestibular nucleus.

Upbeat spontaneous nystagmus

Upbeat spontaneous nystagmus may result from lesions of the posterior fossa which affect the brachium conjunctivum and other nearby fibre pathways (Nakada and Remler, 1981). This vestibulo-ocular reflex finding is produced by interruption of fibre pathways which carry excitatory input to the superior rectus muscle from the anterior semicircular canal through the brachium conjunctivum by way of the superior vestibular nucleus. Ablation of this input leads to unopposed action of the inferior rectus muscle resulting in a downward drift of the eyes with an upward compensatory fast phase.

Perversion of nystagmus

Perversion of nystagmus may be produced by lesions that compress the vestibulo-ocular pathways near the floor of the fourth ventricle in the caudal brain stem. The vestibulo-ocular neurons serving the medial and lateral rectus muscles, as well as interneurons in the abducens nucleus which project to the contralateral medial rectus are located superficially at this level of the brain stem. When the horizontal vestibulo-ocular pathways are interrupted at this point in the posterior brain stem, the intact excitatory vestibulo-ocular pathways in the brachium conjunctivum and the rostral medial longitudinal fasciculus produce vertical and rotatory eye displacement. Therefore vertical and rotatory nystagmus may be observed instead of horizontal nystagmus when the lateral canal is calorically stimulated.

Internuclear ophthalmoplegia

This distinctive oculomotor deficit is produced when a focal lesion (demyelinating) of the medial longitudinal fasciculus interrupts the projection of the abducens interneurons which excite the contralateral medial rectus subnucleus. This interruption of the abducens interneuron results in a dissociated eye displacement on lateral gaze. It is a frequently observed clinical sign in multiple sclerosis.

Conclusion

The preceding anatomicophysiological discussion of the pathology of vertigo is not intended to represent a comprehensive list of pathologies which affect the vestibular system. This presentation provides a description of the various mechanisms by which the normal physiology of the vestibular system may be disrupted producing dysequilibrium or vertigo. An understanding of the mechanism by which asymmetry in the vestibular system is produced not only facilitates diagnosis but allows for logical management. The examples discussed represent the more common disorders encountered in otoneurological practice. It is appreciated that a significant number of unknown pathologies are seen daily in clinical practice. Further information will be necessary in order to clarify the pathophysiology of these disorders. Such documentation may be represented by observations provided by newer clinical technologies (magnetic resonance imaging), and experimental study in the laboratory animal of vestibulopathophysiology using physiological and morphological (ultrastructural or histochemical) techniques. The emphasis in these experimental studies may be directed toward alterations in the make-up and function of the cupula, otoconia, or the ciliary structures of the hair cells in the vestibular receptors. Temporal bone post-mortem material is still a valuable source because of the insight that it provides to disorders that affect the human vestibular system. The acquisition of temporal bone material should be encouraged for study by both light and electron microscopic techniques.

References

ABRAMSON, M. (1969) Collagenolytic activity in middle ear cholesteatoma. *Annals of Otology, Rhinology and Laryngology*, **78**, 112–125

ABRAMSON, M. and GROSS, J. (1971) Further studies on a collagenase in middle ear cholesteatoma. *Annals of Otology, Rhinology and Laryngology*, **80**, 177–185

ALTMANN, F. (1946) Healing of fistulas of the human labyrinth – histopathologic studies. *Archives of Otolaryngology*, **43**, 409–421

ARRAGG, F. and PAPARELLA, M. (1964) Traumatic fracture of the stapes. *Laryngoscope*, **74**, 1329–1332

ARSLAN, M. (1957) The senescence of the vestibular apparatus. *Practica Oto-rhino-laryngologica*, **19**, 475–483

BALOH, R. and SPOONER, J. (1981) Downbeat nystagmus: a type of central vestibular nystagmus. *Neurology*, **31**, 304–310

BÁRÁNY, R. (1921) Diagnose von Krankheit – Serscheinungen im Bereiche des Otolithenapparates. *Acta Otolaryngologica*, **2**, 434–437

BARBER, H. (1984) Positional nystagmus. *Otolaryngology – Head and Neck Surgery*, **92**, 649–655

BERGSTROM, B. (1973) Morphology of the vestibular nerve. III. Analysis of the calibers of the myelinated vestibular nerve fibers in man at various ages. *Acta Otolaryngologica*, **76**, 331–338

BORDLEY, J. E., BROOKHAUSER, P. E. and WORTHINGTON, E. L. (1972) Viral infections and hearing: a critical review of the literature, 1969–1970. *Laryngoscope*, **82**, 557–577

COATS, A. (1969) Vestibular neuronitis. *Transactions of the American Academy of Ophthalmology and Otolaryngology*, **73**, 395–408

DELOZIER, H., GACEK, R. and DANA, S. (1979) Intralabyrinthine schwannoma. *Annals of Otology, Rhinology and Laryngology*, **88**, 187–191

DELOZIER, H., PARKINS, C. and GACEK, R. (1979) Mucocele of the petrous apex. *Journal of Laryngology and Otology*, **93**, 177–180

DIX, M. and HALLPIKE, C. S. (1952) The pathology, symptomatology, and diagnosis of certain common disorders of the vestibular system. *Annals of Otology, Rhinology and Laryngology*, **61**, 987–1016

DOHLMAN, G. (1965) The mechanism of secretion of absorption and endolymph in the vestibular apparatus. *Acta Otolaryngologica*, **59**, 275–288

DROLLER, H. and PEMBERTON, J. (1953) Vertigo in a random sample of elderly people living in their homes. *Journal of Laryngology and Otology*, **67**, 689–694

ERICKSON, L., SORENSON, G. and MCGAVRAN, M. (1965) A review of 140 acoustic neurinomas (neurilemmoma). *Laryngoscope*, **75**, 601–627

FISHER, C., KARNES, W. and KUBIK, C. (1961) Lateral medullary infarction – The pattern of vascular occlusion. *Journal of Neuropathology and Experimental Neurology*, **20**, 323–330

FORGACS, P. (1957) The cochlea and vestibular function at advanced age. *Ful Orr-Gege Gy*, **1**, 5–10

GACEK, R. (1974) The surgical management of labyrinthine fistulae in chronic otitis media with cholesteatoma. *Annals of Otology, Rhinology and Laryngology*, **83** (suppl. 10), 1–19

GACEK, R. (1975) Diagnosis and management of primary tumors of the petrous apex. *Annals of Otology, Rhinology, and Laryngology*, **84** (suppl. 18), 1–20

GACEK, R. (1983) Pathology of jugular foramen neurofibroma. *Annals of Otology, Rhinology and Laryngology*, **92**, 128–133

GACEK, R. (1985) Pathophysiology and management of cupulolithiasis. *American Journal of Otolaryngology*, **6**, 66–74

GOODHILL, V. (1971) Sudden deafness and round window rupture. *Laryngoscope*, **81**, 1462–1474

GREGORIUS, F., CRANDALL, P. and BALOH, R. (1976) Positional vertigo with cerebellar astrocytoma. *Surgical Neurology*, **6**, 183–186

GUSSEN, R. (1977) Polyarteritis nodosa and deafness. A human temporal bone study. *Archives of Otorhinolaryngology*, **217**, 263–271

HALLPIKE, C. and CAIRNS, H. (1938) Observations on the pathology of Menière's syndrome. *Journal of Laryngology and Otology*, **53**, 625–655

HARRISON, M. S. and OZSAHINOGLU, C. (1975) Positional vertigo. *Archives of Otolaryngology*, **101**, 675–678

HILDING, D. A. and HOUSE, W. F. (1965) Acoustic neuroma: comparison of traumatic and neoplastic. *Journal of Ultrastructural Research*, **12**, 611–623

HINOJOSA, R. and KOHUT, R. (1990) Clinical diagnosis of anterior inferior cerebellar artery thrombosis. *Annals of Otology, Rhinology and Laryngology*, **99**, 261–272

HOHMANN, A. (1962) Inner ear reactions to stapes surgery (animal experiments). In: *Otosclerosis: Henry Ford Hospital International Symposium*, edited by H. F. SCHUKNECHT. Boston: Little, Brown & Co. pp. 305–317

HOLDEN, H. and SCHUKNECHT, H. (1968) Distribution pattern of blood in the inner ear following spontaneous subarachnoid hemorrhage. *Journal of Larygology and Otology*, **82**, 321–329

HOSHINO, T., ISHII, T., KODAMA, A. and KATO, I. (1980) Temporal bone findings in a case of sudden deafness and relapsing polychondritis. *Acta Otolaryngologica*, **90**, 257–261

ISHII, T., MURAKAMI, Y., KIMURA, R. S. and BALOGH, K. (1967) Electron microscopic and histochemical identification of lipofuscin in the human inner ear. *Acta Otolaryngologica*, **64**, 17–29

JANETTA, P. (1980) Neurovascular compression in cranial nerve and systemic disease. *Annals of Surgery*, **192**, 518–525

JENKINS, H. A., POLLAK, A. M., and FISCH U. (1981) Polyarteritis nodosa as a cause of sudden deafness. A human temporal bone study. *American Journal of Otolaryngology*, **2**, 99–107

JOHNSSON, L. (1971) Degenerative changes and anomalies of the vestibular system in man. *Laryngoscope*, **81**, 1682–1694

KARMODY, C. S. (1983) Viral labyrinthitis: early pathology in the human. *Laryngoscope*, **93**, 1527–1533

KHETARPAL, U., SCHUKNECHT, H. F., GACEK, R. and HOLMES, L. (1991) Autosomal dominant sensorineural hearing loss. *Archives of Otolaryngology – Head and Neck Surgery*, **117**, 1032–1042

KIMURA, R. (1967) Experimental blockage of the endolymphatic duct and sac and its effect on the inner ear of the guinea pig. *Annals of Otology, Rhinology and Laryngology*, **76**, 664–687

LAWRENCE, M. and MCCABE, B. (1959) Inner ear mechanics and deafness. Special consideration of Menière's syndrome. *Journal of the American Medical Association*, **171**, 1927–1932

LINDSAY, J. (1942) Labyrinthine dropsy and Menière's disease. *Archives of Otolaryngology*, **35**, 853–867

LINDSAY, J. and HEMENWAY, W. (1956) Postural vertigo due to unilateral sudden partial loss of vestibular function. *Annals of Otology, Rhinology and Laryngology*, **65**, 692–706

LINDSAY, J., KOHUT, R. and SCIARRA, P. (1962) Menière's disease – pathology and manifestations. *Annals of Otology, Rhinology and Laryngology*, **76**, 1–22

LINTHICUM, F., ALONSO A. and DENIA, A. (1979) Traumata neurons. A complication of transcanal labyrinthectomy. *Archives of Otolaryngology*, **105**, 654–655

LUNDQUIST, P. and WERSALL, J. (1967) The ototoxic effect of gentamicin – an electron microscopical study in gentamicin. *First International Symposium, Paris*, p. 26

MCCABE, B. F. (1979) Autoimmune sensorineural hearing loss. *Annals of Otology, Rhinology and Laryngology*, **88**, 585–589

MCGEE, T. and OLSZEWSKI, J. (1962) Streptomycin sulfate and dyhydrostreptomycin toxicity. *Archives of Otolaryngology*, **75**, 295–311

MERCHANT, S. N. and SCHUKNECHT, H. F. (1988) Vestibular atelectasis. *Annals of Otology, Rhinology, and Laryngology*, **97**, 565–576

MONEY, K. and MYLES, W. (1974) Heavy water nystagmus and effects of alcohol. *Nature*, **247**, 404–405

NADOL, J. (1977) Positive Hennebert's sign in Menière's disease. *Archives of Otolaryngology*, **103**, 524–530

NADOL, J. B. and SCHUKNECHT, H. F. (1990) Pathology of peripheral vestibular disorders in the elderly. *American Journal of Otolaryngology*, **11**, 213–227

NAGER, G. and HAMMERSMA, H. (1986) Sclerosteosis involving the temporal bone. *American Journal of Otolaryngology*, **7**, 1–16

NAKADA, J. and REMLER, M. (1981) Primary position upbeat nystagmus. *Journal of Clinical Neurophthalmology*, **1**, 185–189

NAUFAL, P. and SCHUKNECHT, H. (1972) Vestibular, facial and oculomotor neuropathy in diabetes mellitus. *Archives of Otolaryngology*, **96**, 468–474

PERLMAN, H. and LINDSAY, J. (1939) Relation of the internal ear spaces to the meninges. *Archives of Otolaryngology*, **29**, 12–23

PULEC, J. L. (1974) Labyrinthectomy: indications, technique and results. *Laryngoscope*, **84**, 1552–1573

PULLEN, F. (1972) Round window membrane rupture: a cause of sudden deafness. *Transactions of the American*

Academy of Ophthalmology and Otolaryngology, **76**, 1444–1450

RAREY, K. E., BICKNELL, J. M. and DAVIS, L. E. (1986) Intralabyrinthine osteogenesis in Cogan's syndrome. *American Journal of Otolaryngology*, **4**, 387–390

REISSER, C. and SCHUKNECHT, H. F. (1991) The anterior inferior cerebellar artery in the internal auditory canal. *Laryngoscope*, **101**, 761–766

RICHTER, E. (1980) Quantitative study of human Scarpa's ganglion and vestibular sensory epithelia. *Acta Otolaryngologica*, **90**, 199–208

RITTER, F. (1970) Chronic suppurative otitis media and the pathologic labyrinthine fistula. *Laryngoscope*, **80**, 1025–1035

ROSENHALL, U. (1973) Degenerative patterns in the aging human vestibular neuro-epithelia. *Acta Otolaryngologica*, **76**, 208–220

SCHUKNECHT, H. (1957) Ablation therapy in the management of Menière's disease. *Acta Otolaryngologica Supplementum*, **132**, 1–42

SCHUKNECHT, H. (1962) Positional vertigo: clinical and experimental observations. *Transactions of the American Academy of Ophthalmology and Otolaryngology*, **66**, 319–332

SCHUKNECHT, H. F. (1969) Cupulolithiasis. *Archives of Otolaryngology*, **90**, 765–778

SCHUKNECHT, H. F. (1974a) Infections. In: *Pathology of the Ear*. Cambridge, Mass: Harvard University Press. Ch. 5, p. 241

SCHUKNECHT, H. (1974b) Disorders of innervation. In: *Pathology of the Ear*. Cambridge, Mass: Harvard University Press. p. 345

SCHUKNECHT, H. (1982) Behavior of the vestibular nerve following labyrinthectomy. *Annals of Otology, Rhinology and Laryngology*, Suppl. 91, 16–32

SCHUKNECHT, H. F. (1991) Ear pathology in autoimmune disease. *Advances in Oto-Rhino-Laryngology*, **46**, 50–70

SCHUKNECHT, H., ALLAM, A. and MURAKAMI, Y. (1968) Pathology of secondary malignant tumors of the temporal bone. *Annals of Otology, Rhinology and Laryngology*, **77**, 5–22

SCHUKNECHT, H., BENITEZ, J. and BEEKHUIS, J. (1962) Further observations on the pathology of Menière's disease. *Annals of Otology, Rhinology and Laryngology*, **71**, 1039–1053

SCHUKNECHT, H. and DAVISON, R. (1956) Deafness and vertigo from head injury. *Archives of Otolaryngology*, **63**, 513–528

SCHUKNECHT, H., IGARASHI, M. and CHASIN, W. (1965) Inner ear hemorrhage in leukemia. *Laryngoscope*, **75**, 662–668

SCHUKNECHT, H., NORTHROP, C. and IGARASHI, M. (1968) Cochlear pathology after destruction of the endolymphatic sac in the cat. *Acta Otolaryngologica*, **65**, 479–487

SCHUKNECHT, H. F. and RUBY, R. (1973) Cupulolithiasis. *Advances in Oto-Rhino-Laryngology*, **20**, 434–443

SHELDON, J. H. (1948) *The Social Medicine of Old Age*. London: Oxford University Press, pp. 1–239

SILVERSTEIN, H. (1970) The effects of perfusing the perilymphatic space with artificial endolymph. *Annals of Otology, Rhinology and Laryngology*, **79**, 754–765

STAHLE, J. (1966) Vestibular neuritis. In: *The Vestibular System and Its Diseases*, edited by R. Wolfson. Philadelphia: University of Pennsylvania Press, pp. 459–470

STENGER, P. (1909) Beitrag zur Kenntnis nach Kopfverletzungen Auftretenden Veranderungen im Inneren Ohr. *Archiv für Ohrenhelkunde*, **79**, 43–52

STEWART, T., LILAND, J. R. and SCHUKNECHT, H. (1975) Occult schwannomas of the vestibular nerve. *Archives of Otolaryngology*, **101**, 91–95

WALL, C. III, BLACK, F. O. and HUNT, A. E. (1984) Effects of age, sex and stimulus parameters upon vestibulo-ocular responses to sinusoidal rotation. *Acta Otolaryngologica*, **98**, 270–278

WANAMAKER, H. (1972) Acoustic neuroma primary arising in the vestibule. *Laryngoscope*, **82**, 1040–1044

WATSON, P., BARBER, H., DECK, J. and TERBRUGGE, K. (1981) Positional vertigo and nystagmus of central origin. *Canadian Journal of Neurological Sciences*, **8**, 133–137

WERSALL, J. and HAWKINS, J. (1962) The vestibular sensory epithelia in the cat labyrinth and their reactions in chronic streptomycin intoxication. *Acta Otolaryngologica*, **54**, 1–23

WILSON, W., BYL, F. and LAIRD, N. (1980) Efficacy of steroids in the treatment of idiopathic sudden hearing loss. *Archives of Otolaryngology*, **106**, 772–778

WOLFF, D., BERNHARD W. G., TSUTSUMI S., ROSS, I. S. and NUSSBAUM, H. E. (1965) The pathology of Cogan's syndrome causing profound deafness. *Annals of Otology, Rhinology, and Laryngology*, **74**, 507–520

6

Diseases of the external ear

David Wright

The auricle

Development

(See Volume 1, Chapter 1.)

Commencing on the 38th day of fetal life, the auricle develops from the first and second branchial arches. Three nodules of mesenchymal proliferation develop on the margins of each arch and by day 41 these nodules have reached maximum size, moved in a dorsolateral direction and begun to fuse to form the auricle. The auricle is anatomically complete by the 20th week (Melnick and Myrianthopoulos, 1979a). In the fully developed ear the first arch contributes only to the tragus and possibly to some of the anterior crus of the helix. The remainder of the auricle is derived from the second arch. The auricle develops initially at the level of the upper part of the neck and migrates into its final position.

It is common to find many minor variations in the shape of the pinna. *Darwin's tubercle* is seen as a small elevation on the posterosuperior part of the helix. This tubercle is homologous with the tip of the mammalian ear and is usually an inherited condition. *Wildermuth's ear* is a distinct entity with prominence of the antihelix and an underdeveloped helix and may be associated with other syndromes and with sensorineural and conductive deafness. Both Mozart and his father had fusion of the helix and antihelix as a dominant inheritance and understandably *Mozart's ear* was thought to indicate musical ability. However, failure of the lobule to separate from the side of the head is more common in females and may affect all females of a family (Potter and Craig, 1975).

Congenital anomalies of the auricle

(See Volume 6, Chapter 9.)

Apart from the minor variations already described many major anomalies may occur. Arrested development of the mesoenchymal nodules leads to anotia, i.e. the total absence of the auricle, or microtia where the pinna is rudimentary and malformed and usually placed lower and more anteriorly than normal (Figure 6.1). These anomalies are often associated with meatal atresia and other abnormalities of the middle ear, the degree of abnormality usually being proportional to the external deformity (Jafek *et al.*, 1975).

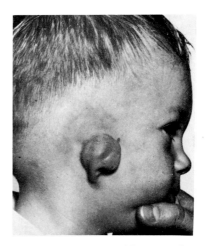

Figure 6.1 Congenital deformity of the pinna. There was no meatal atresia present in this case

Minor dysplasias of the second arch development produce folding or defects in the helix and the typical bat ear appearance produced when the antihelix is poorly formed with an excess of conchal cartilage.

Protruding or bat ears

Varied forms of protruding ear are commonly found in newborn babies although most of these minor deformities disappear spontaneously during the first year of life. Views differ as to whether protruding ears should be considered a variant of the normal ear or a true deformity of the auricle. Hereditary factors are important in the development of the protruding ear (Weerda, 1985). The 'lop ear', in which the crus antihelicis is poorly formed, and the 'cup ear' in which most of the antihelix is undeveloped were differentiated by Luckett (1910). His method of antihelix reconstruction involved an excision of cartilage along the summit of the antihelix and superior crus, with approximation of the cut edges side by side. Numerous techniques have subsequently been described to correct the deformity but, unless there is a complex deformity, the Mustardé (1963) or a simple anterior scoring technique (Rhŷs Evans, 1985) is quite satisfactory.

Auricular appendages

Auricular appendages or accessory auricles occur as small elevations of skin containing a bar of elastic cartilage. They may be single or multiple and most commonly occur just anterior to the tragus or ascending crus of the helix, but may extend along a line from the tragus to the angle of the mouth. They are often associated with macrostomia. They may also be found with other congenital anomalies of the first arch. When excising an auricular appendage it must be remembered that it may contain a bar of elastic cartilage which can extend deep into the underlying soft tissues.

Congenital aural sinuses and fistulae

Congenital sinuses composed of blind tracks lined by squamous epithelium are commonly found in the preauricular region along the ascending crus of the helix (Figure 6.2). Others may open along a line extending from the lower border of the helix to the angle of the mouth. Collaural fistulae open superiorly in the floor of the external auditory meatus and inferiorly at the anterior border of the sternomastoid behind the angle of the jaw. Many authors have found an association between preauricular sinuses, branchial fistulae and deafness (Melnick *et al.*, 1975; Fitch, Lindsay and Srolovitz, 1976).

Congenital sinuses and fistulae do not require treatment unless they cause symptoms. Occasionally they become infected leading to a persistent discharge and sometimes to abscess formation when they require complete excision. During excision, care is required

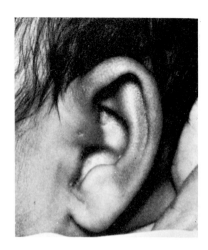

Figure 6.2 Preauricular fistula in an infant

as the tract often extends deep into the soft tissues and can be intimately related to branches of the facial nerve. The tract can be readily identified if injected with gentian violet dye prior to excision.

Congenital syndromes associated with microtia and deformities of the pinna

(See Volume 6.)

Numerous syndromes have been described associating microtia with other congenital defects. The more important of these have been well documented by Melnick and Myrianthopoulos (1979b):

Treacher Collins syndrome: mandibulofacial dysostosis associated with meatal atresia and deafness (autosomal dominant)

Otomandibular syndrome of Konigsmark and Gorlin: folding of the pinna, thin external nares, micrognathia and bilateral stapedial fixation (autosomal dominant)

Branchio-otic dysplasias: a combination of auricular malformation, cervical fistulae, and conductive and sensorineural deafness (autosomal dominant)

LADD syndrome: the lacrimo-auriculodento-digital syndrome of cup-shaped ears with deafness, and anomalies of the digits and the enamel of the teeth (autosomal dominant)

Fraser syndrome: a rare autosomal recessive disorder with consistent features of cryptophthalomos (hidden eye) and meatal stenosis, dysplasia of the pinna, hypoplastic notched nares, choanal stenosis or atresia as well as other abnormalities of the larynx (Ford *et al.*, 1992).

It is important that the otologist appreciates the significance of investigating the renal function of children with familial branchial arch syndromes and conversely the early audiological assessment of children with known renal anomalies. Most of these syndromes have an autosomal dominant inheritance but there is a considerable variation in the manifestations of the syndrome within affected families and among individuals. Melnick and Myrianthopoulos (1979b), in an extensive study of these conditions, concluded that the underlying developmental abnormality was probably a breakdown of neural crest integrity resulting in aberrant crest cell migration.

Potter's syndrome

Potter's syndrome is a well-recognized congenital abnormality of the pinna (Figure 6.3). The auricles are large and flat and may be associated with abnormal limb positioning, pulmonary hypoplasia and compression facies. The syndrome is the result of oligohydramnios leading to flattening and compression of the pinna. By definition, the oligohydramnios is the conse-quence of renal agenesis or dysplasia but may be caused by loss of amniotic fluid. If the infant survives, in most cases the pinna will become normal in time.

Congenital malformation of extrinsic origin

External factors which may affect the development of the fetus and result in abnormalities of the pinna include:

Drugs

Warfarin can lead to microtia, although the most striking and consistent finding produced by this drug is severe hypoplasia of the nose. Auricular abnormalities are also seen following the ingestion of folic acid antagonists such as *methotrexate* and *aminopterin*.

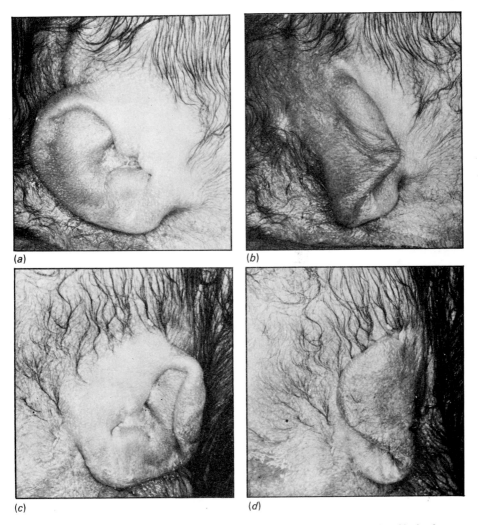

(a)

(b)

(c)

(d)

Figure 6.3 Potter's syndrome. The pinna is large and flattened and can be readily folded. (Reproduced by kind permission of Dr Shawky El-Serafy, 1983, *Atlas of the Ear, Nose and Throat Diseases*, Doha: Ali bin Ali Printing Press)

High alcohol intake during pregnancy, known as the *fetal alcohol syndrome*, can result in microcephaly, maxillary hypoplasia and joint anomalies, and many affected infants show an abnormality of the pinna with a marked ridge running across the concha due to hypertrophy of the crus of the helix.

Thalidomide. Anomalies of the ear including microtia, meatal atresia, and abnormalities of the middle and internal ears occurred when thalidomide was administered to the mother during the first 30–40 days of pregnancy (Takemori, Ishii and Suzuki, 1976).

Fetal hydantoin syndrome, which may include dysplasia of the auricles, occurs as a result of the ingestion of anticonvulsant drugs by epileptic mothers during pregnancy.

Radiation

Radiation of the maternal pelvis during pregnancy can lead to a higher incidence of congenital malformations of the ear (Jafek *et al.*, 1975).

Viruses

Maternal viral infections during the first trimester of pregnancy can be responsible for some isolated cases of external ear deformity, but there has been no conclusive evidence for this.

Steeter bands

Steeter or amniotic bands are bands of connective tissue that stretch across the amniotic space and can result in clefts or deformities of the auricle as well as of the face, skull and limbs.

Congenital tumours

Haemangioma and lymphangioma may involve the auricle. Dermoid cysts are a form of teratoma composed of a fibrous wall lined with stratified squamous epithelium containing hair follicles, sweat and sebaceous glands and usually present as a round spongy growth behind the pinna in the region of the upper part of the sternomastoid or just anterior to the helix.

Pseudocyst of the auricle

Pseudocyst of the auricle is a rare condition found most commonly in China. It presents as a cystic swelling in the upper half of the anterior aspect of the auricle (Engel, 1966). It forms within degenerate cartilage as a cystic space that has no lining but contains straw-coloured fluid, hence, the term pseudocyst (Grabski *et al.*, 1989) (Figure 6.4*a*).

Li-Xiang and Xiu-Yun (1992) examined 42 auricles taken from 18 fetuses and three adults. They found intracartilaginous fibrous tissue with blood vessels

and lymphatics in 12 ears (Figure 6.4*b*) and an interruption of the auricular cartilage in 22 ears (Figure 6.4*c*). These findings support the hypothesis of congenital embryonic dysplasia as the origin of the formation of the pseudocyst of the auricle.

Li-Xiang and Xiu-Yun (1990) recommended the insertion of a drainage tube into the pseudocyst through a guide needle which was left in place for 5 days with a pressure dressing. In their series of 45 cases, only two cases failed to respond. Successful non-surgical treatment has been described by Job and Raman (1992) who gave a high dose of oral prednisolone over a 4-week period, and claimed that the fluid was absorbed and that intracartilaginous fibrosis and granulation was prevented.

Injuries to the auricle

(See Chapter 8.)

Accidental auricular injuries to the ear occur in people of all ages but people participating in high risk activities such as wrestling, boxing and rugby football should wear protective head gear. Auricular injury in a child without a confirmed history of trauma should raise the question of possible child abuse (Willner, Ledereich and de Vreis, 1992). The type and extent of the injury is related to the force of the trauma, so a shearing force of moderate intensity causes haematoma formation whereas a greater force results in lacerations or even amputation. The high ratio of the surface area to the mass makes the pinna vulnerable to extremes of temperature.

Treatment

The aim of treatment should be to restore the normal contours to the pinna and prevent infection. Second degree burns should be treated by regular cleansing and the application of a topical antibiotic. Deeper burns require debridement. Cartilage can be preserved by burying it into subcutaneous tissues for later reconstruction. Simple lacerations should be closed under aseptic technique using either skin-to-skin sutures only or sutures of the skin combined with intercartilage sutures. More extensive and complex lacerations require meticulous care to try to preserve tissue and reconstitute the remaining fragments. Bare cartilage should be covered with vascularized tissue. The treatment of total amputation of the pinna remains controversial, although cosmetically microsurgical reimplantation is the optimal management of the amputated external ear. This requires the use of vein grafts, with heparinization and the alleviation of venous congestion by frequent stab wounds (Turpin, 1990). The amputated pinna can also be dermabraided and re-attached with sutures and then slipped into a pocket of elevated postauricular skin 2 weeks before reshaping. Chondritis, a most

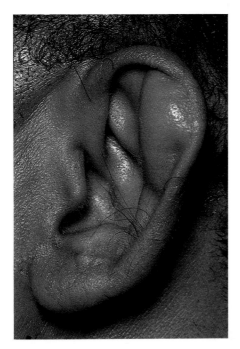

Plate 3/6/I Haematoma of the auricle

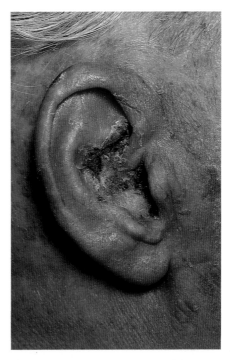

Plate 3/6/III Squamous carcinoma of the pinna

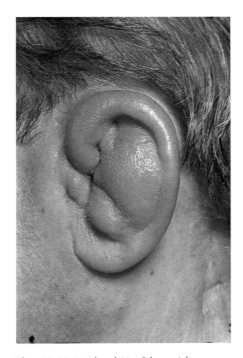

Plate 3/6/II Perichondritis of the auricle

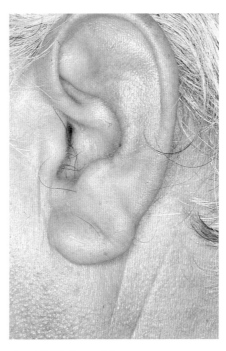

Plate 3/6/IV The ear lobe crease

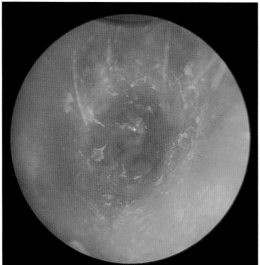

Plate 3/6/V Obliterative otitis externa

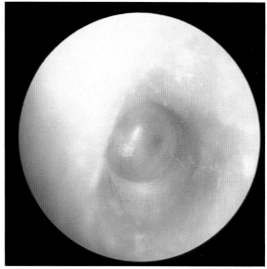

Plate 3/6/VII Deep meatal false membrane

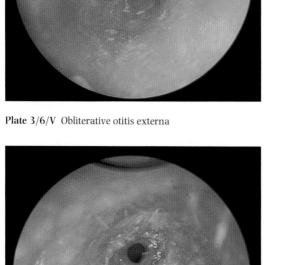

Plate 3/6/VI Deep meatal stenosis

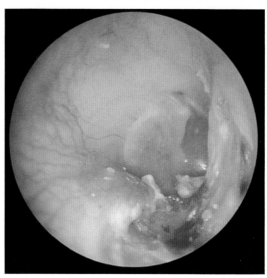

Plate 3/6/VIII Benign necrotizing osteitis of the meatal floor

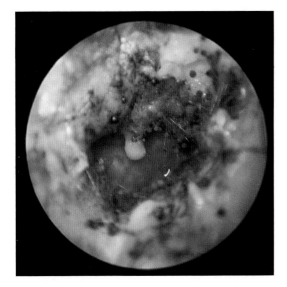

Plate 3/6/IX Otomycosis: *Aspergillus niger* infection of the meatus with an underlying perforation

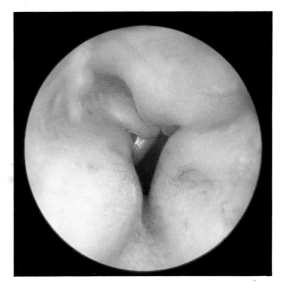

Plate 3/6/XI Meatal exostoses

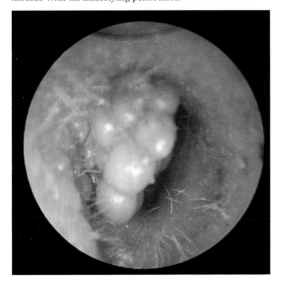

Plate 3/6/X Papilloma of the external auditory meatus

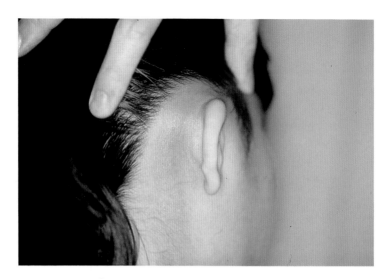

Plate 3/9/I Acute mastoiditis in a young child

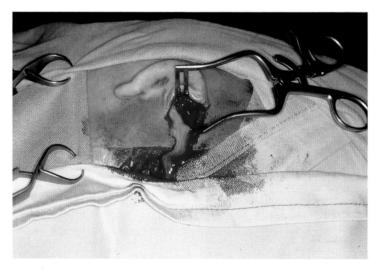

Plate 3/9/II Initial incision for acute mastoiditis in a child

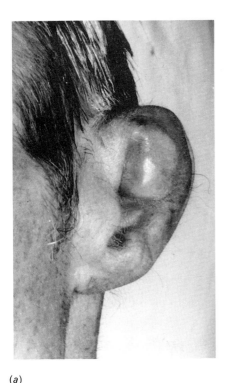

(a)

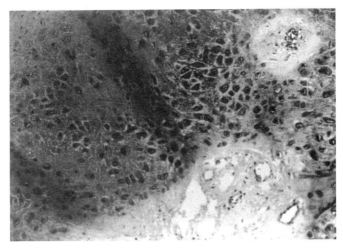

(b)

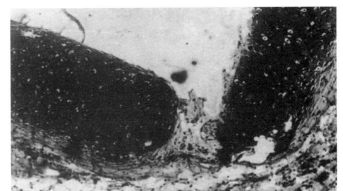

(c)

Figure 6.4 (a) Pseudocyst of the auricle (with kind permission of Mr J. B. Booth). (b) Pseudocyst of the auricle: connective tissue with vessels completely enclosed with auricular cartilage. (c) Pseudocyst of the auricle: interruption of auricular cartilage. (b and c reproduced with kind permission of Z. Li-Xiang and W. Xiu-Yun and Editor of the *Journal of Laryngology and Otology*)

aggressive process, is the most serious complication of injury or surgery of the pinna and requires prompt removal of pus and necrotic cartilage. Exteriorization and the removal of damaged cartilage may be effective but leads to disfigurement. Loss of cartilage and skin can be corrected with composite grafts from the opposite ear, costal cartilage and local pedicle flaps (Templer and Renner, 1990).

Haematoma of the auricle (see Plate 3/6/I)

Haematoma of the auricle is the result of closed trauma and occurs frequently in contact sports such as boxing and rugby football and often results in disfigurement by fibrosis or chondritis. The condition is caused by an extravasation of blood between the cartilage and the perichondrium producing a soft doughy swelling of the pinna. If untreated the blood clot becomes organized and the ear remains permanently thickened, producing the cauliflower ear deformity.

Treatment

Cases seen shortly after the injury should be treated by aspiration using a wide bore needle. Cases of longer standing will require incision and the evacuation of the clot. The incision should be placed along the margin of the helix and any clot sucked out. Strict asepsis is essential for perichondritis may occur if infection is introduced. Following either aspiration or incision, a firm dressing or sheets of silastic can be applied to both surfaces of the pinna and held by a transfixation suture to prevent recurrence of the haematoma. Further aspiration may be necessary should the haematoma recur.

Infections of the auricle

Impetigo

Impetigo is an infection of the superficial layers of the skin by staphylococci. It may involve the whole auricle and sometimes the neck and face but it does not extend into the external auditory meatus. Vesicles filled with serum arise on a reddish-purple base. Later the vesicles burst to exude serum which dries to form semi-adherent amber crusts. The condition is most commonly seen in young children and may be secondary to the otorrhoea of a middle-ear infection.

Treatment

Crusts should be removed by bathing with warm sterile saline. When dried, a topical antibiotic ointment should be applied and the treatment repeated daily for several days. Any otitis media or externa present must be treated at the same time to prevent re-infection of the skin.

Erysipelas

Erysipelas is due to a streptococcal infection of the skin producing a raised red oedematous eruption with a characteristically well-defined edge. The auricle becomes intensely red and swollen and the infection spreads into the adjoining skin of the face usually accompanied by a marked systemic upset with a high temperature and a rapid pulse.

Treatment

The infection usually responds rapidly to the appropriate antibiotic therapy.

Many generalized skin disorders such as psoriasis may involve the pinna but require no separate description.

Perichondritis (see Plate 3/6/II)

Infection of the perichondrium of the auricle occurs most commonly when the cartilage is exposed either by laceration or by surgery. The cartilage may also be injured by frostbite or burns. Infection may be introduced during aspiration or incision of a haematoma auris. At times superficial infections of the meatus or pinna spread deeply to involve the perichondrium.

In the early stages of the infection the pinna becomes red and tender. This is followed by a generalized swelling of the pinna and eventually the formation of a subperichondrial abscess with pus collecting between the perichondrium and the underlying cartilage. The cartilage, deprived of its blood supply, may necrose resulting in marked deformity of the pinna.

Relapsing polychondritis, an episodic inflammatory disease of connective tissue and various cartilages of the head and neck and upper respiratory system, is probably due to an autoimmune reaction and can lead to cauliflower ear deformity. Steroids can be used to control the acute attacks and suppress the recurrences (see Chapter 15).

The insertion of earrings into the pinna is widely practised and when this involves the cartilaginous portion of the auricle it carries a definite risk of perichondritis. The vogue for 'high ear piercing' which traverses cartilage rather than the fatty tissue of the ear lobe increases the risk of infection, particularly with *Pseudomonas* which may produce severe cosmetic deformity (Cumberworth and Hogarth, 1990) as well as fatal septicaemia from *β-haemolytic streptococcal* infection (Lovejoy and Smith, 1970). Subacute bacterial endocarditis has been reported following acupuncture to the ear (Lee and McIlwain, 1985). Ear piercing also carries the risk of spreading viral diseases such as hepatitis and acquired immune deficiency syndrome (AIDS) unless carried out with scrupulous attention to sterility. Septicaemia may also occur.

Treatment

Cases of perichondritis should be treated promptly with a broad-spectrum antibiotic. If there is any discharge from the ear, a swab should be taken for culture and the sensitivities determined. *Pseudomonas aeruginosa* is frequently found in these cases. Treatment should then be commenced immediately. If subperichondrial abscesses form they should be incised and drained, but incision should be delayed until definite fluctuation can be elicited as premature incision may result in a further spread of the infection. Pain and suppuration may continue in some instances, despite these measures, and gross deformity is inevitable. In such cases of extensive disease the whole of the auricular cartilage (except that of the helix) must be excised through a wide incision on the anterolateral aspect of the auricle.

Chondrodermatitis nodularis chronica helicis

Chondrodermatitis nodularis chronica helicis is a painful, persistent erythematous, often crusted papule, most commonly found on the helical rim of the ear of Caucasian men over the age of 40 years. It is caused by trauma, such as frostbite, sun, wind and extremes of temperature. The rounded exposed margin of the helix is particularly susceptible. Ageing is also a factor, resulting in thinning of the skin and cartilage, loss of elastic tissue and degenerative vascular and connective tissue changes. The lesion begins in the dermis and is followed by fibrinoid necrosis, which accumulates a surrounding zone of granulation tissue. The perichondrium then becomes involved leading to degeneration and deformity.

Treatment

The accepted treatment is surgical removal by local excision which should include a small wedge of underlying cartilage. However, the soft necrotic cartilage can be removed more easily by curettage, the end point being reached when the curette is resisted by firm elastic cartilage leaving minimal deformity to the contour of the ear (Colidron, 1991). Alternatively, the CO_2 laser has been used to vaporize the cutaneous nodules and involved cartilage (Taylor, 1991) and the use of injectable collagen implants is described as a conservative treatment (Greenbaum, 1991).

Tophi

Asymptomatic subperichondrial salmon pink deposits of sodium biurate crystals may be found in the helix and antihelix of sufferers from gout. The deposits vary from one millimetre to several centimetres in size and may be confused with rheumatoid nodules and xanthoma tuberosum. Although rarely troublesome, they may occasionally become superficially ulcerated. Gout is familial and related to a defect in the hypoxanthine-guanine phosphorosyltransferase enzyme which involves purine metabolism.

Treatment

Treatment is that of the underlying condition with a colchicine derivative.

Tumours of the auricle

Benign

Benign tumours arise from the pinna much as they do in other skin and subcutaneous areas of the body. Papilloma, fibroma and chondroma do occur but need no special description. Haemangiomas are often seen associated with adjacent involvement of the face and parotid gland.

Malignant

(See Chapter 8.)

Squamous cell carcinoma (see Plate 3/6/III)

The clinical diagnosis of an epithelioma does not usually present any difficulty. Typically the lesion presents as an indurated ulcer with everted margins. The diagnosis is confirmed by biopsy under local anaesthesia. The regional lymph nodes may be involved but this is not usually an early occurrence in tumours confined to the auricle.

Treatment

The primary treatment of small lesions is by local excision or by Mohs' micrographic surgery (1947). Larger tumours need excision with external beam radiation. In advanced cases it is necessary to carry out radical resection of the ear including parotidectomy, neck dissection and mastoidectomy. Unfortunately localized carcinoma of the external ear has a high propensity for local and regional failure and so merits aggressive treatment of the primary lesion with removal of the regional lymph nodes in high risk patients (Yoon *et al.*, 1992).

Basal cell carcinoma (rodent ulcer)

Basal cell carcinoma results from proliferation of the basal cells of the epithelium. It is found less commonly on the auricle than on the skin of the face and forehead. As a rule basal cell growths are sited on the tragus, the border of the helix and the meatal entrance. In late cases, the whole auricle may be destroyed while the underlying bone and parotid gland may be infiltrated. The regional lymph nodes are not involved.

Basal cell carcinoma is more usual in men than women and most likely to occur in those over 50 years of age which is much later than would be expected with squamous cell carcinoma. It is usually asymptomatic and the diagnosis is made by biopsy. The tumour does not metastasize and is usually slow growing but it can be invasive, destroying cartilage and bone. The aetiology is unknown. Basal cell carcinoma develops as an ingrowth which differentiates it from the outward growing squamous cell cancer. First a flat painless slightly raised lesion appears followed by the development of a rolled edge with a penetrating ulcer which bleeds readily. Cystic forms may be encountered which are smooth, often pigmented tumours without any crusting or ulceration and when small may be confused with naevi.

Treatment

The prognosis is excellent in those patients in whom the lesion is small enough to be wholly excised with a wide margin of healthy tissue but, when the tumour has penetrated beyond the reach of surgery, the prognosis is poor. Advanced stages with infiltration of the underlying bone and soft tissues require wide excision and postoperative radiotherapy. However, the combination of surgery and a full dose of radiation often leads to further necrosis of bone and soft tissue.

When extensive infiltration of the deep tissues has occurred it may be impossible to eradicate the tumour and the patient will eventually succumb, although the progress of the disease is usually very slow.

Malignant melanoma

The auricle is rarely affected by this form of malignancy. However, when it occurs it is seen as a nodular pigmented lesion which tends to enlarge rapidly and eventually to ulcerate. Involvement of the regional lymph nodes and distant metastasis may occur when the primary lesion is still quite small.

Treatment

There is no evidence that melanoma of the ear has a worse prognosis or different prognostic factors than melanoma in other cutaneous sites (Cole *et al.*, 1992). Patients with primary tumours less than 2 mm depth have a significantly better prognosis than those with deeper lesions (Hudson *et al.*, 1990).

In selected cases, local disease can be controlled by excision and skin graft, and in larger tumours by wedge excision or wide excision. Excision of the lesion must be sufficiently radical as this offers the best opportunity of cure and may involve complete excision of the pinna and an *en bloc* dissection of the regional nodes. Even with early lesions the prognosis is poor.

Ear lobe crease (see Plate 3/6/IV)

This is a diagonal crease running across the lobule and is frequently present in old age. A relationship between high serum cholesterol and the ear lobe crease has been demonstrated but biopsies of the crease show no abnormalities such as cholesterol deposition. The conclusion of Moraes *et al.* (1992), is that the ear lobe crease should be used as a physical sign predictive of the presence of coronary heart disease rather than as a diagnostic test.

External auditory meatus

Development

The meatus begins development on the 41st day of fetal life at the dorsal end of the first branchial cleft (Melnick and Myrianthopoulos, 1979a). Ectodermal proliferation extends inwards approaching the expanding middle ear cavity forming the meatal plug at about 10 weeks. This extends in a disc-like fashion to fill the lumen of the meatus and in the horizontal plane the meatus is boot-shaped with a narrow neck with the sole of the meatal plug spreading out to form the future tympanic membrane. At the same time the plug in the proximal portion of the neck is reabsorbed.

At 13 weeks, the innermost surface of the plug in contact with the anlage of the malleus is ready to contribute to the formation of the tympanic membrane. At 15 weeks, the innermost portion of this plug splits leaving a thin ectodermal cell layer of immature tympanic membrane. The neck of the boot forms the border between the primary and secondary meatus and is the last part to split. In the 16.5-week fetus, the meatus is fully patent throughout its entire length although the lumen remains narrow and curved. The meatus is fully expanded to its complete form in the 18-week fetus (Nishimura and Kurmori, 1992).

Congenital anomalies

(See Volume 6.)

The association between some deformities of the pinna and congenital meatal atresia or stenosis has already been noted (see above). Meatal atresia and stenosis can occur in the presence of a normal pinna.

Congenital meatal atresia and stenosis

Atresia of the external auditory meatus can occur bilaterally as well as unilaterally and is usually accompanied by auricular deformity. Surgical intervention in bilateral cases should be considered in order to promote normal speech and language development, but with unilateral atresia surgical intervention is not recommended until the patient reaches 18 years of age. Preoperative evaluation should include behavioural audiometry, auditory brain stem evoked response and computerized tomographic scans. It is possible to produce high quality three-dimensional image reconstructions from conventional thin section computerized tomography and to observe the imaged structure from any angle with views and dimensions that are comparable to actual dissections (Figure 6.5). Andrews *et al.* (1992) have applied this technique to the temporal bone to assess congenital aural atresia showing the configuration of the atretic plate and middle ear in relation to the tegmen and glenoid fossa. Most significantly the facial nerve could be accurately and easily identified in its entire intratemporal course.

Jahrsdoerfer *et al.* (1992) have developed a grading scheme to select those patients who have the greatest chance of success based on the preoperative temporal bone CT scan and the appearance of the external ear. Patients are graded on a possible best score of 10. The stapes is assigned the highest rating of 2 points, while all other entries on the scale are 1 point. The grade assigned preoperatively has been shown to correlate well with the patient's chance of success which allows for reasonable prediction of the hearing outcome. Alternatively the hearing impairment associated with congenital external auditory meatal atresia can be managed using a bone conduction hearing aid from an early age. However, many children do not like to wear a bone conduction aid because of physical or social considerations and reconstruction of the external auditory meatus and middle ear may give poor results. Dunham and Friedman (1990) showed that most patients in their series

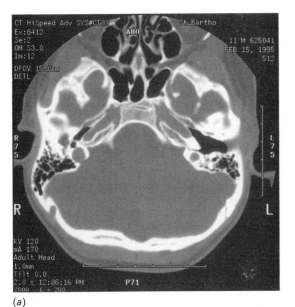

(a)

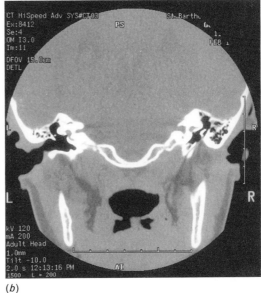

(b)

(c)

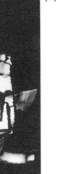

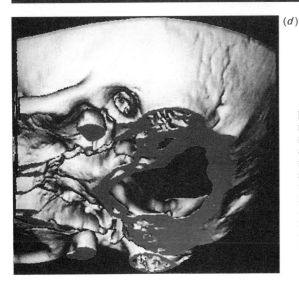

(d)

Figure 6.5 Congenital atresia of right external auditory meatus – evaluation by high resolution CT with 3D reconstructions. (*a*) Axial scan showing apparent bony atresia of the right external auditory meatus with aerated middle ear cleft; the left side is normal. (*b*) Coronal scan showing the malleus in position within the middle ear and the presence of normal inner ear structures. (*c*) 3D surface rendered reconstruction (HU: 190–2500) of right external auditory meatus viewed from the side with lateral tilt. This reveals the relationship of bony and soft tissue components of the atresia. (*d*) 3D surface rendered reconstruction of normal left external auditory meatus for comparison. (Reproduced by kind permission of Dr Michael Charlesworth and Dr Julian Hanson)

experienced a preference for using a bone anchored hearing aid over a standard bone conduction aid.

Congenital meatal stenosis has been found to carry a much greater risk of cholesteatoma development and Cole and Jahrsdoerfer (1990) recommended surgery for patients with stenosis of the external ear canal measuring 2 mm or less. The recommended appropriate time for surgery is during late childhood or early adolescence but before irreversible damage to hearing has occurred.

Acquired meatal atresia and stenosis

Atresia

A true acquired atresia of the cartilaginous meatus is rare but when it occurs it is nearly always traumatic in origin, caused by gunshot wounds, burns, radiation etc. Chronic otitis externa may result in stenosis but is rarely responsible for atresia. Bilateral atresia of the outer meatus following acute otitis externa has been recorded (Marlowe, 1972).

Stenosis

Acquired stenosis of the cartilaginous meatus is not uncommon and can occur as a result of:

Trauma: accidents, lacerations, gunshot wounds, mastoid surgery, burns, thermal and chemical radiation

Infection: chronic otitis externa

Neoplasia: both squamous cell carcinoma and adenocarcinoma may present as a progressive narrowing of the meatus.

The commonest cause of stenosis is chronic otitis externa leading to progressive subepithelial fibrosis resulting in narrowing of the canal. Stenosis may also occur at the junction of the cartilaginous and bony meatus due to keratosis obturans which causes expansion of the bony meatus and exposure of the meatal cartilage at its deep attachment. Infection of the cartilage with the formation of granulation tissue occurs with subsequent fibrosis and stricture formation.

Treatment

The only effective treatment is the creation of a new canal by meatoplasty. Repeated dilatation of the soft tissues of the stenosed canal rarely produces lasting improvement.

Using a postaural incision, the fibrous tissue and thickened meatal skin are excised but where possible preserving a strip of skin along the roof and floor. The outer part of the bony meatus is enlarged using a drill and an ellipse of conchal cartilage is excised so that a flap of conchal skin can be turned back and sutured in place. The meatus is then packed and allowed to re-epithelialize. Split skin grafts may be necessary to cover any denuded areas.

Deep meatus

Bony swellings, either osteomas or exostoses can develop in the bony meatus, representing the commonest form of stenosis (see below).

Obliterative otitis externa

Obliterative otitis externa is a progressive stenosis or atresia of the deep meatus. There is always a preceding otitis externa and in some cases chronic middle ear infection may be present. In most cases there is a history of irritation and discharge, intermittent or continuous over a number of years with an increasing loss of hearing. Infrequently, the condition develops rapidly with deafness persisting after a single episode of otitis externa which may have been present for only a few weeks. Bonding and Tos (1974) used the term 'postinflammatory acquired atresia' to describe the condition.

In the active phase of the disease, the inflammatory changes are usually confined to the deep meatus. The skin is red and thickened and may bleed readily when cleaned. The tympanic membrane is usually obscured by granulation tissue. Some cases of granulating myringitis may represent a more localized form of the same condition.

The deep meatus becomes re-epithelialized as the inflammatory stage settles leaving a mass of connective tissue between the outer surface of the tympanic membrane and a newly formed fundus in the meatus with a resulting conductive deafness (see Plate 3/6/V). No consistent bacteria are found on culture from these cases and histology of tissue obliterating the deep meatus reveals a non-specific vascular connective tissue with inflammatory cells.

At times, instead of atresia, a stenosis or web develops in the deep meatus a few millimetres external to the tympanic membrane (see Plate 3/6/VI). This can progress to complete atresia, in which event, epithelium may persist in the shut-off portion of the meatus and a meatal cholesteatoma may develop (see Plate 3/6/VII).

Why this condition behaves as it does is unknown.

Treatment

In the active granulating phase treatment is best confined to the removal of granulations and packing the meatus with ribbon-gauze soaked in a topical antibiotic/steroid preparation. There is usually a slow response to treatment and a marked tendency to recurrence. Although a few cases respond to treatment, the majority progress to stenosis or atresia. When the atresia is established surgical treatment can be considered but should be postponed until all evidence of increased vascularity has disappeared. This may take many months.

In quiescent cases with conductive deafness, surgical removal of the obstructing tissue may restore hearing. This is best undertaken through a postaural approach. The obliterative fibrous tissue is dissected away from the meatal walls and off the fibrous layer of the tympanic membrane. The deep meatus is enlarged by burring away some bone. If a perforation is present, it should be closed with fascial graft. If the area of exposed bone is no more than a few millimetres, leaving a pack in place for up to 6 weeks will often result in re-epithelialization, but more extensive bare areas should be covered with thin split-skin grafts. A technique recommended by Stucker and Shaw (1991) provides new skin utilizing a postauricular vascularized skin flap rotated into the ear canal to resurface the canal and meatus.

Radical excisional surgery was found to give a 25 dB average hearing gain in the speech frequencies when a successful canalplasty was achieved (Herdman and Wright, 1990).

Radionecrosis

The tympanic plate is highly susceptible to radionecrosis if it is included in the radiation field during treatment of an adjoining area. The process may be very slow with a long latent period between irradiation and the onset of symptoms. Two patterns of temporal bone involvement have been described by Ramsden, Bulman and Lorigan (1975) following radiotherapy in the management of head and neck tumours. *Localized necrosis* principally involves the tympanic plate and leads to spontaneous sequestration of bone, whereas *diffuse necrosis* may involve major adjacent neurovascular structures associated with high morbidity and potentially lethal sequelae.

The underlying pathological process, originally termed 'osteitis' by Ewing (1926), is a slowly progressive avascular necrosis initiated by obliterative endarteritis. In severe radionecrosis the viability of residual bone is difficult to assess and multiple sequestrectomies may be required. However, when radionecrosis is limited to the tympanic ring, small areas of bare bone may appear on the meatal floor, associated with pain and irritation and occasionally with scant discharge. During the process of spontaneous sequestration, conservative treatment is usually all that is required, but the whole process may continue for many years. It may be necessary to remove the remaining dead bone of the tympanic ring and reconstitute the soft tissues of the meatus with a graft.

Benign necrotizing osteitis of the meatus (see Plate 3/6/VIII)

Exposed dead bone may present in the meatal floor for no apparent reason. There is usually a history of previous otitis externa and healing may be delayed until all the sequestrum separates. It has been suggested that the benign necrotizing osteitis is a response to irritation or otitis externa and that constant scratching of the ear with a matchstick, hairpin or some similar object may eventually cause erosion of the skin and periosteum and necrosis of localized areas of bone. While this is true in some cases there are undoubtedly some patients who produce this change spontaneously over a short period of time for no apparent reason. Quite why the tympanic plate has this susceptibility to necrosis remains obscure. The blood supply of the tympanic plate is relatively poor and the additional microangiopathy that accompanies diabetes mellitus appears to predispose towards avascular necrosis with the formation of bony sequestra. The effect of radiation on the tympanic plate is to produce a slow progressive obliterative endarteritis with the suppresion of new bone formation and an apparent attempt at healing by fibrosis (Birzgalis *et al.*, 1993).

Foreign bodies

Foreign bodies in the external auditory meatus are a common and sometimes challenging problem. Insects may enter the meatus accidentally but most foreign bodies are introduced by the patient. A tightly wedged smooth round foreign body remains one of the most difficult to remove, but objects lying medial to the isthmus of the canal are more difficult because they must be brought through the isthmus where the canal wall skin is thin and sensitive. Otitis externa is frequently associated with meatal foreign bodies.

Treatment

Insects should first be killed by instilling oil into the external auditory meatus (Leffler, Cheney and Tandberg, 1993). Small objects are most easily removed by syringing but this method must not be used if the foreign body closely fits the meatus as it may become more deeply impacted. Vegetable foreign bodies may be hygroscopic and swell if syringed with saline. They should either be removed with small forceps or by syringing with alcohol.

Large foreign bodies should be removed under microscopic control using small forceps or a blunt hook, but forceps should not be used for smooth, rounded objects. General anaesthesia is often desirable in children and sometimes in adults. Pride and Schwab (1989) recommended using cyanoacrylate adhesive (Superglue) applied to the blunt end of a cotton swab to make contact and remove a spherical object with safety. Button batteries lodged in the external auditory meatus must be removed as a matter of the utmost urgency. They spontaneously leak alkaline electrolyte solution on exposure to moisture causing liquefaction necrosis of adjacent tissue. Otolaryngological complications include lower motor neuron facial palsy, nasal septal perforation and fatal oesophagoaortic fistula (McRae, Premachandra and Gatland, 1989).

When a large foreign body is impacted in the deep meatus it may be necessary to expose the meatus through a postauricular incision, drilling the bone from the canal wall to facilitate removal.

Cerumen

Ear wax is a mixture of secretions from two different gland types, ceruminous and pilosebaceous glands, together with squames of epithelium, dust and other foreign debris. The ceruminous glands are found deep within the skin of the outer two-thirds of the external auditory meatus which is lined by cuboidal and columnar epithelial cells. Secretion of the cerumen into the lumen is both by eccrine and apocrine function – the latter process being similar to the axillary sweat glands, which accounts for the odour of the cerumen. An unknown stimulus, possibly irritation of the overlying skin acting through adrenergic receptors, causes the surrounding myoepithelial cells to contract, expelling the liquid contents into the external auditory meatus. Once secreted, evaporation occurs allowing the now sticky substance to entrap dust, bacteria, fungi and epithelial squames before being expelled by migration, a process which is aided by jaw movement (Hanger and Mulley, 1992).

The quantity of wax produced varies greatly from one individual to another and its composition varies in different racial groups. Most Caucasians and Negroes have the so-called 'wet' phenotype with moist honey-coloured cerumen; in contrast mongoloid races tend to have grey granular and brittle cerumen, the 'dry' phenotype. Wax may reflect local and systemic disease. In cystic fibrosis there are lower concentrations of most electrolytes and less water which makes the cerumen scanty and very dry. Psoriasis can occasionally cause an increase in waxy material in the ear.

Symptoms of wax impaction include deafness, tinnitus, reflex cough, through stimulation of the auricular branch of the vagus nerve, earache or fullness in the ear and vertigo. The wax may obscure the tympanic membrane and confuse the diagnosis. The role of impacted wax contributing to deafness is disputed, but the superimposition of impacted wax and presbyacusis may significantly alter the ability to function socially and many patients feel a subjective improvement in hearing after its removal. Wax often blocks hearing aid moulds causing unnecessary difficulties to those whose hearing is already compromised.

Treatment

Wax may be removed by ceruminolytics, syringing, suction or hooking it out under direct vision. Syringing should be avoided in patients with a perforation of the tympanic membrane, previous ear surgery or in the presence of middle ear disease, when suction under direct vision under the operating microscope is the safest method.

If syringing is undertaken, normal saline at 37°C is used as the irrigating solution. Any marked variation from body temperature will cause vertigo due to labyrinthine stimulation. Before syringing, the pinna should be pulled upwards and backwards in adults and directly backwards in children in order to straighten the meatus. The stream should be directed onto the roof or posterior wall of the meatus so that it passes around the wax plug forcing it outwards by pressure from behind. Syringing directly onto a mass of wax will only tend to impact it more deeply. When the wax is very hard, it cannot be removed by syringing until it has first been softened. Various softening agents and ceruminolytics, including oils and aqueous preparations have been promoted to soften wax prior to syringing and to disintegrate the wax, to avoid syringing. Syringing is a relatively safe procedure which is easy to learn but damage to an ear drum with subsequent loss of hearing has been known to lead to litigation.

Keratosis obturans

A keratotic mass of desquamating squamous epithelium is found in the bony portion of the external auditory meatus. The aetiology is uncertain but it is probably related to faulty migration of squamous epithelial cells. These epithelial cells arise from the surface of the tympanic membrane and the adjacent canal allowing a mass of squamous epithelium and debris to accumulate and intermix with cerumen. The mass appears pearly white and glistening but may be obscured by overlying wax. Pain is the common presenting symptom and is caused by the erosion of the osseous meatus. Conductive hearing loss and otorrhoea may be present. The histological appearance can be confused with cholesteatoma of the middle ear.

The tympanic membrane is usually intact but perforation may occur as a result of pressure necrosis. The bony canal may become eburnated. Associated contamination with Gram-negative organisms should be treated topically. Keratosis obturans is frequently associated with bronchiectasis and sinusitis in younger patients. Irritation of the efferent vagal nerve endings in the bronchi produces a reflex secretion of wax in the meatus. Armitage *et al.* (1990) reported a case of keratosis obturans associated with the yellow nail syndrome which, besides yellow nails, includes lymphoedema and pleural effusions and which may be a manifestation of this syndrome in the external ear.

Treatment

Treatment consists of removing the keratotic mass. This may be very difficult to achieve, especially in the presence of otitis externa. Syringing is best avoided as it rarely succeeds in shifting the mass and may increase the patient's discomfort. If difficulty is experienced in separating the keratin from the meatal wall it is advisable to complete the removal under general anaesthesia. Refractory cases can require canalplasty.

After successful clearance of the meatus, the patient should be kept under observation as the keratosis may re-form. Local applications do not appear to be of any value in preventing recurrence.

Otitis externa

Otitis externa is the generic term applied to all inflammatory conditions of the external meatal skin. It may arise primarily in the meatus or be a manifestation of a generalized skin condition. Predisposing factors may be *genetically* influenced, i.e. by narrow canal, excessive wax or an inherited tendency to eczema; *environmentally* induced by heat, humidity and swimming; *traumatic* and *self-induced* through matchsticks and hairgrips etc. or *infection* (Peterkin, 1974).

The aetiology can be divided into two broad groups but more than one factor may be present at the same time: either *infective* due to bacterial, fungal and viral infections or *reactive* caused by eczema, seborrhoeic dermatitis or neurodermatitis.

Furunculosis

Furunculosis is due to a Gram-positive infection of the hair follicles of the external meatus, usually caused by *Staphylococcus aureus*. The 'boil' is a painful tender well-circumscribed erythematous pustule around a hair in the outer portion of the ear canal. Discomfort is further aggravated by jaw movement. As the condition progresses, the pain becomes more severe and the meatus becomes occluded by swelling which causes deafness. Several furuncles may become confluent to produce a carbuncle. If the infection progresses untreated, a surrounding cellulitis and regional lymphadenitis may develop. Furunculosis is often coexistent with diffuse external otitis when profuse otorrhoea and accumulation of debris in the meatus lead to infection of the hair follicles.

In severe cases the oedema can spread to the postauricular sulcus producing forward displacement of the auricle. Eventually the furuncle discharges and unless there are multiple lesions present, the condition rapidly resolves.

Difficulties in diagnosis arise when there is gross meatal swelling which prevents examination of the tympanic membrane. The condition must be distinguished from acute mastoiditis as swelling and tenderness can spread to the postauricular region. The main points of distinction are shown in Table 6.1.

Treatment

Management of furunculosis requires careful and gentle cleaning of the ear canal. A wick soaked in a steroid/antibiotic cream, or glycerine (traditionally with ichthamol) inserted into the narrowed meatus will relieve pain by splinting the canal and reducing swelling. The dressing should be changed daily until the lesion is dry. An oral anti-staphylococcal antibiotic should be given, especially if there is accompanying cellulitis. The antibiotics of choice are flucloxacillin or cephradine, each given 500 mg 6 hourly, or erythromycin if there is penicillin sensitivity together with the addition of oral analgesics. Most furuncles drain spontaneously, especially if warm saline dressings are applied. However, if drainage has not occurred over a 24–48-hour period, incision of the boil under local anaesthesia may be necessary. In unresponsive cases or with recurrent infection, culture and sensitivity testing is necessary.

The above methods of treatment are used in *recurrent furunculosis*, but the staphylococci must also be eliminated from the external auditory meatus. The organism is often carried in the nasal vestibule and a cream containing neomycin or gentamicin should be applied to both the meatus and the nasal vestibules twice daily. Tests should always be carried out to exclude diabetes mellitus.

Diffuse otitis externa

Diffuse otitis externa frequently occurs in hot and humid climates, and has been named 'tropical ear' or 'Singapore ear'. Heat, humidity and bathing may be

Table 6.1 Distinguishing features between furunculosis and acute mastoiditis

Sign	Furunculosis	Acute mastoiditis
Postauricular tenderness	Diffuse	Maximal over mastoid antrum
Displacement of pinna	Forwards	Typically forwards and downwards
Enlarged lymph nodes	Present	Absent
Pressure on tragus and moving the pinna	Pain	No pain
Mastoid X-rays	Mastoid air cells clear	Mastoid air cells cloudy

aggravating factors in some cases, but the most important factor is local trauma. Scratching the ears, vigorous drying of the meatus with a dirty towel and unskilled syringing causes minor abrasions of the meatal skin and provide access for the causative organisms. The organisms most commonly found in diffuse otitis externa are *Pseudomonas aeruginosa*, *Bacillus proteus* and *Staphylococcus aureus*.

In some cases, otitis externa is secondary to an underlying chronic suppurative otitis media and this possibility should always be considered and excluded by careful examination of the tympanic membrane.

The condition is seen in two stages – acute and chronic.

The acute stage

In the acute stage the discomfort develops into pain in and around the ear aggravated by movements of the jaw. In severe cases, there may be swelling of the surrounding soft tissues and outward displacement of the pinna. On examination, the meatal skin is red, swollen and very tender. Pus is found in the meatus and as the disease progresses the meatal epithelium desquamates forming a mass of cheesy debris in the deep meatus. The tympanic membrane is often dull and injected in appearance.

Treatment

The most important part of treatment is the meticulous cleaning of the infected meatus. Particular attention should be paid to the deep anteroinferior meatal recess where pus and debris readily accumulate. A swab should be taken and cultured. After cleaning, the meatus is packed with 12-mm ribbon gauze impregnated with a broad-spectrum antibiotic such as neomycin or gentamicin and changed daily or a Pope wick can be inserted and moistened with drops containing similar antibiotic preparations.

There is some evidence that aerosol antibiotic sprays produce better coverage of the external meatus than traditional ear drops (McGarry and Swan, 1992).

Topical antibiotics must be used with caution as sensitization of the skin may occur and may encourage the development of fungal infections. Wilkinson and Beck (1993) have demonstrated that delayed type hypersensitivity reactions to topical corticosteroids and other medicaments should be considered in patients with otitis externa which fails to respond to treatment. Referral to a dermatologist at this stage may allow a more accurate delineation of an individual patient's contact hypersensitivities. The patient must keep the ear dry and avoid rubbing or scratching.

Chronic stage

The chief symptoms of the chronic stage are irritation and discharge. Deafness may occur as a result of the accumulation of debris in the meatus. There is no tenderness but there may be thickening of the meatal skin with a reduced lumen. Pus and debris are found in the meatus. There may be small granulations on the surface of the tympanic membrane denoting a loss of epithelium.

Treatment

As in the acute phase, careful cleaning of the meatus with clearance of the deep anterior meatal recess is the essential part of treatment. This is best achieved under the microscope with the use of suction. If there is marked meatal swelling, this can be reduced by packing the meatus daily with 12-mm gauze wicks impregnated with an antibiotic such as neomycin or gentamicin or an antiseptic (clioquinol) combined with a steroid or as drops applied to a Pope otowick. The addition of the steroid helps both to reduce the inflammatory swelling and to control the irritation. When there is no appreciable meatal swelling the antiseptic and hydrocortisone cream may be applied to the meatus using a syringe. Ear drops such as soframycin or gentamicin combined with hydrocortisone, are often effective in clearing up the infection at this stage but may produce a sensitivity reaction in some individuals. This may be difficult to recognize as it may be masked by the presence of the hydrocortisone in the preparation. Failure to respond to treatment may be due to underlying chronic suppurative otitis media, fungal infection or sensitization of the skin to the topical application being used.

Otomycosis

Fungi are to be found as saprophytes in the external auditory meatus superimposed on an underlying bacterial infection. The presence of bacterial infections with or without treatment by topical or systemic antibiotics appears to change the physiochemical environment of the meatus and facilitate fungal growth. Fungal infections occur more frequently in hot and humid climates. Mycosis is common in patients who have undergone open cavity mastoidectomy and those who wear hearing aids with occlusive ear moulds.

The fungi most frequently isolated in otomycosis are *Aspergillus niger*, *Candida albicans*, *dermatophytes* and *Actinomyces*. They are implanted initially on the stratum corneum and proliferate after a dormant phase.

Itching is the most prominent symptom together with a sense of fullness or deafness with the accumulation of moist debris within the canal. The ear becomes more painful as the deeper tissues become inflamed.

Examination of the ear canal reveals a mass of greyish-white debris resembling wet blotting paper filling the meatus. The conidiophores of *Aspergillus niger* infection will be seen as black specks in the debris or as a mass of fine filaments projecting from the meatal wall (see Plate 3/6/IX). These typical appearances are not always recognizable and if a case of otitis externa fails to respond to treatment, the possibility of a fungal infection should be considered. The diagnosis can always be confirmed by microscopical examination of the debris or by culture.

Treatment

Treatment of saprophytic fungal infections necessitates thorough cleansing of all accumulated debris in the meatus or mastoid cavity as fungi thrive in moist conditions and in the presence of epithelial debris. This is best performed by suction or irrigation unless the tympanic membrane is perforated. A specific antifungal agent can then be applied such as nystatin which is particularly effective against *Candida* species, but less active against the aspergillus group of fungi. Clotrimazole has been shown to be highly effective as an antifungicide when applied as a 1% cream to the ear canal. Gentian violet solution has stood the test of time and still has a place in treatment.

Otitis externa haemorrhagica (bullous myringitis)

This condition is characterized by the formation of purple blebs on the tympanic membrane and the skin of the deep meatus. The purple colour is due to the haemorrhagic effusion filling the vesicles.

Pain, often severe, is the first symptom and serosanguineous discharge may occur as a result of bursting of the blebs. The pain is not relieved by the onset of the discharge. In uncomplicated cases the middle ear is not involved and the hearing remains normal.

The aetiology of the condition is uncertain but it is thought to be the result of a viral infection. In some influenza epidemics many cases of otitis externa haemorrhagica are seen and there does appear to be an association between the two conditions.

Treatment

Treatment consists of prescribing analgesics for the pain and keeping the ear clean and dry. Antibiotics have no influence on the course of the disease. The blebs should not be incised as this is of no value in relieving the symptoms and may only introduce secondary infection.

Herpetic otitis externa

Herpes simplex and herpes zoster are pathogenic viruses known to affect the external ear canal. Herpes simplex occurs most commonly on the lips as the so-called 'cold sore'. Occasionally the skin of the auricle and meatus is affected. The primary form occurs mainly in individuals without a previous history of immunity against the virus, most commonly infants and children. Secondary inflammation occurs in individuals who demonstrate immunity to the virus. The eruption at first consists of a crop of small vesicles which dry up after a few days leaving the skin red and scaly. Treatment by acyclovir, either applied topically or orally should be started within a few hours of the onset of the first prodromal symptoms of an attack but delayed treatment will offer only marginal benefit (Collier, 1992).

Herpes zoster or Ramsay Hunt syndrome (1910) is a viral infection affecting the geniculate ganglion of the facial nerve which presents classically with severe otalgia, a vesicular rash on the concha or pinna of the affected ear in association with a lower motor neuron lesion of the homolateral facial nerve. If facial paralysis occurs, the recovery rate is poor. There also may be labyrinthine symptoms, sensorineural hearing loss and vesicular eruptions in the distribution of the vagus and glossopharyngeal nerves, namely the hypopharynx, buccal mucosa and the hard palate. The severity of the symptoms increases with age. Initially the rash consists of small tense blisters with surrounding erythema. The blisters gradually dry up leaving adherent crusts which usually persist for 7–10 days.

Treatment

Oral acyclovir (800 mg five times daily) started up to 72 hours after the onset of the rash shortens the rash duration and acute symptoms and also reduces the incidence of postherpetic neuralgia (Collier, 1992). However, pain often continues as postherpetic neuralgia for months or years after the rash has healed. Once postherpetic neuralgia has become established, conventional analgesics are ineffective and tricyclic antidepressants seem to be the optimal therapy (Wood, 1991).

Seborrhoeic dermatitis

The main feature of this disease is a scaly condition of the scalp usually referred to as dandruff or scurf. This is often associated with scaling in the external auditory meatus, postauricular sulcus and below the lobe of the auricle. The aetiology of the condition is unknown. When the ear is involved, secondary infection may be introduced by scratching, leading to a diffuse otitis externa.

Treatment

The scalp condition always requires attention. Regular washing with a cetrimide or keratolytic shampoo is an effective method of keeping dandruff under control but there is a tendency for debris to accumulate in the meatus which requires regular removal. The patient should be advised to avoid getting water in the ears and refrain from attempting to remove the waxy debris. Protective ear moulds are commercially available which prevent water from entering the meatus while swimming or bathing.

Eczema

An eczematous reaction occurs as the result of sensitization of the skin cells. This may be produced by an infecting organism or by contact with an allergenic material. Of the latter group, antibiotics most commonly evoke this response, neomycin being by far the most troublesome in this respect, although the topical application of any antibiotic may result in a sensitivity reaction. Clinically the eczematous reaction is characterized by the formation of vesicles. When the vesicles burst, serous discharge exudes from the raw surface with the onset of intense irritation.

Treatment

When the eczematous dermatitis is secondary to an infective process, the condition is best treated by cleaning the meatus and applying a cream containing clioquinol and hydrocortisone.

In cases resulting from the topical application of an antibiotic the preparation responsible must be withdrawn. The ear should be kept dry and cream or lotion containing a topical steroid preparation applied regularly until the condition resolves.

Neurodermatitis

In some cases of otitis externa there is an underlying psychosomatic disturbance which not only initiates the condition but also makes it difficult to clear up. The initial symptom is irritation in the ear, although at this stage the skin will have a normal appearance. However, constant scratching may lead to lichenification of the skin or introduce secondary infection causing a diffuse otitis externa.

Treatment

The secondary infection should be treated and an attempt made to alleviate the irritation with local steroid preparations. In severe cases it may be necessary to bandage the ears to prevent scratching. Due attention should be given to the psychological aspect of the problem.

Malignant otitis externa

Malignant otitis externa is an uncommon but progressive debilitating and sometimes fatal infection of the external meatus, surrounding soft tissues and skull base. This term was first applied by Meltzer and Kelemen (1959) and further described by Chandler (1968). Although it usually occurs in elderly, poorly controlled, diabetic patients, other predisposing conditions include arteriosclerosis, immunosuppression by chemotherapy, high dose steroid administration, hypogammaglobulinaemia (Meyerhoff, Gates and

Montalbo, 1977) and patients with acquired immune deficiency syndrome (AIDS) (Daniels *et al.*, 1992). It should be remembered that it can occasionally occur in otherwise normal patients (Shpitzer *et al.*, 1993). As the incidence of AIDS increases more patients with head and neck manifestations are seen by the otolaryngologist. Marcusen and Sooy (1985) found 41% of patients in their study presented with symptoms relating to the head and neck including Kaposi sarcoma of the auricle and otomycosis of the external canal. Herpes zoster oticus has been reported in a patient with HIV infection (Mishell and Applebaum, 1990).

The infecting organism is *Pseudomonas aeruginosa* in patients with low resistance, but Barrow and Levenson (1992) have reported a case of a 70-year-old diabetic man with *Staphylococcus epidermidis* and Cunningham *et al.* (1988) of an 85-year-old non-diabetic man with *Aspergillus fumigatus*. The infection starts as a cellulitis of the external auditory meatus which may develop in a pre-existing chronic otitis externa, but is often insidious in onset with minimal evidence of meatal infection. As the disease progresses granulomas may appear in the floor of the deep meatus and from overlying areas of osteitis. *Pseudomonas* produces exotoxins and enzymes, including an elastase, which digest vessel walls causing a necrotizing vasculitis that aids the organism by destroying local tissues and resisting phagocytosis.

The disease spreads from the external auditory meatus through the naturally occurring fissures in the meatal cartilage to the adjacent soft tissues either via the tympanomastoid suture or via the clefts of Santorini, spreading to the parotid gland, temporomandibular joint and the soft tissue at the skull base.

Spread from the tympanic plate to the region of the mastoid tip and stylomastoid foramen leads to early facial palsy even though the middle ear and mastoid cells are not involved. Further spread of the infection can lead to thrombosis of the lateral sinus and the superior and inferior petrosal sinuses. Secondary osteomyelitis at the petrous apex can spread to the floor of the middle cranial fossa or to the basisphenoid with the development of sphenoidal sinusitis. Further cranial nerve palsies besides the VIIth nerve may develop with the most frequently affected being the IXth, Xth, XIth at the jugular foramen and the XIIth nerve in the hypoglossal canal. Even after the infection appears well controlled, further deep extension of the disease may appear after many weeks or even months. The progressive cranial polyneuropathy is indicative of a very poor prognosis with impending meningitis and lateral sinus and cavernous sinus thromboses. There is usually granulation tissue at the junction of the cartilaginous and bony external auditory meatus revealing necrotic cartilage. The tympanic membrane is usually intact. *Pseudomonas aeruginosa* will be found on culture. Recurrent pain after apparent control is an ominous sign and warrants further investigation and treatment. Conventional

X-rays are often unhelpful as there may be little involvement of bone, and the middle ear and mastoid air cells may remain clear, but CT scanning will demonstrate abnormalities of the external auditory meatus with or without bone destruction (Rubin *et al.*, 1990) (see Figure 2.32). The response to treatment and the progression of the disease can be monitored by using magnetic resonance scanning to help formulate a management policy (El-Silimand Sharnuby, 1992). Gallium citrate scans have shown that anti-pseudomonas treatment should continue up to 3 months.

Treatment

The success of treatment depends upon the control of the diabetes, administration of antibiotics and debridement of necrotic tissues. The treatment of choice is ciprofloxacin, a highly effective fluoroquinolone which achieves high concentrations in bone and soft tissues and has the advantage of acting not only on dividing but also stationary bacteria. An oral dosage of 1.5 g of ciprofloxacin should be given daily over a period of 6–12 weeks (Brody and Pasak, 1991; Levenson *et al.*, 1991). Treatment with a quinolone has the advantage over previous treatments in that it can be given orally and has a low rate of side effects.

In general, surgery should be confined to debridement of infected tissue. Occasionally necrotic bone, diseased cartilage and if necessary the parotid gland will have to be removed but each case has to be treated on its own merits. Radical mastoidectomy should be avoided if the air cell system is not involved.

Benign tumours of the meatus

Lipomas usually occur in the postauricular sulcus and are extremely rare in the external ear. Fibroma, chondroma, myoma, and angioma may occur in the external auditory meatus but require no special description.

Papilloma (see Plate 3/6/X)

Viral papillomas occur in the outer meatus often associated with similar lesions on the fingers. These viral warts can be removed by curetting under local or general anaesthesia or with the laser. They sometimes disappear of their own accord.

Diffuse papillomas of the meatus are occasionally encountered. These have the typical papilliferous appearance but may extend into the deep meatus and obscure the tympanic membrane. They can be removed permanently in most cases but may recur locally.

Adenoma

There are two types of gland in the skin of the external auditory meatus and both may give rise to adenomas.

Sebaceous adenoma: this tumour arises from the sebaceous glands of the meatus. It is seen as a smooth, painless skin-covered swelling in the outer part of the meatus. It may be treated by local excision.

Ceruminoma: the ceruminous glands are modified apocrine sweat glands present only in the skin overlying the cartilaginous meatus. The adenoma is of sweat gland origin and for this reason the term hidradenoma of the meatus is now generally preferred. Such tumours are rare in humans but common in domestic animals. A ceruminoma appears as a smooth intraverted polypoid swelling in the outer part of the ear canal. The presenting symptom is usually a blocked feeling in the ear with no history of discharge.

Treatment

There is a tendency for the tumour to recur· after removal so the lesion must be widely excised. They may develop into malignant adenocarcinomas (see Chapter 22).

Hyperostosis

Growth of cortical bone in the external auditory meatus can occur in two forms: exostoses and single osteoma.

Exostoses (see Plate 3/6/XI)

Multiple exostoses are the most common tumours of the external bony meatus. Exostoses produce smooth sessile hemispherical elevations in the deep part of the meatus adjacent to the tympanic membrane and usually occur in groups of three. They consist of dense ivory bone covered by a thin layer of normal deep meatal skin producing a V-shaped appearance to the lower part of the canal. Van Gilse (1938) was the first to demonstrate a higher incidence of meatal exostoses in cold water bathers. Fowler and Osman (1942), working with guinea pigs, were able to demonstrate the formation of new bone on the inner surface of the tympanic bulla following irrigation of the external canal with cold water. Harrison (1962) carried out similar experiments, also with guinea-pigs, and found histological evidence of new bone formation in the deep meatus. Umeda, Nakajima and Yoshioki (1989) found that 37% of professional surfers demonstrated stenosis by more than 50% of the diameter of the external canal (*surfer's ear*) and that, in general, it commenced after 5 years and was further aggravated by continued surfing, especially in colder waters.

Meatal exostoses do not cause symptoms when small and are therefore usually discovered accidentally during examination of the ears. However, when large, they may completely occlude the meatus and so significantly reduce the lumen until it becomes readily blocked by small amounts of wax or epithelial debris and cause deafness.

Treatment

When exostoses are small they require no treatment but if they are large enough to cause deafness or hinder the treatment of a chronic middle-ear infection, they should be removed surgically.

Exostoses consist of dense ivory bone, and should be removed through a postaural approach under magnification using a high speed drill with both cutting and diamond burrs, care being taken not to damage the tympanic membrane.

Single cancellous osteoma

This is less common than exostosis and occurs as a smooth, rounded pedunculated tumour attached to the outer part of the bony meatus. It is usually unilateral and arises from the region of either the anteriorly placed tympanosquamous or the more posterior tympanomastoid fissure. If the tumour is causing occlusion of the canal or otitis externa, it can be removed by drilling through its narrow attachment to the meatal wall. Very rarely an osteoma of the temporal bone may impinge on the meatus producing a diffuse swelling in the deep meatus arising from one wall. X-rays will demonstrate the true extent of the lesion. This type of osteoma may be associated with similar lesions arising from other bones and complete removal of these tumours may prove difficult or unwise. Simple burring away of the meatal projection to create an adequate canal may be followed by recurrence. In this case as much of the osteoma should be removed as possible.

Malignant tumours of the meatus

(See Chapter 22.)

References

ANDREWS, J. C., ANZAI, Y., MANKOVICH, N. J., FAVILLY, M., UFKIN, R. B. and JABOUR, B. (1992) Three dimensional CT scan reconstruction for the assessment of congenital aural atresia. *Americal Journal of Otology*, **13**, 236–240

ARMITAGE, J. M., LANE, D. G., STRADLING, J. R. and BURTON, M.

(1990) Ear involvement in the yellow nail syndrome. *Chest*, **98**, 1534–1535

BARROW, H. N. and LEVENSON, M. J. (1992) Necrotizing 'malignant' external otitis caused by *Staphylococcus epidermidis*. *Archives of Otolaryngology – Head and Neck Surgery*, **118**, 94–96

BIRZGALIS, A., RAMSDEN, R., FARRINGTON, W. and SMALL, M. (1993) Severe radionecrosis of the temporal bone. *Journal of Laryngology and Otology*, **107**, 183–187

BONDING, P. and TOS, M. (1974) Post inflammatory acquired atresia of the external auditory canal. *Acta Otolaryngologica*, **79**, 115–123

BRODY, T. and PASAK, M. L. (1991) The fluoroquinolones. *American Journal of Otology*, **12**, 477–479

CHANDLER, J. R. (1968) Malignant external otitis. *Laryngoscope*, **78**, 1257–1294

COLIDRON, B. M. (1991) The surgical management of chondrodermatitis chronica helicis. *Journal of Dermatologic Surgery and Oncology*, **17**, 902–904

COLE, D. J., MACKAY, J., WALKER, B. F., WOODEN, W. W., MURRRAY, D. R. and COLEMAN, J. J. (1992) Melanoma of the external ear. *Journal of Surgical Oncology*, **50**, 110–114

COLE, R. R. and JAHRSDOERFER, R. A. (1990) The risk of cholestatoma in congenital aural stenosis. *Laryngoscope*, **100**, 576–578

COLLIER, J. (1992) Acyclovir in general practice. *Drug and Therapeutics Bulletin*, **30**, 101–104

CUMBERWORTH, V. L. and HOGARTH, T. B. (1990) Hazards of ear piercing procedures which traverse cartilage: a report of Pseudomonas perichondritis and review of other complications. *British Journal of Clinical Practice*, **44**, 512–513

CUNNINGHAM, M., YU, M. L., TURNER, J. and CURTIN, H. (1988) Necrotizing otitis externa due to Aspergillus in an immunocompetent patient. *Archives of Otolaryngology – Head and Neck Surgery*, **114**, 554–556

DANIELS, D. G., NELSON, M. R., BARTON, S. E. and GAZZARD, B. G. (1992) Malignant otitis externa in a patient with AIDS. *International Journal of STD and AIDS*, **3**, 214

DUNHAM, M. E. and FRIEDMAN, H. I. (1990) Audiologic management of bilateral external auditory canal atresia with the bone conducting implantable hearing device. *Cleft Palate Journal*, **27**, 369–373

EL–SILIMY, O. and SHARNUBY, M. (1992) Malignant otitis external otitis: management policy. *Journal of Laryngology and Otology*, **106**, 5–6

ENGEL, D. (1966) Pseudocysts of the auricle in Chinese. *Achives of Otolaryngology*, **83**, 197–202

EWING, J. (1926) Radiation osteitis. *Acta Radiologica*, **6**, 399–412

FITCH, N., LINDSAY, J. R. and SROLOVITZ, H. (1976) The temporal bone in the pre-auricular pit, cervical fistula, hearing loss syndrome. *Annals of Otology, Rhinology and Laryngology*, **85**, 268–275

FORD, G. R., IRVING, R. M., JONES, N. S. and BAILEY, C. M. (1992) ENT manifestations of Fraser syndrome. *Journal of Laryngology and Otology*, **106**, 1–4

FOWLER, E. P. JR and OSMAN P. M. (1942) New bone growth due to cold water in ears. *Archives of Otolaryngology*, **36**, 455–466

GRABSKI, W. J., SALASCHE, S. J., MCCOLLOUGH, M. L. and ANGELONI, V. L. (1989) Pseudocyst of the auricle associated with trauma. *Archives of Dermatology*, **125**, 528–530

GREENBAUM, S. S. (1991) The treatment of chondrodermatits nodularis chronica helicis with injectable collagen. *International Journal of Dermatology*, **30**, 291–294

HARRISON, D. F. N. (1962) The relationship of osteomata of the external auditory meatus to swimming. *Annals of the Royal College of Surgeons of England*, 31, 187–201

HANGER, H. C. and MULLEY, G. P. (1992) Cerumen: its fascination and clinical importance: a review. *Journal of the Royal Society of Medicine*, 85, 346–349

HERDMAN, R. C. and WRIGHT, J. L. (1990) Surgical treatment of obliterative otitis externa. *Clinical Otolaryngology*, 15, 11–14

HUDSON, D. A., KRUGE, J. E., STROVER, R. M. and KING, H. S. (1990) Maligant melanoma of the external ear. *British Journal of Plastic Surgery*, 43, 608–611

HUNT, J. R. (1910) The symptom complex of the acute posterior poliomyelitis of the geniculate, auditory, glossopharyngeal and pneumogastric ganglia. *Archives of Internal Medicine*, 5, 631

JAFEK, B. W., NAGER, G. T., STRIKE, J. and GAYLER, R. W. (1975) Congenital aural atresia: an analysis of 311 cases. *Transactions of the American Academy of Ophthalmology and Otolaryngology*, 88, 588–595

JAHRSDOERFER, R. A., YEAKLEY, J. W., AGUILAR, E. A., COLE, R. R. and GRAY, L. C. (1992) Grading system for the selection of patients with congenital aural atresia. *American Journal of Otology*, 13, 6–12

JOB, A. and RAMAN, R. (1992) Medical management of pseudocyst of the auricle. *Journal of Laryngology and Otology*, 106, 159–161

LEE, R. J. and MCILWAIN, J. C. (1985) Subacute bacterial endocarditis following ear acupuncture. *International Journal of Cardiology*, 7, 62–63

LEFFLER, S., CHENEY, P. and TANDBERG, D. (1993) Chemical immobilization and killing of intraaural roaches: an in-vitro comparative study. *Annals of Emergency Medicine*, 22, 1795–1798

LEVENSON, M. J., PARISIER, S. C., DOLITSKY, J. and BINDRA, G. (1991) Ciprofloxacin: drug of choice in the treatment of malignant external otitis. *Laryngoscope*, 101, 821–884

LI–XIANG, Z. and XIU–YUN, W. (1990) A new technique for treating pseudocyst of the auricle. *Journal of Laryngology and Otology*, 104, 31–32

LI–XIANG, Z. and XIU–YUN, W. (1992) Histological examination of the auricular cartilage and pseudocyst of the auricle. *Journal of Laryngology and Otology*, 106, 103–104

LOVEJOY, F. H. and SMITH, D. H. (1970) Life threatening staphylococcal disease following ear piercing. *Pediatrics*, 46, 301–303

LUCKETT, W. H. (1910) A new operation for prominent ears based on the anatomy of the deformity. *Surgery, Gynecology and Obstetrics*, 10, 635–637

MCGARRY, G. W. and SWAN, I. R. C. (1992) Endoscopic photographic comparison of drug delivery by ear drops and by aerosol spray. *Clinical Otolaryngology*, 17, 359–360

MCRAE, D., PREMACHANDRA, D. J. and GATLAND, D. J. (1989) Button batteries in the ear, nose and cervical oesophagus: a destructive foreign body. *Journal of Otolaryngology*, 18, 317–319

MARCUSEN, D. C. and SOOY, C. D. (1985) Otolaryngologic and head and neck manifestations of acquired immunodeficiency syndrome. *Laryngoscope*, 95, 401–405

MARLOWE, F. I. (1972) Acquired atresia of the external auditory canal. *Archives of Otolaryngology*, 96, 380–383

MELNICK, M., BIXLER, D., SILK, K., YUNE, H. and NANCE, W. E. (1975) Autosomal dominant branchio-otorenal dysplasia. *Birth Defects*, 11, 121–128

MELNICK, M. and MYRIANTHOPOULOS, N. C. (1979) External ear malformations: epidemiology, genetics and natural history. *Birth Defects*, 15, 1–137, (a) p. 8. (b) p. 19–29

MELTZER, P. and KELEMEN, G. (1959) Pyocyaneus osteomyelitis of the temporal bone, mandible and zygoma. *Laryngoscope*, 69, 1300–1316

MEYERHOFF, W. L., GATES, G. A. and MONTALBO, P. J. (1977) Pseudomonas mastoiditis. *Laryngoscope*, 87, 483

MISHELL, J. H. and APPLEBAUM, E. L. (1990) Ramsay–Hunt syndrome in a patient with HIV infection. *Otolaryngology – Head and Neck Surgery*, 102, 177–179

MOHS, F. E. (1947) Chemosurgical treatment of cancer of the ear: a microscopically controlled method of excision. *Surgery*, 21, 605

MORAES, D., MCCORMACK, P., TYRRELL, J. AND FEELY, J. (1992) Ear lobe crease and coronary heart disease. *Irish Medical Journal*, 85, 131–132

MUSTARDÉ, J. C. (1963) The correction of prominent ears using simple mattress sutures. *British Journal of Plastic Surgery*, 16, 170–176

NISHIMURA, Y. and KURMORI, T. (1992) The embryologic development of the human external auditory meatus. *Acta Otolaryngologica*, 112, 496–503

PETERKIN, G. A. G. (1974) Otitis externa. *Journal of Laryngology and Otology*, 88, 15–21

POTTER, E. L. and CRAIG, J. M. (1975) *Pathology of the Foetus and Infant*, 3rd edn. New York: Year Book Publishers

PRIDE, H. and SCHWAB, R. (1989) A new technique for removing foreign bodies of the external auditory canal. *Paediatric Emergency Care*, 5, 135–136

RAMSDEN, R. T., BULMAN, C. H. and LORIGAN, B. P. (1975) Osteoradionecrosis of the temporal bone. *Journal of Laryngology and Otology*, 89, 941–956

RHŶS EVANS, P. H. (1985) The anterior scoring technique. *Facial Plastic Surgery*, 2, 3–99

RUBIN, J. CURTIN, H. D., YU, V. L. and KAMERER, D. B. (1990) Malignant external otitis: utility of CT in diagnosis and follow up. *Radiology*, 174, 391–394

SHPITZER, T., STERN, Y., COHEN, O., LEVY, R., SEGAL, K. and FEINMESSER, R. (1993) *Annals of Otology, Rhinology and Laryngology*, 102, 870–872

STUCKER, F. J. and SHAW, G. Y. (1991) Revision meatoplasty: management emphasizing deepithelialized postauricular flaps. *Otolaryngology – Head and Neck Surgery*, 105, 433–439

TAKEMORI, S., ISHII, T and SUZUKI, J. (1976) Thalidomide anomalies of the ear. *Archives of Otolaryngology*, 102, 425–427

TAYLOR, M. B. (1991) Chondrodermatitis nodularis chronica helicis. Successful treatment with the carbon dioxide laser. *Journal of Dermatologic Surgery and Oncology*, 17, 862–864

TEMPLER, J. and RENNER, G. L. (1990) Injuries of the external ear. *Otolaryngologic Clinics of North America*, 23, 1003–1018

TURPIN, I. M. (1990) Microsurgical replantation of the external ear. *Clinics in Plastic Surgery*, 17, 397–404

UMEDA, Y., NAKAJIMA, M. and YOSHIOKI, H. (1989) Surfers ear in Japan. *Laryngoscope*, 99, 639–641

VAN GILSE, P. H. G. (1938) Des observations ulterieures sur la genese des exostoses due conduit externe par l'irritation d'eau froids. *Acta Otolaryngologica*, 26, 343–352

WEERDA, H. (1985) Embryology and structural anatomy of the external ear. *Facial Plastic Surgery*, 2, 85–89

WILKINSON, S. M. and BECK, M. H. (1993) Hypersensitivity to topical corticosteroids in otitis externa. *Journal of Laryngology and Otology*, **107**, 597–599

WILLNER, A., LEDEREICH, P. S. and DE VREIS, E. J. (1992) Auricular injury as a presentation of child abuse. *Archives of Otolaryngology – Head and Neck Surgery*, **118**, 634–667

WOOD, M. J. (1991) Herpes zoster and pain. *Scandinavian Journal of Infectious Diseases – Supplementum*, **80**, 53–61

YOON, M., CHOUGULE, P., DUFRESNE, R. and WANEBO, H. J. (1992) Localized carcinoma of the external ear is an unreconized aggressive disease with a high propensity for local regional recurrence. *American Jounal of Surgery*, **164**, 574–577

7

Ear trauma

J. G. Toner and A. G. Kerr

Trauma to the ear is on the increase. Society is becoming more violent, urban terrorism with guns and explosives is more widespread, and there are increasing numbers of road and other accidents. Though the advent of compulsory seat-belt legislation has reduced the severity of the injuries to some degree, the improved management of those with severe injuries is contributing to the number of patients surviving to require treatment of aural trauma.

The lesions may range from simple blunt trauma to the pinna, without loss of tissue, through uncomplicated rupture of the tympanic membrane to transverse fracture of the petrous temporal bone with complete loss of inner ear and facial nerve function.

External ear

Traumatic lesions of the outer ear are discussed in Chapter 6.

Tympanic membrane and middle ear

Traumatic perforations of the tympanic membrane

Rupture of the tympanic membrane may be caused by changes in air pressure, by fluids or by solid objects.

Pathogenesis

Air pressure changes

Although gradual changes in air pressure may result in rupture of the tympanic membrane, this most often occurs from a rapid change. The tendency to rupture increases with age (Jensen and Bonding, 1993). Sudden forceful blows on the ear, which seal the external auditory meatus, can result in sufficient increase in the air pressure in the ear canal to rupture the tympanic membrane. The most frequent single cause is a blow on the ear, usually with the open hand. This may occur in sporting and not so sporting situations. A blow on the ear from a ball or a fall on water are not uncommon causes of trauma to the tympanic membrane.

Blast injury of the ear commonly, and barotrauma may uncommonly, cause damage to the tympanic membrane. Blast injury is considered later in this chapter and barotrauma in Volume 1, Chapter 7.

Eustachian tube inflation, either by the Valsalva manoeuvre or by the use of a catheter, rarely results in perforation of a normal, healthy tympanic membrane, but can rupture one weakened by previous disease. Similarly, pressure changes in the middle ear as a result of nitrous oxide anaesthesia may result in rupture of a weakened tympanic membrane. There have been reports of hyperbaric oxygen treatment and lightning, with its associated pressure changes, resulting in perforation of the tympanic membrane.

Perforations due to air pressure changes occur most commonly in the anteroinferior quadrant of the tympanic membrane. Atrophic segments are likely to rupture at pressure changes at least 50% lower than a normal tympanic membrane (Jensen and Bonding, 1993). It is unlikely that they ever cause perforation of the pars flaccida.

Fluid

When syringing an ear, it is important to ensure not only that the fluid is at body temperature, but also that the full force of the jet is not directed onto the tympanic membrane. By directing the jet onto the posterior meatal wall the likelihood of rupture of the tympanic membrane is considerably reduced.

Caloric tests in patients with gossamer-thin tympanic membranes must be undertaken with considerable caution.

In skin-diving, it is possible for perforation of the tympanic membrane to occur not only from air pressure differentials but also from fluid pressure in the ear canal.

Solid objects

Although the usual foreign bodies occurring in children rarely rupture the tympanic membrane, attempts at their removal may do so. Match sticks and hair clips, used to remove wax or relieve itching in the ear canal sometimes cause damage to the tympanic membrane. (It is remarkable how many people stand just inside a door to scratch the ear canal!) Sparks of hot metal, especially in welders, can perforate the tympanic membrane by burning through it. The tympanic membrane may fail to heal after extrusion of a middle ear ventilation tube.

Management

Traumatic perforations often occur in healthy members of the community; generally the prognosis is excellent (Kristensen, 1992). The two main factors leading to failure of the perforation to heal are loss of tissue and secondary infection. Welding injuries usually result in both loss of tissue and secondary infection; water sports injuries frequently result in the latter. Consequently, the prognosis for spontaneous healing is reduced in both.

Small perforations are more likely to close spontaneously than large ones. Nonetheless, in the majority of traumatic perforations, the membrane usually heals and the function of the ear returns to normal.

Generally speaking, the most effective management is to do nothing. Because of the risk of introducing infection, the ear should not be cleaned out unless contaminating material is found in the meatus or there is evidence of active infection. Antibiotic ear drops, in the absence of infection, are of no value and may well introduce organisms. Systemic antibiotics should also not be prescribed in the absence of overt infection unless there is good reason to believe that the ear has been contaminated. The ear must be kept dry.

There are many advocates of an active approach to the tympanic membrane following trauma. They recommend examination under a microscope with eversion of the edges of the perforation. This approach is reasonable so long as it is carried out by a competent person under aseptic conditions and, in fact, could be regarded as the ideal. Inverted edges are certainly undesirable and if infection is not introduced, it is unlikely that any harm will result from this procedure. However, immediate surgical repair with grafting is not indicated because of the excellent prognosis for spontaneous recovery. Even subtotal

perforations often heal with an excellent end result.

If the perforation fails to close spontaneously in 3–6 months, surgical closure is indicated. Special reference should be made to welding injuries. Not only is the perforation unlikely to close spontaneously but the results of surgical closure are disappointing. In addition to the loss of tissue and secondary infection, it is likely that there is also some loss of vascularity of the tissues with dense avascular scarring secondary to the burn.

Complications

The most common complication of a traumatic perforation is secondary infection of the middle ear. The development of squamous epithelial cysts in the middle ear has been seen following perforations caused by blast and is due to implantation or inversion of such tissue. Depending on the force of the injury causing the perforation, there may be ossicular dislocation with conductive deafness, inner ear damage with sensorineural deafness and tinnitus or even facial nerve injury.

Squamous epithelial invasion of the middle ear is a rare but recognized complication of middle ear ventilation tubes, especially when there is a persisting perforation after extrusion.

Blast injury

Explosive material changes suddenly from solid to gaseous form with a massive increase in volume and pressure, resulting in a blast wave spreading outwards from the seat of the explosion (Figure 7.1). There is a short-lived positive pressure phase, usually of the order of a few milliseconds and a longer and less marked negative phase, always less than atmospheric pressure and of the order of tens of milliseconds. The amount of energy in each phase of the wave is approximately equal. The front of the blast wave is irregular and damage may be caused in a capricious fashion.

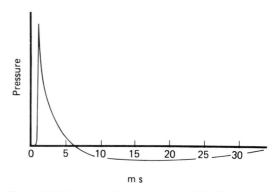

Figure 7.1 Diagrammatic representation of the blast wave

The external factors influencing such damage are:

1 The rise time, i.e. the speed with which the pressure builds up
2 The intensity or height of the peak pressure
3 The duration of the positive pressure wave
4 The site of the explosion and the presence of objects which may reflect or deflect the blast wave.

Patient-related factors include the position of the head, the shape of the external meatus and the state of the tympanic membrane. Some people close to the bomb escape ear damage while others, further away, may be severely deafened. Exposure to blast can result in damage to both middle and inner ears. There may be hyperaemia or even subepithelial bleeding in the tympanic membrane. Perforation due to the blast occurs in the pars tensa and the ear facing the bomb tends to be more seriously damaged. However, reflection of the blast wave from a wall, with augmentation of the pressure, may reverse this situation.

Perforations are probably caused by the positive phase of the blast wave. This conclusion is reached by the demonstration of squamous epithelium in the middle ear in post-mortem specimens and by the occasional finding of epithelial pearls in the middle ear. The latter are also sometimes seen in tympanic membranes which have healed spontaneously. Although everted edges are often seen following blast injury, these are probably caused secondarily by the suction effect of the negative phase.

Most blast injuries of the tympanic membrane heal spontaneously with conservative treatment. Kerr and Byrne (1975) reported spontaneous healing of 83% of 66 perforated tympanic membranes from one explosion.

Radiation injury

The ear is at risk in radiotherapy of any lesion involving the ear itself or in the nasopharynx. The development of middle ear effusion is common in these patients. Osteoradionecrosis has been reported. The management of both these conditions is influenced by the success or otherwise of the radiotherapy in controlling the original malignancy.

There is some circumstantial evidence that sensorineural loss may develop. Although animal experiments have confirmed damage to the inner ear from radiation, the authors are not aware of any controlled prospective study confirming such damage during the treatment of malignant disease and, without this, any aetiological connection between radiotherapy and sensorineural deafness must remain speculative.

Surgical trauma

The chorda tympani nerve

In theory, disorders of taste and salivary secretion should follow every instance of surgical trauma to this structure. In practice, although the nerve is frequently stretched, manipulated, dehydrated and even cut, dysgeusia is an uncommon spontaneous complaint after stapedectomy and hardly ever occurs following tympanoplasty.

However, an abnormal taste, metallic in character, is often described if specifically enquired after both in cases where the chorda has been divided and in cases of bruising. Consequently the surgeon should always handle the chorda tympani with care. There is no unanimity of view on when patients should be warned about possible damage to the chorda. It is not the authors' practice to do so routinely. However, if taste is of particular importance to the patient then preoperative counselling should be considered.

The jugular bulb

This structure is occasionally dehiscent in the posteroinferior quadrant of the mesotympanum. In these cases, it is at risk when the fibrous annulus is being elevated from the sulcus tympanicus in creating a tympanomeatal flap during stapedectomy or transcanal tympanoplasty. Brisk venous bleeding at this stage can usually be controlled by promptly replacing the tympanic membrane and its annulus and applying a small pack. If the bleeding area is then avoided, it is usually possible to complete the procedure with only limited inconvenience (see Figure 2.19).

The facial nerve

In all middle ear surgery, especially for chronic suppurative disease, the safety of the facial nerve will depend upon knowledge of several important landmarks.

In a mesotympanum which is completely filled with granulations or cholesteatoma, it is best to find the landmark which is more resistant to disease than all others – the eustachian tube. From there, it is safe to dissect posteriorly over the promontory as far as the grooves for the tympanic plexus. These grooves can then be followed superiorly to the base of the cochleariform process which marks the junction of the labyrinthine and tympanic segments of the nerve. When the process has been destroyed, a useful alternative guide is the belly of the tensor tympani muscle, which is usually exposed in such cases.

Dissection can then proceed posteriorly following the osseous canal of the tympanic segment of the nerve. In transcanal tympanoplasty, if any doubts develop about the anatomy of the VIIth nerve, it is always wise to increase exposure of the area by converting the procedure into a combined approach tympanoplasty. This permits dissection inferiorly over the medial epitympanic wall and the anterior half of the lateral semicircular canal, exposing the tympanic segment of the nerve from its superior aspect where its bony covering is least likely to be deficient. Once the characteristic pink, rounded bone overlying the nerve is compared with the ivory-white labyrinthine bone, the position of the nerve will be apparent, and dissection can proceed over it in all directions.

It should be remembered that there are several possible abnormalities of the facial nerve in this region which may give rise to confusion and possibly disaster if they are unknown. The most common of these is the facial nerve which is overlying the footplate of the stapes. For this reason, it is important to identify the nerve positively in its normal horizontal canal before removing soft tissue from the surface of the footplate.

In the mastoid segment, the following landmarks are of service: the lateral semicircular canal, the fossa incudis, and the digastric ridge. The posterior semicircular canal lies on the medial aspect of the mastoid segment of the nerve. In performing a mastoidectomy or combined approach tympanoplasty, the first landmark is the mastoid antrum. Korner's septum may give rise to confusion and lead the surgeon in an inferior and anterior route into the mastoid segment of the facial nerve. This can be avoided by:

1 Awareness of the risk
2 Noting the level of the tympanic membrane as compared to the medial wall of the 'false antrum'.

In combined approach tympanoplasty, posterior tympanotomy is performed by cutting a groove downwards from the tip of the short process of incus towards the mastoid tip. In situations where the ossicular chain is intact, early visualization of the incus is particularly important and may be obtained by using the refractive property of an air–water interface (Toner and Kerr, 1987). The groove should be parallel to the expected course of the facial nerve, and the bone should be thinned gradually so that the nerve can be seen before it is uncovered. Bleeding from the nerve sheath is often an excellent warning sign. A cutting burr is probably safe in experienced hands when it is sharp but it would be an unwise recommendation for all, because it can be a disaster if the burr is blunt or with the inexperienced for whom diamond burrs would be safer. Once the facial sinus has been entered, further enlargement of the posterior tympanotomy is carried out by removing bone inferiorly and laterally. For this, the position of the chordal eminence and the chordal ridge should be known and understood. Exposure of the hypotympanum requires removal of the styloid eminence.

Abnormalities of the facial nerve rarely occur in this area but they should be known. The most common of these is the nerve that passes posteriorly, but bifid facial nerves below the genu have been reported. The digastric ridge and the position of the chorda tympani nerve can be used as guides to the nerve when required.

Treatment

Surgical trauma to the facial nerve in temporal bone surgery may result in loss of continuity and loss of substance. In these situations, direct anastomosis does not necessarily produce the best result and it is now agreed that grafting with a piece of the great auricular nerve is the preferred method in most instances. Grafting should be delayed for 3 weeks after the injury by which time axoplasmal regeneration is optimal. The results are better when tension can be avoided. Excessive proliferation of connective tissue in an anastomotic area can be reduced by the removal of several millimetres of epineurium from the stumps. The ends of the stumps should be approximated after they have been cut in order to ensure good contact between the nerve ends. Foreign body reaction with connective tissue proliferation is reduced by the avoidance of suturing material. The natural self-adherence of the nerve tissue is often sufficient to retain the position of the nerve graft in the mastoid and tympanic segments. If there is any doubt about the stability of the graft, however, one or two 8/0 monofilament nylon sutures should be inserted.

In conclusion, avoidance of facial nerve trauma in advanced chronic middle ear disease will be enormously enhanced by the recognition of important landmarks such as the processus cochleariformis, the lateral semicircular canal and the oval window. The great importance of surgical skill, anatomical knowledge and awareness of variations in normal anatomy, were summed up by Fowler (1961) when he said: 'Although traumatic facial palsy is more likely to occur when a surgeon is inexperienced, it can and does occur with the most skilful and experienced otologic surgeon, especially when the course of the nerve is anomalous'.

There is a natural tendency to want to terminate the operation once one is aware of having damaged the facial nerve. This should be resisted. The damage has been done and the patient's interests are not furthered by dealing inadequately with the original disease. The patient has already paid a high price. It is all the more important that the original surgical objectives be attained.

Temporal bone trauma
Fractures

The clinical features of fractures of the temporal bone can only be understood by considering their anatomy and pathology. Fractures involving the temporal bone can be classified into longitudinal, transverse, and mixed, depending on the relationship of the fracture line to the long axis of the petrous temporal bone. In many, the lesion is confined to the squamous temporal bone, in which case it could be regarded as an incomplete or partial longitudinal fracture. Often the diagnosis is made purely on clinical grounds as the fractures do not always show on routine skull radiographs, and may not even be visualized on high resolution CT scanning. Rarely, the diagnosis is delayed until the appearance of discoloration of the skin over the mastoid (Battle's sign).

Pathology

Longitudinal fractures

Most (80%) temporal bone fractures are longitudinal and usually result from blows to the temporal or parietal areas (Proctor, Gurdjian and Webster, 1956). The fracture begins in the squamous temporal bone and extends along the roof of the bony external auditory meatus, tearing the meatal skin and the tympanic membrane and, crossing the roof of the middle ear, reaches the petrous temporal bone. It then runs anterior to the labyrinthine capsule, through the carotid canal, to end near the foramen spinosum or foramen lacerum (Figure 7.2).

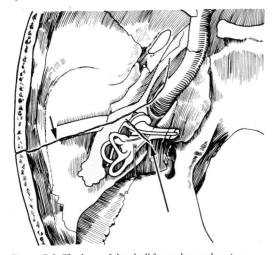

Figure 7.2 The base of the skull from above, showing mainly the middle fossa. The line of the longitudinal fracture is indicated by the small arrow, and runs from the squamous temporal bone along the roof of the external auditory meatus and middle ear, to the region of the carotid artery. The transverse fracture line is indicated by the longer arrow and crosses through the inner ear and facial nerve. (Reproduced from Kerr, 1981 in *Trauma Care* with permission of Academic Press)

Damage to the skin of the external auditory meatus and the tympanic membrane result in bleeding from the ear. In the absence of any other obvious cause, bleeding from the ear following a head injury can be presumed to indicate a fracture of the base of the skull, usually longitudinal despite negative X-ray findings. Displacement of the bone is very rare but a gap may be present at the fracture line (see Figures 2.27 and 2.28).

Middle ear structures are always involved in longitudinal fractures but, in most cases, this is not serious and healing occurs spontaneously without residual conductive deafness. However, should there be persistent conductive deafness, the possibility of ossicular dislocation must be considered (Ballantyne, 1979).

Because a longitudinal fracture usually runs anterior to the dense bone of the labyrinthine capsule, only rarely is the inner ear directly involved, but there may be concomitant inner ear concussion with high tone sensorineural hearing loss. Although the underlying damage in the sensorineural hearing loss of longitudinal fractures is probably more often to be found in the cochlea itself, experimental and clinical evidence has been presented to suggest that some of the deafness is central in origin, secondary to neural damage (Makishima, Sobel and Snow, 1976).

Facial nerve injuries are uncommon in longitudinal fractures and when they occur, are usually delayed in onset.

Transverse fractures

Transverse fractures usually result from frontal or occipital blows and account for approximately 20% of temporal bone fractures (Proctor, Gurdjian and Webster, 1956). These patients usually suffer more severe neurological injury than those with longitudinal fractures.

The fracture line extends transversely across the petrous pyramid, passing through the vestibule of the inner ear (Figure 7.3; see also Figure 5.17). Although the fracture can be demonstrated radiologically in about 50% of cases, the diagnosis is essentially clinical (see Figure 2.29). In a pure transverse fracture there is a haemotympanum but, as the tympanic membrane is not damaged, there is no bleeding from the ear. The severe general injuries of the patient may dominate the clinical picture but, if sought, there is evidence of severe or complete sensorineural deafness on the affected side, usually accompanied by tinnitus. The deafness is usually permanent.

Very severe rotatory vertigo with nausea and vomiting, due to severe damage to the vestibular apparatus on the affected side, occurs initially. Nystagmus is usually present with the fast component to the opposite side. Unfortunately, the significance of the severe dizziness, vomiting and nystagmus, is often missed by those responsible for the management of the head injury. It may not become apparent that the patient has suffered vestibular damage until he is allowed out of bed a week or two after the injury. The patient is then surprised to find that he is extremely unsteady and unable to walk without support. Central compensation develops in the subsequent weeks and months.

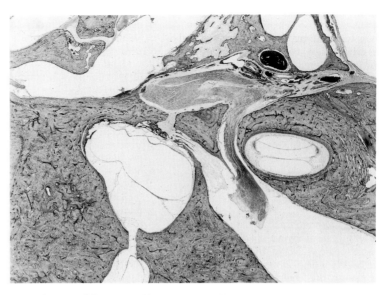

Figure 7.3 Long-standing transverse fracture of the temporal bone (courtesy of H. F. Schuknecht, MEEI Collection)

When the fracture line involves the vestibular aqueduct, delayed secondary endolymphatic hydrops may develop (Rizvi and Gibbin, 1979).

Facial nerve injuries occur in about 50% of these patients and the onset is usually immediate.

Mixed fractures

In severe head injuries there may be a combination of longitudinal and transverse fractures.

Management

The importance of avoiding the introduction of infection into the middle ear cannot be overemphasized and, unless there are signs of active infection, it is better to leave untouched any blood clot in the external auditory meatus. The management of the head injury usually takes precedence and indeed it may be some days before the otolaryngologist is asked to see the patient.

Cerebrospinal fluid leak

The attitude of most neurosurgeons has been changing in recent years and in most units the policy is not to prescribe prophylactic antibiotics.

Most cerebrospinal fluid leaks close spontaneously within 7–10 days. If this does not occur, more active treatment will be necessary. The introduction of a spinal drain at this time may well be all that is required to allow the leak to close but many neurosurgeons are unhappy about this approach. They feel

that, although closure may occur at the time, some leaks will recur later or, even without a recurrence of the leak, there may be an ascending intracranial infection from a subsequent otitis media. If the leak is profuse or if it fails to close promptly, with or without spinal drainage, exploration and surgical closure are indicated. These leaks usually arise from the middle cranial fossa and the help of a neurosurgeon is desirable. The middle cranial fossa is explored, the dura elevated and, after exposure of the tear, the defect is covered with a graft of fascia lata or temporalis fascia.

Some otologists, perhaps chauvinistically, recommend a mastoid approach to this problem. Undoubtedly this is possible and the operation may be shorter and less major. However, access to the site may be impaired and the positioning of the graft is less secure.

In most instances it is advisable to warn these patients of the remote possibility of meningitis in the presence of a middle ear infection, and stress the importance of prompt treatment of any future ear infections.

Meatal damage

Tears in the meatal skin may heal with the formation of fibrous bands in the depths of the meatus, resulting in pockets which collect epithelial debris. If these cannot be cleaned adequately and effectively via the meatus, or if repeated cleaning will be necessary over many years, surgical removal of these bands, perhaps with grafting of the tympanic membrane, may be required.

A wide fracture line predisposes to invasion of the middle ear cleft by squamous epithelium and cholesteatoma development has been reported. However, the vast majority of cholesteatomas diagnosed for the first time after a head injury have not been caused by the trauma. Medico-legal problems can arise but in the absence of a wide fracture line, and especially with a sclerotic mastoid, the cholesteatoma can reasonably be presumed to have been present before the injury. The degree of pneumatization of the temporal bone is usually a guide to the pre-existence of the cholesteatoma. When a cholesteatoma occurs, secondary to a fracture, in a well-pneumatized temporal bone, it can rapidly become very extensive and subsequent surgical control may be difficult.

Deafness

The conductive deafness which follows a longitudinal fracture is, in most instances, due to a tear in the tympanic membrane and blood in the middle ear and it usually recovers spontaneously. Failure to regain normal middle ear transmission is usually due to ossicular dislocation or fracture, or the formation of adhesions. Ossicular damage can also, of course, result from a head injury in the absence of a skull fracture.

The most commonly affected ossicle is the incus, as the malleus and stapes are relatively more stable; the most frequently found defect is a dislocation of the incudostapedial joint (Hough, 1970) (see Figure 2.30). All other lesions are uncommon. These include fracture of the stapedial crura, dislocation of the stapes footplate (see Figure 5.18), total dislocation of the incus, dislocation of the malleus, fracture of the malleus handle, fixation of the malleus head in the epitympanum by fibrous tissue or bone and total destruction of the ossicular chain (Ballantyne, 1979). Delayed necrosis of the long process of the incus has been described.

In these cases there is usually a conductive deafness with an air-bone gap in the region of 40 dB. Exploration of the middle ear is indicated. Ossiculoplasty is carried out applying the general principles of tympanoplasty, usually with better results than in chronic suppurative otitis media.

The sensorineural deafness caused by head injuries is, unfortunately, untreatable. Although there may be some spontaneous recovery of the high tone sensorineural loss that often accompanies longitudinal fracture, there is little likelihood of recovery of any useful hearing following transverse fractures.

Labyrinthine damage can occur without any clinical or radiological evidence of temporal bone fracture. In these cases it is presumed that labyrinthine concussion is responsible for any associated auditory or vestibular symptoms, although there is the possibility of underlying damage in the brain. The deafness usually affects the high frequencies.

Generally speaking, an injury insufficiently severe to cause loss of consciousness does not damage the hearing. However, this is not always the case and

difficult medico-legal problems can arise. These are usually settled on the basis of circumstantial evidence such as when the patient first noticed the deafness and the problems that he describes. For example, the damage due to trauma is usually immediate; a severe hearing loss, first noticed 6 months after the injury, cannot reasonably be attributed to that injury.

Vertigo

Vertigo is common following head injuries and, as with deafness, can occur without a skull fracture. The most common form is that associated with the post-concussional syndrome. These patients have vague unsteadiness, especially when getting up from sitting, and usually associated with frequent severe headaches. The unsteadiness generally settles in a matter of 6–12 months and when it is prolonged beyond this time, the question of a post-concussional neurosis must be considered.

Following transverse fracture of the temporal bone, there is severe incapacitating vertigo making it impossible for the patient to walk unaided for a length of time which varies from 1 to 4 weeks, depending on factors such as age, motivation and other injuries. In the immediate period after a head injury the symptoms can be relieved by labyrinthine sedative drugs. These should not be prescribed for longer than a week as the evidence suggests that they may delay the natural processes of central compensation. There is a slow but gradual improvement; young patients recover to fairly normal balance in a matter of weeks and elderly patients in months. However, the convalescence is often complicated by other injuries and, especially in the elderly, associated brain damage may prevent full compensation.

Benign positional vertigo may follow as a complication of head injuries, with or without fracture of the temporal bone. Schuknecht (1969) has postulated that this results from damage to the utricle with destruction of the otolithic membrane, the otoconia of which become adherent to the cupula of the posterior semicircular canal (see Figure 5.5). This is then stimulated by movement of the head, especially when the affected ear is placed undermost. The dizziness is short-lived, associated with transient and fatiguable rotatory nystagmus, and always precipitated by head movement; between these induced episodes the patient is perfectly steady. This is usually a self-limiting condition, although it often takes up to 2 years before the vertigo settles. Some recent studies have suggested that various habituation excercises may increase the speed of recovery.

When the vestibular aqueduct is involved, delayed secondary endolymphatic hydrops may develop. In the unlikely event that there is any remaining vestibular function this can result, years later, in episodic rotatory vertigo, similar to that seen in Menière's disease (Rizvi and Gibbin, 1979).

A perilymph fistula may also be a cause of post-traumatic vertigo and is discussed later.

Facial paralysis

Facial paralysis following fracture of the temporal bone is classified broadly into two groups – immediate and delayed. Immediate paralysis usually indicates tearing of the facial nerve, impaling of the nerve by bone, or entrapment in a fracture line. Early surgical exploration is indicated if there is to be any reasonable prospect of good functional recovery.

Delayed onset of facial paralysis confirms that, anatomically, the facial nerve is intact, and that there has not been any direct gross trauma. The facial paralysis may be due to oedema within the bony facial canal. The management of delayed traumatic paralysis is similar to that of idiopathic facial paralysis.

Penetrating injuries of the temporal bone

Injuries from bullets, missiles, and explosions may result in lesions involving any part of the body. When the temporal bone is involved, almost any lesion can occur. In most cases, the other injuries predominate and it may be some time after the injury before the otolaryngologist is asked to see the patient.

The lesions of the temporal bone are difficult to classify because of their variability; the management of each patient depends on the specific circumstances. Often the other injuries necessitate compromise in the otological management.

Patients have been reported where gunshot has remained in the temporal bone for many years without any complication. In one patient, the tympanic membrane was largely destroyed, gunshot remained in the middle ear cleft and brain herniated through a damaged tegmen tympani into the attic (Kerr, 1967). The patient lived for 40 years after the injury and died from other causes. Despite such cases, if there is gunshot in the middle ear cleft, with the possibility of infection, surgical exploration and removal are indicated. If, on the other hand, the gunshot has been adequately buried for some time, without any infection or likelihood of infection, and is not causing symptoms, no action is required.

Whiplash

The term 'whiplash injury' used in an unpublished paper in 1928, was first recorded in 1945 and has been a source of controversy ever since. Many object to the name but all agree that it implies an acceleration–extension injury of the neck; some also include deceleration injuries and forward or lateral flexion movements in this syndrome. The diverse symptomatology and prolonged litigation that follows these injuries has led to considerable scepticism about this condition. Nonetheless, it has been shown that many patients continue to have symptoms, sometimes disabling, related to whiplash injuries, not only when other simultaneous severe injuries have become symptom-free, but even years after litigation has ended and compensation has been paid (Gotten, 1956). While symptoms can occur following forward and lateral flexion injuries, the vast majority arise from the acceleration–extension injuries which occur in rear-end collisions. In many instances the initial injury seems trivial, with severe pain in the neck developing only some hours later.

Clinical features

It is not uncommon for the passengers in a car involved in a rear-end collision to be entirely symptom-free immediately after the injury. However, during the succeeding minutes or hours, an ache begins to develop in the neck which increases within a short time to severe pain. Although the most common complaint is pain in the neck, the otolaryngologist becomes involved when the symptoms include dizziness, tinnitus, deafness and dysphagia.

Typically, the onset of dizziness does not occur until some days after the injury. The symptoms tend to be diverse but the most prominent is a generalized sensation of unsteadiness which increases, and may take the form of rotatory vertigo, in association with certain head and neck movements. Routine clinical examination is frequently unremarkable, although positional nystagmus may be demonstrated. However, with the aid of electronystagmography, nystagmus may be demonstrated even when it is not present on clinical examination. Published reports on the findings in the caloric test frequently refer to abnormalities but, unfortunately, many of these do not eliminate those patients with head injuries and, furthermore, do not include controls. However, it is the authors' view that the weight of evidence is that abnormal electronystagmography and caloric tests are often seen following uncomplicated whiplash injury.

There are four theories to explain these features. First, the problem may be neuromuscular with abnormal proprioceptive impulses causing the dizziness. Second, it may be neurovascular with abnormality of the cervical sympathetic nervous system. Third, there may be a mechanical vascular problem with kinking of the vertebral artery. Fourth, brain damage may occur as a result of the whiplash injury. The typical history is of injury followed by a short symptom-free period before the development of pain in the neck. During the next week or so dizziness develops and may persist for years. Although this settles in the vast majority, in Gotten's (1956) series it persisted in 12% for up to 2 years after litigation had ended.

Tinnitus is a frequent complaint in the early stages. It is unlikely that there is any direct damage to the ear. The tinnitus may be due to a concussive effect on the brain; alternatively, and in the authors' opinion more probably, the stress of the injury may result in unmasking or triggering of potential tinnitus due to pre-existing sensorineural deafness. Although deafness has been reported in some publications on this subject there is little substantiating evidence. It seems likely that deafness does not occur in the absence of an associated head injury and that whiplash injuries, of themselves, do not result in hearing loss.

Treatment

In the early days of the recognition of the clinical entity of acceleration–extension injuries of the neck, they were most commonly the result of catapult assisted take-offs from aircraft carriers. The injury was prevented by extending the back of the seat so that the pilot's head was supported. Most modern car seats are now similarly designed and the widespread use of head restraints should reduce the incidence of this syndrome.

Whiplash injuries are best treated during the acute phase. If the nature of the injury and the patient's symptoms suggest this condition, immediate and adequate splinting of the neck is required, accompanied by bed-rest to relieve the neck of the weight of the head. MacNab (1971) has pointed out that the persistent complaints following acceleration–extension injuries do not occur in side collisions where lateral flexion is the predominant lesion. Similarly, wrists and ankles, injured in the same accident become symptom-free long before neck symptoms settle down. He has suggested that the persistence of symptoms in these patients is not because these people are by nature litigious but that the initial injury is inadequately treated. He emphasized that if the neck needs to be splinted, it needs to be done adequately and to have the weight of the head removed from it by bed-rest. Unless the patient is relatively symptom-free within 24 hours he recommended bed-rest for 1 week. The time for a collar is now and not 6 months later. Heat and massage may make the patient feel more comfortable but probably do nothing to speed resolution of the underlying lesion.

Treatment in the chronic phase is difficult. If the patient appears to be developing disabling symptoms due to functional overlay, do not over-treat or over-investigate. There is no evidence that prolonged immobilization is of benefit at this stage, or that heat and massage do more than imprint the symptoms on the patient's mind. Neck traction and muscle strengthening exercises may be of benefit but must not be instituted until it has been established by flexion and extension radiographs that there is no joint instability.

A frank and open discussion with the patient about the possibilities of disordered function is the best approach, once the chronic stage has been reached. The response from tranquillizers and labyrinthine sedative drugs is variable and unpredictable. While many patients improve with time, especially after litigation has been settled, this is not always the case; do not be misled into thinking that all these patients are malingerers.

Perilymph fistula

In a perilymph fistula, not to be confused with a labyrinthine fistula, perilymph may leak from the inner into the middle ear. The leakage may occur either from rupture of the stapediovestibular joint, fracture of the stapes footplate or tearing of the round window membrane. Clinical reports indicate that these are more often from the oval than the round window. Typically, there is a history of a head injury, stapes or other middle ear surgery or some other event associated with raised intracranial pressure, such as coughing, straining or exertion, or sudden changes in middle ear pressure. A certain degree of controversy has arisen over the question of spontaneous perilymph fistula. Most otologists are sceptical about the condition and are agreed that if it does occur it is extremely rare (Shea, 1992).

The clinical features are variable but there are certain characteristics. The most common symptom is unsteadiness, usually with a marked positional element and often with a disproportionate degree of ataxia. The dizziness due to direct trauma to the vestibular apparatus in a head injury usually improves dramatically over a period of weeks. On the other hand, the dizziness associated with a perilymph fistula tends to persist until the fistula is closed either by spontaneous healing or by surgery. The main differential diagnostic problem arises with benign positional vertigo.

Sensorineural deafness and tinnitus often occur in association with a fistula but are not constant features. The deafness may fluctuate.

A high index of suspicion is necessary for the diagnosis of this condition and one must look in the history for a predisposing cause.

Examination of the ear itself is usually unremarkable. The amount of perilymph leaking is usually small and one does not expect to see a fluid level in the middle ear. The fistula test is usually, but not always, negative. (This is not surprising since this test is for a third opening into the inner ear.) However, some authors have reported a positive fistula test in this condition.

Examination of the vestibular system may show a positive Romberg test.

It is in positional testing that the main features are to be seen. Singleton *et al.* (1978) have identified the following characteristics which differentiate the positional nystagmus from that in benign positional vertigo:

1 There is either a short or no latent period
2 The nystagmus is not as violent as in benign positional vertigo
3 The duration tends to be longer with the nystagmus fatiguing slowly or not at all
4 The nystagmus rarely reverses direction when the patient is brought to a sitting position
5 The nystagmus does not necessarily beat towards the involved ear
6 The nystagmus is only occasionally rotatory.

Audiometry confirms a sensorineural hearing loss. Repeated testing, from day to day, may show minor degrees of fluctuation. Fraser and Flood (1982) have reported small improvements in the hearing after 30 minutes in the horizontal position, with the affected ear uppermost. The speech reception threshold and the speech discrimination scores may be depressed more than one would expect from the degree of sensorineural hearing loss.

Diagnosis

The diagnosis of this condition can only be made with certainty by surgical exploration of the ear, however Daspit, Churchill and Linthicum (1980) suggested impedance and ENG recording to assist in the diagnosis. A perilymph fistula may be undiagnosed because it was not considered in the differential diagnosis, because the ear was not explored or because the fistula healed spontaneously before exploration took place. On the other hand, false positive diagnoses may occur because of a failure to understand the anatomy of the round window niche at surgical exploration, because a serious middle ear exudate has been mistaken for perilymph, or because the surgeon has fulfilled his own predictions either by probing or drilling in the region of the round or oval window niches. Unfortunately, it is unlikely that there will ever be a reliable diagnosis of this condition until some foolproof method has been devised for confirming the presence of perilymph in the middle ear. Injection of fluorescein or radioactive substances into the CSF before surgical exploration has been recommended with positive detection in the middle ear at surgery confirming the diagnosis.

Medical management

If the diagnosis is made soon after the injury, bedrest may be all that is required. The patient should be kept in bed for 5 days with the head of the bed elevated 30–40°. Sedation and faecal softeners should be prescribed. After 5 days, if the symptoms have settled, it is recommended that the patient continues to limit his activity for a further 10 days, still sleeping with elevation of the head of the bed and avoiding any exertion.

Surgical management

Surgical intervention is recommended if medical treatment fails or if the symptoms have persisted for over 1 month. After elevation of a tympanomeatal flap it is important to inspect the middle ear carefully before disturbing any of the middle ear structures. Trauma to the middle ear mucosa can, of itself, produce a serous ooze which may be mistaken for a perilymph fistula. If the procedure is performed under local anaesthesia and a fistula is not readily apparent, the Valsalva manoeuvre may help to identify a leak.

It is important to ensure that one does not create a fistula at this stage, thus establishing a self-fulfilling prophecy. Care must be taken in probing the stapes. The round window membrane can never be seen in its entirety without removal of the bone of the round window niche and, in many cases, can barely be seen at all without removing some bone. Once again, at this stage, there is a high risk of creating the fistula for which one is looking.

It is important to remember the anatomy of the round window membrane. It faces inferiorly and care must be taken that one does not confuse mucosal folds in the round window niche for the round window membrane (Figure 7.4; see also Figure 5.19). This is the explanation for some of the published reports which make unreasonable statements such as 'the round window membrane was in tatters'.

Having identified a fistula, the area around it should be denuded of mucosa. In round window membrane fistulae it may be desirable to drill away the bony overhang. A graft, either of fascia or perichondrium, should be applied to the denuded area and packed in place with gelfoam. There is considerable doubt about the efficacy of fat (Seltzer and McCabe, 1986). In some cases of fistula in the oval window, especially with fracture of the stapes footplate, it may be desirable to carry out a total stapedectomy, seal the oval window with a fascial or perichondrial graft and place some sound conductor between the long process of the incus and the graft. This sound conductor may be the stapes itself, which is especially suitable with a thin graft, or it may simply be one of the prostheses used routinely in stapes surgery.

The results of surgery are frequently dramatic in alleviating the patient of his vertigo and ataxia. Unfortunately, the recovery of the sensorineural hearing loss is rarely so dramatic and, with regard to the hearing, the prevention of further deterioration can usually be considered to be a satisfactory outcome.

Blast injury

It has been said in the past that rupture of the tympanic membrane has a significant protective effect

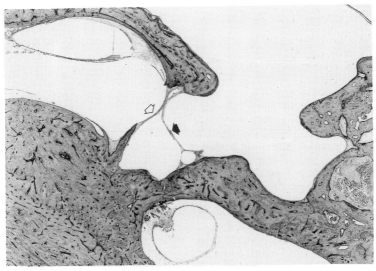

Figure 7.4 Mucosal fold in the round window niche (solid arrow). Round window membrane indicated by hollow arrow (courtesy of H.F. Schuknecht, MEEI Collection)

on the inner ear. This is probably not the case and, although it is difficult to prove, a survey has shown that sensorineural deafness is no less severe in those whose tympanic membranes have been ruptured (Kerr and Byrne, 1975). There is still considerable doubt about the underlying pathology in sensorineural deafness secondary to blast. It tends to be most marked immediately after the explosion with a natural tendency to spontaneous improvement. There may be complete bilateral deafness just after the explosion but there is, in the present authors' experience, always some recovery. Initially, the rate of recovery is rapid so that patients, unable to hear at all at the site of the explosion, are able to understand loud speech without difficulty 1 hour later. In some, the hearing may have returned to its former level within 48 hours, and in others, although there is permanent sensorineural deafness, this may continue to show slight improvement for up to 6 months (Figure 7.5).

In view of the tendency to rapid spontaneous recovery, it is difficult to control any trial of treatment for blast-induced sensorineural deafness. Numerous regimens have been advocated, often without much supporting evidence, including vasodilating drugs, corticosteroids, intravenous low molecular weight Dextran, anticoagulants and carbon dioxide inhalations. Other injuries may preclude some or even all of these forms of treatment. As there is doubt about the efficacy and as some of these treatments carry risks, it is preferable to leave untreated all cases of mild or moderate deafness and to reserve the multi-drug approach only for severe cases where there are no contraindications.

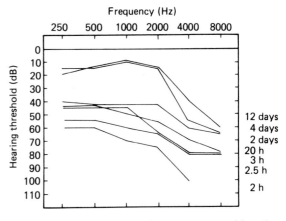

Figure 7.5 Serial audiograms of a young man tested from 2 hours to 12 days after an explosion, demonstrating recovery of hearing. (Reproduced from Kerr, 1978, courtesy of the Editor and Publisher, *The Practitioner*)

Tinnitus is a common complaint in those exposed to blast. The severity of the tinnitus tends to reflect the sensorineural deafness. Initially, the tinnitus may be severe and, although it persists as a big problem to some patients, it tends to decrease. When there is permanent sensorineural deafness the tinnitus may never disappear entirely but usually ceases to be a burden to the patient. In the uncomplicated case where the hearing returns to normal, one can expect complete disappearance of the tinnitus.

Surgical trauma

Injury to any of the structures which lie within the petrous bone is an inherent risk in every ear operation. Although it is certainly true that the introduction of microsurgical techniques in otology has been followed by a reduction in the incidence of surgical accidents such as dislocation of the stapes, opening of the labyrinth and damage to the facial nerve, nevertheless, the possibility of postoperative labyrinthine dysfunction after any operation on the ear, including myringoplasty, is still ever-present, even for the most experienced surgeon. Cochlear losses are reported more frequently than imbalance, but the two can occur together and, indeed, vestibular defects might be recognized more often were they routinely sought.

Although trauma to the facial nerve and major blood vessels is always possible if anatomical knowledge and surgical expertise are lacking, nowadays the majority of surgical injuries to the ear affect the labyrinth and follow the creation of a fistula of the oval window, or hydraulic effects on the membranous inner ear. Cellular damage from infection, circulatory changes and alterations in the dynamics of the inner ear fluids are probably responsible for most of the functional damage which complicates microsurgery of the ear.

Labyrinthine trauma in tympanoplasty

In tympanoplasty the principal causes of cochlear loss are:

1 The removal of cholesteatoma matrix and granulations from a labyrinthine fistula, most commonly involving the lateral semicircular canal, in the presence of infection during an initial procedure. Rupture of the membranous labyrinth, or labyrinthitis, frequently result in total loss of inner ear function.
2 Incautious removal of granulations, tympanosclerosis or cholesteatoma from the oval window, with fracture of the stapes footplate or rupture of its annular ligament creating a fistula between the mesotympanum and the vestibule of the inner ear. Prolonged perilymph loss or labyrinthitis may follow.
3 Excessive movement of the stapes footplate while removing disease from the oval window or from any part of an intact ossicular chain. Similar risks also pertain during reconstruction of the transmission mechanism and the tympanic membrane.
4 Contact between a toothed rotating burr and any part of an intact ossicular chain (most commonly the body of the incus) in combined approach tympanoplasty. Extensive hair cell damage may result (Paparella, 1962).

In a series of 1680 chronic ear operations, Palva, Karja and Palva (1973) reported a 4.5% incidence of sensorineural deafness after operation, mainly limited to the frequency range 4000–8000 Hz. In 81% the ossicular chain was maintained intact throughout the operation.

Smyth (1977) reported various degrees of sensorineural hearing loss in 2.5% of 3000 tympanoplasty operations. Apart from the special risk of cochlear trauma in combined approach tympanoplasty from contact of the burr, transmitted through the intact ossicular chain, which occurred in 5.6% of such ears, labyrinthine trauma did not appear to be related to any particular surgical technique. However, it should be noted that 1.3% of all myringoplasties (transcanal tympanoplasty with an intact chain) were complicated by a depression of cochlear function of greater than 10 dB averaged through the frequencies 500–4000 Hz, or a greater than 10% loss in speech discrimination score. Trauma arising from the removal of diseased tissue from the isolated stapes was considered to be responsible for one-third of the casualties; of these, in one-third the dissection of tympanosclerotic plaques had been noted to cause over manipulation or fracture of the stapes footplate. In another third of the damaged inner ears in this series, the cause appeared to be excessive movement of the stapes footplate during attempts to reconstruct the ossicular chain. Huttenbrink (1993) has explored in detail the forces and mechanisms involved in stapedial luxation.

Tos, Law and Plate (1984) analysed the incidence and characteristics of postoperative sensorineural hearing loss in chronic ear surgery performed in 2303 ears. Sensorineural hearing loss occurred in a total of 1.2% of cases; 0.5% became totally deaf and 0.7% acquired a high tone loss, most often at 4 kHz only. The incidence was highest in congenital malformations, granulating otitis and cholesteatoma, and in mastoidectomy, especially of the canal wall down type. In this series, the most common causes of anacusis were removal of cholesteatoma from the lateral semicircular canal and removal of the membrane covering the fistula.

One of the lessons to be learnt from these reports is that extreme caution is always necessary when instrumentation in the oval window is required in tympanoplasty. Although risks to inner ear function may be considered to be *only* 1%, perhaps this needs to be put into context by remembering that a 1% risk of an air crash at take-off or landing would mean several crashes every day at a major airport! Another lesson is that the considerable risks of severe iatrogenic sensorineural deafness in ears with labyrinthine fistula can only be avoided by the use of a technique in which the matrix over the fistula is meticulously preserved (Gormley, 1986).

Labyrinthine trauma in stapedectomy

This is considered in Chapter 14.

References

BALLANTYNE, J. (1979) Traumatic conductive deafness. In: *Scott-Brown's Diseases of the Ear, Nose and Throat* edited by J. Ballantyne, and J. Groves. Vol. 2. *The Ear.* London: Butterworths. pp. 159–173

DASPIT, P. L., CHURCHILL, D. and LINTHICUM, F. H. (1980) Diagnosis of perilymph fistulae using ENG and impedance. *Laryngoscope*, **90**, 217–223

FOWLER, E. P. (1961) Variations in the temporal bone course of the facial nerve. *Laryngoscope*, **71**, 937–946

FRASER, J. G. and FLOOD, L. M. (1982) An audiometric test for perilymph fistula. *Journal of Laryngology and Otology*, **96**, 513–520

GORMLEY, P. (1986) Surgical management of labyrinthine fistula with cholesteatoma. *Journal of Laryngology and Otology*, **100**, 1115–1123

GOTTEN, N. (1956) Survey of 100 cases of whiplash injury after settlement of litigation. *Journal of the American Medical Association*, **162**, 865–867

HOUGH, J. V. D. (1970) Fractures of the temporal bone and associated middle and inner ear trauma. *Proceedings of the Royal Society of Medicine*, **63**, 245–252

HUTTENBRINK, K. B. (1993) Manipulating the mobile stapes during tympanoplasty: the risk of stapedial luxation. *Laryngoscope*, **103**, 668–672

JENSEN, J. H. and BONDING, P. (1993) Experimental pressure induced rupture of the tympanic membrane in man. *Acta Otolaryngologica*, **113**, 62–67

KERR, A. G. (1967) Gunshot injury of the temporal bone: a histological report. *Journal of the Irish Medical Association*, **60**, 446–448

KERR, A. G. (1978) Blast injuries to the ear. *Practitioner*, **221**, 677–682

KERR, A. G. (1981) Injuries to the ears. In: *Trauma Care*, edited by W. Odling-Smee and A. Crockard. London: Academic Press

KERR, A. G. and BYRNE, J. E. T. (1975) Concussive effects of bomb blast on the ear. *Journal of Laryngology and Otology*, **89**, 131–143

KRISTENSEN, S. (1992) Spontaneous healing of traumatic tympanic membrane perforations in man: a century of experience. *Journal of Laryngology and Otology*, **106**, 1037–1350

MACNAB, I. (1971) The 'whiplash syndrome'. *Orthopedic Clinics of North America*, **2**, 389–403

MAKISHIMA, K., SOBEL, S. F. and SNOW, J. B. (1976) Histopathologic correlates of otoneurologic manifestations following head trauma. *Laryngoscope*, **86**, 1303–1314

PALVA, T., KARJA, J. and PALVA, A. (1973) High-tone sensorineural losses following chronic ear surgery. *Archives of Otolaryngology*, **98**, 176–178

PAPARELLA, M. M. (1962) Acoustic trauma from the bone cutting burr. *Laryngoscope*, **72**, 116–126

PROCTOR, B., GURDJIAN, E. S. and WEBSTER, J. E. (1956) The ear in head trauma. *Laryngoscope*, **66**, 16–59

RIZVI, S. S. and GIBBIN, K. P. (1979) Effect of transverse temporal bone fracture on the fluid compartment of the inner ear. *Annals of Otology, Rhinology and Laryngology*, **88**, 741–748

SCHUKNECHT, H. F. (1969) Cupulolithiasis. *Archives of Otolaryngology*, **90**, 765–778

SELTZER, S. and MCCABE, B. F. (1986) Perilymph fistula: the Iowa experience. *Laryngoscope*, **96**, 37–49

SINGLETON, G. T., KARLAN, M. S., POST, K. N. and BOCK, D. G. (1978) Perilymph fistulas: diagnostic criteria and therapy. *Annals of Otology, Rhinology and Laryngology*, **87**, 797–803

SHEA, J. J. (1992) The myth of spontaneous perilymph fistula. *Otolaryngology – Head and Neck Surgery*, **107**, 613–616

SMYTH, G. D. L. (1977) Sensorineural hearing loss in chronic ear surgery. *Annals of Otology, Rhinology and Laryngology*, **86**, 3–8

TONER, J. G. and KERR, A. G. (1987) Early visualisation of the incus during mastoid surgery. *Laryngoscope*, **97**, 1233–1234

TOS, M., LAW, T. and PLATE, S. (1984) Sensorineural hearing loss following chronic ear surgery. *Annals of Otology, Rhinology and Laryngology*, **93**, 403–409

8

Plastic surgery of the ear

H. Weerda

In the last 20 years, great advances have been made over earlier surgical methods of reconstructing the auricle. Otoplastic surgeons have learned to solve a number of problems inherent in a region that is extremely difficult to reconstruct surgically (Spira, 1974).

The present chapter offers a concise survey of surgical methods now in use for:

1 Auricular malformations
2 Acquired deformities
   (i) tumours
   (ii) trauma.

The body of literature covering the same ground is large, and the standardization of terminology is still awaiting agreement. The usual practice, observed here, is to classify defects, especially auricular deformities, by the surgical methods of treatment (Tanzer, 1974).

Anatomy

The anatomy of the external ear (Figure 8.1) is described in Volume 1. The surfaces of the auricle will be referred to here as anterior and posterior – 'postauricular' will thus mean 'of the posterior surface of the auricle'. The term 'retroauricular region' will signify the mastoid area.

Classification of auricular malformations

The definitions that follow are modifications, by Rogers (1968), of those proposed by Marx (1926).

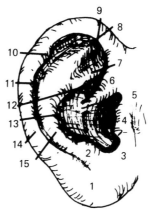

Figure 8.1 Anatomy of the anterior auricular surface: (1) lobule; (2) antitragus; (3) intertragic incisure; (4) tragus; (5) anterior incisure; (6) helical crus; (7) inferior (anterior) crus; (8) superior (posterior) crus; (9) triangular fossa; (10) tubercle of the helix (Darwin); (11) scapha; (12) cymba of the concha; (13) cavum of the concha; (14) helix; (15) antihelix. (Redrawn from Weerda, 1985a; reprinted with permission)

First degree dysplasia

Average definition: most structures of a normal auricle are recognizable (minor deformities).

   Surgical definition: reconstruction normally does not require the use of additional skin or cartilage.

- Macrotia (see Figure 8.3)
- Protruding ears. *Synonyms*: prominent ears, bat ears (see Figures 8.4 and 8.5)
- Cryptotia. *Synonym*: pocket ear
- Absence of the upper helix

- Small deformities: absence of the tragus, satyr ear, Darwin's tubercle, additional folds (Stahl's ear), etc.
- Colobomas. *Synonym*: clefts. Transverse coloboma (see Figure 8.6)
- Lobule deformities (fixed lobule, macrolobule, absence of the lobule, lobule colobomas (bifid lobule), etc.
- Cup ear deformities (see Figures 8.7 and 8.8).
  Type I (Figure 8.7): Cupped upper portion of the helix, hypertrophic concha, reduced height. *Synonyms*: lidding helix, constricted helix, lop ear, minor (mild or moderate) cupping (Tanzer, 1974; Brent, 1980; Weerda, 1988)
  Type II (see Figure 8.8): More severe lopping of the upper pole of the ear. (Rib cartilage is used as support when a short ear has to be expanded or the auricular cartilage is limp (Walter, 1972.)

Second degree dysplasia

Average definition: some structures of a normal auricle are recognizable.

Surgical definition: partial reconstruction requires the use of some additional skin and cartilage (Tanzer, 1974).

Synonym: second degree microtia.

- Cup ear deformity, type III (see Figure 8.9). The severe cup ear deformity is malformed in all dimensions. *Synonyms*: cockleshell ear (Davis, 1987), constricted helix, snail-shell ear (Davis, 1987).
- Mini ear (see Figure 8.10).

Third degree dysplasia (see Figures 8.11 and 8.12)

Average definition: none of the structures of a normal auricle is recognizable.

Surgical definition: total reconstruction requires the use of skin and large amounts of cartilage.

Synonyms: complete hypoplasia (Davis, 1987), peanut ear, third degree microtia.

Normally we will find an atresia auris congenita.

- Unilateral (see Figure 8.11): One ear is normal. No middle ear reconstruction is performed on any child. Auricle reconstruction is begun at the age of 8 or 9 years.
- Bilateral (see Figure 8.12): bone-conducting hearing aid before the first birthday. Middle ear surgery at the age of 9 or 10 years without transposition of the vestige (Brent, 1992). Bilateral reconstruction of the auricle at the age of 8 or 9 years.
- Anotia.

Description of a normal auricle

The different areas of the auricle lie in sharp relief in the normal ear (see Figure 8.1). When the ear is viewed from the front, the helical rim lies slightly further out from the side of the head than the antihelical fold.

An abundant supply of blood is carried to the external ear by the superficial temporal artery and branches of the posterior auricular artery. The sensory supply to the auricle is transmitted by the anterior and posterior branches of the great auricular nerve, which run parallel to the posterior auricular artery. The auriculotemporal nerve supplies roughly the area of the anterior auricular arteries.

The normal protrusion of an ear is about 30°, or between 1.5 and 2 cm (Figure 8.2a). The angle of inclination is measured from the long axis of the auricle to a line through the external auditory canal and parallel to the facial profile line (Figure 8.2c). The inclination of the auricle is between 20° and 30° and is generally parallel to the profile line of the nose. The average length of the pinna is 63.5 mm in men and 59 mm in women (Table 8.1). The normal angle between the concha and scapha is approximately 90°, with deviations of as much as 15° (Figure 8.2a).

Table 8.1 Average length and width of the normal auricle

Age (years)	Males		Females	
	Length (mm)	Width (mm)	Length (mm)	Width (mm)
1	50.0	31.5	46.8	29.1
6	55.3	33.4	53.5	32.5
18	63.5	35.3	59.0	32.5

*After Farkas, 1974.

When the angle at which the auricle protrudes exceeds 40°, or that between the concha and the scapha exceeds 110°, it is known as a protruding ear (Figure 8.2b). In most instances, the distance from the side of the head to the helical rim exceeds 2.0–2.5 cm. The main categories of prominent ear are marked by a prominent helix, lack of a superior antihelical crus, lack of an antihelix and hypertrophy of the concha.

Surgery for auricular malformations
First degree dysplasia
Macrotia

Wedge-shaped excision

A simple way to reduce a macrotic ear is by excising a wedge of skin and cartilage. This method's shortcomings are that it deforms the auricle slightly and leaves conspicuous scars.

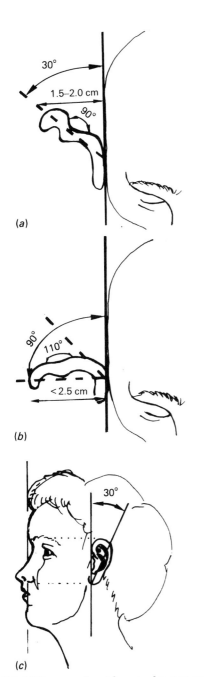

Figure 8.2 (*a*) The normal auricle protrudes at an angle of about 30° or between 1.5 and 2 cm from the head. The conchoscaphalic angle for a normal auricle is roughly 90°. (Redrawn, with modifications, from Farkas, 1974 and Weerda, 1985a). (*b*) A protruding ear has a conchoscaphalic angle greater than 110° or a height of more than 2.5 cm. (From Weerda, 1985a). (*c*) The angle of inclination is about 30°, as measured from the long axis of the ear to a line through the auditory canal and parallel to the facial profile line. (Redrawn, with modifications, from Farkas, 1974 and Weerda, 1985a; reprinted with permission)

A modification of the sliding helix procedure

The reductive procedure recommended combines a sliding helix with a crescent excision (Figure 8.3*a*, *b*) of anterior skin and cartilage (Gersuny, 1903). The author's own otoplastic method is used to form the antihelix (Weerda, 1982a–d). The results are excellent (Figure 8.3*c*, *d*). A multitude of variations on the wedge-shaped and crescent excisions have been described in the literature.

Protruding ears

The synonyms are 'prominent ears', 'bat ears', and 'lop ears'. One of the goals of otoplasty is to invent a single simple operation for correcting all the different types and degrees of protruding ears.

A child's ears grow only slightly after his or her sixth birthday, so that children with the stigma of prominent ears may be operated on about that time without any detrimental effects on the long-term growth of the auricle. Although the size of the ear does not increase significantly, the consistency of the cartilage does change, becoming less flexible as the child grows older. This may influence the method and results of surgical correction (compare Table 8.1).

The main features of protruding ears are under-development or absence of the antihelix and crus superius and an overdeveloped concha (see Figure 8.2*b*). There are three widely used corrective procedures and scores of variants that are preferred by individual surgeons.

Converse procedure

This is the procedure used by most plastic and ENT surgeons (Converse *et al.*, 1955; Converse and Wood-Smith, 1963; Tanzer, 1977). The posterior auricle is incised parallel to the helix and the cartilage underneath is exposed (Figure 8.4*a*). The superior and inferior borders of the antihelix are marked on the posterior aspect of the exposed cartilage with steel cutting needles and blue ink.

Incisions, which should not meet, are made through the exposed cartilage (Figure 8.4*a*). If need be, the surface between the upper and lower incisions can be thinned with an electric diamond drill or rotating wire brush. This last procedure contributes to better results when the antihelix and crus superius are folded with mattress sutures (Figure 8.4*b*). Conchal cartilage and the cauda helicis may have to be removed. An elliptical excision of postauricular skin may also have to be made (Walter, 1972). The incision in the posterior auricle is closed with interrupted or running sutures.

Modification of the Converse procedure

Whereas the Converse procedure uses the incision

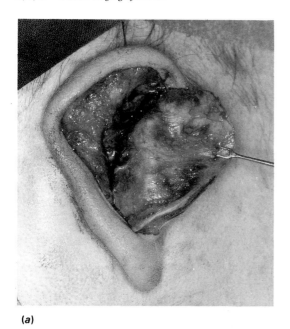

(a)

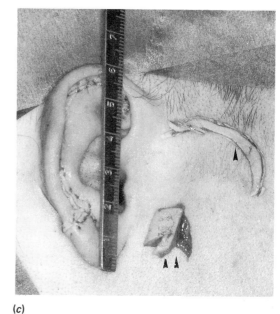

(c)

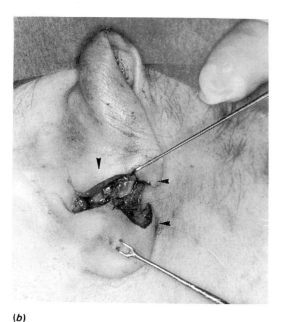

(b)

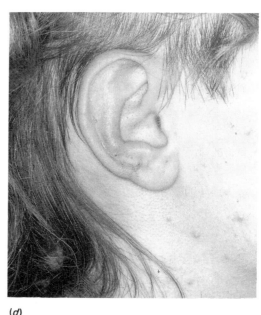

(d)

Figure 8.3 Macrotic ear, auricle length 72 mm. (a) Excision of anterior skin and cartilage; the posterior aspect of the cartilage is exposed as a first step in the otoplastic method. (b) Resection of skin in the postauricular and helical regions. (c) Situation at the end of the operation, auricle length 60 mm: ▲, crescent excision; ▲ ▲, lobule reduction. (d) Two months after surgery

illustrated in Figure 8.4a, in the author's modification (Weerda, 1979, 1982a–d), the cartilage is thinned above and below a new antihelix (Figure 8.5a) with a diamond burr (Figure 8.5b). This method can be applied in correcting other anomalies besides protruding ears, e.g. in dysplasia surgery, in reconstructing

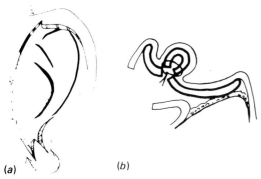

(a) **(b)**

Figure 8.4 (*a*) Converse otoplastic method. (*b*) The auricle is folded with mattress sutures

a missing helical rim, and in elevating a cup ear antihelix (Figures 8.6–8.8).

Mustarde's procedure

When the ear cartilage is thin, Mustarde (1963) prefers to fold the antihelix with mattress sutures without incising or weakening the auricular cartilage. Except in this one respect, Mustarde's procedure is similar to that of Converse.

Stenström procedure

The scapha, conchal rim, and crus superius are marked with straight cutting needles and blue ink after exposure of the posterior auricular cartilage (Stenström, 1963). An incision is made through the cartilage of the scapha, and the anterior cartilage of the antihelical area is freed of skin and perichondrium. The cartilage here is scored parallel to its free margin with a knife or an instrument specially designed for this purpose.

With the tension thus taken out of the cartilage, the antihelix begins to curl back, and assumes a normal curvature without any suturing.

Additional procedures

Rotation of the concha

One way to avoid an elliptical excision of cartilage from the hypertrophic concha is by rotating the concha to the mastoid (Furnas, 1968; Spira and Stal, 1983). The posterior auricular muscle is divided, and the mastoid exposed. The concha is rotated towards the mastoid and fixed with 3–0 Vicryl sutures.

Mild pressure dressings

The ear is carefully packed with a cotton-wool dressing that has been soaked in mineral oil. The dressing

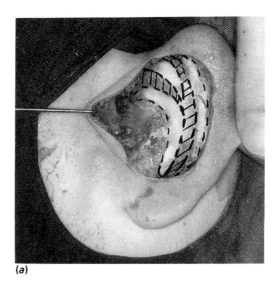

(a)

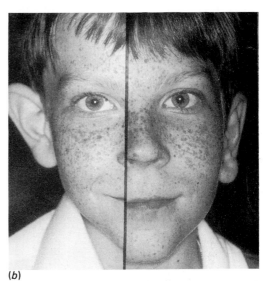

(b)

Figure 8.5 (*a*) The author's otoplastic method. The cartilage is thinned below and above the new antihelix. (*b*) Patient before (right ear) and after (left ear) surgery

is applied for 7 days. From the ninth day after surgery, when the patient's sutures are removed, he should wear a second, elastic dressing or cap for 1 week.

Complications

On the rare occasions when a haematoma or perichondritis occurs, it is treated by coagulation and with antibiotics. Unsatisfactory results are corrected 6 months after surgery. Hypertrophic postauricular scars are treated with pressure and cortisone injections shortly after surgery and again by scar revision

1 or 2 years later if necessary and X-rays with a dose of 10–12 Gy.

Cryptotia (pocket ear)

Definition

The upper part of the auricle is buried beneath the temporal skin.

Procedure

An incision is made along the helical rim, and a flap is incised at the retroauricular hairline. After the auricle has been elevated, the flap is used to cover the postauricular defect. The wounds are closed with sutures.

Colobomas

A small transverse coloboma can be closed by Z-plasty (Figure 8.6). The ear in Figure 8.6 is also protruding; the otoplastic procedure was used to correct the additional anomaly.

Larger defects are closed with a rib cartilage support and retro- and postauricular flaps.

A coloboma of the lobule is closed by excising and adapting skin.

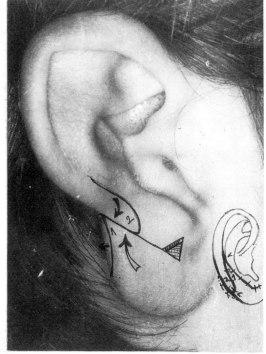

(b)

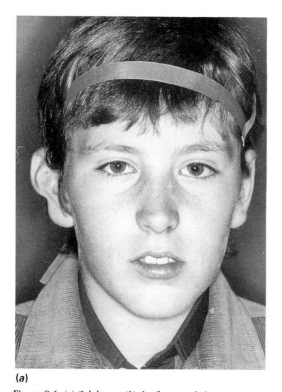

(a)

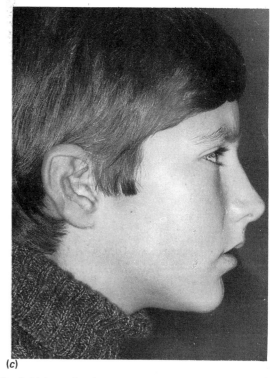

(c)

Figure 8.6 (a) Coloboma; (b) the flaps needed in a Z-plasty are outlined; (c) 6 months after surgery

Cup ear deformities

Type I (Figure 8.7)

Synonyms are 'lop ear', 'lidding helix', 'constricted helix', 'minor (or moderate) cupping'. The otoplastic procedure for treating cup ear deformities of type I (Figure 8.7*a*, *b*) is outlined opposite.

Type II (Figure 8.8)

A more severe lopping of the upper pole of the ear (Figure 8.8*a*) is corrected by a modification of Tanzer's (1974) method. The postauricular skin is incised, and the cupping cartilage is exposed on both sides (Figure 8.8*b*). The cartilage is dissected and turned approximately 180° (Figure 8.8*c*). The otoplastic procedure is used to elevate the scapha (see Figure 8.5).

Rib cartilage is used when a short ear has to be expanded, or for additional support when the auricular cartilage is limp (Weerda and Walter, 1984).

After surgery, the auricle is supported for 14 days by mattress sutures.

Second degree dysplasia (second degree microtia)

Severe type III cup ear deformities

The severe cup ear is malformed in all its dimensions (Figure 8.9).

First stage of reconstruction

The auricle is incised and expanded by a method similar to that described by Davis (1974) (see Figure 8.10*b*). The middle part of the auricle is reconstructed with a rib cartilage support and a retroauricular flap.

Second stage

The ear is raised, and a full-thickness skin graft is sutured and glued* to the rough post- and retroauricular surfaces (Weerda, 1987).

The mini ear

The mini ear (Figure 8.10) is reconstructed in the same way as severe cup ear deformities.

---

* *Manufactured by: Immuno Ltd, Arctic House, Rye Lane, Dunton Green, Near Sevenoaks, Kent TN14 5HB, UK*

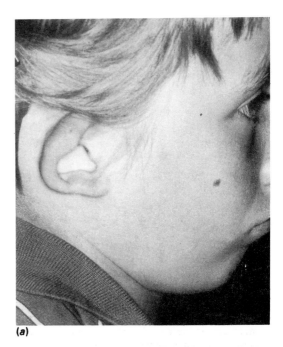

(a)

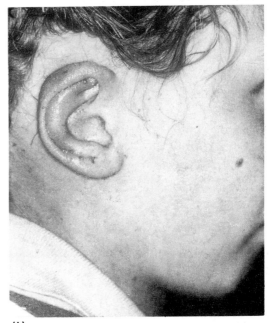

(b)

Figure 8.7 (*a*) Moderate cup ear deformity (type I); (*b*) reconstruction by otoplastic procedure

Lobule reconstruction

This will be discussed in connection with trauma surgery.

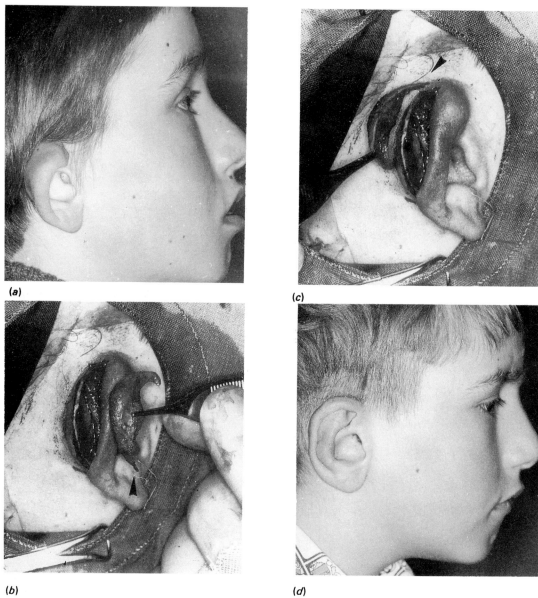

(a)

(b)

(c)

(d)

Figure 8.8 (*a*) More severe, type II, cup ear deformity (corrected by a modification of the Tanzer method, 1974). (*b*) The posterior skin is incised, the cupping cartilage is exposed on both sides. The cartilage is dissected (▲, cauda helicis). (*c*) The antihelix has been folded and the scapha elevated. The excised cartilage has been turned roughly 180° (▲, cauda helicis) and will be sutured to the scapha. (*d*) Auricle 1 year after surgery

Third degree dysplasia (third degree microtia or anotia)

Auricle reconstruction (normal hairline)

The procedure for treating third degree microtia (Figure 8.11*a*) is similar to the procedures described

by Tanzer (1974), Converse and Brent (1977) and Brent (1980).

First stage

Before surgery, a template of the size of the patient's normal ear is cut out of a piece of transparent cellu-

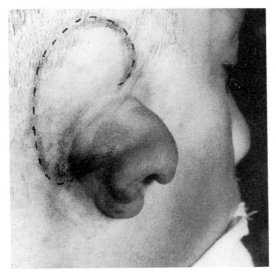

(a)

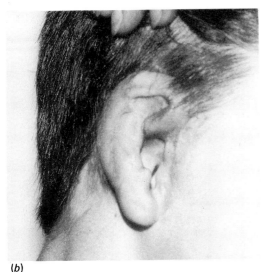

(b)

Figure 8.9 (*a*) Severe, dystopic cup ear deformity, type III. Outline of the normal position of the ear. (*b*) One year after reconstruction in four stages by a method similar to that of Davis (1974). (Compare Figure 8.10*b*)

loid (Figure 8.11). The position of the new auricle is outlined on the mastoid region and a rib cartilage support is carved (Figure 8.11*b*). Remnants of auricular cartilage are removed by a small incision in the vestige. The mastoid skin is tunnelled, and the rib cartilage support inserted (Brent, 1992). With mattress sutures, which are tied over gauze, and fibrin sealant, the thin mastoid skin is snugged into the helical sulcus (Figure 8.11*c*).

Second stage

The auricle is raised from the side of the head, and the postauricular defect is surfaced with a full-thickness skin graft from the buttocks. The lobule can be rotated in the same stage into a transverse position (Figure 8.11*d*).

Third stage

In this stage the scapha is formed, which may require the removal of fibrous tissue and fat. The crus helicis, tragus, antitragus and concha are formed in the third or in a fourth stage according to whether or not the helix is well defined (Figure 8.11*e*). In the last year we started to use Nagata's technique (1993; 1994).

Postoperative care

The reconstructed ear (its concavities in particular) and the auriculocephalic sulcus are packed with fluffed oiled wool. The whole area is then covered with a bulky wool and gauze dressing and bandaged in order to cushion pressure on the ear, especially at night.

Antibiotics may be administered for the first 3 or 4 days after surgery.

Complications

1 A small necrosis exposing cartilage is covered with an antibiotic ointment to prevent the cartilage from drying out.
2 A larger necrosis is excised. The defect created by excision is covered with flaps from the surrounding area.
3 Because fibrin glue* (see footnote on p.3/8/7) is used, bleeding rarely occurs. In the event of a haematoma, the bleeding has to be staunched and the haematoma evacuated.
4 Infection is likewise a very rare complication. When an infection occurs, the surgical wound has to be opened and the affected cartilage removed. An antibiotic appropriate to treating the infection is administered.

Middle ear reconstruction

In Table 8.2 the planning of treatments is outlined. Middle ear surgery is *not performed* on any child with *unilateral microtia* and atresia when one ear is normal. Reconstruction (Weerda, 1984) of the pinna is begun once a child reaches the age of 8 or 9 years (Jahrsdoerfer, 1974; Bellucci, 1980; Weerda, 1985b).

A child with bilateral microtia and atresia is fitted

Table 8.2 Operating schedule for surgery on unilateral and bilateral microtia with atresia auris

Deformity	Operation		Hearing aid	Remarks
	Atresia middle ear	*Microtia*		
Unilateral	Adolescence			Middle ear: by patient's decision good hearing by one ear
		> 8 years	Not required	Auricle: in 3–5 stages
Bilateral			5–7 months	Bone-conduction hearing aid
	> 9–10 years			Good hearing result, second ear as unilateral
		> 8 years		in 5–7 stages
			about 10 years	Air-conducting hearing aid after auricle reconstruction and middle ear reconstruction
	No middle ear surgery possible; disadvantage		> 1–2 years	Bone-anchored hearing aid

with a bone-conduction hearing aid before his or her first birthday. The child has to be at least 9–10 years old before the author will consent to perform middle ear surgery if possible. If there is a score as proposed by Jahrsdoerfer (Aguilar and Jahrsdoerfer, 1988) below five and the middle ear is poorly developed a bone-anchored hearing aid should be attached (Håkansson *et al.*, 1990). Children aged 8 or 9 years are operated on for bilateral microtia; later on they undergo middle ear surgery (Figure 8.12).

Bone-anchored auricular prostheses

In some cases of microtia/anotia, a decision may be made by the patient's parents or surgeon to choose an auricular prosthesis (see Auricular defect prostheses and Figure 8.22).

Surgery for acquired deformities (Figure 8.13)

Often it is irrelevant to one's choice of procedure whether a defect is due to tumour excision or traumatic avulsion.

Tumour surgery

A small defect in the rim from a wedge-shaped excision can be closed by a single operation (Converse and Brent, 1977). A defect in the crus helicis is closed with a preauricular flap. The anterior part of the upper auricle (Figure 8.13) is reconstructed according to a modified version of the sliding helix procedure (Gersuny, 1903; Antia, 1974). Any additional preauricular defect can be closed with a rhomboidal flap (Figure 8.13*a*). The author prefers to reconstruct conchal defects with a full-thickness

skin graft taken from either auriculocephalic sulcus or alternatively a pedicled retroauricular graft may be used.

Subtotal resection with preserved helix

Microscopically controlled surgery allows preservation of parts of the auricle (Figure 8.14) (Weerda, 1978; Weerda and Walter, 1984). Figure 8.14*a* shows a helix and lobule saved in such a fashion; the other parts of the auricle were reconstructed in one stage with a bilobed flap from the neck (Figure 8.14*b*). To prevent shrinkage, a defect-filling support of rib cartilage has to be inserted. Epithelium must be removed preparatory to affixing a folded transposition flap (Figure 8.14*c*).

In reconstructions after ablation or petrosectomy, flaps from the surrounding area, myocutaneous pectoralis major island flaps or radial forearm flaps are used (Weerda, 1994).

Trauma surgery

After removal of a haematoma, seroma, or fibrous tissue (wrestler's ear, cauliflower ear), the thinned skin is readapted with fibrin glue* (see footnote on p. 3/8/7) and sutures (Weerda, 1979, 1980). A deep abrasion of skin from an auricle, or through-and-through laceration, is repaired with thin sutures if the auricle is well supplied with blood. Small defects in the rim or the anterior upper part of the auricle are closed with Burow's triangles or a sliding helix (see Figure 8.13) (Gersuny, 1903; Antia, 1974; Brent, 1978).

Replantation

Replantation of a freshly avulsed auricle or part of one is hazardous work. The largest avulsed parts that

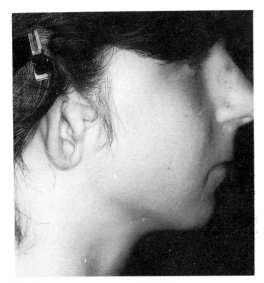

(a)

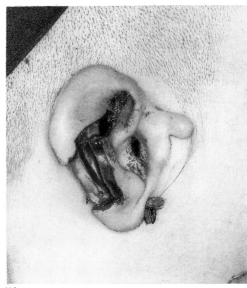

(b)

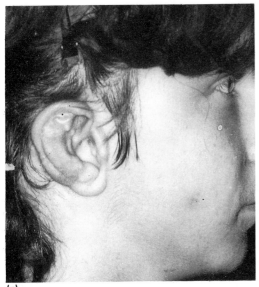

(c)

Figure 8.10 (*a*) A mini ear with an accessory ear tag. (*b*) The auricle is incised and expanded by a method similar to that of Davis (1974). The middle part of the auricle is reconstructed with a rib cartilage support. (*c*) Six months after surgery in four separate stages

have successfully replanted as composite grafts have been under 26 × 10mm (Figure 8.15*a, b*).

Baudet's method of replantation

The only methods that significantly diminish the risks incident to replantation of larger parts of the auricle are replantation by microvascular anastomo-

ses, or those described by Baudet, Tramond and Goumain (1972) and Arfai (after Spira, 1974), (compare Figure 8.17). Ninety per cent (or 31 out of 32) of replantations of larger parts of the auricle by a simple procedure have resulted in loss of the replant (Figure 8.16). By contrast, 90% of the auricles replanted experimentally according to Baudet's method have taken. Replantation should be performed within 24 hours of avulsion (Weerda, 1986). Arfai's modified version of the Baudet operation preserves the postauricular skin (Figure 8.17) of the totally avulsed auricle. The auricle is replanted as a composite graft. The fenestrated cartilage and the postauricular skin are glued* (see footnote on p. 3/8/7) and sutured to the rough surgically enlarged mastoid wound (Figure 8.17) (Spira, 1974). Using Arfai's method, the totally avulsed ear could be reconstructed (Figure 8.17*a*) in four stages – the lobule was repaired with a Gavello flap (Figure 8.17*b, c*).

Microvascular anastomosis

This is discussed in connection with surgery for total avulsion by Buncke and Schultz (1966) and Pennington, Lai and Pelly (1980). Their advice is that auricles should be replanted within 5 hours of avulsion.

Reconstruction of partially avulsed ears

The upper part of the pinna

In tumour and trauma surgery, reconstruction of parts of the auricle is begun by incising and tunnelling the retroauricular skin (Figure 8.18*a*) and

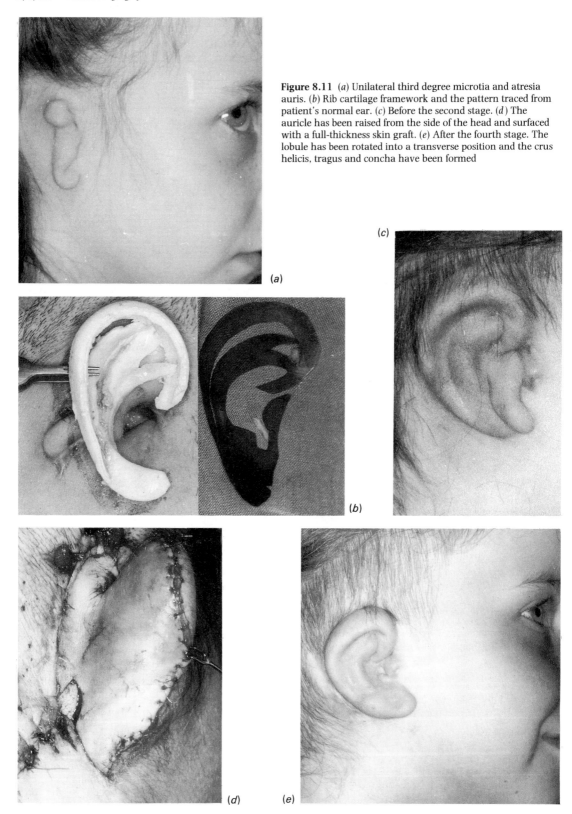

Figure 8.11 (*a*) Unilateral third degree microtia and atresia auris. (*b*) Rib cartilage framework and the pattern traced from patient's normal ear. (*c*) Before the second stage. (*d*) The auricle has been raised from the side of the head and surfaced with a full-thickness skin graft. (*e*) After the fourth stage. The lobule has been rotated into a transverse position and the crus helicis, tragus and concha have been formed

(*a*)

(*c*)

(*b*)

(*d*)

(*e*)

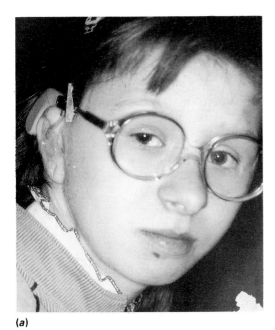

(a)

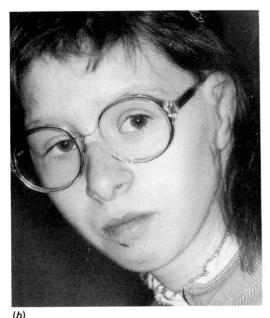

(b)

Figure 8.12 (*a*) Reconstruction of a right middle ear and auricle in surgery to correct bilateral congenital microtia and atresia. A hearing aid was attached to the patient's glasses. (*b*) Reconstruction of the same patient's left auricle

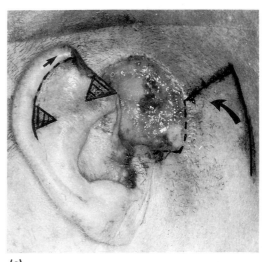

(a)

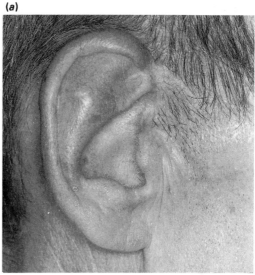

(b)

Figure 8.13 (*a*) Defect in the anterior part of the auricle. Reconstruction according to a modified version of the sliding helix procedure and with a rhomboidal flap. (*b*) One year after reconstruction

inserting a support of rib cartilage. The helix is moulded with fibrin glue* (see footnote on p. 3/8/7) and mattress sutures tied over gauze (Figure 8.18*b*). In a second stage, the auricle is raised, and the post-and retroauricular defects are covered with full-thickness skin grafts. Later on the ear can be corrected, for a satisfactory end result, by deepening the scapha or crus helicis or other parts of the auricle (Figure 8.18*c*).

The middle part of the auricle

This is reconstructed in the same manner as its upper part (Figure 8.19).

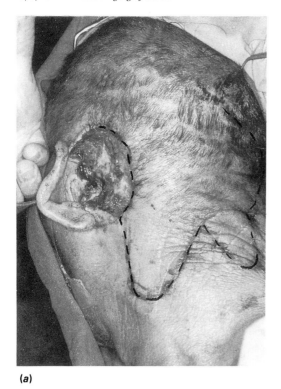

(a)

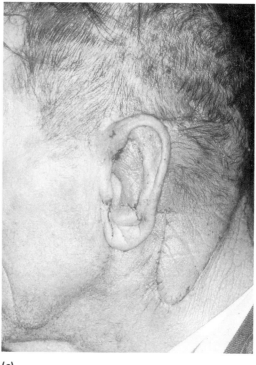

(c)

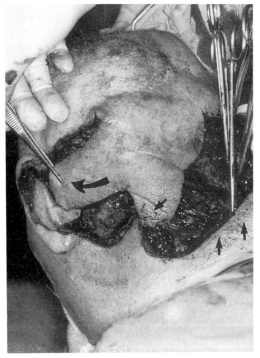

(b)

The lower part of the ear

This and the lobule are both reconstructed by the Gavello-flap technique.

A rib cartilage support is embedded to prevent shrinkage (Figure 8.20*a*). The work of shaping the auricle is completed in a second stage (Figure 8.20*b*).

Reconstruction after the total loss of an avulsed auricle

Retroauricular implantation

A rib cartilage support is embedded under the retroauricular skin in the same way as in the procedure for correcting severe microtia (Figure 8.21). The helix is

Figure 8.14 (*a*) Defect of the auricle and retroauricular regions after tumour extirpation. The helix and lobule were preserved. The transportation flap is outlined and contains two non-hair-bearing transposition flaps, one for the reconstruction of the auricular and postauricular areas, the other for the secondary defect. (*b*) Incision of the flaps. (*c*) Situation after 2 weeks

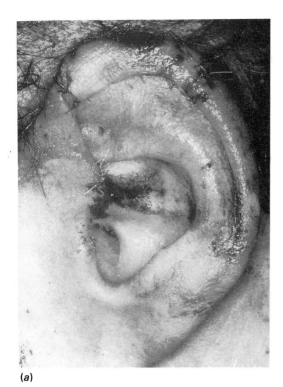

(a)

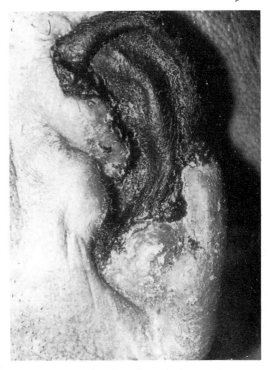

Figure 8.16 Loss of a subtotally avulsed pinna after replantation

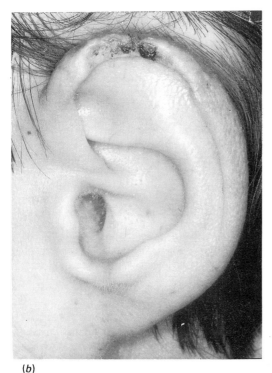

(b)

Figure 8.15 (a) Replanted avulsed helix (26 × 8 mm): (b) the composite graft has taken. A small defect is visible in the middle of the replanted composite graft

moulded with fibrin glue* (see footnote on p. 3/8/7) and mattress sutures (Figure 8.21a, b). The auricle is raised and formed in either three or four stages (Figure 8.21c).

The fan-flap method

When a low hairline makes it impossible to repair a microtic or avulsed auricle by one of the methods outlined so far, a support is embedded under the pedicled temporoparietal fascia. The fascia can be adapted to the support with fibrin glue* (see footnote on p. 3/8/7) and by suction drainage. A full-thickness skin graft is glued to the rough surface. The auricle is raised from the side of the head in a second stage (see Brent and Byrd, 1983).

Auricular defect prostheses

In many cases a defect prosthesis may provide an acceptable alternative for patients who have had surgery for the removal of auricular tumours but who not wish to undergo further surgery for ear reconstruction because of their advanced age or other illness (Figure 8.22a).

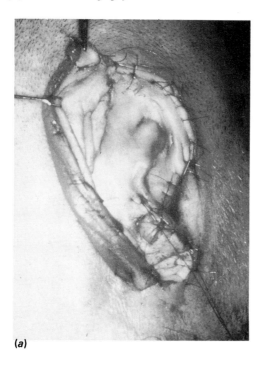

(a)

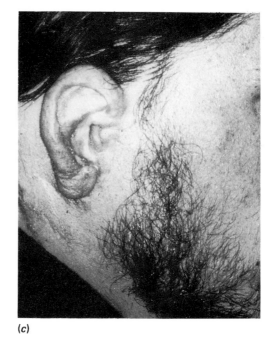

(c)

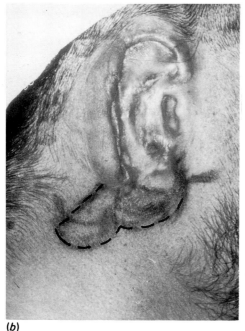

(b)

Figure 8.17 (*a*) Replantation of a totally avulsed auricle as a composite graft according to Arfai's method (after Spira, 1974). The postauricular tissue has been removed and the cartilage fenestrated. The auricular segment is being sutured and glued to the surgically enlarged, rough retroauricular area. (*b*) Situation 6 weeks after implantation of an auricle as a composite graft. The Gavello-flap used to repair the lobule is outlined. (*c*) Reconstructed auricle

In the past, patients with ear prostheses were required to glue them onto the skin every day. Apart from the difficulties involved in such a routine, the regular application of glue to skin will eventually lead to irritations so that the patient may only be able wear his prosthesis part of the time.

Recent advances in this field have now made it possible to fix the prosthesis directly to an anchoring in the bone. This involves implanting screws that permanently perforate the skin directly into bone (Figure 8.22*b*). When carefully placed these screws heal solidly and are irritation-free in 90% of cases. A custom-made metal frame (Figure 8.22*c*) is then attached to the two to four screws required per prosthesis. The prosthesis is fitted onto the frame with clamps and can be put on or taken off by the patient without problem (Figure 8.22 *d*, *e*).

In spite of the often good aesthetic results obtained by defect prostheses, however, many patients never completely lose the feeling of being disfigured, which is especially true among young people. For this reason ear reconstruction remains the preferred method of treatment for children and adolescents.

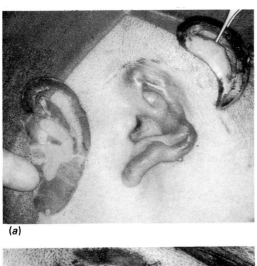

(a)

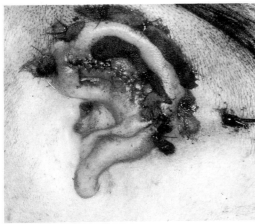

(b)

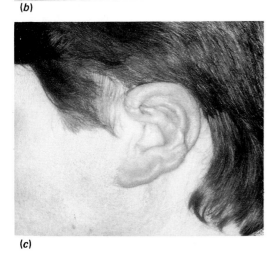

(c)

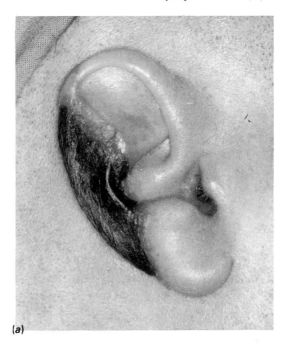

(a)

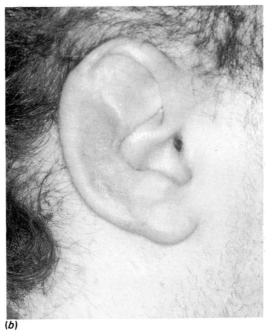

(b)

Figure 8.18 (a) Reconstruction of the upper part of an auricle after loss. The retroauricular skin has been tunnelled and a rib support will be sutured to the auricular stump. (b) The helix is moulded with mattress sutures tied over gauze. (c) End result after 1 year

Figure 8.19 Necrosis of the middle part of an auricle after replantation as a free composite graft. (b) After a two-stage reconstruction

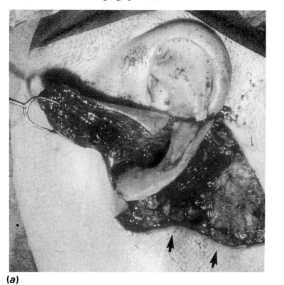

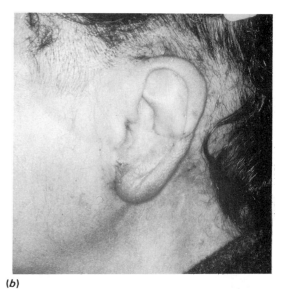

(a)   **(b)**

Figure 8.20 (*a*) Reconstruction of the lower part of the auricle by the Gavello-flap method. (*b*) Four weeks after reconstruction

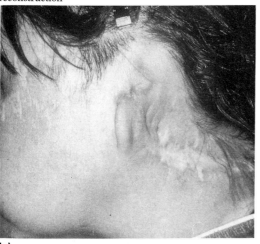

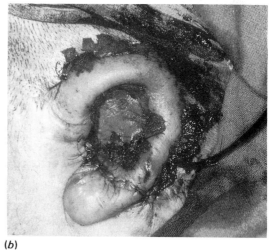

(a)   **(b)**

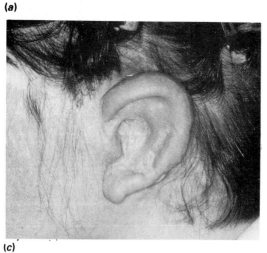

Figure 8.21 (*a*) A totally avulsed auricle. The skin in the ear region is permeated with scars. The auditory canal is closed. (*b*) A rib cartilage support has been embedded, and the helix moulded with mattress sutures. The lobule has been brought into a transverse position. (*c*) Result 6 months after reconstruction

(c)

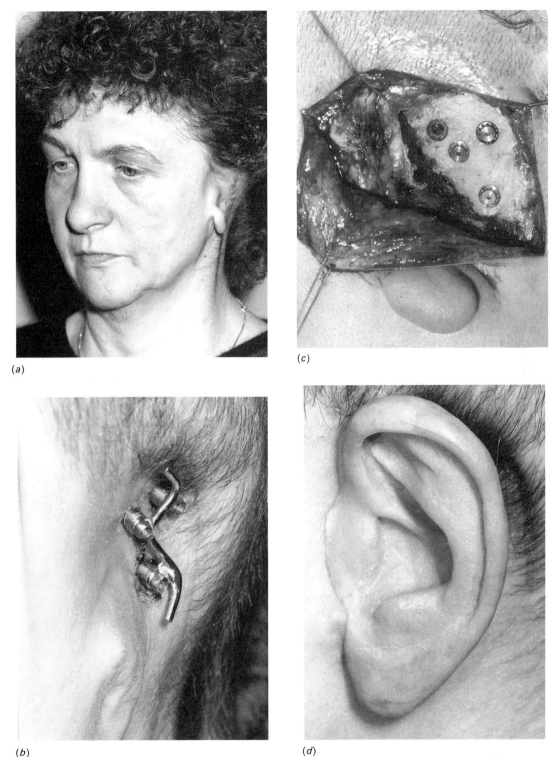

(a)

(c)

(b)

(d)

Figure 8.22 (a) A 55-year-old woman with a third degree dysplasia who did not want an ear reconstruction. (b) Three anchors of tantalum are screwed into the bone. (c) A metal frame is attached to the screws. (d), (e) The ear prosthesis is fitted to the frame

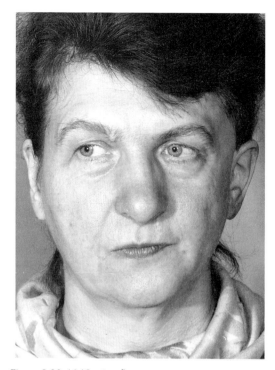

Figure 8.22 *(e) (Continued)*

References

AGUILAR, E. and JAHRSDOERFER, R. I. (1988) The surgical repair of congenital microtia and atresia. *Otolaryngology – Head and Neck Surgery*, **98**, 600–606

ANTIA, H. (1974) Repair of segmental defects of the auricle in mechanical trauma. In: *Symposium on Reconstruction of the Auricle*, edited by R. Tanzer and M. Edgerton, Vol. X, St Louis: C. V. Mosby Co. pp. 218–229

BAUDET, J., TRAMOND, P. and GOUMAIN, A. (1972) A propos d'un procédé original de réimplantation d'un pavillon de l'oreille totalement séparé. *Annales de Chirurgie Plastique*, **17**, 67–72

BELLUCCI, R. J. (1980) The problem of congenital auricular malformation: construction of the external auditory canal. *Transactions of the American Academy of Ophthamology and Otology*, 840

BRENT, B. (1978) Reconstruction of traumatic ear deformities. *Clinics in Plastic Surgery*, **5**, 437–445

BRENT, B. (1980) The correction of microtia with autogenous cartilage grafts: I. the classic deformity; II. atypical and complex deformities. *Plastic and Reconstructive Surgery*, **66**, 1–12; 13–21

BRENT, B. (1992) Auricular repair with autologous rib cartilage grafts: two decades of experience with 600 cases. *Plastic and Reconstructive Surgery*, **90**, 355–374

BRENT, B. and BYRD, H. S. (1983) Secondary ear reconstruction with cartilage grafts covered by axial, random, and free flaps of temporoparietal fascia. *Plastic and Reconstructive Surgery*, **72**, 141–151

BUNCKE, H. J. and SCHULTZ, W. P. (1966) Total implantation in the rabbit using microvascular anastomoses. *Journal of Plastic Surgery*, **19**, 15–22

CONVERSE, J. M. and BRENT, B. (1977) Acquired deformities. In: *Reconstructive Plastic Surgery*, 2nd edn, edited by J. M. Converse, vol. 3. Philadelphia: W. B. Saunders. pp. 1724–1773

CONVERSE, J. M. and WOOD-SMITH, D. (1963) Technical details in the surgical correction of the lop ear deformity. *Plastic and Reconstructive Surgery*, **31**, 118–128

CONVERSE, J. M., NIGRO, A., WILSON, F. A. and JOHNSON, N. (1955) A technique for surgical corrections of lop ears. *Plastic and Reconstructive Surgery*, **15**, 411–418

DAVIS, J. (1987) *Aesthetic and Reconstructive Otoplasty*. Berlin: Springer

DAVIS, J. (1974) Treatment of congenital atresia of the ear and its complications. Repair of severe cup ear deformities. In: *Symposium on Reconstruction of the Auricle*, edited by R. Tanzer and M. Edgerton, Vol. X. St Louis: C. V. Mosby Co. pp. 134–139

FARKAS, L. (1974) Growth of the normal and reconstructed auricles. In: *Symposium on Reconstruction of the Auricle*, edited by R. Tanzer and M. Edgerton, Vol. X. St Louis: C. V. Mosby Co. pp. 24–31

FURNAS, D. W. (1968) Correction of prominent ears by concha-mastoid sutures. *Plastic and Reconstructive Surgery*, **42**, 189–193

GERSUNY (1903) after MÜNDNICH, K. (1962) *Plastische Operationen an der Nase und an der Ohrmuschel*, edited by A. Sercer and K. Mündnich. Stuttgart: Thieme-Verlag. p. 364

HÅKANSSON, B., LIDEN, G., TJELLSTÖM, A., RINGDAHL, A., JACOBSSON, M., CARLSSON, P. *et al.* (1990) Ten years of experience with Swedish bone-anchored hearing system. *Annals of Otology, Rhinology and Laryngology*, **99**, 1–16

JAHRSDOERFER, R. A. (1974) Congenital ear atresia. In: *Symposium on Reconstruction of the Auricle*, edited by R. Tanzer and M. Edgerton. Vol. X. St Louis: C. V. Mosby Co. pp. 150–160

MARX, H. (1926) Die Mißbildungen des Ohres. In: *Handbuch der Hals-Nasen-Ohrenheilkunde*, edited by Denker-Kahler, Bd. VI. Berlin: Springer-Verlag

MUSTARDE, J. C. (1963) The correction of prominent ears using simple mattress sutures. *British Journal of Plastic Surgery*, **16**, 170–176

NAGATA, S. (1993) A new method of total reconstruction of the auricle of microfia. *Plastic and Reconstructive Surgery*, **92**, 187–201

NAGATA, S. (1994) Modification of stages in total reconstruction of the auricle. Parts II, III, IV. *Plastic and Reconstructive Surgery*, **93**, 231–242, 243–253, 254–266

PENNINGTON, D. G., LAI, M. F. and PELLY, A. D. (1980) Successful replantation of a completely avulsed ear by microvascular anastomoses. *Plastic and Reconstructive Surgery*, **65**, 820–823

ROGERS, B. O. (1968) Microtic, lop, cup and protruding ears. *Plastic and Reconstructive Surgery*, **41**, 208–231

SPIRA, M. (1974) Early care of deformities of the auricle resulting from mechanical trauma. In: *Symposium on Reconstruction of the Auricle*, edited by R. Tanzer and M. Edgerton, Vol. X. St Louis: C. V. Mosby Co. pp. 204–212

SPIRA, M. and STAL, D. (1983) The conchal flap. An adjunct in otoplasty. *Annals of Plastic Surgery*, **11**, 291–298

STENSTRÖM, S. J. (1963) A natural technique for correcting congenitally prominent ears. *Plastic and Reconstructive Surgery*, **32**, 509–518

TANZER, R. (1974) Correction of microtia with autogenous costal cartilage. In: *Symposium on Reconstruction of the Auricle*, edited by R. Tanzer and M. Edgerton, Vol. X. St Louis: C. V. Mosby Co. pp. 46–57

TANZER, R. (1977) Congenital deformities. In: *Reconstructive Plastic Surgery*, 2nd edn, edited by J. M. Converse, Vol. 3. Philadelphia: W. B. Saunders. pp. 1671–1719

WALTER, C. (1972) Correction of deformities of the auricle. *Archives of Otorhinolaryngology*, **202**, 203–228; 229–252 (in German)

WEERDA, H. (1978) Covering defects after extirpation of tumours in the ear region. *Laryngologie, Rhinologie, Otologie*, **57**, 93–98 (in German)

WEERDA, H. (1979) Remarks on otoplasty and on total avulsion of the auricle. *Laryngologie, Rhinologie, Otologie*, **58**, 242–251 (in German)

WEERDA, H. (1980) The trauma of the auricle. *HNO*, **28**, 209–217 (in German)

WEERDA, H. (1982a) Our experience with the surgery of the auricle. I. Surgery of small deformities. *Laryngologie, Rhinologie, Otologie*, **61**, 346–349 (in German)

WEERDA, H. (1982b) Our experience with the surgery of the auricle. II. Surgery of the macrotia and the cup ear. *Laryngologie, Rhinologie, Otologie*, **61**, 350–353 (in German)

WEERDA, H. (1982c) Our experience with the surgery of the auricle. III. The mini ear and the severe cup ear deformities. *Laryngologie, Rhinologie, Otologie*, **61**, 493–496 (in German)

WEERDA, H. (1982d) Our experience with the surgery of the auricle. IV. Microtia. *Laryngologie, Rhinologie, Otologie*, **61**, 497–500 (in German)

WEERDA, H. (1984) Surgery of ear deformities in children. *Laryngologie, Rhinologie, Otologie*, **63**, 120–122 (in German)

WEERDA, H. (1985a) Embryology and structural anatomy of the external ear. *Facial Plastic Surgery*, **2**, 85–91

WEERDA, H. (1985b) Middle ear surgery in congenital malformations of the auricle with atresia. Experience with 89 operated ears. *HNO*, **33**, 449–452 (in German)

WEERDA, H. (1986) Fibrinkleber in der Ohrmuschelchirurgie. In: *Neue Techniken in der operativen Medizin*, edited by M. Reifferscheid. Berlin: Springer-Verlag

WEERDA, H. (1988) Classification of congenital deformities of the auricle. *Facial Plastic Surgery*, **5**, 385–388

WEERDA, H. (1994) The auricle. In: *Excision and Reconstruction in Head and Neck*, edited by D. Soutar and R. Tiwari. London: Churchill Livingstone.

WEERDA, H. and WALTER, C. (1984) Surgery of the pinna and surrounding area. In: *Plastic and Reconstructive Surgery of Head and Neck*, edited by P. H. Ward. St Louis: C. V. Mosby Co. pp. 827–846

9

Acute suppurative otitis media

R. J. Canter

A review of the current position of acute suppurative otitis media is a daunting task. The frequency of the condition has meant that it has attracted much interest from the research community and consequently there have been over 500 publications in major journals in the last 10 years. Because of problems in consistently defining acute suppurative otitis media, many of these publications will tend to group together data on serous otitis media and acute otitis media, which leads to particular problems in a review such as this. Furthermore, we all have a different perspective of this condition depending on where we practise, e.g. hospital versus the community; one country versus another. In the UK, a typical consultant otolaryngologist will cover a community of 100 000 people. Very few cases of acute suppurative otitis will be seen by such a consultant, but he or she will be familiar with many of the complications expected for the condition; this practice will generate a particular viewpoint. A colleague in general practice will be seeing such a condition almost daily but will seldom see in his or her life time many of the complications described in this review; this will generate another viewpoint. In the rest of Europe much more of the day-to-day otolaryngological problems are seen by someone with a specific specialist training and this will generate yet another viewpoint. In North America, where we would all recognize that doctors work in a more litigious environment, a further point of view would emerge. A colleague working in the developing world, with less in the way of resources, will see the problem quite differently. All these different viewpoints can be seen in the literature and it means, in my opinion, that it may not be possible to arrive at a 'correct' point of view in answering such questions as treating acute suppurative otitis media with or without antibiotics. At the end of the day it is important to respect each of these viewpoints and

this review is an attempt to provide a few signposts with respect to the condition and should be seen as such.

Definition

At first sight it would seem to be a straightforward task to define acute otitis media, but the topic is made complex by the large number of similar terms employed to encompass the wide pathological and clinical variation that is observed. Classification may be based on duration (Senturia *et al.*, 1980):

1 Acute (up to 3 weeks' duration)
2 Subacute (from 3 weeks to 3 months in duration)
3 Chronic (greater than 3 months in duration).

The Third and Fourth International Symposia on Otitis Media chose to define ear infections on clinical grounds dividing them into four groups (Sadé, 1985a; Klein, Tos and Hussl, 1989):

1 Myringitis
2 Acute suppurative otitis media (ASOM)
3 Secretory otitis media (SOM)
4 Chronic suppurative otitis media (CSOM).

Acute suppurative otitis media in this context was an abrupt infection of the middle ear of short duration.

This classification overlooks 'recurrent otitis media' (Paparella, Kimberley and Alleva, 1991). Paparella and his colleagues also introduced the term 'silent otitis media' to refer to clinically undetected or undetectable middle ear pathology (Paparella, Shea and Meyerhoff, 1980) and reasoned that simple forms of otitis media may progress behind an intact tympanic membrane towards advanced inflammatory disease and the destructive processes associated with these, e.g. granulation tissue, cholesterol granuloma, cholesteatoma and ossicular necrosis (Paparella, Kimberley and Alleva, 1991). This interesting work was developed from findings based on temporal bone pathology research, which probably explains why it has so far not become a popular concept with the practising clinician.

To the otologist, while it might be recognized that there exists a continuous spectrum from acute suppurative otitis media, through serous otitis media to chronic otitis media, the majority would place the distinction between those not operated on (acute suppurative otitis media) and those operated upon (serous otitis media and chronic suppurative otitis media) (Haggard and Hughes, 1991). Despite the confusion that exists when it comes to defining acute suppurative otitis media it is like the man who, when asked to define a 'unicorn', replies that he may have some difficulty in doing so to everyone's satisfaction but we would all recognize one if it walked into the room.

Epidemiology

Otitis media in all its forms is one of the most common diseases world-wide. In North America, in 1986, it accounted for 31 million visits to a physician at a cost of 3.5 billion dollars (Stool and Field, 1989). A review by Pukander, Sipila and Karma (1984) of 4500 Finnish adults and children calculated the annual incidence of acute suppurative otitis media per 100 person years to be 4.44 per cent. An Italian study found that acute suppurative otitis media comprised one third of the problems seen in paediatric practice during the first five years of life (Pestalozza, Romagnoli and Tessitore, 1988), but it was not associated with any other neonatal or prior health problem (O'Shea and Collins, 1987) except wheezy bronchitis (Alho *et al.*, 1990b).

McFadden *et al.* (1985) reported that acute suppurative otitis media in children fell into two distinct patterns. It was much more common in the younger (0–5 years) than in the older group (5–11 years) and factors such as season and sex were much more important and consequently most studies have paid more attention to this younger group, especially those children aged less than 2 years.

Teele, Klein and Rosner (1989) in a prospective cohort study of 877 children in greater Boston found that 62% had experienced one or more episodes of acute suppurative otitis media in the first year of life and 17% had experienced three or more episodes. By the age of three, 83% had experienced one or more episodes and 46% three or more episodes. In a large (*n* = 5356) Finnish birth cohort study for the first year of life, one-third experienced an episode of acute suppurative otitis media, 10% recurrently (more than three episodes) (Kero and Piekkala, 1987). Alho *et al.* (1991) found similar results with a cumulative incidence of 42.4% after the first 12 months and 71.0%

by 2 years with the greatest risks of developing acute suppurative otitis media in the second 6 months of life. They also made the observation that there is simply insufficient consistency in defining acute suppurative otitis media in epidemiological studies. A study (*n* = 129) by Hakansson (1989) in Vaxjo, Sweden reported an incidence of 29% during the first 18 months of life. A Scandinavian review of a number of studies estimated that up to 40% of children were affected in the first year of life and observed that the frequency of the condition may be on the increase (Puhakka, 1991) a view supported by a Far Eastern study (Huang *et al.*, 1991).

Acute suppurative otitis media was more common in males, those with a sibling history of acute suppurative otitis media and those not breast-fed (Kero and Piekkala, 1987; Teele, Klein and Rosner, 1989; Alho *et al.*, 1990b), but Sipila *et al.* (1980), in a Finnish study, found that attendance at a day-care centre was by far the most important risk factor, a finding supported by others (Pukander *et al.*, 1985; Froom and Culpepper, 1991). Low birth weight and prematurity were not felt to be important risk factors in the development of acute suppurative otitis media (Alho *et al.*, 1990a).

Most studies report a seasonal variation, being more common in the winter months, but Williamson, DePra and Sulzberger (1991) made the important observation that in the group with recurrent otitis media this seasonal change was not a feature. A prospective study in Sweden, designed to identify risk factors for children with recurrent acute suppurative otitis media (more than six episodes during a 12-month period), found no association with sex, familial history of allergy, duration of breast feeding, domestic environment or day-care centres (Harsten *et al.*, 1989a). An attempt to identify a genetically determined immunological factor in this group with recurrent acute suppurative otitis media did not meet with success in one study (Prellner *et al.*, 1985), but there is some evidence that, for this subgroup of children with recurrent acute suppurative otitis media, the HLA-A2 antigen was more common (80%) than in controls (56%) (Kalm *et al.*, 1991, 1992). The number of children who developed recurrent acute suppurative otitis media was small (*n* = 13) but it lends credence to the idea that children with recurrent acute suppurative otitis media are a separate group in which the main risk factor is age of first episode (less than 6 months) making it important to have an accurate diagnosis in this young age group.

Anatomical considerations

An assumption has been made by most otologists, a reasonable assumption but an assumption nevertheless, that the eustachian tube plays an important role in the aetiology of acute suppurative otitis media.

This may be summarized by the idea that failure of tubal closure leads to reduced protection against ascending infection from resident organisms in the nasopharynx into the middle ear (Magnuson and Falk, 1984). Unfortunately, the research to date has not really confirmed this assumption to the satisfaction of the scientific community. Careful anatomical studies of temporal bones of controls ($n = 33$) and those with evidence of acute suppurative otitis media ($n = 10$) have shown that the eustachian tube enlarges only a small degree with age, that there are wide variations in cross-sectional area compatible with normal biological function and that there was no difference between the normals and those with acute suppurative otitis media (Sadé *et al.*, 1985a, b, 1986). More detailed analysis of the growth with age of the cartilaginous and bony part of the eustachian tube in a larger series of normals ($n = 115$) was felt by the authors to contradict the hypothesis ascribing the high incidence of acute suppurative otitis media in children because of a wider eustachian tube than adults (Luntz and Sadé, 1988). The elastin content of the tissues surrounding the eustachian tube lumen is known to be less in children than in adults and may account for the relative floppiness of the eustachian tube in children but, while this is thought to play a part in serous otitis media, it may also be relevant in those children with acute suppurative otitis media (Sando, Takahashi and Matsune, 1991).

Experimental tubal occlusion in rats, undertaken as part of a study looking at the pathogenesis of nasal polyps, led after a short time, to the development of acute suppurative otitis media in the majority of animals. Histological examination of the polypoid protrusions of mucosa found in the middle ear revealed accumulation of fluid and inflammatory cells in the lamina propria, although the precise significance of this in relation to acute suppurative otitis media is not as yet clear (Larsen and Tos, 1991).

Any anatomical analysis has serious limitations, but any physiological study may be more difficult still. Jorgensen and Holmquist (1984) investigated middle ear pressures after the Toynbee manoeuvre (swallowing against occluded nostrils) in a control group and those with middle ear disease. They found that 2% of the control group developed a positive middle ear pressure compared with 56% in those with evidence of middle ear disease. Whether this is important in the aetiology of acute suppurative otitis media is unknown. An interesting study by Stenstrom, Bylander Groth and Ingvarsson (1991) examined a variety of measures of eustachian tube function in otitis prone (over 11 episodes) children ($n = 50$) against those with no history ($n = 49$) and found that active tubal function (muscular opening function) was the only measure to reveal any difference between the two groups, but admitted that available techniques of eustachian tube function are not sufficiently refined. The part played by surfactant in lower-

ing opening pressure is also unclear (White, Hermansson and Svinhufvud, 1990). Although otitis media with effusion is now known to be more common in children born and treated for cleft palate, there appears to be only a slight increase in the incidence of acute suppurative otitis media in this group (Rynnel Dagoo *et al.*, 1992). Approximately 5% of children and adolescents with cystic fibrosis will experience an episode of acute suppurative otitis media at some point (Cepero *et al.*, 1987), but perhaps the relative infrequency of this as a problem reflects the fact that many of them are receiving long-term prophylactic antibiotics to prevent pneumonia.

Symptoms and signs

The accurate diagnosis of acute suppurative otitis media depends not on a single piece of information but on the evaluation of a number of factors including fever, pain in the ear, other respiratory symptoms and the appearance and movement of the eardrum.

There may well have been a pre-existing respiratory viral infection typically about 6 days before the onset of acute suppurative otitis media (Arola *et al.*, 1990). The most common symptom is pain in the ear. This may vary greatly in severity and was found in one study ($n = 335$) to be severe in 42%, mild to moderate in 40% and absent in 17 per cent. This last group was found to be especially true of children less than 2 years of age. Fever is usually present and may be severe enough to mimic much more serious disease (Surpure, 1987). Interestingly, despite the presence of local hyperaemia there seems to be no further rise in temperature in the ear canal compared with the rise in body temperature (Terndrup and Wong, 1991).

The appearance of the eardrum in acute suppurative otitis media progresses from injection of the vessels along the handle of the malleus and around the periphery, to reddening with bulging of the drum and finally to perforation and discharge. The discharge may be serous, serosanguineous or mucopurulent. At this stage the diagnosis is obvious but, in the early stages, it is much more difficult to be certain. The International Primary network study involving 3660 children in Australia, Belgium, Great Britain, Israel, Netherlands, New Zealand, Canada, Switzerland and the USA tried to establish certainty of diagnosis of acute suppurative otitis media among primary health care workers. Certainty of diagnosis was related to age. In the youngest group, 0–12 months, the diagnostic certainty was 58 per cent. In the group aged 13–30 months this rose to 66% and in the group aged over 30 months increased still further to 73%. The diagnostic certainty in all age groups was related to the stage of disease and was increased by finding discharging pus or bulging of the tympanic membrane. In the group aged 13–30 months, redness of the tympanic membrane and pain assisted diagnosis and in the older group of over 30 months, reduction in hearing and a recent history of upper respiratory infection was particularly useful (Froom *et al.*, 1990).

Even among otolaryngologists interobserver variation of the appearance of the eardrum in acute suppurative otitis media and its healing phase may be substantial (Holmberg *et al.*, 1985). If tympanometry is undertaken it appears to be better at picking up the reduction in tympanic membrane mobility (Holmberg *et al.*, 1986), but if this practice is formally tested in primary care it is not clear whether this aids the diagnostic certainty in the clinical setting (Lildholdt *et al.*, 1991); this is because the colour and appearance seem to be important in reaching a diagnosis.

The eardrum will eventually perforate in approximately one-third of cases and when it does so, 85% will occur in the anteroinferior quadrant and the remaining 15% in the posterosuperior quadrant (Berger, 1989).

Overall, in approximately one-quarter of patients, there will be a resolution of the inflammatory process with no evidence of remaining effusion within 2 weeks. In approximately 70% of cases a persistent effusion will remain for up to 3 months after the acute inflammatory phase has settled and in 10% of these it may persist beyond this time necessitating the need for insertion of a ventilation tube (Nakajima and Hattori, 1989). Closure of any perforation will occur in more than 90% of cases within 1 month (Berger, 1989).

Microbiology

For a condition that is so common and so universal, only a modest number of studies exists examining the frequency of bacterial pathogens in acute suppurative otitis media. There are obvious difficulties in obtaining material from the middle ear to identify an organism. Aspiration of infected fluid in the middle ear is not routinely made in all parts of the world and, while there may be a modest relationship between the presence of a significant organism in the nasopharynx and the middle ear, it is not close enough to rely on when undertaking studies of the infective agent in the middle ear (Lundgren and Ingvarsson, 1986).

While it is true that many organisms may be responsible for the development of acute suppurative otitis media, essentially only three account for the majority of infections and should, in the absence of bacteriological data, be regarded as the principal organisms. In the largest study to date ($n = 7396$) *Streptococcus pneumoniae* was found to be the most common organism, followed by *Haemophilus influenzae* and *Moraxella (Branhamella) catarrhalis* and ac-

counted for all but 10% of the organisms isolated (Bluestone, Stephenson and Martin, 1992). A recent European study found *Haemophilus influenzae* to be the most common organism followed by *Streptococcus pneumoniae* and *Branhamella catarrhalis* (Gehanno *et al.*, 1992). European studies in general have shown slightly different results recording *Haemophilus influenzae* as more common than *Streptococcus pneumoniae* but observing that as time goes on the pattern is changing towards that reported in the larger American series (Gehanno *et al.*, 1992; Del Castillo Martin, Barrio Gomez de Aguero and Garcia Perea, 1992). Often more than one organism could be cultured from the aspirate from the same ear. Sterile cultures or those producing non-pathogens may account for up to 30% of cultures from aspirates.

Branhamella catarrhalis was originally regarded as a harmless inhabitant of the pharynx, but this was caused by confusion with *Neisseria cinerea* and, until the two could be separately identified bacteriologically, its importance as a pathogen was not appreciated. This interest has largely arisen out of the fact that a high proportion of aspirates in recent years have been beta-lactamase producing organisms and hence resistant to many conventional first-line treatments. The emergence in European studies of *Branhamella catarrhalis* as an important organism seems to be about 4 years after that of North American studies; an earlier study in 1988 did not record it as being significant at that time (Francois *et al.*, 1988). *Branhamella catarrhalis* appears to be seasonal, becoming significantly more common during the winter months (Van Hare *et al.*, 1987; Sarubbi *et al.*, 1990).

Over the last decade or so, the proportion of beta-lactamase producing *Haemophilus influenzae* and *Branhamella catarrhalis* has progressively risen to approximately 20% for the former (Francois *et al.*, 1989; Baron and Begue, 1991; Celin *et al.*, 1991; Bluestone *et al.*, 1992) and up to 75% (Shurin and Van Hare, 1986; Van Hare *et al.*, 1987; Catlin, 1990) or even higher (Suzuki *et al.*, 1988) for the latter. As these beta-lactamase organisms increase it may become more important to obtain accurate local epidemiological data on the frequency of such resistant strains when considering first-line treatment, especially for very young children.

A study of very young infants (less than 3 months) and neonates showed a somewhat different picture with *Streptococcus pneumoniae* accounting for 19%, *Haemophilus influenzae* 9%, *Branhamella catarrhalis* 7%, *Staphylococcus aureus* 17%, coagulase-negative staphylococci 22%, with more than half the organisms producing beta-lactamases (Karma *et al.*, 1987a). An analysis of treatment failures (treatment failures and relapsing acute suppurative otitis media) in a population of young children demonstrated that 52% had a beta-lactamase producing organism but the numbers in the study were small ($n = 21$).

In a further study, looking specifically at acute

suppurative otitis media in adults ($n = 34$), *Haemophilus influenzae* (26%) (22% beta-lactamase producing) was as common as *Streptococcus pneumoniae* (21%) and *Branhamella catarrhalis* less so at 9% (Celin *et al.*, 1991). Other organisms such as *Streptococcus pyogenes* and *Pseudomonas aeruginosa* were also noted.

The importance of anaerobes is unclear. Grampositive cocci were recovered in 25% of aspirates in one study but, at the moment, it does not seem to be important to consider their presence when contemplating treatment (Brook, 1987).

While the common cold is widely thought to be the 'commonest cause of acute suppurative otitis media' formal identification of responsible viruses can prove to be difficult and the role of viral infections would seem to be, on the basis of research carried out to date, only a modest contributor to the aetiology of acute suppurative otitis media. In an analysis of 137 children with acute suppurative otitis media, 15% had respiratory syncytial virus antigen in the middle ear fluid and only 3% were found to have antibody to the adenovirus (Sarkkinen *et al.*, 1985). A more recent study found that rhinovirus infection was more common (24%) (Arola *et al.*, 1990). The bacteriology was the same in both viral and non-viral groups and the clinical outcome was unaffected by the presence or absence of viruses in most studies, but one found that the clinical course was worse when viruses were grown from middle ear fluid (Chonmaitree *et al.*, 1992). The mechanism was unknown. Perhaps the importance of viruses lies in recognition of the fact that in epidemics of respiratory syncytial virus and rhinoviruses, the incidence of acute suppurative otitis media is likely to rise.

Treatment

Controversy in the treatment of acute suppurative otitis media surrounds the decision whether to treat with antibiotics or to rely solely on supportive treatment while the episode is allowed to resolve naturally. Your point of view will depend upon the nature of your practice and the country in which you practice. In the UK, a hospital-based viewpoint would suggest, as Browning (1990) has argued, that antibiotics are not justified in most cases, whereas those in a community-based practice would argue, as Bain (1990) has done, that antibiotic treatment is justified. Certainly this latter view would seem to be supported by studies of day-to-day family practice (Mills, 1984).

This UK view was at variance with a Dutch consensus which suggested that a period of watchful waiting was appropriate in those aged 1 year and over but that antibiotic treatment was important in those in the first year of life (Hordijk, 1992) and this is reflected in studies of the day-to-day practice of this population of doctors (De Melker and Kuyvenhoven, 1991). This practice is supported by an earlier study

which reported that, in 90% of cases, children recover within 3–4 days and, as only 3% develop a severe illness, conservative therapy with nose drops (no longer so popular) and analgesics was acceptable in the early stages of the illness (van Buchem, Peeters and Van't Hof, 1985). The addition of antihistamines and decongestants as part of the treatment rationale is now pretty well discredited (Schnore *et al.*, 1986; Karma *et al.*, 1987b).

In the American literature, there seems to be very little controversy about the use of antibiotics. The arguments have been summarized by Bluestone and are based on the reduction in mortality concomitant with the introduction of antibiotics in the USA, dismissal of the argument that the use of antibiotics leads to an increase in the incidence of serous otitis media, (believing that this is due to the increase in day-care attendance and reduction in breast feeding) and finally the more rapid resolution of the disease (Bluestone, 1990; Canafax and Giebink, 1991).

Much of the controversy will remain unresolved until large double-blind placebo controlled trials with well-defined inclusion criteria and outcome measures have been performed. A comprehensive survey of the English language literature between 1965 and 1989, analysed 50 studies but found that only four fully complied with the above criteria and no formal conclusion could be drawn regarding the treatment with antibiotics from these studies (Claessen *et al.*, 1992). The vast majority of the studies compared the results of treatment with one antibiotic against another and in these studies the 'Polyanna phenomenon' (if efficacy is measured by symptomatic response, drugs with poor antibacterial activity will appear to be clinically effective in the treatment of acute suppurative otitis media) will affect the assessment of results (Marchant *et al.*, 1992).

Oddly enough, if the decision to treat with an antibiotic has been taken, much common ground can be found. There is now widespread acceptance that first-line treatment with amoxycillin is the drug of choice (Mills, 1984; Eichenwald, 1985; Baron and Begue, 1991; De Melker and Kuyvenhoven, 1991; Giebink and Canafax, 1991; Thoene and Johnson, 1991; Bluestone, 1992, 1993; Klass and Klein, 1992; Kligman, 1992) and that this is effective when given rectally (Bergstrom, Bertilson and Movin, 1988), although given by this route gastrointestinal problems were more common. High dose regimens for shorter periods of time (750 mg amoxycillin twice a day for 2 days) have been shown to be equally effective (Bain, Murphy and Ross, 1985).

For those patients who are sensitive to penicillin, cefixime (Principi and Marchisio, 1991) and trimethoprim/sulphamethoxazole combinations (Feldman, Momy and Dulberg, 1988) were shown to be as effective as amoxycillin. However, concern has recently been expressed about the rare but serious adverse reactions such as leucopenia, thrombocytopenia and Stevens–Johnson syndrome seen in trimethoprim/sulphamethoxazole combinations. These are usually attributable to the sulphonamide component. Because of these its use cannot be recommended as a first-line treatment when the antibiotics are available. Trimethoprim alone is not a suitable alternative because of its poor activity against Branhamella catarrhalis (Lewis and Reves, 1995). Erythromycin is popular in the UK as first-line treatment in those who are penicillin sensitive. Penetration into middle ear fluid is much slower than beta-lactam antibiotics but excretion is also delayed; whether one makes up for the other is unclear (Sundberg *et al.*, 1979).

However, it is important to have some knowledge of the prevalence of beta-lactamase producing organisms in the treated population and if this is high then treatment failure may also be unacceptably high. There is a good choice of effective second-line treatment ranging from amoxycillin/clavulanic acid (Baron and Begue, 1991; Giebink and Canafax, 1991; Thoene and Johnson, 1991; Bluestone, 1992; Klass and Klein, 1992; Kligman, 1992; Lambert Zechovsky *et al.*, 1992), trimethoprim/sulphamethoxazole (Feldman, Sutcliffe and Dulberg, 1990; Giebink and Canafax, 1991; Thoene and Johnson, 1991; Bluestone, 1992; Kligman, 1992), cefixime (Kligman, 1992; Rosenfeld *et al.*, 1992; Bluestone, 1993), erythromycin/sulfisoxazole (Giebink and Canafax, 1991; Kligman, 1992), cefuroxime (Kligman, 1992), loracarbef (Gran *et al.*, 1991; Foshee, 1992) and cefaclor (Giebink and Canafax, 1991; Thoene and Johnson, 1991), although recent studies have suggested that there is a higher failure rate with cefaclor than with some of the other antibiotics (Lambert Zechovsky *et al.*, 1992; Berman and Roark, 1993).

What is strikingly absent from the literature is studies involving treatment versus non-treatment for acute suppurative otitis media in adults. Perhaps it is a combination of the frequency of the condition in children, coupled with some reluctance historically to accept that children experience pain in the same way as adults that has resulted in the practice of treating the condition conservatively. It would take a confident physician to prescribe an adult with acute suppurative otitis media nothing but pain relief and no antibiotics.

Treatment failure

This has been shown to be dependent on age and might reflect difficulty in diagnosis and compliance. In an analysis of 300 episodes, failure occurred in 18% in the first year of life, 4.5% in the second and 4.2% in the third year (Harsten *et al.*, 1989b). It was associated with non-compliance or a superimposed viral illness (Harrison and Belhorn, 1991; Prellner, 1992), winter, history of recurrent suppurative otitis

media or an antibiotic administered one month beforehand (Berman and Roark, 1993).

In the event of failure with first-line treatment, there are a number of alternative strategies. These include repeating a course of a first-line antibiotic for 10 days, changing to a second-line antibiotic particularly when practising in an area with a high prevalence of beta-lactamase producing organisms (Harrison and Belhorn, 1991), or undertaking a myringotomy (Harrison and Belhorn, 1991; Bluestone, 1992; Hordijk, 1992). Myringotomy is still considered by some to be important in the first-line treatment of acute suppurative otitis media even with the advent of newer antibiotics because subsequent otitis media with effusion is thought to be less common as a sequel to the acute episode (Mori *et al.*, 1992).

Treatment for recurrent acute otitis media

There is a population of children whose lives are blighted by repeated episodes of acute suppurative otitis media and some form of treatment seems mandatory. Experience with long-term low dose antibiotic has confirmed that it will reduce the number of episodes very satisfactorily and the side effects are mild and reversible (Bergus, 1991; Teele, 1991; Paradise, 1992; Randall, Fornadley and Kennedy, 1992) and anxiety about colonic overgrowth with *Clostridium difficile* was not borne out in clinical practice (Cohen *et al.*, 1992). Adenoidectomy was also effective in this group (Schwartz and Schwartz, 1987; Teele, 1991) as was the insertion of ventilating tubes (Gonzalez *et al.*, 1986). However, there was a price to pay by this latter surgical intervention and in a randomized study of ventilating tubes versus myringotomy/no surgery, tympanosclerosis, retraction and atrophy were more common in the surgically treated ear, which was reflected in a reduction in hearing; although this reduction in hearing was not considered to be significant (Le, Freeman and Fireman, 1991).

Complications

Complications of acute suppurative otitis media of any sort are very uncommon. Surveys of children with a previous history of acute suppurative otitis media show no or only a marginal effect on air conduction and none on inner ear function (Karma, Sipila and Rahko, 1989; Rahko, Karma and Sipila, 1989). There have been reports that hearing thresholds may be elevated in the extended high frequency range (> 8 kHz) following a history of acute suppurative otitis media. These frequencies are not tested in a routine audiogram and the phenomenon may be more frequent than is appreciated at the moment.

Because bone conduction cannot be tested separately at such high frequencies, it is unknown if this is a middle or inner ear effect (Margolis and Hunter, 1991). Animal work suggests that it is likely to be the latter.

Children with recurrent acute suppurative otitis media, treated either by repeated medical intervention or ventilating tubes have been assessed for complicating sequelae (Pichichero, Berghash and Hengerer, 1989). All complications were more frequent in the surgically treated group: tympanosclerosis, 52% versus 7%; atrophy of the tympanic membrane, 40% versus 4%; hearing loss, defined as a hearing threshold greater than 20 dB, according to frequency tested was 9–18% in the surgical group, and 4–9% in the medical group. Unless there are other reasons for considering surgical intervention such as persisting serous otitis media and a hearing loss, treatment of recurrent acute suppurative otitis media by surgical means should not be the automatic first choice.

Facial paralysis in acute suppurative otitis media is rare. In a survey of children aged 1 month to 14.5 years with facial paralysis, 9% were caused by acute suppurative otitis media (Truy *et al.*, 1992). Occasionally facial palsy may be the presenting symptom (Henderson and Baldone, 1989). There is complete agreement that the treatment should consist of appropriate antibiotics and surgical drainage in the form of a myringotomy (Bluestone, 1984; Selesnick and Jackler, 1993) and many would consider adding steroids such as prednisone, although its use has not demonstrated an effect on the rate of recovery (Truy *et al.*, 1992), despite animal work supporting the notion that it speeds the repair of mechanical injury caused by compression (Adour and Hetzler, 1984). Complete recovery of the facial nerve with the above treatment can be expected and other measures such as facial nerve decompression should rarely, if ever, be attempted (Selesnick and Jackler, 1993).

Otogenic intracranial complications in children arise more often from acute rather than chronic suppurative ear disease and have a mortality of about 1% (Grigor'ev, Zagainova and Ternovoi, 1990). The younger child, especially those less than 12 months old, is particularly at risk for this rare complication and accounted for 61% cases in one large series; this reinforces the notion that treatment of the acute episode with antibiotics in this age group is appropriate. There is a high incidence of *Haemophilus influenzae* type B in this age group and any such treatment should include an antibiotic with good activity against this organism (Friedman, McGill and Healy, 1990). The mechanism of spread may be via the oval window in a Mondini-type inner ear deformity or along the horizontal portion of the facial nerve (Barcz *et al.*, 1985) in either a dehiscent segment or via the canniculus for the stapedius muscle or chorda tympani (Takahashi, Nakamura and Yui., 1985), but these routes of spread are not supported by pathological studies. An analysis of 16 temporal bones from children who had died from meningitis, found evidence of acute suppurative otitis media in 14 but no pathway from the tympanomastoid compartment could be found. Inner ear involvement appeared to be retrograde from the meninges (Eavey *et al.*, 1985).

Acute mastoiditis

In a sense every case of acute suppurative otitis media will involve the mastoid chamber, but the clinical picture that we recognize as acute mastoiditis is rare. Palva calculated the annual incidence in a European community as 0.004% (Palva, Virtanen and Makinen, 1985). The common perception is that this complication of acute suppurative otitis media has become much less frequent due to the world-wide use of antibiotics (Faye Lund, 1989; Gaffney, O'Dwyer and Maguire, 1991; Shanley and Murphy, 1992), but better housing and living conditions may have played a greater part than is appreciated. The use of antibiotics may be changing the presenting clinical picture from a more acute episode to one with a more prolonged clinical picture, so-called latent mastoiditis, and this changing pattern has been observed as the medical community changes its prescribing habits (Faye Lund, 1989). Acute mastoiditis can be bilateral (Andreassen and Fons, 1986) and can occur in aural atresia (Zalzal, 1987).

It is still very much a disease of children, especially very young children, and in one study 47% of cases were seen in children aged less than 1 year (Prescott and Malan, 1991), although perhaps this figure is rather high (Zagainova and Nevezhin, 1991). In children, the aetiology is generally after an episode of acute suppurative otitis media (Debruyne and Stoffels, 1985), but in parts of the world where chronic suppurative ear disease in children is common, this may be more important in the aetiology (Ibekwe and Okoye, 1988).

The organisms encountered in acute mastoiditis are, unsurprisingly, much the same as those encountered in acute suppurative otitis media except that pneumococci and beta-haemolytic streptococci may be more likely to cause acute mastoiditis (Prellner and Rydell, 1986). Anaerobic organisms may be present as well (Ogle and Lauer, 1986; Scheibel and Urtes, 1987) and in one study these could be grown in 80% of cases (Maharaj *et al.*, 1987).

It is not always possible to obtain an organism and success seems to be related to the source of material obtained in an effort to cultivate an organism. The most reliable method of obtaining an organism is from the abscess itself (Hawkins and Dru, 1983; Zagainova and Nevezhin, 1991). Cultures from blood were the least successful (14%) followed by mastoid mucosa (68%) and the abscess itself (81%) (Zagainova and Nevezhin, 1991).

It is also important to consider the possibility of infection with *Mycobacterium tuberculosis* and one study reported an incidence of 11% with this particular organism among cases of acute mastoiditis (Hawkins and Dru, 1983). Mastoiditis with *Mycobacterium avis* has also been recognized (Wardrop and Pillsbury, 1984).

Clinical presentation

Tenderness around the ear is generally present but relying on observing changes in the tympanic membrane can be misleading. An abnormality of the eardrum may only be present in one-third of cases (Nadal *et al.*, 1990) particularly as examination in an unwell infant in the first year of life may be very difficult. If the eardrum is intact, it may be associated with a higher incidence of complications, presumably due to the absence of any drainage at all from the infected mastoid air cells (Samuel and Fernandes, 1985).

The classical sign of retroauricular swelling and protrusion of the auricle (see Plate 3/9/I) is still that which alerts the clinician to the development of acute mastoiditis and is the most common sign present in most series (Samuel and Fernandes, 1985; Ogle and Lauer, 1986; Warnaar, Snoep and Stals, 1989; Nadal *et al.*, 1990) although, perhaps with the use of antibiotics, these presenting signs are becoming less common (Zagainova and Nevezhin, 1991).

A classical abscess is present in about half of cases (Samuel and Fernandes, 1985; Nadal *et al.*, 1990). This may track into the posterior fossa to produce meningitis, a posterior fossa abscess, a lateral sinus thrombosis, cerebellitis or a cerebellar abscess, or into the neck to produce a Bezold's abscess. In Bezold's abscess spread is via the mastoid tip into either the sheath of the sternomastoid muscle or the classical route via the digastric muscle to the chin. Bezold's abscess is rarely seen in contemporary otolaryngological practice. A review in 1991 (Gaffney, O'Dwyer and Maguire, 1991) could find only seven cases reported in the literature from 1979 to 1991. All these complications may occur some months after the initial acute episode (Shuster, Chumakov and Chkannikov, 1991). A large series (*n* = 335) of episodes of acute mastoiditis complicated by extension of the disease found that intracranial sepsis was the most common (67%), followed by meningitis (25%), brain abscess (16%), extradural abscess (15%) and lateral sinus thrombosis (12%) (Samuel, Fernandes and Steinberg, 1986).

A facial palsy may develop but appears to be more common in those cases of acute mastoiditis caused by *Mycobacterium tuberculosis*, occurring in 40% in one series (Samuel and Fernandes, 1986).

There is universal agreement that there is no real place any more for the use of plain mastoid X-rays as an aid in the diagnosis and particularly in the management of the condition (Hawkins *et al.*, 1983; Rubin and Wei, 1985; Rosen, Ophir and Marshak, 1986), but that CT scans can be helpful in the early diagnosis and detection of complications. Obtaining good imaging in small unwell children without an anaesthetic may be very difficult.

Treatment

In former days the treatment of acute mastoiditis would centre around surgical drainage of the mastoid, but a more conservative approach is emerging. One-third or more of patients will settle without the need for mastoid surgery (Rubin and Wei, 1985; Ogle and Lauer, 1986; Nadal *et al.*, 1990). Initial treatment should take the form of an appropriate intravenous antibiotic together with a myringotomy, with or without a ventilation tube. If a response is seen it may be possible, in conjunction with the Department of Paediatrics to continue treatment on a carefully supervised outpatient basis (Einhorn *et al.*, 1992). Mastoid surgery should be reserved for those who start to develop a subperiosteal abscess, any complication, or no response after 24–48 hours (Hawkins *et al.*, 1983; Ogle and Lauer, 1986; Nadal *et al.*, 1990). If surgery is undertaken, the vast majority (90%) will require a formal simple mastoidectomy, but a small number will recover with simple incision and drainage of the subperiosteal abscess and a few will require a more extensive mastoidectomy (Hawkins *et al.*, 1983).

Cortical mastoidectomy

Preoperative investigations

In addition to the use of radiological imaging to assess the status of the mastoid (Figure 9.1) the subject's fitness for anaesthesia should be assessed. A record should be made of facial movements, carefully recording any deficit but it is recognized that in small unwell children this may be impossible in practice. If there is any clinical evidence that the central nervous system is involved, a CT scan should establish whether or not there are intracranial collections of pus so that, if necessary, transfer to a neurosurgical unit should be considered prior to the mastroid surgery.

Preparation

As a postauricular incision is employed (see Plate 3/9/II), it may be necessary to shave 1 cm or so of hair behind the ear, in order that the incision can be made close to the hairline. It is hardly ever necessary to shave any hair in children. Intraoperative facial nerve monitoring is becoming more widely available and the needles that record the action potentials can

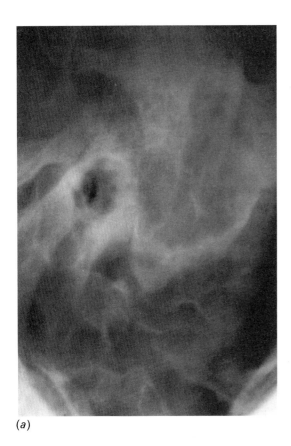

(*a*)

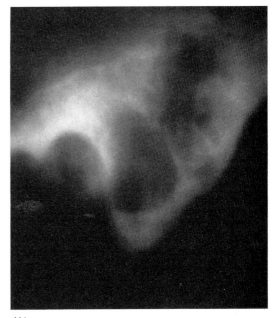

(*b*)

Figure 9.1 (*a*) Lateral x-ray showing coalescent mastoiditis in an adult secondary to cholesteatoma. (*b*) Lateral tomogram of same patient. The cholesteatoma is shown as the erosion with the smooth outline in the mastoid process and the abscess as the irregular cavity above it. (Reproduced by kind permission of the Editor)

be placed into the small muscles of the face before the operative site is towelled and draped.

The operation

The principal complication that needs to be borne in mind is damage to the facial nerve in small infants. At birth, the child has no mastoid process or only the most rudimentary one and so in small children in the first few months of life, the facial nerve may be superficial and higher than expected as it leaves the stylomastoid foramen. Consequently, the standard postauricular incision may sever the facial nerve. In very small infants, in their first month or so of life, it is advisable to make the initial incision above the ear and extend this posteriorly and inferiorly but no lower than the level of the meatus. Any further extension of this incision can be done with careful dissection so that any high facial nerve can be identified and damage avoided.

Any subperiosteal pus can be aspirated with a needle and syringe and inoculated into suitable transport media. Once the cortical bone is uncovered, the bone is removed with a drill and the mastoid air system entered. Not infrequently a communication from the subperiosteum to the mastoid air cell system

will have already been formed and this can be extended to open up the cortical mastoid. In the acute mastoid, simple drainage is usually all that is required but in establishing drainage it is important to be sure that the mastoid antrum has a good communication with the middle ear and that no 'blockage' by membranes, adhesions or granulations exist. This can be assessed by passing a small Dundas-Grant or other suitable probe into the aditus. If this communication is small or absent then a fine bone curette or fine ended drill can be used to enlarge the aditus. Any other collection of infected cells in the sinodural angle, anteriorly into the root of the zygoma, superiorly into the squamous tympanic bone, posteriorly into the occipital bone, inferiorly into the mastoid tip or into cells over the vertical part of the facial nerve should be removed. If the operation becomes technically too difficult because of bleeding or extensive granulations, then it is perfectly acceptable to close the wound with drainage and re-explore the ear a week or so later with the help if necessary of a more experienced colleague. Treatment in the meantime with antibiotics might not only lead to an easier surgical enviroment within the ear but even to complete resolution of the infection.

Extension into the petrous apex

Significant extension of an acute infection from the middle ear or mastoid into the petrous apex is fortunately extremely rare because the patterns and routes of such extensions are variable and complicated. The pneumatized spaces of the temporal bone have been classified by Allam into five regions which are further divided into areas (Allam, 1969):

Middle ear region

Mesotympanic area
Epitympanic area
Hypotympanic area
Protympanic area
Posterior tympanic area

Mastoid region

Mastoid antrum area
Peripheral mastoid areas: tegmental, sinodural, sinal, facial and tip cells

Perilabyrinthine region

Supralabyrinthine area
Infralabyrinthine area

Petrous apex region

Peritubal area
Apical area

Accessory region

Zygomatic area
Squamous area
Occipital area
Styloid area

The air cells within these areas connect with one another to form tracts along which infection can proceed. Figure 9.2 shows the routes that these tracts can take as infection spreads from the middle ear and mastoid region towards the petrous apex. Historical descriptions by various authors have given rise to these various names. These approaches will be used only rarely but may be employed in situations when the middle ear and cortical mastoid disease has responded to surgery and antibiotics, but clinically (e.g. Gradenigo's syndrome) or visible on imaging, there appears to be continuing disease at the petrous apex.

Eagleton's operation

This is a superior approach to the petrous apex that involves removal of the tegmen to the base of zygoma, together with removal of part of the squamous temporal bone. The dura of the middle fossa can now be elevated to expose the petrous apex.

Thornvaldt's operation

This is another superior approach along the supralabyrinthine tracts. As the dissection proceeds it merges with that of Eagleton.

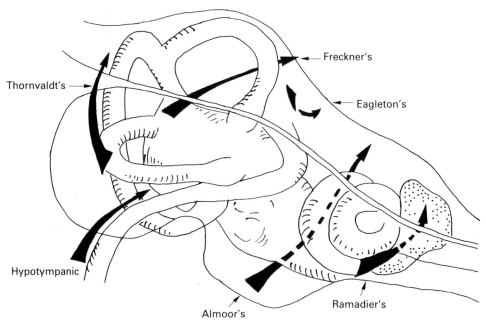

Figure 9.2 Routes of infection to the petrous apex (after Mawson, 1979)

Almoor's operation
This involves an inferior approach to the petrous apex through a space bounded by the cochlea, the carotid artery and the tegmen tympani.

Lempert-Ramadier's operation
This uses an approach slightly anterior to that of Almoor's operation that pursues the peritubal cells to the petrous apex that exist between the cochlea and the carotoid artery.

Frenckner's operation
This is an approach to the petrous apex through the arch of the superior semicircular canal. The blood supply of the arch arises from within this arch and some labyrinthine loss is almost inevitable with this approach. It has to be combined with an inferior approach.

References

ADOUR, K. K. and HETZLER, D. G. (1984) Current medical treatment for facial palsy. *American Journal of Otology*, **5**, 499–502

ALHO, O. P., KOIVU, M., HARTIKAINEN SORRI, A. L., SORRI, M., KILKKU, O. and RANTAKALLIO, P. (1990a) Is a child's history of acute otitis media and respiratory infection already determined in the antenatal and perinatal period? *International Journal of Pediatric Otorhinolaryngology*, **19**, 129–137

ALHO, O. P., KOIVU, M., SORRI, M. and RANTAKALLIO, P. (1990b) Risk factors for recurrent acute otitis media and respiratory infection in infancy. *International Journal of Pediatric Otorhinolaryngology*, **19**, 151–161

ALHO, O. P., KOIVU, M., SORRI, M. and RANTAKALLIO, P. (1991) The occurrence of acute otitis media in infants. A life-table analysis. *International Journal of Pediatric Otorhinolaryngology*, **21**, 7–14

ALLAM, A. F. (1969) Pneumatization of the temporal bone. *Annals of Otology, Rhinology and Laryngology*, **78**, 49–63

ANDREASSEN, U. K. and FONS, M. (1986) [Bilateral acute mastoiditis. A complication which still exists]. Dobbeltsidig akut mastoidit. En stadig eksisterende komplikation. *Ugeskrift For Laeger*, **148**, 961–962

AROLA, M., RUUSKANEN, O., ZIEGLER, T., MERTSOLA, J., NANTO SALONEN, K. *et al.* (1990) Clinical role of respiratory virus infection in acute otitis media. *Pediatrics*, **86**, 848–855

BAIN, J. (1990) Childhood otalgia: acute otitis media. 2. Justification for antibiotic use in general practice. *British Medical Journal*, **300**, 1006–1007

BAIN, J., MURPHY, E. and ROSS, F. (1985) Acute otitis media: clinical course among children who received a short course of high dose antibiotic. *British Medical Journal (Clinical Research Edition)*, **291**, 1243–1246

BARCZ, D. V., WOOD, R. P., STEARS, J., JAFEK, B. W. and SHIELDS, M. (1985) Subarachnoid space: middle ear pathways and recurrent meningitis. *American Journal of Otology*, **6**, 157–163

BARON, S. and BEGUE, P. (1991) [Antibiotic treatment of acute otitis media.] Traitement antibiotique de l'otite moyenne aigue. *Annales de Pediatrie (Paris)*, **38**, 549–555

BERGER, G. (1989) Nature of spontaneous tympanic membrane perforation in acute otitis media in children. *Journal of Laryngology and Otology*, **103**, 1150–1153

BERGSTROM, B. K., BERTILSON, S. O. and MOVIN, G. (1988) Clinical evaluation of rectally administered ampicillin in acute otitis media. *Journal of International Medical Research*, **16**, 376–385

BERGUS, G. R. (1991) Staving off acute otitis media. When is prophylaxis with antibiotics desirable? *Postgraduate Medicine*, **90**, 99–106

BERMAN, S. and ROARK, R. (1993) Factors influencing outcome in children treated with antibiotics for acute otitis media. *Pediatric Infectious Diseases Journal*, **12**, 20–24

BLUESTONE, C. D. (1984) Surgical management of otitis media. *Pediatric Infectious Diseases Journal*, **3**, 392–396

BLUESTONE, C. D. (1990) Rationale for antimicrobial therapy of otitis media. In: *Update on Otitis Media*, edited by J. D. Nelson. London, New York: Royal Society of Medicine Services. pp. 23–32

BLUESTONE, C. D. (1992) Current therapy for otitis media and criteria for evaluation of new antimicrobial agents. *Clinical Infectious Diseases*, **14**, (Suppl. 2), S197–S203

BLUESTONE, C. D. (1993) Review of cefixime in the treatment of otitis media in infants and children. *Pediatric Infectious Diseases Journal*, **12**, 75–82

BLUESTONE, C. D., STEPHENSON, J. S. and MARTIN, L. M. (1992) Ten-year review of otitis media pathogens. *Pediatric Infectious Diseases Journal*, **11**, S7–11

BROOK, I. (1987) The role of anaerobic bacteria in otitis media: microbiology, pathogenesis, and implications on therapy. *American Journal of Otolaryngology*, **8**, 109–117

BROWNING, G. G. (1990) Childhood otalgia: acute otitis media. 1. Antibiotics not necessary in most cases [see comments]. *British Medical Journal*, **300**, 1005–1006

CANAFAX, D. M. and GIEBINK, G. S. (1991) Clinical and pharmacokinetic basis for the antimicrobial treatment of acute otitis media. *Otolaryngologic Clinics of North America*, **24**, 859–875

CATLIN, B. W. (1990) *Branhamella catarrhalis*: an organism gaining respect as a pathogen. *Clinical Microbiology Review*, **3**, 293–320

CELIN, S. E., BLUESTONE, C. D., STEPHENSON, J., YILMAZ, H. M. and COLLINS, J. J. (1991) Bacteriology of acute otitis media in adults. *Journal of the American Medical Association*, **266**, 2249–2252

CEPERO, R., SMITH, R. J., CATLIN, F. I., BRESSLER, K. L., FURUTA, G. T. and SHANDERA, K. C. (1987) Cystic fibrosis – an otolaryngologic perspective. *Otolaryngology – Head and Neck Surgery*, **97**, 356–360

CHONMAITREE, T., OWEN, M. J., PATEL, J. A., HEDGPETH, D., HORLICK, D. and HOWIE, V. M. (1992) Effect of viral respiratory tract infection on outcome of acute otitis media. *Journal of Pediatrics*, **120**, 856–862

CLAESSEN, J. Q., APPELMAN, C. L., TOUW OTTEN, F. W., DE MELKER, R. A. and HORDIJK, G. J. (1992) A review of clinical trials regarding treatment of acute otitis media. *Clinical Otolaryngology*, **17**, 251–257

COHEN, R., DE LA ROCQUE, F., BOUCHERAT, M., BOUHANNA, A., LECOMPTE, M. D., BRAMI, A. *et al.* (1992) [Prevention of acute otitis media. Amoxicillin versus glycoproteins from Klebsiella pneumoniae. Study in children under 5 years of age.] Prevention des otites moyennes aigues. Amoxicilline versus glycoproteines de Klebsiella pneumoniae. Etude chez l'enfant de moins de 5 ans. *Presse Medicale*, **21**, 509–514

DEBRUYNE, F. and STOFFELS, G. (1985) [Acute mastoiditis: 16

clinical cases.] Akute mastoiditis: 16 klinische gevallen. *Acta Oto-rhino-laryngolica Belgica*, **39**, 811–814

DEL CASTILLO MARTIN, F., BARRIO GOMEZ DE AGUERO, I. and GARCIA PEREA, A. (1992) [Acute otitis media in childhood. Clinical and microbiological study of 50 cases.] Otitis media aguda en la infancia. Estudio clinico y microbiologico de 50 casos. *Anales Espanoles de Pediatria (Madrid)*, **37**, 126–129

DE MELKER, R. A. and KUYVENHOVEN, M. M. (1991) Management of upper respiratory tract infection in Dutch general practice [see comments]. *British Journal of General Practice*, **41**, 504–507

EAVEY, R. D., GAO, Y. Z., SCHUKNECHT, H. F. and GONZALEZ PINEDA, M. (1985) Otologic features of bacterial meningitis of childhood. *Journal of Pediatrics*, **106**, 402–407

EICHENWALD, H. (1985) Developments in diagnosing and treating otitis media. *American Family Physician*, **31**, 155–164

EINHORN, M., FLISS, D. M., LEIBERMAN, A. and DAGAN, R. (1992) Otolaryngology and infectious disease team approach for outpatient management of serious pediatric infections requiring parenteral antibiotic therapy. *International Journal of Pediatric Otorhinolaryngology*, **24**, 245–251

FAYE LUND, H. (1989) Acute and latent mastoiditis. *Journal of Laryngology and Otology*, **103**, 1158–1160

FELDMAN, W., MOMY, J. and DULBERG, C. (1988) Trimethoprim-sulfamethoxazole v. amoxicillin in the treatment of acute otitis media. *Canadian Medical Association Journal*, **139**, 961–964

FELDMAN, W., SUTCLIFFE, T. and DULBERG, C. (1990) Twice-daily antibiotics in the treatment of acute otitis media: trimethoprim-sulfamethoxazole versus amoxicillin-clavulanate [see comments]. *Canadian Medical Association Journal*, **142**, 115–118

FOSHEE, W. S. (1992) Loracarbef versus amoxicillin-clavulanate in the treatment of bacterial acute otitis media with effusion. *Journal of Paediatrics*, **120**, 980–986

FRANCOIS, M., BINGEN, E., MARGO, J. N., SICHEL, J. Y., LAMBERT, N. and NARCY, P. (1988) [Bacteriologic study of acute otitis media in hospitals and private practice.] Etude bacteriologique de l'otite moyenne aigue en pratique hospitaliere et en pratique liberale. *Archives Francaises de Pediatrie*, **45**, 471–476

FRANCOIS, M., BINGEN, E., MARGO, J. N., CONTENCIN, P., LAMBERT, N. and NARCY, P. (1989) [Current bacteriologic status and therapeutic results in acute otitis media in children aged over 3 months.] Bacteriologie actuelle des otites moyennes aigues chez l'enfant de plus de trois mois et consequences therapeutiques. *Revue de Laryngologie Otologie Rhinologie (Bord)*, **110**, 17–20

FRIEDMAN, E. M., MCGILL, T. J. and HEALY, G. B. (1990) Central nervous system complications associated with acute otitis media in children. *Laryngoscope*, **100**, 149–151

FROOM, J. and CULPEPPER, L. (1991) Otitis media in day-care children. A report from the International Primary Care Network. *Journal of Family Practice*, **32**, 289–294

FROOM, J., CULPEPPER, L., GROB, P., BARTELDS, A., BOWERS, P., BRIDGES WEBB, C. et al. (1990) Diagnosis and antibiotic treatment of acute otitis media: report from International Primary Care Network. *British Medical Journal*, **300**, 582–586

GAFFNEY, R. J., O'DWYER, T. P. and MAGUIRE, A. J. (1991) Bezold's abscess. *Journal of Laryngology and Otology*, **105**, 765–766

GAN, V. N. et al. (1991) Comparative evaluation of loracarbef and amoxicillin-clavulanate for acute otitis media. *Antimicrobial Agents in Chemotherapy*, **35**, 967–971

GEHANNO, P., BOUCOT, I., SIMOUET, M., BINGEN, F., LAMBERT ZECHOVSKY, N. et al. (1992) [Bacterial epidemiology of acute otitis media.] Epidemiologie bacterienne de l'otite moyenne aigue. *Annales de Pediatrie (Paris)*, **39**, 485–490

GIEBINK, G. S. and CANAFAX, D. M. (1991) Antimicrobial treatment of otitis media. *Seminars in Respiratory Infections*, **6**, 85–93

GONZALEZ, C., ARNOLD, J. E., WOODY, E. A., ERHARDT, J. B., PRATT, S. R., GETTS, A. et al. (1986) Prevention of recurrent acute otitis media: chemoprophylaxis versus tympanostomy tubes. *Laryngoscope*, **96**, 1330–1334

GRIGOR'EV, G. M., ZAGAINOVA, N. S. and TERNOVOI, A. V. (1990) [Otogenic intracranial complications in an urban emergency service hospital.] Otogennye vnutricherepnye oslozhneniia po dannym gorodskoi bol'nitsy skoroi meditsinskoi pomoshchi. *Vestnik Otorinolaringologii (Moskva)*, 65–68

HAGGARD, M. and HUGHES, E. (1991) *Screening Children's Hearing. A review of the literature and the implications of Otitis Media.* London: HMSO. p. 23

HAKANSSON, A. (1989) Health complaints and drug consumption during the first 18 months of life. *Family Practice*, **6**, 210–216

HARRISON, C. J. and BELHORN, T. H. (1991) Antibiotic treatment failures in acute otitis media [see comments]. *Pediatric Annals*, **20**, 600–601 and 603–608

HARSTEN, G., PRELLNER, K., HELDRUP, J., KALM, O. and KORNFALT, R. (1989a) Recurrent acute otitis media. A prospective study of children during the first three years of life. *Acta Otolaryngologica*, **107**, 111–119

HARSTEN, G., PRELLNER, K., HELDRUP, J., KALM, O. and KORNFALT, R. (1989b) Treatment failure in acute otitis media. A clinical study of children during their first three years of life. *Acta Otolaryngologica*, **108**, 253–258

HAWKINS, D. B. and DRU, D. (1983) Mastoid subperiosteal abscess. *Archives of Otolaryngology – Head and Neck Surgery*, **109**, 369–371

HAWKINS, D. B., DRU, D., HOUSE, J. W. and CLARK, R. W. (1983) Acute mastoiditis in children: a review of 54 cases. *Laryngoscope*, **93**, 568–572

HENDERSON, P. E. and BALDONE, S. C. (1989) Facial nerve palsy secondary to acute otitis media. *Journal of the American Osteopathic Association*, **89**, 207–210

HOLMBERG, K., AXELSSON, A., HANSSON, P. and RENVALL, U. (1985) The correlation between otoscopy and otomicroscopy in acute otitis media during healing. *Scandinavian Audiology*, **14**, 191–199

HOLMBERG, K., AXELSSON, A., HANSSON, P. and RENVALL, U. (1986) Comparison of tympanometry and otomicroscopy during healing of otitis media. *Scandinavian Audiology*, **15**, 3–8

HORDIJK, G. J. (1992) [Consensus in the therapy of acute otitis media.] Consensus over therapie bij otitis media acuta. *Nederlands Tijdschrift Voor Geneeskunde*, **136**, 85–88

HUANG, S. E., HUNG, H. Y., WANG, J. H., JOU, W. B. and LIN, W. S. (1991) [An epidemiological study of otolaryngologic emergency diseases.] *Chung. Hua. I. Hsueh. Tsa. Chih. [Chinese Medical Journal]*, **48**, 456–461

IBEKWE, A. O. and OKOYE, B. C. (1988) Subperiosteal mastoid abscesses in chronic suppurative otitis media. *Annals of Otology, Rhinology and Laryngology*, **97**, 373–375

JORGENSEN, F. and HOLMQUIST, J. (1984) Toynbee phenomenon and middle ear disease. *American Journal of Otology*, **5**, 291–294

KALM, O., JOHNSON, U., PRELLNER, K. and NINN, K. (1991) HLA frequency in patients with recurrent acute otitis media. *Archives of Otolaryngology – Head and Neck Surgery*, **117**, 1296–1299

KALM, O., JOHNSON, U., PRELLNER, K. and NINN, K. (1992) HLA antigens and recurrent acute otitis media. *Acta Otolaryngologica*, Suppl. 492, 107–109

KARMA, P., SIPILA, M., and RAHKO, T. (1989) Hearing and hearing loss in 5-year-old children. Pure-tone thresholds and the effect of acute otitis media. *Scandinavian Audiology*, **18**, 199–203

KARMA, P. H., PUKANDER, J. S., SIPILA, M. M., VESIKARI, T. H. and GRONROOS, P. W. (1987a) Middle ear fluid bacteriology of acute otitis media in neonates and very young infants. *International Journal of Pediatric Otorhinolaryngology*, **14**, 141–150

KARMA, P., PALVA, T., KOUVALAINEN, K., KARJA, J., MAKELA, P. H., PRINSSI, V. P. *et al.* (1987b) Finnish approach to the treatment of acute otitis media. Report of the Finnish Consensus Conference. *Annals of Otology, Rhinology and Laryngology*, Suppl. 129, 1–19

KERO, P. and PIEKKALA, P. (1987) Factors affecting the occurrence of acute otitis media during the first year of life. *Acta Paediatrica Scandinavica*, **76**, 618–623

KLASS, P. E. and KLEIN, J. O. (1992) Therapy of bacterial sepsis, meningitis and otitis media in infants and children: 1992 poll of directors of programs in pediatric infectious diseases. *Pediatric Infectious Diseases Journal*, **11**, 702–705

KLEIN, J. O., TOS, M. and HUSSL, B. (1989) Definition and classification. *Annals of Otology, Rhinology and Laryngology*, **98**, (Suppl. 139), **10**

KLIGMAN, E. W. (1992) Treatment of otitis media [see comments]. *American Family Physician*, **45**, 242–250

LAMBERT ZECHOVSKY, N., MARIANI KURKDJIAN, P., DOIT, C., BOURGEOIS, F. and BINGEN, E. (1992) In-vitro bactericidal activity of four oral antibiotics against pathogens responsible for acute otitis media in children. *Journal of Hospital Infection*, **22** (Suppl. A), 89–97

LARSEN, P. L. and TOS, M. (1991) Polyp formation by experimental tubal occlusion in the rat. *Acta Otolaryngologica*, **111**, 926–933

LE, C. T., FREEMAN, D. W. and FIREMAN, B. H. (1991) Evaluation of ventilating tubes and myringotomy in the treatment of recurrent or persistent otitis media [see comments]. *Pediatric Infectious Diseases Journal*, **10**, 2–11

LEWIS, D. A. and REEVES, D. S. (1995) Antibacterial agents: Trimethoprim and co-trimoxazole. *Prescriber's Journal*, **35** (1), 25–31

LILDHOLDT, T., FELDING, J. U., ERIKSEN, E. W. and PEDERSEN, L. V. (1991) [Diagnosis and treatment of ear diseases in general practice. A controlled trial of the effect of the introduction of middle ear measurement (tympanometry).] Diagnostik og behandling af oresygdomme i almen praksis. En kontrolleret undersogelse af virkningen af indforelse af mellemoretrykmaling (tympanometri). *Ugeskrift For Laeger*, **153**, 3004–3007

LUNDGREN, K. and INGVARSSON, L. (1986) Acute otitis media in Sweden. Role of *Branhamella catarrhalis* and the rationale for choice of antimicrobial therapy. *Drugs*, **31** (Suppl. 3), 125–131

LUNTZ, M. and SADE, J. (1988) Growth of the eustachian tube lumen with age. *American Journal of Otolaryngology*, **9**, 195–198

MCFADDEN, D. M., BERWICK, D. M., FELDSTEIN, M. L. and MARTER, S. S. (1985) Age-specific patterns of diagnosis of acute otitis media. *Clinical Pediatrics (Cleveland OH)*, **24**, 571–575

MAGNUSON, B. and FALK, B. (1984) Diagnosis and management of eustachian tube malfunction. *Otolaryngologic Clinics of North America*, **17**, 659–671

MAHARAJ, D., JADWAT, A., FERNANDES, C. M. and WILLIAMS, B. (1987) Bacteriology in acute mastoiditis. *Archives of Otolaryngology – Head and Neck Surgery*, **113**, 514–515

MARCHANT, C. D., CARLIN, S. A., JOHNSON, C. E. and SHURIN, P. A. (1992) Measuring the comparative efficacy of antibacterial agents for acute otitis media: the 'Pollyanna phenomenon'. *Journal of Pediatrics*, **120**, 72–77

MARGOLIS, R. H. and HUNTER, L. L. (1991) Audiologic evaluation of the otitis media patient. *Otolaryngologic Clinics of North America*, **24**, 877–899

MAWSON, S. R. (1979) Acute inflammation of the middle ear cleft. In: *Scott-Brown's Diseases of the Ear, Nose and Throat*, 4th edn, vol 2, edited by J. Ballantyne and J. Groves. London: Butterworths. pp. 189–190

MILLS, R. P. (1984) Policies on antibiotics of south east London general practitioners for managing acute otitis media in children. *British Medical Journal (Clinical Research Edition)*, **288**, 1199–1201

MORI, Y., IWASAKI, S., KUBOTA, K., KINAGA, S. and OCHO, S. (1992) [Evaluation of myringotomy in the treatment of acute otitis media with effusion in infants and children.] *Nippon. Jibiinkoka. Gakkai. Kaiho. (Journal of the Oto-rhino-laryngological Society of Japan)*, **95**, 58–64

NADAL, D., HERRMANN, P., BAUMANN, A. and FANCONI, A. (1990) Acute mastoiditis: clinical, microbiological, and therapeutic aspects. *European Journal of Pediatrics*, **149**, 560–564

NAKAJIMA, Y. and HATTORI, Y. (1989) [Clinical observation of acute otitis media in children.] *Nippon. Jibiinkoka. Gakkai. Kaiho. (Journal of the Oto-Rhino-Laryngological Society of Japan)*, **92**, 347–352

OGLE, J. W. and LAUER, B. A. (1986) Acute mastoiditis. Diagnosis and complications. *American Journal of Diseases of Children*, **140**, 1178–1182

O'SHEA, J. S. and COLLINS, E. W. (1987) Other health problems of children with acute otitis media. *Journal of Otolaryngology*, **16**, 225–227

PALVA, T., VIRTANEN, H. and MAKINEN, J. (1985) Acute and latent mastoiditis in children. *Journal of Laryngology and Otology*, **99**, 127–136

PAPARELLA, M. M., SHEA, D. MEYERHOFF, W. L. (1980) Silent otitis media. *Laryngoscope*, **90**, 1089

PAPARELLA, M. M., KIMBERLEY, B. P. and ALLEVA, M. (1991) The concept of silent otitis media. *Otolaryngologic Clinics of North America*, **24**, 764

PARADISE, J. L. (1992) Antimicrobial prophylaxis for recurrent acute otitis media. *Annals of Otology, Rhinology and Laryngology*, Suppl. 155, 33–36

PESTALOZZA, G. ROMAGNOLI, M. and TESSITORE, E. (1988) Incidence and risk factors of acute otitis media and otitis media with effusion in children of different age groups. *Advances in Otorhinolaryngology*, **40**, 47–56

PICHICHERO, M. E., BERGHASH, L. R. and HENGERER, A. S. (1989) Anatomic and audiologic sequelae after tympanostomy tube insertion or prolonged antibiotic therapy for otitis media [see comments]. *Pediatric Infectious Diseases Journal*, **8**, 780–787

PRELLNER, K. (1992) Is beta-lactamase-producing bacteria of major importance for unfavourable development of acute otitis media? *Acta Otolaryngologica*, Supplement 493, 109–111

PRELLNER, K. and RYDELL, R. (1986) Acute mastoiditis. Influence of antibiotic treatment on the bacterial spectrum. *Acta Otolaryngologica*, **102**, 52–56

PRELLNER, K., HALLBERG, T., KALM, O. and MANSSON, B. (1985) Recurrent otitis media: genetic immunoglobulin markers in children and their parents. *International Journal of Pediatric Otorhinolaryngology*, **9**, 219–225

PRESCOTT, C. A. and MALAN, J. F. (1991) Mastoid surgery at the Red Cross War Memorial Children's Hospital 1986–1988. *Journal of Laryngology and Otology*, **105**, 409–412

PRINCIPI, N. and MARCHISIO, P. (1991) Cefixime vs amoxicillin in the treatment of acute otitis media in infants and children. *Drugs*, **42** (Suppl. 4), 25–29

PUHAKKA, H. J. (1991) [Acute otitis – a problem affecting children, families and health services.] Akut otit – ett problem for barnet, familjen och sjukvarden. *Nordisk Medicin*, **106**, 293–296

PUKANDER, J., LUOTONEN, J., TIMONEN, M. and KARMA, P. (1985) Risk factors affecting the occurrence of acute otitis media among 2–3-year-old urban children. *Acta Otolaryngologica*, **100**, 260–265

PUKANDER, J., SIPILA, M. and KARMA, P. (1984) *Recent Advances in Otitis Media with Effusion.* Philadelphia: BC Decker. pp. 9–13

RAHKO, T., KARMA, P. and SIPILA, M. (1989) Sensorineural hearing loss and acute otitis media in children. *Acta Otolaryngologica*, **108**, 107–112

RANDALL, D. A., FORNADLEY, J. A. and KENNEDY, K. S. (1992) Management of recurrent otitis media. *American Family Physician*, **45**, 2117–2123

ROSEN, A., OPHIR, D. and MARSHAK, G. (1986) Acute mastoiditis: a review of 69 cases. *Annals of Otology, Rhinology and Laryngology*, **95**, 222–224

ROSENFELD, R. M., DOYLE, W. J., SWARTS, J. D., SEROKY, J. and PINERO, B. P. (1992) Third-generation cephalosporins in the treatment of acute pneumococcal otitis media. An animal study. *Archives of Otolaryngology – Head and Neck Surgery*, **118**, 49–52

RUBIN, J. S. and WEI, W. I. (1985) Acute mastoiditis: a review of 34 patients. *Laryngoscope*, **95**, 963–965

RYNNEL DAGOO, B., LINDBERG, K., BAGGER SJOBACK, D. and LARSON, O. (1992) Middle ear disease in cleft palate children at three years of age. *International Journal of Pediatric Otorhinolaryngology*, **23**, 201–209

SADÉ, J. (1985) *International Symposium on Acute and Secretory Otitis Media.* Jerusalem, Israel. Toronto: B.C. Decker Inc

SADÉ, J., WOLFSON, S., SACHS, Z. and ABRAHAM, S. (1985a) The eustachian tube midportion in infants. *American Journal of Otolaryngology*, **6**, 205–209

SADÉ, J., WOLFSON, S., SACHS, Z., LEVIT, I. and ABRAHAM, S. (1985b) The infant eustachian tube lumen – pharyngeal part. *Auris, Nasus, Larynx (Tokyo)*, **12**, (Suppl. 1), S18–S20

SADÉ, J., WOLFSON, S., SACHS, Z., LEVIT, I. and ABRAHAM, S. (1986) The infant's eustachian tube lumen: the pharyngeal part. *Journal of Laryngology and Otology*, **100**, 129–134

SAMUEL, J. and FERNANDES, C. M. (1985) Otogenic complications with an intact tympanic membrane. *Laryngoscope*, **95**, 1387–1390

SAMUEL, J. and FERNANDES, C. M. (1986) Tuberculous mastoiditis. *Annals of Otology, Rhinology and Laryngology*, **95**, 264–266

SAMUEL, J., FERNANDES, C. M., and STEINBERG, J. L. (1986) Intracranial otogenic complications: a persisting problem. *Laryngoscope*, **96**, 272–278

SANDO, I., TAKAHASHI, H. and MATSUNE, S. (1991) Update on functional anatomy and pathology of human Eustachian tube related to otitis media with effusion. *Otolaryngologic Clinics of North America*, **24**, 795–811

SARKKINEN, H., RUUSKANEN, O., MEURMAN, O., PUHAKKA, H., VIROLAINEN, E. and ESKOLA, J. (1985) Identification of respiratory virus antigens in middle ear fluids of children with acute otitis media. *Journal of Infectious Diseases*, **151**, 444–448

SARUBBI, F. A., MYERS, J. W., WILLIAMS, J. J. and SHELL, C. G. (1990) Respiratory infections caused by *Branhamella catarrhalis*. Selected epidemiologic features. *American Journal of Medicine*, **88**, 9S–14S

SCHEIBEL, W. R. and URTES, M. A. (1987) Mastoiditis. *American Family Physician*, **35**, 123–127

SCHNORE, S. K., SANGSTER, J. F., GERACE, T. M. and BASS, M. J. (1986) Are antihistamine-decongestants of value in the treatment of acute otitis media in children? *Journal of Family Practice*, **22**, 39–43

SCHWARTZ, D. M. and SCHWARTZ, R. H. (1987) Validity of acoustic reflectometry in detecting middle ear effusion. *Pediatrics*, **79**, 739–742

SELESNICK, S. H. and JACKLER, R. K. (1993) Facial paralysis in suppurative ear disease. *Operative Techniques in Otolaryngology - Head and Neck Surgery*, **3**, 61–68

SENTURIA, B. H., BLUESTONE, C. D., KLEIN, J. O., LIM, D. J. and PARADISE, J. L. (1980) Report of the ad hoc committee on definitions and classifications of otitis media with effusion. *Annals of Otology, Rhinology and Laryngology*, **89** (Suppl. 68), 3

SHANLEY, D. J. and MURPHY, T. F. (1992) Intracranial and extracranial complications of acute mastoiditis: evaluation with computed tomography. *Journal of the American Osteopathic Association*, **92**, 131–134

SHURIN, P. A. and VAN HARE, G. F. (1986) Therapy of acute otitis media caused by *Branhamella catarrhalis*. Preliminary report. *Drugs*, **31** (Suppl. 3), 122–124

SHUSTER, M. A., CHUMAKOV, F. I. and CHKANNIKOV, A. N. (1991) [Role of computerized tomography in the diagnosis of encapsulated cerebellar abscesses in acute otitis media.] Rol' kompiuternoi tomografii v diagnostike inkapsulirovannykh abstsessov mozzhechka pri ostrykh srednikh otitakh. *Vestnik Otorinolaringologii (Moskva)*, 41–44

SIPILA, M., KARMA, P., PUKANDER, J., TIMONEN, M. and KATAJA, M. (1988) The Bayesian approach to the evaluation of risk factors in acute and recurrent acute otitis media. *Acta Otolaryngologica*, **106**, 94–101

STENSTROM, C., BYLANDER GROTH, A. and INGVARSSON, L. (1991) Eustachian tube function in otitis-prone and healthy children. *International Journal of Pediatric Otorhinolaryngology*, **21**, 127–138

STOOL, S. E. and FIELD, M. J. (1989) The impact of otitis media. *Pediatric Infectious Diseases Journal*, **8** (Suppl. 1), 11–14

SUNDBERG, L., EDEN, T., ERNSTON, S. and PAHLITZSCH, R. (1979) Penetration of erythromycin through respiratory mucosa. *Acta Otolaryngologica*, Suppl. 365, 3–17

SURPURE, J. S. (1987) Hyperpyrexia in children: clinical implications. *Pediatric Emergency Care*, **3**, 10–12

SUZUKI, K., BABA, S., INAGAKI, M. and KOBAYASHI, T. (1988)

The antibiotic susceptibilities and beta-lactamase production of clinical isolated *Branhamella catarrhalis* from acute otitis media in children. *Auris, Nasus, Larynx (Tokyo)*, **15**, 105–111

TAKAHASHI, H., NAKAMURA, H. and YUI, M. (1985) Analysis of fifty cases of facial palsy due to otitis media. *Archives of Otorhinolaryngology*, **241**, 163–168

TEELE, D. W. (1991) Strategies to control recurrent acute otitis media in infants and children. *Pediatric Annals*, **20**, 609–610, 612–614

TEELE, D. W., KLEIN, J. O. and ROSNER, B. (1989) Epidemiology of otitis media during the first seven years of life in children in greater Boston: a prospective, cohort study [see comments]. *Journal of Infectious Diseases*, **160**, 83–94

TERNDRUP, T. E. and WONG, A. (1991) Influence of otitis media on the correlation between rectal and auditory canal temperatures. *American Journal of Diseases of Children*, **145**, 75–78

THOENE, D. E. and JOHNSON, C. E. (1991) Pharmacotherapy of otitis media. *Pharmacotherapy*, **11**, 212–221

TRUY, E., GRANADE, G., BENSOUSSAN, J., KAUFFMAN, I., LANGUE, J. and MORGON, A. (1992) [Acquired peripheral facial palsy in children. Current data illustrated by 66 recent personal cases.] Les paralysies faciales peripheriques acquises de l'enfant. Donnees actuelles illustrees par 66 observations personnelles recentes. *Pediatrie*, **47**, 481–486

VAN BUCHEM, F. L., PEETERS, M. F. and VAN 'T HOF, M. A. (1985) Acute otitis media: a new treatment strategy. *British Medical Journal* (Clinical Research Edition), **290**, 1033–1037

VAN HARE, G. F., SHURIN, P. A., MARCHANT, C. D., CARTELLI, N. A., JOHNSON, C. E., FULTON, D. *et al.* (1987) Acute otitis media caused by *Branhamella catarrhalis*: biology and therapy. *Reviews of Infectious Diseases*, **9**, 16–27

WARDROP, P. A. and PILLSBURY, H. C. (1984) *Mycobacterium avium* acute mastoiditis. *Archives of Otolaryngology*, **110**, 686–687

WARNAAR, A., SNOEP, G. and STALS, F. S. (1989) A swollen cheek, an unusual course of acute mastoiditis. *International Journal of Pediatric Otorhinolaryngology*, **17**, 179–183

WHITE, P., HERMANSSON, A. and SVINHUFVUD, M. (1990) Surfactant and isoprenaline effect on eustachian tube opening in rats with acute otitis media. *American Journal of Otolaryngology*, **11**, 389–392

WILLIAMSON, H. A., JR, DEPRA, J. and SULZBERGER, L. A. (1991) Lack of seasonal variability for recurrent otitis media in very young children. *Journal of Family Practice*, **33**, 489–493

ZAGAINOVA, N. S. and NEVEZHIN, L. V. (1991) [Clinical course of mastoiditis as reported by the specialized emergency care hospital.] Osobennosti klinicheskogo techenia mastoidita po dannym spetsializirovannoi bol'nitsy skoroi meditsinskoi pomoshchi. *Vestnik Otorinolaringologii (Moskva)*, 3–6

ZALZAL, G. H. (1987) Acute mastoiditis complicated by sigmoid sinus thrombosis in congenital aural atresia. *International Journal of Pediatric Otorhinolaryngology*, **14**, 31–39

10

Management of chronic suppurative otitis media

R. P. Mills

Chronic suppurative otitis media (CSOM) has been an important cause of middle ear disease since prehistoric times (Gregg, Steele and Holzhueter, 1965; McKenzie and Brothwell, 1967; Rathbun and Mallin, 1977). Its incidence appears to depend to some extent on race and socioeconomic factors. It is, for example, significantly more common in the Innuit (Eskimos) and American Indians (Fairbanks, 1981), the indigenous population of Alaska (Tschopp, 1977), Australian aboriginal children (McCafferty et al., 1977) and black South Africans (Meyrick, 1951). Poor living conditions, overcrowding and poor hygiene and nutrition have been suggested as a basis for the widespread prevalence of chronic suppurative otitis media in developing countries. Fairbanks (1981) reported a similar incidence of chronic ear disease in poor Caucasians and American Indians in Kentucky. Hinchcliffe (1961) reported a prevalence of 1.1% in an adult rural population in the UK. Rudin et al. (1983) reported that the prevalence of tympanic membrane perforations was 2.1% in a cohort of 60 year olds and 2.3% in a group of 50 year olds. By contrast the prevalence in a cohort of 20 year olds was only 0.8%. This finding might suggest that the prevalence of chronic suppurative otitis media is falling and indeed Thomson (1974) reported a decrease in the incidence of cholesteatoma in the Grampian region of Scotland following the introduction of grommets. However, Padgham, Mills and Christmas (1989) found no change in the incidence of cholesteatoma in Tayside, which lies immediately south of Grampian, over a 20-year period, despite a 60-fold increase in the use of ventilation tubes. The most recent investigation of the prevalence of chronic ear disease in the UK was carried out by the MRC Institute of Hearing Research (Browning and Gatehouse, 1992). A stratified sample of 2708 adults was studied in four different centres. Otoscopic findings indicated that 2.6% had evidence of inactive chronic otitis media while 1.5% had active disease. Of the patients with active chronic otitis media, 86% had not undergone surgery.

Classification

Chronic suppurative otitis media is usually classified into two main groups; tubotympanic and atticoantral disease.

Tubotympanic disease is characterized by a perforation of the pars tensa. Patients with this form of otitis media are generally not considered to be at risk of developing complications such as intracranial sepsis. This view has been challenged by Browning (1984a) who reported that some cases of intracranial abscess were associated with active tubotympanic disease. None-the-less the term 'safe' otitis media is often applied to this condition. Perforations vary in size and position (Figure 10.1). Marginal perforations are considered to be more sinister, because they may, in some cases, be associated with the formation of cholesteatoma.

Atticoantral disease most commonly involves the pars flaccida and is characterized by the formation of a retraction pocket in which keratin accumulates to produce cholesteatoma. *Cholesteatoma* may be divided into congenital and acquired types. Derlaki and Clemis (1965) have proposed three criteria for the diagnosis of congenital cholesteatoma:

1 Development behind an intact tympanic membrane
2 No previous history of otitis media
3 An origin from embryonal inclusion of squamous epithelium, or from undifferentiated epithelium which changes into squamous epithelium during development.

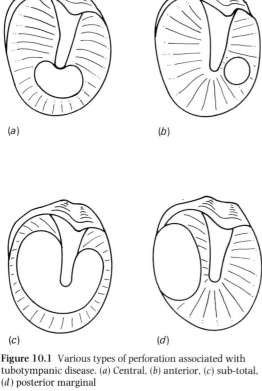

(a)   (b)

(c)   (d)

Figure 10.1 Various types of perforation associated with tubotympanic disease. (*a*) Central, (*b*) anterior, (*c*) sub-total, (*d*) posterior marginal

Congenital cholesteatoma is most commonly found either in the middle ear or within the temporal bone, particularly at the petrous apex. Expansion of these lesions may lead to secondary infection and this, together with the frequency of a past history of otitis media in the population, makes it difficult to be certain that some lesions are genuine congenital cholesteatomas. Cholesteatomas may also develop in association with congenital atresia of the ear (Jahrsdoefer, 1980; Haberman and Werth, 1981; Miyamoto, Fairchild and Daugherty, 1984; Mills and Graham, 1986).

This approach to classification is pathologically correct, but difficult to apply clinically. For this reason Tos (1988) has proposed an alternative otoscopic classification. Mills and Padgham (1991) have proposed a modification of this scheme to include cholesteatomas behind an intact tympanic membrane (Figure 10.2). Lesions occurring within the temporal bone cannot be included, as they cannot be diagnosed otoscopically. Attic cholesteatoma is the commonest type, but tensa cholesteatoma is also common.

Retraction pockets of the tympanic membrane may involve either the pars tensa or the pars flaccida. Retraction pockets of the pars tensa have been classified into four stages or grades by Sadé (1979) (Figure

10.3). In grade 3, the tympanic membrane is not adherent and can be seen to move on pneumatic otoscopy, while in grade 4 it is adherent to the promontory. Attic retraction pockets have been classified into four types or grades by Tos (1988) (Figure 10.4).

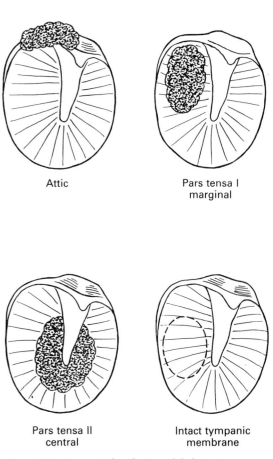

Attic   Pars tensa I
                         marginal

Pars tensa II   Intact tympanic
central   membrane

Figure 10.2 Otoscopic classification of cholesteatoma. (Reproduced by courtesy of the Editor of the *Journal of Laryngology and Otology*)

Clinical assessment

History

The principal symptoms of chronic suppurative otitis media are hearing loss and aural discharge. In tubotympanic disease the discharge tends to be profuse and is frequently mucoid rather than frankly purulent. It is seldom malodorous and frequently intermittent. It may be precipitated by the passage of water through a perforation.

In atticoantral disease the discharge is generally scanty, foul smelling and tends to be more chronic.

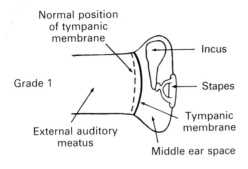

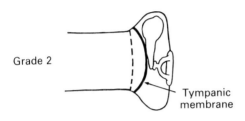

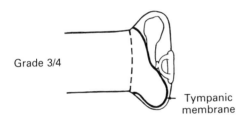

Figure 10.3 Classification of retraction pockets of the pars tensa. (Reproduced by courtesy of the Editor of the *Journal of Laryngology and Otology*)

Occasionally there is nó history of discharge and the diagnosis may only be made when the ear is explored because of conductive hearing loss. Alternatively there may be hardly any hearing loss because the cholesteatoma is itself transmitting sound. When there is formation of granulation tissue or an aural polyp, blood-stained discharge may occur. Otalgia is uncommon, but may occasionally occur in cholesteatoma cases. The development of headache, vertigo or facial palsy is evidence of complications.

Examination

The pinna should be inspected, and it is important to look at both sides to exclude the presence of a scar from previous ear surgery. Otoscopic examination will reveal the presence and position of any perforations and retraction pockets. In the presence of a per-

foration, the condition of the middle ear mucosa can be assessed. A polyp may be observed though if this is large it may completely obstruct the ear canal precluding adequate assessment of the disease. Similarly wax crusts may obscure the opening of an attic retraction pocket.

Most cases benefit from further assessment under the operating microscope and this allows discharge and attic crusts to be removed. In some cases a second examination after a course of medical treatment will help to clarify the details of the pathology. In others, especially in children, it is necessary to examine the ear under general anaesthesia in order to make a proper assessment. A labelled diagram of the findings can be very helpful. Rinne's and Weber's tests should be performed to establish the nature of the hearing loss. Valuable information may also be obtained from examination of the nose and throat. Preoperative assessment of eustachian tube function is unhelpful (Smyth, 1980; Sheehy, 1981).

Bacteriology

A wide range of organisms, both aerobic and anaerobic may be isolated from cases of chronic suppurative otitis media. The proportions of different organisms isolated vary from study to study, but *Proteus* species and *Pseudomonas aeruginosa* most frequently predominate (Palva and Hallstrom, 1965; Ojala *et al.*, 1981; Sugita *et al.*, 1981; Constable and Butler, 1982; Sweeney, Picozzi and Browning, 1982; Brook, 1985). *Staphylococcus aureus* (Friedmann, 1952; Karma *et al.*, 1978) and *Escherichia coli* (Constable and Butler, 1982; Sweeney, Picozzi and Browning, 1982) are also frequently isolated. The predominance of Gram-negative aerobes indicates that the source of infection is not the nasopharynx, which does not contain these organisms. A 'faecal–aural' route of infection has been proposed by Fairbanks (1981). However, Senior and Sweeney (1984) reported that most of the *Proteus* strains which they isolated from cases of chronic suppurative otitis media were of 'non-faecal' types.

The role of anaerobes in chronic suppurative otitis media has been the subject of speculation. *Bacteroides melaninogenicus*, *Bacteroides fragilis* and other species can be isolated from 30 to 50% of cases (Jokipii *et al.*, 1977; Karma *et al.*, 1978; Sweeney, Picozzi and Browning, 1982). According to Sugita *et al.* (1981), they are most frequently detected in ears with extensive cholesteatoma or granulation tissue formation. Anaerobes and aerobes are often found together and it has been suggested this is because the aerobic organisms create an environment in which the anaerobes can grow in mixed infections by lowering the local oxygen concentration (Onderdonk *et al.*, 1976; Karma *et al.*, 1978). Kelly (1978) has demonstrated that the combination of aerobic and anaerobic organisms can produce a more marked inflammatory

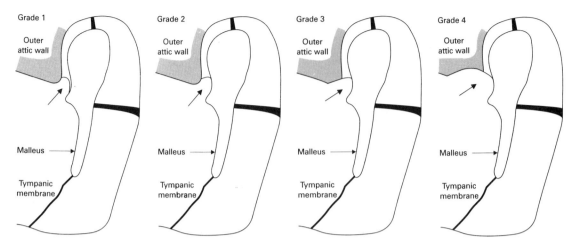

Figure 10.4 Classification of attic retraction pockets (Tos, 1988) Grade 1: Pars flaccida not in contact with malleus neck. Grade 2: Pars flaccida in contact with malleus neck. Grade 3: Limited outer attic wall erosion. Grade 4: Severe outer attic wall erosion

response than the same organisms alone in an experimental animal. However, the elimination of anaerobic bacteria from active ears does not necessarily render them inactive (Browning *et al.*, 1983).

Audiological assessment

Audiometric evaluation

A pure tone audiogram including air and bone conduction with full masking is essential to evaluate the degree of hearing loss and to determine the air–bone gap. In cases in which an attempt to improve hearing is being considered, a speech audiogram is valuable to check that the speech reception threshold is in line with the mean hearing loss as assessed by pure tone audiometry. While there is generally good agreement between the results of speech audiometry and mean hearing losses calculated using the frequencies 500, 1000 and 2000 Hz, occasionally the speech discrimination proves to be so poor and therefore no useful hearing improvement can be anticipated following surgery.

Hearing loss in chronic suppurative otitis media

Hearing thresholds vary considerably in cases of chronic suppurative otitis media. Some patients will be found to have virtually normal hearing, while others have a severe mixed hearing loss or even a dead ear. Perforations of the tympanic membrane reduce the efficiency of the drum component of the middle ear impedance matching transformer. When the perforation directly exposes the round window niche, the protection which is normally afforded to the round window membrane by the drum is lost

and this has an adverse effect on cochlear mechanics. The loss of the 'round window baffle' effect is associated with a greater hearing loss than might otherwise be expected. Destruction of the ossicular chain leads to more severe hearing losses. Hearing losses in cases with loss of the stapes arch are generally more severe than those in which the arch is intact. Other factors such as the presence of active mucosal disease, reduction of ossicular chain mobility by fibrosis or tympanosclerosis and the presence of a cholesteatoma also play their part in determining the degree of hearing loss present. Patients who have undergone open cavity mastoidectomy frequently have a tympanic remnant which is significantly smaller than a normal drum and which lacks its normal conical shape. These factors, together with the tendency to have a shallow middle ear space and extensive destruction of the ossicular chain, further undermine the efficiency of the impedance matching transformer. The development of attachments between the tympanic membrane and the stapes or stapes footplate can result in good hearing in some cases, though in others these arrangements are inefficient and are associated with a significant conductive loss (Mills, 1991).

In addition to the conductive hearing loss, many patients have a degree of sensorineural hearing loss (Paparella, Brady and Hoel, 1970). Patients with unilateral chronic suppurative otitis media were found to have significantly greater hearing thresholds in the affected ear compared with the normal ear in a multicentre trial reported by Paparella *et al.* (1984). However, Dumich and Harner (1983) failed to demonstrate any evidence of sensorineural hearing loss in a series of 200 patients. Cochlear damage has been attributed to the diffusion of the toxic products of inflammation through the scala tympani via the

and reported the presence of inflammatory cells in the cochlea in four of them. However, they failed to demonstrate the loss of hair cells. Walby, Barrer and Schuknecht (1983) reported elevated bone conduction thresholds as compared to those on the contralateral side in 87 patients with unilateral chronic suppurative otitis media. In the same study they also examined 12 temporal bones from patients with chronic suppurative otitis media and failed to demonstrate any abnormality of the hair cells. They postulated that the elevated bone conduction thresholds were due to changes in the mechanics of sound conduction. In most cases of chronic suppurative otitis media treated surgically, the postoperative bone conduction thresholds are the same as those found preoperatively. However, overclosure of the air–bone gap, a phenomenon more usually associated with stapes surgery, has been observed following tympanoplasty (Wehrs, 1985).

Radiological assessment

Conventional radiology

Some surgeons feel that plain radiographs are of value in cholesteatoma cases, either as a means of demonstrating pathology, or to identify variations in temporal bone anatomy. In expert hands both can be achieved (Figures 10.5 and 10.6). However, other specialists do not routinely use radiology in such cases.

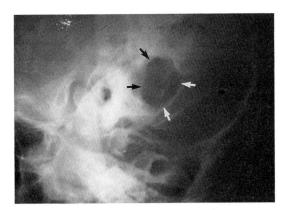

Figure 10.5 Plain film, lateral view, showing more extensive bone erosion (arrows). (Reproduced by courtesy of Dr P. D. Phelps)

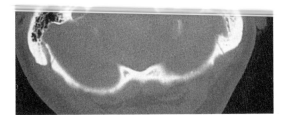

Figure 10.6 Axial CT scan showing soft tissue in the mastoid with cell wall breakdown (arrows). (Reproduced by courtesy of Dr P. D. Phelps)

CT scanning

The anatomy of the temporal bone can be more effectively demonstrated by CT scanning and cholesteatoma can be demonstrated (Jackler, Dillon and Schindler, 1984; O'Donoghue *et al.*, 1987). However, the findings are unlikely to influence decisions about the management of most cases. It may be of some value in children, medically unfit patients and those with only one hearing ear (Leighton *et al.*, 1993). It is not an adequate substitute for the 'second look' operation in the assessment of cases which have undergone intact canal surgery for cholesteatoma (Wake *et al.*, 1992). CT scanning is of vital importance in the detection of intracranial complications. The role of MRI scanning in otitis media is currently being evaluated (see Figures 2.34 and 2.41).

Medical management

The basic principles of medical management of chronic suppurative otitis media can be summarized as follows:

1 Clean the ear adequately
2 Instil a topical antimicrobial agent in such a way that it reaches the disease in adequate amounts.

Aural toilet

This can be achieved by mopping the ear or by suction. Removal of small polyps can often be achieved at the same time and granulation tissue can be cauterized to good effect with silver nitrate applied with care. Improvement can also be achieved by dry mopping alone (Browning, 1984b).

Topical antimicrobial therapy

It is generally considered that antibiotic or antibiotic/steroid eardrops are effective in reducing aural discharge in chronic suppurative otitis media (Fairbanks, 1981). Picozzi, Browning and Calder (1983) compared gentamicin/hydrocortisone ear drops with placebo. The success rate for gentamicin/hydrocortisone was 65%, compared with 18% with placebo. However, the choice of preparation has to be based on experience as there are no data from controlled trials on which to base this decision. Alternatively various types of powder, including boric acid with or without iodine, nystatin or cicatrin can be used.

Most of the antibiotics used in topical preparations are potentially ototoxic and have been shown to cause cochlear damage when applied topically in guinea pigs (Kohonen and Tarkanen, 1969; Brummett, Harris and Lindgren, 1976). Proud, Mittelman and Seiden (1968) applied chloramphenicol powder to the round window of the guinea pigs and reported cochlear damage, despite the fact that this drug is not generally considered to be ototoxic in normal usage. There is, however, no evidence that the use of ear drops causes sensorineural deafness in patients with chronic otitis media (Fairbanks, 1981). Brummett, Harris and Lindgren (1976) have postulated that this may be because the round window niche in humans is relatively deep and often protected by a pseudomembrane, while in the guinea pig the round window is completely exposed.

Surgical management: (general principles)

Tympanic membrane perforations

There is no overwhelming need to close a perforation of the tympanic membrane. The decision whether to operate or not is therefore based on the potential benefits to the patients in terms of:

1 Prevention of recurrent discharge
2 Hearing improvement
3 The ability to swim without the fear of aural discharge.

Ideally the ear should be free of infection at the time of surgery, but in some cases the only way to control discharge is to repair the perforation. The presence of infection at the time of surgery has not been found to have an adverse affect on success rate (Smyth, 1980; Glasscock *et al.*, 1982; Sheehy, 1983; Browning, 1984b). A less favourable outcome may, however, be expected in larger perforations (Booth, 1974; Smyth, 1980; Sadé *et al.*, 1981) and in those placed anteriorly (Sadé *et al.*, 1981).

Most published series have not demonstrated any relationship between age and outcome (Lee and Schuknecht, 1971; Booth, 1974; Sadé *et al.*, 1981). However, Raine and Singh (1983) reported that operations were more likely to fail in children under 12 years of age. Russell and Kleid (1991) found that failures were more likely in patients under 10 and over 50 years of age. This finding is not supported by the experience of Lee and Schuknecht (1971) or Lau and Tos (1988). It appears reasonable to operate on bilateral cases with significant hearing loss, while waiting until the age of 12 in cases with unilateral perforations and adequate hearing. The greater maturity of the child at that age enables them to cope better with the surgery and to cooperate in their postoperative care.

The operation can be carried out permeatally or via an endaural or postaural incision. An endaural approach provides a better view of the ossicular chain, while a postaural approach allows the anterior margin of the perforation to be seen more easily in some ears. The graft can be introduced medial to the tympanic membrane (underlay), or lateral to it (onlay). Both approaches have their advocates. The middle ear space must be entered if an underlay technique is to be used. While this could be viewed as a disadvantage, it allows inspection of the ossicular chain and middle ear mucosa. The onlay technique does not require opening the middle ear space, but may be complicated by intratympanic keratin pearl formation, due to inadequate removal of squamous epithelium from the outer surface of the drum, and blunting of the angle between the anterior portion of the drum and the canal wall with impairment of drum function (Smyth, 1980).

The most popular material for tympanic membrane grafts is autologous temporalis fascia. This material has provided good results over a considerable period of time and is readily available when either an endaural or postaural incision is made. Other autograft tissues, including perichondrium, can also be used. Homograft dura has enjoyed considerable popularity in the past and produces results comparable with those obtained using temporalis fascia (Smyth, 1980). However, more recently concerns about transmission of viral infection has led many surgeons to abandon dura. One case of Creutzfeldt-Jacob disease following the use of homograft dura has been described (JAMA Update, 1987).

Cholesteatoma

Surgery is the treatment of choice for the majority of cases. There is, however, a small group of elderly and medically unfit patients who are best managed by regular suction clearance of keratin in the outpatient department. In the early days of chronic ear surgery radical mastoidectomy, with removal of the incus, malleus and tympanic membrane, was the operation of choice. This proved to be effective as a means of eradicating or at least exteriorizing the disease, but was associated with poor hearing and a high inc' dence of chronic or intermittent discharge. The mo' fied radical operation, with preservation of the r leus handle and a remnant of drum tissue was de to overcome these disadvantages. This operat' mains the most commonly performed proce the UK, but elsewhere intact canal wall sv mains popular. Intact canal wall mastoidect' bined approach tympanoplasty) was int the late 1950s by Jansen (1968). The ain

1 To avoid an open cavity with its inhereⁿ of retention of wax and recurrent discharge
2 To facilitate functional reconstruction of the miuu.. ear
3 To improve the chances of being able to fit a hearing aid in a dry ear with a suitable external auditory meatus.

In some cases these aims can be achieved, but all those who have reported the results of such operations have experienced residual and recurrent disease. Residual cholesteatoma represents failure to eradicate the original disease and occurs in 13–36% of cases (Wright, 1977; Charachon, 1978; Sheehy and Robinson, 1982; Cody and McDonald, 1984; Sanna et al., 1984). Recurrent cholesteatoma arises as a result of postoperative drum retraction and has been reported in 5–13% of cases (Charachon, 1978; Sheehy and Robinson, 1982; Cody and McDonald, 1984; Sanna et al., 1984). It is therefore mandatory to re-explore ears which have undergone intact canal wall surgery approximately one year after the original operation. At this stage an ossiculoplasty can be carried out if appropriate. If residual disease is present a modified radical conversion can be performed.

Cholesteatoma occurring in childhood is often said to be more aggressive than that developing in adult life. Palva, Karma and Karja (1977) studied the extent of cholesteatoma at surgery and reported 'more rapid and expansive growth' in childhood cases, but a lower incidence of lateral semicircular canal fistula. The same authors confirmed that the mastoid process tends to be more extensively pneumatized in paediatric cholesteatoma cases than in adults. This means that when the disease is treated by an open cavity technique a large cavity which is difficult to manage may result. This is one reason for the predominance in the literature of reports of intact canal wall surgery for children (Sheehy, 1978; Glasscock, Dickens and Weit, 1981; Charachon and Gratacap, 1985; Sanna et al., 1988). However, those authors who have compared the frequency of residual disease in adults and children report a higher rate in children (Sheehy, 1978; Glasscock, Dickens and Weit, 1981). In view of these findings, open cavity surgery appears a particularly attractive option in childhood. It is possible to obtain good hearing results using modified radical mastoidectomy with ossiculoplasty

lar ui uic masioid uowi sump. Variations in the anatomy of the temporal bone, such as an anteriorly placed lateral venous sinus, low middle cranial fossa dura or a prominent Körner's septum create additional difficulties, especially for the inexperienced surgeon. When Körner's septum is breached by the drill, the operator may think that the mastoid antrum has been entered, rather than the antral group of mastoid air cells. A densely sclerotic mastoid process also makes the approach to the antrum more difficult because there are fewer landmarks to follow.

Ossicular chain pathology

Ossicular chain damage is found in all types of chronic suppurative otitis media, but tends to be more extensive in cholesteatoma cases. The decision as to whether or not to attempt reconstruction of the ossicular chain must be based on the chances of success. In patients with serviceable hearing in the other ear, the bone conduction thresholds at 500, 1000 and 2000 Hz should be 30 dB or better. However, in cases of bilateral hearing loss improvement in the hearing thresholds, such that they are within 15 dB of those of the unoperated ear, will generally provide subjective improvement in hearing acuity (Smyth and Patterson, 1985). In cases with severe hearing loss, a modest improvement in hearing thresholds may be valuable in that it allows an adequate hearing level to be achieved with a hearing aid.

Patients with loss of the stapes arch, particularly those in whom a drum to stapes footplate assembly is the only option, obtain significantly poorer hearing results than those with an intact stapes arch (Mills, 1993).

Retraction pockets

Shallow, self-cleansing retraction pockets are common incidental findings and require no treatment. Attic pockets in particular require a period of observation to confirm that they are stable. Some retraction pockets of the pars tensa discharge intermittently and develop granulation tissue within them. A small number are sufficiently troublesome to require intervention. The pocket can be everted and the drum reinforced with a soft tissue graft, such as temporalis fascia. This procedure can be combined with a cortical mastoidectomy to provide a larger air reservoir or the insertion of a ventilation tube (Arnvig, 1963; Palva, 1963; Sirala, 1963; Grahne, 1964). A stiffer graft can be produced using tragal cartilage and perichondrium (Glasscock *et al.*, 1982; Mills, 1991). Alternatively the thin retracted segment of drum can be excised and the resulting perforation can be left to heal (Sharpe and Robinson, 1992). The early results with all these approaches are satisfactory, but further retraction of the tympanic membrane occurs in a proportion of cases over the longer term.

Mastoid revision surgery

According to Beales and Hynes (1958), 20% of mastoid cavities remain unhealed 6 months after surgery and of the remainder some begin to discharge again subsequently. The reported frequency of discharge varies between 30 and 60% (Beales, 1959; Palva 1982; Mills, 1988). Cavities are more likely to be dry if they are not excessively large, have a low facial ridge, an adequate meatal opening and a closed middle ear space (Sadé *et al.*, 1982).

A number of different surgical approaches to the discharging cavity have been described. Cavity revision alone is likely to result in a dry ear in 57% of cases, while the combination of this approach with a meatoplasty increases the success rate to 83% (Mills, 1988). Good results can also be obtained with meatoplasty alone (Osborne, Terry and Gandhi, 1985). Various techniques for obliteration of mastoid cavities have been described using a pedicled muscle flap (Kisch, 1928), or a musculoperiosteal flap (Palva, 1962). An alternative approach uses a mixture of bone dust and water (bone paté) to fill in the mastoid bowl (Palva, 1973). This technique results in a dry ear in 63–94% of cases (Mills, 1988; Soloman and Robinson, 1988). An alternative method of eliminating the cavity is the technique of tympanomastoid re-aeration described by Bennett (1981). In some cases discharge arises from a perforation of the tympanic membrane remnant and in these cases a myringoplasty may eliminate the problem.

Tuberculosis

The incidence of tuberculous otitis media has fallen dramatically since the beginning of this century. At that time 3–5% of cases of otitis media were due to the tubercle bacillus, whereas today the condition is rare (Glover, Tranter and Innes, 1981). Tuberculosis is also overall less common than before, though more recently there has been a resurgence of cases, some of them occurring in association with AIDS.

The typical clinical features are painless otorrhoea which fails to respond to topical treatment in a patient with evidence of tubercle infection elsewhere (Windle-Taylor and Bailey, 1980; Glover, Tranter and Innes, 1981). Pale exuberant granulations are present and the hearing loss tends to be greater than might otherwise be expected. Complications include facial palsy, mastoiditis, sensorineural hearing loss and labyrinthitis (Singh, 1991). In some cases there may be multiple perforations of the tympanic membrane. However, in a significant proportion of cases the typical picture is not seen. For example, there may be otalgia associated with the otorrhoea and there may not be evidence of tuberculosis elsewhere (Windle-Taylor and Bailey, 1980). The clinician must therefore suspect the diagnosis in any atypical case of chronic suppurative otitis media not responding to conventional treatment, particularly those in at risk groups such as members of the Asian ethnic minority. It must be made by culturing the discharge for tubercle bacilli and histological examination of the granulation tissue.

The treatment consists of systemic antituberculous chemotherapy, usually with multiple agents to avoid resistance. Surgery may be required in some cases to remove sequestra and improve drainage (Singh, 1991). When combined with adequate chemotherapy, there is a good chance of healing with a dry ear.

Unusual presentations
Immune deficiency

Immune deficiency may be idiopathic or secondary to the use of drugs which depress the immune response. Deficiency of IgG or IgA may be associated with an increased incidence of upper respiratory infections and otitis media. If surgery is required in such a patient, cover with the appropriate immunoglobulin fraction may be appropriate (Sasaki *et al.*, 1981). Chronic ear disease may also be observed in Job's syndrome ('lazy leucocyte syndrome').

Wegener's granuloma

This condition is characterized by the development of granulomatous lesions in the kidneys, lungs and at various sites in the head and neck, notably the nose and sinuses. Middle ear involvement also occurs not infrequently and may be the presenting feature of the disease (Kornblut, Wolff and Fauci, 1982). It may take the form of a subacute otitis media, otitis media with effusion or chronic suppurative otitis media. In some cases it may present with a mixed hearing loss of sudden onset which can be improved by steroid therapy (Clements *et al.*, 1989).

The diagnosis must be considered in cases of atypical otitis media, particularly with a significantly raised ESR. Confirmation depends on the recognition of involvement of the kidneys and lungs, detection of the antineutrophil cytoplasmic antibody (ANCA) and histological examination of material from the nose or middle ear.

Treatment is by a combination of cyclophosphamide and prednisolone (Fauci *et al.*, 1983). The middle ear disease improves in parallel with the systemic response to treatment and deteriorates if the disease ceases to be controlled.

Histiocytosis X

This disease, which is also known as Langerhan's cell histiocytosis, is an uncommon granulomatous condition characterized by the idiopathic proliferation of Langerhan's cells or their marrow precursors. Ear disease is a reasonably common feature of the disease and may be the presenting feature (Quraishi, Blayney and Brearnach, 1994). The most common manifestation is aural discharge, but there may also be lesions within the temporal bone. The involvement of other body systems and elevation of the ESR are suggestive of the diagnosis. Treatment involves chemotherapy, radiotherapy and steroids.

References

ARNVIG, J. (1963) Some problems concerning the prognosis and treatment of chronic adhesive otitis media. *Acta Otolaryngologica*, Supplement 188, 75–76

BEALES, P. H. (1959) The problem of the mastoid segment after tympanoplasty. *Journal of Laryngology and Otology*, 73, 527–531

BEALES, P. H. and HYNES, W. (1958) Rapid healing after mastoid surgery by the use of the post-auricular flap. *Journal of Laryngology and Otology*, 72, 888–901

BENNETT, R. J. (1981) The operation of tympanomastoid re-aeration: physiological repair of the radical mastoid cavity. *Journal of Laryngology and Otology*, 95, 1–10

BOOTH, J. B. (1974) Myringoplasty: the lessons of failure. *Journal of Laryngology and Otology*, 88, 1223–1236

BROOK, I. (1985) Prevalence of beta-lactamase-producing bacteria in chronic suppurative otitis media. *American Journal of Diseases of Children*, 139, 280–283

BROWNING, G. G. (1984a) The unsafeness of 'safe' ears. *Journal of Laryngology and Otology*, 98, 23–26

BROWNING G. G. (1984b) Medical management of chronic mucosal otitis media. *Clinical Otolaryngology*, 9, 141–144

BROWNING, G. G. and GATEHOUSE, S. (1992) The prevalence of middle ear disease in the adult British population. *Clinical Otolaryngology*, 17, 317–321

BROWNING, G. G., PICOZZI, G., SWEENEY, G. and CALDER, I. T. (1983) Role of anaerobes in chronic otitis media. *Clinical Otolaryngology*, 8, 47–51

BRUMMET, R. E., HARRIS, R. F. and LINDGREN, J. A. (1976) Detection of ototoxicity from drugs applied topically to the middle ear space. *Laryngoscope*, 86, 1177–1187

CHARACHON, R. (1978) Cholesteatoma, epidermization: choice between closed and obliteration technique. *Clinical Otolaryngology*, 3, 363–367

CHARACHON, R. and GRATACAP, B. (1985) The surgical treatment of cholesteatoma in children. *Clinical Otolaryngology*, 10, 177–184

CLEMENTS, M. R., MISTRY, C. D., KEITH A. O. and RAMSDEN, R. T. (1989) Recovery from sensorineural hearing loss in patients with Wegner's granulomatosis. *Journal of Laryngology and Otology*, 103, 515–518

CODY, D. T. R. and MCDONALD, T. J. (1984) Mastoidectomy for acquired cholesteatoma: follow up to 20 years. *Laryngoscope*, 94, 1027–1030

CONSTABLE, L. and BUTLER, I. (1982) Microbial flora in chronic otitis media. *Journal of Infection*, 5, 57–60

DERLAKI, E. L. and CLEMIS, J. D. (1965) Congenital cholesteatoma of the middle ear and mastoid. *Annals of Otology, Rhinology and Laryngology*, 74, 706–727

DUMICH, J. and HARNER, S. G. (1983) Cochlea function in chronic otitis media. *Laryngoscope*, 93, 583–586

FAIRBANKS, D. N. F. (1981) Anti-microbial therapy for chronic otitis media. *Annals of Otology, Rhinology and Laryngology*, 90, (suppl. 94), 58–62

FAUCI A., HAYNES, B. F., KATZ, P. and WOLFF, S. M. (1983) Wegener's granulomatosis: prospective clinical and therapeutic experience with 85 patients for 21 years. *Annals of Internal Medicine*, 98, 76–85

FRIEDMANN, I. (1952) Bacteriological studies in otitis. *Journal of Laryngology and Otology*, 66, 175–180

GLASSCOCK, M. E., DICKENS, J. R. E. and WEIT, R. (1981) Cholesteatoma in children. *Laryngoscope*, 91, 1743–1753

GLASSCOCK, M. E., JACKSON, C. G., NISSEN, A. J. and SCHWABER, M. K. (1982) Post-auricular undersurface tympanic membrane grafting: a follow-up report. *Laryngoscope*, 92, 718–727

GLOVER, S. C., TRANTER, R. M. D. and INNES, J. A. (1981) Tuberculous otitis media: a reminder. *Journal of Laryngology and Otology*, 95, 1261–1264

GOYCOOLEA, M. V., PAPEARELLA, M. M., JUHN, S. K. and CARPENTER, A. M. (1980) Oval and round window changes in otitis media: potential pathways between the middle and inner ear. *Laryngoscope*, 90, 1387–1390

GRAHNE, B. (1964) Simple mastoidectomy with air chamber creation in progressive adhesive otitis. *Acta Otolaryngologica* 58, 258–270

GREGG, J. B., STEELE, J. P. and HOLZHUETER, A. (1965) Roentgenographic evaluation of temporal bones from South Dakota Indian burials. *American Journal of Physical Anthropology*, 23, 51–62

GUERRIER, T. (1988) Open cavity mastoidectomy in children. Hearing results at 5 years. In: *Pediatric Otology*, edited by C. Cremers and G. Hoogland. Basel: Karger. pp. 138–141

HABERMAN, R. S. and WERTH, J. L. (1981) Recurrent acquired atresia of the external auditory canal and associated canal cholesteatoma. *American Journal of Otology*, 21, 269–271

HINCHCLIFFE, R. (1961) Prevalence of the commoner ear, nose and throat conditions in the adult rural population of Great Britain: a study by direct examination of two random samples. *British Journal of Preventative and Social Medicine*, 15, 128–140

JACKLER, R. K., DILLON, W. P. and SCHINDLER, R. A. (1984) Computed tomography in suppurative disease: a correlation of surgical and radiographic findings. *Laryngoscope*, **94**, 746–752

JAHRSDOEFER, R. (1980) Congenital atresia of the ear. *Laryngoscope*, **88** (Supplement 13), 1–48

JAMA Update (1987) Creutzfeldt-Jacob disease in a patient receiving a cadaveric dura mater graft. *Journal of the American Medical Association*, **258**, 309–310

JANSEN C. (1968) The combined approach for tympanoplasty (report on 10 years experience) *Journal of Laryngology and Otology*, **82**, 779–793

JOKIPII, A. M. M., KARMA, P. OJALA, K. and JOKPII, L. (1977) Anaerobic bacteria in chronic otitis media. *Archives of Otolaryngology*, **103**, 278–280

KARMA, P., JOKIPII, L., OJALA, K. and JOKIPII, A. M. M. (1978) Bacteriology of the chronically discharging middle ear. *Acta Otolaryngologica*, **86**, 110–114

KELLY, M. J. (1978) The quantitative and histological demonstration of pathogenic synergy between *Escherichia coli* and *Bacteroides fragilis* in guinea pig wounds. *Journal of Medical Microbiology*, **11**, 513–523

KISCH, H. (1928) Temporalis muscle grafts in the radical mastoid operation. *Journal of Laryngology and Otology*, **43**, 735–736

KOHONEN, A., and TARKANEN, J. (1969) Cochlea damage by ototoxic antibiotics by intratympanic application. *Acta Otolaryngologica*, **68**, 90–97

KORNBLUT, A. D., WOLFF, S. M. and FAUCI, A. S. (1982) Ear disease in patients with Wegener's granulomatosis. *Laryngoscope*, **92**, 713–717

LAU, T. and TOS, M. (1988) When to do tympanoplasty in children? In: *Pediatric Otology*, edited by C. Cremers and G. Hoogland. Basel. Karger: pp. 156–161

LEE, K. and SCHUKNECHT, H. F. (1971) Results of tympanoplasty and mastoidectomy at the Massachusetts Eye and Ear Infirmary. *Laryngoscope*, **81**, 529–543

LEIGHTON, S. E. J., ROBSON, A. K., ANSLOW, P. and MILFORD, C. A. (1993) The role of CT imaging in the management of chronic suppurative otitis media. *Clinical Otolaryngology*, **18**, 23–29

McCAFFERTY, C. J., COMAN, W. B., SHAW, E. and LEWIS, N. (1977) Cholesteatoma in Australian Aboriginal children. In: *Cholesteatoma: First International Conference*, edited by B. F. McCabe, J. Sade and B. Abramson. Birmingham: Aesculapius. p. 293

McKENZIE, W. and BROTHWELL, D. (1967) Diseases of the ear. In: *Diseases of Antiquity*, edited by D. Brothwell and T. Sandison. Springfield: Charles C. Thomas. pp. 464–473

MEYRICK, P. S. (1951) The incidence of diseases of the ear, nose and throat: A survey of a remote native reservation. *South African Medical Journal*, **25**, 701–704

MILLS, R. P. (1988) Surgical management of the discharging mastoid cavity. *Journal of Laryngology and Otology*, Supplement **16**, 1–6

MILLS, R. P. (1991) Management of retraction pockets of the pars tensa. *Journal of Laryngology and Otology*, **105**, 525–528

MILLS, R. P. (1993) The influence of technical and pathological variables on outcome in ossiculoplasty. *Clinical Otolaryngology*, **18**, 202–205

MILLS, R. P. and GRAHAM, M. D. (1986) The development of cholesteatoma in association with congenital abnormalities of the ear. *Journal of Laryngology and Otology*, **100**, 1063–1066

MILLS, R. P. and PADGHAM, N. D. (1991) The management of childhood cholesteatoma. *Journal of Laryngology and Otology*, **105**, 343–345

MIYAMOTO, R. T., FAIRCHILD, T. H. and DAUGHERTY, H. S. (1984) Primary cholesteatoma in the congenitally atretic ear. *American Journal of Otology*, **51**, 283–285

O'DONAHUGHE, G. M., BATES, G. J., ANSLOW, P. and ROTHERA, M. P. (1987) The predictive value of high definition computerised tomography scanning in chronic suppurative otitis media. *Clinical Otolaryngology*, **12**, 89–96

OJALA, J. K., SORRI, M., RIIHKANGAS, P. and SIPILA, P. (1981) Comparison of pre- and postoperative bacteriology of chronic ears. *Journal of Laryngology and Otology*, **95**, 1023–1029

ONDERDONK, A. B., BARTLETT, J. G., LOUIE, T., SULLIVAN, N. and GORBACH, S. L. (1976) Microbial synergy in experimental intra-abdominal abscess. *Infection and Immunity*, **13**, 22–26

OSBORNE, J. E., TERRY, R. M. and GANDHI, A. G. (1985) Large meatoplasty technique for mastoid cavities. *Clinical Otolaryngology*, **10**, 357–360

PADGHAM, N. D., MILLS, R. P. and CHRISTMAS, H. E. (1989) Has the increasing use of grommets influenced the frequency of surgery for cholesteatoma? *Journal of Laryngology and Otology*, **103**, 1034–1035

PALVA, A., KARMA, P. and KARJA, J. (1977) Cholesteatoma in children. *Archives of Otolaryngology*, **103**, 74–77

PALVA, T. (1962) Reconstruction of the ear canal in surgery for chronic ear. *Archives of Otolaryngology*, **75**, 329–334

PALVA, T. (1963) Surgical management of adhesive tympanum. *Acta Otolaryngologica*, Supplement 188, 70–74

PALVA, T. (1973) Operative technique in mastoid obliteration. *Acta Otolaryngologica*, **75**, 289–290

PALVA, T. (1982) Obliteration of the mastoid cavity and reconstruction of the canal wall. In: *International Medical Reviews; Otolaryngology 1: Otology*, edited by A. G. Gibb and M. F. Smith . London Butterworths. pp. 19–29

PALVA, T. and HALLSTROM, O. (1965) Bacteriology of chronic otitis media. *Archives of Otolaryngology*, **82**, 359–364

PAPARELLA, M. M., BRADY, D. R. and HOEL, R. (1970) Sensorineural hearing loss in chronic otitis media and mastoiditis. *Transactions of the American Academy of Ophthalmology and Otolaryngology*, **741**, 108–115

PAPARELLA, M. M., HIRAIDE, O. M. and BRADY D. R. (1972) Pathology of sensorineural hearing loss in otitis media. *Annals of Otology, Rhinology and Laryngology*, **81**, 632–647

PAPARELLA, M. M., MORIZONO, T., LE, C. T., MANCINI, F., SIPILA, P., CHOO, Y. B. *et al.* (1984). Sensorineural hearing loss in otitis media. *Annals of Otology, Rhinology and Laryngology*, **931**, 623–629

PICOZZI, G. L., BROWNING, G. G. and CALDER, I. T. (1983) Controlled trial of gentamicin and hydrocortisone ear drops in the treatment of active chronic otitis media. *Clinical Otolaryngology*, **8**, 367–368

PROUD, G. O., MITTELMAN, H. and SEIDEN, G. D. (1968) Ototoxicity of topically applied chloramphenicol. *Archives of Otolaryngology*, **87**, 580–587

QURAISHI, M. S., BLAYNEY, A. W. and BREARNACH, F. (1994) Aural symptoms as primary presentation of Langerhan's cell histiocytosis. *Clinical Otolaryngology*, **18**, 317–323

RAINE, C. H. and SINGH, S. D. (1983) Tympanoplasty in children: a review of 144 cases. *Journal of Laryngology and Otology*, **97** 217–221

RATHBUN, T. A. and MALLIN, R. (1977) Middle ear disease in

a prehistoric Iranian population. *Bulletin of the New York Academy of Medecine*, **531**, 901–905

RUDIN, R., SVARSUDD, K., TIBBLIN, G. and HALLEN, O. (1983) Middle ear disease in samples from the general population: Prevalence and incidence of otitis media and its sequelae, the study of men born in 1913–23. *Acta Otolaryngologica*, **96**, 237–246

RUSSELL N. W. and KLEID, S. (1991), Myringoplasty: factors influencing results. *Journal of the Society of Otolaryngology of Australia*, **6**, 365–367

SADÉ, J. (ed.) (1979) The atelectatic ear. In: *Secretory Otitis Media and its Sequelae*. London. Churchill-Livingstone. pp. 64–88

SADÉ, J., BERCO, E., BROWN, M., WEINBERG, J. and AVRAHAM, S. (1981) Myringoplasty. *Journal of Laryngology and Otology*, **95** 653–665

SADÉ, J., WEINBERG, J., BERCO, E., BROWN, M., and HALVEY, A. (1982) The marsupialised (radical) mastoid. *Journal of Laryngology and Otology*, **96**, 869–875

SANNA M., ZINI, C., SCANDERELLI, R. and JEMMI, G. (1984) Residual and recurrent cholesteatoma in closed tympanoplasty. *American Journal of Otology*, **5**, 277–282

SANNA, M., ZINI, C., GAMOLETTI, R., RUSSO, A., SCANDERELLI, R. and TAIBAH, A. (1988) Surgery for congenital and acquired cholesteatoma in children. In: *Pediatric Otology*, edited by C. Cremers and G. Hoogland. Basel: Karger. pp. 124–130

SASAKI, C. T., ASKENASE, P., DWYER, J. and YANAGISAWA, E. (1981) Chronic ear infections in the immune deficient patient. *Archives of Otolaryngology*, **107**, 82–86

SENIOR, B. W. and SWEENEY, G. (1984) The association of particular types of proteus with chronic suppurative otitis media. *Journal of Medical Microbiology*, **17**, 201–205

SHARPE, J. F. and ROBINSON, J. M. (1992) Treatment of tympanic membrane retraction pockets by excision. A prospective study. *Journal of Laryngology and Otology*, **106**, 882–886

SHEEHY, J. L. (1978) Management of cholesteatoma in children. *Otorhinolaryngology*, **23**, 58–64

SHEEHY, J. L. (1981) Testing Eustachian tube function. *Annals of Otology, Rhinology and Laryngology*, **90**, 562–564

SHEEHY, J. L. (1983) Tympanoplasty with mastoidectomy: Present status. *Clinical Otolaryngology*, **8**, 391–403

SHEEHY, J. L. and ROBINSON, J. V. (1982) Cholesteatoma surgery at the Otologic Medical Group: residual and recurrent disease. A report on 307 revision operations. *American Journal of Otology*, **3**, 209–215

SINGH, B. (1991) Role of surgery in tuberculous mastoiditis. *Journal of Laryngology and Otology*, **105**, 907–915

SIRALA, U. (1963) Pathogenesis and treatment of adhesive otitis. *Acta Otolaryngologica*, Suppl. 188, 9–18

SMYTH, G. D. L. (1980) *Chronic Ear Disease*. Edinburgh: Churchill Livingstone

SMYTH, G. D. L. and PATTERSON, C. C. (1985) Results of middle ear reconstruction: do patients and surgeons agree? *American Journal of Otology*, **6**, 276–279

SOLOMAN, N. B. and ROBINSON, J. M. (1988) Obliteration of mastoid cavities using bone pate. *Journal of Laryngology and Otology*, **102**, 783–784

SUGITA, R., KAWAMURA, S., ICHIKAWA, G., GOTO, S. and FUJIMAKI, Y. (1981) Studies on anaerobic bacteria in chronic otitis media. *Laryngoscope*, **91**, 816–821

SWEENEY, G., PICOZZI, G. L. and BROWNING, G. G. (1982) A quantitative study of aerobic and anaerobic bacteria in chronic suppurative otitis media. *Journal of Infection*, **5**, 47–55

THOMSON, I. (1974) Exudative otitis media, grommets and cholesteatoma. *Journal of Laryngology and Otology*, **88**, 947–953

TOS, M. (1988) Incidence, etiology and pathogenesis of cholesteatoma in children. In: *Pediatric Otology*, edited by C. Cremers and G. Hoogland. Basel: Karger: pp. 110–117

TSCHOPP, C. F. (1977) Chronic otitis media and cholesteatoma in Alaskan native children. In: *Cholesteatoma, First International Conference*, edited by B. F. McCabe, J. Sadé and B. Abramson. Birmingham: Aescapulus. p. 290

WAKE, M., ROBINSON, J. M., WHITCOMBE, J. B., BAZERBACHI, S. STANSBIE, J. M. and PHELPS, P. D. (1992) Detection of recurrent cholesteatoma by computerised tomography after 'closed' cavity mastoid surgery. *Journal of Laryngology and Otology*, **106**, 393–395

WALBY, A. P., BARRERA, A. and SCHUKNECHT, H. F. (1983) Cochlea pathology in chronic suppurative otitis media. *Annals of Otology, Rhinology and Laryngology*, **92** (Supplement 103), 3–19

WEHRS, R. E. (1985) Hearing results in tympanoplasty. *Laryngoscope*, **95**, 1301–1306

WINDLE-TAYLOR, P. C. and BAILEY, C. M. (1980) Tuberculous otitis media: a series of 22 patients. *Laryngoscope*, **901**, 1039–1044

WRIGHT, W. K. (1977) Management of otic cholesteatoma. *Archives of Otolaryngology*, **103**, 144–147

YOUNGS, R. (1992) The histopathology of mastoid cavities, with particular reference to persistent disease leading to chronic otorrhoea. *Clinical Otolaryngology*, **17**, 505–510

11

Reconstruction of the middle ear

Nicholas J. Frootko

In this chapter the evolution of surgical techniques of tympanoplasty with and without mastoidectomy in chronic suppurative otitis media is outlined, the terminology defined and the biological and biomaterials used to reconstruct the middle ear transformer mechanism are described.

Definitions of operative terms currently used in middle ear and mastoid surgery

Skin incisions

These are named according to the anatomical site in which they are made, that is *meatal, endaural* and *postaural* and can be combined and fashioned in a variety of ways to provide the access, exposure and other requirements (e.g. meatal skin flaps, muscle flaps and meatoplasty) of the operation to be performed.

Meatoplasty

(Synonym: *canalplasty*). An operation performed to widen the cartilaginous and/or bony external auditory meatus. The procedure may be limited, e.g. removal of bone from the deep anterior canal wall to gain access to the anterior recess, or may be more extensive, i.e. when cartilage and bone are removed as an integral part of many of the mastoidectomy and tympanoplasty with mastoidectomy procedures.

Myringoplasty

An operation performed to repair or reconstruct the tympanic membrane, often incorrectly referred to as type I tympanoplasty (because myringoplasty

does not imply removal of disease from the middle ear).

Tympanoplasty

An operation performed to 'eradicate disease in the middle ear and to reconstruct the hearing mechanism, without mastoid surgery, with or without tympanic membrane grafting' (Committee on Conservation of Hearing of the American Academy of Ophthalmology and Otolaryngology, 1965).

Ossiculoplasty

An operation performed to repair or reconstruct the ossicular chain.

Mastoidectomy

Open or canal wall-down procedures

Atticotomy

An operation performed to remove all or part of the outer attic wall (scutum) and adjacent deep posterior meatal wall, to expose the attic (epitympanum) and, when necessary, the aditus ad antrum in order to gain access to these sites and their contents and/or remove disease limited to these sites.

Radical mastoidectomy

An operation performed to eradicate all middle ear and mastoid disease, in which the mastoid antrum and air cell system (when present), aditus ad antrum, attic and middle ear (mesotympanum and hypotympanum) are converted into a common cavity, exteriorized to the external auditory meatus. During the course of removal of all diseased tissues the tympanic membrane, malleus and incus are removed, leaving only the stapes *in situ* (footplate alone, or with the superstructure, if intact and healthy).

Modified radical mastoidectomy

This operation differs from the radical mastoidectomy in that the tympanic membrane or remnants thereof and ossicular remnants (usually the malleus handle and stapes) are retained (synonym: *attico-antrostomy* if the operation is performed by the anterior-posterior technique, i.e. by exposing the attic first and then proceeding backwards into the aditus ad antrum and mastoid antrum).

Closed or canal wall-up procedures

Cortical mastoidectomy

This is an operation performed to remove disease from the mastoid antrum and air cell system (when present) and the aditus ad antrum, with preservation of an intact posterior bony external auditory canal wall, without disturbing the existing middle ear contents.

Combined approach tympanoplasty

(Synonym: *intact canal wall tympanoplasty with mastoidectomy*.) This is an operation performed to remove disease from the middle ear and mastoid by way of (a) the mastoid, (b) a posterior tympanotomy, and (c) the transcanal route, followed by reconstruction of the middle ear transformer mechanism (Figures 11.1 and 11.2).

Tympanoplasty with mastoidectomy

This is an operation performed to eradicate disease from the middle ear and mastoid and to reconstruct the hearing mechanism with or without tympanic membrane grafting; e.g:

1. Combined approach tympanoplasty or cortical mastoidectomy with tympanoplasty (*closed cavity or canal wall-up techniques*)
2. Muscle or other obliteration of an open mastoid cavity with tympanoplasty (*obliteration techniques*)
3. Reconstruction of the outer attic and posterior canal wall of an open mastoid cavity, with tympanoplasty (*canal wall reconstruction techniques*)
4. Open or canal wall-down mastoidectomy with tympanoplasty (*open cavity techniques*).

NB: Cavity obliteration and canal wall reconstruction techniques convert an open cavity into a closed cavity.

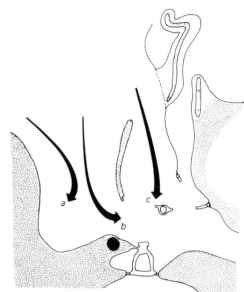

Figure 11.1 Combined approach tympanoplasty in which disease is removed from the middle ear and mastoid via: (*a*) the mastoid; (*b*) a posterior tympanotomy; and (*c*) the transcanal route. ●: facial nerve

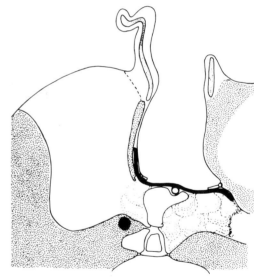

Figure 11.2 In this example the malleus handle and an intact and mobile stapes remain after the excision of disease, requiring reconstruction of the tympanic membrane and a malleus/stapes assembly. ●: facial nerve

The evolution of surgical techniques of tympanoplasty with and without mastoidectomy

The fundamental techniques and concepts of modern reconstructive middle ear surgery in chronic suppurative otitis media with and without cholesteatoma, came into being when Moritz (1952), Zöllner (1953, 1955) and Wullstein (1953, 1956) in Germany, introduced the tympanoplasty operations. These operations were designed to restore or conserve hearing and promote healing, after the excision of disease from the middle ear and mastoid. Skin grafts were used to repair the tympanic membrane and close the tympanum and were positioned as free 'onlay' grafts over the tympanic membrane remnant and whatever elements of the ossicular chain remained after the surgical excision of disease. If only a mobile stapes footplate remained, this was left exteriorized and the skin graft was positioned so as to create a round window baffle (an air-containing tunnel, in continuity with the eustachian tube and incorporating the round window). If the stapes was fixed by tympanosclerosis or otosclerosis, a fenestration operation was performed (Figure 11.3).

Prior to this pioneering work, the surgery of chronic suppurative otitis media had been wholly orientated to the eradication of chronic infection and cholesteatoma and the prevention of intracranial infection. The radical mastoid operation (Stacke, 1893), the Heath modification of this operation (Heath, 1904), the modified radical mastoid operation (Bondy, 1910) and the more conservative modifications of the Bondy operation, such as the atticotomy (Tumarkin, 1948) were all operations designed to *expose*, *excise* and *exteriorize* disease to the external auditory meatus. Although attempts had been made by a few surgeons to obliterate open mastoid cavities with muscle, and thus promote healing (Kisch, 1928; Meurman and Ojala, 1949), no attempt had been made by these surgeons to close the tympanum and repair the ossicular chain after the excision of disease. (For further reading, the author would refer you to a short historical review by Briggs and Luxford, 1994.)

The concepts and final execution of the classical tympanoplasty operations by Moritz, Zöllner and Wullstein had not come about by chance, but were influenced by other events. Berthold (1878), in Germany, had successfully repaired the tympanic membrane with full thickness skin and called the operation 'myringoplastik'. In 1921, Nylen, working in the Stockholm University Ear Clinic, introduced a monocular operating microscope and a year later Holmgren, Nylen's teacher, was the first to introduce the binocular operating microscope and magnifying ocular loop.

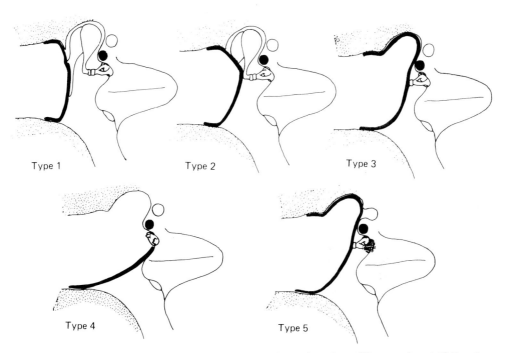

Figure 11.3 Wullstein's five tympanoplasty techniques after removal of disease from the middle ear and mastoid. Type 1, reconstruction of the tympanic membrane (ossicular chain intact and mobile). Type 2, malleus handle absent, reconstruction of the tympanic membrane over the malleus remnant and long process of incus. Type 3, malleus and incus absent, reconstruction of the tympanic membrane over an intact and mobile stapes (myringostapediopexy) with stapes acting as a columella. Type 4, mobile stapes footplate exteriorized with reconstruction of the tympanic membrane as a round window baffle. Type 5, stapes fixed, fenestration

There had also been a re-orientation of otological surgery from operations for infection towards reconstruction, when Lempert (1938) in America, successfully carried out the one-stage fenestration operation. Rosen (1953) revived the stapes mobilization procedure for otosclerosis and Juers (1953) had noted that, in some patients with cholesteatoma and erosion of the long process of the incus, pathological approximation of the pars tensa with an intact mobile stapes, produced excellent hearing. He created a similar conduction mechanism surgically, using a meatal skin flap and called the operation 'myringodermostapediopexy'. The dental drill rapidly replaced the hammer and gouge previously used for mastoid exenteration, sulphonamides and antibiotics in the form of penicillin were now available and there had been significant improvements in general and local anaesthetic techniques. Leading otologists such as Simson Hall in Edinburgh, Cawthorne in London and Shambaugh in America had operating microscopes which incorporated light sources and were developing new otological techniques, but were largely ignorant of developments in Germany at that time. In 1948, Wullstein had his own binocular microscope built by Leitz and from 1948 to 1953 performed over 1000 ear operations (Wullstein, 1981).

In 1953, the Zeiss operating microscope became available commercially and, in the same year, Wullstein and Zollner launched their tympanoplasty methods at the Fifth International Congress of Otorhinolaryngology in Amsterdam.

These methods were soon adopted vigorously by otologists all over the world, but many experienced difficulty and disappointment with skin grafts used to repair the tympanic membrane and line open mastoid cavities and with the hearing results obtained from the classic tympanoplasties. Full thickness skin fared badly in the ear. The grafts were bulky, continued to secrete sebum, became infected and necrotic (Wright, 1960). Eleven per cent of the grafts perforated; epithelial cysts and graft cholesteatomas complicated 3% of cases (Guilford, 1962; Wright, 1963), and the formation of fibrous adhesions between the undersurface of the graft and promontory resulted in obliteration of the middle ear space (Thorburn, 1960; Palva, 1963). Similar problems were encountered with split skin grafts, 30% of which perforated, and surgeons were encouraged to find alternative grafting materials for tympanic membrane repair.

In 1956, Zollner (Zollner, 1963) successfully used autologous fascia lata. Hall (1956) introduced autologous cheek mucosa and Claros-Domenech (1959) introduced autologous periosteum. Shea (1960a) accidentally tore the tympanic membrane during a stapedectomy procedure and repaired the tear successfully with a free autologous vein graft placed medial to the tympanic membrane, thus introducing the 'underlay' technique of myringoplasty. Heermann (1960) reported successful myringoplasty results using autologous temporalis fascia 'onlay' grafts and successful results were also reported using tragal perichondrium (Goodhill, Harris and Brockman, 1964) and free autologous fat grafts (Ringenberg, 1962). These grafts were stable and easy to handle, only a small percentage perforated and they could be positioned lateral to the tympanic membrane remnant (onlay) or medial to it (underlay) (Figure 11.4). Chalat (1964) was the first to use tympanic membrane allografts (thus paving the way for the introduction of tympanomeatal and tympano-ossicular allografts) and 2 years later Albright and Leigh (1966) published their preliminary report on allograft dura mater myringoplasty. As an alternative to tympanomeatal allografts for the repair of large perforations, Perkins (1975) introduced the moulded formaldehyde preserved autologous temporalis fascia graft. Small perforations of the tympanic membrane may also be repaired by stimulating or enhancing reparative processes, by topical application of weak acids, sodium hyaluronate (Hellstrom *et al.*, 1991) and basic fibroblast growth factor (Vrabec *et al.*, 1994).

The surgery of otosclerosis was yet again to have a profound effect on tympanoplasty techniques. In 1956, Shea performed the first stapedectomy, covered the oval window with subcutaneous connective tissue and replaced the stapes with a Teflon replica (Shea, 1956). He later introduced the vein graft-polyethylene tube method of stapes replacement (Shea, 1960b). Soon other implant materials including titanium, tantalum, platinum and stainless steel were used as stapes replacement prostheses and, as such, were well tolerated in the middle ear. These materials were, therefore, applied to ossicular chain reconstruction in tympanoplasty, but early enthusiasm for these techniques soon waned when it became apparent that many prosthetic assemblies were unstable and became displaced in the middle ear. If the prosthesis came into contact with the undersurface of the tympanic membrane, extrusion was common, despite the ingenuity of design, such as that shown by the polyethylene-tube umbrella (Oppenheimer and Harrison, 1963), the polyethylene tube-wire mesh 'sunflower' columella (House and Sheehy, 1963) and the Teflon 'umbrella' (Austin, 1963), and these prostheses were, therefore, abandoned.

From this catalogue of disasters, enormous experience was gained with microsurgical techniques, together with a more comprehensive understanding of the reparative processes in the middle ear and mastoid and the realization that successful ossicular chain reconstruction could only be achieved in a closed air-containing middle ear cavity (Rambo, 1961; Tabb, 1963). To promote growth of new, healthy middle ear mucosa, to maintain a middle ear free of adhesions and to support the neotympanic membrane, absorbable and non-absorbable materials were placed in the middle ear. Wullstein (1960) advocated the use of absorbable gelatin sponge known today as Gel-

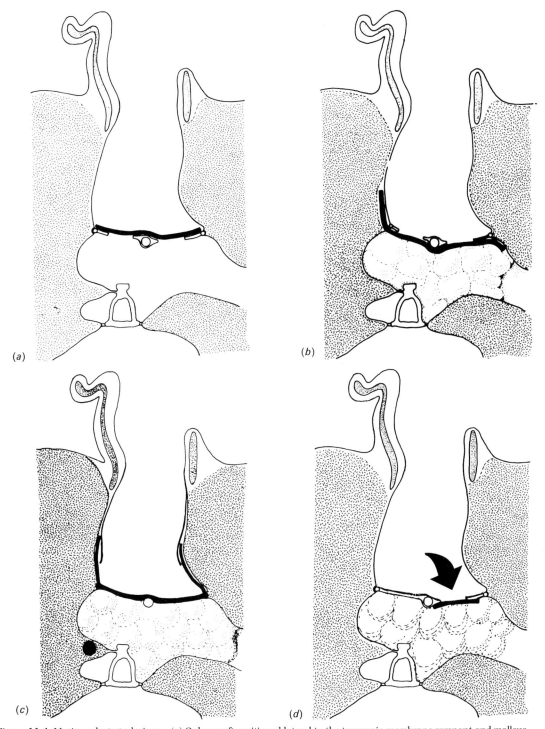

Figure 11.4 Myringoplasty techniques. (*a*) Onlay graft positioned lateral to the tympanic membrane remnant and malleus handle after removing all squamous epithelium from these structures. (*b*) Underlay graft positioned medial to the tympanic membrane remnant and malleus handle or medial to the tympanic membrane remnant and lateral to the denuded malleus handle as in Figure 11.2. (*c*) Tympanomeatal allograft positioned underneath the deep meatal skin cuff and lateral to the malleus handle. (*d*) 'Pop in' underlay technique for small central perforations. Autologous fat, tragal perichondrium or temporalis fascia inserted through the perforation onto a gel-foam bed after excising the perforation margins and scarifying the undersurface of the adjacent tympanic membrane

foam or Gel-film. Non-absorbable polymer sheeting made of polyethylene (House, 1960), Teflon, Silastic (see Shea, 1981) and paraffin wax (Rambo, 1961; Tabb, 1963) were introduced for use in ears where the excision of disease included removal of most of the middle ear mucoperiosteum. These materials needed to be removed from the ear 3–6 months postoperatively and the concept of 'staged tympanoplasty' was born, i.e. in these 'severely damaged' ears, no attempt was made to reconstruct the sound-conducting mechanism until a healthy, ventilated middle ear cavity and an intact, healthy tympanic membrane existed (Tabb, 1963; Farrior, 1966; Austin, 1969; Sheehy and Crabtree, 1973).

Leading otologists had also come to realize that no single operation was pertinent to the surgical treatment of chronic suppurative otitis media. The two opposing demands of tympanoplasty, namely radical and complete removal of disease and reconstruction of the sound-conducting mechanism posed a major problem. Every case needed to be evaluated on the basis of whether disease excision required a purely transcanal operation, or whether, in addition, some form of mastoidectomy was needed together with a tympanoplasty.

When a mastoidectomy is necessary, two basic surgical techniques have evolved, namely, the canal wall-down and the canal wall-up procedures.

In the *canal wall-down* procedures, the posterior bony meatal wall and the outer attic wall are removed and the attic, aditus ad antrum together with the mastoid antrum and air cell system are exteriorized to the external auditory meatus. Small 'open cavities' thus created usually epithelialize rapidly and are healthy and stable postoperatively.

Large cavities, however, are often prone to recurrent infection due to incomplete epithelialization (despite complete excision of disease, a low facial ridge, the presence of a wide meatus and closure of the middle ear space isolating the eustachian tube from the mastoid cavity) and this, in turn, prejudices the reconstruction of the middle ear sound-conducting mechanism. To avoid this, cavity lining, cavity obliteration and posterior canal wall reconstruction techniques were introduced.

When incomplete epithelialization of an open cavity is the cause of recurrent infection and discharge, Premachandra *et al.* (1993) have used cultured epithelial keratinocytes, prepared from autologous epidermal cells, to form a healthy protective lining of the open mastoid cavity. This technique has been more successful than cavity lining techniques using split skin grafts, dura mater and free fascial grafts.

Obliteration techniques to line and reduce the size of the mastoid cavity, or obliterate it completely, have been successfully achieved using autologous cancellous iliac crest bone grafts (Schiller and Singer, 1960), allogeneic femoral cortical bone chips (Shea,

Gardner and Simpson, 1972) and hydroxylapatite ceramic powders and particles (see Table 11.5). More popular, however, are the muscle obliteration techniques using local 'random pattern' muscle-periosteal transposition and rotation flaps of sternomastoid muscle (Meurman and Ojala, 1949), temporalis muscle (Rambo, 1958), postauricular muscle-periosteal flaps based on the sternomastoid muscle (Hilger and Hohmann, 1963) and the anteriorly based postauricular muscle-periosteal transposition flap together with bone paté (Palva, 1963, 1982, 1993). Mastoid cavity obliteratiion has also been successfully achieved using local 'axial pattern' flaps, based on the superficial temporal vessels, i.e. the temporoparietal fascia flap (Byrd, 1980; East, Brough and Grant, 1991) and the temporalis fascia flap, known as the 'Hong Kong flap' (van Hasselt, 1994).

Posterior canal wall and outer attic wall reconstruction techniques using autologous or allogeneic cartilage grafts (Jansen, 1972; Smyth, 1972a; Wehrs, 1972, 1982a; Adkins, 1990), allogeneic external auditory meatus bone (Smith, 1970) or autologous mastoid bone (Marquet, 1976a) and mastoid bone paté (Pulec, 1976; Moffat, Gray and Irving, 1994) have been introduced as an alternative to cavity obliteration.

The *canal wall-up* techniques of tympanoplasty with mastoidectomy preserve the posterior bony external auditory canal wall and the tympanic sulcus, avoid a postoperative mastoid cavity and allow for reconstruction of the tympanic membrane in its normal anatomical position.

With the passage of time, increasing evidence has accumulated indicating that many surgeons fail to eradicate cholesteatoma (residual disease) in about 25% of all 'closed' operations at primary surgery (Smyth and Hassard, 1981) and in all forms of combined approach tympanoplasty there is a high incidence of retraction pocket formation (recurrent disease) (Austin, 1977; Smyth, 1982a). Of necessity, therefore, all 'closed' operations must be staged and 'second look' revision procedures need to be continued until the surgeon is confident that the tubotympanic cleft is free of cholesteatoma. Alternatively, the ear with recurrent or residual disease must be converted into an 'open cavity'.

Enormous controversy surrounds the merits and demerits of 'open cavity' and 'closed cavity' (cavity obliteration, posterior canal wall reconstruction and intact canal wall techniques) (Kohut, 1980; Sheehy, 1980; Smyth, 1982a). Despite this, these operations produce two distinctly different types of middle ear space, namely, 'shallow' and 'deep', depending on whether the tympanic membrane is reconstructed in its normal anatomical position or at the level of the facial ridge (Figures 11.5, 11.6, 11.7 and 11.8). Consequent upon this, different techniques of ossicular chain reconstruction needed to be found.

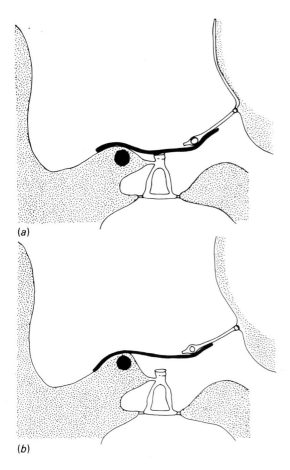

(a)

(b)

Figure 11.5 (*a*) Open mastoid cavity, low facial ridge, shallow middle ear space enabling type 3 reconstruction – myringostapediopexy. (*b*) Open mastoid cavity, high facial ridge, shallow middle ear space requiring reconstruction of the tympanic membrane and a malleus/stapes assembly

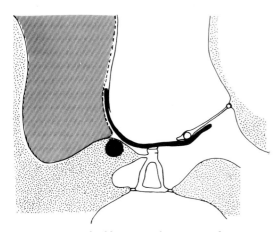

Figure 11.6 Muscle obliteration of open mastoid cavity, low facial ridge, shallow middle ear space enabling type 3 reconstruction – myringostapediopexy

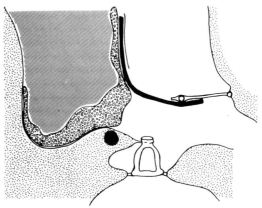

Figure 11.7 Reconstruction of the posterior canal wall and obliteration of the mastoid cavity with muscle and bone paté, with reconstruction of the tympanic membrane in its normal anatomical position creating a deep middle ear space in which a malleus/stapes assembly is required to establish ossicular chain continuity

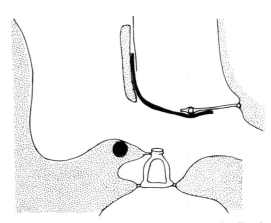

Figure 11.8 Reconstruction of the posterior canal wall and outer attic wall using sculptured autologous bone from the outer mastoid table, with reconstruction of the tympanic membrane in its normal anatomical position thus creating a deep middle ear space and requiring a malleus/stapes assembly to establish ossicular chain continuity

Grafts used in tympanoplasty and mastoidectomy

Otologists using tissue transplants to reconstruct the middle ear have, like other transplant surgeons, needed to add a number of new words to their vocabulary in order to describe the types of graft they use. This jargon has been called 'transplantese' and there has been much debate over the terminology that will prove to be most appropriate, informative and etymologically accurate. Nonetheless, a new terminology has evolved and this can and should be applied to tympanoplasty and mastoidectomy (Frootko, 1985a).

Four types of graft can be defined according to the genetic relationship between the donor and the host (Table 11.1).

Grafts of any genetic origin may be further defined according to their new anatomical site, pattern of vascularization and functional capacity. Grafts placed in an anatomical position normally occupied by such tissue are *orthotopic grafts* (Greek orthos = right or correct), e.g. a tympano-ossicular allograft used to reconstruct the tympanic membrane and ossicular chain. Sculptured ossicular bone grafts used to reconstruct the ossicular chain, placed in their normal anatomical site, but not usually into their normal anatomical position, should probably also be called 'orthotopic' to avoid confusion. Those grafts placed in an unnatural recipient location are *heterotopic grafts* (Greek heteros = other or different), e.g. a sculptured nasal septal cartilage allograft used to reconstruct the ossicular chain or outer attic wall.

A graft placed directly onto a vascular pedicle is a *vascularized graft*, e.g. a kidney transplant, whereas a *free* or *non-vascularized graft* vascularizes indirectly from the recipient bed, e.g. a preserved dura mater graft used to repair the tympanic membrane.

Those grafts expected or intended to fulfil their normal physiological functional capacity are *vital grafts*, e.g. a kidney transplant, while *static grafts*, serve a mechanical function that does not require 'physiological viability'. Such grafts act as a scaffolding or matrix onto, and into, which host tissues extend. At present, all tissue grafts used in tympano-plasty and tympanoplasty with mastoidectomy, are free, non-vascularized static grafts and these latter distinctions do not therefore have to be made (Table 11.2).

Reconstruction of the ossicular chain
Ossicular bone autografts

Reticent to use metal and polymer prostheses in the middle ear, Hall and Rytzner (1957) performed the first ossicular chain reconstruction using autologous ossicular bone. Having, accidentally, fractured the stapes superstructure performing a stapes mobilization for otosclerosis, they successfully *interposed* the patient's own sculptured incus between the tympanic membrane and the mobilized stapes footplate. The immediate postoperative air-bone gap closure was short-lived because the incus slipped off the footplate. To prevent this complication in subsequent cases of otosclerosis, a small fenestration was made in the footplate or the stapes was removed, and the short process of the autologous incus placed directly into the oval window. In cases of chronic suppurative otitis media with erosion of the long process of the incus, Hall and Rytzner removed the incus, malleus and stapes superstructure. The autologous malleus was then sculptured and interposed between the neo-tympanic membrane and stapes footplate. They reported no serious cochlear damage but, in some cases, the interposed ossicle became displaced, or bony fixation occurred in the oval window niche. Three interposed ossicles removed at revision surgery showed histological evidence of vascularization of marrow spaces, some viable osteocytes in the lacu-

Table 11.1 Transplant terminology

Old terminology		New terminology		
Noun	*Adjective*	*Noun*	*Adjective*	*Definition*
Autograft	Autogenous	Autograft	Autologous or autogeneic	Tissue transplanted from one part of the body to another in the same individual, e.g. a temporalis fascia or tragal perichondrial graft used to repair the tympanic membrane
Isograft	Isologous or isogenic	Isograft	Isogeneic or syngeneic	Tissue transplanted between genetically identical individuals, e.g. an incus graft between rats of the same inbred strain
Homograft	Homologous	Allograft	Allogeneic	Tissue transplanted between genetically non-identical members of the same species, e.g. a preserved human cadaver-acquired tympanomeatal graft used to reconstruct the tympanic membrane, or a preserved human cadaver-acquired incus used to repair an ossicular chain defect
Heterograft	Heterologous	Xenograft	Xenogeneic	Tissue transplanted between members of different species, e.g. a preserved bovine vein graft used to repair a human tympanic membrane

Table 11.2 Grafts currently used in middle ear and mastoid reconstructive surgery

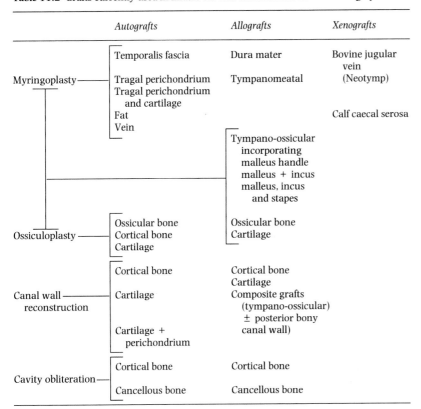

	Autografts	*Allografts*	*Xenografts*
Myringoplasty	Temporalis fascia Tragal perichondrium Tragal perichondrium and cartilage Fat Vein	Dura mater Tympanomeatal Tympano-ossicular incorporating malleus handle malleus + incus malleus, incus and stapes	Bovine jugular vein (Neotymp) Calf caecal serosa
Ossiculoplasty	Ossicular bone Cortical bone Cartilage	Ossicular bone Cartilage	
Canal wall reconstruction	Cortical bone Cartilage Cartilage + perichondrium	Cortical bone Cartilage Composite grafts (tympano-ossicular) ± posterior bony canal wall)	
Cavity obliteration	Cortical bone Cancellous bone	Cortical bone Cancellous bone	

nae, but no obvious new bone formation or bone resorption apart from minor reduction of the calcified matrix on the surface (Hall and Rytzner, 1960, 1961). This work led directly to the application of ossicular bone grafting for reconstruction of the ossicular chain in tympanoplasty.

Autologous ossicles were also repositioned using *transposition* techniques. In these operations the incus remnant and/or malleus were partially mobilized from their normal anatomical positions and transposed onto the stapes head or footplate.

When the long process of the incus was missing, Bell (1958) removed the incus and transposed the malleus, attached to the tympanic membrane by its umbo, onto the stapes head (tympanomalleostapediopexy). Similar malleus transpositions were described by Hall and Rytzner (1957), Farrior (1960) and Portmann (1963). Other transposition techniques used when the long process of the incus was missing involved mobilizing the incus out of the fossa incudis, dislocating the incudomalleal joint and transposing the necrosed long process onto the stapes head. In such cases Farrior (1960) mobilized the incus/malleus complex leaving the incudomalleal joint intact and transposed either the short process of the incus,

or its eroded long process, onto the stapes head. Long-term hearing results achieved with these transposition procedures were not published, but Farrior (1969) reported that many transpositions had failed because of ankylosis of the transposed ossicles to the bony walls of the tympanum.

Throughout the 1960s, therefore, most surgeons focused their attention on the more successful *interposition* techniques using a sculptured autologous incus or malleus (Farrior, 1960, 1966; Portmann, 1963; Chandler, 1965; Guilford, 1965; Sheehy, 1965; Szpunar, 1967; Wright, 1967).

The usefulness of autologous ossicular bone grafts in tympanoplasty was challenged by Jongkees (1957) when he stressed that failure to control infection in chronic suppurative otitis media might be due to occult osteitis in the ossicles retained in the middle ear after the surgical removal of mucosal disease and/or cholesteatoma. These suspicions were confirmed when Grippaudo (1958) reported histological evidence of infection in 92% of incus and malleus bones removed from 42 cases of chronic suppurative otitis media. Grippaudo emphasized that the use of these diseased autologous ossicles in tympanoplasty may prejudice the results of reconstruction. Similar evidence of osteitis in ossicles removed from cases of chronic suppurative otitis media was reported by Bellucci and Wolff (1966), and Steinbach and Hildmann (1972). Austin (1971) warned about the use of autologous ossicles that showed any evidence of erosion macroscopically and advised that any such ossicles with adherent squamous epithelium or cholesteatoma should never be used in reconstruction.

Ossicular bone allografts

Realizing the need to find a new material to reconstruct the ossicular chain in patients without a malleus, and/or incus, and/or stapes superstructure, or with severe infection or cholesteatoma involving the ossicles, House, Patterson and Linthicum (1966) introduced the incus allograft. These incus allografts, acquired from the healthy middle ears of patients undergoing surgery for the removal of an acoustic neuroma were preserved in 70% ethyl alcohol prior to use. Twenty-eight ossiculoplasties were performed using an alcohol-preserved allograft incus interposition technique, but only 10 were followed up. Of five tympanic membrane-to-stapes head interpositions, only two achieved a postoperative air-bone gap of less than 20 dB and, in five tympanic membrane-to-footplate interpositions, only one was successful. One incus extruded 9 months postoperatively and was examined histologically. No inflammatory response was found in or around the graft, the marrow spaces were vascularized but there was no new bone formation. House's (1969) impression was that these grafts remain in the middle ear as dead bone and he recommended that ossicles could be acquired post-mortem provided the donor did not have malignant disease, hepatitis, syphilis or chronic suppurative otitis media. Pulec (1966) found no evidence of resorption or change in shape of three alcohol-preserved incus allografts removed at revision surgery 3–21 months postoperatively. Histologically, these grafts were found to be covered by mucous membrane and there were no signs of an inflammatory response. In the bony matrix 'no evidence of any living cell was discerned'. Linthicum (1966) compared the histological findings in nine autograft incudes and two alcohol-preserved allograft incudes used in tympanic membrane-to-stapes interpositions removed 9–12 months after surgery, because of lateral displacement of the graft off the stapes head. He found no evidence of inflammation in the middle ears of these cases at the time of revision surgery. In all specimens, host vascularization and connective tissue infiltration of marrow spaces was seen. New endosteal bone formation was found at a single site in only one specimen; in all the others, no new bone formation was found and most lacunae were empty. There was no difference in the macroscopic or histological appearance between the autografts and allografts. Austin (1971)

found histological evidence of limited osteoblastic activity with new bone formation in one alcohol-preserved incus removed one year postoperatively; in another, 'massive absorptive erosion' was seen and Austin questioned whether or not this represented a rejection phenomenon. Kerr and Smyth (1971a) examined 19 incudes (nine autografts and 10 alcohol-preserved allografts) and four mallei (one autograft and three alcohol-preserved allografts) removed at revision surgery 3–39 months postoperatively; no macroscopic evidence of erosion was found. Histologically, both the allografts and autografts were similar, with vascularization and plasma cell infiltration of marrow spaces together with small areas of new bone formation. It was noted that most new bone was formed in those grafts which had been longest in the middle ear. The authors concluded that there was no evidence of allograft ossicular bone rejection in the middle ear and that in time the grafts would be incorporated into the ossicular chain as vital structures. In a later report, however, Smyth, Kerr and Hassard (1977) concluded that new bone formation in alcohol-preserved ossicular bone allografts was not directly proportional to the time in the middle ear and that complete replacement of these grafts by new bone would be rare.

Preservation of cadaver-acquired ossicular bone by autoclaving was introduced by Hildyard (1967). Having observed no adverse reactions and no morphological changes in autoclaved allogeneic incudes placed in the hypotympanum of six patients with central tympanic membrane perforations, Hildyard used an autoclaved incus allograft as a tympanic membrane-to-footplate interposition in one case. Ten months postoperatively, the incus was removed because of poor hearing gain; histologically the graft was found to be acellular with no evidence of revascularization, new bone formation or inflammatory response.

Encouraged by the apparent lack of immune or inflammatory response and the ability of these ossicular bone allografts to remain in the middle ear without resorption, many surgeons started using allograft ossicular bone preserved in alcohol (Pulec, 1966; Wehrs, 1967; Smyth and Kerr, 1967) or by autoclaving (Hildyard, 1967; English *et al.*, 1971) for ossiculoplasty when healthy ossicular autografts were not available.

Otologists now began to concentrate on designing stable ossicular interpositions. The popular 'loose' interposition techniques, i.e. tympanic membrane-to-stapes head interposition or tympanic membrane-to-footplate interposition did not produce consistently good results (Guilford, 1966; Hildyard, 1967; Armstrong, 1969; Szpunar, 1969; Hough, 1970). The problems encountered included displacement of the graft, lateral retraction off the stapes head or footplate, consequent on lateral retraction of the neotympanic membrane during healing, and fibrous and bony ankylosis between graft and posterior bony annulus, facial canal or promontory (Hough, 1970; Austin, 1971). The grafts were also often too bulky (Goodhill, Westerbergh and Davis, 1974) and filled the space between the facial canal and the annulus, blocking the epitympanic isthmus and therefore obstructing air flow into the aditus ad antrum with resulting mucus accumulation and continued inflammation (Austin, 1971).

By surgical trial and error, coupled with careful postoperative observation, Guilford (1966) found that interpositions between the malleus handle and stapes head, i.e. malleus-stapes interposition or malleus-footplate interposition were more stable and produced better postoperative hearing gains than tympanic membrane-to-stapes head or tympanic membrane-to-footplate interposition. These sentiments were strongly supported by the experiences of Hildyard (1967), Armstrong (1969), Szpunar (1969) and Hough (1970) and confirmed by Elbrond and Elpern (1965) in an experimental study of the stability and acoustic properties of various incus interposition techniques in cadaver temporal bone models.

In 1971, Austin presented his classification of the anatomical defects found in the ossicular chain in 1151 consecutive ears with chronic suppurative otitis media at the Abraham Lincoln School of Medicine in Chicago. Isolated loss of the malleus handle (2% of ossicular defects) and isolated loss of the stapes superstructure (1.7% of ossicular defects) were not classified because of their rarity. In all other cases, the incus was deficient either wholly or in part and four types of ossicular defect were therefore described depending on the presence or absence of the malleus handle and the presence or absence of the stapes superstructure (Austin, 1971) (Figure 11.9).

When the malleus handle and stapes superstructure were present, Austin sculptured an autologous or allogeneic malleus head or incus body to fit between the malleus handle and stapes head. A cup-shaped depression was drilled into the graft to receive the stapes head and a concave depression carved to fit snugly against the malleus handle. This interposition technique was called the 'malleus/stapes assembly' and was more stable, less bulky, and less affected by lateral movement of the tympanic membrane during healing than was tympanic membrane-to-stapes head interposition (Figure 11.10).

When the malleus handle was present/stapes superstructure absent, Austin sculptured an autologous or allogeneic incus and interposed the graft precisely between the malleus handle and a small connective tissue pad placed on the stapes footplate. As with malleus/stapes assembly, the malleus handle was used as an energy coupler and lateral fixing point, and the small connective tissue pad on the stapes footplate helped centre the graft in the oval window niche and prevent slipping. This interposition tech-

Malleus handle

Present   Absent

Present

Stapes superstructure

Absent

(i)   (a)   (b)   (c)   (d)

Figure 11.9 (i) Modification of Austin's classification of ossicular chain defects. (Incus absent in all cases and tympanic membrane reconstruction required in all cases.) (*a*) Malleus handle present, stapes superstructure present, requiring reconstruction of the tympanic membrane and reconstruction of the ossicular chain from the malleus handle to the stapes head. (*b*) Malleus handle absent, stapes superstructure present, requiring reconstruction of the tympanic membrane, malleus and incus. (*c*) Malleus handle present, stapes superstructure absent, requiring reconstruction of the tympanic membrane and reconstruction of the ossicular chain from the malleus handle to the stapes footplate. (*d*) Malleus handle absent, stapes superstructure absent, requiring reconstruction of the tympanic membrane, malleus, incus and stapes superstructure

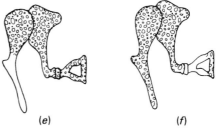

(e)   (f)

Malleus handle absent   Stapes superstructure absent
(ii)

Figure 11.9 (ii) Rare ossicular chain defects. (*e*) Isolated loss of the malleus handle, requiring reconstruction of the tympanic membrane and malleus, removal of the incus and its reconstruction. (*f*) Isolated loss of the stapes superstructure, requiring reconstruction of the tympanic membrane and reconstruction of the stapes superstructure

nique was called the 'malleus/footplate assembly' and was more stable than tympanic membrane-to-footplate interposition and produced better hearing results (Figure 11.11). Similar techniques were described by Hildyard (1967) and Hough (1970).

Pennington (1973) improved the design of the Austin malleus/stapes assembly to deal with the two

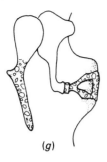
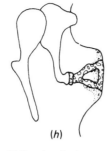

(g) **(h)**

Malleus handle present   Malleus handle absent
Stapes fixed   Stapes fixed

(iii)

Figure 11.9 (iii) The fixed stapes. (*g*) Malleus handle present, incus and stapes fixed, requiring reconstruction of the tympanic membrane and when possible, removal of the stapes, sealing of the oval window with a vein or tragal perichondrial autograft and reconstruction of the ossicular chain from the oval window to the malleus handle (malleolabyrinthopexy). (*h*) Malleus handle absent, incus absent, stapes fixed, requiring reconstruction of the tympanic membrane and malleus and when possible, removal of the stapes, sealing of the oval window with a vein or tragal perichondrial autograft and reconstruction of the ossicular chain from the oval window to the neomalleus handle. Note: in (*g*) and (*h*) an intact tympanic membrane and a healthy well-ventilated middle ear space must be achieved before the fixed stapes is removed, i.e. the procedure must be staged. In (*a*)–(*f*) the reconstruction may or may not be staged

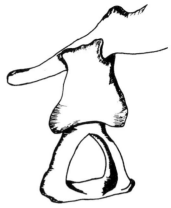

Figure 11.10 Malleus/stapes assembly – MSA (after Austin)

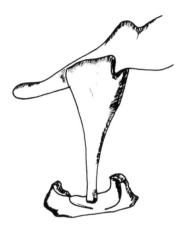

Figure 11.11 Malleus/footplate assembly – MFA (after Austin)

basic anatomical malleus/stapes relationships encountered in tympanoplasty. He designated the vertical malleus/stapes head relationship 'type 1a' and 'type 1b' and the horizontal malleus/stapes head relationship 'type 2' (Figure 11.12). In type 1a and 1b the incudomalleal joint surface of the incus was grooved to a deep yoke or 'mortice' to receive the malleus neck or handle, the incus short process was amputated and the long process dowelled or cupped to fit over the stapes head (Figure 11.13). In the type 2 cases, a double dowel technique was used over the stapes head (Figure 11.14). Using these malleus/stapes assembly techniques, Pennington reported closure of the air-bone gap to less than 16 dB in 69% of 216 ears followed up for 2–5 years.

Wehrs (1974) introduced the notched incus autograft or allograft technique. For malleus/stapes assembly, the incus long process was amputated, a notch was drilled into the short process to accommodate the malleus neck or handle and the incus body was dowelled to fit the stapes head ('notched incus with short process'). For malleus/footplate assembly, the incus short process was drilled in a similar fashion and the long process placed directly onto the stapes footplate ('notched incus with long process'). To deal with the varying spatial relationships between the malleus handle and the stapes head or footplate, appropriate sculpturing of the notch and dowel was

found to be applicable to most anatomical situations encountered (Figure 11.15).

These basic sculpturing techniques for malleus/stapes and malleus/footplate assemblies using allograft or autograft incudes or mallei with minor modifications are used by most surgeons today (Smyth, 1972b; Goodhill, Westerbergh and Davis, 1974; Marquet, 1976a; Ironside, 1979; Smith, 1980a,b; Hough, 1982; Smith and McElveen, 1982) (Figure 11.16).

The least common of the ossicular defects encountered, namely the absent malleus handle but with stapes superstructure present and the absent malleus handle with absent stapes superstructure, pose the most difficult reconstructive problems. The number of solutions proposed testify to this fact, but fundamentally the problem has been tackled in two ways.

The first was to establish a link between the neotympanic membrane and the stapes using a sculptured allograft malleus or incus, i.e. tympanic membrane-to-stapes head or tympanic membrane-to-

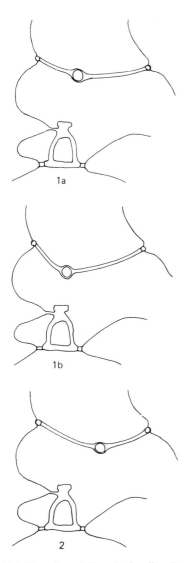

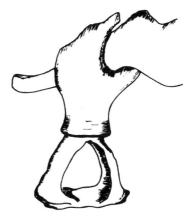

Figure 11.13 Vertical malleus/stapes assembly (after Pennington)

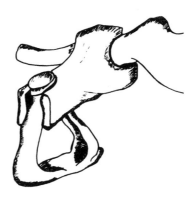

Figure 11.14 Horizontal malleus/stapes assembly (after Pennington)

Figure 11.12 Types 1a and 1b vertical malleus/stapes relationships and type 2 horizontal malleus/stapes head relationship (after Pennington)

footplate interposition (Austin, 1971, 1982; McGee, 1979; Smyth, 1980). In a shallow middle ear space, myringostapediopexy has been recommended by Lee and Schuknecht (1971), Goodman (1980) and Smyth (1980) if the stapes superstructure is intact. If the stapes superstructure is absent, Smith and Dobie (1976) and Marquet (1976a) recommended myringostapediopexy using an allograft stapes positioned onto the footplate. Gotay-Rodriguez and Schuknecht (1977) were able to achieve a 30 dB postoperative air-bone gap in 59% of 72 ears treated by open mastoidectomy and the use of autologous temporalis fascia to create a round window baffle and small

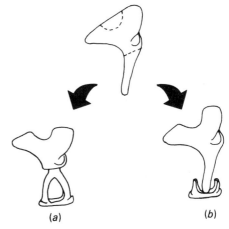

Figure 11.15 (*a*) Notched incus with short process. (*b*) Notched incus with long process (after Wehrs)

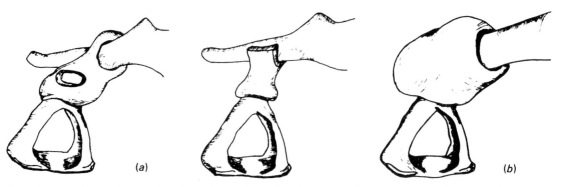

Figure 11.16 (*a*) Other reliable sculpturing techniques for malleus/stapes assembly and (*b*) for incus/stapes assembly when only the lenticular process of the incus is absent

split-skin grafts to cover the exteriorized mobile footplate (type IV tympanomastoidectomy).

The second method was to reconstruct a neomalleus in the neotympanic membrane to form the main building block upon which a link could be established with the stapes head or footplate. Early attempts by Guilford (1966) to suture a rod-shaped autologous cortical bone graft to the undersurface of the neotympanic membrane were unsuccessful. Schiller (1979) was able to achieve a postoperative air-bone gap of less than 15 dB in only 30% of 33 cases using his two-stage malleomyringoplasty procedure. Hough (1982) has reported successful results using autologous cortical bone, shaped like the malleus handle or an allogeneic malleus placed on the undersurface of the neotympanic membrane and held in place by a sculptured allograft ossicle interposed between the neomalleus and the stapes head or footplate. Using a two-ossicle (allograft stapes-incus) assembly in ears without a tympanic membrane, malleus, incus and stapes superstructure, Tos (1978) has reported early postoperative closure of the air-bone gap to 18 dB or less in 67% of 23 cases.

Tympanomeatal and tympano-ossicular allografts

A major contribution to the problem of reconstruction of the malleus handle in the neotympanic membrane developed as an evolution of the pioneering work with orthotopic cadaver-acquired allograft tympanic membrane transplants by Chalat, Betow and Marquet in the early 1960s.

Chalat (1964) used fresh, unpreserved tympanic membrane allografts to repair central perforations in three patients; two of these grafts perforated early and the procedure was abandoned. In 1959, Betow (1982) used an unpreserved tympanic membrane allograft to repair a perforation and noted graft resorption and necrosis on the twenty-eighth day postoperatively. In the same year, Brandow (1973) had observed similar necrosis and perforation of unpreserved tympanic membrane allografts in 11 patients. Both Betow and Brandow recognized that this graft necrosis was probably an immunological rejection phenomenon. Betow (1982) subsequently preserved tympanic allografts preoperatively in an antibiotic solution at −24°C, but the majority of these grafts perforated. Smyth and Kerr (1969) using tympanic membrane allografts which included a 6 mm cuff of meatal skin (tympanomeatal grafts), preserved in 5% chlorhexidine and 10% framycetin solution at −20°C preoperatively, reported necrosis and perforation in 65% of cases, and Glasscock and colleagues (Glasscock and House, 1968; Glasscock, House and Graham, 1972) reported a similarly high incidence of necrosis in tympanic membrane grafts preserved preoperatively in propriolactone or benzalkonium chloride or by freeze-drying techniques. Preservation in 70% ethyl alcohol, however, increased the graft take rate to 70%. House, Glasscock and Sheehy (1969) then conceived the idea of alcohol preserved composite allografts, consisting of *en-bloc* tympanic membrane with ossicles attached (tympano-ossicular monoblock grafts) for use in ears without a tympanic membrane, malleus and incus, with or without a stapes superstructure. Sixteen tympano-ossicular transplants were performed but the hearing results were poor.

Working independently in Antwerp, Marquet had noted that bone and tendon allografts preserved in the organomercuric compound Cialit (sodium 2-ethyl mercurithiobenzoxazole-5-carboxylate, Hoechst Pharmaceuticals) had been used successfully in orthopaedic procedures. Inspired by the reported lack of an immune response to these grafts, Marquet used Cialit to preserve cadaver-acquired de-epithelialized tympanic membranes to repair perforations and reported successful myringoplasties using this technique in 15 out of 17 cases (Marquet, 1966). Other surgeons (Brandow, 1969; Morrison, 1970; Smyth, Kerr and Goodey, 1971; Smyth, 1976) were less successful with Cialit-preserved tympanic membrane grafts. Marquet's excellent results coupled with the experiences of House, Glasscock and Sheehy (1969) with tympano-ossicular grafts, offered a potentially reliable method for reconstruction of the middle ear transformer, in those ears where radical excision of disease was necessary. With the recent introduction of combined approach tympanoplasty (Jansen, 1963), Marquet was now able to transplant and position accurately tympanomeatal allografts with attached ossicles via a posterior tympanotomy (Marquet, 1968, 1969, 1976a,b).

Perkins (1970a,b) reported successful myringoplasty surgery in 23 out of 24 subtotal perforations repaired with allogeneic tympanic membranes preserved preoperatively in buffered formaldehyde solutions. Glasscock, House and Graham (1972) reported a 90% graft take rate and Lesinski (1982) has reported an 85% graft take rate in 100 consecutive tympanomeatal allografts with and without attached ossicles using the formaldehyde preservation technique. Marquet then combined his method of preservation with that of Perkins by fixing tympano-ossicular grafts in 4% buffered formaldehyde for 2–3 weeks and then preserving the grafts in aqueous Cialit 1:2000 at 2°C prior to use. His immediate postoperative graft take rate in 1912 ears improved progressively from 73% in 1964 to 97% in 1976 (Marquet, 1977). This improvement has been attributed to refinements in surgical technique (Marquet, 1976a,b) and to the introduction of the Marquet/Perkins method of preservation (Marquet, 1977; Plester and Steinbach, 1977).

Wehrs froze cadaver temporal bone cores prior to preservation of the 'dissected out' tympanic membranes and tympano-ossicular grafts in 70% ethyl alcohol. Using 'de-epithelialized' tympanic membranes preserved in this manner (with or without an attached malleus) as onlay grafts, covered by autologous temporalis fascia or pedicled meatal skin, Wehrs (1982b) has reported successful closure of perforations in over 90% of 920 cases operated on between 1968 and 1980.

In 1976, Smith introduced the technique of freeze-drying and ethylene oxide gas sterilization for the preoperative preservation of otologic allografts (Smith, 1980a, b). Tympanomeatal, tympano-ossicular and ossicular bone allografts prepared by this technique appear to be successful in the short term, but long-term results have not been published (Smith, 1982; Smith and McElveen, 1982).

The Hyogo Ear Bank of Japan adopted the method of freeze drying and ethylene oxide gas sterilization for tympano-ossicular allografts but early necrosis of the tympanic allografts was observed and this bank has now changed its method of preservation of these grafts. Tympano-ossicular allografts are fixed in 4% buffered formaldehyde followed by freeze drying and ethylene oxide gas sterilization. Using this method of

preservation and sterilization Minatogawa *et al.* (1990) reported tympanic membrane allograft necrosis or perforation in 16 of 68 operations.

In those ears without a tympanic membrane, malleus or incus, with or without an intact stapes superstructure, composite tympano-ossicular allografts have been used by some surgeons as the main building block for middle ear reconstruction. In combined approach tympanoplasty procedures, tympano-ossicular allografts (comprising tympanic membrane and meatal skin cuff, malleus and incus) have been transplanted successfully into ears where only an intact mobile stapes remains (Marquet, 1977) (Figure 11.17*a*). Tympano-ossicular allografts (comprising tympanic membrane and meatal skin cuff, malleus, incus and stapes crura) have been less successful in those ears where only a mobile stapes footplate remains. This is primarily because of problems inherent in making adequate and lasting contact between the donor stapes crura and the recipient stapes footplate (Marquet, 1982, personal communication). Another major problem encountered with these types of reconstruction is fibrous and bony ankylosis of the short process of the transplanted incus to the lateral semicircular canal (Ironside, 1979) or to the bony margins of the posterior tympanotomy (Figure 11.17*b,c*).

In order to adapt these tympano-ossicular grafts to both the shallow and deep middle ear and to try to avoid postoperative discontinuity and fixation of the reconstructed ossicular chain, a two-stage tympanoplasty method has been advocated by Ironside (1979), Lesinski (1982), Smith (1982), Wehrs (1982b), Foggia and McCabe (1990) and Campbell (1990). In stage I, a composite tympanic membrane and meatal skin cuff with incorporated malleus is transplanted to act as the main building block for the middle ear reconstruction. At the second stage, 6 months later, a sculptured preserved ossicular bone allograft can be used as a malleus-to-stapes assembly or malleus-to-footplate assembly (Figure 11.18) according to whether or not the stapes superstructure is intact.

Autologous and allogeneic cortical and cancellous bone grafts

Sculptured columellae of autologous cortical bone from the outer mastoid cortex, bony external auditory meatus and spine of Henle have been used in tympanic membrane-to-stapes head and tympanic membrane-to-footplate interpositions, malleus-to-stapes and malleus-to-footplate assemblies by Hough (1958), Zollner (1960, 1969), Farrior (1960, 1966), Kley and Draf (1965), Bauer (1966), Guilford (1966), Wright (1967) and Tos (1974), but long-term hearing results have not been reported by these authors. Pulec and Sheehy (1973) reported resorption of autologous cortical bone columellae in the middle ear

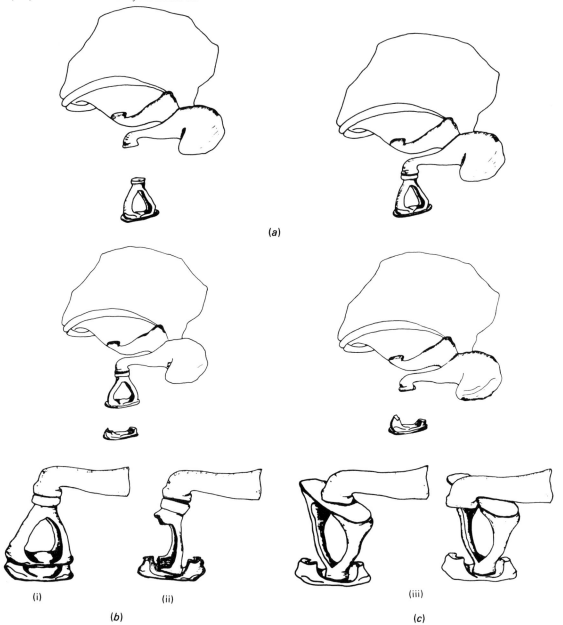

Figure 11.17 (*a*) Reconstruction of the middle ear using a tympano-ossicular allograft comprising meatal skin cuff, tympanic membrane, malleus and incus when only an intact recipient stapes is present. (*b*) When only the recipient stapes footplate is present, the middle ear may be reconstructed using a tympano-ossicular allograft comprising meatal skin cuff, tympanic membrane, malleus, incus and stapes. The donor stapes may be: (i) positioned to lie 'piggy-back' on the recipient stapes crural remnants; (ii) partially removed, so that one crus and part of the footplate lie on the recipient stapes footplate, or (*c*) (iii) inverted and interposed between the donor incus and recipient stapes footplate. This latter method has proved the most successful of the three techniques

but Robin, Bennett and Gregory (1976) were unable to comment on surface resorption of cortical bone grafts removed at revision surgery 12–48 months postoperatively, because such features were masked by preoperative sculpturing of the grafts. Berkovits *et al.* (1978) have performed 200 ossiculoplasties using autologous cortical bone, precisely modelled on a Micro-fraize machine for malleus-to-stapes and

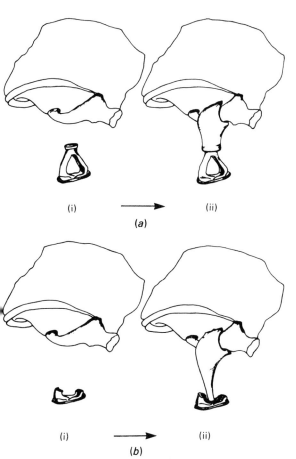

(i) → (ii)

(a)

(i) → (ii)

(b)

Figure 11.18 Two stage reconstruction in those ears where the tympanic membrane, malleus and incus are absent, (*a*) with or (*b*) without an intact stapes superstructure. In stage one, a meatal skin cuff, tympanic membrane and malleus handle allograft are transplanted. At stage two, a malleus/stapes assembly is performed if the stapes is intact or a malleus/footplate assembly is performed if the stapes superstructure is absent

malleus-to-footplate assemblies. Eight grafts removed because of recurrent cholesteatoma, showed histological evidence of vascularization of marrow spaces with some viable osteocytes in the lacunae, but there was 'rounding off' of the edges of these grafts due to surface resorption of bone. Graft resorption was also seen in those ears in which chronic infection persisted postoperatively (Berkovits, 1982, personal communication).

Ojala *et al.* (1983) compared the hearing results in 51 ears in which autologous mastoid bone struts were used, and 113 ears in which autologous or preserved allogeneic ossicular bone had been used to reconstruct the ossicular chain. They concluded that the early (one year postoperatively) and late (5–12 years postoperatively) hearing results were the same

for ossicular and cortical bone grafts in tympanic membrane-to-stapes head interposition and malleus-to-stapes assembly.

In animal experiments, Beck and Franz (1961) have demonstrated resorption of fresh allogeneic cortical bone grafts in the middle ear of guinea-pigs and Musebeck and Falck (1963) reported similar results in rabbits. Fresh cortical bone allografts used to reconstruct the ossicular chain in dogs (Guilford, Shortreed and Halpert, 1966) and in cats (Benitez, Bejar and McIntire, 1971) showed new bone formation, good vascularization of marrow spaces and no histological evidence of resorption. Cialit-preserved cortical bone allografts induced an inflammatory response associated with osteoclastic resorption of the grafts in the middle ear of non-inbred rabbits (Hildmann, Steinbach and Koburg, 1974; Steinbach, 1982, personal communication). As a result of these experiments preserved cortical bone allografts have not been used extensively in tympanoplasty.

Maisin, Munting and Gersdorff (1989) have used cadaver-acquired human long bone defatted in 1:1 methanol-chloroform, decalcified in 0.6 M HCl solution and lyophilized, for ossiculoplasty, canal wall reconstruction and mastoid cavity obliteration procedures, but long-term results with these allografts have not been published.

Autologous and allogeneic cartilage grafts

Utech (1960) introduced sculptured auricular cartilage autografts for tympanic membrane-to-stapes head and tympanic membrane-to-footplate interpositions and Jansen (1963) found autologous tragal cartilage and autologous or preserved allogeneic nasal septal cartilage suitable for tympanic membrane-to-stapes head interposition (short columella) and tympanic membrane-to-footplate interposition (long columella) reconstructions in combined approach tympanoplasty procedures. Jansen (1972) soon found the long cartilage columellae too flimsy and reinforced them with stainless steel wire, a procedure also adopted by Smyth (1969) in his 'boomerang' strut (Figure 11.19). To increase the stability of tympanic membrane-to-footplate interposition, Brockman (1965) designed a composite autologous tragal cartilage-perichondrial columella. Using this technique, he reported postoperative closure of the air-bone gap to less than 16 dB in 30 cases. Encouraging hearing results were also achieved by Portmann (1963) and Shea and Glasscock (1967) using similar techniques with autologous cartilage/perichondrial grafts.

Altenau and Sheehy (1978) found that the most common cause of failure of autologous and alcohol-preserved allogeneic cartilage struts assessed at revision surgery was that they were 'too short' and

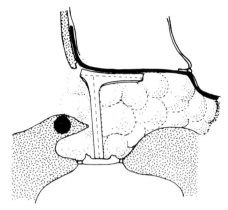

Figure 11.19 'Boomerang' nasal septal cartilage allograft reinforced with stainless steel wire (tympanic membrane to footplate interposition – 'long columella')

became displaced. No obvious resorption of cartilage was found in these grafts or in the cartilage grafts removed from the middle ear and studied histologically by Don and Linthicum (1975). Goodhill *et al.* (1979) noted postoperative softening of autologous tragal cartilage used in tympanic membrane-to-footplate interpositions and Smyth (1980) reported displacement of 'boomerang' struts in 22 revision operations, with erosion of the medial limb of the strut in three cases. Notching of the medial limb of the strut was also noted in some ears where the strut had come into contact with Silastic sheeting placed over the promontory and oval window niche.

Seventy-six alcohol-preserved nasal septal cartilage allografts which had been in the middle ear for up to 9 years were studied histologically by Kerr, Byrne and Smyth (1973). In most cases the morphology of the grafts was retained. Variable amounts of fibrous tissue replacement of cartilage together with erosion and thinning of the medial limb were seen particularly in those grafts present for longest in the middle ear. Kuijpers and van den Broek (1975) have also reported resorption of alcohol-preserved cartilage columellae and Smyth (1980) found resorption of the medial limb of 3% of 'boomerang' struts removed at revision surgery. Other causes of failure were lateral displacement of the columella off the stapes footplate and immobilization of the columella by middle ear adhesions.

A most significant histological study of the fate of cartilage in ossicular reconstruction was undertaken by Steinbach and Pusalkar (1981). Fifty-two cartilage struts (39 tragal cartilage autografts and 13 Cialit-preserved nasal septal cartilage allografts) were removed 1–15 years postoperatively. Forty-four of these grafts were removed because of failure of hearing improvement and eight because of recurrent disease. In the vast majority of cases, deterioration in hearing

occurred between the third and seventh year postoperatively. There were no obvious differences in the macroscopic or histological appearance in the removed allografts and autografts. Thirty-eight grafts had become soft and spongy, 25 grafts had decreased in size and, in seven, the medial limb had been resorbed completely. In three ears revised because of recurrent cholesteatoma, the grafts had disappeared.

Total or partial resorption of alcohol-preserved cartilage columellae with or without stainless steel wire reinforcement has been a common finding at revision surgery by the author (unpublished data) and Austin (1982) has used the term 'creeping resorption' to describe the behaviour of cartilage columellae in the middle ear.

Glues and adhesives

To aid in stabilizing ossicular bone assemblies and tympano-ossicular allografts, stainless steel microscrews and wire have been employed by Marquet (1969) and Jako (1972) and the properties of different glues have also been evaluated. Mecrylate (COAPT-1), Bucrylate (COAPT) and Eubucrylate (Histo-Acryl) cause inflammatory responses including foreign body reactions and osteitis in the middle ear (Kerr and Smyth, 1971b; Heumann and Steinbach, 1980) and have therefore been abandoned by most otologists. The two component fibrin-sealant, Tissucol/Tisseel (Seelich, 1982), forms a stable adhesive by combining concentrated human fibrinogen and factor XIII with a thrombin calcium chloride/aprontinin solution. The resulting adhesive retains its properties in a moist field and does not induce an inflammatory response (Marquet, 1982; Portmann, 1982; Katzke, Pusalkar and Steinbach, 1983). This commercially manufactured fibrin adhesive does, however, carry potential risk of contamination with hepatitis viruses and human immunodeficiency viruses (HIV).

The most promising adhesive for use in otology is autologous fibrin tissue adhesive, but problems preparing this adhesive preoperatively or intraoperatively have precluded its widespread use.

Otological tissue banks

Many surgeons using allografts in tympanoplasty secure their own cadaver donor material from the hospitals in which they work and the 'dissecting out' and preservation of these allografts is performed by themselves or their staff. In the USA, the passing of the Universal Donor Act in 1969, made it possible to obtain donor material easily and, in 1970, Perkins created the first ear bank under the sponsorship of Project Hear (Palo Alto, California). Other ear banks have subsequently been established in the USA (under the auspices of the American association of tissue banks) and elsewhere. Most function as non-profit-making organizations to provide high quality, preserved, sterile otological allografts. These banks are currently preserving otological allografts in chemical agents, i.e. formaldehyde, glutaraldehyde, Cialit, alcohol or by freeze-drying and ethylene oxide sterilization (Table 11.3). Grafts are distributed on demand, nationally and internationally, to surgeons who do not have the time or facilities to acquire their own donor tissues or cannot do so because of the medicolegal or religious restrictions of the countries in which they work (Chiossone, 1977; Lesinski, 1977, 1982; Smith 1980b).

Table 11.3 Preservation techniques for otological allografts

1	70% Ethyl alcohol
2	0.02% Aqueous Cialit, (sodium 2-ethylmercurithiobenzoxazole-5-carboxylate)
3	4% Buffered formaldehyde fixation and 0.5% buffered formaldehyde preservation
4	4% Buffered formaldehyde fixation and 0.02% aqueous Cialit preservation
5	0.5% Buffered glutaraldehyde fixation and 0.02% aqueous Cialit preservation
6	Freeze-drying and ethylene oxide gas sterilization
7	4% Buffered formaldehyde fixation followed by freeze drying and ethylene oxide gas sterilization

Transmission of human immunodeficiency viruses (HIV) and the acquired immunodeficiency syndrome (AIDS) has been reported in recipients of infected donor tissues and organs. For this reason rigid protocols have been established to ensure that all allografts are acquired from low risk, HIV-negative donors. In the 'static' allografts used in otology, HIV is inactivated by tissue preservation in 70% alcohol, buffered formaldehyde and buffered glutaraldehyde, thus adding to the safety of these allografts. The author is unaware of transmission of any disease to a recipient of an otologic allograft provided by the registered American tissue banks.

The fatal spongiform encephalopathy of Creutzfeldt-Jakob disease (CJD) was, however, diagnosed in a 28-year-old woman in the USA, 19 months after lyophilized, irradiated human cadaveric dura mater 'Lyodura' (Lot # 2105 processed in 1982 by B. Braun Melsungen AG of the Federal Republic of Germany) had been used to reconstruct her tympanic membrane after removal of a cholesteatoma. This case prompted hazard warnings from Government departments of health, that there is a small risk that the agent (generally considered not to be a virus but an abnormal prion glycoprotein) responsible for CJD may be carried in allogeneic dura mater and that current methods of sterilization and preservation of allogeneic dura mater cannot guarantee complete inactivation of the CJD agent. Tange, Troost and Limburg (1990) reported the case of a 54-year-old man who died

from CJD 4 years after a successful myringoplasty with homograft pericardium preserved in Cialit. The pericardium had been obtained peroperatively from a patient undergoing open heart bypass surgery; there was no known history of CJD in this donor or his family. There is also currently no laboratory investigation that will positively identify the CJD agent in donors or donor tissues.

It is ultimately the responsibility of the surgeon to guarantee the recipient of an allograft that the graft is free of a transmittable disease.

Biomaterials

In recent years, collaborative efforts between biomaterial scientists and surgeons have led to the manufacture of new materials specifically designed for implantation. As a result of these efforts, metals, solid and porous polymer materials, together with a vast range of ceramic materials have been developed for use in tympanoplasty and mastoidectomy. These biomaterials (also known as alloplastic materials) used in otology can be conveniently and broadly subdivided into four groups based on their interface reactions with bone, i.e. biotolerant, bio-inert, bioreactive and bioactive.

Solid and porous polymers and metallic implants are biotolerant, i.e. they do not bond with bone and a layer of fibrous tissue forms in the interface between implant and bone (Table 11.4).

Proplast 1 prepared by the combination of two polymer families, namely polytetrafluoroethylene and vitreous carbon was first used by Janeke and Shea (1975) as a total ossicular replacement prosthesis in 23 cases in whom the malleus, incus and stapes superstructure were missing. Proplast prostheses subsequently became available for tympanic membrane-to-stapes head and tympanic membrane-to-footplate interpositions, and malleus-to-stapes, and malleus-to-footplate assemblies, but foreign body reactions to the prostheses and extrusion of these prostheses through the tympanic membrane have occurred (Kerr, 1981; Palva and Makinen, 1983; Babighian, 1985).

The second plastic implant material, Plastipore (porous polyethylene) reported to have non-reactive properties and sufficient porosity to encourage host tissue ingrowth to stabilize the implant in the middle ear, was first used successfully by Shea (1976) for tympanic membrane-to-footplate interposition and malleus-to-footplate assembly and was called the total ossicular replacement prosthesis (TORP). For tympanic membrane-to-stapes head interposition and malleus-to-stapes assembly, a Plastipore partial ossicular replacement prosthesis (PORP) was introduced (Figure 11.20) (Richards Technical Publication, 1980).

Shea, Emmett and Smyth (1977) and Hicks,

Table 11.4 Biotolerant biomaterial implants used in middle ear and mastoid reconstructive surgery

Metals	Polymers	
Stainless steel	*Solid*	
Tantalum	Polyethylene	
Platinum	Polytetrafluoroethylene (Teflon)	
Titanium	Polydimethylsiloxane (Silastic)	
	Porous	
	Polytetrafluoroethylene-carbon fibre composite	(Proplast 1)
	Polytetrafluoroethylene-aluminium oxide composite	(Proplast 2)
	High density polyethylene	(Plastipore)
	Ultra-high molecular weight polyethylene	(Polycel)
	Light Harness satin-weave carbon fibre impregnated with phenolic resin	(Carbon-carbon)

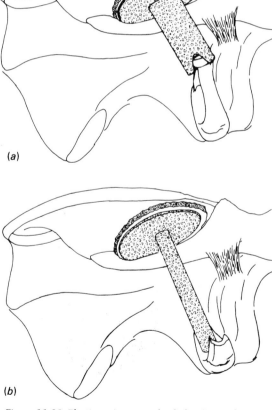

(a)

(b)

Figure 11.20 Plastipore (porous polyethylene) partial ossicular replacement prosthesis (PORP) and total ossicular replacement prosthesis (TORP) with cartilage interposed between the prosthesis head and tympanic membrane to protect against extrusion

Wright and Wright (1978) reported encouraging short-term hearing results and only a small percentage of extrusions using partial and total ossicular replacement prostheses. Smyth (1982b), however, reported a 5-year follow up of 28 ears in which partial ossicular replacement prostheses were used and 116 ears in which total ossicular replacement prostheses were used. Fifty-seven per cent of the partial and 78% of the total prostheses failed to maintain closure of the air-bone gap (preoperative bone conduction and postoperative air conduction) to 10 dB or less at 0.5–2 kHz. Using the same criteria, Frootko (1983) reported a 3–5 year follow up of 78 ears in which partial ossicular replacement prostheses and 41 ears in which total ossicular replacement prostheses were used; the failure rates were 72% and 83% respectively. Extrusion of the prosthesis through the tympanic membrane was the major cause of failure (40% partial, 32% total). This was not prevented by the interposition of connective tissue between the prosthesis head and the undersurface of the tympanic membrane, nor was extrusion prevented by placing the prosthesis under the malleus handle or chorda tympani nerve, when present. At the present time, it appears that autologous tragal or conchal cartilage interposed between the prosthesis and the tympanic membrane is the best method of protection against extrusion, reducing this complication to less than 5% of cases (Sheehy, 1984; Brackmann, 1986). Other causes of failure include postoperative migration and displacement of the prosthesis. With partial ossicular replacement prostheses, necrosis and fracture of the stapes superstructure has been observed (Belal and Odnert, 1982; Frootko, 1983) and with total ossicular replacement prostheses single cases of foreign body granuloma on the stapes footplate (Palva and Makinen, 1983) and perforation of the stapes footplate with resultant perilymph fistula (Myer and Cotton, 1982) have occurred. There is also conclusive light and electron microscopic evidence that biodegradation of Plastipore occurs in the middle ear, albeit at microscopic level (Kerr, 1981; Belal and Odnert, 1982) and the prostheses evoked a local but sustained foreign body reaction (Kerr, 1981; Frootko, 1983; Palva and Makinen, 1983).

The third plastic implant material, Polycel (thermofusion formed ultra-high-molecular-weight porous polyethylene; Treace Medical Inc.) offers design advantages over other porous plastic implants. The prostheses for both tympanic membrane-to-stapes head and tympanic membrane-to-footplate interpositions offer a variety of platforms onto which the cartilage interposition can be secured and incorporation of a stainless steel core into the slim shaft of these prostheses enables the shaft and the platform head to be bent to the desired configuration required. Using these pros-

theses Chuden (1985), Brackmann (1986) and Moretz *et al.* (1986) have reported encouraging hearing results and low extrusion rates. Foreign body reactions to Polycel, however, do occur in the middle ear and long-term follow-up results of cases in which these prostheses have been used are awaited.

Carbon-carbon made from Light Harness satin weave carbon fibre impregnated with phenolic resin has been used as an ossicular replacement prosthesis (Podoshin, Fradis and Gertner, 1988) with encouraging short-term follow-up results. Long-term follow-up results, however, have not been published.

The most recent materials available for ossiculoplasty, posterior canal wall and outer attic wall reconstruction and mastoid obliteration, are the bioceramics (Grote, 1984a) (Table 11.5). These bioceramics are classified as follows:

Table 11.5 Bioceramics used in middle ear and mastoid reconstructive surgery

Product	Appearance	Prostheses
I Bioinert aluminium oxide ceramics		
Frialit	Dense white	Partial and total ossicular replacement prostheses
Bioceram	Dense white	Partial ceramic ossicular replacement prosthesis (CORP-P) and total ceramic ossicular replacement prosthesis (CORP-T)
Macor	Dense white	Partial and total ossicular replacement prostheses
II Bioreactive glass ceramics		
Bioglass	Dense transparent	Partial and total ossicular replacement prostheses
Ceravital	Dense white	Partial and total ossicular replacement prostheses Canal wall prostheses
III Bioactive calcium phosphate ceramics		
Hydroxylapatite	Macroporous white	Canal wall prostheses
	Dense white	Partial and total ossicular replacement prostheses
Tricalcium phosphate	White powder or particles	
Hydroxylapatite + purified fibrillar collagen (Collagen Corp. California)	White powder or particles and collagen	Used for mastoid obliteration
Hydroxylapatite + fibrin glue	White powder or particles and fibrin glue	
Tricalcium phosphate + fibrin glue		
Tricalcium phosphate + hydroxylapatite + fibrin glue		

1 *Bio-inert aluminium oxide ceramics.* These ceramics are bio-inert because there is no measurable exchange of calcium and phosphate ions at the implant/bone interface and although contact between bone and these ceramics is maintained, bonding osteogenesis of the ceramic to bone does not occur.

2 *Bioreactive glass ceramics.* These ceramics will bond with bone. Calcium and phosphate ions found in the interface between the ceramic and bone are thought to be derived principally from the ceramic itself (forming ionic and covalent type bonds).

3 *Bio-active calcium phosphate ceramics.* These ceramics induce chemical reactions at the interface with bone resulting in strong bonding osteogenesis.

The very hard bio-inert aluminium oxide ceramic *Frialit* has been used in ossiculoplasty by Jahnke and Plester (1981). Polycrystalline dense aluminium oxide ceramic *Bioceram* prostheses (CORP-P and CORP-T) designed by Yamamoto (1985) have proved successful in ossicular chain reconstruction. These aluminium oxide ceramics induce no foreign body reactions in the middle ear, are soon covered by a thin mucous membrane and biodegradation of the prostheses has not been reported. Nonetheless, Yamamoto (1988) reported displacement of some prostheses and where the prosthesis made direct contact with the tympanic/neotympanic membrane, extrusion occurred in 8.3% of CORP-P and 5.2% of CORP-T prostheses. The extrusions were thought to be due primarily to poor eustachian tube function and tympanic membrane retraction postoperatively. Extrusions of Frialit prostheses may also occur under the above circumstances (Jahnke, personal communication).

The bioreactive glass ceramic, *Ceravital*, in which a crystal fraction of hydroxylapatite is embedded into a polycrystalline glassy network, has the consistency of 'mother of pearl'. This ceramic has been used very successfully in ossiculoplasty and posterior canal wall reconstruction in over 1000 operations by Reck (1981, 1985). Malleus/stapes head and malleus/footplate interpositions (Figure 11.21) proved very successful and, when the malleus was absent, autologous cortical bone paste was placed over the disc shaped portion of the prosthesis under the tympanic membrane or temporalis fascia graft.

Posterior canal wall prostheses were placed into preformed bony grooves and covered with autologous bone paste, temporalis fascia and meatal skin flaps; 78% of all operations were not staged. In a long-term follow-up review of these operations, Reck, Storkel and Meyer (1988) reported excellent hearing results and no prosthesis extrusions. Sixty-one implants removed at revision operations were examined histologically. Most were covered by a single epithelial layer with a poorly vascularized tunica propria and circumscribed zones of lysis were seen in some implants removed 7 years postoperatively. In infected ears,

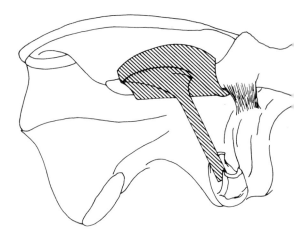

Figure 11.21 Ceravital prosthesis in malleus/stapes footplate assembly

more severe lysis of implants was found. A thin bony mantle covered those areas on which autologous bone paste had been placed and inflammatory responses to the implants were minimal.

Lysis or biodegradation of these ceramics occurs and this process is exacerbated by chronic middle ear infection. Autologous bone paste interposed or sandwiched between the ossicular implants and the tympanic membrane protects against extrusion (less than 8% extrusions 2 years postoperatively) and implant lysis was observed at soft tissue/implant interfaces (Babighian, 1985; Gersdorff, Maisin and Munting, 1986; Niparko *et al.*, 1988). When autologous bone paste is not interposed between the implant and the tympanic membrane, extrusion rates as high as 29% 1 year postoperatively have been reported (Austin, 1985).

The bioactive ceramic, *hydroxylapatite*, is one of the crystallographic forms of calcium phosphate that closely mimics the mineral matrix of human bone. The application of this ceramic in ossiculoplasty and posterior canal wall reconstruction has been subject to extensive experimental and clinical evaluation in recent years (Grote, 1984a,b; van Blitterswijk *et al.*, 1990). This ceramic has low tensile strength and is easily sculptured with a diamond paste burr. For posterior canal wall reconstruction, macroporous hydroxylapatite prostheses with a macroporosity of 26% and a microporosity of less than 5% are used. Ossicular replacement prostheses are made of dense hydroxylapatite with a microporosity of less than 5% and no macropores. Macroporous and dense prostheses removed at revision surgery have been found to be very biocompatible in that they induce a very small inflammatory response. Biodegradation or lysis of the macroporous ceramic appears roughly to parallel the process of bonding osteogenesis, in which vascularization of the ceramic macropores is followed by the 'laying down' of collagen-rich fibrous tissue and bone resulting in an integration of the ceramic into the bony implantation bed. The dense ossicular replacement prostheses are enveloped by fibrous tissue covered by a thin epithelial layer. New bone formation was not seen on or in these prostheses (van Blitterswijk *et al.*, 1990).

Grote (1984b, Grote, van Blitterswijk and Kuijpers, 1986) and Wehrs (1989a, b) have designed dense

hydroxylapatite prostheses for malleus/stapes and malleus/footplate assembly (Figures 11.22 and 11.23). These prostheses have proved as successful as sculptured autologous and allogeneic bone grafts where the malleus is present in the tympanic membrane to act as the lateral building block for the ossicular chain reconstruction.

Combinations of dense hydroxylapatite 'heads' with porous and dense polymer 'shafts' are also avail-

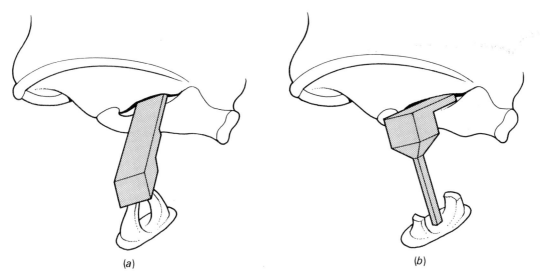

(a)   (b)

Figure 11.22 Dense hydroxylapatite prostheses (after Grote). (*a*) Incus prosthesis; (*b*) incus/stapes prosthesis. Note the prosthesis head or platform is anchored laterally in a pouch created between the malleus handle and the undersurface of the tympanic membrane

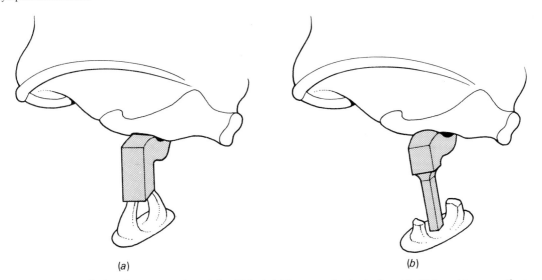

(a)   (b)

Figure 11.23 Dense hydroxylapatite prostheses (after Wehrs). (*a*) Incus prosthesis, single notch; (*b*) incus/stapes prosthesis, single notch. These prostheses have similar design characteristics as the notched incus with short process and the notched incus with long process (see Figure 11.15). Both the Grote and Wehrs hydroxylapatite prostheses are available commercially in a variety of different sizes to accommodate the various spatial relationships found between malleus and stapes (see Figure 11.12)

able commercially. Black (1990) has designed an ossicular replacement prosthesis with a flattened egg-shaped dense hydroxylapatite head set on a Teflon shaft for interposition between the tympanic membrane and stapes head (PORP) or stapes footplate (TORP). With this prosthesis a malleus handle is not required as a lateral building block and the dome or head of the prosthesis follows the contour of the posterior superior tympanic segment. Black, however, has reported extrusion of these prostheses if the tympanic membrane is atrophic and he advises the interposition of tragal perichondrium or temporalis fascia between the prosthesis head and tympanic membrane to prevent extrusion in such cases.

Many other 'combination' ossicular chain prostheses have been designed incorporating an hydroxylapatite, autologous ossicular bone or allogeneic ossicular bone head with a porous or dense polymer shaft.

New biomaterials continue to be introduced to the otological and neuro-otological arena. The most recent of these is Ionogran, a glass-ionomer cement produced by a combination of calcium aluminosilicate glass with unsaturated carboxylic acids (Ionos Medizinische Produkte GmbH Co., K. G. Seefeld, Germany). This cement has been used in ossicular chain and canal wall reconstruction and mastoid obliteration. Short-term results are encouraging (Geyer and Helms, 1990, 1992). However, two cases of subacute aluminium myoclonic encephalopathy have been reported in France following the use of Ionocem – calcium aluminium fluorosilicate and polyalkenoic acid (Ionos-D8031, Seefeld/OBB, Germany) for bone reconstruction following translabyrinthine vestibular schwannoma surgery (Renard, Felten and Béquet, 1994) and, pending further investigation, the use of Ionocem has been stopped in France by the Director General of Health.

Conclusions

The ear surgeons of today, have at their disposal, a wide range of surgical procedures for the treatment of chronic suppurative otitis media, both with and without cholesteatoma. The fundamental prerequisite for this type of surgery to be successful, is the meticulous and complete removal of disease from the middle ear and/or mastoid.

This has been made easier in recent years by technical advances in operating microscopes, the instrumentation available and by the introduction of carbon dioxide, argon Nd/Yag and KTP lasers. These lasers have proved to be an extremely useful adjuvant to the surgeons' instrument armamentarium by virtue of their cutting, vaporizing, coagulating and 'tissue welding' ability, allowing the surgeon to avoid manual pulling and tugging dissection techniques that may transmit unwanted mechanical energy to the cochlea causing cochlear damage.

Ideally, every ear surgeon should be accomplished and competent enough to perform all of the surgical procedures that have evolved and should have a thorough knowledge of temporal bone anatomy and physiology and of the pathogenesis of chronic suppurative otitis media, but this ideal has and probably never will be achieved. The surgery of chronic suppurative otitis media must, therefore, not only be tailored to the patient's presenting pathology and requirements, but also to the level of competence of the surgeon and the surgical and follow-up facilities available. It is, to take the extreme example, quite wrong for an unaccomplished ear surgeon to perform a combined approach tympanoplasty on a patient who will be lost to follow up postoperatively.

The debate as to whether the open techniques of mastoidectomy with tympanoplasty are better or worse than the closed techniques will continue. There is no short cut to successful excision of disease and the operation of choice must be that in which all the disease can be excised. Once this is achieved, the surgeon can decide on the type of middle ear and/or mastoid reconstruction procedure to be used, whether this should be staged or not, and what the reconstruction should ultimately achieve.

Preoperative evaluation of eustachian tube function has been found to be of little value in predicting the outcome of surgery in patients with chronic suppurative otitis media. Nonetheless, for tympanoplasty with and without mastoidectomy to be successful in the long term, the middle ear must be air containing and adequately ventilated via the eustachian tube. Cholesteatoma and mucosal disease together with infected osteitic bone must be removed and the middle ear must become lined by a healthy mucous membrane. The tympanic membrane must be intact, healthy and mobile, and the ossiculoplasty must be secure and stable.

Inadequate eustachian tube function, recurrent and residual cholesteatoma and persistent mucous membrane disease remain the most important causes of surgical failure. (The catch 22 situation, is that abnormal eustachian tube function is probably the single most important cause of chronic suppurative otitis media. It must not be forgotten that even after complete removal of disease from the middle ear and/or mastoid, abnormal eustachian tube function remains the most common cause of failure of middle ear reconstruction procedures.)

Grafts and biomaterials chosen for use in middle ear and mastoid reconstruction, should ideally, not induce a sustained foreign body reaction, extrude or biodegrade.

If an 'open' canal wall down operation is performed, the facial ridge must be lowered to the level of the floor of the external auditory canal, to create an 'hemispherical' or 'round', rather than a 'bean' or 'kidney' shaped cavity, and the ear must be adequately aerated (and easy to access postoperatively) by fashioning a wide meatoplasty.

There is one situation that permits special mention in this chapter: the patient who has lost all useful hearing in one ear and requires surgical removal of cholesteatoma in the other. In this situation, the surgeon must be aware that any surgical technique or manoeuvre that may endanger the cochlea must be avoided. The best method of management is by open mastoidectomy and the stapes superstructure and/or footplate must *not* be manipulated. Tympanic membrane reconstruction should only be considered if ossicular discontinuity already exists, thus protecting the stapes and cochlea, and the middle ear must be free of disease.

Many grafts and biomaterials are available for middle ear reconstruction. Most ear surgeons prefer to use healthy, fresh, autologous tissues whenever possible and, in the main, these have proved most successful. Their second choice has been preserved allogeneic tissues and their use has only been possible, because the deep external auditory meatus and middle ear are sites where immune rejection responses to a tissue allograft across major histocompatibility barriers are somewhat muted (Frootko, 1985b). These sites may therefore be regarded as sites favourable to graft acceptance, that is immunologically privileged sites (van den Broek, 1968; Frootko, 1984, 1987). Current preoperative otological allograft preservation techniques (see Table 11.3), also appear to make these tissues less susceptible to rejection after grafting across major histocompatibility barriers, by altering, to a greater or lesser extent, the molecular configuration of antigenic determinants of transplantation antigens. This appears to diminish the graft's ability to immunize the recipient, but does not alter their specificity (Frootko, 1985b). It is presumably for similar reasons that successful tympanic membrane reconstruction has been achieved using preserved bovine connective tissue xenografts.

The polymer biomaterials have enjoyed widespread usage by otologists over the past 15 years, but have not gained universal acceptance by the otological fraternity and the ceramics have yet to prove their superiority over autografts and preserved allografts in middle ear and mastoid reconstruction.

References

ADKINS, W. Y. (1990) Composite autograft for tympanoplasty and tympanomastoid surgery. *Laryngoscope*, **100**, 244–247

ALBRIGHT, J. P. and LEIGH, B. G. (1966) Dural homograft (allostatic) myringoplasty. *Laryngoscope*, **76**, 1687–1693

ALTENAU, M. M. and SHEEHY, J. L. (1978) Tympanoplasty: cartilage prostheses – a report of 564 cases. *Laryngoscope*, **88**, 895–904

ARMSTRONG, B. W. (1969) Experiences with the ossicular chain. *Annals of Otology, Rhinology and Laryngology*, **78**, 939–949

AUSTIN, D. F. (1963) Vein graft tympanoplasty: 2 year report. *Transactions of the American Academy of Ophthalmology and Otolaryngology*, **67**, 198–208

AUSTIN, D. F. (1969) Types and indications of staging. *Archives of Otolaryngology*, **89**, 235–242

AUSTIN, D. F. (1971) Ossicular reconstruction. *Archives of Otolaryngology*, **94**, 525–535

AUSTIN, D. F. (1977) The significance of the retraction pocket in the treatment of cholesteatoma. In: *Cholesteatoma. First International Conference*. Birmingham, Alabama: Aesculapius Publishing Co. pp. 379–383

AUSTIN, D. F. (1982) Avoiding failures in the restoration of hearing with ossiculoplasty and biocompatible implants. *Otolaryngologic Clinics of North America*, **4**, 763–771

AUSTIN, D. F. (1985) Columellar tympanoplasty. *American Journal of Otology*, **6**, 464–467

BABIGHIAN, G. (1985) Bioactive ceramics versus proplast implants in ossiculoplasty. *American Journal of Otology*, **6**, 285–290

BAUER, M. (1966) Bone autograft for ossicular reconstruction. *Archives of Otolaryngology*, **83**, 335–338

BECK, C. and FRANZ, H. (1961) Das verhalten im mittelohr implantiertter auto-und homoioplastischer knochenspane in teirexperiment. *Archiv für Ohren Nasen Kehlkopfheilkunde*, **179**, 111–122

BELAL, A. and ODNERT, M. S. (1982) Torps and Porps: a transmission and scanning electron microscopic study. *Journal of Laryngology and Otology*, **96**, 49–55

BELL, H. L. (1958) A technique of tympanoplasty (tympanomallear stapediopexy). *Transactions of the American Laryngological, Rhinological and Otolaryngological Society*, 572–576

BELLUCCI, R. J. and WOLFF, D. (1966) The incus, normal and pathological. *Archives of Otolaryngology*, **83**, 413–419

BENITEZ, J. T., BEJAR, I. R. and MCINTIRE, C. L. (1971) Ossiculoplasty: experimental studies of cortical bone grafts for replacement of the incus in cats. *Journal of Laryngology and Otology*, **85**, 1177–1182

BERKOVITS, R. N. P., KRUITHOF, C., BOS, C. E. and VAN DER BERG, J. (1978) Reconstruction of the ossicular chain with an autologous bone cylinder, produced with a hollow drill. *Journal of Laryngology and Otology*, **92**, 969–978

BERTHOLD, E. (1878) Über Myringoplastik. *Wien Med Bl.* **1**, 627

BETOW, C. (1982) 20 years of experience with homografts in ear surgery. *Journal of Laryngology and Otology*, Suppl. 5

BLACK, B. (1990) Design and development of a contoured ossicular replacement prosthesis: clinical trials of 125 cases. *American Journal of Otology*, **11**, 85–89

BONDY, G. (1910) Totalaufmeisselung mit erhaltung von trommelfell und gehorknochelchen. *Monatsschrift für Ohrenheilkunde*, **44**, 15–23

BRACKMANN, D. E. (1986) Porous polyethylene prosthesis: continuing experience. *Annals of Otology, Rhinology and Laryngology*, **95**, 76–77

BRANDOW, E. C. (1969) Homograft tympanic membrane transplant in myringoplasty. *Transactions of the American Academy of Ophthalmology and Otolaryngology*, **73**, 825–835

BRANDOW, E. C. (1973) Tympanic transplants – panel discussion. *Archives of Otolaryngology*, **97**, 68

BRIGGS, R. J. S. and LUXFORD, W. M. (1994) Chronic ear surgery: a historical review. *American Journal of Otology*, **15**, 558–567

BROCKMAN, S. J. (1965) Cartilage graft tympanoplasty Type III. *Laryngoscope*, **75**, 1452–1461

BYRD, H. S. (1980) The use of subcutaneous axial fascial flaps in reconstruction of the head. *Annals of Plastic Surgery*, **4**, 191–198

CAMPBELL, E. E. (1990) Homograft tympanoplasty: a long-term review of 477 ears. *American Journal of Otology*, **11**, 66–70

CHALAT, N. I. (1964) Tympanic membrane transplant. *Harper Hospital Bulletin*, **22**, 27–34

CHANDLER, J. R. (1965) The incus in tympanoplasty. *Laryngoscope*, **75**, 793–804

CHIOSSONE, E. (1977) The establishment of an ear bank. *Otolaryngologic Clinics of North America*, **10**, 599–612

CHUDEN, H. G. (1985) Total ossicular replacement with a porous ultra-high molecular weight prosthesis. *American Journal of Otology*, **6**, 461–463

CLAROS-DOMENECH, A. (1959) 100 tympanoplasties practised with the aid of the use of free periosteal membrane graft. *Revue de Laryngologie, Otologie, Rhinologie (Bordeaux)*, **80**, 917–921

COMMITTEE ON CONSERVATION OF HEARING OF THE AMERICAN ACADEMY OF OPHTHALMOLOGY AND OTOLARYNGOLOGY (1965) Standard classification for surgery of chronic ear infection. *Archives of Otolaryngology*, **81**, 204–205

DON, A. and LINTHICUM, F. H. (1975) The fate of cartilage grafts for ossicular reconstruction in tympanoplasty. *Annals of Otology, Rhinology and Laryngology*, **84**, 187–193

EAST, C. A., BROUGH, M. D. and GRANT, H. R. (1991) Mastoid obliteration with the temporoparietal fascia flap. *Journal of Laryngology and Otology*, **105**, 417–420

ELBROND, O. and ELPERN, B. S. (1965) Reconstruction of ossicular chain in incus defects. An experimental study. *Archives of Otolaryngology*, **82**, 603–608

ENGLISH, G. M., HILDYARD, V. H., HEMENWAY, W. G. and DAVIDSON, S. (1971) Autograft and homograft incus transplantations in chronic otitis media. *Laryngoscope*, **81**, 1434–1447

FARRIOR, J. B. (1960) Ossicular repositioning and ossicular prostheses in tympanoplasty. *Archives of Otolaryngology*, **71**, 443–449

FARRIOR, J. B. (1966) Principles of surgery in tympanoplasty and mastoidectomy. *Laryngoscope*, **76**, 816–841

FARRIOR, J. B. (1969) Tympanoplasty (ossicular repositioning in reconstruction). Spine of Henle and supporting attic grafts. *Archives of Otolaryngology*, **89**, 220–225

FOGGIA, D. A. and MCCABE, M. D. (1990) Homograft tympanoplasty: The Iowa experience. *American Journal of Otology*, **11**, 307–309

FROOTKO, N. J. (1983) Causes of ossiculoplasty failure using porous polyethylene (Plastipore) prostheses. *Proceedings of the First International Congress of Biomaterials in Otology*, edited by J. J. Grote. The Hague, Holland: Martinus Nijhoff Publishers. pp. 169–176

FROOTKO, N. J. (1984) Allograft rejection in the middle ear of the rat. *MSc. Thesis*, University of Oxford

FROOTKO, N. J. (1985a) Applying the language of 'transplantese' to tympanoplasty. *Acta Oto-Rhino-Laryngologica (Belgica)*, 374–376

FROOTKO, N. J. (1985b) Immune responses in allograft tympanoplasty. In: *Immunobiology, Auto-immunity and Transplantation in Otorhinolaryngology*, edited by J. E. Veldman, B. F. McCabe, E. Huizing and N. Mygind. Amsterdam/Berkeley: Kugler Publications. pp. 171–176

FROOTKO, N. J. (1987) Immune responses in allograft tympanoplasty. In: *Otoimmunology*, edited by J. E. Veldman

and B. F. McCabe. Amsterdam/Berkeley: Kugler Publications. pp. 119–124

GERSDORFF, M., MAISIN, J. and MUNTING, E. (1986) Comparative studies of the clinical results obtained by means of Plastipore and ceramic ossicular prostheses and bone allografts. *American Journal of Otology*, **7**, 294–296

GEYER, G. and HELMS, J. (1990) Reconstructive measures in the middle ear and mastoid using a biocompatible cement – preliminary clinical experience. In: *Clinical Implant Materials*, edited by G. Heimme, U. Soltész and A. J. C. Lee. *Advances in Biomaterials*, vol. 9. Amsterdam: Elsevier Science Publishers BV. pp. 529–536

GEYER, G. and HELMS, J. (1992) Reconstruction of the posterior canal wall and obliteration of the mastoid cavity using glass-ionomer cement. Two and a half years of experience. In: *Transplants and Implants in Otology II, Proceedings of the Second International Symposium on Transplants and Implants in Otology, Matsuyama, Ehime, Japan, April 1991*, edited by N. Yanagihara and J. Suzuki. Amsterdam/New York: Kugler Publications. pp. 165–170

GLASSCOCK, M. E. and HOUSE, W. F. (1968) Homograft reconstruction of the middle ear. *Laryngoscope*, **78**, 1219–1225

GLASSCOCK, M. E., HOUSE, W. F. and GRAHAM, M. (1972) Homograft transplants to the middle ear. A follow up report. *Laryngoscope*, **82**, 868–881

GOODHILL, V., HARRIS, I. and BROCKMAN, S. J. (1964) Tympanoplasty with perichondral graft. *Archives of Otolaryngology*, **79**, 131–137

GOODHILL, V., WESTERBERGH, A. M. and DAVIS, C. (1974) Prefabricated homografts in ossiculoplasty. *Transactions of the American Academy of Ophthalmology and Otolaryngology*, **78**, 411–422

GOODHILL, V., BROCKMAN, S. J., HARRIS, I., SHULMAN, J. B. and COOPER, S. H. (1979) Otomastoiditis surgery – mastoidectomy and tympanoplasty. In: *Ear Diseases, Deafness and Dizziness*, edited by V. Goodhill. Hagerstown, Maryland: Harper and Row

GOODMAN, W. S. (1980) Tympanoplasty – 25 years later. *Journal of Otolaryngology*, **9**, 155–168

GOTAY-RODRIGUEZ, V. M. and SCHUKNECHT, H. F. (1977) Experiences with type IV tympanomastoidectomy. *Laryngoscope*, **87**, 522–528

GRIPPAUDO, M. (1958) Histopathological studies of the ossicles in chronic otitis media. *Journal of Laryngology and Otology*, **72**, 177–189

GROTE, J. J. (1984a) Biomaterials in otology. *Proceedings of The First International Symposium, 1983*. Leiden, The Netherlands: Martinus Nijhoff Publishers

GROTE, J. J. (1984b) Tympanoplasty with calcium phosphate. *Archives of Otolaryngology*, **110**, 197–199

GROTE, J. J., VAN BLITTERSWIJK, C. A. and KUIJPERS, W. (1986) Reconstruction of the middle ear with hydroxyapatite implants. *Annals of Otology, Rhinology and Laryngology*, **95** (Suppl.)

GUILFORD, F. R. (1962) Tympanic grafts: personal experiences with surgical repair of tympanic perforations. *Laryngoscope*, **72**, 1028–1053

GUILFORD, F. R. (1965) Repositioning of the incus. *Laryngoscope*, **75**, 236–242

GUILFORD, F. R. (1966) Tympanoplasty: repair of the sound conduction mechanism. *Laryngoscope*, **76**, 709–718

GUILFORD, F. R., SHORTREED, R. and HALPERT, B. (1966) Implantation of autogenous bone and cartilage into bullae of dogs. *Archives of Otolaryngology*, **84**, 144–147

HALL, A. (1956) Central tympanic perforations: treatment with prosthesis or free transplantation? *Svenska Läkartidningen*, **53**, 140–145

HALL, A. and RYTZNER, C. (1957) Stapedectomy and autotransplantation of ossicles. *Acta Otolaryngologica*, **47**, 318–324

HALL, A. and RYTZNER, C. (1960) Vitality of autotransplanted ossicles. *Acta Otolaryngologica Supplementum*, **158**, 335–340

HALL, A. and RYTZNER, C. (1961) Autotransplantation of ossicles: stapedectomy and biological reconstruction of the ossicular chain mechanism. *Archives of Otolaryngology*, **74**, 42–46

HEATH, C. J. (1904) The restoration of hearing after removal of the drum and ossicles by a modification of the radical mastoid operation for suppurative ear disease. *Lancet*, ii, 1767–1769

HEERMANN, H. (1960) Frommelfillplastik mit faszrengewebe von muskulus temporalis nach. Begradrgung der vorderen gehorgangsward. *HNO*, **9**, 136–137

HELLSTROM, S., BLOOM, G. D., BERGHEM, L., STENFORD, L. E. and SODERBURG, O. (1991) A comparison of hyaluronan and fibronectin in the healing of tympanic membrane perforations. *European Archives of Oto-Rhino-Laryngology*, **248**, 230–235

HEUMANN, H. and STEINBACH, E. (1980) The effects of an adhesive in the middle ear. *Archives of Otolaryngology*, **106**, 734–736

HICKS, G. W., WRIGHT J. W. and WRIGHT, J. W. (1978) Use of Plastipore for ossicular chain reconstruction: an evaluation. *Laryngoscope*, **88**, 1024–1033

HILDMANN, H., STEINBACH, E. and KOBURG, E. (1974) The fate of bone transplants in the middle ear. *Journal of Laryngology and Otology*, **88**, 531–537

HILDYARD, V. H. (1967) Transplant of incus homograft in the human. *Archives of Otolaryngology*, **86**, 294–297

HILGER, J. A. and HOHMANN, A. (1963) The pedicle graft in tympanomastoid surgery. *Laryngoscope*, **73**, 1121–1141

HOUGH, J. V. D. (1958) Malformations and anatomical variations seen in the middle ear during the operation for mobilization of the stapes. *Laryngoscope*, **68**, 1337–1379

HOUGH, J. V. D. (1970) Tympanoplasty with the inferior fascial graft technique and ossicular reconstruction. *Laryngoscope*, **80**, 1385–1413

HOUGH, J. V. D. (1982) Experience in tympanoplasty – avoiding revisions and complications. *Otolaryngologic Clinics of North America*, **15**, 845–860

HOUSE, H. P. (1960) Polyethylene in middle ear surgery. *Archives of Otolaryngology*, **71**, 926–931

HOUSE, W. F. (1969) Round table on ossicular autografts and homografts. *Archives of Otolaryngology*, **89**, 232–234

HOUSE, H. P. and SHEEHY, J. L. (1963) Functional restoration in tympanoplasty. *Archives of Otolaryngology*, **78**, 304–309

HOUSE, W. F., PATTERSON, M. E. and LINTHICUM, F. H. (1966) Incus homografts in chronic ear surgery. *Archives of Otolaryngology*, **84**, 148–153

HOUSE, W. F., GLASSCOCK, M. E. and SHEEHY, J. L. (1969) Homograft transplants of the middle ear. *Transactions of the American Academy of Ophthalmology and Otolaryngology*, **73**, 836–841

IRONSIDE, W. M. S. (1979) Homograft ossicular reconstruction. *Journal of Laryngology and Otology*, **93**, 1055–1061

JAHNKE, K. and PLESTER, D. (1981) Aluminium oxide Ceramic implants in middle ear surery. *Clinical Otolaryngology*, **6**, 193–195

JAKO, G. J. (1972) Biomedical engineering in ear surgery. *Otolaryngologic Clinics of North America*, **5**, 173–182

JANEKE, J. and SHEA, J. J. (1975) Self stabilizing total ossicular replacement prosthesis in tympanoplasty. *Laryngoscope*, **85**, 1550–1556

JANSEN, C. (1963) Cartilage tympanoplasty. *Laryngoscope*, **73**, 1288–1302

JANSEN, C. (1972) Methods of ossicular reconstruction. *Otolaryngologic Clinics of North America*, **5**, 97–109

JONGKEES, L. B. W. (1957) On reoperation on patients treated by reconstructive middle ear surgery. *Practica Otorhinolaryngologica*, **19**, 532–548

JUERS, A. L. (1953) Modified radical mastoidectomy. Indications and results. *Archives of Otolaryngology*, **57**, 245–256

KATZKE, D., PUSALKAR, A. and STEINBACH E. (1983) The effects of fibrin tissue adhesive on the middle ear. *Journal of Laryngology and Otology*, **97**, 141–147

KERR, A. G. (1981) Proplast and Plastipore. *Clinical Otolaryngology*, **6**, 187–191

KERR, A. G. and SMYTH, G. D. L. (1971a) The fate of transplanted ossicles. *Journal of Laryngology and Otology*, **85**, 337–347

KERR, A. G. and SMYTH, G. D. L. (1971b) Bucrylate (isobutylcyanoacrylate) as an ossicular adhesive. *Archives of Otolaryngology*, **94**, 129–131

KERR, A. G., BYRNE, J. E. T. and SMYTH, G. D. L. (1973) Cartilage homografts in the middle ear – a long term histological study. *Journal of Laryngology and Otology*, **87**, 1193–1199

KISCH, J. (1928) Temporal muscle grafts in the radical mastoid operation. *Journal of Laryngology and Otology*, **43**, 735

KLEY, W. and DRAF, W. (1965) Histologische untersuchungen über autotransplantierte gehörknochelchen und knochenstückchen in mittelohr beim menschen. *Acta Otolaryngologica*, **59**, 593–603

KOHUT, R. I. (1980) Cholesteatoma: the advantages of modified radical and radical mastoidectomy. In: *Controversy in Otolaryngology*, edited by J. B. Snow. London: W. B. Saunders. pp. 223–227

KUIJPERS, W. and VAN DEN BROEK, P. (1975) Biological considerations for the use of homograft tympanic membranes and ossicles. *Acta Otolaryngologica*, **80**, 283–293

LEE, K. and SCHUKNECHT, H. F. (1971) Results of tympanoplasty and mastoidectomy at the Massachusetts Eye and Ear Infirmary. *Laryngoscope*, **81**, 529–543

LEMPERT, J. (1938) Improvement in hearing in cases of otosclerosis. A new one-stage surgical technique. *Archives of Otolaryngology*, **28**, 42–97

LESINSKI, S. G. (1977) Availability of homograft otologic tissue. *Otolaryngologic Clinics of North America*, **10**, 613–616

LESINSKI, S. G. (1982) Complications of homograft tympanoplasty. *Otolaryngologic Clinics of North America*, **15**, 795–811

LINTHICUM, F. H. (1966) Postoperative temporal bone histopathology. *Laryngoscope*, **76**, 1232–1241

MCGEE, T. M. (1979) Management of the totally disabled middle ear. *Laryngoscope*, **89**, 730–734

MAISIN, J. P., MUNTING, E. and GERSDORFF, M. (1989) New perspectives on lyophilized bone allografts. *Archives of Oto-Rhino-Laryngology*, **246**, 283–285

MARQUET, J. (1966) Reconstructive microsurgery of the eardrum by means of a tympanic membrane homograft. *Acta Otolaryngologica*, **62**, 459–464

MARQUET, J. (1968) Myringoplasty by eardrum transplantation. *Laryngoscope*, **78**, 1329–1336

MARQUET, J. (1969) Ossicular chain homografts. *Proceedings of the International Congress of Oto-rhino-laryngology, Mexico.* Amsterdam: Excerpta Medica. pp. 151–162

MARQUET, J. (1976a) Homografts in tympanoplasty and other forms of middle ear surgery. In: *Operative Surgery: Ear*, 3rd edn, edited by J. Ballantyne. London: Butterworths. pp. 100–115

MARQUET, J. (1976b) Ten years experience in tympanoplasty using homologous implants. *Journal of Laryngology and Otology*, **90**, 897–905

MARQUET, J. (1977) Twelve years experience with homograft tympanoplasty. *Otolaryngologic Clinics of North America*, 581–593

MARQUET, J. (1982) The fibrin seal in otorhinolaryngology. *Journal of Head and Neck Pathology*, **3**, 71–72

MEURMAN, Y. and OJALA, L. (1949) Primary reduction of a large operation cavity in radical mastoidectomy with a muscle periosteal flap. *Acta Otolaryngologica*, **37**, 245–252

MINATOGAWA, T., KUMOI, T., INAMORI, T., OKI, K. and MACHIZUKA, H. (1990) Hyogo ear bank experience with allograft tympanoplasty – review of tympanoplasties on 68 ears. *American Journal of Otology*, **11**, 157–163

MOFFAT, D. A., GRAY, R. F. and IRVING, R. M. (1994) Mastoid obliteration using bone paté. *Clinical Otolaryngology*, **19**, 149–157

MORITZ, W. H. JR, EMMETT, J. R., SHEA, J. J. and SHEA, J. J., III (1986) Ossicular prostheses with peg-top fixation of interposed tissue. *Otolaryngology – Head and Neck Surgery*, **94**, 407–409

MORITZ, W. (1952) Plastiche eingriffe am mittelohr zur wiederherstellung der innenchr-schalleitung. *Zeitschrift für Laryngologie*, **31**, 338–351

MORRISON, A. W. (1970) Homograft tympanoplasty and myringoplasty. *Acta Oto-Rhino-Laryngologica (Belgica)*, **24**, 45–52

MÜSEBECK, K. and FALCK, P. (1963) Über knöcherne druckstructuren in reponierten und homologen steigbügeln und in knochenspänen. *Archiv für Ohren, Nasen Kehlkopfheilkunde*, **181**, 279–290

MYER, C. M. and COTTON, R. T. (1982) Total ossicular replacement prosthesis. Unusual cause of a perilymph fistula. *American Journal of Otology*, **4**, 123–125

NIPARKO, J. K., KEMINK, J. L., GRAHAM, M. D. and KARTUSH, J. M. (1988) Bioactive glass ceramic in ossicular reconstruction: a preliminary report. *Laryngoscope*, **98**, 822–825

OJALA, K., SORRI, M., VAINIO-MATILLA, J. and SIPILA, P. (1983) Late results of tympanoplasty using ossicle or cortical bone. *Journal of Laryngology and Otology*, **97**, 19–25

OPPENHEIMER, P. and HARRISON, W. (1963) The missing lenticular process. *Archives of Otolaryngology*, **78**, 143–150

PALVA, T. (1963) Middle ear surgery in Northern Europe. *Archives of Otolaryngology*, **78**, 363–370

PALVA, T. (1982) Obliteration of the mastoid cavity and reconstruction of the canal wall. *Otolaryngology* Vol. I *Otology*, edited by A. G. Gibb and M. F. W. Smith. London: Butterworths. pp. 19–29

PALVA, T. (1993) Cholesteatoma surgery today. *Clinical Otolaryngology and Allied Sciences*, **18**, 245–252

PALVA, T. and MAKINEN, J. (1983) Histopathological observations on polyethylene-type materials in chronic ear surgery. *Acta Otolaryngologica*, **95**, 139–146

PENNINGTON, C. L. (1973) Incus interposition techniques. *Annals of Otology, Rhinology and Laryngology*, **82**, 518–531

PERKINS, R. (1970a) Human homograft otologic tissue transplantation. Buffered formaldehyde preparation. *Transactions of the American Academy of Ophthalmology and Otolaryngology*, **74**, 278–282

PERKINS, R. (1970b) Homograft tympanic membrane with suture sling. *Laryngoscope*, **80**, 1100–1108

PERKINS, R. (1975) Formaldehyde-formed autogenous fascia graft tympanoplasty. *Transactions of the American Academy of Ophthalmology and Otolaryngology*, **80**, 565–572

PLESTER, D. and STEINBACH, E. (1977) Histological fate of tympanic membrane and ossicle homografts. *Otolaryngologic Clinics of North America*, **10**, 487–499

PODOSHIN, L., FRADIS, M. and GERTNER, R. (1988) Carbon-carbon middle ear prosthesis: a preliminary clinical human trial report. *Otolaryngology – Head and Neck Surgery*, **99**, 278–281

PORTMANN, M. (1963) Tympanoplasty. *Archives of Otolaryngology*, **78**, 7–19

PORTMANN, M. (1982) The use of 'Tissucol' in ossicular chain reconstruction. *Journal of Head and Neck Pathology*, **3**, 96

PRAMACHANDRA, D. J., WOODWARD, B., MILTON, C. M., SERGEANT, R. J. and FABRE, J. W. (1993) Long term results of mastoid cavities grafted with cultured epithelium prepared from autologous epidermal cells to prevent chronic otorrhoea. *Laryngoscope*, **103**, 1121–1125

PULEC, J. L. (1966) Symposium on tympanoplasty. 1. Homograft incus. *Laryngoscope*, **76**, 1429–1438

PULEC, J. L. (1976) Conversion of the radical mastoid cavity for obliteration or reconstruction. In: *Operative Surgery: Ear*, 3rd edn, edited by J. Ballantyne. London: Butterworths. pp. 116–124

PULEC, J. L. and SHEEHY J. L. (1973) Tympanoplasty: ossicular chain reconstruction. *Laryngoscope*, **83**, 448–465

RAMBO, J. H. T. (1958) Musculoplasty: a new operation for suppurative middle ear deafness. *Transactions of the American Academy of Ophthalmology and Otolaryngology*, **62**, 166–177

RAMBO, J. H. T. (1961) The use of paraffin to create a middle ear space in musculoplasty. *Laryngoscope*, **71**, 612-619

RECK, R. (1981) Tissue reactions to glass ceramics in the middle ear. *Clinical Otolaryngology*, **6**, 63–65

RECK, R. (1985) The bioglass ceramic ceravital in ear surgery. Five years experience. *American Journal of Otology*, **6**, 280–283

RECK, R., STORKEL, S. and MEYER, A. (1988) Bioactive glass ceramics in middle ear surgery. *Annals of the New York Academy of Sciences*, **523**, 100–106

RENARD, J. L., FELTEN, D. and BÉQUET, D. (1994) Post-otoneurosurgery aluminium encephalopathy. *Lancet*, **ii**, 63–64

RICHARDS TECHNICAL PUBLICATION (1980) no. 4240. Memphis: Richards Manufacturing Co. Inc.

RINGENBERG, J. C. (1962) Fat graft tympanoplasty. *Laryngoscope*, **72**, 188–192

ROBIN, P. E., BENNETT, R. J. and GREGORY, M. (1976) Study of autogenous transposed ossicles, bone and cartilage in man. *Clinical Otolaryngology*, **1**, 295–308

ROSEN, S. (1953) Mobilisation of the stapes to restore hearing in otosclerosis. *New York Journal of Medicine*, **53**, 2650–2653

SCHILLER, A. (1979) Middle ear reconstruction by malleo-myringoplasty. *Journal of Laryngology and Otology*, **93**, 1063–1073

SCHILLER, A. and SINGER, M. (1960) Mastoid osteoplasty using autogenous cancellous bone. A new procedure. *South African Medical Journal*, **34**, 645–650

SEELICH, T. (1982) Tissucol (Immuno, Vienna): biochemistry and methods of application. *Journal of Head and Neck Pathology*, **3**, 65–69

SHEA, J. J. (1956) Symposium on the operation for mobilization of the stapes in otosclerotic deafness. *Laryngoscope*, **66**, 729

SHEA, J. J. (1960a) Vein graft closure of eardrum perforations. *Journal of Laryngology and Otology*, **74**, 358–362

SHEA, J. J. (1960b) Fenestration of the oval window. *Archives of Otolaryngology*, **71**, 257–264

SHEA, J. J. (1976) Plastipore total ossicular replacement prosthesis. *Laryngoscope*, **86**, 239–240

SHEA, J., EMMETT, J. and SMYTH, G. D. L. (1977) Biocompatible implants in otology. *Otorhinolaryngology Digest*, **39**, 9–15

SHEA, M. C. (1981) The use of Silastic in tympanoplasty surgery. *Clinical Otolaryngology*, **6**, 125–126

SHEA, M. C. and GLASSCOCK, M. E. (1967) Tragal cartilage as an ossicular substitute. *Archives of Otolaryngology*, **86**, 308–317

SHEA, M. C., GARDNER, G. and SIMPSON, M. E. (1972) Mastoid obliteration with bone. *Otolaryngologic Clinics of North America*, **5**, 161–172

SHEEHY, J. L. (1965) Ossicular problems in tympanoplasty. *Archives of Otolaryngology*, **81**, 115–122

SHEEHY, J. L. (1980) Intact canal wall tympanoplasty with mastoidectomy. In: *Controversy in Otolaryngology*, edited by J. B. Snow. London: W. B. Saunders & Co. pp. 213–222

SHEEHY, J. L. (1984) TORPS and PORPS: causes of failure – a report on 446 operations. *Otolaryngology – Head and Neck Surgery*, **92**, 583–587

SHEEHY, J. L. and CRABTREE, J. A. (1973) Tympanoplasty: staging the operation. *Laryngoscope*, **83**, 1594–1621

SMITH, M. F. W. (1970) Composite reconstruction of the open mastoidectomy ear. *Transactions of the American Academy of Ophthalmology and Otolaryngology*, **74**, 1166–1182

SMITH, M. F. W. (1980a) Freeze-dried otologic implants. *Journal of Otolaryngology*, **9**, 222–227

SMITH, M. F. W. (1980b) Allograft ossicular chain transplantation. In: *Controversy in Otolaryngology*, edited by J. B. Snow. London: W. B. Saunders & Co. pp. 178–183

SMITH, M. F. W. (1982) Middle ear transformer reconstruction. In: *Otolaryngology* Vol. 1, *Otology*, edited by A. G. Gibb and M. F. W. Smith. London: Butterworths. pp. 49–57

SMITH, M. F. W. and DOBIE, R. (1976) The use of homograft stapes. *Laryngoscope*, **86**, 1196–1202

SMITH, M. F. W. and MCELVEEN, J. T. (1982) Lyophilised partial ossicular replacement allografts. *Annals of Otology, Rhinology and Laryngology*, **91**, 538–540

SMYTH, G. D. L. (1969) Combined approach tympanoplasty. *Archives of Otolaryngology*, **89**, 250–251

SMYTH, G. D. L. (1972a) Outline of surgical management in chronic ear disease. *Otolaryngologic Clinics of North America*, **5**, 59–77

SMYTH, G. D. L. (1972b) Tympanic reconstruction. *Otolaryngologic Clinics of North America*, **5**, 111–125

SMYTH, G. D. L. (1976) Tympanic reconstruction. *Journal of Laryngology and Otology*, **90**, 713–741

SMYTH, G. D. L. (1980) Ossiculoplasty. In: *Chronic Ear Disease, Monographs in Clinical Otolaryngology*. Edinburgh: Churchill Livingstone. pp. 146–174

SMYTH, G. D. L. (1982a) Tympanomastoid disease. In: *Otolaryngology*, Vol. 1. *Otology*, edited by A. G. Gibb and M. F. W. Smith. London: Butterworths. pp. 3–18

SMYTH, G. D. L. (1982b) Five year report on partial ossicular replacement prostheses and total ossicular replacement prostheses. *Otolaryngology – Head and Neck Surgery*, **90**, 343–346

SMYTH, G. D. L. and HASSARD, T. H. (1981) The evaluation of policies in the surgical treatment of acquired cholesteatoma of the tubotympanic cleft. *Journal of Laryngology and Otology*, **95**, 767–773

SMYTH, G. D. L. and KERR, A. G. (1967) Homologous grafts for ossicular reconstruction in tympanoplasty. *Laryngoscope*, **77**, 330–336

SMYTH, G. D. L. and KERR, A. G. (1969) Tympanic membrane homografts. *Journal of Laryngology and Otology*, **83**, 1061–1066

SMYTH, G. D. L., KERR, A. G. and GOODEY, R. J. (1971) Tympanic membrane homograft: further evaluation. *Journal of Laryngology and Otology*, **85**, 891–895

SMYTH, G. D. L., KERR, A. G. and HASSARD, T. H. (1977) Homograft materials in tympanoplasty. *Otolaryngologic Clinics of North America*, **10**, 563–580

STACKE, L. (1893) Stacke's Operation Methode. *Archiv für Ohren-Nasen-Kehlkopfheilkunde*, **35**, 145

STEINBACH, E. and HILDMANN, H. (1972) Zur wiederverwendung des autologen Ambossess loeim Cholesteatem und bei der chronischen Schleimhauteiterung. *Laryngologie, Rhinologie, Otologie*, **51**, 659–664

STEINBACH, E. and PUSALKAR, A. (1981) Long term histological fate of cartilage in ossicular reconstruction. *Journal of Laryngology and Otology*, **95**, 1031–1039

SZPUNAR, J. (1967) Biological reconstruction of the ossicular chain. *Archives of Otolaryngology*, **86**, 303–307

SZPUNAR, J. (1969) Autografts of the ossicular chain. *Proceedings of the Ninth International Congress of Otorhino-laryngology*. Mexico, 1969. Amsterdam: Excerpta Medica. pp. 147–150

TABB, H. G. (1963) The surgical management of chronic ear disease, with special reference to staged surgery. *Laryngoscope*, **73**, 363–383

TANGE, R. A., TROOST, D. and LIMBURG, M. (1990) Progressive fatal dementia (Creutzfeld-Jakob disease) in a patient who received homograft tissue for tympanic membrane closure. *European Archives of Oto-Rhino-Laryngology*, **247**, 199–201

THORBURN, I. B. (1960) A critical review of tympanoplastic surgery. *Journal of Laryngology and Otology*, **74**, 453–474

TOS, M. (1974) Late results in tympanoplasty. *Archives of Otolaryngology*, **100**, 302–305

TOS, M. (1978) Allograft stapes-incus assembly. A new ossiculoplasty. *Archives of Otolaryngology*, **104**, 119–121

TUMARKIN, A. (1948) Transmeatal attico-antrotomy in chronic tympanomastoid suppuration. *Journal of Laryngology and Otology*, **62**, 316–330

UTECH, H. (1960) Better final hearing after tympanoplasty. Modification of the method. *Zeitschrift für Laryngologie, Rhinologie, Otologie*, **39**, 367–371

VAN BLITTERSWIJK, C. A., HESSELING, S. C., GROTE, J. J., KOERTEN, H. K. and DE GROOT, K. (1990) The biocompatibility of hydroxyapatite ceramic: a study of retrieved human middle ear implants. *Journal of Biomedical Materials Research*, **24**, 433–453

VAN DEN BROEK, P. (1968) The fate of incus grafts in rats. *PhD Thesis*, University of Nijmegen, The Netherlands

VAN HASSELT, C. A. (1994) Toynbee Memorial Lecture 1993. Mastoid surgery and the Hong Kong flap. *Journal of Laryngology and Otology*, **108**, 825–833

VRABEC, J. T., SCHWABER, M. K., DAVIDSON, J. H. and CLYMER, M. A. (1994) Evaluation of basic fibroblast growth factor in tympanic membrane repair. *Laryngoscope*, **104**, 1059–1063

WEHRS, R. E. (1967) The borrowed ossicle in tympanoplasty. *Archives of Otolaryngology*, **85**, 371–379

WEHRS, R. E. (1972) Reconstructive mastoidectomy with homograft knee cartilage. *Laryngoscope*, **82**, 1177–1188

WEHRS, R. E. (1974) The homograft notched incus in tympanoplasty. *Archives of Otolaryngology*, **100**, 251–255

WEHRS, R. E. (1982a) Homograft tympanoplasty. *Otolaryngologic Clinics of North America*, **15**, 781–793

WEHRS, R. E. (1982b) The homograft tympanic membrane after 12 years. *Annals of Otology, Rhinology and Laryngology*, **91**, 533–537

WEHRS, R. E. (1989a) Ossicular reconstruction in ears with cholesteatoma. *Otolaryngologic Clinics of North America*, **22**, 1003–1013

WEHRS, R. E. (1989b) Incus replacement prostheses of hydroxylapatite in middle ear reconstruction. *American Journal of Otology*, **10**, 181–182

WRIGHT, W. K. (1960) Myringoplasty. *Archives of Otolaryngology*, **71**, 369–375

WRIGHT, W. K. (1963) Tissues for tympanic grafting. *Archives of Otolaryngology*, **78**, 291–296

WRIGHT, W. K. (1967) Reconstruction of the middle ear with fascia and bone. *Archives of Otolaryngology*, **85**, 492–496

WULLSTEIN, H. (1953) Die tympanoplastik als gehörverbessernde operation bei otitis media chronica und ihre resultate. *Proceedings of the Fifth International Congress of Oto-Rhino-Laryngology*, Amsterdam. pp. 104–118

WULLSTEIN, H. (1956) Theory and practice of tympanoplasty. *Laryngoscope*, **66**, 1076–1093

WULLSTEIN, H. (1960) Tympanoplasty. The problem of the free graft and the mucous membrane graft. *Archives of Otolaryngology*, **71**, 363–368

WULLSTEIN, H. (1981) In retrospect of a surgeon. In: *Zeiss Microscopes for Microsurgery*, edited by W. H. Lang and F. Muchel, Berlin: Springer-Verlag

YAMAMOTO, E. (1985) Aluminium oxide ceramic ossicular replacement prosthesis. *Annals of Otology, Rhinology and Laryngology*, **94**, 149–152

YAMAMOTO, E. (1988) Long term observations on ceramic ossicular replacement prosthesis (CORP). *Laryngoscope*, **98**, 402–404

ZÖLLNER, F. (1953) Hörverbessernde eingriffe am schalleitungsapparat. *Proceedings of the Fifth International Congress of Oto-Rhino-Laryngology*, Amsterdam. pp. 119–126

ZÖLLNER, F. (1955) The principles of plastic surgery of the sound-conducting apparatus. *Journal of Laryngology and Otology*, **69**, 637–652

ZÖLLNER, F. (1960) Tecknik der formung einer columella aus knochen. *Zeitschrift für Laryngologie, Rhinologie und Otologie*, **39**, 536–540

ZÖLLNER, F. (1963) Panel on myringoplasty (2nd Workshop, Reconstructive middle ear surgery). *Archives of Otolaryngology*, **78**, 301–302

ZÖLLNER, F. (1969) Round table on ossicular autografts and homografts. *Archives of Otolaryngology*, **89**, 230

12

Complications of suppurative otitis media

Harold Ludman

Complications of suppurative otitis media develop if infection spreads from the middle ear cleft to structures from which this mucosa-lined space is usually separated by bone. Before antibiotics were regularly available, these complications followed acute suppuration more often than chronic middle ear disease. Nowadays chronic middle ear infection is the greater hazard, although some writers, exceptionally, (Gower and McGuirt, 1983) have still found a higher incidence of intracranial complications from acute infections. This may reflect the high proportion of young patients in their series, and illustrates the fact that complications of acute otitis media are commoner in the young. In a more recent series of over 1400 patients with chronic ear disease and cholesteatoma, followed over 15 years, nearly 7.5% developed intracranial complications and, of those, meningitis was the commonest (Maksimovic and Rukovanjski, 1993). Although the overall incidence of complications has fallen greatly with antibiotic treatment, the mortality from intracranial complications was still high even a decade ago (Lancet, 1982).

The complications (Figure 12.1) to be discussed fall into two main categories:

1 Those within the cranial cavity

Extradural abscess
Subdural abscess (empyema)
Sigmoid sinus thrombophlebitis
Meningitis
Brain abscess
Otitic hydrocephalus

2 Those within the temporal bone

Facial paralysis
Labyrinthine infections.

Rarer complications, e.g. subclavian vein thrombo-

sis, and internal carotid artery aneurysm (Kimmelman and Grosman, 1983) have also been reported. Petrositis, which may be considered an unusual extension of mastoiditis, is described in Chapter 9.

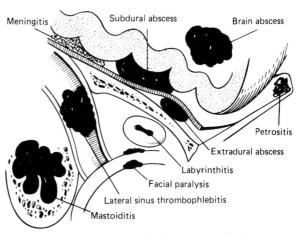

Figure 12.1 Diagram of sites of infection in complications of otitis media. (From Ludman, 1988, *Mawson's Diseases of the Ear*, 5th edn, London: Edward Arnold, by kind permission)

Whether acute or chronic, infection may spread by a number of possible routes (Figure 12.2).

1 By extension through bone that has been demineralized during acute infection, or suffered resorption by cholesteatoma or osteitis in chronic disease (see Figure 5.2).
2 By the spreading of infected clot within small veins through bone and dura to venous sinuses – the lateral and the superior petrosal – and so to intracranial structures. Apparently intact bone may be transgressed by thrombophlebitis within its haver-

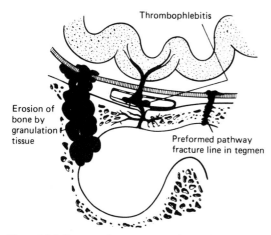

Figure 12.2 Diagram showing routes of spread of infection from the middle ear cavity. (From Ludman, 1988, *Mawson's Diseases of the Ear*, 5th edn, London: Edward Arnold, by kind permission)

sian vascular system. Thrombophlebitic spread from the lateral sinus to the cerebellum and from the superior petrosal sinus to the temporal lobe explains the frequent association between these complications.

3 Through normal anatomical pathways – the oval or round windows into the internal auditory meatus, the cochlear and vestibular aqueducts, dehiscence of the thin bony covering of the jugular bulb, dehiscence of the tegmen tympani, and dehiscent suture lines of the temporal bone (see Figures 5.7, 5.8 and 5.9).

4 Through non-anatomical bony defects caused by trauma – accidental or surgical – or by neoplastic erosion.

5 Through other surgical defects; in particular, the vestibular opening deliberately created at a stapedectomy operation, and possibly through a fenestration opening into the lateral semicircular canal.

6 Into brain tissue along the periarteriolar spaces of Virchow-Robin. This spread does not affect the cortical arterioles themselves and explains abscess development in the white matter with no apparent continuity of infection to the brain surface. Chronic middle ear disease extends slowly and many of its complications are caused by the progressive and relentless erosion of bone, thus exposing the structures at risk to damage – the facial nerve, the labyrinth, the dura. Acute infections cause complications earlier, through the thrombophlebitic mechanisms and the anatomically available pathways. Despite the apparent 'skipping' of a brain abscess into the white matter, the general pattern of infective spread, through the mechanisms described, is progressive from one structure and tissue plane to the next. Progress is from the middle ear

cleft to extradural spaces and venous sinuses, through dura to the cerebrospinal fluid spaces, and into brain tissue. It should not then be surprising that multiple complications are common, arising in one-third of cases, and that certain associations such as those between lateral sinus thrombosis and cerebellar abscess, are frequent. The propensity for spread of infection, and the development of complications depend on:

a patient attributes – age, immune state, intercurrent chronic disease such as diabetes mellitus or leukaemia

b bacterial attributes – virulence, susceptibility to chemotherapeutic elimination. For example in acute suppurative infection, *Streptococcus pneumoniae* type III and *Haemophilus influenzae* type B have sinister reputations

c efficacy of treatment of the underlying middle ear disease. Infecting bacteria predominantly responsible for infections have varied in accounts over the years, and still do from one report to another. One explanation is the difference in the nature of bacteria associated with acute and with chronic cholesteatomatous disease. Some variations may represent genuine differences in the pattern of microbial infections in different parts of the world, while others indicate changes that have taken place in patterns of infection over the years. Lastly, previously unidentified bacteria such as obligatory anaerobes (Ingham, Selkon and Roxby, 1977) were recognized by newer bacteriological techniques. These explanations for apparent inconsistencies should be remembered when reading the sections below on the individual complications. Although cholesteatoma, with posterior marginal or attic disease, is considered to be the hallmark of an ear with a poor prognosis, Browning (1984), in a study of patients in the West of Scotland, showed that a brain abscess may arise from ears with mucosal disease, and from ears previously treated by modified radical mastoidectomy. Nunez and Browning (1990), in a further study of Scottish patients have assessed that the annual risk in an adult with active chronic otitis media, of developing a brain abscess, is 1 in 10 000. They commented that this means that the life-time risk for a 30 year old is as high as 1 in 200.

General principles

Certain aspects of the presentation, diagnosis and management of intracranial complications are common to all; so it is pertinent to make some general comments concerned with principles here, before considering individual features under separate headings below. This may help to avoid unnecessary repetition, and should emphasize that these complications have to be considered as a group, since they are multiple in about one-third of instances. The symptoms of intracranial spread of infection are those of infection, and those of brain tissue compression. Headache, malaise, fever, drowsiness are all suspicious symptoms. Otalgia is never a symptom of uncomplicated cholesteatoma. Any of these should alert the otologist to the possibility of a complication, and provoke initiation of appropriate investigation and treatment. More specific features of individual complications will be discussed under the appropriate headings. At any time one complication may be clinically dominant, with others emerging from the investigative findings. Investigation and treatment must run concurrently. To delay treatment until investigation is complete may allow disease to proceed beyond the chance of recovery. The principles of treatment, common to all intracranial complications include:

1 Systemic antibiotic therapy.
2 Local neurosurgical attention to the complication(s) identified.
3 Treatment of the ear lesion.

Antibiotics

The choice of an effective antibiotic regimen depends first on understanding the bacteriology of intracranial infections. In the pre-antibiotic era, most were caused by *Streptococcus pyogenes* and *Staphylococcus aureus*, and complications were usually sequelae to acute infections. Today, most follow chronic infections, and are caused by multiple organisms. Acute infections are likely to yield *Haemophilus influenzae* or *Strep. pneumoniae*. Chronic ear diseases cause complications infected by Gram-negative organisms, sometimes by staphylococci that may be β-lactamase producers, and by obligate anaerobes such as *Bacteroides fragilis*. The recognition of anaerobic infections as an explanation for apparently sterile abscesses (Ingham, Selkon and Roxby, 1977) was an important development in the understanding and improved management of intracranial sepsis.

The use of antibiotics has certainly reduced the incidence of complications, but has had a less dramatic effect on the mortality of established ones. Antibiotics have also changed the pattern of clinical presentation, introducing an element of 'masking' with much less florid and less typical development. It is indicative of this problem that Pfaltz and Griesemer (1984) found normal otoscopic appearances in 10% of children with mastoiditis, and there are other reports of normal looking ears with serious complications (Samuel and Fernandez, 1985; Oyarzabal, Patel and Tolley, 1992).

It is not wise to offer rigid recommendations for antibiotic regimens, for several reasons. First, the armamentarium of available drugs is changing rapidly, so that suggestions at the time of writing may be obsolete within a short period. Secondly, the pattern of infecting organisms is also changing. Finally, bacterial resistance will vary from time to time and from place to place. Microbiologists are usually familiar with the drugs available locally, and have often developed policies for treating particular types of infection. Advice from the pathologist in the hospital where treatment is undertaken should assist the otologist's selection of drugs. Certain general principles can, however, be addressed.

It is, first of all, important to know of the ability of antibiotics to penetrate infected lesions, and particularly abscesses. At one time it was thought that penicillin would not easily pass the blood–brain barrier, but it is now recognized that most drugs will readily enter the cerebrospinal fluid in high doses if the meninges are inflamed. Abscess pus will absorb significant levels of many antibiotics, including chloramphenicol, penicillin, ampicillin, metronidazole, rifampicin and some cephalosporins (Ingham *et al.*, 1991). Interestingly though, no studies have correlated outcome results with drug levels within pus.

Antibiotics must be chosen on an empirical basis on the grounds of infection probabilities, before culture and sensitivity information is available. They must be given in large doses, in combinations, and usually by intravenous administration. A typical regimen should include a broad-spectrum antibiotic effective against Gram-negative organisms in chronic infections and against *Haemophilus influenzae* in acute ones, a penicillin – possibly one capable of destroying β-lactamase secreting staphylococci – and metronidazole as the most efficient drug against the anaerobic *Bacteroides* organisms.

In acute infective complications, then, chloramphenicol, to which *Haemophilus influenzae* is sensitive, even when it is resistant to ampicillin, may be combined with methicillin, flucloxacillin or ampicillin, and with metronidazole. The recommended dose of chloramphenicol is generally 100 mg/kg per day (Brand, Caparosa and Lubic, 1984). The risk of agranulocytosis and aplastic anaemia demand that its adminstration be repeatedly monitored by blood counts every second day. Metronidazole is given in a dose of 400–600 mg 8-hourly, and is a standard component of every regimen for the treatment of infective complications.

A similar cocktail may be used for the treatment of chronic infective complications, but chloramphenicol is inactivated by *Bacteroides fragilis* groups of organisms, and the most useful broad-spectrum antibiotics effective against *Pseudomonas aeruginosa* and other Gram-negative aerobes are the aminoglycosides, of which gentamicin is the most favoured. Other options include azlocillin and ticarcillin and some of the cephalosporins. A basic regimen of gentamicin, ampicillin and metronidazole is favoured as the first line of empirical medication by Ingham and his co-workers (Ingham *et al.*, 1991) for the treatment of brain abscesses, lateral sinus thrombophlebitis and subdural abscess. Gentamicin, when used as an alternative to chloramphenicol, supplements the activity of ampicillin against facultative anaerobes and provides an effective combination against *Staph. aureus*. These authors, with wide experience over the past 15 years, accept chloramphenicol as a reasonable alternative to gentamicin in lateral sinus thrombosis and in subdural abscesses in infancy. Gentamicin is generally given in a dose of 4.5 mg/kg per day, after a loading dose of about 1.5 mg/kg. The precise dose depends on the patient's serum creatinine and lean body mass. The risks of ototoxicity and nephrotoxicity must be minimized by measuring peak (20 minutes after intravenous administration) and trough (pre-dose) serum levels. Acceptable are peak levels of 5–10 mg/l, and trough levels of less than 1 mg/l.

Cephalosporins also include some that are bactericidal for Gram-negative rods and β-lactamase producing cocci; Taylor (1987) has achieved the low mortality of 6% in 50 patients with brain abscesses using cefuroxime and cefotaxime.

Treatment of the ear

Acute otitis media will usually be cured by the antibiotic selected for the treatment of its complications, but occasionally a myringotomy will be needed. If cortical mastoidectomy becomes necessary, it is customary to advise removal of the bony covering of the sigmoid sinus, and also of the middle fossa dura, since extradural pus or granulation tissue can exist deep to intact bone.

Chronic middle ear disease poses the eventual need for some form of radical or modified radical mastoidectomy. Timing is important. Generally, with exceptions that will be noted, it is advisable to wait until the intracranial complications have been controlled before operating on the ear. Deterioration of the state of a complication, despite appropriate treatment could, however, impose the need for earlier intervention.

Investigations

The advent of CT scanning and, in particular, the introduction of the latest generation of high resolution scanners with the ability to reconstruct images in different planes, has revolutionized the investigation of intracranial complications to the same dramatic extent that antibiotics have affected the

incidence and prognosis. By the use of CT scanning, intracranial masses – extradural abscesses, subdural abscesses and brain abscesses – can be identified, localized and monitored during treatment. Before the advent of these techniques, masses could be suspected from straight X-rays, which might show shift of a calcified pineal gland, and by EEG. Arteriography offered the best way to demonstrate supratentorial masses by distortion of the vascular pattern. Air encephalography and ventriculography were also valuable, but had certain risks.

Magnetic resonance imaging (MRI) may offer advantages over CT scanning, but few centres have yet had extensive experience with this form of investigation for intracranial sepsis. MRI does show soft tissue in the posterior fossa and temporal lobes well, because of the absence of bone artefacts, and its ability to show cuts in different planes without mechanical adjustment is also a benefit. It has already been shown to be useful in the recognition of early infections (Schroth *et al.*, 1987), and it can accurately diagnose early brain abscesses (Figure 12.3), distinguishing between abscess capsule oedema and central pus without enhancement (Haimes *et al.*, 1989). Enhancement with gadolinium DTPA is a valuable additional aid, for instance in recognizing changes in the dura and arachnoid in meningitis.

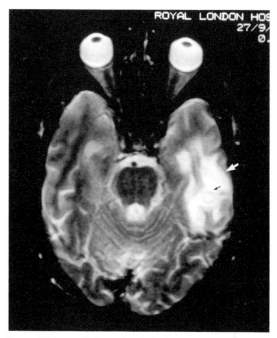

Figure 12.3 Axial T2 weighted (dual echo image) level of upper pons. The temporal lobe shows the focal area of an early abscess (black arrow) surrounded by vasogenic oedema (white arrow). (Reproduced by kind permission of the Editor)

Lumbar puncture, to provide cerebrospinal fluid for examination, still has an essential role in diagnosing meningitis, but its risks in the presence of raised intracranial pressure must be recognized. Its contribution to the diagnosis of lateral sinus thrombosis is discussed under that heading. Specialized forms of angiography, e.g. digital subtraction venography, are also mentioned below.

Extradural abscess (Figure 12.4)

Involvement of the dura mater by spreading disease constitutes pachymeningitis. Most often such spread is preceded by bone loss, through demineralization in

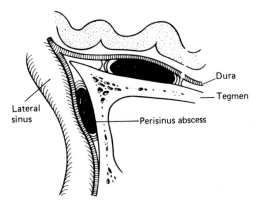

Figure 12.4 Extradural abscess. (From Ludman, 1988, *Mawson's Diseases of the Ear*, 5th edn, London: Edward Arnold, by kind permission)

acute infection, or erosion by cholesteatoma in chronic disease. Non-infected cholesteatoma may expose and coat the dura with matrix, without inflammatory reaction, but more often an inflammatory response produces granulation tissue on the surface of the dura. Fortunately the dura is tough, and resistant to invasion and destruction. Often the result of infection reaching its outer surface is the development of a collection of pus between it and the more superficial bone. This constitutes an extradural abscess, and is the commonest of all intracranial complications arising from middle ear infections. A middle fossa extradural abscess may strip dura from bone extensively on the inner surface of the squamous temporal bone, even to the extent of producing a sizeable intracranial mass, which, by raising intracranial pressure can, albeit rarely, cause focal neurological signs and papilloedema. Erosion through the skull to the exterior from there would produce a subperiosteal abscess – the classical but rare 'Pott's puffy tumour' (Figure 12.5). Most middle fossa extradural abscesses are confined to the upper surface of tegmen tympani, with much less dramatic results, since firm attachment of the dura to the arcuate eminence prevents separation of a large area from the bone, and impedes the development of a large volume of pus. More rarely, an extradural abscess may develop medially to the arcuate eminence, over the petrous apex (see Figure 5.34). Irritative involvement there of the Gasserian ganglion of the trigeminal nerve, and of the VIth cranial nerve (Figure 12.6), produces the characteristic features of Gradenigo's syndrome – facial pain, diplopia, and aural discharge. Posterior fossa extradural abscesses are limited anatomically

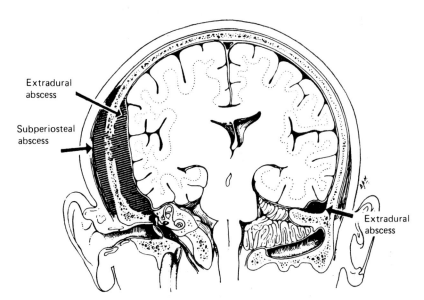

Figure 12.5 Diagram of middle fossa extradural abscesses showing enlargement of the abscess and erosion through the vault of the skull to produce a subperiosteal abscess

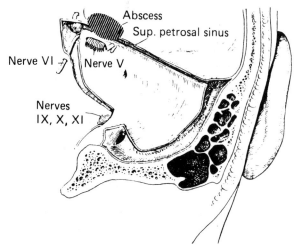

Figure 12.6 Diagram of the relations of the petrous apex to show proximity of an apical extradural abscess to the Vth and VIth cranial nerves

by the attachments of the dura laterally to the groove for the sigmoid sinus, and medially to the region of the internal auditory meatus and the subarcuate fossa. Posterior extension around the sigmoid sinus produces a sigmoid sinus-perisinus abscess. This may contribute to the development of, and may be associated with, thrombophlebitis developing within the sigmoid and transverse sinuses. Very rarely such a perisinus abscess may extend through the jugular foramen into the neck.

Clinical features

The clinical pattern depends on the site of the abscess, its size, duration and the rate of its development. The discussion above touched on some of the features associated with the more unusual patterns of extradural pus but, in most instances, the features are vague and rather non-specific. Indeed, many times an extradural abscess is an incidental finding uncovered during mastoid surgery. With chronic ear disease, a complaint of headache, broadly spread on the side of the affected ear, especially when accompanied by malaise, is suspicious. If the abscess communicates freely with the middle ear, there is, characteristically, intermittent relief from pain during episodes of aural discharge.

Diagnosis

Ultimately, diagnosis depends on operative findings. Suspicion may be confirmed by the appearances of a CT scan, and this investigation is essential to exclude a possible brain abscess in those unusual patients presenting with raised intracranial pressure.

Management

Suspicion of dural inflammation or an extradural abscess is an indication for surgical exploration. Released pus is evacuated, and enough bone should be removed for an area of healthy dura to be exposed all the way round the diseased portion. Granulation tissue attached to the dura should not be disturbed, for fear of breaching the dura and infecting the subdural spaces. The possibility of other coexisting complications must always be considered. Appropriate antibiotic treatment will be needed, especially when the extradural abscess complicates acute otitis media. In the absence of other complications, recovery should be as rapid and as complete as after uncomplicated mastoid surgery.

Subdural abscess (empyema) (Figure 12.7)

Spread of infection through the dura exposes the subdural space to the hazards of infection, which become manifest as widespread leptomeningitis or, if the accumulating fluid is contained, as subdural effusions or abscesses (subdural empyemas). The rate of spread probably determines the clinical and pathological pattern; the type of organisms may also be important. Dawes (1979) described the predominance of non-haemolytic streptococci, especially the microaerophilic or anaerobic *Strep. milleri*, in subdural abscess. As is the case with other intracranial complications, the condition is frequently, if not usually, associated with other complications, and that should be expected from an understanding of the way in which it develops.

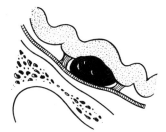

Figure 12.7 Subdural abscess. (From Ludman, 1988, *Mawson's Diseases of the Ear*, 5th edn, London: Edward Arnold, by kind permission)

As has been noted, the dura is very resistant to destruction, and granulation tissue developing on its inner surface as an inflammatory reaction tends to obliterate the adjacent space. This granulation tissue may eventually be converted to fibrous tissue. Eventual necrosis of the dura may lead to infection of the subdural compartment. At first, a seropurulent effusion collects. Gower and McGuirt (1983) identified sterile effusions in the subdural space in a small proportion of patients with subdural fluid collections, and observed that none had been recorded before the advent of CT scanning. Eventually, a seropurulent effusion becomes frankly purulent, and extends over the surface of the cerebral hemisphere to an extent limited by the granulation tissue obliteration of the space. Continuing granulation tissue invasion loculates the developing abscess.

The abscess may remain small near the site of dural penetration, or it may extend widely, with the production of a volume of pus large enough to act as a space-occupying lesion. Adjacent cortical veins may become involved with thrombophlebitis, which is responsible for some of the clinical features. This process may produce multiple small abscesses within the brain adjacent to the preceding subdural infection. The subdural pus tends to accumulate near the falx cerebri, and particularly where that structure joins the tentorium cerebelli. Healing may be accompanied by fibrosis in the limiting granulation tissue, with obliteration of subdural space. The established pathological pattern is commonly one of numerous multiloculated abscesses over the convex surface of the cerebral hemisphere, and between the hemispheres along the falx. Although non-haemolytic streptococci are often the infecting organisms, Gower and McGuirt (1983) reported the finding of *Haemophilus influenzae* in all of eight non-sterile effusions, although only one of these was of the sinister type B.

Clinical features

The development of a subdural empyema is heralded by the development of severe headache, fever and drowsiness, which is followed by the onset of focal neurological symptoms, both irritative as fits, and paralytic. The course is much more rapid than that of a brain abscess. The mortality used to be 100%. Recent reports with the use of modern antibiotics are of rates between 8 and 25% (Shearman, Lees and Taylor, 1987; Bok and Peter, 1993). Drowsiness may develop over a few hours and proceed quickly to coma. Paralysis of one upper or lower limb may rapidly extend to hemiplegia. Hemianopia and hemianaesthesia occur and, if the lesion is on the dominant side, aphasia develops. Epileptic fits of Jacksonian type, starting locally and spreading to affect one side of the body, may precede the weakness. These fits sometimes increase in frequency, and are probably the result of the cortical thrombophlebitis. Papilloedema is uncommon, as are cranial nerve palsies, but they have been described in the fully developed picture. The site of the fits, and the pattern of weakness indicate the position of the empyema.

Diagnosis

Meningism may accompany the headache. The clinical picture can usually be distinguished from that of meningitis by virtue of the characteristic neurological localizing features. The rate of development, over hours rather than days, is much faster than would be expected from a typical brain abscess. In children suspected of having meningitis, subdural empyema should be seriously considered if there is no response to treatment, or if motor seizures occur (Gower and McGuirt, 1983). Nowadays, a definitive diagnosis relies on enhanced CT scanning (Figure 12.8), but pictures may be equivocal or normal and MRI may prove to be more reliable (Feuerman *et al.*, 1989). Lumbar puncture is helpful, but risky. The cerebrospinal fluid pressure is raised, but its sugar content is normal, and cultures are sterile. The fluid may occasionally be turbid if there is marked pleocytosis. If CT scanning is not available, angiography and exploratory burr holes may be needed to clinch the diagnosis.

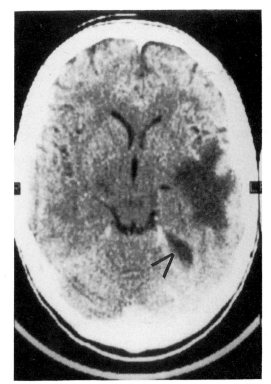

Figure 12.8 CT scan showing subdural abscess in middle fossa

Management

This complication must be managed in close cooperation with a neurosurgeon. Treatment comprises the administration of massive doses of systemic antibiot-

ics, removal of the subdural fluid, and treatment of
the ear disease. The choice of antibiotic will probably
now include intravenous penicillin and chloramphenicol, because of the increasing presence of *Haemophilus
influenzae* in acute infections. The possibility of Gram-
negative organisms from chronic ear disease imposes
a response by the use of aminoglycosides. Acute ear
infection will almost always require myringotomy
and sometimes cortical mastoidectomy, while appropriate surgical treatment to the mastoid will be
needed to treat chronic infection, but not usually
until the patient's general state has been stabilized by
neurosurgical treatment. Traditional neurosurgical
management involves at least one burr hole to sample
the fluid, with several subsequent ones to establish
an irrigation system. In earlier times, when disease
was often more advanced before diagnosis, it was
common practice to advise burr holes on both sides
of the skull, since the abscess can track under the
falx to the opposite hemisphere. An alternative form
of treatment favoured now by many neurosurgeons
is craniotomy and abscess excision (Feuerman *et al.*,
1989). As with other complications the otologist
must depend on local neurosurgical opinion and
practice.

After recovery antiepileptic medication is prescribed to suppress fits, and it may need to be continued for many months after recovery from the acute
complication.

Lateral sinus thrombophlebitis

Thrombophlebitis may develop in any of the veins
adjacent to the middle ear cleft. Of these the lateral
sinus, comprising the sigmoid and transverse sinuses,
is the largest, threatening the greatest risks when it
is filled with suppurating blood clot. The process is
usually, but not always, preceded by the development
of an extradural perisinus abscess (Figure 12.9).
Mural thrombus then partly fills the sinus. Progressive expansion of this clot eventually occludes its
lumen. The clot may become partly organized, and

may be partly broken down and softened by suppuration. From this stage on, the release of infecting
organisms and infected material into the systemic
venous circulation causes bacteraemia, septicaemia,
and septic embolization. Extension or propagation of
the thrombus upwards may reach the confluence of
the sinuses – the torcula Herophili – and even the
superior sagittal sinus beyond. Invasion of the superior or inferior petrosal sinuses may lead the disease
to the cavernous sinus. Venous thrombophlebitis extending into brain substance accounts for the very
high association of this complication with brain abscesses. Downward propagation of thrombus into and
through the internal jugular vein can reach the
subclavian vein (Surkin *et al.*, 1983; Albert and
Williams, 1986).

The patient is then harmed by the release of infective emboli into the circulation, and by the haemodynamic disturbances caused to venous drainage from
inside the cranial cavity.

The use of antibiotics has greatly reduced the
incidence of lateral sinus thrombosis. Formerly, most
instances were associated with acute otitis media in
childhood; now the incidence is much higher in
chronic ear disease (Teichgraber, Per-Lee and Turner,
1982; Ingham *et al.*, 1991), although in one series,
(Gower and McGuirt, 1983), acute infections dominated. The mortality from lateral sinus thrombosis
before the days of operative treatment was 100%.
This fell to 50% in the early 1900s (Gower and
McGuirt, 1983).

Before the use of antibiotics, the commonest infecting organisms were the *β*-haemolytic streptococcus
and *Staphylococcus aureus*, and the former could reliably be cultured from the blood. Its propensity for red
cell destruction caused progressive anaemia, which
was a characteristic feature of the disease in the preantibiotic era. Nowadays, a large variety of mixed
flora may be found. Aural cultures by Venezio and
colleagues (Venezio, Naidich and Shulman, 1982)
grew *Proteus mirabilis*, staphylococci, *Streptococcus
pneumoniae*, and *Bacteroides oralis*, and in only one of
14 cases were blood cultures positive. Southwick

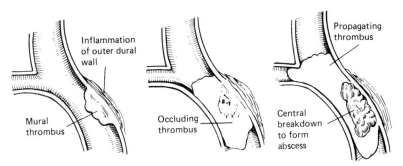

Figure 12.9 Progression of venous sinus thrombophlebitis. (From Ludman, 1988, *Mawson's Diseases of the Ear*, 5th edn,
London: Edward Arnold, by kind permission)

found *Proteus*, staphylococci, and *Escherichia coli* and anaerobic bacteria as principal organisms (Southwick, Richardson and Swartz, 1986). Similar floral diversity, with cultures producing *Bacteroides*, streptococci, enterobacteriaceae and other Gram-negative rods, has been reported (Teichgraber, Per-Lee and Turner, 1982). This last account described many negative cultures.

Clinical features

The classical picture before antibiotic modification is worth recalling. There was a severe pyrexial wasting illness in a patient with middle ear infection. Usually this would develop over several weeks, but occasionally a fulminating infection by virulent organisms arose soon after the onset of an acute otitis media. Fever was high and swinging, following a so-called 'picket-fence' pattern. Rigors, with profuse sweating, occurred as the temperature rose rapidly to 39–40°C and then fell. The shivering during these rigors has been described as so violent as to shake the bed, but few otologists practising today will have seen this phenomenon. Headache and neck pain were the rule. Emaciation was accompanied by progressive anaemia.

Many clinical features depended on the gradual extension of thrombus, effectively limiting the systemic dissemination of infection. As clot extended down the internal jugular vein, it would be accompanied by perivenous inflammation, with tenderness along its course. This tenderness descended the neck with the clot, and might be accompanied by perivenous oedema, or even suppuration in jugular lymph nodes. Perivenous inflammation around the jugular foramen occasionally caused paralysis of the lower three cranial nerves. Raised intracranial pressure produced papilloedema and visual loss. Hydrocephalus could develop if the larger or only lateral sinus was occluded, or if the clot reached the superior sagittal sinus. Extension to the cavernous sinus, along the superior petrosal sinus, presented with chemosis and proptosis of one eye. This could spread to the other eye if the circular sinus became involved.

Embolic propagation of infected clot and organisms produced infiltrates in the lung fields and septic spread to large joints and subcutaneous tissues. Other viscera and the pleuroperitoneal cavity were also targets for embolization. Although these distant effects usually developed late in the course of the disease, they could be presenting features if the insidious nature of the sinus disease had prevented its earlier recognition. Even in the modern era, there are reports of chest disease caused by septic pulmonary emboli from a completely inapparent lateral sinus thrombosis (Hawkins, 1985). This is even more likely to occur nowadays, perhaps because of the 'masking' effects of antibiotics on the primary ear disease.

This masking by antibiotic treatment has muted the more dramatic and often diagnostic clinical character of the disease (Teichgraber, Per-Lee and Turner 1982; O'Connell, 1990).

The clinical picture has so far been described in the past tense, to indicate that the disease has changed, but it is important to remember these dramatic features as they may still be encountered occasionally. What follows is an attempt to describe the clinical pattern more likely to be seen today, in those patients who have been treated with antibiotics before coming to the attention of the otologist.

Patients always feel ill and persisting fever is still usual, but often without the violent swings and rigors of pre-antibiotic times. Otalgia and neck pain with mastoid tenderness and stiffness along the sternomastoid muscle are universal features. These, together with fever, should be recognized nowadays as the most consistent clinical features of lateral sinus thrombosis. Anaemia is now rare. Cases have even been described with no evidence of ear infection (Hawkins, 1985). Papilloedema is still a common finding, as it was when described in 50% of instances by Wolfowitz (1972). The state of mental awareness may be impaired, with drowsiness, lethargy and coma. Other intracranial complications should be expected in nearly 50% of patients with lateral sinus thrombosis. Of these, meningitis and brain abscess are the most common, and their symptoms can so dominate the illness that the lateral sinus thrombosis may be inadvertently overlooked.

Extension of infected clot down the internal jugular vein is always accompanied by tenderness extending along its course in the neck, and localized oedema over the thrombosing internal jugular vein may still be seen.

Very rarely, thrombosis may extend to the subclavian vein (Surkin *et al.*, 1983; Albert and Williams, 1986). In the latter report, engorged collateral veins developed over the shoulder, and intravascular clotting was so extensive that it mopped up platelets and caused thrombocytopenia.

The clinical examination will usually, but not always, indicate middle ear infection. Tenderness over the mastoid process and along the sternomastoid muscle is almost always apparent, and must be regarded seriously as an important sign exciting suspicion of this complication. Examination of the fundi may show papilloedema. A rare finding is pitting oedema over the occipital region, well behind the mastoid process, caused by clotting within a large mastoid emissary vein; this constitutes Griesinger's sign. Physical signs of other associated complications are often present.

There is no single pathognomonic sign of lateral sinus thrombophlebitis. Vigilance, a high level of suspicion, and investigation along the lines suggested below should secure recognition of this dangerous complication.

Investigation

A full blood count may show anaemia with a raised white cell count and raised erythrocyte sedimentation rate, but none of these possible abnormalities is sufficiently specific to be reliable in making or excluding the diagnosis.

Blood cultures, with specimens taken as the temperature rose to its swinging peak, used to be considered a most important diagnostic step, but their value nowadays has become greatly diminished, since bacteraemia with rigors is so much less common, and because of the development of more reliable diagnostic tests.

A lumbar puncture should be performed, if papilloedema does not suggest that raised intracranial pressure might precipitate coning. Examination of the cerebrospinal fluid is the most important way of identifying meningitis. In uncomplicated lateral sinus thrombosis, the white blood count in the cerebrospinal fluid will be low when the cause is chronic middle ear disease, but perhaps somewhat raised in acute otitis media (Gagnon, Sierra-Dupont and Huot, 1976). The cerebrospinal fluid pressure is usually normal. Variations in protein and sugar levels in the cerebrospinal fluid are not sufficiently consistent to be useful.

The Queckenstedt, or Tobey-Ayer test was traditionally recommended whenever a lumbar puncture for possible intracranial infection is indicated and is described here for its historical interest. Queckenstedt (1916) had described the manoeuvre as a means for recognizing spinal cerebrospinal fluid obstruction, but Tobey and Ayer (1925) declared it diagnostic of lateral sinus thrombosis. The test involves measurement of the cerebrospinal fluid pressure and observing its changes on compression of one or both internal jugular veins by fingers on the neck (Figure 12.10). In the normal subject, compression of each internal jugular vein in turn is followed by a rapid rise of cerebrospinal fluid pressure of 50–100 mmHg, above the normal level. There is an equally rapid fall on release of pressure. It is normal for there to be a difference in rise on the two sides, but unusual for it to exceed 50 mmHg. In a typical case of lateral sinus thrombosis, pressure over the vein draining the occluded sinus causes either no rise, or a very slow one of 10–20 mmHg. Compression of the normal internal jugular vein, on the other hand, produces a rapid pressure rise to two or three times the normal level. Unfortunately, the Tobey-Ayer test is of low sensitivity and specificity. There are instances in which it may suggest lateral sinus thrombosis when there is none, and false-negative results with a normal finding in the presence of lateral sinus thrombosis. The false-negative results have been blamed on collateral channels draining the dural venous sinuses (Albert and Williams, 1986). False-positive results appear if a normal lateral sinus is very small or absent, giving an erroneous impression of occlusion by disease.

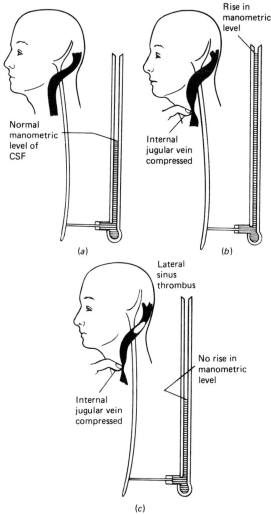

Figure 12.10 The Tobey-Ayer test. (From Ludman, 1988, *Mawson's Diseases of the Ear*, 5th edn, London: Edward Arnold, by kind permission)

Before the advent of CT scanning and angiography, the Tobey-Ayer test, combined with blood cultures, was considered of high diagnostic importance. Now the emphasis has changed.

CT scanning

A CT scan is an essential investigation for any patient with suspected intracranial complications. It may show the increased density of fresh clot (Venezio, Naidich and Shulman, 1982). Filling defects within the sinus can often be exposed with meglumine iothalamate (Conray) enhancement, and failure of opacification may be evident. Septic thrombosis shows as intense inflammatory enhancement of the sinus walls and of the adjacent dura. This enhancement of the

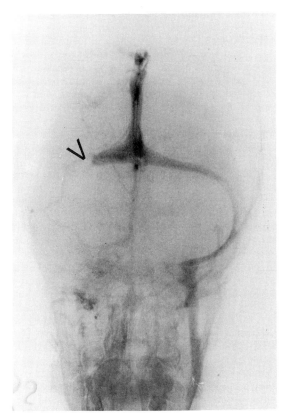

Figure 12.11 Subtraction angiogram showing obstruction of the right transverse sinus

walls, but not of the contents of the sinus constitutes the empty triangle or 'delta' sign (Irving *et al.*, 1991). Other findings, which are non-specific, include cerebral oedema, reduced ventricular size because of oedema, parasagittal haemorrhages, and tentorial enhancement from collateral venous flow. CT scanning is essential also to identify or exclude accompanying complications, such as brain abscess and subdural empyema.

Angiography

Despite the help available from CT scanning and its literally vital role in exposing other complications, the definitive investigations for lateral sinus thrombosis (before operative exposure) involve angiography, to demonstrate the obstruction and its site and extent, and the anatomical arrangement of the individual's venous drainage. There is a possible risk of displacing loose infected thrombus, but the consensus view is that vascular studies should be undertaken whenever a lateral sinus thrombophlebitis is suspected.

Arteriography, with radiopaque dye in the carotid artery can show the venous outflow during the venous phase. The demonstration is made clearer by subtraction angiography. This technique involves precisely registered superimposition of a negative arteriogram on a positive film of the bone structures. The effective cancellation of the skeletal image leaves the vascular pattern clearly exposed (Figure 12.11).

Digital subtraction venography is the preferred vascular imaging technique available at present. The contrast material is administered intravenously, and so without anaesthesia, and without any of the risks of arteriography. The imaging is produced by digital computer techniques. These allow the much diluted agent to be traced even after passing through the heart and onwards into the systemic circulation for a second systemic venous transit.

Magnetic resonance imaging

MRI may be sufficiently suggestive for angiography to be avoided (Figure 12.12). Typically, established thrombus shows increased signal intensity in both T1 and T2-weighted images (Stein, Cunningham and Weber, 1992). MRI can be used to show venous flow, which will be restricted in the presence of thrombus, by using gradient echo images. Special sequences can enhance signal from inflowing venous blood while suppressing signals from stationary tissue (Irving *et al.*, 1991). Gadolinium enhancement may show a 'delta' sign comparable with that seen on CT scans (Irving *et al.*, 1991).

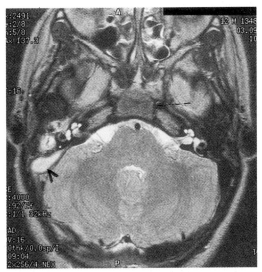

Figure 12.12 T2 weighted axial MRI – patient with right lateral sinus thrombophlebitis. The bright signal on the right side (arrow), represents reduced or absent flow in the sigmoid sinus, to be compared with the black area of the sinus on the other side, where flow is normal. A slightly higher cut showed a similar high signal from the thrombosed transverse sinus. (Reproduced by kind permission of the Editor and Dr M. Charlesworth)

For completeness, radioisotope scanning with gallium should be mentioned. This is a technique that can show the 'hot spots' of sepsis. Radionuclide scanning may show blocked venous flow (Stein, Cunningham and Weber, 1992).

Treatment

Treatment consists of the administration of antibiotics together with exposure of the lateral sinus and incision and removal of its contents.

The principles involved in the choice of an antibiotic for treating any intracranial infection have been discussed in the introductory remarks to this chapter, and those guiding rules should govern the selection of the most appropriate agents for managing a patient with lateral sinus thrombophlebitis. Intravenous administration will generally be recommended. Most patients should receive a combination of two or more of the following: ampicillin, chloramphenicol, a cephalosporin and an aminoglycoside (Teichgraber, Per-Lee and Turner, 1982). Ingham and coworkers (Ingham *et al.*, 1991) considered ampicillin, gentamicin and metronidazole to constitute a sensible regimen.

In the past, anticoagulants were recommended, with prevention of clot propagation to be balanced against the risk of cerebral haemorrhage. Some neurologists still recommend the use of heparin but their reports are influenced by assessment of non-septic thrombosis (Einhaupl *et al.*, 1991). Most writers agree that there is no regular place for anticoagulation except in those very rare instances where spreading thrombus has reached the cavernous sinus (Hawkins, 1985).

Surgical

Of all intracranial complications, lateral sinus thrombophlebitis is the most important for which operation should be undertaken early, in order to expose and treat the infected lesion. The same could be argued for extradural abscess, but this is a much less serious condition, and one often discovered incidentally at the time of operative exploration. This recommendation for early intervention contrasts with the principles governing the otological surgical management of other intracranial complications, which dictate that it is almost always advisable for the complication to be treated, medically or with neurosurgical intervention, first, and for the infecting ear to receive operative attention later, when the patient's condition has greatly improved. Exceptions to this principle, when treating the other complications, usually arise if the ear continues to infect the intracranial contents, preventing the expected improvement in the brain abscess or meningitis. Lateral sinus thrombophlebitis, however, like an extradural abscess, is a localized, often purulent, lesion to which easy access is available only through the mastoid region. Drainage of the infected site requires a mastoidectomy operation.

Before operation intensive medical treatment must be started, and the timing of mastoidectomy should depend to some extent on the response. During this early period under otological care, the temperature chart should be watched every 4 hours, and the central nervous system should be examined once or preferably twice daily. Unless there is a very rapid improvement, and certainly if there is deterioration, mastoid exploration should be carried out within the first 2 days.

If the lateral sinus thrombophlebitis follows acute otitis media and coalescent mastoiditis, cortical mastoidectomy is needed. In chronic otitis media, a radical mastoidectomy is undertaken through a postaural incision. With the temporal bone drill the mastoid is opened and the region of the sinus plate approached. A perisinus abscess may declare itself with an outflow of pus through a tract in necrotic bone over the sinus. That necrotic plate can be separated from the underlying sinus with probes and curettes.

Often, there is no bone necrosis and the sinus plate is firm, healthy and intact. The sinus must then be deliberately uncovered, by drilling the plate, at first with a fast cutting burr, and later, as the soft tissue becomes visible through the thinning bone, with a diamond paste burr. When the bone is tissue-paper thin, it can be lifted off the underlying sinus with flat blunt dissectors. At this stage, the sinus should be fairly widely exposed upwards towards the sinodural angle and downwards towards the jugular bulb. Its appearance determines further action.

The normal healthy sinus is soft, bluish in colour and compressible with a blunt probe. If this is the case, a small needle should be inserted through the wall to seek a free flow of venous blood. This would indicate that the diagnosis of lateral sinus thrombophlebitis was incorrect and, apart from stopping the bleeding by placing a small piece of free muscle tissue on the puncture, no further action is needed. The sinus might feel firm, and appear white and opaque. This would suggest that its lumen was occluded with fibrosing clot or fibrous tissue. In these circumstances it should be opened with a sharp instrument, and the absence of blood or necrotic debris confirmed by inspection. Lund (1978) pointed out that an obliterated cord of scar tissue is sometimes found as testimony to a 'silent' lateral sinus thrombophlebitis. If the sinus wall is covered with granulation tissue or if it is necrotic, the sinus must also be opened and the abscess and necrotic tissue within it removed.

This evacuation must extend in both directions – upwards towards the confluence of the sinuses, and downwards if necessary as far as the jugular bulb. Pus and any unorganized thrombus should be removed. In the past, it was advised that clot removal should be extended in each direction until blood flowed freely from either end of the opened sinus. It is now generally agreed (Teichgraber, Per-Lee and Turner, 1982; Hawkins, 1985) that it is unnecessary to remove organized thrombus, and that it is no longer desirable to follow clot centrally until free blood flow is established. If profuse venous bleeding is encountered, the lumen of the sinus should be obliterated with a ribbon gauze pack, impregnated with an antibacterial agent, inserted between the bone and sinus wall; bismuth iodoform paraffin paste (BIPP) should be avoided since it is radiopaque.

Whenever a cortical mastoidectomy is performed for coalescent mastoiditis, even if intracranial complications are not suspected, the sigmoid sinus should be exposed and needled. This is a routine measure to avoid missing an unsuspected lateral sinus thrombophlebitis. The same investigation of the sinus is not recommended during radical mastoidectomy for chronic ear disease, unless the operation is being conducted during the management of an intracranial complication.

Internal jugular vein ligation used to be considered important to prevent dissemination of infected clot. The consensus view, as summarized by Teichgraber, which is still valid (Teichgraber, Per-Lee and Turner, 1982), is that ligation should be reserved for the very rare cases in which septicaemia does not respond to initial antibiotic treatment and surgery and that it should be considered for children showing signs of embolization.

Meningitis (leptomeningitis)

This is a major and serious complication of middle ear infection, and probably still the commonest intra-cranial complication (Maksimovic and Rukovanjski, 1993). Before the days of antibiotics most sufferers died. Nowadays, recovery is usual provided that recognition is prompt, and treatment expeditious. The patients at greatest risk are those with other complications, which may be overlooked because of the severe symptoms of the meningitis. As with all other otogenic complications, the incidence, particularly that from acute otitis media, has fallen greatly with the use of antibiotics. Although most reports indicate that it is more frequently now a complication of chronic ear disease, childhood otogenic meningitis is seen most often as a complication of acute middle ear infection (Gower and McGuirt, 1983). In adults, it is now more commonly a complication of chronic disease.

Although spread may be through any of the channels previously described, such as preformed pathways, otogenic meningitis usually arises by direct spread through necrosing bone from the middle ear cleft (Figure 12.13). The rate of development depends on factors discussed in the introduction to this chapter, and particularly on the virulence of the organism, the resistance of the host, and the development of preformed access by bone erosion. Suppurative labyrinthitis, described later, offers access to the cerebrospinal spaces through the internal auditory meatus and through the vestibular and cochlear aqueducts. Rarely, rupture of an established brain abscess into the subarachnoid space may lead to meningitis. At its most virulent meningitis can develop within hours of the onset of acute suppurative otitis media.

The organisms usually responsible for acute infection are *Haemophilus influenzae* especially type B, and *Streptococcus pneumoniae*, of which type III has a vicious reputation for causing rapid complications.

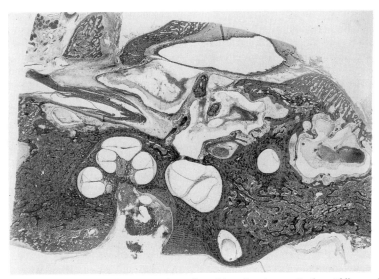

Figure 12.13 Otogenic meningitis: midmidiolar section through cochlea, showing pus in the middle ear cleft and in the internal auditory meatus (courtesy H. F. Schuknecht, MEEI collection)

Infection from chronic ear diseases may be caused by any of the organisms normally found in those conditions (Lampe and Edwards, 1984), including Gram-negative enteric organisms, *Proteus*, and *Pseudomonas*. Anaerobes such as *Bacteroides* species have also been reported (Siegler, Faiers and Willis, 1982).

The initial inflammatory response of the pia-arachnoid to infection is an outpouring of fluid into the subarachnoid space, with a rise in cerebrospinal fluid pressure. This fluid soon becomes permeated with white blood cells, and then with rapidly multiplying bacteria. The organisms feed on glucose, and thereby reduce its level in the cerebrospinal fluid, producing the characteristic biochemical feature of pyogenic meningitis. Once purulent, a sticky exudate is formed. This accumulates at first in the basal cisterns, and more rarely at the vertex. Free flow of cerebrospinal fluid is impeded by exudate obstructing the ventricular foramina to cause a non-communicating hydrocephalus. Obstruction to cerebrospinal fluid flow in the subarachnoid spaces may cause communicating hydrocephalus. Irritation of upper cervical nerve roots by inflammatory exudate is the basis for the classical features of this condition – neck pain and neck stiffness. Exudate collecting around exit foramina of cranial nerves can cause palsies in the late stages of the disease. Spread of infection along the Virchow-Robin spaces into the brain substance sometimes leads to brain abscesses, while accumulations of the exudate in loculated masses on the cerebral surface are no different from those found in subdural empyema, which has been discussed under that heading.

Clinical features

The two most constant and reliable early clinical features are headache and neck stiffness. At first the headache may be localized to the side of the infected ear, but soon becomes generalized and 'bursting'. There is malaise and pyrexia, often to 39°C. Initial neck stiffness shows as resistance to flexion; later, rigidity or retraction develop. Mental hyperactivity usually colours this early stage with restlessness and fretfulness in children. Anxiety, punctuated by periods of drowsiness is usual in adults. At this stage, the tendon reflexes may be exaggerated. Photophobia is a constant characteristic symptom and, before neck stiffness is marked, the patient may lie curled up away from the light. Vomiting, caused by raised intracranial pressure is also a feature.

As the condition proceeds, all these symptoms become more severe. The headache may be excruciating, and neck rigidity is marked, with a positive Kernig's sign, retraction and, later on, opisthotonus. The temperature remains uniformly raised with none of the swinging pattern which used to characterize lateral sinus thrombosis. Gradually, the tendon re-

flexes become less marked, and the abdominal reflexes may be lost.

Deterioration is marked by alternating delirium and stupor, passing finally into coma. The tendon reflexes disappear, and cranial nerve palsies develop. Eventually Cheyne-Stokes respiration follows, with fixed dilated pupils, then coma and death.

Any focal neurological signs, especially in the early stages, should raise suspicion of a subdural or cerebral abscess. Similarly epileptic fits do not occur with otherwise uncomplicated meningitis. The neck stiffness, which is so typical of the disease may be delayed for several days from the onset, especially if the first accumulation of exudate is vertical, rather than in the basal cisterns.

Diagnosis

The diagnosis is made by examination of cerebrospinal fluid. Any patient with middle ear infection, headache and neck stiffness must undergo a lumbar puncture. At the same time, suspicion of other complications must always be entertained, and possible brain abscesses and subdural empyemas need to be excluded, preferably by CT scanning. In the earliest stages of otogenic meningitis the only abnormality on lumbar puncture is a rise in fluid pressure above the normal 100–150 mmHg. As the infection proceeds white cells accumulate in the cerebrospinal fluid, and the fluid becomes cloudy and then turbid in appearance. On histological inspection, most of these cells will be found to be polymorphonuclear leucocytes, which are not normally present in cerebrospinal fluid. They increase in number to reach the range of $0.1–10 \times 10^9/l$ (100–10 000/mm^3), although with *Staphylococcus epidermidis*, counts below $0.1 \times 10^9/l$ may be met. As the inflamed blood–brain barrier allows free passage into the cerebrospinal fluid, its constitution approximates more closely to that of serum, and this can be demonstrated by biochemical tests. Thus the protein content may rise from a normal 150–400 mg/l to a raised level of 2–3 g/l. The chloride content may fall from the normal 120 mmol/l to 80 mmol/l. The appearance of bacteria in the cerebrospinal fluid is accompanied by a fall of cerebrospinal fluid glucose levels from the normal value of 1.7–3.0 mmol/l to zero. Bacteriological examination of cerebrospinal fluid is first undertaken by direct examination after Gram staining, and then by culture of the fluid. Despite positive diagnostic findings on cellular and biochemical testing, positive bacteriological diagnosis is by no means the rule, and so treatment cannot wait for, nor depend upon, it. The lumbar puncture findings are decisive when no mass shows on CT scanning, even without bacteriological identification. There is no other complication in which the cerebrospinal fluid sugar level is lowered, and few in which the white cell count is so high. A brain abscess, if leaking into the subarachnoid space may cause a huge rise of cerebrospinal fluid white cell count even to more than $50 \times 10^9/l$, ($50\,000/mm^3$), and a subdural abscess to counts over $0.1 \times 10^9/l$. In both of these the cerebrospinal fluid pressure may be raised, but in neither is the cerebrospinal fluid sugar level reduced. In the presence of cerebrospinal fluid pleocytosis, CT scanning should exclude either form of abscess, leaving a diagnosis of meningitis unchallenged.

MRI may show typical signal changes in meningitis, although a CT scan will be normal. Exudate and adhesions in the basal cisterns produce a high signal intensity on T2-weighted images and abnormal enhancement with gadolinium (Ingham *et al.*, 1991).

Recently polymerase chain reactions (PCR) have been used to detect bacterial DNA in apparently sterile CSF (Kristiansen *et al.*, 1991) and similar techniques may become more widely used in future.

Treatment

Surgical

As with most other complications, treatment of the intracranial sepsis should take precedence over management of the otitis media. Medical treatment of the meningitis is of paramount importance, and any operation for the ear condition should, if possible, be deferred for several days until the patient's general condition has improved. Years ago, before antibiotics offered hope of cure, appropriate ear surgery was undertaken as soon as the diagnosis had been made. Nowadays, urgent surgical intervention should be advised only if the expected response to treatment does not appear. Certainly deterioration or failure of response over 48 hours implies loculated infection in the mastoid, needing surgical drainage. In acute otitis media, early middle ear drainage is advised, with myringotomy, either repeatedly, or possibly assisted by insertion of a ventilation tube (Gower and McGuirt, 1983). Coalescent mastoiditis is an indication for cortical mastoidectomy but in many, if not most, instances, cure of the meningitis by antibiotics eliminates the preceding acute infection. As with other complications, chronic middle ear disease needs eradication by some form of radical mastoidectomy, but again that should be deferred if possible until the dangerous meningitis is under control.

Medical

The lumbar puncture used for diagnosis may be repeated several times to reduce intracranial pressure, possibly a second time in the first 24 hours, and then daily until improvement is assured. Subsequent punctures are needed to check the state of the patient, and discharge from hospital must not be considered until the cerebrospinal fluid characteristics have returned to normal. Differential white cell counts are needed, since improvement may be indicated by a change from polymorphs to macrophages, even though the total count persists at, say, the $0.2 \times 10^9/l$ level. In earlier days, the initial and subsequent lumbar punctures were used to instil intrathecal antibiotics, and in particular pure crystalline penicillin in a dose not exceeding $5000–10\,000$ units in 5 ml of normal saline. Intrathecal antibiotics pose a risk of epilepsy, and their use now has largely been abandoned.

The mainstay of medical treatment rests with large doses of systemic antibiotics. A few years ago a standard choice was intramuscular penicillin, intrathecal penicillin, and sulphadiazine (which, of all sulphonamides, most readily crosses the blood-brain barrier). Streptomycin might have been recommended as an occasional adjunct because of its efficacy against *Haemophilus influenzae*. Today, as has been discussed in the introduction to this chapter, it is more difficult to be dogmatic. Because of its frequent role as a causative agent, *Haemophilus influenzae* must be a target of any regimen, and since more and more strains are becoming resistant to ampicillin, chloramphenicol is considered the first choice (Pecoul *et al.*, 1991), combined with ampicillin or penicillin. The risk of toxic effects from chloramphenicol must be minimized by regular blood cell counts.

Rifampicin has recently been shown to an effective agent against *Haemophilus influenzae* type B that has previously not responded to chloramphenicol (Lewis and Priestley, 1986). This drug has the unique ability to penetrate pus and kill phagocytosed organisms – even after oral administration.

Agents likely to be effective against Gram-negative organisms must also be considered when the infection is secondary to chronic middle ear disease. In these categories are azlocillin, ticarcillin, and some newer cephalosporins such as ceftazidime. All are less toxic than aminoglycosides like gentamicin. Whichever combination is selected, the preferred route is intravenous. Systemic therapy must be continued for at least 10 days after apparent clinical recovery. If *Bacteroides* are found on anaerobic culture, metronidazole should be administered in a dose of 400 mg 8-hourly (Siegler, Faiers and Willis, 1982).

Dexamethasone is nowadays considered to be useful adjunctive therapy in the treatment of bacterial meningitis (Lebel *et al.*, 1989). There is also evidence for reduction of neurological sequelae, and in particular of bilateral hearing loss (Geiman and Smith, 1992).

Failure of an adequate response to antimicrobial therapy may be the result of:

1 Organisms resistant to the chosen antibiotics: a change should be planned, guided as far as possible by bacteriological data
2 Persisting leakage of infected material into the

cerebrospinal fluid: urgent surgical treatment of the ear must then be considered
3 Presence of a previously unidentified other complication: CT scanning will be needed urgently for its recognition
4 Leakage into the cerebrospinal fluid from an unrecognized brain abscess.

Brain abscess

Otogenic brain abscesses almost always develop in the temporal lobe (Figure 12.14) or the cerebellum (Figure 12.15) of the same side as the infected ear from which they arise. They are found in the temporal lobe approximately twice as often as in the cerebellum. In children, 25% of all brain abscesses are otogenic, while in the adult, with a greater predominance of chronic ear disease, the proportion of brain abscesses caused by ear infection is greater than 50%. In one recent series, 73% of intracranial abscesses were caused by chronic middle ear disease (Kulai, Ozatik and Topçu, 1990). Of the various routes of spread previously described, the commonest responsible for brain abscess is by direct extension of infection through an osteitic tegmen tympani, with formation of a middle fossa extradural abscess. Although the dura is very resistant to infective invasion, a local pachymeningitis may be followed by thrombophlebitis penetrating the cerebral cortex of the temporal lobe, or by extension of infection along periarteriolar Virchow-Robin spaces into the cerebral white matter. Cerebellar abscesses are frequently preceded by lateral sinus thrombophlebitis. They usually lie within the lateral lobe of the cerebellum, which may be adherent to the lateral sinus or to a patch of dura underneath Trautmann's triangle. That intracranial complications are often multiple is explained by this pattern of progressive involvement.

Formation of an abscess starts with an area of cerebral oedema and encephalitis. Rarely, this oedema is poorly contained and proceeds to massive cerebral oedema with spreading encephalitis. More often the development and extension of the abscess is contained by the formation of a capsule. This fibrous tissue restriction depends on a microglial and blood vessel mesodermal response to the inflammatory process, and is variable in its rate of development. In general, capsular formation takes 2–3 weeks and, while it proceeds, the central part of the affected brain liquefies. After these stages of initial encephalitis and abscess localization, there may be a period of abscess enlargement, as renewed or continuing infection increases the volume of contained pus. Now, the features of a space-occupying lesion dominate, with rising intracranial pressure and focal neurological damage. Abscesses in the posterior fossa – in the cerebellum – cause raised intracranial pressure earlier than those above the tentorium, and rapidly rising

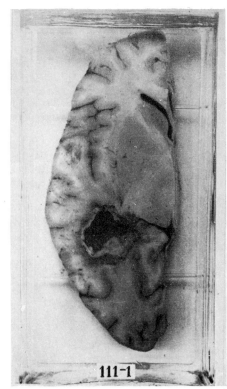

Figure 12.14 Acute temporal lobe abscess showing a poorly developed capsule and surrounded by marked hyperaemia

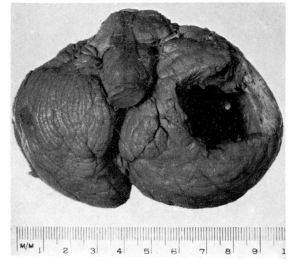

Figure 12.15 Large cerebellar abscess with marked thinning of the cerebellar cortex

intracranial pressure may cause 'coning' or impaction of the flocculus and brain stem into the foramen magnum, followed by fatal disruption of vital centres in the brain stem. If capsular development is slow, softening of brain around the developing abscess may allow further spread of infection into the relatively avascular white matter, with the formation of secondary abscesses, separate from the original or connected by a narrow stalk. In this way a multilocular abscess is formed. Eventually, an abscess may rupture into the ventricular system or subarachnoid space, with overwhelming meningitis and death.

Like other complications the incidence of otogenic brain abscess has fallen. The mortality rate was 60–70% before the days of antibiotics, and had declined to 40% by the 1960s (British Medical Journal, 1977). A report by Fischer, McLennan and Suzuki (1981) of their experiences during the 1970s described a mortality of 14% and this is a typical figure in recently reported series. Taylor (1987) achieved a figure of 6% in 50 patients. This gradual decline in mortality can be attributed to the introduction of broad-spectrum antibiotics, but more to the recognition of the role of anaerobic organisms. The earlier diagnosis by CT scanning, and the use of steroids to control cerebral oedema, are other propitious factors.

Bacteriology

The bacterial flora is usually a complex mixture of aerobes and obligate anaerobes. Anaerobic streptococci are the commonest organisms (Maurice-Williams, 1983). Pyogenic staphylococci are also common, especially in children, and *Streptococcus pneumoniae* and *Strep. haemolyticus* are often found. Gram-negative bacilli – *Proteus mirabilis*, *Escherichia coli* and *Pseudomonas aeruginosa* – are cultured with increasing frequency. This may reflect the higher incidence of otogenic abscesses from chronic ear disease, or the fact that the Gram-positive organisms are so often sensitive to, and therefore eradicated by, the most commonly prescribed systemic antibiotics. Indeed there are reports of brain abscesses with intact tympanic membranes where an acute infection has presumably been treated effectively with antibiotics (Samuel and Fernandez, 1985). The recognition of obligate anaerobes, first suggested as infecting agents by McFarlan (1943) has shown that many supposedly sterile abscesses are infected by organisms of the *Bacteroides* genus, especially *B. fragilis*, an organism that produces a highly active β-lactamase (British Medical Journal, 1977; Ingham, Selkon and Roxby, 1977).

Clinical features

The earliest stage of 'encephalitis', when brain tissue is invaded, causes headache, fever, malaise and vomiting, followed by drowsiness. The symptoms may be slight, and are easily masked by those of an acute otitis media, but drowsiness should always provoke suspicion. These early features may be hidden completely by a dramatic complication such as meningitis, or even by lateral sinus thrombophlebitis. The cerebral disturbance is sometimes so slight as to be ignored, and in chronic otitis media, headache must be considered the most important symptom. Persistent headache with chronic middle ear infection suggests intracranial spread and, although it may be caused by a much less sinister cause such as an extradural abscess, the possibility of local encephalitis must be entertained.

If this phase of localized encephalitis progresses rapidly to a generalized form before containment by encapsulation, drowsiness may progress to stupor and then coma and death from tentorial herniation. More often, the period of local encephalitis is followed by a 'latent period' during which the pus becomes contained within a developing fibrous capsule. Throughout this stage, which may last from 10 days to several weeks, there are no symptoms, and the preceding encephalitic illness may be forgotten, if indeed it ever attracted the patient's attention.

The next stage of an enlarging abscess causes clinical events, first as a result of changes in cerebrospinal fluid dynamics, common to abscesses in any part of the brain, and secondly as site-specific features from focal neurological impairment. Naturally, the neurological effects of damage to the temporal lobe are different from those in the cerebellum.

Abscesses are surrounded by an area of cerebral oedema and low grade encephalitis, and this fluctuates in size with variation in the severity of the symptoms. There is malaise and anorexia, weakness and lethargy. With rising intracranial pressure the pulse rate slows and the temperature may fall to subnormal levels. Constant headache is usual, and vomiting of cerebral type occurs in many patients. The drowsiness varies and may alternate with irritability. Thought processes may become slow. Papilloedema is often found, but only if cerebrospinal fluid pressure remains raised for 2 or 3 weeks. As explained before, papilloedema appears earlier with an abscess in the cerebellum than in the temporal lobe. A long-standing abscess is often associated with emaciation. If intracranial pressure continues to rise, the patient eventually lapses into coma, the ipsilateral pupil dilates, and finally both become fixed and dilated. Death eventually supervenes, either from the effects of raised intracranial pressure, or from overwhelming meningitis following intraventricular rupture of the abscess contents.

These phenomena are common to all abscesses, and during their development specific neurological signs must be sought to try to localize the site of the space-occupying lesion.

Cerebral-temporosphenoidal abscesses

A cerebral abscess in the dominant (usually left) hemisphere often causes so-called 'nominal aphasia'.

The patient cannot name a common everyday object such as a key, a pen or a screwdriver, but he or she is able to demonstrate its use correctly. Visual field defects arise from involvement of the optic radiations. Most commonly there is a quadrantic homonymous hemianopia, affecting the upper part of the temporal visual fields, or much more rarely the lower quadrants (Figure 12.16). The fields lost are on the side opposite to that of the lesion, because of damage to fibres arising from both retinae of the same side. Although best examined by formal perimetry, the patient's state of consciousness may prevent adequate cooperation. Simple clinical testing by confrontation can then be useful. Motor paralysis develops as the abscess enlarges. Upward development affects facial movement on the opposite side, and then, progressively, paralysis of the upper and lower limb (Figure 12.17). Inward expansion affects first the leg, then the arm, and finally the face.

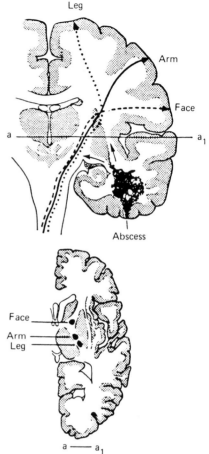

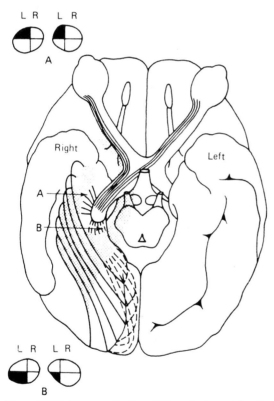

Figure 12.16 Diagram of optic radiations. Lesions at A or B produce field defects shown in the insets. (Note, the brain is viewed from below and the lesion is on the right side)

Figure 12.17 Diagram illustrating sequence of paralysis caused by an abscess in the temporosphenoidal lobe. When the abscess extends superficially the face is first affected, then the arm and the leg, but if the abscess spreads inwards towards the posterior part of the internal capsule the order of paralysis is reversed, the leg is affected first, then the arm and lastly the face

Cerebellar abscesses

The focal signs of cerebellar involvement include weakness and muscle incoordination on the same side as the lesion. Ataxia causes a tendency to fall to the side of the lesion. Clinical tests for cerebellar defects reveal ipsilateral ataxia, with a tendency to past-pointing when attempting to touch a target with a finger. The finger-nose test exposes intention tremor and past-pointing, and dysdiadochokinesis is demonstrated by attempts at rapid alternating supination and pronation of forearm, and by difficulty in rapidly touching each finger to the thumb tip. Spontaneous nystagmus may be present; this is coarse and irregular, but very variable in its appearance. Generally, it beats to the side of the lesion, which contrasts with the paralytic jerk nystagmus of suppurative labyrinthitis. As mentioned previously, intracranial pressure rises early and rapidly with a cerebellar abscess, and the effects of this rising pressure may dominate the clinical pattern before focal signs can be recognized clinically.

Investigations

The investigations and management of brain abscess require a team approach, and at the earliest stage of clinical suspicion, advice should be sought from neurosurgical colleagues in order to plan the most expedient way of investigating the possible complication, and of treating both it and the underlying ear disease.

Radiological

CT scanning with and without intravenous meglumine iothalamate (Conray) enhancement is without question the most important investigation in the diagnosis of brain abscess (Figure 12.18). Not only can the position and size of the abscess be identified, but the appearances of localized encephalitis can be distinguished from those of an encapsulated abscess. A CT scan will also help to identify associated complications such as subdural abscesses, and lateral sinus thrombophlebitis. Scanning is also the most valuable method for observing the progress of an abscess during treatment.

The increasing role of MRI for the diagnosis of intracranial masses has been reviewed recently (Haimes *et al.*, 1989). Unenhanced appearances are characteristic and it is possible to distinguish between pus, abscess capsule, oedema and normal brain (see Figure 12.3). Spread to ventricles and subarachnoid spaces is more obvious on MRI than CT scanning.

Before CT scanning became available, supratentorial masses were best demonstrated by carotid arteriography. Upward and medial displacement of the middle cerebral artery was seen as an indication of a temporal lobe mass. Plain X-rays of the skull are of virtually no value – they may show displacement of a calcified pineal gland but little else. Ventriculography was necessary in the past to demonstrate posterior fossa masses. Electroencephalography is now of historical interest only.

Lumbar puncture

Great care is needed when cerebrospinal fluid is removed in the presence of raised intracranial pressure, because there is a risk of coning. If a patient is stuporose, has violent headache, or papilloedema, sampling should be performed only in a neurosurgical unit with immediate availability for intervention. Before this terminal phase of brain abscess development, lumbar puncture is valuable, particularly to exclude meningitis, for which it is the definitive investigation. A lumbar puncture in a patient with a brain abscess may show some rise of cerebrospinal fluid pressure, with raised protein content. A rise in white cell count, if any, is much less than that expected in meningitis, except when an abscess is leaking into the cerebrospinal fluid, and then very high cell counts can be expected. The glucose content of the cerebrospinal fluid remains at a normal level.

Burr hole needling

The definitive diagnosis used to be established by needling the brain through a burr hole and finding pus. This is a neurosurgical manoeuvre, for consideration by neurosurgical colleagues. With modern CT scanning, it is no longer necessary.

Differential diagnosis

A brain abscess must be suspected during the course of any other intracranial complication. The conditions to be differentiated include meningitis, subdural abscess, lateral sinus thrombophlebitis, otitic hydrocephalus, and other masses such as brain tumours.

In meningitis, there is high sustained fever and neck stiffness, and the cerebrospinal fluid findings are abnormal and diagnostically typical. A subdural abscess is suggested by much more rapid evolution of focal neurological signs. Lateral sinus thrombophlebitis is often a precursor of cerebellar abscess, and an abscess is a possibility even when most features are typical of a thrombosed sinus. Otitic hydrocephalus is easily distinguishable by the absence of focal neurological signs, the CT scan findings, and the cerebro-

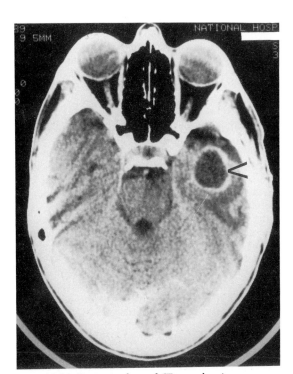

Figure 12.18 Contrast enhanced CT scan showing encapsulated lobe abscess

spinal fluid findings on lumbar puncture. Finally, evidence of a space-occupying lesion in a patient with middle ear disease requires exclusion of a coincidental brain tumour. The CT scan appearance, especially with reconstruction in different planes, available on the most advanced scanners, usually makes the distinction, and MRI is likely to offer diagnostic differentiation. If not, neurosurgical exploration may be necessary.

Treatment

Historically several phases have been recognized in the management of otogenic brain abscesses (Brand, Caparosa and Lubic, 1984). Until this century, most patients died when all that was available was craniotomy. During the next phase, in the early part of the 20th century, intracranial pus was evacuated during the mastoidectomy operation, by opening the dura and needling the brain along the tract established by the inward extension of the infection. There must now rarely, if ever, be a place for that form of management. Today, the treatment of the abscess involves the use of large doses of systemic antibiotics, combined with a surgical approach to the abscess through a clean field. Treatment of the ear disease must take second place, in accordance with the principles discussed previously. Ideally, the abscess should be completely controlled neurosurgically and with antibiotics, and predisposing chronic ear disease dealt with by radical mastoidectomy 10–14 days later. As is the case with most of the other intracranial complications discussed, acute ear infections may well resolve with the antibiotics used for the abscess treatment, and only rarely will myringotomy or cortical mastoidectomy be needed.

The first step must be urgent consultation with neurosurgical colleagues. If raised intracranial pressure has caused coma or rapid deterioration, it may be lowered temporarily by the administration of dexamethasone, 4 mg intravenously every 6 hours, or intravenous 20% mannitol, in a dose of 0.5 g/kg. This can be a life-saving measure until neurosurgical help is available. Corticosteroids may also be used after surgical treatment of an abscess if cerebral oedema persists. The administration of steroids to patients with brain abscesses does not have adverse effects (Chun *et al.*, 1986; Ingham *et al.*, 1991). Antibiotics must be given intravenously in large doses. For reasons already discussed, the initial choice should include chloramphenicol, which is effective against *Haemophilus* and many enterococci, and which passes readily into the cerebrospinal fluid in high doses (Brand, Caparosa and Lubic, 1984). This is combined with a penicillin, often chosen from those active against β-lactamase-producing organisms. Both chloramphenicol and penicillin penetrate the capsule in effective concentrations. If *Pseudomonas*

or *Proteus* species are suspected, because of a primary source in a chronically infected mastoid, an aminoglycoside will probably be added. Metronidazole should be administered from the start, in view of the strong likelihood of *Bacteroides* infections. This drug, too, penetrates abscess capsules and high concentrations have been found in the pus within abscesses after administration in doses of 400–600 mg 8-hourly (Ingham, Selkon and Roxby, 1977). A soundly based cocktail of gentamicin, metronidazole and ampicillin can be recommended (Ingham *et al.*, 1991). Antibiotics should be administered for at least 3 or 4 weeks, with careful regard to their various potential toxic effects.

Surgical

The current neurosurgical options are to drain the abscess repeatedly through burr holes, or to excise it completely with its capsule. Opinion is divided on the choice of technique (Maurice-Williams, 1983). Repeated needle aspiration involves a smaller operation than excision and, since it can be performed under local anaesthetic, it is safer for very ill patients. There are, however, several disadvantages. It may do little to reduce the mass effects of the abscess, especially if the pus is thick. Forty per cent of abscesses are multilocular (Stephanor, 1978) and total removal of pus is not always possible by aspiration. Aspiration involves repeated procedures, and as the capsule collapses, it thickens so that there is a risk of the cannula glancing off to damage adjacent white matter. If the abscess does not collapse, excision may eventually be necessary after all. There is also a risk of late recurrence, which may be as high as 8 per cent.

Aspiration offers access to the pus for bacteriological examination. In order to identify obligatory anaerobes, such as *Bacteroides fragilis*, which has increasingly been shown to cause apparently 'sterile' abscesses, cultures must be set up rapidly (within an hour) in a low oxygen tension medium, and preferably one containing nalidixic acid to inhibit the growth of Gram-negative organisms. With each aspiration antibiotics can be instilled into the cavity of the abscess. Before the advent of CT scanning, it was also usual to put 2 ml of thorotrast into the abscess on the first aspiration. This radiopaque agent is taken up by the fibrous wall of the abscess capsule, and allowed subsequent changes in the lesion to be watched by straight X-ray examinations.

Some workers now consider that aspiration of pus under CT stereotactic control to be the treatment of choice (Stapleton, Bell and Uttley, 1993).

Primary excision is favoured by other neurosurgeons. It offers a means of decompressing the brain immediately. Its main disadvantage is that the operation can cause extensive damage to cerebral tissue, especially if the abscess is multiloculated with tentacular extensions. Excision is then possibly associated with a higher incidence of residual neurological deficit. It is a more major operation than repeated aspiration, and one demanding a higher level of neurosurgical skill to minimize brain damage, and to avoid rupture into the ventricle. Despite excellent survival results from excision (Taylor, 1987) there is nonetheless a strongly supported view that surgical removal is only rarely indicated (Bidzinski and Koszewski, 1990).

Although the otologist will be interested in arguments about the relative merits of aspiration and excision, the plan for abscess management must be a neurosurgical one, and it will be determined by the preferences and facilities of the neurosurgical colleague cooperating in the patient's care.

After successful treatment of a temporal lobe abscess, there is a high risk of epileptic seizures. If followed up for long enough, 70% of patients will have a fit, so anticonvulsant medication is needed, and should be continued indefinitely.

Otitic hydrocephalus (benign intracranial hypertension)

This is the rarest complication of middle ear infection. First described over 60 years ago (Symonds, 1931), it is a misnomer; it is a syndrome of raised intracranial pressure during or following middle ear infection. The most frequent victims are children and adolescents. In a review of 60 patients with benign intracranial hypertension, Foley (1955) uncovered a history of preceding acute otitis media in thirteen. 'Pseudotumor cerebri' occasionally appears in the literature as an unhelpful synonym for the condition.

Pathogenesis

The aetiology is unknown, but most accounts recognize a relationship with lateral sinus thrombosis (Isaacman, 1989). The inference is either that obstruction of the lateral sinus affects cerebral venous outflow, or that extension of thrombus to the superior sagittal sinus impedes cerebrospinal fluid resorption by Pacchionian bodies (Pfaltz and Griesemer, 1984). However, it has been argued that superior sagittal sinus thrombosis should be associated with more neurological deficits than are found in otitic hydrocephalus. Seid and Sellars (1973) found only one case among 13 with sinus thrombosis and, indeed, ligation of the internal jugular vein in the neck does not cause hydrocephalus; so that mechanism must also be suspect. Gower and McGuirt (1983) considered that otitic hydrocephalus should be accepted as an idiopathic benign intracranial hypertension associated with ear disease, and argued that raised intracranial pressure following lateral sinus thrombosis is a different entity. Any attempt to make this distinction is probably unhelpful since most writers accept that the syndrome to which the name of otitic hydrocephalus is properly attached most often follows lateral sinus thrombosis. Thus, Foley with a large series of 44 cases, described lateral sinus disease in 27 out of 34 cases explored surgically (Foley, 1955); Wright and Grimaldi (1973) described three cases, all with lateral sinus thrombosis. Lenz and McDonald (1984) reviewed the literature to disclose 10 patients of whom only one, with bilateral ear disease, had normal lateral sinuses. Some of the problems in explaining pathophysiology may depend on variations in venous arrangement in the skull. Clemis and Jerva (1976) described the venous patterns, showing that there is a right predominance in 35% of subjects and a left predominance in 13%; 24% show disproportion, while there is poor cross circulation at the confluence of the sinuses in just over 10%, and an absent sinus in 4 per cent. Foley's series indicated more cases with right-sided ear disease, and a higher incidence of sinus thrombosis in right than in left-sided cases (Foley, 1955). These lateralizing relationships were also evident in the rather smaller review by Lenz and McDonald (1984).

Clinical features

The leading symptoms are headache, drowsiness, blurred vision, nausea and vomiting, and sometimes diplopia. The onset may be many weeks after an acute otitis media, or many years after the start of chronic middle ear disease. Clinical examination reveals papilloedema and drowsiness. Lateral rectus palsy due to VIth cranial nerve stretching (a false localizing sign in raised intracranial pressure) may be found on one or both sides. These signs are associated with evidence of acute or chronic middle ear infection, or with a history of acute or chronic middle ear infection, or with a history of a recent acute middle ear infection since recovered.

The differential diagnosis includes any other cause for raised intracranial pressure, and in particular a brain abscess. Investigations to exclude that possibility should include CT scanning, which will show normal ventricles.

Treatment

The ear disease, if acute, may have recovered. Persisting middle ear infection has to be treated on its own merits. Management of the complication entails reduction of the raised intracranial pressure in order to prevent visual impairment by papilloedema. Treatment includes the use of steroids, diuretics, and hyperosmolar dehydrating agents. Repeated lumbar puncture has been advocated, but this is not free from risk in the presence of raised intracranial pressure. Long-term thecoperitoneal shunting may occasionally be needed.

Prognosis

The outlook for survival is good, but treatment may be needed over many weeks or even months. Permanent deficits such as visual impairment are uncommon (Pennybacker, 1961), but recurrences have been reported, albeit rarely (Johnston and Paterson, 1974).

Facial paralysis

The management of the paralysed facial nerve is discussed fully in Chapter 24. Here, mention will be made of aspects of facial palsy only as a complication of middle ear infection.

Acute otitis media

Facial palsy occurs in acute otitis media in that small proportion of patients (less than 10%) with a congenital dehiscence of the thin bony wall normally separating the horizontal part of the facial nerve canal from the middle ear mucosa. Infection of the mucosa may cause an inflammatory reaction in the subjacent epineurium and perineurial spaces. The diagnosis is usually straightforward, but the Ramsay Hunt syndrome (see Chapter 24) can cause confusion, since the pain and facial palsy of that condition is sometimes associated with blistering of the surface of the tympanic membrane, which may be mistaken for evidence of acute otitis media.

Treatment

The affection of the nerve is invariably a neuropraxia, and full recovery of facial muscle function is to be expected after recovery from the preceding infection. This can usually be achieved by appropriate systemic antibiotic treatment, but occasionally myringotomy or, more rarely, cortical mastoidectomy could be needed. Operative decompression of the facial nerve is unnecessary (Alford and Cohn, 1980).

Chronic otitis media

In chronic destructive middle ear disease, the facial nerve trunk may be exposed if its bony covering is eroded by cholesteatoma, or by granulation tissue and osteitic disease in ears without cholesteatoma (Djeric and Savic, 1989; Harker and Pignatari, 1992). Pressure by a cholesteatoma sac may also be a factor, since uninfected congenital cholesteatoma of the petrous apex invariably presents with a slowly progressive facial paralysis. Almost always the tym-panic portion of the nerve, on the medial wall of the middle ear, is affected (Savic and Djeric, 1989).

Diagnosis

Facial paralysis of slow onset must always suggest erosive disease in the temporal bone. An association with aural discharge should raise the possibility of chronic middle ear infection, although a similar clinical story may be caused by neoplasms, such as carcinoma of the middle ear. Pain is usually a feature of that disease, but it is not a symptom of otherwise uncomplicated cholesteatoma. Absence of discharge does not exclude the possibility of cholesteatoma; meticulous examination of the tympanic membrane, preferably under the binocular operating microscope, is essential in all patients with a lower motor neuron facial palsy. If there is no sign of attic or posterior marginal disease, radiological examination with high definition CT scanning may provide an alternative explanation for a progressive facial nerve lesion. Sometimes it may not be possible to examine the tympanic membrane fully without general anaesthesia. Surgical exposure of the nerve in the middle ear and mastoid region should always be advised if there is any suspicion of middle ear disease.

Treatment

Urgent operative exploration of the middle ear and mastoid region is mandatory to treat the chronic middle ear disease, proceeding if necessary to a radical mastoidectomy. The facial nerve should be carefully exposed especially throughout its horizontal course in the middle ear but also in its vertical mastoid segment, by following cholesteatoma, granulation tissue and osteitic bone. Cholesteatoma matrix may be removed carefully from the surface of the 'soft' nerve, but any attached granulation tissue should be left untouched to avoid further neural injury. Healthy bone should be removed from the nerve on either side of the diseased segment, to allow space for oedema of the nerve without further compression. Naturally, any packing in the cavity, at the end of the operation, must be inserted gently and with care to avoid pressure on the nerve. The management of the problems caused by the facial paralysis are discussed in Chapter 24. Good recovery should be expected if no axonal degeneration had preceded treatment, but prognosis should be temperate; Savic and Djemic (1989) have reported recovery full to normal in no more than 70% of 64 patients.

Labyrinthine complications
Pathogenesis
Acute middle ear suppuration

Acute middle ear suppuration may extend to the labyrinth through the round window. The round window membrane is thinner in acute than in chronic otitis media and its permeability may be increased. Pus cells can pass into the perilymph of the scala tympani by diapedesis from adjacent inflamed labyrinthine blood vessels. A fibrillary precipitate then accumulates in both perilymphatic and endolymphatic spaces, and developing endolymphatic hydrops is followed by destruction of the membranous labyrinth. Experimental work on chinchillas has shown that bacteria can pass through the layers of the round window into the cochlea with subsequent neuronal damage (Schachern *et al.*, 1992). Preformed fistulae into the labyrinth from the middle ear, as for example, after a stapedectomy operation offer another route for infective spread. The process may stop at any stage and, if the inflammatory changes induced in the labyrinth by the transgression are reversible, the clinical condition is retrospectively called serous labyrinthitis. Should the intralabyrinthine suppuration destroy cochlear and vestibular function in the affected ear, the complication is later called suppurative labyrinthitis (see Figures 5.7 and 5.8).

Chronic destructive ear disease

Chronic destructive ear disease can erode the bony labyrinth by cholesteatoma or by osteitis, leading to similar inner ear destruction, but fully developed intralabyrinthine inflammation is usually preceded by thinning of the bony labyrinthine wall and the development of a fistula of the labyrinth (see Figure 5.1). Labyrinthine damage from slowly eroding cholesteatomas is often followed by new bone deposition. This allows destruction of part of the labyrinth with partitioning and preservation of the rest. Bony fistulae also are often closed by new bone deposition after the eroding disease has been eliminated (see Figures 5.10 and 5.11).

Vestibular irritation by inflammatory disease close to the endosteum of the bony labyrinthine lumen has been termed 'paralabyrinthitis'. Very rarely, chronic osteitis around the bony labyrinth causes necrosis of the whole otic capsule, a condition described as sequestration of the labyrinth. The term 'perilabyrinthitis' is also encountered in writings on this topic, and its correct usage is discussed below.

Suppurative labyrinthitis is now a rare complication of acute otitis media, probably because of the use of antibiotics, but the development of labyrinthine fistulae has remained as common, at 10% of all cases of chronic otitis media, as it was in the pre-antibiotic days (McCabe, 1984). Because of this high incidence, labyrinthine fistula should be considered the most important of the labyrinthine complications.

Suppurative labyrinthitis and serous labyrinthitis

As has been indicated, the distinction between these depends on the retrospective recognition of recovery of cochlear and vestibular function; so the term serous labyrinthitis has little clinical value. The method of spread of infection has been described, but should be amplified by the observation that, on rare occasions, infection extends from meningitis to the labyrinth through the internal auditory meatus (see Figure 5.9), or through the cochlear or vestibular aqueducts. Much more rarely, the infection may be blood borne.

Clinical features

A patient suffering from acute or chronic middle ear infection presents with violent prostrating vertigo and vomiting. Severe hearing loss of a sensorineural type is to be expected, but will be adumbrated by the severe disabling vertigo, especially if there has been a preceding conductive impairment from middle ear disease. The patient lies immobile, on the side with the infected labyrinth upwards, avoiding any head movement. Examination demonstrates evidence of the preceding ear disease. The complication itself causes no systemic infective disturbance. Pyrexia and leucocytosis appear only as features of accompanying acute suppurative otitis media. At first there may be a spontaneous 'irritative' jerk nystagmus beating with quick component towards the infected ear; but this is soon replaced by a 'paralytic' jerk nystagmus, beating towards the healthy side. The direction of this nystagmus probably dictates the preference for lying on the unaffected ear. In that position the patient's efforts to look at a bedside visitor involve turning the eyes towards the damaged labyrinth, and in this direction of gaze, the violence of the nystagmus is least. In the earliest, irritative phase, when subsequent progress may happily confirm that serous labyrinthitis was the appropriate label, tests of cochlear function by masked bone conduction should indicate retained hearing. Loss of cochlear function, as the condition is watched, is evidence of transition to the irreversible suppurative state. The paralytic jerk nystagmus is initially third degree in its severity. Provided no additional problems develop, recovery takes place by the mechanisms common to recovery from any cause of vestibular failure. There is gradual subsidence of the nystagmus through a second to a first degree state, and then to absence of spontaneous nystagmus with fixation. At this stage, after perhaps 2–3 weeks, the patient will have gained fairly good balance, but will still be unsteady when trying to walk in the dark, or with the eyes closed, and will still be unhappy to make sudden head movements. Since this improvement in equilibrium depends on central compensatory changes, it may be upset later in life long after the original infection by other general illnesses, impaired central nervous system function, drugs or psychiatric illness. The hearing loss in the damaged ear is inevitably total and permanent.

Diagnosis

The clinical pattern described above is the same as that of sudden vestibular failure from any cause, and suspicion of suppurative labyrinthitis primarily rests with precise recognition of the underlying middle ear infection. Examination of the ears with the binocular microscope is necessary, and occasionally examination under general anaesthesia will be needed to inspect the attic fully, and to remove obscuring crusts, secretions or debris. Haemorrhagic, or bullous, myringitis with varicella zoster infection can cause sudden vestibular failure with acute pain and inflammatory changes on otoscopic examination. Mastoid radiological imaging confirming a clear air cell system would help to support that diagnosis but, if in doubt, the safest course must be to treat as if the cause is suppurative labyrinthitis. Once a middle ear infection has been recognized the diagnosis poses little difficulty, although traditionally a cerebellar abscess has always been considered to offer a source of confusion. With that complication, the patient appears far more ill, shows cerebellar signs on neurological examination, and demonstrates nystagmus persisting longer after the time of the severest vertigo. Nowadays, a CT scan will provide a definitive distinction.

Sequelae

During the course of the acute illness there is a continuing danger of intracranial spread of infection with the development of meningitis. In the long term, the labyrinth may remain filled with sequestered pus, and classical teaching suggested the occasional need to drain such a labyrinth surgically. The long-term effects on balance and hearing have been mentioned above.

Management

As with all complications, separate attention must be given to the management of the complication itself, and to the antecedent ear disease.

Treatment of suppurative labyrinthitis requires complete bed rest. Head movements should be avoided as much as possible. Any hearing tests must be carried out at the bedside, and not in a chair in the audiology department. Vestibular function tests inevitably excite endolymphatic movement and must be eschewed. (In any case they add nothing useful to the clinical examination.) Vertigo and vomiting may be controlled by parenteral prochlorperazine or cinnarizine. If vomiting prevents hydration, intravenous fluids must be infused. It is has been customary to recommend the administration of parenteral antibiotics. These will be needed to treat acute otitis media as the cause, but it is doubtful whether penetration into the labyrinth itself can affect the course of the labyrinthitis. The development of meningitis, however, may possibly be prevented by antibiotics. The choice of antibiotic may be influenced by bacteriological examination of any available secretions. Broad-spectrum drugs such as ampicillin should be used, and if there is any worry about infection with *Haemophilus influenzae* type B, then intravenous chloramphenicol should be included. Immobility must be maintained throughout treatment, and observations are arranged to recognize the earliest signs of meningitis.

Treatment of an acute ear infection may require myringotomy, and more rarely cortical mastoidectomy but, in most instances, the otitis media will recover with antibiotic therapy alone. Chronic middle ear infections will require formal exploration of the mastoid to make the ear safe. Premature surgical trauma to the temporal bone can promote dissemination of infection, so mastoid exploration should be deferred until the acute symptoms of the suppurative labyrinthitis have subsided. This policy involves conservative medical treatment with continuing observation for 7–10 days before mastoid exploration is performed. Nowadays, it is not considered necessary, nor is it advisable, to drain a 'dead' labyrinth during that mastoidectomy operation.

After full recovery from the acute infective illness, vestibular head exercises (Cawthorne-Cooksey, see Appendix 12.1) will accelerate central compensation for the vestibular deficit.

Labyrinthine fistula

As has been explained, this is a complication of chronic otitis media. An ear in which the endosteum of the labyrinth has been exposed by bony erosion is continuously threatened by suppurative labyrinthitis, and so urgent treatment is essential. The incidence of 10% of all cases of chronic mastoid disease with mastoidectomy has probably not changed since an important report covering a 20-year-period (Sheehy, Brackmann and Graham, 1977). Fistulae occur most commonly in the dome of the lateral semicircular canal, but other parts of the bony labyrinth including the promontory may be eroded.

A labyrinthine fistula may be silent, with no symptoms, and then its discovery at operation is unexpected. Suspicion should be aroused by any patient with chronic middle ear disease complaining of brief episodes of vertigo or unsteadiness. Even if longer attacks of vertigo are a complaint, and even if they seem to fit the pattern of another disorder (such as

Ménière's disease), an infected middle ear and possible labyrinthine fistula should be suspected until operative exploration proves otherwise. *It is safer to explore an ear with an intact otic capsule than to miss exploration of one with a fistula.* CT scanning can demonstrate the lateral semicircular canal (see Figures 2.38 and 2.39), but coronal sections may incorrectly suggest the presence of a fistula from volume averaging artefacts; 30° tilted axial scans produce fewer false positives (Jackler, Dillon and Schindler, 1984).

Assessment of a dizzy patient with chronic middle ear disease must include a careful examination of auditory function. The state of hearing in the apparently healthy ear bears heavily on treatment decisions. Although cold air caloric stimulation may be used as an indication of vestibular function, water must never be used for caloric testing in the presence of chronic ear disease especially with a suspected fistula.

The fistula sign

This is an important physical sign, which depends on transmission of air pressure changes from the external ear canal to a fistula in the labyrinth, causing perilymph movement. Raised air pressure may be produced by pressure with a finger on the tragus, but more reliably by the use of a pneumatic otoscope fitted with a speculum large enough to fit securely into the meatus to produce an air-tight seal. Specific responses to pressure changes are provoked if the fistula test is positive. The nature of these positive findings has often been incorrectly described in textbooks. The sign is not simply one of nystagmus induced by the increased pressure. McCabe (1984) has explained the features of the fistula sign in detail. Increased pressure causes conjugate deviation of the eyes away from the examined side. If the pressure is maintained, a jerk nystagmus develops beating towards the examined, and affected ear. As the pressure is released, the eyes return to the mid-line. Pulsation of pressure in the meatus causes repeated deviation of the eyes to the unaffected side with each pressure rise, and return to the primary position of gaze when the pressure falls (McCabe, 1984). The patient feels dizzy during these events, and accompanying head movements away from the examiner may make continuous inspection of the eyes difficult. McCabe has also shown that the direction of deviation of the eyes on raised pressure depends on the site of the fistula. The description of deviation towards the normal ear is the commonest finding and is associated with a fistula in the most usual site – the dome of the lateral semicircular canal. A lateral canal fistula anterior to the ampulla however causes deviation towards the side of the fistula, while an erosion into the vestibule is indicated by rotatory horizontal deviation towards the diseased ear. Raised pressure on a fistula in the superior canal causes rotatory movement towards the normal ear. Finally, vertical deviation of the eyes suggests a fistula into the posterior canal.

It is important to perform a fistula test in any vertiginous patient, and in every patient with chronic middle ear disease. There are, however, both false-positive and false-negative results. The fistula sign can be positive (misleadingly in the context of chronic ear disease) with an apparently normal tympanic membrane and middle ear. This so-called Hennebert's sign was initially believed to indicate syphilitic disease, and that misconception has been iterated through generations of editions of textbooks. More recently some workers have related a positive fistula sign to evidence of the possible presence of a perilymph fistula (Kohut, 1992). This is a controversial issue. Hennebert's sign is occasionally found in association with other forms of pressure induced vertigo – with Valsalva-induced vertigo and the Tullio phenomenon. One suggested explanation relies on transmission of pressure through a subluxed stapes footplate to the otolith organ of the saccule (Dietrich, Brandt and Fries, 1989). A false-negative fistula sign, when there is actually a fistula with cholesteatoma, may come about because there has been inadequate sealing of the speculum in the meatus, or because a mass of cholesteatomatous debris is protecting the inner ear from the transmission of the raised air pressure, or yet again if the vestibular labyrinth has previously succumbed to the disease and cannot be stimulated.

Treatment of labyrinthine fistula

Whenever chronic destructive middle ear disease is identified in a vertiginous patient, labyrinthine erosion must be presumed. This is so no matter how slender the available evidence for middle ear disease and no matter how characteristic of another disorder the pattern of vertigo may seem to be. The patient's safety demands surgical exploration of the middle ear. Only if inspection during operation fails to reveal erosion of the labyrinth, should other possible explanations be accepted.

During surgical exploration of the middle ear cleft, the possibility of a labyrinthine fistula must be suspected whenever cholesteatoma is encountered, since asymptomatic fistulae are not rare. Preoperative demonstration of a positive fistula sign can alert the surgeon to the risk, and its characteristics may suggest where the fistula may be found. Great care is needed while peeling cholesteatoma matrix off the dome of the lateral semicircular canal, and away from areas where fistula is suspected. Matrix should be removed from other sites first, and then dissection carried out slowly under high power magnification. A slight change in colour at the junction of the matrix and subjacent bone suggests a possible fistula.

Eventually a small sheet of cholesteatoma matrix over a possible fistula will have been isolated. Its management requires careful consideration, for if the endosteum of the bony labyrinth is breached, a 'dead ear' with total deafness may be expected, although Palva and Ramsay (1989) mentioned two instances of accidental opening of the horizontal canal with no sensorineural damage. This probably reflects the fact that slow destruction of the labyrinth by cholesteatoma can compartmentalize it allowing functional survival of the cochlea despite extensive destruction of the semicircular canal system. The options are to remove the matrix, or to leave it in place (see Figure 5.1). There are staunch proponents of the view that matrix should be removed (Palva and Ramsay, 1989; Parisier *et al.*, 1991), but others advocate a more cautious conservative approach with matrix preservation in most circumstances (Vartiainen, 1992). The state of hearing in the other ear is important, and if poor may commend a more cautious attitude with preservation of matrix over the fistula.

If an open cavity operation, such as a radical mastoidectomy, is in hand the matrix can usually be left safely undisturbed unless there is any suspicion of vascular infected granulation tissue deep to it. That is unlikely if the fistula is clearly demarcated as a bluish area through the matrix. A bony fistula left under cholesteatoma matrix will close by new bone growth if the surface inflammatory condition is controlled (see Figures 5.10 and 5.11). If matrix is completely removed from a fistula, the defect should be closed with connective tissue material such as temporalis fascia or perichondrium and fibrin glue to avert the problems of perilabyrinthitis discussed below. During intact canal wall tympanoplasty, as opposed to an open cavity operation, any fistula will remain protected from the exterior, so vertigo caused by perilabyrinthitis will not become a problem. However, remaining cholesteatoma matrix over a fistula, whether left deliberately or accidentally, does require a second exploration after an interval of 6–12 months. By that time, the abandoned matrix will have formed a small epithelial pearl, which can easily be removed. Most surgeons would contemplate intact canal wall procedures only when the other ear has good hearing and is free from disease, and only when the patient will accept a second operation, and may be relied upon to honour that obligation.

Whatever procedure is undertaken, accurate documentation about the state of hearing and vestibular function before operation, about the findings and events during the procedure, and about any postoperative vertigo that may have been caused by vestibular damage during operation, is of paramount importance. Investigation of vestibular symptoms after mastoid surgery is very difficult if such records are not available.

Perilabyrinthitis

This term should be reserved for the particular condition for which it was appropriated by Cawthorne (1957). It denotes the problems caused by a fistula into the labyrinth after mastoidectomy, in the presence of retained vestibular function. The fistula may have preceded the mastoidectomy, or have been caused by it. The vertigo arises through the Tullio phenomenon, since the stapes footplate in the affected ear is mobile. Giddiness is provoked by pressure changes near the fistula, and cold air blown into the ear at windy street corners may cause imbalance. Sometimes the symptoms can be prevented by occluding the external meatus. Operative relief comprises exploration, removal of skin from the fistula and protection by a connective tissue graft. Occasionally, deliberate labyrinthine destruction, or vestibular nerve section may be needed to prevent vertigo.

Vertigo after mastoid surgery

Vertigo and imbalance may develop for many reasons after mastoid surgery (Ludman, 1984, 1986). Analysis of an individual problem is greatly helped by access to reliable information about the state of the ear before operation, the findings at operation, and subsequent progress. The causes include:

1 Unrelated vestibular disease
2 Persisting middle ear disease with further bone erosion
3 Perilabyrinthitis (Cawthorne, 1957)
4 Delayed endolymphatic hydrops (Nadol, Weiss and Parker 1975; Schuknecht, 1978; Ludman, 1986)
5 Breakdown of central compensation, after loss of labyrinthine function (Ludman, 1984)
6 Cerebellar abscess
7 Vestibular nerve neuroma activity, after labyrinthectomy (Ludman, 1971, 1986).

Cochlear complications

When discussing labyrinthine complications of middle ear infections emphasis has usually been placed on vestibular symptoms. It is probable, however, that sensorineural hearing loss can follow middle ear infection, without overt balance disturbance (Paparella *et al.*, 1972). Experimental work with chinchillas and *Strep. pneumoniae* has shown penetration of the cochlea by bacteria passing through the round window membrane, with subsequent neuronal degeneration and hair cell loss (Schachern *et al.*, 1992). The transmission of macromolecular toxic substances through the round window membrane, into the basal turn of the cochlea has been well documented (see Figures 5.7 and 5.26). Serous labyrinthitis induced in this way may be confined to that region, causing first a temporary, and later a permanent, high frequency threshold shift. High frequency sensorineural hearing losses have been shown in chronic otitis media (Walby, Barrera and Schuknecht, 1983). The risk to hearing may be greater in acute than in chronic infection, because the round window membrane is demonstrably thicker in the latter condition, and pus may accumulate under pressure when the tympanic membrane is intact.

Appendix 12.1. The Cawthorne/Cooksey regimen of head exercises

The Cawthorne/Cooksey system of exercises is designed to restore balance and to train the eyes and muscles and joint sense by performing many exercises with the eyes closed. The movements are carried out in the following graduated stages:

Stage 1: head kept still – in bed or sitting

Eye movements only are practised, looking up and down and from side to side and then focusing. The patient focuses on the instructor's finger held three feet (1 m) away and follows the finger to one foot (30 cm) from the eyes.

Stage 2: head and eye movements while sitting

Head movements bending forwards and backwards and then from side to side are at first slow, then quick. The movements are then repeated with the eyes closed.

Stage 3: head and body movements while still sitting

Movements of shoulder shrugging and circling are first practised. The patient then picks up an object from the ground and looks right up with it. Bending forwards, he then passes an object (such as a ball) from hand to hand under the knees. It is important that he should relax between the various movements.

Stage 4: standing exercises

The following manoeuvres are carried out in turn:
1 The patient gets up and stands without support first with the eyes open and later closed
2 The above exercise is repeated turning round while standing
3 A large ball is thrown from hand to hand while standing.

Stage 5: moving about

1 Walking across the room and around a chair with the eyes open. The exercise is repeated with the eyes closed
2 Circling around a centre person who throws a large ball and to whom it will be returned
3 Standing back to back with an instructor who passes a large ball to the patient between the legs, receiving the ball back above the head. This manoeuvre is performed as quickly as possible
4 Walking up and down a slope with the eyes open and later closed
5 Walking up and down steps with the eyes open and later closed
6 Games involving stooping, stretching, and aiming, such as skittles, bowls or basketball.

The principles of the Cawthorne/Cooksey exercises – instructions for patients

The balance parts of the two ears complement each other, sending equal impulses to the brain which are essential for the maintenance of equilibrium of the head and body.

If either or both balance centres are damaged, equilibrium is upset. The result of this is vertigo or giddiness which may be accompanied by nausea and vomiting. Although this condition may be very frightening it is not serious in that it does not, in itself, threaten life. It can, furthermore, be overcome by carrying out special exercises.

The purpose of the exercises is to build up a tolerance mechanism in the brain which compensates for the unequal balance of the two ears. The exercises stimulate the development of this tolerance mechanism and the more diligently and regularly they are performed, the sooner will vertigo disappear.

The exercises should be carried out persistently for at least 5 minutes three times daily and for as long as vertigo persists. This may be for 1–3 months. A conscious effort should be made to seek out the head positions and movements that cause vertigo insofar as one can be tolerated, because the more frequently vertigo is induced the more quickly is the brain compensation mechanism built up.

Certain medications help to control the vertigo while brain compensation is being achieved and any such tablets should be taken regularly during the course of exercises.

As normal a life as possible is, meanwhile, to be recommended. Early return to work and sports are helpful in rehabilitation.

Diligence and perseverance will be required but the earlier and more regularly the balance exercise regimen is carried out the faster and more complete will be recovery to normal activity.

References

ALBERT, D. M. and WILLIAMS, S. R. (1986) Clinical and anatomical considerations of the Tobey-Ayer test in lateral sinus thrombosis. *Journal of Laryngology and Otology,* **100**, 311–313

ALFORD, B. R. and COHN, A. M. (1980) Complications of suppurative otitis media and mastoiditis. *Otolaryngology,* 2nd edn, edited by M. M. Pararella and D. A. Shumnick. Philadelphia: W. B. Saunders. pp. 1490–1509

BIDZINSKI, J. and KOSZEWSKI, W. (1990) The value of different methods of treatment of brain abscess in the CT era (see comments). *Acta Neurochirurgica,* **105**, 117–120

BOK, A. P. and PETER, J. C. (1993) Subdural empyema: burr holes or craniotomy? A retrospective computerized tomography-era analysis of treatment in 90 cases. *Journal of Neurosurgery,* **78**, 574–578

BRAND, B., CAPAROSA, R. J. and LUBIC, L. G. (1984) Otorhinological brain abscess therapy – past and present. *Laryngoscope,* **94**, 483–487

British Medical Journal (1977) Treatment of cerebral abscess. **283**, 978

BROWNING, G. G. (1984) The unsafeness of safe ears. *Journal of Laryngology and Otology,* **98**, 23–26

CAWTHORNE, T. E. (1957) Perilabyrinthitis. *Laryngoscope,* **67**, 1233–1236

CHUN, C. H., JOHNSON, J. D., HOFSTETTER, M. and RAFF, M. J. (1986) Brain abscess. A study of 45 consecutive cases. *Medicine,* **65**, 415–431

CLEMIS, J. D. and JERVA, M. J. (1976) Hydrocephalus following translabyrinthine surgery. *Journal of Otolaryngology,* **5**, 303–309

DAWES, J. D. K. (1979) Complications of infections of the middle ear. In: *Scott Brown's Diseases of the Ear, Nose and Throat,* vol. 2, 4th edn, edited by J. Ballantyne and J. Groves. London, Butterworths. pp. 305–384

DIETRICH, M., BRANDT, T. and FRIES, W. (1989) Otolith function in man – results from a case of otolith Tullio phenomenon. *Brain,* **112**, 1377–1392

DJERIC, D. and SAVIC, D. (1989) Characteristics of a pathological process in the destroyed tympanic part of the facial canal in chronic otitis media with cholesteatoma. *Revue de Laryngologie Otologie Rhinologie,* **110**, 449–451

EINHAUPL, K. M., VILLRINGER, A., MEISTER, W., MEHRAEIN, S., GARNER, C., PELLKOFER, M. *et al.* (1991) Heparin treatment in sinus venous thrombosis (published erratum appears in *Lancet* 1991 Oct 12; ii 958). *Lancet,* ii 597–600

FEUERMAN, T., WACKYM, P. A., GADE, G. F. and DUBROW, T. (1989) Craniotomy improves outcome in subdural empyema. *Surgical Neurology,* **32**, 105–110

FISCHER, E. G., MCLENNAN, J. I. and SUZUKI, Y. (1981) Cerebral abscess in children. *American Journal of Diseases of Children,* **135**, 746–749

FOLEY, J. (1955) Benign forms of intracranial hypertension – 'toxic' and 'otitic' hydrocephalus. *Brain,* **78**, 1–41

GAGNON, N. B., SIERRA-DUPONT, S. and HUOT, L. A. (1976) Thrombosis of the lateral sinus. *Journal of Otolaryngology,* **61**, 257–261

GEIMAN, B. J. and SMITH, A. L. (1992) Dexamethasone and bacterial meningitis. A meta-analysis of randomized controlled trials. *Western Journal of Medicine,* **157**, 27–31

GOWER, D. and MCGUIRT, W. F. (1983) Intracranial complications of acute and chronic infectious ear disease: a problem still with us. *Laryngoscope,* **93**, 1028–1033

HAIMES, A. B., ZIMMERMAN, R. D., MORGELLO, S., WEINGARTEN,

K., BECKER, R. D., JENNIS, R. *et al.* (1989) MR imaging of brain abscesses. *Journal of Radiology,* **10**, 279–291

HARKER, L. A. and PIGNATARI, S. S. (1992) Facial nerve paralysis secondary to chronic otitis media without cholesteatoma. *American Journal of Otology,* **13**, 372–374

HAWKINS, D. B. (1985) Lateral sinus thrombosis: a sometimes unexpected diagnosis. *Laryngoscope,* **95**, 674–677

INGHAM, H. R., SELKON, J. B. and ROXBY, C. M. (1977) Bacteriological study of otogenic cerebral abscesses: chemotherapeutic role of metronidazole. *British Medical Journal,* **283**, 991–993

INGHAM, H. R., SISSON, P. R., MENDELOW, A. D., KALBAG, R. M. and MCALLISTER, V. L. (1991) *Pyogenic Neurosurgical Infections.* London, Edward Arnold

IRVING, R. M., JONES, N. S., HALL-CRAGGS, M. A. and KENDALL, B. (1991) CT and MR imaging in lateral sinus thrombosis. *Journal of Laryngology and Otology,* **105**, 693–695

ISAACMAN, D. J. (1989) Otitic hydrocephalus: an uncommon complication of a common condition. *Annals of Emergency Medicine,* **18**, 684–687

JACKLER, R. K., DILLON, W. P. and SCHINDLER, R. A. (1984) Computer tomography in suppurative ear disease: a correlation of surgical and radiographic findings. *Laryngoscope,* **94**, 746–752

JOHNSTON, I. and PATERSON, A. (1974) Benign intracranial hypertension. *Brain,* **97**, 289–312

KIMMELMAN, C. P. and GROSMAN, R. (1983) Intratemporal carotid aneurysm as a complication of chronic otitis media: treatment. *Otolaryngology – Head and Neck Surgery,* **91**, 306–308

KOHUT, R. I. (1992) Perilymph fistulas – clinical criteria. *Archives of Otolaryngology, Head and Neck Surgery,* **118**, 687–692

KRISTIANSEN, B. E., ASK, E., JENKINS, A., FERMER, C., RADSTROM, P. and SKOLD, O. (1991) Rapid diagnosis of meningococcal meningitis by polymerase chain reaction. *Lancet,* i, 1568–1569

KULAI, A., OZATIK, N. and TOPÇU, I. (1990) Otogenic intracranial abscesses. *Acta Neurochirurgica,* **107**, 140–146

LAMPE, R. M. and EDWARDS, M. S. (1984) Intracranial complications in children with chronic middle ear disease. *Texas Medicine,* **80**, 52–54

LANCET (1982) Lateral sinus thrombosis. ii, 806

LEBEL, M. H., HOYT, M. J., WAAGNER, D. C., ROLLINS, N. K., FINITZO, T. and MCCRACKEN, G. J. (1989) Magnetic resonance imaging and dexamethasone therapy for bacterial meningitis. *American Journal of Diseases of Children,* **143**, 301–306

LENZ, R. P. and MCDONALD, G. A. (1984) Otitic hydrocephalus. *Laryngoscope,* **94**, 1451–1454

LEWIS, R. and PRIESTLEY, B. L. (1986) Addition of rifampicin in persistent *Haemophilus influenzae* type B meningitis. *British Medical Journal,* **292**, 448–449

LUDMAN, H. (1971) Destruction of the labyrinth and perilabyrinthitis. *Proceedings of the Royal Society of Medicine,* **64**, 849–852

LUDMAN, H. (1984) Surgical treatment of vertigo. In: *Vertigo.* Chichester: John Wiley & Sons, pp. 113–131

LUDMAN, H. (1986) Neuronal activity in otology. *Journal of Laryngology and Otology,* **100**, 989–1007

LUDMAN, H. (1988) *Mawson's Diseases of the Ear,* 5th edn. London: Edward Arnold

LUND, W. S. (1978) A review of 50 cases of intracranial complications from otogenic infection between 1961 and 1977. *Clinical Otolaryngology,* **3**, 495–501

MCCABE, B. F. (1984) Labyrinthine fistula in chronic mastoiditis. *Annals of Otology, Rhinology and Laryngology*, Suppl. 112, 138–141

MCFARLAN, A. M. (1943). The bacteriology of brain abscess. *British Medical Journal*, 2, 643

MAKSIMOVIC, Z. and RUKOVANJSKI, M. (1993) Intracranial complications of cholesteatoma. *Acta Oto Rhino Laryngologica Belgica*, 47, 33–36

MAURICE-WILLIAMS, R. S. (1983) Open evacuation of pus: a satisfactory surgical approach to the problem of brain abscess? *Journal of Neurology, Neurosurgery and Psychiatry*, 46, 697–703

NADOL, J., WEISS, A. and PARKER, S. (1975) Vertigo of delayed onset after sudden deafness. *Annals of Otology, Rhinology and Laryngology*, 84, 841–846

NUNEZ, D. A. and BROWNING, G. G. (1990) Risks of developing an otogenic intracranial abscess. *Journal of Laryngology and Otology*, 104, 468–472

O'CONNELL, J. E. (1990) Lateral sinus thrombosis: a problem still with us. *Journal of Laryngology and Otology*, 104, 949–951

OYARZABAL, M. F., PATEL, K. S. and TOLLEY, M. D. (1992) Bilateral acute mastoiditis complicated by lateral sinus thrombosis. *Journal of Laryngology and Otology*, 106, 535–537

PALVA, T. and RAMSAY, H. (1989) Treatment of labyrinthine fistula. *Archives of Otolaryngology, Head and Neck Surgery*, 115, 804–806

PAPARELLA, M., ODA, M., HIRAIDE, F. and BRADY, D. (1972) Pathology of sensorineural hearing loss in otitis media. *Annals of Otology, Rhinology and Laryngology*, 81, 632–647

PARISIER, S. C., EDELSTEIN, D. R., HAN, J. C. and WEISS, M. H. (1991) Management of labyrinthine fistulas caused by cholesteatoma. *Otolaryngology – Head and Neck Surgery*, 104, 110–115

PECOUL, B., VARAINE, F., KEITA, M., SOGA, G., DJIBO, A., SOULA, G. *et al.* (1991) Long-acting chloramphenicol versus intravenous ampicillin for treatment of bacterial meningitis. *Lancet*, ii, 862–866

PENNYBACKER, J. (1961) Discussion on intracranial complications of otogenic origin. *Proceedings of the Royal Society of Medicine*, 54, 309–320

PFALTZ, C. R. and GRIESEMER, C. (1984) Complications of acute middle ear infections. *Annals of Otology, Rhinology and Laryngology*, 93, (suppl. 112), 133–137

QUECKENSTEDT (1916) Zur diagnose der Ruckenmarkskompression. *Zeitschrift für Nervenheilkunde*, 55, 325–333

SAMUEL, J. and FERNANDEZ, C. M. C. (1985) Otogenic complications with an intact tympanic membrane. *Laryngoscope*, 95, 1387–1390

SAVIC, D. L. and DJERIC, D. R. (1989) Facial paralysis in chronic suppurative otitis media. *Clinical Otolaryngology*, 14, 515–517

SCHACHERN, P. A., PAPARELLA, M. M., HYBERTSON, R., SANO, S. and DUVALL, A. (1992) Bacterial tympanogenic labyrinthitis, meningitis, and sensorineural damage. *Archives of Otolaryngology, Head and Neck Surgery*, 118, 53–57

SCHROTH, G., KRETZSCHMAR, K., GAWEHN, J. and VOIGT, K. (1987) Advantage of magnetic resonance imaging in the diagnosis of cerebral infections. *Neuroradiology*, 29, 120–126

SCHUKNECHT, H. (1978) Delayed endolymphatic hydrops. *Annals of Otology, Rhinology and Laryngology*, 87, 743–748

SEID, A. B. and SELLARS, S. L. (1973) The management of otogenic lateral sinus disease at Groote Schuur Hospital. *Laryngoscope*, 83, 397–403

SHEARMAN, C. P., LEES, P. D. and TAYLOR, J. C. (1987) Subdural empyema: a rational management plan. The case against craniotomy. *British Journal of Neurosurgery*, 1, 179–183

SHEEHY, J. L., BRACKMANN, D. E. and GRAHAM, M. D. (1977) Complications of cholesteatoma: a report on 1024 cases. *The First International Conference on Cholesteatoma*. Birmingham, Alabama, Aesculapius Press. pp. 420–429

SIEGLER, D., FAIERS, M. C. and WILLIS, A. T. (1982) Bacteroides meningitis complicating chronic mastoiditis. *Postgraduate Medical Journal*, 58, 560–561

SOUTHWICK, F. S., RICHARDSON, E. P. and SWARTZ, M. N. (1986) Septic thrombosis of the dural venous sinuses. *Medicine*, 65, 82–106

STAPLETON, S. R., BELL, B. A. and UTTLEY, D. (1993) Stereotactic aspiration of brain abscesses: is this the treatment of choice? *Acta Neurochirurgica*, 121, 15–19

STEIN, E. H., CUNNINGHAM, M. J. and WEBER, A. L. (1992) Noninvasive radiologic options in evaluating intracranial complications of otitis media. *Annals of Otology, Rhinology and Laryngology*, 101, 363–366

STEPHANOR, S. (1978) Experience with multiloculated brain abscess. *Journal of Neurosurgery*, 49, 199–203

SURKIN, M. I., GREEN, R. P., KESSLER, S. M. and LUCENTE, F. E. (1983) Subclavian vein thrombosis secondary to chronic otitis media. *Annals of Otology, Rhinology and Laryngology*, 92, 45–48

SYMONDS, C. P. (1931) Otitic hydrocephalus. *Brain*, 54, 55–71

TAYLOR, J. C. (1987) The case for excision in the treatment of brain abscess. *British Journal of Neurosurgery*, 1, 173–178

TEICHGRABER, J. F., PER-LEE, J. H. and TURNER, J. S. (1982) Lateral sinus thrombosis: a modern perspective. *Laryngoscope*, 92, 744–751

TOBEY, G. L. and AYER, J. B. (1925) Dynamic studies on the cerebrospinal fluid in the differential diagnosis of lateral sinus thrombosis. *Transactions of the American Otological Society*, 17, 174–188

VARTIAINEN, E. (1992) What is the best method of treatment for labyrinthine fistulae caused by cholesteatoma? *Clinical Otolaryngology*, 17, 258–260

VENEZIO, F. R., NAIDICH, T. P. and SHULMAN, S. T. (1982) Complications of mastoiditis with special emphasis on venous sinus thrombosis. *Journal of Pediatrics*, 101, 509–513

WALBY, A., BARRERA, A. and SCHUKNECHT, H. (1983) Cochlear pathology in chronic suppurative otitis media. *Annals of Otology, Rhinology and Laryngology*, 92 (suppl.103), 3–19

WOLFOWITZ, B. (1972) Otogenic intracranial complications. *Archives of Otolaryngology*, 96, 220–222

WRIGHT, J. L. W. and GRIMALDI, P. M. B. (1973) Otogenic intracranial complications. *Journal of Laryngology and Otology*, 87, 1085–1096

13

Otalgia

Carol Wengraf

Most episodes of earache are caused by pathology in the ear itself. The diagnosis should be simple once an accurate history has been taken and a full examination of the ears, nose and throat carried out. Previous chapters in this volume have described in detail the signs, symptoms and pathology of painful ear diseases and Table 13.1 lists these for clarity.

This chapter describes the diseases which appear to cause pain in the ear but which are actually referred from other sites which share the same nerve supply, or those in which the nerves themselves are inflamed or irritated.

Innervation of the ear

The ear is not only served by the Vth, VIIth, IXth and Xth cranial nerves but also by the second and third branches of the cervical plexus. Presumably this richness of innervation explains why pain referred to the ear is so common.

The exact distribution of the nerves is subject to variation and some overlap occurs (Last, 1984). Briefly, the pinna is supplied by:

1 The great auricular nerve, C2 and C3, which supplies most of the cranial surface, and the posterior part of the lateral surface.
2 The lesser occipital, C3, which supplies the upper part of the cranial surface.
3 The auricular branch of the vagus nerve which supplies much of the concavity of the concha and the posterior and inferior walls of the meatus.
4 The auriculotemporal branch of the mandibular nerve which supplies the tragus, the crus and adjacent parts of the helix and the anterior and superior walls of the meatus.
5 The facial nerve which probably supplies small areas on both aspects of the auricle and in the depression of the concha.

The tympanic membrane is supplied by the auriculotemporal branch of the vagus nerve, tympanic branches of the glossopharyngeal nerve and possibly branches of the facial nerve. The middle ear cavity and lateral portion of the eustachian tube are supplied by the glossopharyngeal nerve via the tympanic plexus and the mastoid air cells by a meningeal branch of the trigeminal nerve (Gray, 1989).

In summary therefore, the pinna is supplied by V, VII, X, C2 and C3, the meatus by cranial nerves V, VII and X, the drum by VII, IX and X and the middle ear by V, VII and IX.

The temporomandibular joint is supplied by the auriculotemporal and the masseteric branches of the mandibular division of the trigeminal nerve. The skin over the joint and the parotid gland is supplied by C2 and C3.

Referred pain

Pain is one of the most disturbing of human experiences and it must be remembered that individuals vary widely in their appreciation of, and reaction to it, and the same individual may react in different ways to a similar pain at different times. Pain is a warning and is always real to the patient. If it is not possible to find the cause of the pain, this should be regarded as the physician's inadequacy rather than the patient's fault.

The physiological explanation for referred pain is uncertain (Walton, 1985a), but the phenomenon can probably be explained by a central summation mechanism in relation to the gate theory (Melzack and Wall, 1965; Verrill, 1990). There is a widespread

Table 13.1 Conditions of the outer, middle and inner ear associated with pain

Pinna
1   Trauma – tears, lacerations, bites
2   Haematoma, which may lead to perichondritis
3   Infected eczema
4   Infected preauricular sinus
5   Erysipelas
6   Frostbite
7   Sunburn
8   Chondrodermatitis nodularis chronica helicis
9   Infected basal or squamous cell carcinoma

Meatus
1   Impacted wax. Misguided attempts at removal with blunt instruments, wax solvents. Failed syringing
2   Keratosis obturans
3   Impacted foreign bodies
4   Boils (furunculosis)
5   Otitis externa. Pain suggests fungal infection
6   Hypersensitivity to local antibiotics
7   Malignant otitis externa. Persistent pain indicates activity and requires continuing systemic antibiotics
8   Necrotizing osteitis
9   Herpes zoster oticus
10 Exostoses, when wax and debris are impacted medially
11 Tumours, mainly carcinoma. Pain should alert suspicion

Middle ear
1   Bullous myringitis
2   Traumatic perforations
3   Haemotympanum
4   Otitic barotrauma
5   Acute otitis media
6   Otitis media with effusion
7   Carcinoma
8   Acoustic reflex (Painton and Shaw, 1988)

Mastoid
1   Acute mastoiditis. Persistent pain is an indication for drainage
2   Bezold abscess – torticollis
3   Zygomatic mastoiditis
4   Exacerbations of chronic granulomatous mastoiditis
5   Complications of cholesteatoma. Pain is usually an indication for surgery
6   Cholesterol granuloma. Again pain is an indication for surgery
7   Wegener's granuloma
8   Eosinophilic granuloma (Fradis *et al.*, 1985)

Inner ear
1   Noise. In noise-sensitive people this may cause pain
2   Tinnitus may be described as a throbbing pain
3   Menière's disease. Attacks may be preceded by pain and fullness in and behind the ear
4   Vestibular schwannoma – 30% complain of otalgia (Moffat *et al.*, 1989)

diffuse monosynaptic input to the cells of the substantia gelatinosa of the spinal cord, often from relatively distant afferents, and it is suggested that this diffuse input is normally inhibited by presynaptic gate mechanisms, but may be triggered if the stimulus is sufficiently intense.

A good example of referred pain is that in which there is irritation of the diaphragm – innervated by the phrenic nerve cervical branches 3 and 4 – and this is then appreciated as pain in the tip of the shoulder, whose cutaneous innervation is C3 and C4.

Tonsillitis

Tonsillitis must be one of the commonest causes of pain referred to the ear. Children find localization of pain difficult and there is often an associated otitis media.

Post-tonsillectomy pain varies considerably between individuals and seems to be less severe in children than adults. The average length of time for which pain was experienced in a group of 95 children was 4.9 days (Paradise *et al.*, 1984). It is important not to assume that the pain in the ear is referred pain and to check that there is not a concomitant ear infection.

Peritonsillar, retropharyngeal and parapharyngeal abscesses will all cause earache too, but should be easy to distinguish from simple tonsillitis if considered. If trismus makes it impossible to examine the throat adequately, then 12 hours of intravenous broad-spectrum antibiotics plus rehydration should reduce this sufficiently to allow visualization. It is most important that these abscesses are drained promptly to prevent the development of complications, such as respiratory obstruction.

Nasal polyps

Antrochoanal and nasal polyps, which are large enough to protrude through the posterior choanae and obstruct the eustachian tube orifice will give rise to a feeling of blockage and discomfort in the ear. Sinusitis may also cause a feeling of blockage in the ear when purulent secretions flow past the orifice of the eustachian tube. A secondary serous otitis may also develop thereby adding to the discomfort.

Mumps

Mumps is one of the major viral infections which usually affects children. Pain in the ear is very common and may well appear before the swelling and if only one gland is affected may cause diagnostic problems. When the infection is associated with mumps labyrinthitis it is most important that a bacterial ear infection be excluded.

Parotitis

Postoperative parotitis in adults, with pain in front of, and in, the ear was not uncommon, but now with better hydration, dental hygiene and aftercare it is usually confined to the debilitated, very elderly and those who are immunocompromised. The causative organism was commonly *Staphylococcus aureus* (Lundgren, Kylen and Odkvist, 1976), but more recently *Pseudomonas aeruginosa* (Pruett and Simmons, 1984), and strict anaerobes (Lewis, Lamey and Gibon, 1989) have been cultured from Stensen's duct, which means that metronidazole should be included in the therapy. In South-East Asia acute parotitis in children is caused relatively commonly by *Pseudomonas pseudomallei* (Dance *et al.*, 1989). Juvenile recurrent parotitis is probably related to the Epstein-Barr virus (Akaboshi *et al.*, 1983), is often self-limiting at puberty (Ericson, Zetterlund and Ohman, 1991) but, in severe cases, parotidectomy may have to be considered.

Thyroid

Earache has been described as the presenting symptom of acute thyroiditis (Stevenson, 1990) and up to 64% of subacute (de Quervain's) thyroiditis may have ear and jaw ache which is not at first obviously due to the thyroid (McDougall, 1990). There is usually a small firm diffusely tender goitre with a high ESR. The pain will usually respond to aspirin but severe cases may require steroids (*Lancet*, 1986). These do not alter the natural history of the disease, however, and 10% of patients will become hypothyroid. Occasionally Hashimoto's thyroiditis is painful, though thyroxine will usually alleviate this if the dose is high enough to suppress thyrotropin secretion (Zimmermann *et al.*, 1986). Haemorrhage into a cyst or nodule will cause acute pain but this will only last a few days. Fibrosis (Reidel's struma) must be differentiated from malignancy and biopsy of the isthmus should confirm this when this is split to relieve pressure symptoms (DeGroot *et al.*, 1984).

Tuberculosis of the larynx

Pain in the ear is sometimes found in tuberculous disease of the larynx (Tilley, 1919). The disease is now uncommon in the UK (Bailey and Windle-Taylor, 1981), but at the first world conference on tuberculosis in 1992 it was stated that nearly one-third of the world's population was infected by the mycobacterium, that the disease was commonly associated with AIDS and that multiresistant strains were an increasing problem (*Lancet*, 1992). Manni (1983) found one-third of pulmonary cases to have laryngeal involvement, but in Soda *et al.*'s (1989) 19 cases of laryngeal tuberculosis, none had earache. This may

well revert to the old picture with the increasing incidence of the disease.

Styloid process

'The styloid process has been blamed for pain within the ear but we have never been satisfied that this is true' (Edwards, 1973). Syme (1915) described a patient who had a stabbing pain in the ear plus throat discomfort which was relieved by tonsillectomy and removal of an elongated styloid process. Eagle (1937, 1958) re-described this syndrome and attempted to popularize this operation, but as between 13% (Kaufman, Elzay and Irish, 1970) and 29% (Lengele and Dhem, 1988) of patients have a styloid process which is longer than 30 mm, the vast majority of these cannot cause pain (Figure 13.1). Russell (1977) advocated infiltrating the tonsillar fossa with local anaesthetic and if this cured the ear pain temporarily, then one would be justified in removing the styloid process. This can be done either via the tonsillar fossa or externally, when the great vessels can be visualized and should be safer (Loeser and Cardwell, 1942; Strauss, Zohar and Laurian, 1985). There does seem to be the occasional patient who may

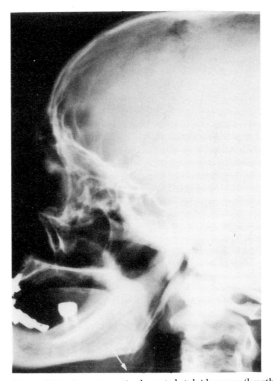

Figure 13.1 Asymptomatic elongated styloid process (length 5.0 cm) (with kind permission of Mr J. B. Booth)

have suffered pain for years, who is cured by this procedure (Baddour, McAnear and Tilson, 1978).

Teeth

Pain caused by diseased teeth is commonly referred to adjacent structures; the fifth and sixth lower and upper fifth molars are most frequently implicated in pain referred to the ear (Sharav, 1989). Erupting teeth, caries causing exposure of the dentine, periodontal and dental abscesses, may all cause 'earache' as well as pain in the tooth itself. Episodic pain arising in teeth is rare and if there is doubt, infiltration around the tooth with local anaesthetic will abolish the pain and thus prevent unnecessary and ineffective extraction of an otherwise healthy tooth.

Oral ulceration

Oral ulcers are painful locally but if they involve the posterior third of the tongue, tonsil or pharynx will give rise to earache. Primary herpetic stomatitis, caused by the herpes simplex virus, usually affects children aged between 1 and 3 years (Bissett, 1992), is self-limiting within 7–10 days and rarely recurs. Recurrent aphthous stomatitis (RAS) (Tyldesley, 1989a) can be classified as minor, major – where the ulcers are larger than 1 cm, last more than a week and may therefore need to be biopsied (Daniels, 1992) – and herpetiform. There is evidence that recurrent aphthous stomatitis is related to autoimmunity (Lehner, 1968), trauma (Wray, Graykowski and Notkins, 1981), nutritional deficiencies (Tyldesley, 1989a), altered hormonal levels, coeliac disease (Fergusson *et al.*, 1975) and may become more frequent and severe in associaton with HIV infection (Daniels, 1992). Behçet's syndrome (Behçet, 1937) is characterized by oro-genital ulceration and uveitis and may be an autoimmune disease (Wray, 1984). These ulcers can be treated with local steroids and topical analgesics, dapsone, colchicine (Scully, 1989), or tetracycline mouthwashes (Tyldesley, 1989a). Severe cases and those with Behçet's syndrome may require thalidomide (Bowers and Powell, 1983), azathioprine (Yazici *et al.*, 1990) or chlorambucil (Ball, 1992).

Temporomandibular joint

The temporomandibular joint, as any other joint in the body, is subject to trauma, infection and arthritis. Not only is the joint the immediate anterior relation of the external auditory meatus, but it is supplied by an articular branch of the auriculotemporal nerve which also supplies cutaneous sensation to a large portion of the pinna. Not surprisingly, disorders of this joint are frequently misinterpreted by the patient as earache. Rheumatoid arthritis can affect this joint in both children and adults (Gardner, 1986), as can osteoarthritis, which develops relatively frequently following trauma to the jaw (Norman, 1982). About 60% of these people have otalgia and condylectomy will usually relieve their pain. Gout occasionally occurs but rarely in the absence of other affected joints. Ten per cent of those with ankylosing spondylitis have pain in the joint and trismus (Scully and Cawson, 1987).

Chronic pain in the temporomandibular joint or the pain dysfunction syndrome is common – affecting 15–20% of the population at some time in their life (Howe, 1983) – but 80% of those affected are young females (Tyldesley, 1989b), a large proportion of whom have other physical illnesses with pain and who lack emotional support (Marbach, Lennon and Dohrenwend, 1988). Children can be affected however (Blake, Thorburn and Stewart, 1982). A separate group of patients are those who have worn full dentures for years and have lost alveolar bone which creates an increase in the freeway space between the dentures and overclosure of the jaw, causing pain (Mumford, 1987). Short-lived pain can often occur following extractions or prolonged restorative dentistry and is common in those who grind or clench their teeth (Every, 1960).

Treatments for this condition are many and varied and depend upon one's particular theory of causation. They include aspirin, local heat, physiotherapy (Hargreaves and Wardle, 1983), acrylic splints, restorative dentistry to alter the bite (Thomson, 1959) and muscular exercises (Howe, 1983). A large proportion of patients will become pain free either because of, or in spite of the treatment, but a small number will persist. The recent introduction of arthroscopy (McCain, de la Rua and LeBlanc, 1989) and probably even more accurately MRI (Katzberg, 1989), should help to find the exact cause of the pain and direct treatment accordingly. It is most important that those offered operative treatment should be distinguished from patients with atypical facial pain, which is related to emotional stress and adverse life events and is more effectively treated with antidepressants (Feinmann and Harris, 1984). A very small number of these patients may have a peripherally placed intracranial tumour, but they will usually also have an area of sensory loss, which will distinguish them (Bullitt, Tew and Boyd, 1986). Costen's syndrome (Costen, 1934) still appears in many textbooks and consists of pain and fullness in the ear, associated with tinnitus and vertigo. This was attributed to wearing of the glenoid fossa and pressure on the auriculotemporal nerve. This has been largely discredited; Brookes, Maw and Coleman (1980), in a series of 45 patients, were unable to find one case who satisfied the criteria.

Myocardial ischaemia

Pain in the ear related to episodes of stress and exercise has been described (Bryhn and Hindfelt, 1984). The patient had angiographic evidence of coronary artery disease and a treadmill test brought on the ear pain, but no angina.

Malignant disease

The most important cause of referred pain to the ear which must be excluded in all cases, is a malignant tumour. The commonest 'silent' neoplasm causing earache is one in the pyriform fossa (Trotter, 1926), but those in the glottis, supraglottis, postcricoid region, posterior pharyngeal wall, posterior third of the tongue, parotid and nasopharynx may all do so. All these sites must be inspected carefully, and if necessary examined under general anaesthesia with any suspicious areas biopsied, if necessary more than once, to exclude a neoplastic cause for the earache.

Unfortunately, one of the most difficult types of earache to treat is that caused by a mass of malignant glands in the neck. A radical neck dissection should be performed, if possible, to include the parotid gland where indicated. If an area of skin is involved, this should be excised and cover provided by a flap. If the carotid artery is involved this should be excised, if possible, and replaced by a graft (Collins, 1987). Radical neck surgery is justified, even when cure is not expected as the pain from a mass of neck glands is so very difficult to control.

Pain of nervous origin

Herpes zoster oticus

Ramsay Hunt (1907) was the first to describe this disease, consisting of a herpetic eruption on the pinna, facial palsy and hearing loss. Herpetic inflammation of the geniculate ganglion was the suggested cause. Dawes (1963) disagreed with this site as often more than one cranial nerve may be affected. In a typical case, however, post-mortem examination showed unequivocal changes in the geniculate ganglion consistent with previous herpetic inflammation (Aleksic, Budzilovich and Leibermann, 1973).

Hunt also described pre-herpetic pains in and around the ear for 3–4 days before the eruption, although they have been described as arising up to 3 weeks before vesicles appear (Juel-Jensen *et al.*, 1970). The diagnosis at this stage may be extremely difficult, but if repeated examination shows no other pathology, this in itself should suggest the diagnosis, which will become obvious when the vesicles appear. The pain will sometimes subside when the eruption appears but usually continues to be severe for many days. There is good evidence that oral acyclovir, if given within 3 days of the onset of the rash, in doses of 800 mg five times a day, will not only reduce the severity of the pain, but will reduce the extent and number of the vesicles that appear (Huff *et al.*, 1988; Morton and Thomson, 1989).

Glossopharyngeal zoster

This has been described (Clark, 1979) in a patient who was exposed to varicella, developed vesicles on the posterior third of the tongue only, with pain in the ear and rising varicella virus titres.

Postherpetic neuralgia

Postherpetic neuralgia, defined as pain persisting for more than a month after the original eruption, will develop in about 10% of patients, one-third of whom will still have pain a year later. The proportion of those affected will rise to 50% in those over 70 years of age (*Lancet*, 1990). The exact cause of the continuing pain is still uncertain, but a careful post-mortem study on a patient with a T7–8 lesion has shown atrophy of the dorsal horn from T4 to 8 and fibrosis and cell loss in the ganglion of T8 (Watson *et al.*, 1988). It was suggested that the pain may result from the uninhibited activity of unmyelinated primary afferents as a result of the loss of myelinated afferent fibres and the possible presence of hypersensitive neurons in the dorsal horn. Nurmikko and Bowsher (1990) have shown that in a large group of cases with postherpetic neuralgia there were significant changes in all sensory thresholds on the affected side and suggested that all primary afferent fibres, both large and small, are damaged, plus major central involvement. Certainly the continuing pain in and around the ear, especially if associated with an ipsilateral facial palsy and sensorineural hearing loss is a very major problem for the patient. Much work therefore has been done to try to prevent the development of postherpetic neuralgia but as yet there is no evidence that oral steroids (Esmann, Kroon and Brown, 1987) or acyclovir (McKendrick, McGill and Wood, 1989; Freestone and Brigden, 1990), reduce the incidence significantly. Numerous treatments have been used to try to control the pain and disordered sensation of postherpetic neuralgia. They include ethyl chloride spray (Taverner, 1960), prolonged electrical stimulation (Nathan and Wall, 1974), amitriptyline (Watson *et al.*, 1982), vibratory stimulation at 100 Hz (Lundeberg *et al.*, 1983) and topical capsaicin (Watson, Evans and Watts, 1988). Unfortunately each of these is only effective in a relatively small proportion of cases.

Trigeminal neuralgia

Trigeminal neuralgia is characterized by frequent paroxysms of lancinating pain, involving the same part of the face on each occasion and may include the auricle, meatus and tragus. Attacks last 10–30 seconds and are often triggered by moving or touching a particular part of the face. It is commoner in women than in men, in the old rather than the young and on the right rather than the left (*Lancet*, 1984). Carbamazepine in doses up to 200 mg q.d.s., will usually control the pain, but if this fails further investigation is required as some cases of trigeminal pain are due to carcinomatous infiltration along the nerve (Trobe *et al.*, 1982) and some are associated with multiple sclerosis (Harris, 1921). If no cause can be found and the patient is not too frail, surgery is indicated. This can be alcohol injection of the trunk at the foramina or of the ganglion (Harris, 1921), or section of the trunk, or thermocoagulation of the ganglion (Sweet and Wepsic, 1974). These procedures all have the major disadvantage of producing anaesthesia of the affected area which may become as distressing as the original pain – anaesthesia dolorosa (Walton, 1985b). There is increasing evidence that in many cases the pain is related to compression of the nerve by vascular loops (Richards, Shawdon and Illingworth, 1983; Hamlyn and King, 1992). Operations to relieve this compression, first described by Gardner and Miklos (1959), are becoming commoner and do appear to be successful in a large proportion of cases. There is however a significant mortality rate and they are less successful if the vessel transfixes the nerve (Tashiro *et al.*, 1991).

Glossopharyngeal neuralgia

This condition was first described by Harris in 1921, occurs only about 1% as frequently as trigeminal neuralgia (Giorgi and Broggi, 1984) and is often a less discrete syndrome. The pain mainly affects the tonsil, root of tongue and ear and can be either lancinating or continuous. When paroxysmal, it usually lasts at most a minute but may be repeated for several hours without a break (Chawla and Falconer, 1967). The pain radiates in front of and into the ear and even down the neck and is often precipitated by swallowing. Patients may even become cachectic by trying to avoid the pain (Jennett and Galbraith, 1983). Frequently there is a trigger zone in the pharynx; if this is anaesthetized and the pain temporarily abolished then the diagnosis is established (Miles, 1987). Occasionally, attacks are accompanied by asystole, syncope and even convulsions and these are thought to include the vagus nerve (St. John, 1982). The trigeminal nerve can also be included (Rushton, Stevens and Miller, 1981) and some cases

are caused by carcinomatous infiltration of the glossopharyngeal nerve (Giorgi and Broggi, 1984).

Carbamazepine in doses from 100 mg b.d. to 200 mg q.d.s. will control the pain in many cases, but if this does not happen or control escapes then surgery is required. This may consist of section and avulsion of the glossopharyngeal nerve in the neck as first described by Sicard and Robineau in 1920, or section of the nerve in the posterior cranial fossa as first described by Dandy in 1927. Recurrence of pain is relatively common following these proceedures so Jennett and Galbraith (1983) suggested that the upper rootlets of the vagus nerve should also be divided as they carry sensory fibres to those areas in which the pain arises. Laha and Jannetta (1977) described compresssion of the glossopharyngeal nerve by tortuous vertebral or posterior inferior cerebellar vessels in a similar manner to those in trigeminal neuralgia and decompression again relieves the pain.

Intermedius (geniculate) neuralgia

This rare condition presents as severe, brief episodes of pain deep in the external auditory meatus. It may be relieved by dividing the nervus intermedius of Wrisberg (Harris, 1921). Attacks may be triggered by touching the meatus and a dull background pain may persist between attacks (Dubuisson, 1989a).

Carcinoma of the bronchus

In 1983, Des Prez and Freemon reported a patient who had had pain in the right ear and face for 4 months without satisfactory explanation. This pain had disappeared when he woke following removal of a carcinoma of the right lower lobe bronchus, which was encasing the vagus and phrenic nerves, which were sacrificed. There was no alteration in sensation in the face or ear postoperatively. Bindoff and Heseltine (1988) reported eight similar cases and Nestor (1991) one, all of whom had relief of pain after either radiotherapy or surgery for their lung tumours. Unrelieved pain had usually been present for several months before the diagnosis was made. Bindoff and Heseltine (1988) suggested that this pain is referred via the vagus to Arnold's nerve (Figure 13.2).

Cervical spine

In degenerative or neoplastic disease of the upper cervical spine, when C1, C2 or C3 roots are compressed or distorted, pain may be felt in the neck, occiput or mastoid area (Dubuisson, 1989b). The pinna, but not the meatus, and the lower border of the jaw may be affected on one or both sides, depending on the site and severity of the disease.

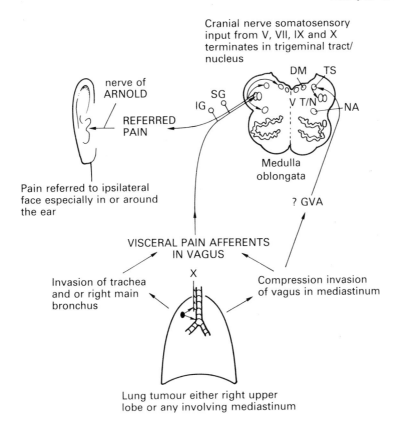

Figure 13.2 Schematic representation of how facial pain may be referred from an ipsilateral lung tumour. TS = tractus solitarius; NA = nucleus ambiguus; DM = dorsal motor nucleus of vagus; V T/N = trigeminal tract and nucleus; 0 = olivary nucleus; GVA = general visceral afferents; IG = inferior ganglion; SG = superior ganglion. (Reproduced with kind permission from the editor, *Lancet*)

Upper cervical or occipital migraine is usually associated with upper cervical root damage and causes either paroxysms of pain lasting from minutes to hours, or constant pain. Tenderness or hyperaesthesia in the occiput or over the mastoid region is sometimes present.

Migraine

Classical migraine with its aura, followed by a throbbing unilateral headache, associated with nausea, is easy to diagnose (Blau, 1991). Less clear cut are those cases where the temple or postauricular areas are involved (Delessio, 1989), and which may be preceded by tinnitus or rarely by auditory hallucinations. Again, the episodic nature with complete freedom from pain and lack of signs between attacks should confirm the diagnosis.

Periodic migrainous neuralgia

This was first described in 1936 by Harris and is also known as cluster headache, Horton's syndrome (Horton, 1956) or alarm clock neuralgia. It affects mainly men and the pain is usually severe and mainly retro-orbital. It can also be situated in the nose, cheek or spread into the ear or temple and is often associated with an ipsilateral red eye and blocked nose, and sometimes a Horner's syndrome. The attacks usually occur one to ten times daily for several weeks and then there is a period of freedom of months, they last from 30 minutes to 3 hours and mainly occur at night. Many patients will develop individual repetitive movements, e.g. kneeling and rocking, while holding the affected side of the head. These will separate this condition from other types of headache where the patient attempts to keep as still as possible (Blau, 1993). Effective prophylaxis can be obtained by ergot, pizotifen, methysergide or lithium.

Acoustic neuroma

'Pain, pressure or numbness around the ear are common complaints in acoustic tumours' (Ramsden, 1987). Moffat *et al.* (1989) in a series of 100 patients noted that 30% had otalgia as a secondary symptom and 25% had a dull ache in the mastoid region. These symptoms should be an added indication for examination of the patient with MRI.

Thalamic syndrome

The thalamic syndrome is usually caused by an infarct or tumour in the posterolateral thalamus, which produces a diminution in sensation on one side of the body. During recovery some patients will develop a peculiar unpleasant burning pain, often with additional grinding or tearing qualities (thalamic pain) most often felt in the side of the face and in the hand and foot on the affected side (Walton, 1987).

School avoidance

Occasionally an older child will be seen with recurrent earache necessitating absence from school. There is often a long history of previous, well documented ear infections, but in some cases when seen during an 'attack' the drums and hearing are perfectly normal. When this is pointed out to the child and parents, the excuse for school absence is lost and the problem usually resolves itself.

References

AKABOSHI, I., KATSUKI, T., JAMAMOTO, J. and MATSUDA, I. (1983) Unique pattern of Epstein-Barr virus specific antibodies in recurrent parotitis. *Lancet*, ii, 1049–1051

ALEKSIC, S., BUDZILOVICH, G. N. and LIEBERMANN, A. N. (1973) Herpes zoster oticus and facial paralysis. *Journal of Neurological Sciences*, **20**, 149–159

BADDOUR, H. M., MCANEAR, J. J. and TILSON, H. B. (1978) Eagle's syndrome: report of a case. *Oral Surgery, Oral Medicine, Oral Pathology*, **46**, 486–494

BAILEY, C. M. and WINDLE-TAYLOR, P. C. (1981) Tuberculous laryngitis: a series of 37 cases. *Laryngoscope*, **91**, 93–100

BALL, E. V. (1992) Behçet's disease. In: *Cecil Textbook of Medicine*, 19th edn, edited by J. B. Wyngarden, L. H. Smith and J. C. Bennett. Philadelphia: W. B. Saunders and Co. p. 1550

BEHÇET, H. (1937) Uber Rezidivierende Aphthose durch ein Virus verursachte Geschwure am Mund am Auge und an den Genitalien. *Dermatologie Wochenschrifte*, **36**, 1152–1157

BINDOFF, L. A. and HESELTINE, D. (1988) Unilateral facial pain in patients with lung cancer: A referred pain via the Vagus? *Lancet*, i, 812–815

BISSETT, W. M. (1992) The oral mucosa. In: *Forfar and Arneil's Textbook of Paediatrics*, 4th edn, edited by A. G. M. Campbell and N. McIntosh. Edinburgh: Churchill Livingstone. p. 493

BLAKE, P., THORBURN, D. N. and STEWART, I. A. (1982) Temporo-mandibular joint dysfunction in children presenting as otalgia. *Clinical Otolaryngology*, **7**, 237–244

BLAU, J. N. (1991) The clinical diagnosis of migraine: the beginning of therapy. *Journal of Neurology*, **238**, S6–11

BLAU, J. N. (1993) Behaviour during a cluster headache. *Lancet*, **342**, 723–725

BOWERS, P. W. and POWELL, R. J. (1983) Effect of thalidomide on orogenital ulceration. *British Medical Journal*, **287**, 779–780

BROOKES, G. B., MAW, R. A. and COLEMEN, M. J. (1980) Costen's syndrome – correlation or coincidence? *Clinical Otolaryngology*, **5**, 23–26

BRYHN, M. and HINDFELT, B. (1984) Ear pain due to myocardial ischaemia. *American Heart Journal*, **107**, 186–187

BULLITT, E., TEW, J. M. and BOYD, J. (1986) Intracranial tumours in patients with facial pain. *Journal of Neurosurgery*, **64**, 865–871

CHAWLA, J. C. and FALCONER, M. A. (1967) Glossopharyngeal and vagal neuralgia. *British Medical Journal*, **3**, 529–531

CLARK, J. (1979) Herpes zoster of the glossopharyngeal nerve. *Lancet*, i, 38–39

COLLINS, S. L. (1987) Management of the carotid artery and residual neck disease. In *Comprehensive Management of Head and Neck Tumours*, edited by S. E. Thawley and W. R. Panje. Philadelphia: W. B. Saunders. p. 1424

COSTEN, J. B. (1934) A syndrome of ear and sinus symptoms dependent upon disturbed function of the temporo-mandibular joint. *Annals of Otology, Rhinology and Laryngology*, **43**, 1–15

DANCE, D. A. B., DAVIS, T. M. E., WATTANAGOON, Y., CHAOWAGUL, W., SAIPHAN, P., LOOAREESUWAN, S. *et al.* (1989) Acute suppurative parotitis caused by *Pseudomonas pseudomallei* in children. *Journal of Infectious Diseases*, **159**, 654–660

DANDY, W. E. (1927) Glossopharyngeal neuralgia (tic douloureux). Its diagnosis and treatment. *Archives of Surgery*, **15**, 198–214

DANIELS, T. E. (1992) Oral ulceration. In: *Cecil Textbook of Medicine*, 19th edn, edited by J. B. Wyngarden, L. H. Smith and J. C. Bennett. Philadelphia: W. B. Saunders, pp. 635–636

DAWES, J. D. K. (1963) Virus lesions of the cranial nerves with special reference to the VIIIth nerve. *Proceedings of the Royal Society of Medicine*, **56**, 777–780

DEGROOT, L. J., LARSEN, P. R., REFETOFF, S. and STANBURY, J. B. (eds) (1984) Thyroiditis. In: *The Thyroid and its Diseases*, 5th edn. New York: John Wiley and Sons. pp. 717–731

DELESSIO, D. J. (1989) Headache. In: *Textbook of Pain*, 2nd edn, edited by P. D. Wall and R. Melzack. Edinburgh: Churchill Livingstone. pp. 392–396

DES PREZ, R. D. and FREEMON, F. R. (1983) Facial pain associated with lung cancer: a case report. *Headache*, **23**, 43–44

DUBUISSON, D. (1989a) Intermedius (geniculate) neuralgia. In: *Textbook of Pain*, 2nd edn, edited by P. D. Wall and R. Melzack. Edinburgh: Churchill Livingstone. pp. 545–546

DUBUISSON, D. (1989b) Nerve root damage and arachnoiditis. In: *Textbook of Pain*, 2nd edn, edited by P. D. Wall and R. Melzack. Edinburgh: Churchill Livingstone. pp. 437–438

EAGLE, W. W. (1937) Elongated styloid processes: report of two cases. *Archives of Otolaryngology*, **25**, 584–587

EAGLE, W. W. (1958) Elongated styloid process: symptoms and treatment. *Archives of Otolaryngology*, **67**, 172–176

EDWARDS, C. H. (1973) Other local causes of head and face pain. In: *Neurology of Ear, Nose and Throat Diseases*. London: Butterworths. pp. 59–60

ERICSON, S., ZETTERLUND, B. and OHMAN, J. (1991) Recurrent parotitis and sialectasia in childhood. *Annals of Otology, Rhinology and Laryngology*, **100**, 527–535

ESMANN, V., KROON, S. and BROWN, J. A. (1987) Prednisolone does not prevent post-herpetic neuralgia. *Lancet*, ii, 126–129

EVERY, R. C. (1960) The significance of extreme mandibular movement. *Lancet*, ii, 37–38

FEINMANN, C. and HARRIS, M. (1984) The diagnosis and management of psychogenic facial pain disorders. *Clinical Otolaryngology*, **9**, 199–201

FERGUSSON, R., BASN, M. K., ASQUITH, P. and COOKE, W. T. (1975) Jejunal abnormalities in patients with recurrent aphthous lesions. *British Medical Journal*, **1**, 11–13

FRADIS, M., PODOSHIN, L., BEN-DAVID, J. and GRISHKAN, A. (1985) Eosinophil granuloma of the temporal bone. *Journal of Laryngology and Otology*, **99**, 475–479

FREESTONE, D. S. and BRIGDEN, W. D. (1990) Acyclovir and post herpetic neuralgia. *Lancet*, **336**, 1279

GARDNER, D. L. (1986) Pathology of rheumatoid arthritis, the temporomandibular joint. In: *Copeman's Textbook of the Rheumatic Diseases*, 6th edn, edited by J. T. Scott. Edinburgh: Churchill Livingstone. p. 622

GARDNER, W. J. and MIKLOS, M. V. (1959) Response of trigeminal neuralgia to 'decompression' of sensory root. *Journal of the American Medical Association*, **170**, 1773–1776

GIORGI, C. and BROGGI, G. (1984) Surgical treatment of glossopharyngeal neuralgia and pain from carcinoma of the nasopharynx. *Journal of Neurosurgery*, **61**, 952–955

GRAY, H. (1989) Innervation of the ear. In: *Gray's Anatomy*, 37th edn, edited by: P.L. Williams, R. Warwick, M. Dyson and L. H. Bannister, London: Churchill Livingstone. pp. 1221–1222

HAMLYN, P. J. and KING, T. T. (1992) Neurovascular compression in trigeminal neuralgia: a clinical and anatomical study. *Journal of Neurosurgery*, **26**, 948–954

HARGREAVES, A. S. and WARDLE, J. J. M. (1983) The use of physiotherapy in the treatment of temporo-mandibular disorders. *British Dental Journal*, **155**, 121–124

HARRIS, W. (1921) Persistent pain in lesions of the peripheral and central nervous system. *Brain*, **44**, 557–571

HARRIS, W. (1936) Ciliary (migrainous) neuralgia and its treatment. *British Medical Journal*, **1**, 457–460

HORTON, B. T. (1956) Histamine cephalgia. *Journal of the American Medical Association*, **160**, 468–469

HOWE, G. L. (1983) Disorders of the masticatory apparatus. *British Dental Journal*, **155**, 405–411

HUFF, J. C., BEAN, B., BALFOUR, H. H., LASKIN, O. L., CONNOR, J. D., COREY, L. *et al.* (1988) Therapy of herpes zoster with oral acyclovir. *American Journal of Medicine*, **85**, (2A)84–89

HUNT, J. R. (1907) Herpetic inflammation of the geniculate ganglion. A new syndrome and its complications. *Journal of Nervous and Mental Diseases*, **34**, 73–96

JENNETT, B. and GALBRAITH, S. (1983) Glossopharyngeal neuralgia. In: *An Introduction to Neurosurgery*, 4th edn. London: Heinemann Medical Books Limited. pp. 344–345

JUEL-JENSEN, B. E., MACCALLUM, F. O., MACKENZIE, A. M. R. and PIKE, M. C. (1970) Treatment of zoster with idoxuridine

in dimethyl sulphoxide: results of two double-blind controlled trials. *British Medical Journal*, **4**, 776–780

KATZBERG, R. W. (1989) Temporomandibular joint imaging. *Radiology*, **170**, 297–307

KAUFMAN, S. M., ELZAY, R. P. and IRISH, E. F. (1970) Styloid process variation: radiologic and clinical study. *Archives of Otolaryngology*, **91**, 460–463

LAHA, R. K. and JANNETTA, P. J. (1977) Glossopharyngeal neuralgia. *Journal of Neurosurgery*, **47**, 316–332

LANCET (1984) Management of trigeminal neuralgia. i, 662–663

LANCET (1986) The painful thyroid. i, 1308–1309

LANCET (1990) Post herpetic neuralgia. **336**, 537–538

LANCET (1992) Burden of tuberculosis worldwide. **340**, 1403

LAST, R. J. (1984) Innervation of the ear. In: *Anatomy*, 7th edn. Edinburgh: Churchill Livingstone. pp. 451–460

LEHNER, T. (1968) Autoimmunity in oral disease with special reference to recurrent oral ulceration. *Proceedings of the Royal Society of Medicine*, **61**, 515–524

LENGELE, B. G. and DHEM, A. J. (1988) Length of the styloid process of the temporal bone. *Archives of Otolaryngology*, **114**, 1003–1006

LEWIS, M. A. O., LAMEY, P-J. and GIBON, J. (1989) Quantitative bacteriology of a case of acute parotitis. *Oral Surgery, Oral Medicine, Oral Pathology*, **68**, 571–575

LOESER, L. H. and CARDWELL, E. P. (1942) Elongated styloid process. A cause of glossopharyngeal neuralgia. *Archives of Otolaryngology*, **36**, 198–202

LUNDEBERG, T., OTTOSON, D., HAKANSSON, S. and MEYERSON, B. A. (1983) Vibratory stimulation for the control of chronic orofacial pain. In: *Advances in Pain Research and Therapy*, edited by J. J. Bonica. New York: Raven Press. pp. 555–561

LUNDGREN, A., KYLEN, P. and ODKVIST, L. M. (1976) Nosocomial parotitis. *Acta Otolaryngologica*, **82**, 275–278

MCCAIN, J. P., DE LA RUA, H. and LEBLANC, W. G. (1989) Correlation of clinical, radiographic and arthroscopic findings in internal derangements of the TMJ. *Journal of Oral and Maxillofacial Surgery*, **47**, 913–921

MCDOUGALL, I. R. (1990) Sub-acute thyroiditis. In: *Thyroid Disease in Clinical Practice*. London: Chapman and Hall. pp. 263–268

MCKENDRICK, M. W., MCGILL, J. I. and WOOD, M. J. (1989) Lack of effect of acyclovir on postherpetic neuralgia. *British Medical Journal*, **298**, 431

MANNI, H. (1983) Laryngeal tuberculosis in Tanzania. *Journal of Laryngology and Otology*, **97**, 565–570

MARBACH, J. J., LENNON, M. C. and DOHRENWEND, B. P. (1988) Candidate risk factors for temporomandibular pain and dysfunction syndrome: psychosocial, health behaviour, physical illness and injury. *Pain*, **34**, 139–151

MELZACK, R. and WALL, P. D. (1965) Pain mechanisms: a new theory. *Science*, **150**, 971–979

MILES, J. B. (1987) Glossopharyngeal neuralgia. In: *Northfield's Surgery of the Central Nervous System*, 2nd edn, edited by J. D. Miller. Edinburgh: Blackwell Scientific Publications. pp. 678–679

MOFFATT, D. A., BAGULEY, D., EVANS, R. A. and HARDY, D. G. (1989) Mastoid ache in acoustic neuroma. *Journal of Laryngology and Otology*, **103**, 1043–1044

MORTON, P. and THOMSON, A. N. (1989) Oral acyclovir in the treatment of herpes zoster in general practice. *New Zealand Medical Journal*, **102**, 93–95

MUMFORD, J. M. (1987) Trigeminal neuralgia and possible orofacial causes. *Hospital Update*, March, 231–238

NATHAN, P. W. and WALL, P. D. (1974) Treatment of post-herpetic neuralgia by prolonged electrical stimulation. *British Medical Journal*, **3**, 645–647

NESTOR, J. J. (1991) Unilateral facial pain in lung cancer. *Lancet*, ii, 1149

NORMAN, J. E. DE B. (1982) Post-traumatic disorders of the jaw joint. *Annals of the Royal College of Surgeons of England*, **64**, 29–36

NURMIKKO, T. and BOWSHER, D. (1990) Somatosensory findings in postherpetic neuralgia. *Journal of Neurology, Neurosurgery and Psychiatry*, **53**, 135–141

PARADISE, J. L., BLUESTONE, C. D., BACKMAN, R. Z., COLBORN, D. K., BERNARD, B. S., TAYLOR, F. H. *et al.* (1984) Efficacy of tonsillectomy for recurrent throat infections in severely affected children. *New England Journal of Medicine*, **310**, 674–683

PAINTON, S. W. and SHAW, M. B. (1988) Aural pain resulting from acoustic reflex. *Annals of Otology, Rhinology and Laryngology*, **97**, 131–132

PRUETT, T. L. and SIMMONS, R. L. (1984) Nosocomial gram-negative, bacillary parotitis. *Journal of the American Medical Association*, **251**, 252–253

RAMSDEN, R. T. (1987) Acoustic tumours. In: *Scott Brown's Otolaryngology*, 5th edn, edited by A. G. Kerr, vol. 3 *Otology*, edited by J. B. Booth, London: Butterworths. pp. 500–533

RICHARDS, P., SHAWDON, H. and ILLINGWORTH, R. (1983) Operative findings on microsurgical exploration of the cerebello-pontine angle in trigeminal neuralgia. *Journal of Neurology, Neurosurgery, and Psychiatry*, **46**, 1098–1101

RUSHTON, J. G., STEVENS, J. C. and MILLER, R. H. (1981) Glossopharyngeal (vagoglossopharyngeal) neuralgia. A study of 217 cases. *Archives of Neurology*, **38**, 201–205

RUSSELL, T. E. (1977) Eagle's syndrome: diagnosis and report of a case. *Journal of the American Dental Association*, **93**, 548–550

ST JOHN, J. N. (1982) Glossopharyngeal neuralgia associated with syncope and seizure. *Neurosurgery*, **10**, 380–383

SCULLY, C. (1989) Management of aphthous ulcers. In: *The Mouth and Perioral Tissues*. Vol.2 of *Clinical Dentistry in Health and Disease*, edited by C. Scully and R. A. Cawson, Oxford: Heinemann Medical Books. pp. 164–165

SCULLY, C. and CAWSON, R. A. (eds) (1987) Ankylosing spondylitis. In: *Medical Problems in Dentistry*, 2nd edn. Bristol: Wright P. S. G. p. 307

SHARAV, Y. (1989) Orofacial pain. In: *Textbook of Pain*, 2nd edn, edited by P. D. Wall and R. Melzack, Edinburgh: Churchill Livingstone. pp. 441–454

SICARD, R. and ROBINEAU, M. (1920) Algie velo-pharyngée essentielle. Traitment chirugical. *Revue Neurologique*, **36**, 256–257

SODA, A., RUBIO, H., SALAZAR, M., GANEM, J., BERLANGER, D. and SANCHEZ, A. (1989) Tuberculosis of the larynx – clinical aspects in 19 patients. *Laryngoscope*, **99**, 1145–1150

STEVENSON, J. (1990) Acute bacterial thyroiditis presenting as otalgia. *Journal of Laryngology and Otology*, **105**, 788–789

STRAUSS, M., ZOHAR, Y. and LAURIAN, N. (1985) Elongated styloid process syndrome: intra-oral versus external approach for styloid surgery. *Laryngoscope*, **95**, 976–979

SWEET, W. H. and WEPSIC, J. G. (1974) Controlled thermo-coagulation of trigeminal ganglion and rootlets for differ-ential destruction of pain fibres. *Journal of Neurosurgery*, **40**, 143–156

SYME, W. S. (1915) Abnormally long styloid process causing throat symptoms. *Journal of Laryngology*, **30**, 303–304

TASHIRO, H., KONDO, A., AOYAMA, I., NIN, K., SHIMOTAKE, K., NISHIOKA, T. *et al.* (1991) Trigeminal neuralgia caused by compression from arteries transfixing the nerve. *Journal of Neurosurgery*, **75**, 783–786

TAVERNER, D. (1960) Alleviation of post-herpetic neuralgia. *Lancet*, ii, 671–673

THOMSON, H. (1959) Mandibular joint pain: a survey of 100 treated cases. *British Dental Journal*, **107**, 243–251

TILLEY, H. (1919) Tuberculosis of the larynx. In: *Diseases of the Nose and Throat*, 4th edn. London: H. K. Lewis & Co Ltd. pp. 629–650

TROBE. J. D., HOOD, I., PARSONS, J. T. and QUISLING, R. G. (1982) Intracranial spread of squamous carcinoma along the trigeminal nerve. *Archives of Ophthalmology*, **100**, 608–611

TROTTER, W. (1926) The surgery of malignant disease of the pharynx. *British Medical Journal*, **1**, 269–272

TYLDESLEY, W. R. (1989a) Recurrent oral ulceration. In: *Oral Medicine*, 3rd. edn. Oxford: Oxford Medical Publications. pp. 70–82

TYLDESLEY, W. R. (1989b) The temporomandibular joint. In: *Oral Medicine*, 3rd. edn. Oxford: Oxford Medical Publications. pp. 221–226

VERRILL, P. (1990) Does the gate theory of pain supplant all others? *British Journal of Hospital Medicine*, **43**, 325

WALTON, J. N. (ed.) (1985a) Referred pain. In: *Brain's Diseases of the Nervous System*, 9th edn. Oxford: Oxford University Press. pp. 598–599

WALTON, J. N. (ed.) (1985b) Trigeminal neuralgia. In: *Brain's Diseases of the Nervous System*, 9th edn. Oxford: Oxford University Press. pp. 110–112

WALTON, J. N. (1987) Thalamic syndrome. In: *Introduction to Clinical Neuroscience*, 2nd edn. London: Ballière Tindall. pp. 201–202

WATSON, C. P., EVANS, R. J., REED, K., MERKSEY, H., GOLDSMITH, L. and WARSH, J. (1982) Amitriptyline versus placebo in postherpetic neuralgia. *Neurology*, **32**, 671–673

WATSON, C. P., EVANS, R. J. and WATTS, V. R. (1988) Post-herpetic neuralgia and topical capsaicin. *Pain*, **33**, 333–340

WATSON, C. P., MORSHEAD, C., VAN DERKOOY, D., DECK, J. and EVANS, R. J. (1988) Post-herpetic neuralgia: post-mortem analysis of a case. *Pain*, **34**, 129–138

WRAY, D. (1984) Aphthous ulceration. *Journal of the Royal Society of Medicine*, **77**, 1–3

WRAY, D., GRAYKOWSKI, E. A. and NOTKINS, A. L. (1981) Role of mucosal injury in initiation of recurrent aphthous stomatitis. *British Medical Journal*, **283**, 1569–1570

YAZICI, H., PAZARLI, H., BARNES, C. G., TUZUN, Y., OZYAGAN, Y., SILMAN, A. *et al.* (1990) A controlled trial of azothioprine in Behçet's syndrome. *New England Journal of Medicine*, **322**, 281–285

ZIMMERMANN, R. S., BRENNAN, M. D., MCCONAHEY, W. M., GOELLNER, J. R. and GHARIB, H. (1986) Hashimoto's thyroiditis: an uncommon cause of painful thyroid unresponsive to corticosteroid therapy. *Annals of Internal Medicine*, **104**, 355–357

14

Otosclerosis

Gordon D. L. Smyth †

The bone of the otic or labyrinthine capsule may be affected by many conditions of diverse aetiology and the majority of these are generalized diseases affecting the skeletal system as well as the temporal bone.

Otosclerosis is confined to the otic capsule and gives rise to deafness and vestibular symptoms.

Definition

Otosclerosis is an hereditary localized disease of the bone derived from the otic capsule characterized by alternating phases of bone resorption and formation. Mature lamellar bone is removed by osteoclasis and replaced by woven bone of greater thickness, cellularity and vascularity. The characteristic lesion is a deposit of new bone with a different fibrillar and cellular pattern which is laid down at certain sites in the temporal bone. Known sites of predilection are the oval and round windows, in areas where cartilaginous rests are normally found.

The otosclerotic focus may be asymptomatic or, if in the area of the stapes footplate, may give rise to ankylosis and conductive deafness. Other parts of the labyrinthine capsule may be involved, resulting in sensorineural deafness and vestibular abnormalities. The focus is believed to produce enzymes which may give rise to these symptoms, whether or not the stapes footplate is affected. A combination of effects may thus be produced by the otosclerotic lesion, sometimes referred to as 'histological', 'stapedial', 'cochlear' and 'combined otosclerosis'. The commonest manifestation seen clinically is of the combined variety where there is both a conductive and sensorineural hearing loss.

Many European otologists use the term 'otospongiosis' when referring to the active vascular focus, but in North America and in the UK the term 'otosclero-sis' is used and this refers to the final inactive stage of the lesion where the bone is sclerotic or hardened; neither of these terms is strictly accurate.

History

The first description of ankylosis of the stapes is attributed to Antonio Valsalva who, in 1741, carried out a post-mortem examination on the body of a patient who was believed to be deaf (Politzer, 1907). In 1861, Joseph Toynbee noted ankylosis of the stapes footplate in 39 out of a total of 1959 temporal bone dissections.

In 1894, Adam Politzer introduced the term 'otosclerosis' and gave the first account of the histopathology of this condition. He described bony deposits developing in and around the stapes footplate, leading to its progressive ankylosis in the oval window niche and a progressive conductive deafness.

Siebenmann introduced the term 'otospongiosis' in 1912, which referred to the active and vascular stage of the process and this term is widely used in Europe. It is more accurate as it indicates that an active lesion may be present. The belief that the process is inactive, or soon becomes so, has delayed understanding that sensorineural deafness is often an integral part of the disease. Politzer's work was of fundamental importance as he demonstrated, for the first time, that the stapedial ankylosis was not secondary to 'chronic middle ear catarrh', but was the result of a primary disease of the labyrinthine capsule. It was not until nearly 50 years later, when the fenestration operation allowed direct inspection of the oval window in the living patient, that the concept of a chronic catarrhal condition causing secondary fixation of the stapes footplate, was finally abandoned.

Aetiology

Otosclerosis is a disorder affecting the growth of collagen and it is seen only in the human species. Despite intensive research, the cause of the development of the disease process remains obscure.

Many theories of the aetiology of otosclerosis have been proposed and these include metabolic and immune disorders, vascular disease, infection, trauma, and anatomical and histological anomalies of the temporal bone.

Several aetiological theories relate to the presence of unstable rests of embryonic cartilage within the labyrinthine capsule and fissurae, and it has been proposed that enzyme activity derived from inflammatory monocytes recruited by an immune reaction in these rests, results in otospongiotic changes. Yoo (1984) has measured elevated levels of antitype II collagen antibodies in patients with otosclerosis and in otosclerotic-like lesions in rats induced by type II collagen immunization. Petrovic, Stutzmann and Shambaugh (1985) hypothesized that, in the absence of physiological tissue renewal (characteristic of the otic capsule), cell degeneration in labyrinthine bone produces antigens to which certain possibly genetically predisposed individuals have intolerance. More recent research suggests a possible relationship between prior infection with the measles virus and later development of clinical otosclerosis (Arnold and Friedmann, 1988). A more detailed antigen study of 24 otosclerotic stapes removed at surgery failed to detect any viral antibodies (Roald *et al.*, 1992). Although histological studies of focal changes in otosclerosis have shown features in common with bone dystrophies, such as Paget's disease and osteogenesis imperfecta, studies of the mineral content of the temporal bone and ossicles have shown variable results. Jensen, Neilson and Elbrond (1979) reported a study of the mineral content of skeletal bone in patients with and without otosclerosis and showed no difference between the two groups. This work supports the assumption that otosclerosis is a localized disease of the labyrinthine capsule.

Incidence

Guild (1944) first pointed out the importance of making a distinction between clinical and non-clinical, or histological otosclerosis; the latter is about 10 times more common than the former. The results of other workers (Weber, 1935; Engstrom, 1940; Soifer *et al*, 1970; Huer *et al.*, 1991) supported those of Guild, giving an incidence of histological otosclerosis of up to 13% in white adults but much less in the African races. Friedmann (1974) has estimated that 2% of all white persons suffer from deafness caused by otosclerosis. This incidence is identical to that more recently reported in a large population study of adults in the UK (Browning and Gatehouse, 1991). Shambaugh (1949) in North America estimated the frequency of otosclerosis to be at least 0.5%.

The variation in the figures produced by different authorities makes it obvious that the true incidence of the disease is unknown. In recent years, it has become quite clear that the number of patients seen in clinics and operated on by stapedectomy has fallen dramatically and this is unlikely to be the result of patients failing to attend for treatment as the results of surgery are good and widely known to be highly successful. The most likely explanation is that the original pool of patients has been reduced by energetic otologists, keen to operate on those patients who came to them with a conductive deafness caused by otosclerosis. Greater stringency in the selection of patients suitable for operation is also likely to have been contributory. If the measles virus is confirmed as an aetiological agent, the effect of vaccination on the incidence of otosclerosis may already be in progress.

Racial incidence

Otosclerosis is most frequently encountered in the Caucasian races and is a common cause of hearing loss in Europe, the Balkans, the Middle East, and the subcontinent of India, together with the Caucasian peoples of North and South America, Australia, New Zealand, South Africa and elsewhere. It is rarely found in Mongoloid or Negroid men, although it is encountered in the Black population of America and the West Indies, presumably as a consequence of hybridization. In the latter group, the disease is about 10 times less frequent than among Caucasians (Morrison, 1967).

The disease also occurs, less frequently, in the Negrito populations of Malaya, New Guinea and the Philippines, and in the Japanese, a mixed race of Mongul, Ainu and Negrito blood (Joseph and Fraser, 1964).

Sex incidence

In clinical practice, otosclerosis is seen more often in women than men, and a sex ratio of 2:1 has been noted by many authorities. However, the incidence is likely to be the same in both sexes, although hormonal influences may cause the disease to advance more rapidly in women. This is confirmed in histological reports where bilateral otosclerosis is more frequent in women (Huer *et al.*, 1991) and in clinical population reports where the incidence was similar, but women were three times more likely to have an air–bone gap of 30 dB or greater (Browning and Gatehouse, 1992). Asymmetric deafness caused by otosclerosis is more common in men and those working in a noisy environment are less likely to be aware of this because of the phenomenon of paracusis.

Genetic factors

Although Toynbee (1861) noticed the familial pattern of deafness and ear disease, it was not until nearly a century later that a comprehensive investigation into the genetics of otosclerosis was conducted by Larsson (1962). Larsson carried out a field investigation into 357 otosclerotic families between 1956 and 1958. His analysis pointed to a simple autosomal dominant inheritance with incomplete 'penetrance' or manifestation.

Larsson's views were confirmed by Morrison (1979) who concluded that otosclerosis, like osteogenesis imperfecta, belonged to a group of hereditary disorders of collagen, with a similar mode of inheritance, incomplete manifestation, varying degrees of expressivity, and possibly an abnormal enzyme system (Figure 14.1).

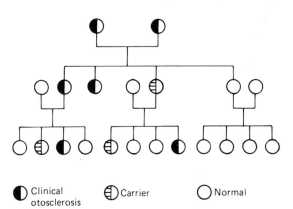

Figure 14.1 Inheritance of otosclerosis. Diagrammatic representation of a typical family tree. Dominant inheritance with manifestation of clinical otosclerosis in half the expected ratio. 'Carriers' can transmit the disease

Age of onset of hearing impairment

Symptoms rarely become apparent before the late teens and are very uncommon before the age of 5 years.

The rate of progression is variable and there are periods of extension alternating with quiescent phases in some patients, while in others the progress of the disease continues relentlessly and, in a small proportion, may be rapid. During periods of endocrine activity, such as pregnancy and the menopause, the disease may progress; in the majority of patients, signs of hearing loss are complained of between the ages of 20 and 30 years, but sometimes not until 50 years of age or even later.

The effect of prolonged exposure to industrial noise on patients with otosclerosis

Alberti *et al.* (1980) reported on the results of an investigation of 135 cases of otosclerosis among men referred for compensation for industrial deafness, all of whom had been exposed to high level industrial noise for a prolonged period of time. When compared to cases without otosclerosis, following similar exposure, both groups showed the typical audiogram of high frequency sensorineural hearing loss associated with acoustic trauma. Most otologists who are experienced in examining patients with industrial deafness will have noticed that the bone conduction audiograms of patients with a marked conductive loss probably caused by otosclerosis, show a high frequency sensorineural deafness which is typical of noise-induced hearing loss. The explanation of this phenomenon is that it is likely that the person was exposed to damaging levels which gave rise to the sensorineural deafness before the conductive loss developed. The conductive loss developed later and so the audiometric pattern is the combined result of the otosclerosis and the noise deafness present when the person was younger. As otosclerosis may also give rise to sensorineural deafness it can be difficult to arrive at a definite conclusion from the medicolegal point of view.

It is inconceivable that a marked conductive deafness does not protect the individual from the damaging effects of a high level of industrial noise (McShane *et al.*, 1991), although it is also possible that otosclerosis may make the cochlea of the affected person more sensitive to the damaging effects of noise in the early stages of the disease with minimal hearing loss.

Otosclerosis and pregnancy

In 1967, Shambaugh studied 475 mothers who had received surgical treatment by the fenestration operation. He found that 50% had not observed any noticeable effect on their hearing from any of the pregnancies but, in 42%, there was an associated increase in hearing loss. He estimated the risk of increased hearing loss from any one pregnancy in a woman with stapedial otosclerosis to be about one in 24. Elbrond and Jensen (1979) studied the influence of pregnancy on the hearing threshold, before and after stapedectomy, and found that the operation afforded some protection from further hearing loss.

Gristwood and Venables (1975) studied 479 women who were deaf from otosclerosis. They found that in bilateral cases, pregnancy aggravated the deafness and this incidence ranged from 33% after one, to 63% after six pregnancies. In unilateral cases, it was found that the pregnancy-related deterioration of hearing was much less common.

Site of otosclerosis in the temporal bone

Although any part of the bony labyrinth may be affected by otosclerosis, the most common site is between the anterior part of the stapedial footplate, the processus cochleariformis and the bulge of the promontory (Figure 14.2).

About 85% of lesions are situated in the oval window area. The focus extends, infiltrates and reduces the mobility of the footplate in the oval window niche and eventually firm bony ankylosis results. It is more common for the new bone to affect the anterior part of the footplate leaving the centre free. Less frequently, the focus originates in the footplate itself and as it expands gives rise to the 'biscuit' or 'rice-grain' footplate with delineated margins. Less frequently still, a large mass of new bone fills the oval window niche and totally obscures the footplate, a condition termed 'obliterative otosclerosis' (Figure 14.3). The second most common site for the focus is in the region of the round window, and here, evidence of otosclerosis has been found in up to 50% of cases.

In the majority of cases (70–80%) both temporal bones are affected, and a characteristic feature of the disease is the striking similarity of the localization and extent of the lesion in the two ears.

Although both temporal bones are usually affected, unilateral otosclerosis has been described by various authorities as occurring in 10–15% of patients with this disease (Nager, 1939; Cawthorne, 1955).

Obliterative otosclerosis

In this condition the oval window is filled with a mass of unusually dense new bone. The footplate rim cannot be identified and the crura are often enveloped. Frequently, conductive hearing loss becomes apparent during childhood or adolescence. Gristwood (1966) has reported obliterative otosclerosis in 30% of operated patients and attributes this high incidence to low levels of fluorine in South Australian drinking water. In Europe and North America a lower incidence (10%) is usually cited.

Histopathology of otosclerosis

Although it is usual on light microscopy to describe several stages, there is no orderly progression from one to another and it is a feature of the otosclerotic lesion that one focus may contain areas at different stages of activity. The stages may be described as active, intermediate, and inactive (final stage).

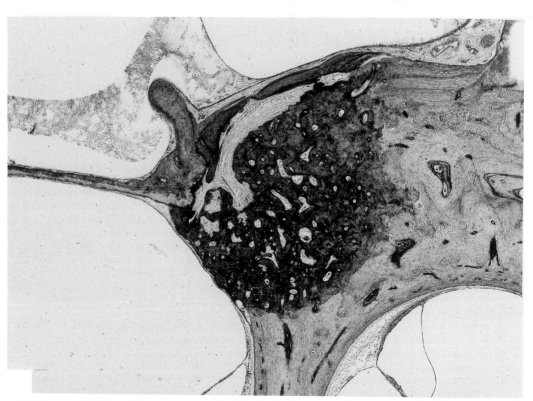

Figure 14.2 Otosclerotic fixation of the stapes at site of predilection in the oval window niche (reproduced by permission of Y. Murakami and H. F. Schuknecht and the Editor of *Archives of Otolaryngology*)

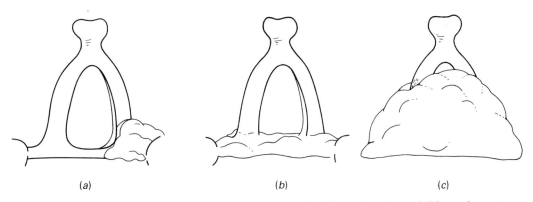

Figure 14.3 Types of oval window otosclerosis. (*a*) Rim fixation anteriorly; (*b*) biscuit footplate with delineated margins; (*c*) obliterative otosclerosis

The term 'otospongiosis' refers to the active phase of the disease and the characteristic feature is the presence of vascular spaces containing highly cellular fibrous tissue. Mononuclear histiocytes together with osteocytes and osteoclasts are prominent. These cells contain a large number of enzymes which are expelled into the surrounding tissue resulting in its absorption (Bretlau *et al.*, 1982). A clearly defined boundary between normal and abnormal bone is a feature. There may be finger-like processes, which are spaces produced by resorption of perivascular bone. These spaces become filled with projections of remodelled bone along and around blood vessels which are sometimes referred to as 'blue mantles'. These are also seen in chronic mastoiditis and other bone diseases (Friedmann, 1974), but Weber (1935) believed that the 'blue bone' was abnormal and otosclerotic foci might be formed through its fusion.

The term 'otosclerosis' refers to the final stage consisting of highly mineralized bone with a mosaic appearance. Osteoclasts have disappeared but osteocytes and/or osteoblasts may still be seen in the peripheral areas. The vascular spaces are narrowed, or obliterated, by new bone formation and the lamellar bone which is formed is thicker and more cellular when compared to normal bone.

As has been stated previously, there is no orderly development from the active to the inactive stage and all stages may be seen together in one focus which may become quiescent or reactivated at any time.

Clinical features

Deafness

The typical features of otosclerotic deafness are a bilateral, gradually increasing hearing loss, most frequently occurring between the third and fifth decade, the presence of paracusis and tinnitus.

The deafness is often unnoticed by the patient until the loss reaches 25–30 dB, when difficulty in understanding speech becomes apparent. The patient may remark that the hearing is better in the presence of background noise. This phenomenon (paracusis Willisii) is frequently present if there is a predominantly conductive deafness without a sensorineural loss. One explanation of this is that, in general, people with normal hearing raise their voices above the noise level, so that they can overcome the masking effects of the noise, and this level of speech sound is above the threshold of the patient with conductive deafness. Although paracusis is seen in other forms of conductive deafness, it is most often seen in stapedial fixation caused by otosclerosis.

The patient with otosclerotic deafness has a characteristically quiet voice, of good tone, and the change in speech pattern may be detected by close relatives who often notice the hearing loss before the patient becomes aware of it. The deafness is generally progressive, occurring in a direct linear form; alternatively there may be a plateau-like period, or both features may occur together.

The hearing loss may be almost equal in each ear but often one ear shows a greater loss, and this ratio is usually maintained. Unilateral otosclerosis occurs in approximately 15% of patients. The deafness can remain confined to one ear, or the second ear may become affected later. Many patients with a pure conductive loss will, in later years, develop a sensorineural deafness that is greater than that to be expected as the result of ageing.

Tinnitus

Tinnitus is a common symptom and occasionally the presenting feature. It is sometimes seen in patients without cochlear degeneration when it is the result of an abnormal degree of vascularity of the otosclerotic bone; more often, tinnitus is an indication of sensorineural degeneration.

Tinnitus may be unilateral or bilateral, and of a roaring, hissing or pulsatile character. Fluctuation of tinnitus is not uncommon and this can be related to metabolic and endocrine disturbances, pregnancy or menstruation. It is more common in the early stages of the disease and it may disappear as the lesion matures and the spongy vascular bone is replaced by the hard sclerotic bone.

Vertigo

Attacks of dysequilibrium, usually of a transient nature, are not uncommon, and they are possibly the result of the action of toxic enzymes, which are liberated by the lesion, on the vestibular labyrinth (Causse *et al.*, 1977a). A variety of vestibular symptoms have been described in otosclerosis and the most common is true benign positional vertigo (Colman, 1979). If vertigo occurs, although it may be due to vestibular hydrops secondary to capsular otosclerosis, or involvement of the vestibular aqueduct (Franklin, Pollak and Fisch, 1990; Yoon, Paparella and Schachern, 1990), the coexistence of Menière's disease must also be considered, as both disorders are common and will be seen from time to time in the same patient.

When taking a history, former episodes of ear disease, head injury, exposure to noise, administration of ototoxic drugs, bone or joint disease must be enquired into, as these factors may be of importance in diagnosis and management.

Morrison (1979) has called attention to the importance of a detailed family history in the assessment of the prognosis when other members of the family are affected.

Diagnosis

Examination

The examination of the tympanic membranes will include inspection at rest, and testing with a Siegle's speculum for mobility. The tympanic membranes in otosclerotic patients are sometimes described as being in 'mint condition' but they may be atrophic, thickened, rigid or immobile due to prior inflammatory disease. The 'flamingo flush', or Schwartze sign, is uncommon. It is said to be a result of vascular bone on the promontory, or prominent blood vessels in the submucosal layer of the mucous membrane of the promontory. When seen, it may indicate active disease which might progress rapidly.

In every case, examination of the nose, nasopharynx and nasal accessory sinuses is necessary to exclude infection, which may need treatment.

Clinical assessment of hearing loss

A rapid estimation of the hearing loss is made in the clinic by simple speech tests, using conversational and whispered voice, using a Bárány noise box to mask the other ear, the effect of trying a hearing aid, and

tuning fork tests. Patients with otosclerosis do not usually show recruitment and are able to hear amplified sounds clearly, unless there is a marked sensorineural deafness.

The tuning fork tests, which will include the Rinne, Weber and Schwabach tests, must be carried out before the more complex tests of auditory function are performed. They are of particular value in two instances:

1 When there is a predominantly unilateral otosclerosis, with poor bone conduction simulating sensorineural deafness. Here the Weber test will show lateralization to the deaf side.
2 When there is a severe combined (stapedial and cochlear) otosclerosis where the bone conduction cannot be recorded as there is more than 60 dB hearing loss (which is beyond the limit for the majority of clinical audiometers). If the Rinne test is negative with a 256 Hz tuning fork and the patient's voice has reasonable quality, good results can still nevertheless be obtained from operation (Morrison, 1979).

Audiometric testing is the most important method of evaluating the otosclerotic patient. Pure tone audiometry will establish the degree of hearing disability and the suitability of treatment, either by surgical means or by amplification. However, difficulties can arise in the assessment when hearing loss is relatively minor or when both ears are affected. For guidance in the avoidance of misleading and false information, the reader should see Volume 2, Chapter 12. When clinical and audiometric findings indicate that a conductive or mixed hearing loss may not be due to otosclerosis, radiological examination is mandatory to detect conditions such as Paget's disease or vestibular schwannoma. Details of appropriate investigations will be found in Chapter 2.

Differential diagnosis

The diagnosis of otosclerosis is usually straightforward and is made on the history of progressive hearing loss, often bilateral, an intact mobile tympanic membrane and evidence of conductive deafness. Evidence of similar symptoms and possibly an ear operation in relatives should be enquired for. The possibility that a conductive hearing loss has a cause other than otosclerosis must always be considered. Otosclerosis should also be considered in the differential diagnosis of sensorineural deafness.

Middle ear lesions

Secretory otitis media (otitis media with effusion)

This is a common condition giving rise to a conductive hearing loss which may persist for many years. Tinnitus and vertigo are usually absent and careful examination of the tympanic membrane shows loss of translucency – fluid may or may not be seen. The tympanogram is usually typical in this condition (see Figure 1.30) and a plain X-ray of the mastoids will show haziness or reduced pneumatization. In a comparison between healthy controls and patients with clinical otosclerosis, Sadé *et al.* (1989) have shown a link between otosclerosis and extensive mastoid pneumatization. In adults, secretory otitis media is often unilateral and may be associated with a lesion in the postnasal space.

Middle ear fibrosis (chronic adhesive process)

In this condition, the tympanic membrane may appear normal, but it is usually retracted, or thickened, and show lack of mobility and one or all of the ossicles may also be affected. A tympanogram and mastoid X-rays will establish the diagnosis.

Tympanosclerosis

Tympanosclerosis, with only minor changes in the tympanic membrane, may result in a severe conductive deafness if the deposits immobilize the stapes, or the malleus and incus. Tympanometry will show reduced compliance and an X-ray may show lack of translucency of the mastoid air cells.

Congenital footplate fixation

It is important to recognize this condition as stapedectomy carries a risk of perilymph flooding ('gusher') and a consequent sensorineural hearing loss. Deafness from this cause is not progressive but the audiogram with an up-sloping curve and best air conduction at 2 kHz is strongly suggestive (Cremers, Hombergen and Wentges, 1983). If the condition is bilateral, speech will be affected. Unilateral cases are usually diagnosed in late childhood or early adult life.

Ossicular discontinuity

Traumatic dislocation of the incus is seen after injuries. It is not uncommon as a result of road traffic accidents where the injuries are severe with loss of consciousness, and bleeding from the ear and not infrequently facial palsy. Less commonly, traumatic dislocation of the incus also occurs after minor head injuries. A blow on the ear, or an unskilful attempt to remove a foreign body when it is pushed through the tympanic membrane, may also lead to dislocation.

Tympanometry is of importance in the diagnosis of these lesions and it will show an absent stapedial reflex, an abnormal compliance and low impedance system (see Figure 1.31).

Polytomography may demonstrate ossicular chain abnormalities, but radiography cannot be relied upon if there is only a very small gap, even though the hearing loss may be profound (see Figure 2.30).

Tympanotomy will often be required to make the exact diagnosis, but it is essential for the otologist to recognize the presence of these lesions, as in most cases stapedectomy is not indicated and the deafness will be treated by some form of ossiculoplasty. It should also be remembered that injury can also result in ossicular fixation.

Malleus and incus lesions

The fixed malleus–incus syndrome

This lesion was described by Goodhill in 1960, and Morrison (1979) found it in 2% of tympanotomies.

In this condition, there is stiffness, or fixation, of the malleus, incus, or both, but the stapes is not immediately involved. This lesion may be missed if the surgeon who has made a diagnosis of otosclerosis proceeds to remove the stapes without a preliminary testing of the mobility of the malleus and incus. Following stapedectomy there will be no improvement in hearing and this is attributed to a failure of the stapedectomy.

Tympanometry may help to distinguish this lesion and if the mobility of the ossicular chain is tested at every operation, a wrong surgical procedure will be avoided.

Congenital cholesteatoma

A primary cholesteatoma may occur behind an intact tympanic membrane, producing a conductive deafness. Careful examination of the drum with magnification will usually reveal this condition before operation. Tympanotomy and removal of the cholesteatoma with or without mastoidectomy, depending on its extent, with, if necessary, ossicular chain reconstruction will be required.

Fluid in the middle ear: cerebrospinal fluid or perilymph

The most common cause of fluid in the middle ear is secretory otitis media and this has already been described.

A patient at operation for otosclerosis may show the presence of clear fluid in the middle ear and this fills up again after aspiration. The fluid may be cerebrospinal fluid, the result of a fracture of the tegmen tympani caused by a previous head injury, or via congenital communications between the subarachnoid and mastoid air cell systems (Hyrtl's fistula).

Alternatively, fluid accumulating in the middle ear may be perilymph leaking from the scala vestibuli when there has been a fracture or dislocation of the stapes. Rupture of the round window membrane usually heals spontaneously but this does not always occur and perilymph can leak from an unsuspected fistula of both round and oval windows due to rapidly developing implosive and explosive forces affecting the labyrinthine fluids. Fistula of the oval or round windows also occurs in association with the Mondini deformity and with congenital middle ear malformations.

Persistent stapedial artery

A persistent stapedial artery is occasionally seen at operation and stapedotomy, as opposed to stapedectomy, may be possible if the whole footplate is not covered. Rarely, a large artery may cover the footplate and immobilize the stapes, giving rise to a conductive deafness without footplate fixation. Operation is contraindicated in the presence of this condition.

Paget's disease (osteitis deformans)

Woodhouse (1973) estimated that about 750 000 people have this disease in the UK and that the temporal bone is involved in about 50% of those with clinical evidence of the disease. Paget's disease rarely gives rise to conductive deafness but, if it occurs, it usually starts after the age of 45 years. In the early stages, there is a conductive type of loss associated with a high tone sensorineural loss (see Chapter 15).

The cause of the conductive deafness is ossicular fixation, mainly of the malleus head. As there is no histological evidence of stapedial fixation, the operation of stapedectomy is illogical, although ossicular mobilization may cause temporary improvement in hearing for a few years before the sensorineural deafness neutralizes the hearing gain.

Osteogenesis imperfecta (fragilitas osseum, van der Hoeve's and de Kleijn's syndrome)

This is a rare disease belonging to a group of hereditary disorders of collagen (see Figures 4.37 and 4.38). The otological features of osteogenesis imperfecta are a progressive conductive and sensorineural deafness, the absence of a Schwartze sign and the absence of vertigo. Tympanometry shows absence of the acoustic reflex with a very high compliance value.

The deafness of osteogenesis imperfecta may be treated surgically but operation must be delayed until all spontaneous fractures have ceased. A high incidence of floating footplate has been found at operation and increased likelihood of sensorineural deafness arising from progression in the disease process occurs after surgery for this condition (Garritsen and Cremers, 1991).

Sensorineural deafness in otosclerosis

Sensorineural deafness is frequently associated with the conductive hearing loss of otosclerosis, but there is still argument about the exact mechanism by which it occurs. There is controversy about the concept of 'cochlear otosclerosis' which is a sensorineural hearing loss caused by otosclerosis of the labyrinth in the absence of stapes fixation. Shambaugh (1965), Derlacki and Valvassori (1965) and Balle and Linthicum (1985) have produced strong arguments for supporting the theory of cochlear otosclerosis while, on the other hand, Gross (1969), and Schuknecht and Kirschner (1974), and Schuknecht (1983) have failed to show otosclerotic foci of significant size or incidence in the temporal bones of patients with pure sensorineural deafness of unknown cause.

The possible causes of the cochlear degeneration seen in otosclerosis are:

1 Bony invasion of the scala tympani of the cochlea (Politzer, 1894)
2 Circulatory changes in the cochlea as a result of abnormal bony foci (Mayer, 1911; Ruedi, 1965)
3 Damage to the cochlea by toxic metabolites from abnormal bone (Siebenmann, 1912; Witmaak, 1919; Chevance *et al.*, 1970).

Bony invasion of the scala tympani of the cochlea

In the very early descriptions of the disease by Politzer (1894), Habermann (1904) and Siebenmann (1912), sporadic cases are mentioned showing bone formation in the scala tympani which were thought to be caused by otosclerosis. In 1921, Lange found the scala tympani to be partially filled with newly formed bone tissue into which the otosclerotic process of the labyrinthine wall had penetrated.

Nager and Fraser (1938), in their paper on bone formation in the scala tympani in otosclerosis, stated that the main change occurs in the labyrinthine capsule with the inner ear showing only minor alterations. After the examination of a large number of temporal bones, they found that in rare cases there was extensive bone formation in the scala tympani, and in the more advanced cases it was almost filled with new bone. They believed that the cause of this in the scala tympani was the result of the otosclerotic focus in the wall of the labyrinth producing a certain alteration, or irritation, of the endosteal layer and perilymphatic spaces leading to circumscribed fibrosis and bone production. This type of bone formation in the inner ear is found only in otosclerosis, but it is a rare and uncommon cause of the inner ear deafness which is so common in this condition.

Circulatory changes in the cochlea as a result of abnormal bony foci

Ruedi (1965) re-examined Otto Mayer's theory that venous obstruction caused by invasion of the root of the spiral lamina in the basal turn of the cochlea by otosclerotic bone, gave rise to incompetence of the venous drainage of the anterior and middle spiral veins, leading to neuroepithelial degeneration of the inner ear. Ruedi described how the actively growing otosclerotic focus advanced, giving rise to thrombosis in the vessel adjacent to it. The vessels became walled in, so that a sharp demarcation was apparent between the new vascular channels of the otosclerotic focus and the old vessels of the otic capsule. It was noticed that each focus developed its own self-contained, largely autonomous vascular system, and it was found that a connection between a wide capillary of the old otic capsule and the vascular space of an active otosclerotic focus could develop. When the otosclerotic lesion had penetrated the region of the promontory to appear under the mucous membrane, shunts were often seen between the blood vessels of the otosclerotic deposit and those of the mucosa. These vascular shunts are well known clinically as the 'flamingo blush' first described by Schwartze, and when seen on examination, are an indication of active otosclerosis.

Ruedi also demonstrated vascular shunts between otosclerotic blood vessels and spiral capillaries, which caused marked congestion in the region of the modiolus and he was of the opinion that the formation of new lamellar bone within the inner ear was caused by this stasis, as opposed to Nager's theory that it was the stimulation of the osteoblastic activity of the endosteal capsule.

Ruedi's final investigation, after establishing the presence of the shunts, was to determine whether the atrophy of the labyrinth could be the result of the disturbances in the inner ear brought about by the otosclerosis. He found, in seven out of 10 temporal bones examined, that the organ of Corti had disintegrated or was missing altogether, with a degeneration of the corresponding nerve fibres and ganglion cells. In the majority (six out of seven bones), he detected a shunt in the region of the spiral capillary and the inferior spiral vein. In one of these there was no sign of a venous shunt but an obliterated artery, thought to be the vestibulocochlear, and thrombosis of this accounted for the disintegration of the neuroepithelium and atrophy of the stria vascularis, within the basal turn, seen in the specimen.

Although Ruedi believed that a vascular aetiology accounted for all the inner ear changes seen in otosclerosis, it is only in advanced disease that such abnormalities are seen. The sensorineural hearing loss so common in otosclerosis cannot be explained, in all cases, as being the result of venous congestion alone and his theory is only applicable to some cases.

It is necessary to examine the other theory, of a humoral factor, to explain more satisfactorily the phenomenon of sensorineural degeneration in otosclerosis.

Damage to the cochlea by toxic metabolites from the abnormal bone

In 1912, Siebenmann postulated that the abnormal bone of a focus of otosclerosis, which was invading the labyrinth, poured out inflammatory products into the fluid and these contained toxic metabolites which caused the labyrinthine lesions. Witmaak (1919) also assumed that degeneration of the labyrinth was caused by the diffusion into the labyrinthine fluids of an acid liberated by otosclerotic lesions dissolving the bone.

The actively growing deposit of otosclerosis, as it erodes the endosteum, comes into close relationship with the perilymph of the basal scala tympani. Such active foci have a rich blood supply and extensive marrow tissue; the spaces of the latter may communicate directly with the scala tympani, so that the perilymph flows, not only over the otosclerotic bone, but also into the spaces, allowing mixing of their contents.

It is surprising that, until recently, so little attention has been paid to the humoral theory, for there is such a close relationship between the actively growing deposit of otosclerosis and the perilymphatic spaces. In 1958, Harrison and Naftalin formulated a theory of the active circulation of the labyrinthine fluids which suggested that the inner ear damage in otosclerosis is humoral in origin. They believed that perilymph is formed by ultrafiltration from blood vessels in the perilymphatic space. The perilymph, as a result of the hydrostatic pressure in the general circulatory system, passes across Reissner's membrane and the basilar membrane as a plasma transudate and reaches the scala media. The plasma transudate is then converted into endolymph by a specific process of the stria vascularis, which replaces sodium from the plasma transudate with potassium, by a low energy exchange mechanism analogous to the resorption process of the renal tubules.

If metabolites and other breakdown products of the otosclerotic process were to contaminate the perilymph they could in fact pass across Reissner's membrane and the basilar membrane, with the perilymph, and on reaching the scala media cause damage to the organ of Corti. A simpler explanation of the route of entry of toxic products is through the canaliculi.

In 1970, a research project was undertaken by a biochemist, two histopathologists, an enzymologist and an otologist from three different centres (Paris, Copenhagen and Béziers), which has led to further development of the theory that the inner ear damage in otosclerosis may be humoral in origin (Chevance *et al.*, 1970).

They found that osteoclasts are rarely, and only exceptionally, found in the extension zone of the focus, or in the marrow spaces that constitute the active or otospongiotic focus. This confirms the observations of Ogilvie and Hall (1953) who had noted that in the diffuse form of otosclerosis 'the osteoclasts were remarkable for their scarcity, small size with degenerate cytoplasm and nuclei, and loss of direct application to the bone . . .'. It has been generally believed that these cells are responsible for the entire bony resorption which takes place in the lytic phase of the otosclerotic lesion.

Chevance *et al.* have been able to demonstrate that apart from fibroblasts, fibrocytes, osteoblasts, and osteocytes there is, in addition, a special type of cell, containing lysosomes which are dense vesicular bodies in the cytoplasm. The frequency of this cell, its location and morphology indicated that, in their opinion, it was a histiocyte taking an active part in bone resorption.

These cells were most often found in the 'front' of the otosclerotic process and the bone surrounding them showed the presence of lysis. It is well known that lysosomes contain a number of hydrolases with a very high enzymatic content and the activity of acid phosphatases is generally considered to be the best index of lysosomal content. It was found that the histiocytes exhibited strong acid phosphatase activity and these workers are of the opinion that the histiocytes play the decisive role in the process of otosclerotic resorption.

In addition to the demonstration of the presence of histiocytes in the active focus, otosclerotic microfoci have been found beyond the advancing edge of the lesion, and in these the lytic and rebuilding phases were found to be proceeding simultaneously.

The perilymph of patients subjected to stapedectomy operations, with the presence of otosclerosis confirmed by biopsy, has been examined; six enzymes have been identified: phosphatasic acid, collagenase, alpha-chymotrypsin, lactic dehydrogenase, ribonuclease and trypsin. These enzymes control the evolution of the otosclerotic microfoci and they also pass into the labyrinthine fluids through the cochlear barrier, previously thought to be impassable, entering through the canaliculi.

The actual passage of these enzymes has been demonstrated in a series of perilymph specimens, first studied by Adam's method (Adams and Tuqan, 1961), later by qualitative study and finally by quantitative methods using a microelectrophoretic technique.

Perilymph specimens were studied by multiple statistical analysis and it was found that:

1 Proteases or hydrolases enter the labyrinthine fluids in about 75% of cases of otosclerosis and this corresponds to the 75% incidence of cochlear degeneration which is seen in patients with clinical stapedial otosclerosis
2 Statistical correlations have been arrived at by standard tests, and binary and threefold correlations have been established between the proteolytic activity of the perilymph and the progressive sen-

sorineural hearing loss which is seen in 75% of the cases with stapedial fixation from otosclerosis.

A correlation was also seen between the proteolytic activity of the perilymph and impairment of the posterior labyrinth, shown by the torsion swing test and electronystagmography, in patients without clinical symptoms of vertigo.

The enzymatic concept of otosclerosis

The experimental findings of Chevance, Causse and their co-workers have led them to postulate the theory of the enzymatic concept of otosclerosis.

The process begins in one or more of the numerous cartilaginous rests scattered through the enchondral layer of the otic capsule. Hydrolytic enzymes and proteases, causing cellular destruction, spread from the original focus to the different parts of the cochlea. If the focus is close to the stapediovestibular joint the process of bone rebuilding may produce a fixation of the stapes footplate and a conductive hearing loss. If the proteases and proteolytic enzymes reach the inner ear a sensorineural hearing loss occurs, and if the enzymes reach the posterior labyrinth vertigo may be caused. If the focus is situated far from these sites, the disease may never be detected clinically.

It is well recognized that conductive deafness in otosclerosis may exist without substantial hearing loss, but a sensorineural hearing loss that is disproportionate to the age of the patient is commonly associated with the conductive deafness. The sensorineural hearing loss may precede fixation, although it is usually associated with it. It is also recognized that a gradually developing sensorineural deafness occurs in many patients who have had a successful stapedectomy operation, and this also is often disproportionate to the patient's age.

If otosclerosis of the cochlear capsule can cause sensorineural hearing loss when there is stapedial otosclerosis, it can cause sensorineural hearing loss when there is no stapedial fixation and when this occurs, the condition is known as cochlear otosclerosis.

The enzymatic concept of otosclerosis, elaborated by Chevance and Causse and their colleagues, is of considerable interest as it explains many facets of the disease which still remain obscure, and it explains the long, slow and variable progress of the disease.

These workers believe that otosclerosis is a local disease in which there is an upset of the equilibrium between enzymes and antienzymes in the microfoci of otosclerosis and this gives rise to variable clinical results; e.g. if the focus is stapedial a conductive loss occurs, but if the focus is outside the region of the footplate a sensorineural deafness may result, and if the focus is in the region of the vestibule, vertigo may result. This theory gives strong support to those who believe that medical treatment, by antienzymes or enzyme inhibitors, is important in the treatment of this disease.

The belief that sensorineural hearing loss can occur in a pure form, as the result of otosclerosis without a conductive hearing loss, has been strongly criticized (Schuknecht and Kirschner, 1974; Schuknecht, 1983; Huer *et al.*, 1991). The criticism is based entirely on histological examination of temporal bones, is dogmatic, and does little to help in the explanation of the obscure aspects of this disease.

Audiometric studies were carried out by Glorig and Gallo (1962) who compared bone conduction levels of patients with otosclerosis with air conduction levels in the general population. The assumption was made that, because the hearing losses found in the general population are largely sensorineural, the comparisons would be valid. Their results indicated that otosclerosis does not increase the sensorineural hearing loss above that to be expected in the general population and audiometric patterns for higher frequencies, in those with otosclerosis, resemble those found in general populations. In patients over the age of 60 years, it was found that the sensorineural hearing loss in high frequencies was greater in patients with otosclerosis than in the general population. This finding contradicts their conclusions.

Although otologists are in agreement that gross lesions cause sensorineural deafness in otosclerosis by direct invasion of the scala tympani of the cochlea, and gross lesions interfere with the circulation of the stria vascularis and this may also give rise to sensorineural deafness, there is still controversy concerning the humoral theory.

Causse and Chevance have developed the humoral theory, first postulated by Siebenmann in 1912, and their theory of the enzymatic concept of otosclerosis is the only one that attempts to explain many of the enigmas of this disease.

Diagnosis of sensorineural deafness in otosclerosis

In 1978, Shambaugh pointed out that, before Lempert's fenestration operation for otosclerosis came into general use, few clinicians in North America were able to diagnose stapedial ankylosis caused by otosclerosis. As recently as 1931–1932, not one patient coming to the Massachusetts Eye and Ear Infirmary during those 2 years was diagnosed as having otosclerosis. He believes that the situation concerning pure cochlear otosclerosis is similar today in that this diagnosis is denied in some large clinics and is made with hesitation in others.

Shambaugh (1966) gave six reasons for suspecting that otosclerosis may be the cause in cases of pure sensorineural deafness:

1 A positive Schwartze sign, in one or both ears
2 A family history of surgically confirmed stapedial otosclerosis

3 The presence of symmetrical sensorineural hearing loss in both ears, one of which has stapes fixation
4 A flat, rising, or a 'cookie-bite' audiometric air conduction curve with unusually good speech discrimination for someone with a pure sensorineural loss
5 Pure sensorineural hearing loss beginning insidiously in early, or middle, adult life and progressing with no apparent cause
6 The demonstration of stapes fixation in a patient with previous pure sensorineural deafness of no apparent cause.

Radiological demonstration of cochlear otosclerosis

Conventional radiography is of little value in the diagnosis of otosclerosis and linear tomography does not give adequate information about the very small structures in the temporal bone. However, multi-directional hypocycloidal polytomography may be of value and Derlacki and Valvassori (1965) have developed this technique.

It is necessary for the lesion to be greater than 1 mm for it to be visible and the density of the focus must be different from that of the normal capsule for it to be detected. The normal capsule of the labyrinth is the densest bone and cannot become more sclerotic, but it can become thicker when mature otosclerotic bone increases the thickness of the capsule, which then appears roughened, or scalloped on its edges caused by the irregular outline of the new bone. Derlacki and Valvassori have shown that capsular changes can be demonstrated in 65% of patients with confirmed stapedial otosclerosis and in 30% of patients with clinical findings suggestive of cochlear otosclerosis.

Applebaum and Shambaugh (1978) stated that: 'Caution must be exercised in the interpretation of subtle polytomographic changes in the cochlear capsule and restraint used in the X-ray diagnosis of pure cochlear otosclerosis until there is evidence of correlation with pathological material'.

High resolution computerized tomography

This method has proved to be valuable in assessing the pathology and extent of chronic suppurative otitis media, and precise information concerning the normal anatomy of the ossicles, facial nerve, tegmen and semicircular canals. More recently, it has been possible to demonstrate such changes by CT scanning using densitometry (de Groot, 1985) (see Figures 2.64 and 2.69).

Treatment of otosclerosis

The majority of patients with otosclerotic deafness can be helped by surgical or non-surgical methods and with the improvements in the design and construction of hearing aids, there are few that cannot be given some help.

Medical treatment

The place of fluoride treatment

In 1964, Shambaugh and Scott suggested that sodium fluoride, in moderate doses, might promote recalcification and reduce bone remodelling in an actively expanding otosclerotic lesion. In the human subject, fluoride is most effective on the active focus and less so on the mature lesion.

Otosclerotic foci show a tendency to be more active in young persons and less active in older people, although all stages can be found at any age. It should be appreciated that a mature focus can become active again and this may be the result of hormonal activity such as pregnancy or the menopause. The natural tendency for the active lesion in otosclerosis to become recalcified is inconstant and may be feeble. Shambaugh believed that sodium fluoride, in moderate doses, assists this natural tendency of the focus to become recalcified and inactive, and the evidence in favour of this is given as: fading of the injection of the mucous membrane over an active focus (Schwartze sign); stabilization of the progressive sensorineural deafness which is so often found in otosclerosis; reduction of tinnitus; improvement of mild vestibular symptoms; and X-ray demonstration of recalcification of the focus. Bretlau *et al.* (1985 and 1989) reported on an experimental and clinical evaluation of sodium fluoride treatment. The results showed that using the calcium/phosphorus ratio as an indication for bone maturity, sodium fluoride could stabilize otospongiotic lesions in retaining calcium relative to phosphorus. The results supported the view that sodium fluoride can change otospongiotic, active lesions to more dense, inactive otosclerotic lesions.

Fluoride is a trace element found in widely varying concentrations of ground water, that is between 0.1 and 16 parts per million. Some local authorities add fluoride to the drinking water to bring the concentration to one part per million and this has proved to be very beneficial in the prevention of dental caries in school children. Bernstein, Sadowsky and Hagstead (1966) studied the incidence of osteoporosis in rural communities in North Dakota, where the farming population remained in the area for a lifetime, and it was found that where there was an abnormally low fluoride content in the drinking water, osteoporosis was four times more common than in areas with a high content. A similar study of otosclerosis by Daniel (1969) showed that stapedial fixation was four times as high in the low area compared with that in the high fluoride area.

Gristwood (1966), in Australia, reported on the unusually high incidence of the truly obliterated footplate, and it has been the experience of most Australian otologists, that the incidence of the thick and obliterated footplate is in the region of 30%. Gristwood and Venables (1975) have pointed out that the surface water in the most densely populated areas of South Australia is deficient in fluoride ions and it was not until 1971 that fluoridation of metropolitan water supplies was commenced.

Action of fluoride

Fluoride reduces osteoclastic bone resorption and increases osteoblastic bone formation. The work of Causse and colleagues (1977a and 1980) suggested, in addition, that in otosclerosis fluorides have an antienzymatic action on proteolytic enzymes which are cytotoxic to the cochlea and produce sensorineural deafness. In a series of over 4000 patients treated with fluorides, in Chicago, USA and Béziers, France, very few have experienced improvement of the sensorineural element of their deafness, but it has become stabilized in over 80%.

Indications for sodium fluoride therapy

Sodium fluoride therapy is indicated in the following groups of patients (Shambaugh and Scott, 1964):

1 Patients with surgically confirmed otosclerosis who show progressive sensorineural deafness disproportionate to age
2 Patients with pure sensorineural deafness whose family history, age of onset, audiometric pattern and good auditory discrimination indicate the possibility of cochlear otosclerosis
3 Patients with radiological demonstration by polytomography of spongiotic changes in the cochlear capsule
4 Patients with a positive Schwartze sign.

Preoperative treatment

When the patient has an otosclerotic focus which shows activity, as evidenced by a positive Schwartze sign, progressive sensorineural hearing loss, and radiological evidence of a demineralized focus in the cochlear capsule, both Shambaugh and Causse believed that a substantial reduction in vascularity and remodelling of the focus will result from fluoride treatment.

Postoperative treatment

If patients are found to have an active focus at operation, fluoride therapy is prescribed for 2 years or longer (Causse and Causse, 1979).

Contraindications to sodium fluoride therapy

Sodium fluoride therapy is contraindicated in the following groups of patients:

1 Patients with chronic nephritis with nitrogen retention
2 Patients with chronic rheumatoid arthritis
3 Patients who are pregnant or lactating
4 In children before full skeletal growth has been completed
5 Patients who show an allergy, as demonstrated by an itching rash
6 Patients with skeletal fluorosis. This is a rare condition seen in certain areas of India.

Dosage and administration of sodium fluoride

When there is evidence of an active lesion, a daily dose of sodium fluoride 50 mg is given for 2 years and this can be increased to 75 mg daily in very active cases with a positive Schwartze sign. When there is evidence of stabilization of hearing, fading of the Schwartze sign, and radiological signs of recalcification of the focus, a daily maintenance dose of 25 mg is given for the rest of the patient's life. In the UK, imported enteric coated capsules of 40 mg can be used and may be supplemented with calcium and vitamin D (BPC).

Adverse effects of sodium fluoride therapy

Gastric disturbance is the most common side effect which is largely prevented by taking enteric-coated capsules of sodium fluoride after meals. Patients with a peptic ulcer may complain of a flare up of their symptoms and the treatment must be stopped. An increase of joint symptoms may occur in those with chronic arthritis. A return to the previous state is rapid after cessation of treatment.

There is the remote possibility of skeletal fluorosis being produced and a skeletal survey should be made at the beginning of treatment and repeated at intervals.

There is still a widespread prejudice and almost an emotional dislike of fluoride therapy by some members of the medical profession, which is not justified and is the result of ignorance about the facts of this form of treatment. At the present time, fluoride therapy is the only known method of promoting recalcification and inactivation of an actively expanding focus of otosclerosis. There is also evidence that sensorineural deafness may be stabilized or even improved in patients who receive fluoride medication.

Hearing aids

The modern transistorized hearing aid with an air conduction receiver gives good results in the great majority of patients with otosclerotic deafness. Although a standard bone conduction aid is rarely prescribed, an osseous implanted aid may be of value in those with bilateral fenestration cavities. Auditory training and rehabilitation are helpful and those with poor discrimination and severe hearing loss should be advised to have instruction in lipreading.

Many patients prefer natural hearing to the use of a hearing aid and there is evidence that stapedectomy may reduce the rate of cochlear dysfunction which affects all patients with otosclerosis and, although surgery is the best method of treatment for otosclerosis if it is successful, there is a high price to pay in the event of failure.

Surgical treatment

Historical

It is interesting to remember that although the first attempt at mobilization of the stapes was carried out over 100 years ago, it was not until 1958 that John Shea, in Memphis, described the operation of stapedectomy.

The first stapedectomy operations were carried out by Jack of Boston, Massachusetts in 1893, with reportedly good results. However, in other hands, this operation proved to be dangerous and was strongly condemned by leading authorities of the time, including Politzer, almost certainly because of serious complications.

Subsequently, interest in the surgical treatment of hearing loss due to otosclerosis lapsed until the introduction of an indirect method that allowed the inner ear fluids to move again, under the influence of sound stimuli. The fenestration operation started around 1913 by Jenkins, was developed by Holmgren (1923), Bárány (1924) and Sourdille (1930) and later by Lempert (1938). However, the results with fenestration were often less than optimal because of the limiting effect of reduced cochlear function and potential instability of open surgical cavities. Fenestration lasted until 1952 when the operation of mobilization of the stapes was described by Rosen in New York. Early results were good but refixation was common. Comprehending the relentless and aggressive nature of active otosclerosis and the inevitability of recurrent ankylosis after mobilization in most patients, Shea introduced the modern operation of stapedectomy in 1958, which is the basis of all the operations developed since that time. Shea's contribution to the surgery of otosclerosis was monumental and he is rightly regarded as the originator of modern surgery for otosclerosis.

Indications for surgery

The majority of patients with a conductive deafness caused by otosclerosis can be treated surgically and, in general, a patient who will benefit from an operation will also hear satisfactorily with a hearing aid.

The average patient with otosclerosis and a bone conduction level of 0–25 dB in the speech range, and an air conduction of 45–65 dB, is a suitable candidate for surgery (Goodhill, 1979). The air-bone gap should be at least 15 dB and there should be a speech discrimination score of 60% or more for a good hearing improvement.

In the era of fenestration surgery, patients with very severe hearing losses were not suitable for operative treatment, but with the advent of stapedectomy this was no longer the case and patients with hearing losses in the 90–100 dB range and no measurable cochlear reserve on speech discrimination, may still be suitable for operative treatment to enable them to use a hearing aid which was previously of no help. This last group of patients, although small, is the only one where operative treatment is essential as there is no alternative method available. 'The ultimate aim is restoration of available cochlear function, even though this may not carry with it the possibility of unaided hearing' (Goodhill, 1979).

Contraindications to surgery

Morrison (1979) listed 16 contraindications to operation in otosclerosis which remain appropriate:

1 The presence of general medical disease when the patient is unfit for surgery, or where the expectation of life is limited. Patients with diabetes mellitus or bleeding disorders are entirely unsuited for operation.
2 Old age; in those over the age of 70 years there is a 40% chance of discrimination becoming worse, and the risk of fistula formation is greater in the older age group. Unless there is some special reason for operation, a hearing aid should be advised.
3 Most surgeons would not advise operation in children, but Robinson (1983) and von Haacke (1985) have reported good results in young people between the ages of 16 and 21 years.
4 In conductive losses from other causes, the stapes should not be touched. This applies particularly to stapes fixation caused by tympanosclerosis as stapedectomy carries with it a high incidence of sensorineural loss.
5 If other conditions are present, such as otitis externa, or a perforation, stapedectomy is contraindicated until they have been successfully treated.
6 If there is early fixation with a small degree of hearing loss, operation is probably unnecessary, although some surgeons might consider stapes mobilization in such cases.
7 In unilateral otosclerosis, surgery may not be necessary, but many patients find loss of binaural hearing a great handicap, and in these cases operation is justified.
8 If the patient has only one hearing ear, operation

is not justified unless a hearing aid does not give relief.

9 In stapedial and cochlear otosclerosis, with a poor air-bone gap, operation is not advised if a hearing aid can be used.
10 The presence of vertigo and clinical evidence of labyrinthine hydrops, especially fluctuating hearing loss, is a contraindication to operation as there is an increased risk of a 'dead ear' from damage to a distended saccule during operation.
11 Morrison is of the opinion that revision stapedectomy is dangerous because fine adhesions may exist between the footplate area and the saccule or cochlear duct. If the small fenestra operation was previously carried out, this criticism does not apply and good results are possible in the hands of the expert.
12 Second ear stapedectomy is still controversial because of the risk of immediate and delayed sensorineural hearing loss which, in rare cases, can be bilateral. Vestibular damage can occur with permanent loss of coordination. The advantages of bilateral stapedectomy, if it is successful, are the restoration of binaural hearing and the ability to localize the direction from which sound is coming. A sloping high frequency sensorineural hearing loss, as seen in bone conduction thresholds in older patients, indicates a considerable likelihood that postoperative speech discrimination will be inadequate.

Technical difficulties at the first operation and abnormalities in caloric response are contraindications to operating on the second ear (Smyth, Kerr and Singh, 1975). The advantages of stapedotomy over stapedectomy in regard to better preservation of cochlear function and greatly reduced fistula incidence support the concept of second ear operations for optimum auditory rehabilitation. However, many surgeons, especially those who do not specialize in the surgical treatment of otosclerosis, feel that the patient should be allowed the safeguard of being able to wear a hearing aid, if necessary, in the second ear.

Additional support for operations on the second ear in carefully selected patients derives from reports of better maintenance of bone conduction thresholds in operated as opposed to unoperated ears (Smyth, Hassard and El Kordy, 1980; Karjalainen, Karja and Harma, 1984; Marquet, 1985).

13 In the young adult with rapidly spreading stapedial and cochlear otosclerosis and a positive Schwartze sign, surgery should be delayed until the activity is controlled by sodium fluoride.
14 Stapedectomy is contraindicated in pregnancy, and operation should be delayed for 12 months after parturition.
15 Stapedectomy may be inadvisable on those whose occupations demand considerable physical strain,

in those engaged in sport and in airmen, especially those flying small unpressurized aircraft, as there is an increased risk of perilymph fistula.

16 If there is evidence of poor eustachian tube function in one ear, detected by tympanometry, and there is bilateral otosclerosis, it is advisable to operate on the ear with normal atmospheric middle ear pressure rather than the poorer hearing ear.

Preoperative counselling of the patient

As there is an alternative method of treatment, a hearing aid, which in most cases is satisfactory, it is essential to explain to the patient the advantages and possible disadvantages of surgery. In many clinics where stapes surgery is performed, patients are told that there is at least an 85% chance of obtaining a good hearing improvement, that about 10% of patients gain only slight improvement of hearing and that the remaining 5% may expect some degree of sensorineural loss after operation, which may become total. The validity of this advice will be reviewed later in this chapter. It should be explained to the patient that the operated ear may fail after an initially good result, and this can occur many years later.

Patients should also appreciate the possibility of additional slowly developing deterioration in their auditory acuity which may eventually result in a return of the kind of incapacity of which they initially complained. Long-term deterioration is mainly sensorineural and may be the result of presbyacusis or cochlear otosclerosis or be a delayed result of trauma caused by the surgical intervention. Should it occur in due course, amplification may become necessary, and patients will want to know for how long surgical treatment is likely to postpone their need for a hearing aid. Slight vertigo for a few days after operation may be experienced, and a transient weakness of the facial muscles can occur. If bilateral stapedectomy is carried out the possibility of alteration of taste from chorda tympani damage must be mentioned. The patient must be warned against violent nose blowing at all times, as this can lead to a fistula. Flying is contraindicated for at least 2 weeks after surgery, and strenuous exercise, and the lifting of heavy weights, must also be avoided for a similar period.

The surgeon who does not tell the patient of the risks of operative treatment, including the possibility of a 'dead ear', is, today, likely to become involved in litigation. To ensure, as far as possible, that patients fully comprehend the realities of surgical treatment, it is advisable that they are also given this information in written form.

Surgery

Fenestration of the lateral semicircular canal and stapes mobilization were superseded by the reintroduction of stapedectomy by Shea in 1958. Safety and success lacking in the methods attempted 50 years previously were enhanced by sealing the oval window with connective tissue and reconstruction of the sound conducting mechanism. In obliterative disease, Shea gained access to the vestibule by drilling a small hole through the footplate to accommodate a piston prosthesis. The observation that patients treated by this method experienced minimal vestibular symptoms led some surgeons to adopt the small fenestra technique for virtually all patients (Marquet, Creten and van Camp, 1972; Smyth, Kerr and Singh, 1972; McGee, 1981; Bailey, Pappas and Graham, 1981; Fisch, 1982). Thus, out of stapedectomy evolved stapedotomy.

Stapedectomy

Immediate preoperative debridement and cleansing of the ear canal is mandatory in all stapes operations. Ototoxic alcohol-based solutions must be rigorously avoided. Although many surgeons prescribe antibiotic cover, many do not and there is little documented evidence for either choice.

Exposure

Although in Europe an endaural incision was initially popular, from the outset North American surgeons have usually favoured a speculum approach using the triangular tympanomeatal flap introduced for stapes mobilization. More recently, although an endaural incision is of benefit when the ear canal is unusually narrow, in most major otological centres a tympanomeatal flap is preferred, using either local or general hypotensive anaesthesia, depending on availability and the surgeons' choice. Local anaesthesia is specifically recommended for revision operations because an awake patient may be able to report disturbance of equilibrium if the procedure is endangering the vestibular membranes. Elevation of the flap proceeds anteriorly until identification of the fibrous annulus of the tympanic membrane which is displaced from its sulcus allowing the posterior half of the tympanic membrane to be folded forwards over the handle of the malleus. The chorda tympani nerve is freed from mucosal attachments and gently displaced anteriorly to permit removal of canal wall bone using curettes or diamond burrs sufficient to provide wide exposure of the long process of the incus, the stapes and the pyramid as far posteriorly as its base. The importance of avoiding instrumental trauma or stretching of the chorda nerve cannot be overemphasized to avoid distressing and often permanent disorders of taste and salivary secretion, especially in operations on the second ear.

Preparation of the oval window

Before removing the stapedial crura the existence of footplate fixation should be confirmed by gentle palpation of the stapes head, and the location and extent of the otosclerotic focus determined visually. Using a microscissor, the stapedius tendon is divided and the stapes head separated from the lenticular process with a right-angled knife. The posterior crus is then fragmented near its base with a sharp straight pick or crurotomy scissors, followed by the application of inferiorly directed pressure with a curved mobilization needle against the anterior crus. Fracture of the crura by applying pressure sharply against the stapes head should be avoided because of its leverage effect which may cause footplate dislocation. The crura having been removed, a measuring rod is used to determine the length of the prosthesis which is later to be used. After removing a 2 mm strip of mucosa from around the margins of the oval window, the footplate is then transected transversely with sharp angled and straight picks into two or three separate pieces which are then gently extracted from the oval window using right-angled hooks or a microforceps. In ears with a pronounced anterior otosclerotic focus, this is left undisturbed, resulting in partial footplate removal.

Restoration of the sound conduction mechanism

In order to limit loss of perilymph and prevent subsequent fistula formation, a soft tissue graft is used to cover or fill the oval window. This may be previously prepared compressed vein (Shea and Sanabria, 1963) or ear lobe fat (Schuknecht, 1971). If vein is used this should extend over the margins of the oval window for 2–3 mm. Using small pieces of moistened gelfoam, the graft is indented into the oval window niche in such a way that its margins are clearly apparent. The prosthesis, usually a piston made of

Teflon or steel, or a combination of both, is then centred on the graft and articulated with the long process of the incus (Figure 14.4). If a stainless steel wire prosthesis is used, its loop is then tightened around the incus with crimping forceps, avoiding excessive pressure which can cause fracture of the bone. Small pieces of gelfoam are packed around the medial end of the piston to support its position on the centre of the graft.

If ear lobe fat is used as the grafting material, this is tied to a stainless steel wire by the surgeon using a special jig to ensure correctness of length and shape. This type of reconstruction is probably best suited to ears in which the footplate is totally removed (Figure 14.5).

Stapedotomy

Exposure is achieved in the same way as for stapedectomy. Thereafter, an exact order of steps has been proposed (Fisch, 1982; Smyth, 1982) so as to minimize pressure changes within the labyrinth which might occur as a result of fenestrating the footplate and implanting a prosthesis (Figure 14.6). Having gained visual access to the footplate, a defect is created 1 mm larger in its diameter than that of the preferred prosthesis. This defect can be made either with a penetration needle (Fisch, 1982), a small diamond drill (Causse and Causse, 1984) or a laser (Perkins, 1980; McGee, 1983).

The prosthesis, gripped by alligator forceps, is then placed so that it enters the fenestra and encircles the incus simultaneously. Its loop is gently tightened so that it will remain on the incus until later it is crimped in its final position near the tip of the long process. Next, after sectioning the stapedius tendon, the posterior crus is cut at its midpoint with crurotomy scissors, using a two-handed technique and the anterior crus fractured with a mobilization needle.

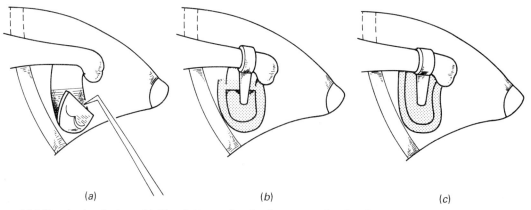

(a)   (b)   (c)

Figure 14.4 Steps in stapedectomy. (*a*) After division with picks, the posterior footplate fragment is removed; (*b*) if the anterior fragment remains fixed the partial oval window defect is covered with vein or fascia and the prosthesis positioned; (*c*) if the anterior footplate fragment has become unstable it is removed and a larger graft used to cover the oval window

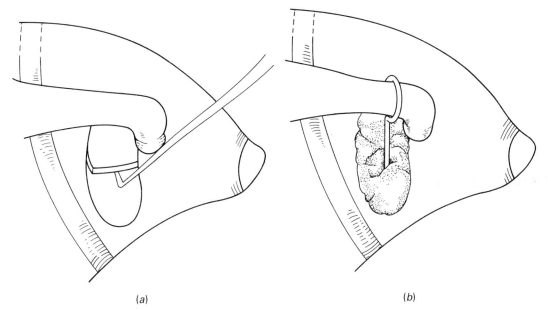

Figure 14.5 The fat–wire operation. (*a*) Removal of the footplate in two or more parts; (*b*) insertion of composite ear lobe fat, stainless steel wire prosthesis

In the laser technique, division of the stapedius tendon and removal of the posterior crura are achieved with the laser beam. The stapes head with the attached fragments of crura is then turned inferiorly, severed from the lenticular process with microscissors and removed. The procedure is completed by moving the prosthesis caudally to the desired position on the incus where it is then crimped firmly, and two small pledgets of gelatin sponge placed around the fenestra.

The use of a connective tissue seal in the oval window has been advocated as a means of preventing postoperative fistula. There is, as yet, no convincing evidence to support the use of this step which is technically difficult when the diameter of the fenestra is 5 mm or less.

It is proposed that by performing the steps of stapedotomy in this sequence, cochlear trauma and stimulation of the otosclerotic focus which might provoke the release of tryptotic enzymes into the vestibule (Causse and Causse, 1984) are reduced to the utmost possible degree. The fenestra is created to its desired final size before any leverage on the crura occurs. The prosthesis is positioned, almost closing the fenestra and limiting loss of perilymph and the entry of blood into the vestibule before any problems such as over-mobility or fracture of the footplate can occur. The extent of penetration of the prosthesis into the vestibule (0.1 mm) and its stability and control within the fenestra margins can be checked visually. Finally, the crura are divided by cutting with scissors, a drill or laser beam rather than lever-

age, the safety of this step being enhanced by the supporting strength of the still-present medial and lateral attachments of the crura. The final adjustment of the prosthesis involves no further risks and the operation is completed immediately.

A detailed study of distance between the medial surface of the footplate and the utricle, saccule and cochlear duct confirms that a 0.4 mm prosthesis can be introduced to a depth of 0.5 mm into the vestibule over the entire surface of the stapedial footplate without risk (Pauw, Pollak and Fisch, 1991) (see Figure 2.63). Recently, Causse has been advocating the use of a polycell collar around the prosthesis which is glued to the cut stapedius tendon (Causse, Causse and Parahy, 1985). Whether this restores stapedial function remains to be proven. An alternative is to preserve the tendon and this has been reported to result in better long-term hearing, which may be due to the protective effect of the stapedius on the inner ear from noise trauma (Collette and Fiorino, 1994).

The laser in stapedotomy

Perkins, in 1980, introduced the argon laser for stapes operations and successful results with argon and KTP lasers have been reported by other surgeons (Silverstein, Rosenberg and Jones, 1989; Bartels, 1990; Hodgson and Wilson, 1991). The advantages claimed are better ability to prepare a bloodless fenestra, reduced risk of footplate subluxation with equally good or better hearing results than reported with other techniques, although Gantz *et al.* (1982) reported saccular damage

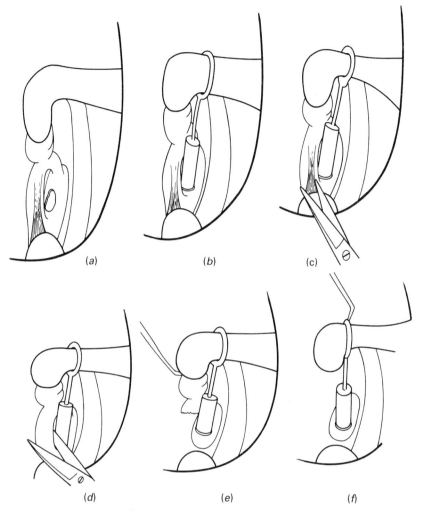

Figure 14.6 Steps in stapedotomy. (*a*) Calibrated fenestra in centre or posterior half of footplate; (*b*) the prosthesis is placed in the fenestra and around the incus long process; (*c*) section of the stapedius tendon; (*d*) the posterior crus is divided using crurotomy scissors; (*e*) the stapes head and crural remnants are removed; (*f*) final adjustment of the prosthesis

in cats following footplate fenestration with the argon laser. Although Silverstein, Rosenberg and Jones (1989) have reported vestibular symptoms postoperatively in 39% of patients, which they attributed to an increase in perilymph temperature, the occurrence of serious inner ear trauma has not yet been reported.

Problems found at operation

Although many stapes operations are straightforward and present little technical difficulty, anatomical and pathological variations can be encountered which may present great difficulty, and while the experienced surgeon may be able to overcome them with a successful result, the less experienced may be wiser to abandon the operation.

The most common abnormalities are discussed below.

Abnormalities of the facial nerve

Dehiscences of the facial nerve are not uncommon and in about 0.5% of middle ears there is a sizeable dehiscence, so that the nerve bulges down and obscures the arch and footplate. In some cases, it is possible to displace the nerve upwards and complete the operation, but if footplate surgery is likely to be blind, it is safer to abandon the operation. Very rarely, the facial nerve takes an anomalous course, either splitting to surround the stapes or coursing inferior to the oval window (Hoogland, 1977).

Persistent stapedial artery

A persistent stapedial artery of sufficient size to prevent the completion of the operation is very rare and is found in 0.2% of operations. Troublesome bleeding from a small vestigial vessel, which is not uncommon, is avoidable with the stapedotomy technique.

Perilymph flooding

This is a rare complication and is seen in an ear with an unusually patent cochlear aqueduct. Polytomography before operation may show an abnormally-shaped vestibule. The existence of this abnormality is suggested by an upward sloping air conduction audiogram with best response at 2 kHz (Cremers, Hombergen and Wentges, 1983). The complication is more common in ears with congenital fixation of the footplate. In stapedectomy, if a small safety hole is made in the footplate before the crura are detached, the condition will be detected and it may then be possible to close it by a connective tissue graft packed between the footplate and the crura. The advantages for surgeons who perform stapedotomy are obvious.

In other cases, it may be possible to seal the 'perilymph gusher' with a soft tissue graft and the prosthesis put into position in order to hold the graft in contact with the oval window. The flow of cerebrospinal fluid may last for several days and a severe sensorineural hearing loss is likely to occur with this complication. Clearly, if such ears can be identified, operation is contraindicated.

Floating and submerged footplate

This is a potentially serious complication of stapedectomy as opposed to stapedotomy and may result in a 'dead' ear if attempts are made to extract the footplate, which in some cases becomes hinged on itself, or even disappears from view. A preliminary drill hole in the footplate, before attempts to remove the crural arch are made, is a wise precaution and will often prevent the complication. If the footplate is visible within the vestibule it may be possible to remove it by manipulation and extraction with a fine hook, after drilling a small hole at the inferior margin of the oval window. Such measures are extremely hazardous to the inner ear and are inadvisable. If a floating footplate cannot be removed without excessive manipulation it should be left in place, a soft tissue graft placed over the oval window and the operation abandoned. At re-operation in not less than 6 months, it is may be possible to remove the graft and footplate as one unit. Some authorities apply a prosthesis from the incus to a floating footplate, if it remains slightly hinged inwards, and good results have been reported from this procedure.

Presence of blood in the vestibule

Excessive bleeding during operation is a hazard. The benefits of a dry field cannot be overemphasized, and if the surgeon cannot persuade his anaesthetist to provide this he would be best advised to use local anaesthesia. There is still some disagreement about the possible serious effects of leaking blood into the vestibule. Linthicum and Sheehy (1969) could find no evidence of any detectable ill effects from this complication, while Smyth and Hassard (1978) believed that labyrinthine trauma due to suctioning blood (and inevitably perilymph) cannot be dismissed. Preoperative fluoride therapy may help in reducing the activity and thus the vascularity of otosclerotic bone. Aspirin should not be taken for at least 3 weeks before operation.

Tympanic membrane tear

If a small tear of the drum is found at the end of the operation and it is only a slit, it is underlaid with gelatin sponge. A large tear is closed by rotating the flap and covering it with gelatin sponge. Healing almost always occurs. If inadequate flaps have been made and this is associated with excessive bone removal, a defect may be left at the end of the operation and this should be repaired with temporalis fascia and, if necessary, tragal cartilage, placed beneath the edge of the drum and on to the adjoining meatus.

Obliterative otosclerosis

Radical removal of foci filling the oval window and saucerization incurs serious risk of anacusis. Surgeons with limited experience would be well advised not to proceed with the operation. The condition is best treated by stapedotomy.

Using a microdrill and diamond burr, bone is removed over an area 1.5 mm in diameter until proximity to the vestibule is indicated by a blue shadow and seepage of perilymph. Sharp picks are then used to create a fenestra, just large enough to accommodate freely a Teflon or steel piston, and a small amount of areolar tissue or gelfoam is placed around the fenestra (Figure 14.7).

Narrowed oval window niche

Otosclerotic foci around the oval window may lead to a marked narrowing of the niche which produces a slit-like effect at the oval window. Attempts to remove the footplate or make a fenestra within it should not be made until the overhanging bone has been removed and there is adequate exposure of the footplate.

Damage to the chorda tympani nerve

During a stapedectomy operation, it is frequently necessary to displace the chorda tympani nerve to

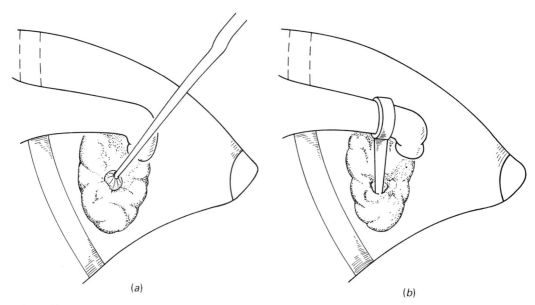

(a)   (b)

Figure 14.7 Obliterative otosclerosis. (*a*) Preliminary saucerization of central area by drilling until blue area is seen; (*b*) after fenestration with picks the prosthesis is positioned

gain adequate exposure, and there is controversy concerning the advisability of stretching the nerve or cutting it. It should be appreciated that if the nerve is cut, it will produce permanent loss of sensation of taste in the anterior two-thirds of the tongue on the same side and no re-innervation of the taste buds can take place, either from the chorda tympani nerve of the opposite side or the posterior third of the tongue supplied by the glossopharyngeal nerve. Permanent loss of chorda tympani innervation results in atrophy of the taste receptors in the anterior two-thirds of the tongue; the dorsum of the tongue becomes smooth and pale. The patient may not complain of the loss of taste sensations, if one nerve is cut, as the tongue retains sensation in 66% of its surface (Diamond and Frew, 1979).

If the nerve is stretched during operation, a persistent abnormal sensation in the tongue may occur, described by the patient as salty, or metallic, and this is caused by paraesthesia of this sensory nerve. Cutting the nerve may also produce these unpleasant sensations of taste. If the nerve is displaced but not divided the taste disturbance is less (Bull, 1965).

Bilateral loss of the chorda tympani nerve produces marked symptoms in the majority of patients and, in addition to the loss of taste, there is loss of the secretomotor supply to the submandibular and sublingual salivary glands which produces an uncomfortable dry mouth. If at all possible, the surgeon must preserve the chorda tympani nerve, and this is essential in bilateral operations.

Results of surgical treatment

Although reports published over 20 years ago indicated that not all initially successful stapedectomy results were likely to be maintained indefinitely (Hough, 1969; House and Greenfield, 1969; McGee, 1969), there has been little information in the subsequent otological literature to substantiate that warning. Although recommendations for modifications in technique, principally to do with dimensions of the fenestra and prosthesis, have been made on the grounds of less trauma to the labyrinth and consequently less postoperative sensorineural deterioration, little has been published to indicate how well and for how long good results, obtained with any procedure, will withstand the passage of time. Notwithstanding the few longer-term reports which originate from specialized centres with a great number of operations by very experienced surgeons, which tend to be reassuring (Robinson, 1985; Shea, 1985), the experience of some surgeons, who are by comparison 'occasional operators', must cause some concern (Doyle and Woodham, 1980).

Experience of a growing number of patients requiring assistance with amplification 10 or more years postoperatively suggests that a reappraisal of the prognosis previously given to many patients may be both appropriate and necessary. In addition to warnings that, in spite of an excellent chance of an immediate successful outcome, a hearing aid will eventually be needed by many patients, there is evidence that the criteria for surgical treatment have narrowed in the light of the experience of those who have systematically related preoperative and interoperative findings with results. Factors such as age, preoperative cochlear function, and oval window pathology, have been highlighted as important considerations in advising for a stapes operation as opposed to the prescription of a hearing aid. This trend has certainly been encouraged by recent developments in microchip technology. Because, unfortunately, experience has shown that a less than optimum result with stapes surgery cannot necessarily be retrieved by the subsequent application of even highly sophisticated amplification, the initial decision by both patient and surgeon as to primary treatment with hearing aid or operation has now become more crucial than it was in the 1960s.

Although many patients will receive surgical treatment at centres of excellence, many more will be advised and treated in departments where the surgeon has considerably less experience. The growth of training programmes and teaching courses in many countries, coupled with a greatly diminished number of new patients, make any alternative unlikely. Hopefully, surgeons in smaller areas of population will assume the responsibility to perform stapedectomy only when their skills in otological microsurgery are maintained by regular experience with tympanoplastic operations. Nevertheless, an apparent lack of awareness of the actual long-term results achieved by stapes operations in terms of the patients' auditory status overall, should cause concern among medical professionals (Coker *et al.*, 1988).

An additional factor in the difficulty of providing realistic advice to patients lies in the usual methods of measuring results which have remained virtually unchanged since the fenestration era. Changes in air-bone gap do not necessarily correlate with patients' experience (Smyth and Patterson, 1985).

Most reports on the success or failure of reconstruction of the ossicular chain in otosclerosis and chronic otitis media employ air-bone gap closure as the main method of measurement. This parameter is useful when comparing the performance of one material or technique with another, but it is inappropriate from the perspective of the patient. The request from the patient with a hearing loss is never 'Can you close my air-bone gap?' This method of evaluation also suffers from the fact that the transmission element of bone conduction measured by standard methods will be enhanced by an efficient reconstructed ossicular mechanism, and therefore bone conduction thresholds may be improved postoperatively (Smyth and Hassard, 1981). Alternatively, bone conduction thresholds may have deteriorated due to intraoperative trauma; the most effective way of closing the air-bone gap is to produce a dead ear. As will be proposed below it is more useful to plot the air conduction changes which are achieved by various reconstructive techniques. This measure provides a more realis-

tic indication of the prospects of improving the patient's overall auditory performance because the aim of stapes surgery is not to close the air-bone gap but to reduce the patient's auditory disability. In general, the degree of disability is determined by the status of the better ear. The ideal of bilateral normal hearing is often unattainable, and so in advising patients regarding surgery for hearing gain, it is important not to forget the contribution of the other ear. Hearing is a bilateral sense and the central auditory pathways receive input from both cochleae. Unless the contribution of the operated ear to the activity in the central auditory centres is sufficiently increased postoperatively, surgery will be of limited benefit to the patient. In most cases the worse hearing ear will be selected for surgical treatment, but unless the proposed operation can restore symmetrical hearing or convert the operated ear into a better hearing ear, the patient is unlikely to experience a reduction in disability.

The requirements for patient benefit were assessed by Smyth and Patterson (1985) (Belfast 'rule of thumb'). They concluded that for significant benefit to be achieved the postoperative air conduction average over the speech frequencies must be close to 30 dB or the interaural difference reduced to <15 dB. This figure of 15 dB corresponds to the cross-attenuation effect of the skull (Browning, 1986).

The Glasgow plot devised by Browning, Gatehouse and Swan (1991) is a valuable elaboration using a pair of coordinate axes. The pre- and postoperative plots of the air conduction thresholds in both ears are used as a method of presenting the results. First, the proportion of patients that fall into each of three main preoperative impairment groups are identified. This is important, as the potential benefits from surgery are not the same in each group. Thereafter, the percentages of patients that achieve various postoperative hearing categories can be calculated, allowing surgeons to audit their results and make comparisons between series. Therefore, if the surgeon is aware of his success rates in stapes surgery in terms of air conduction change then, using either the Belfast 'rule of thumb' or the Glasgow plot, he will be able to advise the patient realistically as to the potential benefit of the surgery proposed.

It should also be remembered that if preoperative bone conduction thresholds, even with correction of the Carhart (1962) effect are used in predicting outcomes, the effect of alterations in cochlear function, whether due to presbyacusis, cochlear otosclerosis, or delayed effects of surgical intervention, fails to be taken into account.

Regardless of which surgical technique is used in patients with clinical otosclerosis, failure to achieve a technically optimal result (total closure of the air-bone gap using preoperative bone conduction) or a technically acceptable result (closure of the air-bone gap to 10 dB) is due either to the development of a postoperative sensorineural hearing loss or the persist-ence of a greater than 10 dB conductive loss. Both may be either immediate or delayed.

There have been numerous published reports on the results of stapedectomy and stapedotomy. Closure of the air-bone gap to 10 dB or less in more than 90% of patients has been reported from specialized centres by very experienced surgeons (Schuknecht, 1971; Bailey, Pappas and Graham, 1981; McGee, 1981; Fisch, 1982; Causse and Causse, 1984; Shea, 1985; Cremers, Bensen and Huygen, 1991). How-ever, it should be clearly understood that many re-ports have incomplete follow up and few are extended – most are short term. The dangers inherent in the use of short-term reports as a basis for prognostic advice to patients, many of whom will have consider-able life expectancies, are self-evident. From a study of 750 patients aimed at establishing a long-term prog-nosis of such patients (Smyth and Hassard, 1978), the following categories of failure were assembled.

Immediate severe sensorineural losses

An average loss of 20 dB or more (many were very severely affected) occurred in 1.5% of stapedectomy operations, but not in any stapedotomy ears. The surgical notes indicated likely traumatic events, such as excessive perilymph loss due to difficulties in remov-ing the footplate, hydraulic effects due to prematurely mobile footplates, or prolonged drilling in 75% of affected ears. Because such events had been recorded in only 23% of those ears in which sensorineural losses exceeding 10 dB did not occur, it was con-cluded that surgical trauma was a major cause of cochlear deficits in stapedectomy ($P < 0.001$).

To provide a means of identifying patients at risk of severe sensorineural hearing loss, especially from stape-dectomy, other possible factors were considered. When age, oval window pathology, and the audiograms were related to the overall outcome, it was seen that patients aged 50 years or more, with either a type C Juers (1948) bone conduction threshold (greater than 35 dB) or obliterative otosclerosis, ran a one in three risk of severe sensorineural loss ($P < 0.001$).

Delayed sensorineural hearing losses

Sudden onset

An averaged sensorineural loss of 10 dB or more due to surgically confirmed fistulae occurred in 2% of stapedectomy and 0.6% of stapedotomy operations. Re-operation resulted in restoration of hearing to pre-fistula levels in one half of these ears.

Chronic progressive

In addition to acute losses due to fistulae, slowly developing progressive sensorineural losses with dete-

rioration in speech discrimination scores have been recognized since the introduction of stapedectomy. A consistent pattern of linear deterioration in mean hearing threshold has emerged at a rate of 5.5 dB per decade in the group as a whole (Smyth, Hassard and El Kordy, 1980). Although patients aged 50 years or more were consistently worse throughout the early follow-up period, this was no longer statisti-cally significant after 10 years, and both age groups had almost identical estimated times of reaching the critical 40 dB threshold at 18.5 years postoperatively. This level was categorically chosen as that at which amplification would become desirable. During the first 5 years, stapedotomy ears had a significantly poorer averaged response than the others, because of less effective closure of the air-bone gap at 0.5 and 1 kHz, but by 7 years the stapedectomy group exhibited a significantly poorer mean response.

On the basis of a predicted deterioration rate of 9.5 dB per decade for stapedectomy (which is similar to that reported by Causse and Causse, 1980) and that calculated from data from Ginsberg, Hoffman and White (1981) and by Marquet (1985) compared with 3.2 dB per decade for stapedotomy, it was estimated that a typical stapedectomy patient would be expected to reach the critical 40 dB level at which amplification would be beneficial 13 years postopera-tively, whereas stapedotomy patients would not be expected to reach this level for 21 years.

Using deterioration gradient estimates of changes in bone conduction, the percentage of initially success-ful ears likely to have developed a mean air conduc-tion threshold at or shortly after 5 years greater than 10 dB relative to the preoperative bone conduction threshold, has been calculated. This suggests that while 26% of stapedectomy ears have become failures only 10% of stapedotomy ears will do so, according to generally accepted criteria.

Immediate and delayed conductive losses

An estimate of the contribution of mechanical failures to the overall incidence of unsatisfactory results can be made from findings at revision operations. Loose articulations between the incus and prosthesis were detected in 1.15% of 0.8 mm Teflon, 4.25% of 0.8 mm Teflon wire and 1.9% of 0.3 mm Teflon prostheses. Secondary incus necrosis was detected in 1.7% of 0.8 mm Teflon, 3.5% of 0.8 mm Teflon wire, and 3.2% of 0.3 mm Teflon prostheses (Smyth and Hassard, 1978) (Figure 14.8).

Revision of loose articulations and incus necrosis ears restored hearing to previous levels in 65% and 77% respectively, but in some cases the duration of follow up was insufficient to verify their per-manence.

When the above categories of postoperative loss in hearing are assembled (Table 14.1) it is obvious that the results may be much less frequently 'successful'

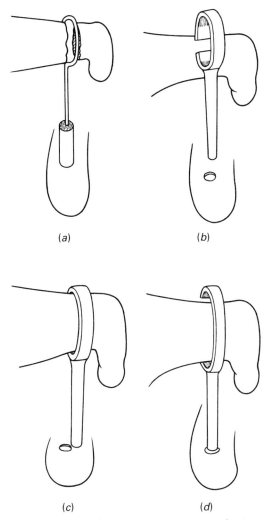

(a)   *(b)*

(c)   *(d)*

Figure 14.8 Causes of persistent postoperative conduction hearing loss. (*a*) Incus necrosis; (*b*) disarticulated prosthesis; (*c*) medially displaced prosthesis; (*d*) loosely articulated prosthesis

at 5 years than is generally assumed using the 10 dB air-bone gap criterion.

Continued analysis of results in the groups studied by Smyth and Hassard (1978) has provided information which may make it necessary to modify the information given to patients in the future about their auditory status as time passes postoperatively. In addition to the possible early losses about which council is given when stapedectomy is under consideration, it is of vital importance that patients appreciate the possibility of additional, slowly developing deteriorations in their auditory acuity which may eventually result in a return of the kind of incapacity of which they initially complained. Long-term deterioration is mainly sensorineural and may be the result of presbyacusis and cochlear otosclerosis or result from trauma caused by the surgical intervention. Should it occur in due course, amplification may become necessary, and patients will want to know for how long stapedotomy is likely to postpone their need for a hearing aid (Smyth and Hassard, 1986).

This evidence suggests that the deteriorations in cochlear function, which many patients experience, can be reduced by limiting surgical trauma as far as possible by means of stapedotomy, which is less likely to produce superimposed defects due to fistulae. Although the most frequent mechanical problem at the incus articulation occurred with wire-loop prostheses, this is in conflict with the experience of other surgeons and may have been due to faulty technique (McGee, 1983).

The conclusion which emerges most forcefully from this study relates to the eventual prognosis for maintenance of socially adequate hearing. It seems likely that many patients will eventually require amplification. They should be made aware of this when contemplating surgical treatment of their hearing loss. In addition, because the time-honoured method of reporting results appears to be no longer appropriate, a system which would include thresholds at 4 kHz and relate results both to social adequacy and also

Table 14.1 Causes and percentage of patients having air-bone gap > 10 dB at 5 years postoperatively

	Stapedectomy *0.8 mm* *Teflon*	*0.8 mm* *Tefwire*	*Stapedotomy* *0.3 mm* *Teflon*
Immediate sensorineural	3.50	3.50	0
Disarticulation of prostheses	2.85	7.75	4.10
Fistula	0.60	3.50	0.60
Predicted delayed sensorineural	27.00	25.00	10.00
Total	33.95	39.75	14.70

Smyth and Hassard, 1986

to contralateral hearing is preferable and more realistic.

By virtue of a small number of otosclerotic ears in this study operated over a 15-year period, the surgeon involved must rate as an 'occasional' stapedectomist. However, there is still a place for the provision of this service by surgeons who maintain their microsurgical skills by continued experience in tympanoplasty and otoneurosurgery, provided they are comfortable with their stapedectomy technique. In this respect stapedotomy is recommended.

As against the disappointing but hardly surprising findings in this study, it is reassuring to know that stapedotomy can, on average, effectively postpone the need for a hearing aid for longer than 20 years, a period which in the opinion of some surgeons may possibly be extended by means of sodium fluoride therapy. Additional support for stapedotomy derives from reports of better maintenance of bone conduction thresholds in operated as opposed to unoperated ears (Smyth and Hassard, 1978; Karjalainen, Karja and Harma, 1984).

Complications of surgical treatment

Perilymph fistula

This serious complication is potentially dangerous due to the risk of meningitis. It may give rise to dysequilibrium and hearing loss, which will progress if the fistula does not close either by spontaneous healing or as the result of a revision operation.

The signs and symptoms of perilymph fistula were first described by Lewis (1961) and by Farrior (1962), and the complication, at one time thought to be unusual, is now accepted as being the most common single complication of stapedectomy.

Aetiology of perilymph fistula

Primary fistula

The surgeon creates a fistula at every stapedectomy operation and relies on the natural process of healing, or in some techniques a graft of soft tissue, to seal the opening which has been made into the vestibule. In most operations, there is enough surgical trauma to the oval window mucoperiosteum to lead to the production of an inflammatory repair envelope around the prosthesis sealing the opening into the oval window. A fistula is more common with a plastic prosthesis than with an interposition technique; however, the hearing result using a prosthesis is better.

There is no doubt that a small fistula remains after many stapedectomy operations with incomplete closure of the air-bone gap and the hearing result may be acceptable to the patient. Although a perilymph fistula usually leads to a sensorineural hearing loss this is not always the case and a persisting conductive

loss after an operation, which appeared to be satisfactory at the time, should warn the surgeon that there may be a perilymph fistula and a revision operation to close it will be the best line of treatment. It must be appreciated that a small fistula may become larger under the influence of barotrauma; a sensorineural hearing loss will follow and it may then be too late to save the hearing.

Secondary or acquired fistula

A secondary perilymph fistula is usually the result of barotrauma which breaks the fragile seal and can occur at any time after operation. In most cases, the stapedius tendon has been cut and a sudden change of intratympanic pressure may produce an abnormal movement of the prosthesis, giving rise to a rupture of the oval window seal (Figure 14.9).

The reported incidence of a fistula with stapedotomy is very much less than with stapedectomy (Smyth and Hassard, 1978; McGee, 1983; Causse and Causse, 1984).

Prevention of perilymph fistula

The very thin membrane which will develop to close the oval window if fat or gelfoam is used in stapedectomy, can be avoided if the oval window is covered with a vein graft. If the greater part of the footplate is removed, not only is there a greater risk of sensorineural deafness being produced by such a traumatic procedure, but there is a greater risk of a fistula developing later.

Clinical experience has shown that the stapedotomy operation is an advance on techniques where a large opening is made in the footplate. This view is supported by engineering preference for smaller diameter windows in supersonic aircraft design.

Opinions are divided over the value of soft tissue grafts in stapedectomy. According to Marquet (1985), vestibular endothelium regenerates medial to the piston and forms a seal which does not benefit from the addition of any other material. In his opinion, the functional result depends only upon a close contact between the prosthesis and the perilymph.

Advice given to the patient after operation

It is important to warn the patient who has had a stapedectomy operation that:

1 Nose blowing should be avoided and the mouth should be kept open on coughing and sneezing
2 Flying or going over a mountain pass should be avoided for at least 10 days after operation, or when an upper respiratory tract infection develops
3 Diving when swimming should be avoided
4 Lifting heavy objects should be avoided
5 Any hearing loss, vertigo or ear infection must be reported immediately.

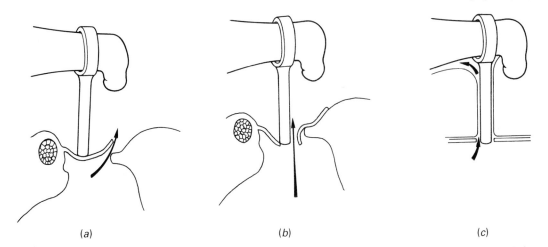

(a)   (b)   (c)

Figure 14.9 Routes of perilymph leak in fistula. (*a*) At oval window margin; (*b*) through defect in soft tissue graft at medial end of prosthesis; (*c*) along track between prosthesis and mucosal capsule

When eustachian tube dysfunction develops after operation, Hemenway, Hildyard and Black (1968) placed ventilation tubes in the tympanic membrane.

Diagnosis of a perilymph fistula

The symptoms of a perilymph fistula are a fluctuating hearing loss, tinnitus, a feeling of fullness in the ear and vertigo. The symptoms are those of endolymphatic hydrops, which is the underlying cause of symptoms in this condition.

The fistula may be primary, dating from the time of operation when there is failure of the oval window to seal, or it may be secondary, when it can appear many months or even years after the original operation.

Primary perilymph fistula

When the opening, created by the surgeon in the oval window region, fails to heal after the operation, a disturbance of equilibrium persists in the days and weeks after operation, until vestibular paralysis and compensation occur. In other patients, there may be brief periods of vertigo continuing over a long period.

Secondary perilymph fistula

The characteristic symptom of secondary perilymph fistula is a change of hearing coming on after an interval, which may be months or years after a successful operation; associated with this are feelings of fullness, tinnitus and dysequilibrium. There may be considerable variation in the symptoms but a conductive deafness may be the early sign of a fistula and this may precede a serious irreversible labyrinthine lesion (Goodhill, 1979).

The symptoms and findings in a review of 49 cases of perilymph fistula are given in Table 14.2 (Moon, 1970). Sometimes the patient may give a history of symptoms developing after an incident such as severe nose blowing, strenuous exercise or flying in an unpressurized aircraft, but often no precipitating factor may present and the patient may not seek advice until there is a considerable degree of sensorineural deafness.

Table 14.2 Hearing loss

	Primary fistula	Secondary fistula
Sensorineural	16 (52%)	7 (39%)
Mixed	13 (42%)	5 (28%)
Conduction	2 (6%)	3 (17%)
None	0	3 (17%)
	31	18

(Reproduced from Moon (1970) by kind permission of the Editor of *The Laryngoscope*)

Clinical findings in perilymph fistula

The clinical examination of the ear is usually normal, rarely the tympanic membrane may be retracted or there is evidence of fluid in the middle ear.

Audiometric tests

Hearing tests carried out soon after the onset of a fistula will show findings similar to those seen in labyrinthine hydrops, i.e. a pure tone sensorineural hearing loss, in the low frequencies initially, followed by a flat loss which fluctuates. There may be recruitment. In the early stages, discrimination scores fluctuate with the pure tone threshold, but later they may be disproportionally lower than expected when compared with the stapedius reflex threshold. In some cases, and particularly when vertigo is the main complaint with little or no depression of pure tone levels, there may be a markedly diminished speech discrimination score. It has already been pointed out that a variable conductive loss may occur without a sensorineural component, and this is characteristic of dislocation of the prosthesis from the incus.

Vestibular tests

Hallpike caloric test The characteristic finding is canal paresis, or hypoactive response, and this may be present at an early stage of the condition. It must be appreciated that after stapedectomy there is a high incidence of diminished caloric response (Smyth, Kerr and Singh, 1975) and so the significance of the caloric test is difficult to evaluate and of little value in the diagnosis of a fistula.

Electronystagmography Electronystagmography may reveal a directional fixed positional nystagmus but this cannot be relied upon as an indication of a fistula.

Fistula tests Fistula tests with the pneumatic otoscope may be helpful but have been found to be negative in one-third of cases. The negative pressure fistula test with electronystagmography produces nystagmus with the quick phase away from the affected ear. Fistula tests with electronystagmography and the impedance bridge have superseded the older methods as they give a higher degree of accuracy, but the results are inconsistent and a negative response does not rule out the presence of a fistula (Seltzer and McCabe, 1986).

Diagnosis by radioactive tracer method Radioactive indium-111 DTRA is injected into the lumbar subarachnoid space. The demonstration of increased radioactivity in nasopharyngeal secretions strongly supports the diagnosis of fistula (Weider, Saunders and Musiek, 1991).

Treatment of a perilymph fistula

The treatment of a perilymph fistula is a tympanotomy at the earliest possible moment, with an attempt to close the fistula.

When the leak is detected the fistulous track is excised and the prosthesis removed with great care. The opening in the vestibule is covered with a soft tissue graft which is held in place by another prosthesis. A disadvantage of a two-stage method of closing a fistula is that the graft may float off with a recurrence of the fistula as there is no prosthesis to hold it in place.

Results of treatment of a fistula

Unless early treatment is instituted, the changes of restoration or improvement of hearing are small and in some cases a troublesome dysequilibrium may remain. It is imperative that the surgeon is fully aware of this complication and realizes that some techniques are safer than others. The use of gelatin sponge to seal the oval window in stapedectomy produces a very thin membrane and gives the highest incidence of fistula formation. Most surgeons have abandoned this technique. Stapedotomy is a safe method and the small fenestra stapedectomy, with vein graft and Teflon piston, as practised by Causse, has also proved to be relatively free from this complication.

If the results of treatment of perilymph fistula are to show improvement, early diagnosis and immediate revision surgery are essential.

Revision operations

Conductive deafness may occur after any successful stapes operation. There are four principle causes: necrosis of the tip of the incus; loose attachment between the incus and the prosthesis; detachment of the prosthesis from the incus; and displacement or dislodgement of the prosthesis from the oval window area.

Recurrence of otosclerosis may spread from the anterior footplate area and recurrence of the lesion can lead to closure of the oval window area even if the whole footplate has been removed.

With the passage of time, poor results from attempts to correct residual conductive hearing loss after stapedectomy have become apparent (Sheehy, Nelson and House, 1981; Glasscock, 1987; Farrior and Sutherland, 1991). Profound sensorineural hearing loss has been reported in up to 14% of ears (Crabtree, Button and Powers, 1980). Histopathological studies of temporal bones from post-stapedectomized patients have demonstrated adhesions between the prosthesis or the neomembrane of the oval window and the utricle and saccule (Hohmann, 1962; Linthicum, 1971). Many surgeons are prepared to do revision procedures only under local anaesthesia. If manipulation of the prosthesis causes vertigo the surgeon will be aware of this and may feel obliged to discontinue attempts at improving the hearing in the interests of preserving inner ear function.

In order to identify and rectify the cause of surgical failure, blind tissue manipulation in the oval window may be unavoidable. The risks to the membranous inner ear and of consequent imbalance and anacusis are obvious. Otospongiotic closure of the oval window is a contraindication for further surgery. In other ears, in order to minimize the risk of re-operation, the use of the KTP laser (Bartels, 1990) or the CO_2 laser (Lesinski and Stein, 1989) has been advocated. Indeed, many surgeons would now regard the laser as indispensable in this situation.

Immediate sensorineural deafness after operation

Sensorineural deafness after operation may occur in the immediate postoperative period, in the intermediate period weeks or months after operation, or be delayed for months or even years after surgery.

The reported incidence of severe sensorineural deafness following stapedectomy varies from 0.5 to 4% and it is important to realize that these are the figures from a series of operations by expert surgeons with a special interest in stapedectomy. The results of the occasional operator are rarely reported and it is likely that the incidence of cochlear damage is much higher when the surgeon is inexperienced (Doyle and Woodham, 1980).

The causes of cochlear loss produced by operation are numerous – they are the direct result of trauma of varying types to the inner ear at the time of, or soon after, operation.

All operations involve the possibility of trauma to the inner ear; some techniques are more traumatic than others and the pathology of the lesion will influence this. In addition, a small group of patients is particularly sensitive to the creation of a window in the footplate of the stapes and so there is always the risk of this disaster after every operation, even by the most expert surgeon. This risk is small and indeed almost non-existent with some techniques, if correctly managed.

The causes of immediate sensorineural deafness include: acoustic trauma from drilling; excessive movement of the stapes producing a hydraulic effect; rupture of the membranous inner ear; rapid loss of perilymph; footplate fragments or bone dust in the vestibule; and the floating footplate. Attempts at removal of the last of these may result in a 'dead ear' and it is essential that this complication is correctly managed.

Acoustic trauma

The modern microdrill is a safe instrument if it is used correctly. The drill must be light, preferably fixed to a small motor which allows slow rotary motion, and the drill ends must not be toothed unless there is an obliterative footplate.

Excessive movement of the stapes

In stapedectomy, if an attempt is made to remove a prematurely mobilized footplate, and this can occur when there is minimal fixation, a hydraulic effect can be produced which is damaging to the membranous structures in the vestibule. It is a wise precaution to make a small opening in the footplate, with a sharp pick or slowly rotating microdrill before attempting to detach the crura from the footplate. This precaution may prevent the hydraulic effect.

Rupture of the membranous inner ear

Meticulous technique and the making of a small fenestra should prevent this complication, but if small particles of bone do enter the vestibule, *no* attempt should be made to remove them either by instruments or suction.

Rapid loss of perilymph

This may be caused by the use of suction in the oval window which must therefore be avoided. It is occasionally seen in an ear with an abnormally patent cochlear aqueduct, when cerebrospinal fluid will enter the ear.

Presence of blood in the vestibule

This condition has already been discussed. It is unlikely that blood in the vestibule *per se* will cause any damage to the inner ear. The problem is the difficulty in dealing with the pathology found at operation when the operative field is obscured. In clinics which specialize in the surgery of otosclerosis, a dry field is achieved by suitable anaesthetic techniques.

Preoperative cochlear impairment, obliterative otosclerosis and increased age all independently increase the risks of immediate postoperative cochlear dysfunction. This may be due to associated changes in vascular status and the additional possibility of advanced *cochlear* otosclerosis, both of which are likely to be reflected in the audiometric pattern. Therefore, older patients in the Juers type C group must be considered in an 'at risk' category, especially when an obliterated oval window is also found at operation. It would therefore seem sensible to avoid stapedectomy in these patients, remembering that, as in all forms of otosclerosis, a hearing aid can frequently offer a great deal and carries no risk of worsening the auditory status.

Under no circumstances should the other ear be operated upon when the first ear has suffered a significant cochlear loss because the possibility of delayed total hearing loss in the second ear can never be ruled out. This is because both ears are likely to be affected by the same problems initially during the operation, because of the high incidence of symmetrical footplate pathology (Ludman and Grant, 1973) and also permanently thereafter because the threat of upper respiratory infection and abrupt changes in atmospheric and cerebrospinal pressure are always likely to affect *both ears*.

An operation which limits trauma to the minimum should be used in every case. Thus, all large fenestra techniques (stapedectomy) are to be avoided if possible. Wide removal of the stapes footplate must predispose to contamination of the vestibule by bone dust and blood, produce a large hydraulic effect in the vestibule of the inner ear, lead to prolonged perilymph drainage and threaten the vascular sufficiency of the membranous labyrinth.

The very low incidence of severe sensorineural hearing loss reported in ears treated by stapedotomy supports the claim that this operation carries much less risk of serious damage to hearing than any other currently available.

A connection between influenzal viral infection and unexplained sensorineural hearing loss immediately after stapes surgery has been postulated (Pedersen and Felding, 1991). Although without serological evidence this cannot be proven, it would seem prudent to avoid operations when respiratory viral infections are prevalent, especially in the patient, the patient's family or the surgeon.

Treatment of immediate postoperative cochlear loss

If a technique is adopted which does not lead to a fistula after operation, e.g. 'vein graft interposition' or the true small fenestra technique, it is possible to obtain complete closure of the air-bone gap and avoid postoperative high tone loss.

Causse *et al.* (1970) were of the opinion that careful monitoring of the hearing after operation is of vital importance since it may be possible, if a sensorineural hearing loss is detected within a few hours of its appearance, to reverse the hearing loss by medical treatment.

The monitoring of the patient involves strict audiometric surveillance by means of effectively masked (modified Rainville method) bone conduction audiometry and Weber tests of the pure tone and speech variety. Speech and pure tone audiometry are carried out later and the final speech and pure tone audiogram is made on the twentieth postoperative day. After discharge the patient is instructed to report immediately to the surgeon, by telephone, if there is any sudden hearing drop, or the onset of tinnitus or vertigo.

The treatment of sensorineural deafness after operation is similar to that given for Menière's disease, although in both disorders its rationale is unproven. Bed rest and diuretic therapy are usual. Hydrocortisone is also used, in gradually decreasing doses, as it is believed that it protects cell membranes, and has an anti-inflammatory, antioedematous and antihaemorrhagic action. Treatment with inhalation of 5% CO_2 and 95% O_2 has also been recommended. Sodium fluoride is added to this basic treatment for its anti-enzymatic action on cochlear lesions.

However, investigation of inner ear function after stapes surgery is carried out by few surgeons. Diagnosis is difficult as there is loss of discrimination for a time after most techniques. This is caused by the fistula created at surgery which usually closes spontaneously. Audiometry often shows an incomplete closure of the air-bone gap and a high tone loss in the immediate postoperative period. The audiometric pattern improves during the course of a few weeks after operation but the high tone loss takes longer and may never recover completely, especially after stapedectomy.

If medical treatment can lead to recovery of sensorineural hearing loss after stapes surgery, it should be tried more frequently, although it will remain difficult to say if a successful outcome is the result of therapy, or due to the remarkable power of the inner ear to recover after injury.

Delayed sensorineural hearing loss after operation

A comparison of changes (at yearly intervals over 10 years) in the bone conduction response and speech discrimination with stapedotomy and stapedectomy, corrected for the effects of age and Juers grouping by the technique of orthogonalized analysis of variance has been reported (Smyth and Hassard, 1978). Stapedotomy caused significantly less depression of bone conduction thresholds with the passage of time at 4 kHz. This effect was conspicuously absent at 0.5 kHz and was reversed at 1 and 2 kHz. Better speech discrimination scores were achieved with stapedotomy (statistically significant at 1, 2 and 7 years) in all but one postoperative evaluation. This general profile is similar to that of most other series which have been reported in detail (Bailey, Pappas and Graham, 1981; McGee, 1981).

Stapedotomy is now seen to be an important advance in the surgical treatment of otosclerosis, but it must not be forgotten that, although it significantly lessens the loss of high tone response with time, it certainly does not eliminate the problem. In addition, it should be noted that stapedotomy frequently does not provide better bone conduction at 0.5 kHz and provides less satisfactory thresholds at 1 and 2 kHz than does stapedectomy.

In order to explain the lack of uniformity in results, the possible ways in which one operation might influence bone conduction more than the other can be considered under the following headings:

1 Energy transmission to the cochlea
2 Effects on the sensory apparatus.

Energy transmission to the cochlea

The response of the cochlea to bone conduction stimuli has three components, all of which may be influenced by the size of the oval window fenestration.

1 The contribution of translatory and especially transmitted factors in bone conduction is directly related to the overall efficiency of the ossicular chain. In stapedectomy, a mesothelial membrane develops on the vestibular aspect of the prosthesis and forms a tent anchored at the fenestral rim, having its apex at the prosthesis. This system works first, by producing a good fluid-tight seal in the vestibule proper and, second, because the membrane, owing

to its diameter being greater than that of a piston has less impedance. The acoustic impedance (Z_a) in the plane of the piston is the ratio of the mechanical impedance (Z_m) and the square of the area of the acting surface of the piston: $Z_a = \frac{Z_m}{S^2}$ (Moller, 1974). This transmission system being less rigid than the footplate entails some losses. Nevertheless, it is more efficient than one would obtain with a very narrow piston projecting through a very narrow opening and giving rise to a much smaller membrane than that occurring in stapedectomy. Therefore, better overall hearing should be provided by stapedectomy if only by virtue of its being a better mechanical system than stapedotomy. Although this effect may account for the significantly better bone conduction response at 1 and 2 kHz, the lack of better response with stapedectomy at 0.5 kHz presents a problem. It is proposed that a better match between the surface area of the oval window membrane and the diameter of the scala vestibuli is provided by stapedectomy as compared to stapedotomy. Consequently, in theory, stapedectomy would deliver more energy to the low frequency receptors at the furthest end of the cochlear duct. The explanation as to why this is not apparent in practice may be that the impedance of the cochlea, which is much greater for the lower frequencies, masks the differences in the respective responses with stapedectomy and stapedotomy in such a way as to render them too small to show significance. Again, cochlear impedance may override the theoretical advantage arising from removal of the rigid footplate, which would be expected to reduce middle ear impedance for low frequencies.

2 Compressional bone conduction depends upon differential mobility of the oval and round windows. Footplate fixation is responsible for an impairment of bone conduction response which is maximum for 2 kHz. Stapedectomy will provide a much better restoration of compressional bone conduction when most or all of the footplate is removed. One would not expect a fenestra of 0.4 mm to do much to reverse a Carhart notch. Herein appears to be at least part of the explanation for significantly better bone conduction thresholds at 1 and 2 kHz with stapedectomy.

Effects on the sensory apparatus

In spite of its undoubted mechanical deficiencies, stapedotomy provides a significantly better bone conduction response at 4 kHz. This may be because stapedotomy causes less trauma to the higher frequency receptors, which are already vulnerable to high intensity noise and ageing. If an explanation for this can be found, it will be based on a better understanding of the events which occur in the labyrinth at, and shortly following, oval window fenestration and the changes which subsequently develop in the components of the cochlea as a consequence of those earlier events.

The problem basically concerns the multiplicity of possible responses to trauma. In tissues generally, there would appear to be an inverse relationship between cell complexity and reparative potential. Therefore, in an organ as highly specialized as the cochlea, we would expect a less complete recovery than we might after a simple skin incision. Every organ has its own specific ability to survive trauma; however, once the upper limits of tolerance have been passed, the outcome will depend upon:

1 The specific potential of that organ tissue for repair. Reports on experimental stapedectomy have recorded outer hair cell loss postoperatively. It has been postulated that some of the high frequency losses which follow stapedectomy may be the result of surgically-induced stimulation injury (Schuknecht and Tonndorf, 1960). Similar lesions possibly account for some or all of the hearing losses in this series. The inability of hair cells to regenerate (fixed postmitotic state) is an example of the special vulnerability of the cochlea to trauma.
2 The functional reserve of the organ. In the cochlea this factor is important and most valuable, as illustrated by the maintenance of bone conduction thresholds in the face of a loss of up to 75% of the first order neurons (Schuknecht and Woellner, 1955).
3 The ability of the organ *as a whole* to compensate for functional loss. It is frequently possible to demonstrate subclinical defects in vestibular function by caloric testing after stapedectomy (Stroud, 1963; Ali and Groves, 1964; Smyth, Kerr and Singh, 1975).

Although the response of the ear to stapedectomy is as yet poorly understood, studies of long-term effects of diseases of the otic capsule on labyrinthine function strongly suggest that progressive accumulative degenerative processes may be initiated whose clinical manifestations may be delayed possibly for long periods. In order to find an explanation for delayed sensorineural loss following stapedectomy, we can extrapolate from what we know about another type of delayed loss due to trauma, i.e. noise deafness, and postulate a theory which takes into account the mechanical aspects of the problem. Although the modes of action in these two mechanisms may not be identical, i.e. overstimulation compared to membrane distortion, they could have a common denominator such as vascular sludging and spasm occurring as a basic response to trauma. The general principle that trauma causes vasospasm which, if prolonged, leads to thrombosis, is in line with the findings of Lawrence, Gonzales and Hawkins (1967) and Schnieder (1975) which suggest that the damaging effect of high intensity noise has a vascular and simultaneous biochemical and humoral basis.

Noise exposure data

At present much of our knowledge about the effects of excess energy on the cochlea is based on noise exposure experiments. It has been shown experimentally that exposure to high levels of noise results in:

1 Distortion of hair cells and swelling of their nuclei (Spoendlin, 1971)
2 Degenerative changes within the hair cell cytoplasm, with eventual membrane rupture and lysis (Mizukoshi, Konishi and Nakamura, 1957; Lim and Melnick, 1971)
3 Reduction of ribonucleic acid (Misrahy, Shenabarger and Arnold, 1958), endolymphatic oxygen tension (Vosteen, 1958) and succinic dehydrogenase (Zorzoli and Boriani, 1958) and glycogen levels (Ruedi and Furrer, 1946).

It is tempting to reason that hair cell damage in the experimental animal is due to vascular changes and that these may be similar to those vascular changes observed in the human inner ear and interpreted as being part of the ageing process (Johnsson and Hawkins, 1972). If abnormal energy input, in this case loud prolonged noise which can occur during stapes surgery, can cause irreparable damage by virtue of exceeding the reserve capacity of the cochlea, then it may be possible that other forms of energy, in excess, regardless of their nature, could also be traumatic.

Mechanical aspects

That a sudden loss of perilymphatic pressure occurs at the moment of footplate fenestration is indicated by the flow of perilymph which quickly fills the oval window niche in many stapedectomies. The immediate distortion of the membranous labyrinth which would appear to be inevitable, can be expected to affect ionic transport and microcirculation and the overall problem will be aggravated by the release of histamine (Schnieder, 1975).

If partial or total removal of the stapes footplate can cause vasospasm and metabolic disturbance because of its hydraulic effect, the outcome must be related to the *size* of the defect which in turn determines the volume and rate of perilymph loss. It is to be expected therefore that stapedectomy would be more traumatic than stapedotomy.

It is argued therefore that considerable hydraulic effects on the labyrinth must follow decompression of the perilymphatic space causing membrane distortion and an effect on the cochlea similar to that produced by excessive noise exposure. When structural loss occurs from both or either cause, this is the end result of primary vasospasm. If the effect of the pro-

gressive phases of vascular disease which have been attributed to ageing (Johnsson and Hawkins, 1972) is similar to the degenerative process which follows trauma, then the clinical picture will resemble presbyacusis but will be related more to the postoperative interval than specifically to age. Attempts to explain the particular susceptibility of the basal turn to delayed degenerative changes have been based on mechanical (Hilding, 1953), vascular (Crowe, Guild and Polvogt, 1934) and enzymatic theories (Thalmann, Matschinsky and Thalmann, 1970). Possibly all these factors, together with a poverty of reserve due to other disease, including genetic defects, play a part in the development of this serious complication of stapedectomy.

However, there is no indication that the cochlea of ears undergoing uncomplicated stapedectomy suffer undue *generalized* degenerative changes as a direct result of operation (provided a clearly defined at risk group is excluded). The finding that generalized degenerative changes do not appear to advance more rapidly in the operated ear argues strongly in favour of both stapedectomy and stapedotomy as a better treatment than amplification through the use of a hearing aid in the younger patient with good cochlear function.

The size of fenestra should be limited to the least possible in each operation in order to minimize the inevitable loss of high tone response which complicates all types of stapes surgery and which is very significantly greater following total removal of the footplate.

Final conclusions

Throughout the world at the present time stapedectomy, as opposed to stapedotomy, is still performed. Its advantages are obvious, namely, that it is easier technically and provides a good overall early result in most instances. Its disadvantages are not so often apparent because difficulties in obtaining accurate and comprehensive follow-up information may lead to a lack of real awareness of the incidence of serious sensorineural loss occurring in the early postoperative period. Additionally, because there have been few studies of sufficient duration to reveal the long-term effects on high tone cochlear response and speech discrimination, the eventual effects on the patient's auditory capacity are not widely recognized.

However, it is clear that stapedotomy has not been the panacea for all otosclerotic patients, possibly because of mechanical inefficiency for the lower frequencies and a tendency to disarticulation from the incus due to faults in the characteristics of the prostheses. In all other respects, this technique does have an enormous advantage to recommend it. This is that the risk of immediate or delayed inner ear complications is significantly reduced. In addition, and most importantly, balanced frequency response is preserved and with it speech discrimination for assistance by amplification, if this is eventually required. Although the available evidence necessary to support the use of sodium fluoride in the treatment of otospongiosus is so far restricted, its possible future role in the treatment of both surgical and non-surgical patients should not be overlooked or dismissed.

Acknowledgement

During the 9 years which have passed since Philip Beales wrote his chapter on otosclerosis for the fifth edition of *Scott Brown's Otolaryngology* there have been some additions to our knowledge of this disease and its treatment.

My acceptance of the Editor's invitation to update this chapter was conditional on the preservation of much of Mr Beale's work. The reader will find that the excellent historical, pathological and diagnostic sections remain largely as they were. Most of what has been added concerns recent advances in surgical treatment and the long-term results which can be anticipated.

Postscript by the General Editor

This chapter is special in two different ways. First, it probably will be the last to be written by a British otologist who was practising at the onset of modern stapes surgery and who therefore had a really large series of stapes operations. Those who follow in the current British system are very unlikely ever to have the opportunity of such wide experience. Secondly, Gordon Smyth was working on this chapter when he became seriously ill and he completed it in 1992 during a remarkably productive terminal illness, knowing that he would never see it in print. He had been aware that the publication date of 1996 was 4 years ahead and he expressed fears that it might be out of date. However, John Booth and I were keen to have his experience recorded and prevailed upon him to remain as the author and he produced this excellent chapter based on his very extensive experience. John Booth and George Browning have both surveyed this chapter in detail, along with the literature of the past 4 years, and have added relevant up to date references, but the text remains essentially that which Gordon Smyth submitted.

It was Gordon Smyth who taught me how to perform stapes surgery and I am delighted to have this chapter in the sixth edition. I wish to acknowledge my indebtedness to him for so many aspects of my otological career and to express my appreciation to John Booth and George Browning for the time and effort they have put into ensuring that a chapter written 4 years ago is still significant and up to date.

AGK

References

ADAMS, C.W. and TUQAN, N.A. (1961) The histochemical demonstration of protease by a gelatin substrate. *Journal of Histochemistry and Cytochemistry*, **9**, 469–472

ALBERTI, P.M., HYDE, M.L., SYMONS, B.A. and MILLAR, R.B. (1980) The effect of prolonged experience to industrial noise on otosclerosis. *Laryngoscope*, **90**, 407–413

ALI, Y. and GROVES, J. (1964) Vestibular disorders after stapedectomy. *Journal of Laryngology and Otology*, **78**, 1102–1113

APPLEBAUM, E.J. and SHAMBAUGH, G.E. (1978) Otospongiosis (otosclerosis). Polytomographic and histological correlation. *Laryngoscope*, **88**, 1761–1768

ARNOLD, W. and FRIEDMANN, I. (1988) Otosclerosis – an inflammatory disease of the otic capsule of viral aetiology. *Journal of Laryngology and Otology*, **102**, 865–871

BAILEY, H.A.T., PAPPAS, J.P. and GRAHAM, S.S. (1981) Small fenestra stapedectomy. A preliminary report. *Laryngoscope*, **91**, 1308–1320

BALLE, V. and LINTHICUM, F.H., JR (1985) Histologically proven otosclerosis with pure sensorineural hearing loss. *Annals of Otology, Rhinology and Laryngology*, **93**, 105–111

BARANY, R. (1924) Die Indikationen zur Labyrinthoperation. *Acta Otolaryngologica*, **6**, 260–288

BARTELS, L.J. (1990) KTP laser stapedotomy: Is it safe? *Otolaryngology – Head and Neck Surgery*, **103**, 685–692

BERNSTEIN, D.S., SADOWSKY, N. and HAGSTEAD, D.M. (1966) The prevalence of osteoporosis in high and low fluoride areas of North Dakota. *Journal of the American Medical Association*, **198**, 499–504

BRETLAU, P., CHEVANCE, G.L., CAUSSE, J. and LORGANSEN, M.B. (1982) Bone resorption in otospongiosis. *American Journal of Otology*, **3**, 284–289

BRETLAU, P., CAUSSE, J., CAUSSE, J.-B., HANSEN, H.J., JONSEN, N.J. and SALOMON, G. (1985) Otospongiosis and sodium fluoride. A blind experimental and clinical evaluation of the effect of sodium fluoride treatment in patients with otospongiosis. *Annals of Otology, Rhinology and Laryngology*, **94**, 103–107

BRETLAU, P., SALOMON, G. and JOHNSEN, N.J. (1989) Otospongiosis and sodium fluoride: A clinical double-blind, placebo-controlled study on sodium fluoride treatment in otospongiosis. *American Journal of Otology*, **10**, 20–22

BROWNING, G.G. (ed.) (1986) *Clinical Otology and Audiology*. London: Butterworths. p. 181

BROWNING, G.G. and GATEHOUSE, S. (1992) The prevalence of middle ear disease in the adult British population. *Clinical Otolaryngology*, **17**, 317–321

BROWNING, G.G., GATEHOUSE, S. and SWAN, R.C. (1991) The Glasgow Benefit Plot: a new method for reporting benefits from middle ear surgery. *Laryngoscope*, **101**, 180–185

BULL, T.R. (1965) Taste and the chorda tympani. *Journal of Laryngology and Otology*, **79**, 479–493

CARHART, R. (1962) Effect of stapes fixation on bone conduction response. In: *Otosclerosis*, edited by H. F. Schuknecht. London: Churchill Livingstone. pp. 175–197

CAUSSE, J. and CAUSSE, J-B. (1979) Medical management of otospongiosis and NaF therapy. 13th Annual Colorado Otology-Audiology Workshop, Vail. Corti's Organ, **4**, no. 3

CAUSSE, J. and CAUSSE, J-B. (1980) Problems of stapedial fixation. *Clinical Otolaryngology*, **5**, 49–59

CAUSSE, J., BEL, J., MICHAUX, P., CANUT, Y. and TAPON, J. (1970) Otospongiosis surgery. Sudden deafness after stapedectomy. *Annales d'Oto-Laryngologie (Paris)*, **87**, 751–778

CAUSSE, J., CHEVANCE, L.G., BRETLAU, P., JORGENSEN, M.B., URIEL, J. and BERGES, J. (1977) Enzymatic concept of otospongiosis and cochlear otospongiosis. *Clinical Otolaryngology*, **2**, 23–32

CAUSSE, J., SHAMBAUGH, G.E. and CHEVANCE, L.G. (1977) Cochlear otospongiosis: etiology, diagnosis and therapeutic implications. *Advances in Oto-Rhino-Laryngology*, **22**, 43–56

CAUSSE, J.R., SHAMBAUGH, G.E., CAUSSE, J.B. and BRETLAU, P. (1980) Enzymology of otospongiosis and NaF therapy. *American Journal of Otology*, **1**, 206–214.

CAUSSE, J.B. and CAUSSE, J.R. (1984) Stapedectomy technique and results. *American Journal of Otology*, **5**, 68–71

CAUSSE, J.B., CAUSSE, J.R. and PARAHY, C. (1985) Stapedotomy technique and results. *American Journal of Otology*, **6**, 68–75

CAWTHORNE, T. (1955) Otosclerosis. *Journal of Laryngology and Otology*, **69**, 437–456

CHEVANCE, L.G., BRETLAU, P., JORGENSEN, M.B. and CAUSSE, J. (1970) Otosclerosis. An electron microscope and cytological study. *Acta Otolaryngologica Supplementum*, **272**, 1–44

COKER, N.J., DUNCAN, N.O., WRIGHT, G.L., JENKINS, H.A. and ALFORD, B.R. (1988) Stapedectomy trends for the resident. *Annals of Otology, Rhinology and Laryngology*, **97**, 109–113

COLLETTE, V. and FIORINO, F.G. (1994) Stapedotomy with stapedius tendon preservation: Technique and long term results. *Otolaryngology – Head and Neck Surgery*, **111**, 181–188

COLMAN, B.H. (1979) Otosclerosis. In: *Clinical Otolaryngology*, edited by A. G. Maran and P. M. Stell. Oxford: Blackwell. pp. 189–206

CRABTREE, J.A., BUTTON, W.H. and POWERS, B. (1980) An evaluation of revision stapes surgery. *Laryngoscope*, **90**, 224–227

CREMERS, C.W.R.J., BENSEN, J.M.S. and HUYGEN, P.L.M. (1991) Hearing gain after stapedotomy, partial platinectomy or total stapedectomy for otosclerosis. *Annals of Otology, Rhinology and Laryngology*, **100**, 959–961

CREMERS, C.W.R.J., HOMBERGEN, G.C.J.H. and WENTGES, R.T.L.R. (1983) Perilymphatic gusher and stapes surgery. A predictable complication. *Clinical Otolaryngology*, **8**, 235–240

CROWE, S., GUILD, S. and POLVOGT, L. (1934) Observation on pathology of high tone deafness. *Bulletin of the Johns Hopkins Hospital*, **54**, 315–379

DANIEL, H.J. (1969) Stapedial otosclerosis and fluorine in the drinking water. *Archives of Otolaryngology*, **90**, 585–589

DE GROOT, J.A. (1985) Labyrinthine otosclerosis studied with a new computed tomography technique. *Annals of Otology, Rhinology and Laryngology*, **94**, 223–225

DERLACKI, E. and VALVASSORI, G. (1965) Clinical and radiological diagnosis of labyrinthine otosclerosis. *Laryngoscope*, **75**, 1293–1306

DIAMOND, D. and FREW, I. (1979) In: *The Facial Nerve*. Oxford: Oxford University Press. p. 178

DOYLE, P.J. and WOODHAM, J. (1980) Results of stapes surgery – subjective and objective. *Journal of Otolaryngology*, **9**, 381–386

ELBROND, O. and JENSEN, J.J. (1979) Otosclerosis and pregnancy: a study of the influence of pregnancy on the hearing threshold before and after stapedectomy. *Clinical Otolaryngology*, **4**, 259–266

ENGSTROM, H. (1940) Uber das Vorkommen der Otosklerose nebst experimentellen Studien uber Chirurgische Behandlung der Krankheit. *Acta Otolaryngologica Supplementum*, **43**, 1–49

FARRIOR, J.B. (1962) Abstruse complications of stapes surgery. Diagnosis and treatment. In: *Otosclerosis*, edited by H. F. Schuknecht. Boston: Little, Brown Co. pp. 509–521

FARRIOR, J.B. and SUTHERLAND, M.S. (1991) Revision stapes surgery. *Laryngoscope*, **101**, 1155–1161

FISCH, U. (1982) Stapedotomy versus stapedectomy. *American Journal of Otology*, **4**, 112–117

FRANKLIN, D.J., POLLAK, A. and FISCH, U. (1990) Menière's symptoms resulting from bilateral otosclerotic occlusion of the endolymphatic duct: an analysis of a causal relationship between otosclerosis and Menière's disease. *American Journal of Otology*, **11**, 135–140

FRIEDMANN, I. (1974) *Pathology of the Ear*. Oxford: Blackwell.

GANTZ, B.J., KISHIMOTO, S., JENKINS, H.A. and FISCH, U. (1982) Argon laser stapedotomy. *Annals of Otology, Rhinology and Laryngology*, **91**, 25–26

GARRITSEN, T.J.M. and CREMERS, C.W.R.J. (1991) Stapes surgery in osteogenesis imperfecta. Analysis of postoperative hearing loss. *Annals of Otology, Rhinology and Laryngology*, **100**, 120–130

GINSBERG, I.A., HOFFMAN, S.R. and WHITE, T.P. (1981) Hearing changes following stapedectomy: a six year follow-up. *Laryngoscope*, **91**, 87–92

GLASSCOCK, M.E. (1987) Revision stapedectomy surgery. *Otolaryngology – Head and Neck Surgery*, **96**, 141–148

GLORIG, A. and GALLO, R. (1962) Comments on sensorineural loss in otosclerosis. In: *Otosclerosis*, edited by H.F. Schuknecht. Boston: Little, Brown & Co. pp. 63–78

GOODHILL, V. (1960) Pseudo-otosclerosis. *Laryngoscope*, **70**, 722–757

GOODHILL, V. (1979) *Ear Diseases, Deafness and Giddiness*. New York: Harper and Row

GRISTWOOD, R.E. (1966) Obliterative otosclerosis: an analysis of the clinical and audiometric findings. *Journal of Laryngology and Otology*, **80**, 1115–1126

GRISTWOOD, R.E. and VENABLES, W.N. (1975) Otosclerotic obliteration of the oval window niche: an analysis of the results of surgery. *Journal of Laryngology and Otology*, **89**, 1185–1217

GROSS, C. (1969) Sensorineural hearing loss in clinical and histologic otosclerosis. *Laryngoscope*, **79**, 104–112

GUILD, S.R. (1944) Histologic otosclerosis. *Annals of Otology, Rhinology and Laryngology*, **53**, 246–266

HABERMANN, J. (1904) Zur Pathologie der sogenannenten Otosklerose. *Archivs für Ohrenheilkunde*, **60**, 37–96

HARRISON, M.S. and NAFTALIN, L. (1958) The circulation of labyrinthine fluids. *Journal of Laryngology and Otology*, **72**, 118–136

HEMENWAY, W.G., HILDYARD, V.H. and BLACK, F.O. (1968) Post stapedectomy perilymph fistulas in the Rocky Mountain Area. *Laryngoscope*, **78**, 1687–1715

HILDING, A.C. (1953) Studies on the otic labyrinth. Anatomic explanation for hearing dip at 4096 characteristic of acoustic trauma and presbycusis. *Annals of Otology, Rhinology and Laryngology*, **62**, 950–956

HODGSON, R.S. and WILSON, D.F. (1991) Argon laser stapedotomy. *Laryngoscope*, **101**, 230–233

HOHMANN, A. (1962) Inner ear reactions to stapes surgery (animal experiments). In: *Otosclerosis*, edited by H.F. Schuknecht. Boston: Little, Brown Co. pp. 305–317

HOLMGREN, G. (1923) Some experiences in surgery for otosclerosis. *Acta Otolaryngologica*, **5**, 460–466

HOOGLAND, G.A. (1977) The facial nerve coursing across the promontory with a persistent stapedial artery. *Otorhinolaryngology*, **39**, 338–342

HOUGH, J.V.D. (1969) Long-term results in partial stapedectomy. *Archives of Otolaryngology*, **89**, 414–419

HOUSE, H.P. and GREENFIELD, E.C. (1969) Five-year study of wire loop-absorbable gelatin sponge technique. *Archives of Otolaryngology*, **89**, 420–421

HUER, M.M., GOYCOOLEA, M.V., PAPARELLA, M.M. and OLIVEIRA, J.A. (1991) Otosclerosis: The University of Minnesota temporal bone collection. *Otolaryngology – Head and Neck Surgery*, **105**, 396–405

JACK, F.L. (1893) Remarkable improvement of the hearing by removal of the stapes. *Transactions of the American Otological Society*, **284**, 474–489

JENKINS, G.J. (1913) Otosclerosis: certain clinical features and experimental operative procedures. *Transactions of the XVIIth International Congress of Medicine, London*, **16**, 609

JENSEN, K.J., NEILSON, H.E. and ELBROND, O. (1979) Mineral contents of skeletal bone in otosclerosis. *Clinical Otolaryngology*, **4**, 339–342

JOHNSSON, L. and HAWKINS, J.E. (1972) Vascular changes in the human inner ear associated with ageing. *Annals of Otology, Rhinology and Laryngology*, **81**, 364–376

JOSEPH, R.B. and FRASER, J.P. (1964) Otosclerosis incidence in Caucasians and Japanese. *Archives of Otolaryngology*, **80**, 256–262

JUERS, A.L. (1948) Observations on bone conduction in fenestrated cases. *Annals of Otology, Rhinology and Laryngology*, **57**, 28

KARJALAINEN, S., KARJA, J. and HARMA, R. (1984) Otosclerotic ears not subjected to operation. *Journal of Laryngology and Otology*, **98**, 255–257

LANGE, W. (1921) Ueber die Morphologie und Genese der otosklerotischen Kwockenerkrankung. *Beitrag zur Anatomie, Physiologie, Pathologie und Therapie des Ohres, der Nase und der Halses*, **xvi**, 189–213

LARSSON, A. (1962) Genetic problems in otosclerosis. In: *Otosclerosis*, edited by H. F. Schuknecht. London. Churchill Livingstone. pp. 109–117

LAWRENCE, M., GONZALES, G. and HAWKINS, J.E. (1967) Some physiological factors in noise induced hearing loss. *American Industrial Hygiene Association Journal*, **28**, 425–430

LEMPERT, J. (1938) Improvement of hearing in cases of otosclerosis: new one stage technique. *Archives of Otolaryngology*, **28**, 42–97

LESINSKI, S.G. and STEIN, J.A. (1989) Stapedectomy revision with the CO_2 laser. *Laryngoscope*, **99** (Suppl. 46), 13–19

LEWIS, M.L. (1961) Inner ear complications of stapes surgery. *Laryngoscope*, **71**, 377–384

LIM, D. and MELNICK, W. (1971) Acoustic damage of the cochlea. A scanning and transmission electron microscopic observation. *Archives of Otolaryngology*, **94**, 294–305

LINTHICUM, F. (1971) Histologic evidence of the cause of failure in stapes surgery. *Annals of Otology, Rhinology and Laryngology*, **80**, 67–77

LINTHICUM, F. and SHEEHY, J.L. (1969) Blood in the vestibule at stapedectomy. Human case report with histological findings. *Annals of Otology, Rhinology and Laryngology*, **78**, 425–429

LUDMAN, H. and GRANT, H. (1973) The case against bilateral stapedectomy and problems of postoperative follow-up. *Journal of Laryngology and Otology*, **87**, 833–844

MCGEE, T.M. (1969) Fat-and-wire stapedectomy surgery. *Archives of Otolaryngology*, **89**, 423–424

MCGEE, T. M. (1981) Comparison of small fenestra and total stapedectomy. *Annals of Otology, Rhinology and Laryngology*, **90**, 633–636

MCGEE, T.M. (1983) The argon laser in surgery for chronic ear disease and otosclerosis. *Laryngoscope*, **93**, 1177–1182

MCSHANE, D.P., HYDE, M.L., FINKELSTEIN, D.M. and ALBERTI, P.M. (1991) Unilateral otosclerosis and noise-induced occupational hearing loss. *Clinical Otolargyngology*, **16**, 70–75

MARQUET, J. (1985) Stapedotomy technique and results. *American Journal of Otology*, **6**, 63–67

MARQUET, J., CRETEN, W.L. and VAN CAMP, K.J. (1972) Considerations about the surgical approach in stapedectomy. *Acta Otolaryngologica*, **74**, 406–410

MAYER, O. (1911) *Otosklerose*. Wien: Halder

MISRAHY, G., SHENABARGER, W. and ARNOLD, I. (1958) Changes in cochlear endolymphatic oxygen availability, action potential and microphonics during and following asphyxia, hypoxia and exposure to sounds. *Journal of the Acoustical Society of America*, **30**, 701–704

MIZUKOSHI, O., KONISHI, T. and NAKAMURA, F. (1957) Physiochemical process in hair cells of the organ of Corti. *Annals of Otology, Rhinology and Laryngology*, **66**, 106–126

MOLLER, A.R. (1974) *Handbook of Sensory Physiology. Function of the Middle Ear*. Berlin, Springer-Verlag

MOON, C.N. (1970) Perilymph fistula complicating the stapedectomy operation. A review of 49 cases. *Laryngoscope*, **80**, 515–531

MORRISON, A.W. (1967) Genetic factors in otosclerosis. *Annals of the Royal College of Surgeons of England*, **41**, 202–237

MORRISON, A.W. (1979) Diseases of the otic capsule – 1. Otosclerosis. In: *Scott Brown's Diseases of the Ear, Nose and Throat*, 4th edn, vol. 2 edited by J. Ballantyne and J. Groves. London: Butterworths. pp. 405–464

NAGER, F.R. (1939) Zur klinik und pathologischen Anatomie der Otosklerose. *Acta Otolaryngologica*, **27**, 542–551

NAGER, F.R. and ARNVIG, J.S. (1938) On bone formation in the scala tympani of otosclerotics. *Journal of Laryngology and Otology*, **53**, 173–180

OGILVIE, R.F. and HALL, I.S. (1953) Observations on the pathology of otosclerosis. *Journal of Laryngology and Otology*, **67**, 497–535

PAUW, B.K.H., POLLAK, A.M. and FISCH, U. (1991) Utricle, saccule and cochlear duct in relation to stapedotomy. A histologic human temporal bone study. *Annals of Otology, Rhinology and Laryngology*, **100**, 966–970

PEDERSEN, C.B. and FELDING, J.U. (1991) Stapes surgery: complications and airway infection. *Annals of Otology, Rhinology and Laryngology*, **100**, 607–611

PERKINS, R.C. (1980) Laser stapedotomy for otosclerosis. *Laryngoscope*, **90**, 228–240

PETROVIC, A.G., STUTZMANN, J.J. and SHAMBAUGH, G.E. (1985) Experimental studies on pathology and therapy of otospongiosis. *American Journal of Otology*, **6**, 43–50

POLITZER, A. (1894) Über primare Erkrankung der Knockernen Labyrinthkapsel. *Zeitschrift für Ohrenheilkunde*, **25**, 309–327

POLITZER, A. (1907) *History of Otology*, Vol. 1, translated by S. Milstein, C. Portnoff and A. Coleman, 1981. Phoenix: Columella Press. p. 141

ROALD, B., STORVOLD, G., MAIR, I.W.S. and MJOEN, S. (1992) Respiratory tract viruses in otosclerotic lesions. An immunohistochemical study. *Acta Otolaryngologica*, **112**, 334–338

ROBINSON, M. (1983) Juvenile otosclerosis. A twenty year study. *Annals of Otology, Rhinology and Laryngology*, **92**, 561–562

ROBINSON, M. (1985) Robinson stainless steel prosthesis: technique and results. *American Journal of Otology*, **6**, 72–73

ROSEN, S. (1952) Palpation of the stapes for fixation, preliminary procedure to determine suitability for fenestration in otosclerosis. *Archives of Otolaryngology*, **56**, 610–615

RUEDI, L. (1965) Histopathologic confirmation of labyrinthine otosclerosis. *Laryngoscope*, **75**, 1582–1609

RUEDI, L. and FURRER, W. (1946) Das akustische Trauma. *Otorhinolaryngology (Basel)*, **8**, 177–372

SADÉ, J., SHATZ, A., KREMER, S. and LEVIT, I. (1989) Mastoid pneumatisation in otosclerosis. *Annals of Otology, Rhinology and Laryngology*, **89**, 451–454

SCHNIEDER, E.A. (1975) A contribution to the physiology of the perilymph. Part IV. Effect of histamine on the cochlear microcirculation. *Annals of Otology, Rhinology and Laryngology*, **84**, 228–232

SCHUKNECHT, H.F. (1971) *Stapedectomy*. Boston: Little, Brown Co

SCHUKNECHT, H.F. (1983) Cochlear otosclerosis, an intractable absurdity. *Journal of Laryngology and Otology*, Suppl. 8, 81–83

SCHUKNECHT, H.F. and KIRSCHNER, J. (1974) Cochlear otosclerosis: fact or fantasy? *Laryngoscope*, **84**, 766–781

SCHUKNECHT, H.F. and TONNDORF, J. (1960) Acoustic trauma of the cochlea from ear surgery. *Laryngoscope*, **70**, 479–505

SCHUKNECHT, H.F. and WOELLNER, R.C. (1955) An experimental and clinical study of deafness from lesions of the cochlear nerve. *Journal of Laryngology and Otology*, **69**, 75–97

SELTZER, S. and MCCABE, B.F. (1986) Perilymph fistula: the Iowa experience. *Laryngoscope*, **96**, 37–49

SHAMBAUGH, G.E. JR (1949) The fenestration operation for otosclerosis, experimental investigations and clinical observations over a period of ten years. *Acta Otolaryngologica Supplementum*, **79**, 1–107

SHAMBAUGH, G.E. JR (1965) Clinical diagnosis of cochlear (labyrinthine) otosclerosis. *Laryngoscope*, **75**, 1558–1562

SHAMBAUGH, G.E. JR (1966) Therapy of cochlear otosclerosis. *Annals of Otology, Rhinology and Laryngology*, **75**, 579–583

SHAMBAUGH, G.E. JR (1967) *Surgery of the Ear*, 2nd edn. Philadelphia: W. B. Saunders

SHAMBAUGH, G.E. JR (1978) Sensorineural deafness due to cochlear otosclerosis. Pathogenesis, clinical diagnosis and therapy. *Otolaryngologic Clinics of North America*, **11**, 135–154

SHAMBAUGH, G.E. JR and SCOTT, A. (1964) Sodium fluoride for the arrest of otosclerosis. *Archives of Otolaryngology*, **80**, 263–270

SHEA, J.J. (1958) Fenestration of the oval window. *Annals of Otology, Rhinology and Laryngology*, **67**, 932–951

SHEA, J.J. (1985) Stapedectomy techniques and results. *American Journal of Otology*, **6**, 61–62

SHEA, J.J. and SANABRIA, F. (1963) A critical appraisal of stapes surgery after ten years. *Journal of Laryngology and Otology*, **77**, 101–114

SHEEHY, J.L., NELSON, R.A. and HOUSE, H.P. (1981) Revision stapedectomy. A review of 258 cases. *Laryngoscope*, **91**, 43–51

SIEBENMANN, F. (1912) Totaler knocherner Verschluss beider Labyrinthfester und Labyrinthitis serosa infolge progressiver Spongiosierung. *Verhandlungen Deutschen Otologischen Gesellschaft*, **6**, 267–283

SILVERSTEIN, H., ROSENBERG, S. and JONES, R. (1989) Small fenestra stapedotomies with and without KTP laser. A comparison. *Laryngoscope*, **99**, 485–488

SMYTH, G.D.L. (1982) Practical suggestions on stapedotomy. *Laryngoscope*, **92**, 952–953

SMYTH, G.D.L. and HASSARD, T.H. (1978) Eighteen years experience in stapedectomy. The case for the small fenestra operation. *Annals of Otology, Rhinology and Laryngology*, Suppl. 49, Part 2, 1–36

SMYTH, G.D.L. and HASSARD, T.H. (1981) A reconsideration of the parameters for evaluating tympanic reconstruction. *American Journal of Otology*, **2**, 365–367

SMYTH, G.D.L. and HASSARD, T.H. (1986) Hearing aids post-stapedectomy: incidence and timing. *Laryngoscope*, **96**, 385–388

SMYTH, G.D.L. and PATTERSON, C.C. (1985) Results of middle ear reconstruction. Do patients and surgeons agree? *American Journal of Otology*, **6**, 276–279

SMYTH, G.D.L., HASSARD, T.H. and EL KORDY, A.F.A. (1980) Long term hearing performance after stapedectomy. *Journal of Laryngology and Otology*, **94**, 1097–1105

SMYTH, G.D.L., KERR, A.G. and SINGH, A.K.P. (1975) Second ear stapedectomy – a continued controversy. *Journal of Laryngology and Otology*, **89**, 1047–1056

SOIFER, N., WEAVER, K., ENDAHL, G.L. and HOLDSWORTH G.E. (1970) Otosclerosis: a review. *Acta Otolaryngologica Supplementum*, **269**, 1–25

SOURDILLE, M. (1930) Surgical treatment of otosclerosis. *Proceedings of the Royal Society of Medicine*, **23**, 89–101

SPOENDLIN, H. (1971) Primary structural changes in the organ of Corti after acoustic overstimulation. *Acta Otolaryngologica*, **71**, 166–176

STROUD, M.H. (1963) Permanent vestibular dysfunction in surgery for otosclerosis. *Laryngoscope*, **73**, 474–481

THALMANN, I., MATSCHINSKY, F. M. and THALMANN, R. (1970) Quantitative study of selected enzymes involved in energy metabolism of the cochlear duct. *Annals of Otology, Rhinology and Laryngology*, **79**, 12–29

TOYNBEE, J. (1861) Pathological and surgical observations on the diseases of the ear. *Medico Chirurgical Transactions*, **24**, 190–211

VON HAACKE, N.P. (1985) Juvenile stapedectomy. *Clinical Otolaryngology*, **9**, 223–225

VOSTEEN, K.H. (1958) Fatigue of phonoreceptors after functional stress; experimental histochemical study on the problem of sound transformation in the inner ear. *Archiv für klinische und experimentelle Ohrenheilkunde Nasen Kehlkopfheilkunde*, **172**, 489–512

WEBER, M. (1935) *Otosklerose und Umbau der Labyrinthkapsel*. Leipzig: Offizin Poeschel und Treptel

WEIDER, D.J., SAUNDERS, R.L. and MUSIEK, F.E. (1991) Repair of a cerebrospinal perilymph fistula primarily through the middle ear and secondarily by occluding the cochlear aqueduct. *Otolaryngology – Head and Neck Surgery*, **105**, 35–39

WITMAAK, K. (1919) *Die Otosklerose auf Grund eigener Forschungen*. Jena: Fischer

WOODHOUSE, N.J.V. (1973) Paget's disease and calcitonin therapy. *Ninth Symposium on Advanced Medicine*, edited by G. Walker. London: Pitman. pp. 202–208

YOO, T.J. (1984) Etiopathogenesis of otosclerosis: a hypothesis. *Annals of Otology, Rhinology and Laryngology*, **93**, 28–33

YOON, T.H., PAPARELLA, M.M. and SCHACHERN, P.A. (1990) Otosclerosis involving the vestibular aqueduct in Meniere's disease. *Otolaryngology – Head and Neck Surgery*, **103**, 107–112

ZORZOLI, G.C. and BORIANI, A.V. (1958) Histochemical research on ciliated cells of Corti's organ submitted to acoustic stimulations. *Revue de Laryngologie Otologie Rhinologie (Bordeaux)*, **79**, 213–220

Further reading

A selection of helpful articles published since this article was first written.

Awengen, D. F. (1993) Change of bone conduction thresholds by total footplate stapedectomy in relation to age. *American Journal of Otolaryngology*, **14**, 105–110

Causse, J. B., Gherini, S., Lopez, A., Juberthie, L., Oliver, J.-C. and Bastianelli, G. (1993) Impedance transfer: acoustic impedance of the annular ligament and stapedial tendon reconstruction in otosclerosis surgery. *American Journal of Otology*, **14**, 613–617

Causse, J. R., Causse, J. B., Uriel, J., Berges, J., Shambaugh, G. E., Jr. and Bretlau, P. (1993) Sodium fluoride therapy. *American Journal of Otology*, **10**, 482–490

Colletti, V., Fiorino, F. G., Sittoni, V. and Policante, Z. (1993) Mechanics of the middle ear in otosclerosis and stapedoplasty. *Acta Otolaryngologica*, **113**, 637–641

Cook, J. A., Krishnan, S. K. and Fagan, P. A. (1995) Quantifying the Carhart effect in otosclerosis. *Clinical Otolaryngology*, **20**, 258–261

Farrior, J. and Sutherland, A. (1991) Revision stapes surgery. *Laryngoscope*, **101**, 1155–1161

Franklin, D. J., Pollak, A. and Fisch, U. (1990) Menière's symptoms resulting from bilateral otosclerotic occlusion of the endolymphatic duct: an analysis of a causal relationship between otosclerosis and Menière's disease. *American Journal of Otology*, **11**, 135–140

Frattali, M. A. and Sataloff, R. T. (1993) Far-advanced otosclerosis. *Annals of Otology, Rhinology and Laryngology*, **102**, 433–437

Holmgren, G. (1992) The surgery of otosclerosis. *Annals of Otology, Rhinology and Laryngology*, **101**, 546–555 (reproduced from 1937, **46**, 3–12)

Horn, K. L., Pai, V. and Beauparlant, P. A. (1990) Stapedotomy in Larsen's syndrome. *American Journal of Otology*, **11**, 205–206

House, J. W. (Guest Editor) (1993) *Otolaryngologic Clinics of North America*, **26**, No. 3

Iurato, S., Ettorre, G. C., Onofri, M. and Davidson, C. (1992) Very far-advanced otosclerosis. *American Journal of Otology*, **13**, 482–487

Kveton, J. F. and Bartoshuk, L. M. (1994) The effect of unilateral chorda tympani damage on taste. *Laryngoscope*, **104**, 25–29

McGee, T. M., Diaz-Ordaz, E. A. and Kartush, J. M. (1993) The role of KTP laser in revision stapedectomy. *Otolaryngology – Head and Neck Surgery*, **109**, 839–843

McShane, D. P., Hyde, M. L., Finkelstein, D. M. and Alberti, P. W. (1991) Unilateral otosclerosis and noise-induced occupational hearing loss. *Clinical Otolaryngology*, **16**, 70–75

Pedersen, C. B. (1994) Revision surgery in otosclerosis – operative findings in 186 patients. *Clinical Otolaryngology*, **19**, 446–450

Perkins, R. and Curto, F. S. (1992) Laser stapedotomy; a comparative study of prostheses and seals. *Laryngoscope*, **102**, 1321–1327

Prasad, S. and Kamerer, D. B. (1993) Results of revision stapedectomy for conductive hearing loss. *Otolaryngology – Head and Neck Surgery*, **109**, 742–747

Robinson, M. (1993) Otosclerosis regrowth. *Laryngoscope*, **103**, 1383–1384

Rosenberg, G. D. and Tubergen, L. B. (1993) Composition of the otosclerotic stapes: electron microprobe analyses. *Annals of Otology, Rhinology and Laryngology*, **102**, 353–357

Shambaugh, G. E. Jr. (1995) Julius Lempert and the fenestration operation. *American Journal of Otology*, **16**, 247–252

Shea, J. J. (1994) How I do primary and revision stapedectomy. *American Journal of Otology*, **15**, 71–73

Silverstein, H., Bendet, E., Rosenberg, S. and Nichols, M. (1994) Revision stapes surgery with and without laser: a comparison. *Laryngoscope*, **104**, 1431–1438

Vartiainen, E, and Karjalainen, S. (1992) Bone conduction thresholds in patients with otosclerosis. *American Journal of Otolaryngology*, **13**, 234–236

Vartiainen, E., Karjalainen, S., Nuutinen, J., Suntioinen, S. and Pellinen, P. (1994) Effect of drinking water fluoridation on hearing of patients with otosclerosis in a low fluoride area: a follow up study. *American Journal of Otology*, **15**, 545–548

Welling, D. B., Glasscock, M. E. and Gantz, B. J. (1992) Avulsion of the anomalous facial nerve at stapedectomy. *Laryngoscope*, **102**, 729–733

15

Diseases of the temporal bone

Gerald B. Brookes and John B. Booth

Many different systemic diseases may involve the temporal bone. They invariably result in a sensory hearing loss, occasionally there are associated vestibular symptoms and, in some instances, middle ear function is also compromised.

Several diseases have been excluded from this chapter, or considered only briefly, as they are covered more appropriately in other sections. Thus, the many causes of severe childhood deafness, in particular teratogenic, hereditary and metabolic, are largely excluded. Secondary involvement of the temporal bone by neoplasms, reticuloses, or by the leukaemias are also described elsewhere, together with diseases of the cardiovascular, haemopoietic, respiratory and renal systems (Chapter 17). This chapter concentrates upon disorders of bone which may involve the petrous temporal structures and those caused by infective, granulomatous, metabolic and dietary-induced diseases. The contemporary field of auto-immune inner ear disease is also considered.

Structure of the temporal bone

The bony labyrinth differs histologically and biologically from all other skeletal tissues. The otic capsule is unique in that it retains its fetal structure into adult life. As a result its response to pathological stimuli differs from that seen in other bones (Figure 15.1). Histologically the labyrinth consists of three layers of bone (Milroy and Michaels, 1990a). The outer periosteal or intramembranous layer corresponds to the circumferential lamellae of long bones. The inner or 'endosteal' layer is essentially another periosteal layer. The middle or 'endochondral' layer has a unique structure. It is composed of bone inti-

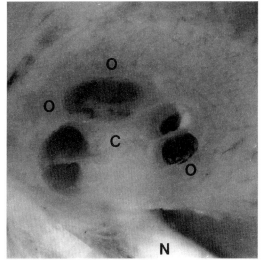

Figure 15.1 Microsliced temporal bone showing normal otic capsule. C = cochlea; N = VIIIth nerve; O = otic capsule. (Reproduced by kind permission of Milroy and Michaels, 1990a and the Editor, *Journal of Laryngology and Otology*)

mately mixed with calcified cartilaginous cells, called globuli interossei. In other bones this calcified cartilage is resorbed by phagocytosis, but in the otic capsule it remains unchanged throughout life. There are fundamental differences between the response of endochondral and periosteal (intramembranous) bone to pathological influences. For example Chole (1993) has recently studied the effect of increased pressurization on localized bone resorption in these bony layers. The osteoclast surface is increased in the intramembranous bone, but not in the endochondral bone, which is therefore more resistant to pressure-induced localized resorption.

Maurer (1967) studied the mineral content of the bone of the otic capsule and ossicles, and compared it to the composition of bone from the mastoid cortex and general skeleton. He found that the calcium and phosphorus content of the former was significantly greater than that of the ordinary haversian bone of the mastoid cortex and other regions. In addition, alkaline phosphatase activity was one-third to one-sixth lower in this woven bone, indicating that there are fundamental metabolic differences compared to general skeletal bone. Animal studies have shown that otic bone takes up radioactively-labelled calcium significantly slower than does femoral bone, a reflection of its reduced metabolic rate (Ross, 1979). It is also relevant that the metabolic regulation of the entry of calcium into bone varies with both sex and age (Bronner, 1973; Preston *et al.*, 1975). There is reduced entry of calcium in women, compared with men and with increasing age. These basic physiological differences between otic capsule and other bone will clearly affect the likelihood of preferential involvement of the petrous temporal bone as a localized manifestation of a more generalized bone disorder.

Temporal bone imaging

Since the introduction of high resolution thin section computerized tomography, CT has become the optimum imaging technique for studying the temporal bone. Better contrast resolution and freedom from blurring, which is inherent to multidirectional tomography from incomplete cancellation of structures outside the focal plane, enables areas of rarefaction and increased thickening of the bone of the labyrinthine capsule to be demonstrated more readily. Recent technical developments are now providing quantitative data on bone density and mineralization in cases where local disturbances in bone metabolism are present. This is not only facilitating earlier diagnosis, but is also improving our ability to monitor the effects of a variety of newer biochemical drug treatments.

Phelps and Lloyd (1989) have emphasized the difficulties involved in obtaining readings at constant and reliably reproducible points. Partial volume averaging must also be avoided at the edge of the otic capsule. Valvassori and Dobben (1985) described a protocol in which two sections, one at the level of the round window and another through the level of the oval window, are used. Multiple measurements of bone density compared to the point of maximum density are then made to give two profiles around the

coils of the cochlea. De Groot and Huizing (1987) defined six points around the basal turn of the cochlea using four imaginary lines (Figure 15.2). Unfortunately partial volume averaging significantly affects readings at points one and six. Phelps and Lloyd have therefore subsequently recommended a regimen in which several attenuation readings are obtained at four points equivalent to points two, three, four and five and their mean values compared to the maximum capsular density. Normal values are approximately 2300–2400 Hounsfield units (HU) for the maximum capsular density, and 1800–2200 HU for the four points, though slight variations will occur depending on other scanning variables. Phelps and Lloyd have also recommended plotting a histogram through the middle of the modiolus and central bony spiral as this is a constant landmark, and may graphically reflect changes in bone mineralization.

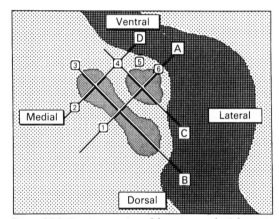

Figure 15.2 Density mapping of the otic capsule. Schematic view of right ear of the construction of six measuring points in the transverse plane at a level of 1.5 mm caudally from the lateral semicircular canal. (Reproduced by kind permission of the Editor, *Acta Otolaryngologica*)

Monsell, Cody and Bone (1993) have recently reported a further refinement. They are critical of conventional CT densitometry on the grounds that calculated mean values are based on relative measures within a subject. Likewise, density values as measured in Hounsfield units also represent only relative densities. Their modified CT software, used in combination with fixed external density standards, allows collection of a three dimensional array of precise, accurately reproducible bone density values as well as high quality CT images.

In view of the sensitivity of CT imaging and densitometry in the recognition of temporal bone abnormalities, it would seem appropriate to include this assessment as part of a screening protocol to investigate patients with progressive symmetrical bilateral sensorineural hearing loss of unknown aetiology. One of the authors has studied 69 patients of mean age 38.0 years (range 12–64) in this manner over a 6-year period (Harcourt *et al.*, 1996). Only two patients were found to have a radiological abnormality of the cochlear capsule. An area of low mineralization around the cochlea was observed in a young Asian man with severe hearing loss, slightly low vitamin D levels and presumed osteomalacia. Another patient had florid Paget's disease. This study therefore reflects the relatively low incidence of temporal bone diseases in clinical practice.

Systemic bone disease

The temporal bone may be affected by many specific conditions (Table 15.1). Table 15.2 summarizes the biochemical, radiological and other characteristics encountered in the most important of these conditions. Somewhat paradoxically, however, the temporal bone is relatively infrequently involved in many of the generalized systemic bone diseases. Perhaps the lower metabolic rate of the bony labyrinth confers some degree of protection, although it must be appreciated that any cochleovestibular symptoms are probably often overshadowed by other more generalized features.

Table 15.1 Systemic bone diseases

1 Osteogenesis imperfecta (van der Hoeve syndrome)
2 Osteitis deformans (Paget's disease)
3 Fibrous dysplasia
4 Osteopetrosis
5 Neurofibromatosis
6 Genetic craniotabular hyperostoses
   a hyperostosis corticalis generalisata
   b sclerosteosis
   c congenital hyperphosphatasia
   d progressive diaphyseal dysplasia
7 Genetic craniotabular dysplasias
   a craniometaphyseal dysplasia
   b frontometaphyseal dysplasia
8 Craniofacial dysostosis
9 Osteopathia striata

Direct involvement of the otic bone which supports and protects the delicate cochlear and vestibular neuroepithelial structures, by other rarefractive or sclerotic processes, can lead to secondary degenerative changes in the spiral ligament, stria vascularis and cochlear hair cells, either by local ischaemia or by the toxic effect caused by the release of enzymes, as has been postulated and generally accepted in cochlear otosclerosis. This is the likely pathogenesis in

most conditions although, in addition, sustained biochemical aberrations may cause adverse effects in other ways. Calcium is involved with many cellular functions, including the regulation of membrane permeability and the control of neuromuscular excitability. Active transport mechanisms, which maintain the differential biochemical integrity of the inner ear fluids which is vital for normal cochlear function, are probably calcium dependent. Deficiency of ionized calcium may also adversely affect transmission of the nerve action potentials generated by the cochlea by inhibiting the release of transmitter substances at the neural synapses.

Otosclerosis

Otosclerosis is a localized disease of the bony labyrinth which is unique to the human species. Most frequently it causes ankylosis of the stapes footplate and a conductive hearing loss (see below). Less commonly, the bone surrounding the cochlea is affected, causing sensorineural hearing impairment. 'Capsular' otosclerosis is usually associated with stapedial fixation, and results in a mixed hearing loss which is invariably progressive in nature (Figure 15.3). It is, however, now accepted that pure cochlear otosclerosis can occur, albeit rarely (Nager, 1993). Schuknecht (1983) estimated that otosclerosis is the cause of 1% of cases of progressive sensorineural

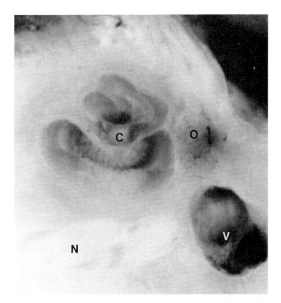

Figure 15.3 Microslice showing an otospongiotic focus (O) in the otic capsule. C = cochlea; N = VIIIth nerve; V = vestibule. (Reproduced by kind permission of Milroy and Michaels, 1990a and the Editor, *Journal of Laryngology and Otology*)

Table 15.2 Summary of features of specific conditions affecting the temporal bone

Condition	Type of hearing loss	Biochemistry		Radiology	General features
Osteogenesis imperfecta	Conductive and/or sensorineural	Ca PO$_4$	} normal	Varied – demineralization and sclerosis produce mottled appearances	Spontaneous fractures Excess callus formation Blue sclerae Joint hypermobility
		Alkase	occasionally raised		
		Acidase	normal		
Paget's disease (osteitis deformans)	Conductive and/or sensorineural	Ca PO$_4$	usually normal hypercalcaemia – immobilization	Varied – lytic, sclerotic and mixed phases Skull – great increase in thickness of both tables, particularly outer ? patchy sclerosis – woolly appearance Platybasia; basilar impression	X-ray pelvis including femoral heads Osteoporosis circumscripta – patch of reduced density resembling bony defect Pathological fracture
		Alkase	elevated in active disease		
		Acidase	may be raised		
		Urinary HDP elevated in active disease			
Fibrous dysplasia	Conductive Rarely sensorineural	Ca PO$_4$ Alkase	usually normal always normal may be raised in active disease, especially polyostotic form	Monostotic/polyostotic appearances – same Multiloculated cystic lesion (bone frequently expanded) Occasionally lesion more diffuse ground-glass appearance due to multiple fine trabeculae Occasionally diffuse sclerotic appearance	Skeletal survey to exclude polyostotic Pathological fracture Café-au-lait pigmentation may be present (either type)
		Acidase	normal		
Osteopetrosis a Albers-Schönberg	Conductive Occasionally mixed	Ca PO$_4$	} normal	Symmetrical increase in bone density; bones appear structureless Sclerotic foci – 'bones within bone' Thickening of vertebral end-plates ('rugger jersey')	Thick dense brittle bones Pathological fracture Facial palsy Occasional osteomyelitis of mandible after dental extraction Mild anaemia
		Alkase Acidase	} may be markedly elevated		
		Urinary HDP usually normal			
b Malignant recessive	Sensorineural	As above		Transverse bands in metaphyseal regions of long bones and longitudinal striations Proximal humerus and distal femur – flask-shaped Vertebrae – 'rugger jersey'	Facial palsy Blindness Pathological fracture Mental retardation Liver and spleen enlargement Haemolytic anaemia and thrombocytopenia

EAM: external auditory meatus; ICP: intracranial pressure; HDP: hydroxyproline. (Reproduced from Booth, J. B. (1982) Medical

hearing loss and may progress to total deafness. Thus each cochlear implant programme will inevitably contain a few patients with previously untreated end-stage cochlear otosclerosis.

The mature hard lamellar bone of the otic capsule becomes replaced by immature woven bone of increased thickness, vascularity and cellularity, similar to that seen elsewhere in healing fractures. The new bone is initially spongy, hence the descriptive term 'otospongiosis', but these foci subsequently become denser and sclerotic. It is generally accepted that gradual spread to involve surrounding bone is responsible for the progressive symptoms. Although the aetiology is unknown, there is increasing evidence to suggest that immunological factors may be important (Schrader, Poppendieck and Plester, 1987; Arnold

Table 15.2 (*Continued*)

Condition	Type of hearing loss	Biochemistry		Radiology	General features
Genetic craniotabular hyperostoses					
a van Buchem's (autosomal recessive)	Conductive and /or sensorineural	Ca PO$_4$ Alkase	normal frequently raised (50–250%)	Diffuse, symmetrical increase in bone density Cortical bone – abnormally thick but bones not increased in size Hyperplasia diaphysis long and short bones Endosteal thickening diaphysis – tubular bones	Normal stature Facial palsy Clavicles – thickened and palpable Overgrowth of brow and mandible
b Sclerosteosis (autosomal recessive)	Conductive and/or sensorineural	Ca PO$_4$ Alkase Acidase normal	normal markedly elevated in nearly all patients	Bones show increased density but only minor degree of bony modelling, if present Progressive bony thickening Tubular bones markedly undermodelled with lack of usual diaphyseal constriction	Syndactyly and digital malformation Facial paralysis Tall stature Distortion of face and jaw Chronic headache Raised ICP Anosmia Majority Afrikaners
c Congenital hyper-phosphatasia (autosomal recessive)	Conductive with decreased bone conduction	Ca PO$_4$ Alkase Acidase Urine-HDP high	normal both consistently elevated	Similar to Paget's Marked irregular thickening of skull ?Narrowing of EAM Tubular bones – width greatly increased, bowing and lack of modelling	Multiple fractures Dwarfing Blue sclerae (?increased serum uric acid and leucine aminopeptidase)
d Progressive diaphyseal dysplasia (autosomal dominant)	Combined with big air-bone gap	Ca PO$_4$ Alkase Acidase	usually normal	Generalized sclerosis of skull base; vault less commonly severely affected	Marked thickening of cortices of leg bones and medullary canals narrowed; external bony contours irregular

management of sensorineural hearing loss. Part II Musculoskeletal system. *Journal of Laryngology and Otology*, **96**, 773–795)

and Friedmann, 1988), in conjunction with a pre-existing genetic susceptibility.

The use of high resolution CT to study mineralization of the labyrinthine capsule in otosclerosis was first reported by Damsma and colleagues in 1984. Subsequent studies have confirmed the efficacy of this imaging modality, though there are wide variations in the reported incidence of 'radiological otospongiosis' in patients with audiological evidence of cochlear involvement, which has varied from 42 to 75% (Mafee *et al.*, 1985; Swartz *et al.*, 1985b, c; Blakeley *et al.*, 1986). Severe cochlear otospongiosis appears as a double ring effect due to confluent foci within the capsule (Figure 15.4). The modiolar histogram will show a dip for any zone of decreased bone density.

Valvassori and Dobben (1985) found that CT densitometry was more sensitive than visual evaluation

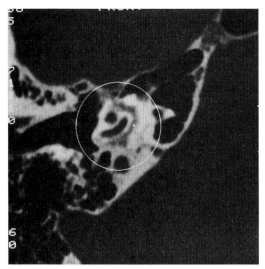

Figure 15.4 High resolution CT scan showing marked labyrinthine otospongiosis. The small white dot denotes a site where a densitometry reading has been made

alone. Thus abnormalities were only seen in 84% of ears with low densitometry readings. De Groot and Huizing (1987) observed density loss in the labyrinthine capsule in only about 20% of 84 patients with surgically confirmed otosclerosis. With CT densitometry, however, density loss was found in 56% of 134 affected ears. One of the authors has studied an unselected series of patients with mixed otosclerosis (Brookes, Porter and Phelps, 1992); 22% of 67 ears had severely reduced densities below 1500 Hounsfield units, and 3% moderately reduced readings of 1500–1700 units. A weak correlation between minimum capsular density and maximum bone conduction loss in affected ears was apparent ($P < 0.5$). This discrepancy in the radiological incidence of otospongiosis with earlier studies is most likely to be due to case selection.

Various theories have been proposed to explain the pathogenesis of cochlear degeneration. Rüedi (1965) suggested that the vascular foci preferentially shunted oxygenated blood away from the stria vascularis resulting in hair cell ischaemia. Parahy and Linthicum (1984) proposed that hyalinization of the endosteal layer of the otic capsule adjacent to the spiral ligament causes strial atrophy. If these theories were correct one would expect to find regularly qualitative and quantitative otic capsule abnormalities. Because most patients with impaired bone conduction have normal labyrinths in the author's experience, it would seem that the enzymatic theory proposed by Causse *et al.* (1977) is a more plausible pathogenesis in the majority of cases.

Treatment

Evidence has been gradually accumulating over the last 25 years which now strongly supports the contention that the progressive sensorineural hearing loss in otosclerosis can be prevented or at least retarded by medical treatment. Sodium fluoride has been the primary agent while calcium and vitamin D play a supporting role.

In 1964, Shambaugh and Scott suggested that sodium fluoride could promote recalcification and reduce bone remodelling in an actively expanding otospongiotic lesion. Fluoride acts at several points of the bone remodelling cycle. It reduces osteoclastic bone resorption leading to more calcium deposition, and increases osteoblastic bone formation. In addition Causse and colleagues (Causse, Shambaugh and Chevance, 1977; Causse *et al.*, 1977) suggested that it has an antienzymatic action on proteolytic enzymes which are toxic to the cochlea. The rationale for fluoride usage is generally based on the premise that recalcification of the otospongiotic focus reduces its activity and limits possible spread to involve other adjacent sites. However, Causse *et al.* (1977) and Forquer, Linthicum and Bennett (1986) working independently consider that the primary effect is one of neutralization of hydrolytic enzymes.

There are a number of experiments which have contributed to our understanding of the specific mechanism of the effect of fluoride on the otospongiotic focus. Petrovic and Shambaugh (1966) conducted organ culture studies using otospongiotic bone. In one study the uptake of radioactive calcium-45 from the medium was measured. Immature osteoporotic bone takes up calcium at a much higher rate than the mature type, and this rate is significantly reduced after more than 1 year of fluoride treatment. Acid phenylphosphatase activity provides a good assessment of osteoclastic bone resorption, and is reduced progressively under the same laboratory conditions. In 1973, Linthicum, House and Althaus conducted a similar experiment using radioactive strontium. They also demonstrated reduced uptake by the otospongiotic footplate bone following fluorides, indicating reduced bone-modelling activity, and enhanced maturation of the focus.

Causse *et al.* (1977) considered the effect of fluoride treatment on the concentration of hydrolytic enzymes in the perilymph which they removed at stapedectomy surgery. They found a very much higher incidence of cytotoxic enzymes in patients with a sensorineural loss (89%), compared with ears with pure stapedial otosclerosis (11%). Treatment with 45 mg of fluoride daily reduced the incidence of elevated toxic enzymes to 2.6%. These corroborative reports support the continuing clinical usage of fluoride in certain cases.

Shambaugh and Scott (1964) initially recommended fluoride therapy in the following patients:

1 Progressive sensorineural loss with surgically confirmed otosclerosis
2 Pure sensorineural loss with family history and audiology consistent with cochlear otosclerosis
3 Radiological spongiotic changes in the cochlear capsule
4 Positive Schwartze sign.

Contraindications to therapy consisted of chronic nephritis, rheumatoid arthritis, pregnancy, children with incomplete skeletal growth, systemic fluorosis and those patients with known sensitivity. Despite these apparently specific criteria for treatment, the selection of cases for category 2 will, in many instances, be rather subjective. The advent of CT densitometry should, however, certainly facilitate earlier diagnosis.

Evaluation of treatment for most types of inner ear hearing loss is far from straightforward, because success is usually measured in terms of absence of further progression, as sustained hearing gains are infrequent. Clinical experience with very large numbers of patients receiving moderate dosages of sodium fluoride shows that this treatment can be helpful in most cases of progressive sensorineural loss in otosclerosis.

Shambaugh and Causse (1974) described the results of treatment of more than 4000 patients over a 10-year period. Progressive sensorineural hearing loss was halted in some 80% of patients, while only 3% actually improved. Forquer, Linthicum and Bennett (1986) reported similar results in their study of 94 patients with cochlear involvement, when fluoride halted or slowed the progression of sensorineural loss in 63%. They found that those patients with more rapid rates of hearing loss responded better. The criticism of these studies is that they are retrospective, and that there are very few controls, who have not necessarily even been selected randomly. Bretlau *et al.* (1985) reported the results of the first prospective placebo-controlled double blind study of 95 patients, conducted over a 12–24 month period. Only 10% of fluoride-treated patients were worse compared to nearly 27% of the placebo group, and this difference was statistically significant ($P < 0.025$).

Vitamin D and calcium supplements have been recommended in conjunction with fluorides since the encouraging clinical report by Cody and Baker in 1978. Fluoride increases the requirement for calcium to allow satisfactory mineralization, while vitamin D plays an essential role in the regulation of calcium and bone metabolism and in particular facilitates gastrointestinal absorption of calcium (see later). One of the authors has reported the results of a prospective study of vitamin D status in a population of 47 patients with otosclerosis (Brookes, 1985c). Cochlear involvement was present in 84%, the mean age was 46 years, and the mean duration of symptoms was 17 years. Abnormally low 25-hydroxy vitamin D levels were found in just over 20%, and elevated alkaline phosphatase levels in 32%. This study was carried out at The London Hospital, which has a relatively socially deprived local population and a large Asian immigrant community. This latter group is particularly susceptible to vitamin D undernutrition in the UK, which may have artificially increased the incidence of biochemical anomalies. Nevertheless, one patient showed a spectacular response to vitamin D and calcium replacement therapy given over a 3-month period (Figure 15.5). Perhaps therefore a criticism of the Bretlau study is that the placebo used

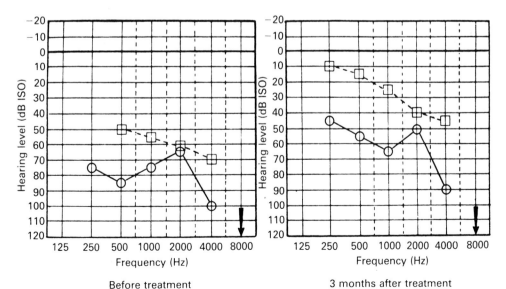

Before treatment   3 months after treatment

Figure 15.5 Pure tone audiogram of right ear of a 51-year-old man with mixed otosclerosis before and 3 months after vitamin D and calcium treatment

may have had a beneficial effect in some patients, thereby tending to offset any efficacious effect of the fluoride-treated group.

The recommended dose of sodium fluoride is 50 mg daily for 2 years, and thereafter a daily maintenance of 25 mg. In North America two or three capsules of Florical (8.5 mg sodium fluoride and 364 mg of calcium carbonate) three times a day are prescribed. Vitamin D can be given as a separate supplement with both regimens. The first author prescribes enteric coated sodium fluoride 50 mg daily in conjunction with calcium and vitamin D BPC tablets (calcium lactate 450 mg, calcium phosphate 150 mg and 500 units vitamin D) twice daily for 3 years initially and thereafter for 6 monthly periods interspersed with a 6 month drug-free interval. Despite the use of enteric coated capsules, experience shows that about 25% of patients still complain of dyspepsia and unpleasant nausea, which undoubtedly affects drug compliance. These effects are largely attributable to conversion to hydrofluoric acid in the stomach, and can be reduced by taking the drug with food.

Since the advent of the diagnostic confidence provided by CT densitometry, the author has tended to prescribe biochemical treatment only for those patients with 'radiological' capsular otosclerosis. De Groot and his colleagues (1987) described a case of florid juvenile labyrinthine otosclerosis where they were able to demonstrate markedly progressive increased radiodensity of the cochlear capsule lesion by serial scanning, following fluoride therapy over a period of 3 years. Despite following several patients with serial CT imaging, the authors have yet to observe demonstrable remineralization. Recent researches have shown that the stimulation of osteoblasts by fluorides results in a parallel increase in serum osteocalcin (Dandona, Gill and Khokher, 1989), which can provide a valuable index of therapeutic efficacy. This may also be helpful in defining a patient's optimum treatment protocol.

Those who are intolerant of sodium fluoride may be suitable for treatment with some of the newer bone metabolism modifying drugs. Diphosphonates such as etidronate also inhibit bone resorption primarily by inhibiting osteoclastic activity, and were first advocated in the long-term management of Paget's disease (see below). Petrovic, Stutzmann and Shambaugh (1985) have investigated their effects in otospongiosis, and believe that the mechanism of their action is primary enzymatic inhibition. Their preliminary results suggested a clear tendency towards stabilization of both conductive and sensorineural hearing losses following regular treatment with diphosphonates for one year. Kennedy, Hoffer and Holliday (1993) have reported a double-blind placebo controlled study of oral etidronate (20 mg/kg) in 26 patients with sensorineural hearing loss due to mixed otosclerosis over a 2-year period. A trend towards stabilization or improvement of bone conduc-

tion thresholds at 500, 1000 and 2000 Hz was noted, though the results were not statistically significant. Perhaps more importantly the incidence of side effects was low, and only one patient developed significant adverse effects on etidronate necessitating withdrawal from the trial. Boumans and Poublon (1991), however, cautioned against the use of biphosphonates intravenously. They reported two patients with otosclerosis who developed sudden profound bilateral sensorineural hearing loss within a few weeks of systemic aminohydroxypropylidene biphosphonate (APD), which they believe was a direct result of drug administration by this route.

Other newer agents may be effective in otospongiosis at least on theoretical grounds, and have been developed as a result of increasing contemporary knowledge of bone physiology. There is now convincing evidence that the hormone calcitonin has a direct inhibitory effect on osteoclasts, even in low concentrations. Chambers and Azria (1988) studied the inhibitory effect of various types of calcitonin on osteoclast resorption by electron microscopic analysis of cortical bone preparations. Calcitonin is now available as a nasal spray, a far preferable mode of administration than parenteral injection. The plasma wall of the osteoclast contains energy rich ATPases which prime both sodium and proton pumps. These two pump systems are both vital for cell function. The proton pump is supplied with protons by carbonic anhydrase, which catalyses the fundamental conversion of carbon dioxide and water to bicarbonate and hydrogen ions. Carbonic anhydrase is now known to play a role in bone resorption, and congenital absence of one specific type found in bone causes osteopetrosis, a condition of deficient bone resorption (Sly *et al.*, 1983). Carbonic anhydrase inhibitors such as acetazolamide can therefore inhibit bone resorption, and may, as a result, have an adjunctive role in therapy.

Osteogenesis imperfecta

Osteogenesis imperfecta or fragilitas ossium is a relatively rare disease. Its incidence varies between 2 and 15 per 100 000 births (Smärs, 1961; Morrison, 1967; Pedersen, 1984). It is an hereditary disorder of collagen synthesis due to a cross-linking defect (Smith, Francis and Haughton, 1983) and occurs in two main forms. In the *congenita* (type II) form, multiple fractures occur *in utero* and early death is commonplace. In the *tarda* form (types I,III,IV) multiple fractures occur with relatively minor trauma in childhood but tend to become less frequent after puberty. Abnormal fracture alignment frequently results in excess callus formation and skeletal deformity of the limbs. It is generally accepted that the tarda form has a dominant mode of inheritance with variable penetrance, resulting in three degrees of severity of the condition. Asymptomatic 'carriers' exist in some families, and sporadic cases have also been encountered. The congenita form has a recessive mode of inheritance.

The chief manifestation is spontaneous fractures which occur in more than 95% of cases (Smärs, 1961). These usually follow relatively minor trauma and may exceed 60 in number in any one individual. Eighty-five per cent of cases have blue sclerae, due to mutations in the two genes for type I collagen (Prockop, 1992) (see Plate 3/15/I). There is both a quantitative reduction in the number of collagen fibres and a qualitative reduction in the actual diameter of the fibres. These changes in molecular structure result in abnormally thin transparent sclera, thus allowing the underlying pigmented uvea, plus its vasculature to show through (Chan *et al.*, 1982). Blue sclerae may also be seen in other conditions, where a collagen differentiation defect is present, e.g. Ehlers–Danlos syndrome and Marfan's syndrome. Many healthy children under 3 years of age also have blue sclerae because their collagen is immature, so that scleral colour is an unreliable diagnostic feature in the young.

Approximately 50–60% of affected individuals eventually develop a hearing loss (Smärs, 1961; Morrison, 1975; Quisling *et al.*, 1979; Pedersen *et al.*, 1985; Stewart and O'Reilly, 1989). When multiple fractures, blue sclerae and deafness occur together they constitute the syndrome ascribed to van der Hoeve and de Kleyn (1918). It is now known that this eponymous association is rather unsatisfactory because the syndrome was in fact described 6 years earlier by Adair–Dighton (1912), while Bronson (1917) independently published 19 cases of the same triad at an earlier date. In some family members, hearing impairment and blue sclerae are present without the tendency to fractures (Morrison, 1979; Stoller, 1982).

Altered collagen synthesis results in defective connective tissue with a tendency to hypermobility and laxity of joints, 'thin' skin and subcutaneous bruising. The abnormal formation of dentine and cracking of the overlying enamel results in yellow-stained irregular teeth, the so-called amelogenesis imperfecta. The appearances are reminiscent of tetracycline staining of the permanent teeth. This feature is found in about 15% of patients with osteogenesis imperfecta and may be the only manifestation. This can be confirmed radiologically by demonstration of obliteration of the root canals.

Otological features

Characteristic features of the hearing loss in osteogenesis imperfecta are its age of onset and progression. Although only 10–20% of affected individuals will be deaf in childhood or adolescence, by middle age the figure exceeds 50% (Smärs, 1961; Pedersen, 1985; Stewart and O'Reilly, 1989) and usually progresses significantly from the third decade. The hearing loss may increase during pregnancy, while rather surprisingly, there is no correlation between its severity and that of the disease as indicated by the degree of physical handicap.

The hearing loss in osteogenesis imperfecta is clinically indistinguishable from otosclerosis. Characteristically it commences soon after puberty when fractures become less frequent. A conductive component is present in nearly 80% of cases, although more often than not this is part of a mixed loss. The deafness can be entirely sensorineural and total deafness may result in a few instances.

Tympanometry studies, using a probe tone of 220 Hz, show a tendency to high normal or raised compliance values. Although fixation of the stapes footplate is invariably present in cases with a conductive loss, hypermobility of the tympanic membrane (Carruth, Lutman and Stephens, 1978; Pedersen, 1984), fracture or aplasia of the stapedial crura, or distal atrophy or absence of the long process of the incus may coexist (Shea and Postma, 1982; Pederson, 1985). Carruth, Lutman and Stephens (1978) suggested that the reduced stiffness of the fibrous layer of the tympanic membrane, which has the same embryological origin as the sclera, was the more important factor leading to increased membrane mobility, possibly due to defective cross linkage between the circular and radial fibres. In ears with a fracture of the stapedial arch or loss of the incus long process, very high compliance values are present combined with a stapedius reflex of high amplitude providing there is not too large a contralateral conductive hearing loss. Carhart notches are not seen, and despite the widespread changes in the temporal bone neither is the Schwartze sign.

Vestibular symptoms have been reported as rare (Smärs, 1961; Morrison, 1979; Quisling *et al.*, 1979) or as frequently as 20% of affected cases (Shea and Postma, 1982; Pedersen, 1984). Stewart and O'Reilly (1989) reported an incidence of 9%. Johnsson *et al.* (1982) described extensive bilateral endolymphatic hydrops in a case in which temporal bone microdissection was undertaken. Morrison (1979) described two patients with amelogenesis imperfecta and Menière's syndrome, in whom abnormal sclerosis of the otic capsule was demonstrated on polytomography. However, secondary hydrops appears to be an unusual feature of the condition.

Changes in the labyrinthine capsule on petrous temporal bone tomography are virtually indistinguishable from those of labyrinthine otosclerosis. Demineralization, which is perhaps more widespread, and sclerosis produce a mottled appearance which is, however, not so marked as in Paget's disease of bone. Ross *et al.* (1993) have recently studied nine patients from three families with osteogenesis imperfecta by high resolution CT and by high resolving scintigraphy of the labyrinthine capsule. In four out of the six cases with osteogenesis imperfecta and a mixed hearing loss, severely decreased pericochlear bone density was established by CT. In these cases increased bone metabolism in the cochlear region was shown by tympanocochlear scintigraphy.

Histologically, there are some similarities to otosclerosis. Nager (1988) suggested that the two conditions may coexist, although the disorders are usually considered distinct entities (Wullstein, 1960; Bretlau, Jorgensen and Johansen, 1970; Shea and Postma, 1982; Pedersen, 1985) (see Figures 4.37 and 4.38). It is of interest that immunohistochemical studies by Arnold and Friedmann (1988) offered some evidence to support a possible role of paramyxoviruses in the aetiology of both these bony dyscrasias. In about two-thirds of cases stapedial fixation is due to a focal lesion in the footplate which, histologically, resembles the early active stages of otosclerosis. However, there is a greater degree of disorganization in the new bone formation in the osteogenesis imperfecta footplate compared with that seen in otosclerosis (Brosnan *et al.*, 1977). In other cases, fixation is the result of a diffuse structural alteration of the entire footplate. Biochemical assays of serum calcium, phosphorus and calciferol are normal, while alkaline phosphatase levels may occasionally be elevated. Photon absorptiometry has demonstrated that patients with osteogenesis imperfecta have a reduced thickness of cortical bone, while other generalized features include reduced dermal and central corneal thickness (Pedersen, 1985). These features are not found in otosclerosis. It is considered very likely, therefore, that the temporal bone features in osteogenesis imperfecta represent a local manifestation of the generalized skeletal and connective tissue disorder.

Treatment

There is no known curative treatment for the condition. In a typical case, new fractures cease to occur in adolescence, but skull involvement continues causing the characteristic 'soldier's helmet' appearance and deafness. Rehabilitation using an appropriate hearing aid is often the mainstay of treatment, although there may also be a place for surgery. More recently various medical treatments have been tried. Pedersen *et al.* (1985) evaluated human calcitonin but were unable to demonstrate any increase in bone mineral content in a small pilot study after 2–12 months; though perhaps the duration of treatment was just too short. Side effects were common, and two of their seven patients had to discontinue treatment. Because of the histological similarities with cochlear otospongiosis, Ross *et al.* (1993) advocated fluoride treatment, though as yet there is no evidence to support its efficacy.

Stapedectomy may well have a place in patients with a large air-bone gap and good cochlear function. Surgical results are generally satisfactory and can give hearing improvement similar to that obtained in otosclerosis if delayed until several years after the cessation of fractures (Patterson and Stone, 1970; Kosoy and Maddox, 1971; Shea and Postma, 1982; Stoller, 1982; Pedersen, 1985). Thus Garretsen and Cremers (1990) found hearing improvement in 85% of 58 ears undergoing stapedectomy, and an immediate increased sensorineural hearing loss due to the surgery in 9%. Some hearing loss was observed with long-term follow up to 9 years, but this was always due to progression of the coexistent sensorineural component. The fixed footplate is often very thick and soft, while middle ear mucosa around the oval window appears to be more vascular than normal. A high risk of a 'floating' footplate has been reported (Kosoy and Maddox, 1971; Brosnan *et al.*, 1977), although this is not the experience of others (Pederson, 1985). Extra care is required not to fracture the long process of the incus when crimping a wire prosthesis.

Paget's disease (*osteitis deformans*)

Sir James Paget described the detailed clinical and pathological features of this bone disease in 1877. The alternative term *osteitis deformans*, introduced by Czerny in 1873, is inappropriate because there is no evidence that the basic pathology is inflammatory, and marked skeletal deformity rarely occurs. The disease is characterized by spreading osteolytic and osteoblastic changes, most frequently affecting the pelvis, lumbar spine, skull, femur and tibia. However, the archetypal patient displaying the full clinical picture with an enlarged skull, progressive kyphosis, bowed legs and short stature is now rarely seen. It affects men four times more often than women and has a curious racial and geographical distribution, being very common in the UK (Woodhouse, 1973; Detheridge, Guyer and Barker, 1982), where estimates suggest that some three-quarters of a million people have the disease. The incidence is also high in Australia and New Zealand and in other populations of Anglo-Saxon origin, such as North America and South Africa. Surveys have revealed a marked geographical disease variation, and within the UK the prevalence has been shown to be considerably higher in Lancashire than elsewhere, but decreasing from high to lower levels over short distances (Barker *et al.*, 1980).

As described by Paget himself, the onset of the disease occurs in middle age. It is rarely seen before the age of 40 years and is more commonly encountered after the age of 55 years. Hereditary aspects are not easy to evaluate because of this relatively late age of onset, but it is has been thought to be inherited by a simple autosomal mendelian dominant gene (McKusick, 1972).

Three-quarters of patients with the disease have pelvic involvement, while the skull is affected in some 28% (Figure 15.6). An increased tortuosity and hypertrophy of the anterior terminal branch of the superficial temporal artery may be seen in many patients with skull involvement in Paget's disease, but it is by no means characteristic of the condition. Of those with widespread active disease, bone pain is a troublesome symptom, and probably is sufficient to warrant treatment in as many as 20%. Expansion of bones around foramina at the base of the skull and in the orbit can lead to neurological defects and optic atrophy. Early workers suggested that narrowing of the internal auditory meatus and the nerve channels in the bony modiolus with compression of the nerve fibres might account for the sensorineural loss, but this is not supported by histological evidence (Schuknecht, 1974). Monsell *et al.* (1995) carried out a comprehensive assessment of 64 ears with Paget's disease involving the skull by CT and auditory brain stem response recordings. There were no auditory brain stem response abnormalities, while the diameter of the internal auditory meatus did not show any correlation with hearing thresholds. This recent study therefore also supports a pathogenesis involving a primary cochlear site of lesion (Figures 15.7).

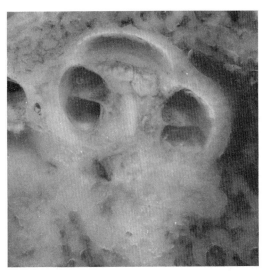

Figure 15.7 Paget's disease. Microslice of temporal bone with marked erosion of the otic capsule by pagetic bone. (Reproduced with kind permission of Milroy and Michaels, 1990a and the Editor, *Journal of Laryngology and Otology*)

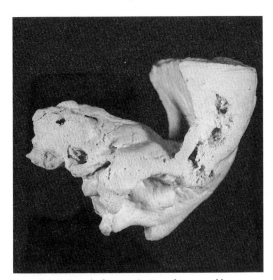

Figure 15.6 Paget's disease. Sectioned temporal bone showing gross thickening of cortex and petrous areas

While the exact aetiology is unknown, it is now widely accepted that Paget's disease is an example of primary osteoblast dysfunction in which the pathogenesis involves increases in the number and activity of osteoblasts. The stimulus for these increases is unknown, but as a result of the bone resorption, leading to a greatly enhanced rate of bone turnover, the normal lamellar structure of the collagen of the ground substance becomes grossly disordered and replaced by adjacent areas of osteolytic and sclerotic bone of increased vascularity. This results in bone softening, a tendency to fractures and deformity and typical biochemical changes. The serum calcium is usually normal, even though the rate of turnover of calcium in bone is enormously increased. Immobilization as a result of this disease, however, causes even greater bone resorption and formation so that both hypercalcaemia and hypercalciuria can occur. Serum alkaline phosphatase activity is elevated in active disease particularly if it is widespread. Activity of this enzyme is related to bone formation by osteoblasts and probably also by osteocytes. Serum acid phosphatase is an index of osteoclastic activity and is often increased in Paget's disease, particularly when the alkaline phosphatase is quite high, but its measurement is of little diagnostic value. Urinary hydroxyproline is an amino acid found exclusively in collagen and levels may be greatly elevated in Paget's disease, when the condition is active, reflecting the breakdown of bone collagen.

The most interesting recent hypothesis is that the disease results from a slow virus infection of the osteoblasts. Rebel *et al.* (1980) demonstrated inclusion bodies only in the osteoblasts, which are morphologically analogous to those seen in proven paramyxovirus infections – measles or respiratory syncytial virus. The work of Mills and his colleagues (1984) also support this association. Clinicopathological aspects of Paget's disease have several features in common with other proven slow virus disorders, and both Harvey (1984) and Mirra (1987) have reviewed the evidence for this proposed association. If a viral aetiology is confirmed, co-factors are almost certainly necessary, perhaps on a genetically susceptible background.

Otological features

Despite the frequency of Paget's disease, it is only rarely recognized as a cause of deafness in clinical practice. In many instances the disease may be asymptomatic apart from the otological features and the diagnosis can therefore easily be missed. However, in other cases, although hearing loss is present it may not be directly due to the disease. In patients with deafness due to Paget's disease. one would normally expect to see obvious signs in the plain skull X-rays (Figure 15.8). Davies (1968) reviewed 236 patients with the disease, finding skull involvement in 70% and deafness in 41%. Of the 97 patients with deafness, there was no radiological skull abnormality in 14. Vertigo and tinnitus, which was characteristically pulsatile, were present in 36% and 32% respectively. Harner, Rose and Facer (1978) studied 1066 patients with objective evidence of Paget's disease over a 5-year period. More than 43% had a hearing loss which was usually sensorineural. However, when the records were carefully reviewed they concluded that the hearing loss was not usually part of the disease process and most patients had no direct evidence of temporal bone involvement. In their series, 17% of patients had tinnitus and 22% dizziness. The most common vestibular symptoms were postural and positional unsteadiness. However, in those with radiological evidence of skull involvement, the incidence of mixed hearing loss was statistically greater than expected and the incidences of tinnitus and dizziness were also higher than in the group as a whole.

The type of hearing loss most commonly encountered is progressive and mixed with both conductive and sensorineural components (Davies, 1968). It is usually fairly symmetrical. In the earlier stages of the disease, conductive deafness is present in more than two-thirds of affected ears. Davies found that the air-bone gap averaged 30 dB for women and 20 dB for men, and was most marked at the 500 Hz frequency. The stapedius reflex is often present and preserved with moderate conductive hearing losses. By contrast, in patients with otosclerosis and in osteogenesis imperfecta, as little as 15 dB of hearing loss due to stapedial fixation abolishes the reflex. The greater age of onset also helps to distinguish Paget's disease from otosclerosis.

There are still relatively few histological studies of the temporal bone in Paget's disease (see Figures 4.39 and 4.40). Changes are rarely present in the stapes footplate, while pagetic changes in the other ossicles (Figure 15.9) and the formation of bony spurs in the epitympanum interfering with incudomalleal mobility are the common findings which have been suggested to account for the conductive hearing loss (Davies, 1970; Schuknecht, 1974; Proops, Bayley and Hawke, 1985). However, Khetarpal and Schuknecht (1990) have recently performed histological studies on 26 temporal bones from 16 patients with Paget's disease of the temporal bone, many with audiometric data. In the seven ears with a documented conductive hearing loss there was no

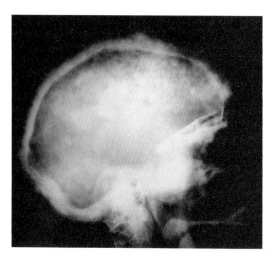

Figure 15.8 Paget's disease. Lateral skull X-ray showing the typical 'moth-eaten' appearance of the thickened cortical bone. (Reproduced by kind permission of Dr S. Murray, Royal London Hospital)

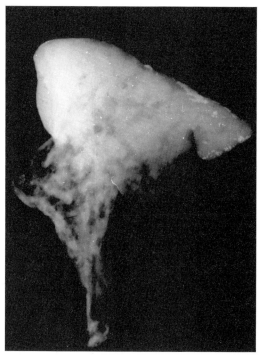

Figure 15.9 Paget's disease. 'Moth-eaten' involvement of incus bone. (Reproduced by kind permission of Dr Robert L. Davis)

evidence of ossicular fixation, nor could they define a clear alternative cause. These workers therefore suggested that the conductive loss, as well as a sensorineural component, could be caused by changes in bone density, mass and form that dampen the finely tuned motion mechanics of the middle and inner ears.

A progressive sensorineural hearing loss mainly affecting the higher frequencies, that is greater than normal for age, is seen in 20% of patients and can also be associated with a conductive element (Davies, 1968). Pagetoid osteitis involving the endosteal layer of the otic capsule results in degenerative changes in the stria vascularis with atrophy of both the cochlear duct and vestibular labyrinth (Kornfield, 1967; Rüedi, 1968; Lindsay and Lehman, 1969; Schuknecht, 1974). The basal turns of the cochlea are most severely affected and Schuknecht initially suggested a local toxic effect caused by pagetic disease of the bony labyrinth, similar to that observed in cochlear otosclerosis. More recently Khetarpal and Schuknecht (1990) have conducted more comprehensive histological studies. They found that pagetic lesions in the periosteal layer extended to the endosteal layer in only 54% of cases with temporal bone involvement, while neither invasion of the inner ear spaces nor compression of the nerves in the internal auditory meatus was seen. Occasionally microfractures of the bony labyrinth are present, which reflect the considerable stresses that develop as the pagetic bone replaces normal bone. Secondary endolymphatic hydrops of the cochlear duct and saccule, and atrophy of the membranous semicircular canals have been described. The vascular shunts connecting vessels of diseased pagetic bone with those of the spiral ligament described by Rüedi (1968) have not been confirmed by others. Thus, in the early stages, the inner ear loss is mainly sensory with relatively well preserved speech discrimination, but later, secondary neuronal degeneration occurs. Bony softening and deformity of the skull base can lead to acquired basilar impression and possibly sensorineural hearing loss by torsion of the VIIIth nerve or its associated vasculature. Vestibular symptoms are usually rather non-specific, taking the form of transient vertigo or imbalance, although exceptionally they assume a Menière-like character when secondary hydrops has occurred.

In the early stages, small areas of lucency and dense patches which fade into one another are seen on X-ray. There is often a typical mixture of lytic and sclerotic areas and the skull is thick where it is affected, predominantly over the vertex. Some coarse trabeculae are nearly always visible except in the most advanced cases. Osteoporosis circumscripta is a different manifestation of the disease causing a total radiographic disappearance of bone which always stops short of involving the whole structure (Kasabach and Gutman, 1937; du Boulay, 1980). The radiological appearance of the temporal bone in the established disease is pathognomonic and variations from minimal demineralization of the petrous apex to demineralization of the entire petrous pyramid including the otic capsule are encountered.

The temporal bone changes frequently correlate with the degree of skull involvement. In the initial stage when extensive demineralization primarily affects the medial aspect of the petrous pyramid, the labyrinthine capsule stands out more clearly than normal. Involvement of the internal auditory meatus consists of demineralization of the walls without evidence of narrowing and, when surrounded by featureless homogeneous pagetoid bone, it may no longer be identifiable as a distinct structure. The otic capsule is spared until advanced changes are present. Involvement of the labyrinthine capsule begins in the outer periosteal layer; the middle endochondral layer is more resistant and the greatest resistance is present in the endosteal layer, but with extensive involvement these three layers can no longer be distinguished. Eventually the medial ends of the petrous pyramids become tilted upwards due to bone softening causing acquired basilar impression. High resolution computerized tomography may yield additional information about bone architecture (Figure 15.10) (Lloyd, Phelps and du Boulay, 1980; Swartz *et al.*, 1985a). (See also Figure 2.65.)

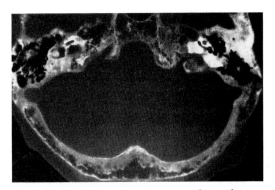

Figure 15.10 Paget's disease. CT scan; axial view showing disease affecting the skull base (woven bone)

Treatment

It is generally agreed that the results of reconstructive middle ear surgery are unsatisfactory in Paget's disease. There are several reasons for this surgical pessimism. There is no consistent defect responsible for the conductive loss and, indeed, several may coexist in some cases. Stapedial ankylosis is probably very uncommon. The frequently associated sensorineural hearing loss is another significant factor mitigating against the prospects of a successful surgical outcome. Perhaps it sensitizes the cochlea to further impairment of function during the footplate manipulations of a stapedectomy procedure. Finally, and probably most important, the long-term results in most reported cases are poor.

Morrison (1975) performed stapedectomies on two patients with 40–50 dB air-bone gaps. In each case the stapes was found to be normal. Both patients experienced a hearing gain which was unfortunately only temporary and was followed by progressive conductive and sensorineural hearing loss. This experience has been shared by others (Sparrow and Duval, 1967; Davies, 1968). Stapes or ossicular mobilization has also generally produced a less than favourable long-term outcome. Morrison (1975) described two good hearing results after mobilization which reverted to preoperative levels within a few months.

The effects of medical treatment with calcitonin on hearing loss have been studied by several groups, although with conflicting results. Calcitonin causes a rapid inhibition of osteoblast activity, while continued therapy leads to a reduction in the rapid turnover of calcium and a gradual remineralization of bone (Woodhouse, 1973). Successful treatment results in a fall in the serum alkaline phosphatase and urinary hydroxyproline excretion by an average of 50%. A typical protocol consists of daily subcutaneous injections of 10–50 mg calcitonin which can be reduced to an alternate day regimen when biochemical parameters become normal, after about 2 weeks. Shai, Baker and Wallach (1971), Morrison (1975) and Moffat, Morrow and Simpson (1977) all reported hearing improvement following calcitonin treatment, while Grimaldi, Mohamedally and Woodhouse (1975) and Walker *et al.* (1979) found no significant differences between treated and untreated groups. The Otologic Medical Group of Los Angeles reported the results of a comprehensive study of calcitonin therapy in this disorder (El Sammaa *et al.*, 1986). Twenty-six patients with hearing loss due to Paget's disease seen by one clinician received calcitonin regularly for periods ranging from 5 to 8 years and were compared to 19 patients, seen concurrently by other colleagues, who received no treatment. They found that, although there was no significant hearing improvement in the treatment group, their hearing thresholds were effectively stabilized, in contrast to the untreated group in whom a mean increase hearing loss of more than 25 dB was observed. Such long-term treatment is certainly expensive and may be affected by antibody formation with calcitonin of porcine or salmon origin.

Disodium etidronate (EHDP) is a biphosphonate which seems to possess all the biological properties of pyrophosphate including the ability to inhibit bone resorption. The drug appears to inactivate osteoclasts and osteoblasts and these effects have led to its clinical usage in Paget's disease (Kanis and Russell, 1981). Although the drug is effective, long-term or short-term high dose administration may result in histological osteomalacia. It has the distinct advantage that it may be taken orally, though absorption is relatively poor and unpredictable. A suggested starting regimen is 400 mg per day for not more than 6 months. There are still few published reports of its use in the deafness of Paget's disease. Gennari and Sensini (1975) treated five patients and their pure-tone audiograms showed a significant improvement in the air conduction threshold of greater than 15 dB in three cases. It has been shown that short-term high dosage treatment with EHDP may well maximize suppression of disease activity but decrease exposure to unwanted secondary effects (Preston *et al.*, 1986). Lando, Hoover and Finerman (1988) have suggested that combined treatment with both calcitonin and etidronate may improve efficacy and reduce the incidence of side effects when treating patients with progressive hearing loss.

Severe hearing loss, particularly in younger adults, with evidence of rapidly progressive disease would seem a clear indication for medical treatment, while the enhanced patient acceptability of EHDP, as a result of oral administration, makes the decision for a therapeutic trial in other cases easier to make. Second-generation biphosphonates have the major advantage over etidronate that remineralization is not inhibited resulting in fewer side effects, and clinical evaluation appears promising. In the study by Cantrill, Buckler and Anderson (1986), intravenous 3-amino-1-hydroxypropylidene-1,1-biphosphonate (APD) resulted in an alkaline phosphatase reduction and symptomatic improvement in 95% of 20 cases with Paget's disease, and was associated with minimal side effects. Intravenous administration is essential as poor and unpredictable gastrointestinal absorption occurs with oral ingestion. Third generation biphosphonates, such as risedonate, also markedly reduce bone absorption. Richardson, Tinling and Chole (1993) conducted tests *in vitro* and *in vivo* using a neonatal mouse model, and showed that they act by inhibiting parathormone-activated calcium release from bone. They commended this drug for clinical trials on the basis of its high level of potency and low level of observed cellular toxicity.

Such treatments are clearly not devoid of risk and must be undertaken in close conjunction with a metabolic physician. The reader is reminded of the possible adverse side effect of delayed significant sensorineural hearing loss (see cochlear otosclerosis treatment).

Fibrous dysplasia

Fibrous dysplasia is a fairly common benign disorder of fibro-osseous tissue of unknown aetiology which was not recognized as a specific disease entity until the 1940s. It can affect one or several bones and while the dominant features are skeletal, occasionally certain endocrinopathies, abnormal pigmentation of skin and mucous membrane and other abnormalities may form part of the disease process. The craniofacial skeleton is a predilective site and the temporal bone is affected in more than 15% of cases with skull involvement. For many years, fibrous dysplasia of bone was not distinguished from primary hyperparathyroidism, and both kinds of osseous lesions were described pathologically and radiologically as osteitis fibrosa cystica.

Three separate types of fibrous dysplasia are now described.

Type I: monostotic

This type is limited to one bone, usually the femur, tibia, ribs or facial bones. The mandible and maxilla are the most frequent sites of facial bone involvement.

Type II: polyostotic

In this type more than one bone is involved, most frequently of the lower limbs. In the skull, the lesser and greater wings of the sphenoids, and the vertical and horizontal processes of the frontal bones are mainly affected. The frontal and sphenoid sinuses are frequently obliterated.

Type III: disseminated and extraskeletal manifestations

This is also known as the McCune-Albright syndrome (McCune, 1936; Albright *et al.*, 1937). Bone distribution is similar to the polyostotic form but is commonly unilateral, with areas of skin hyperpigmentation and endocrine disturbances, particularly hyperthyroidism. The disorder primarily affects women who characteristically display precocious puberty.

The monostotic form, which accounts for about 70% of cases (van Tilberg, 1972), generally becomes arrested at puberty. The polyostotic form, on the other hand, may progress beyond the third or fourth decades. Initial clinical symptoms usually appear during childhood or early adolescence – a period of active skeletal growth (Lichtenstein and Jaffe, 1942) – and include pain, deformity and recurrent fractures.

In the disease, normal bone is replaced by fibrous tissue consisting of spindle cells and poorly formed trabeculae of immature woven bone. Increased osteoblastic and osteoclastic activity is usually present and islands of cartilage may be observed. It primarily involves the cancellous bone, although tissue expansion may give rise to distortion and structural weakness. As the lesions enlarge, the overlying bony cortex becomes thinner, although its histological structure usually remains normal. The disease has been considered variously as an arrest of bone maturation (Reed, 1963), as a disturbance of postnatal cancellous bone maintenance (Aegerter and Kirkpatrick, 1968), or as a misdifferentiation of the bone-forming mesenchyme (Lichtenstein and Jaffe, 1942). Carcinomatous degeneration is very rare (Schwartz and Alpert, 1964) and has never been reported in the temporal bone.

Otological features

In 1982, Nager, Kennedy and Kopstein reviewed the literature and summarized the findings in 69 cases of fibrous dysplasia involving the temporal bone. The male to female sex incidence was 2:1 and a majority of the patients had the monostotic form of the disease. The mean age of onset of the clinical symptoms was 15 years, although the range extended to 59 years. The mean age at clinical presentation was 28 years.

The commonest presenting symptoms were progressive hearing impairment (57%), localized swelling of the temporal bone (51%) and progressive bony occlusion of the external auditory meatus (42%). About 15% of the patients with hearing loss had a total or profound sensorineural deafness and the remainder had an early conductive loss. Vestibular symptoms and tinnitus were uncommon. In 11 cases, marked constriction or obliteration of the external auditory meatus was associated with an underlying epidermoid inclusion cyst or cholesteatoma. The pathogenesis is similar to other situations with acquired stenosis of the meatus, when desquamation of normal meatal skin and tympanic membrane continues medial to an obstruction (Brookes and Graham, 1984). Labyrinthine involvement was present in three of the cases; five developed facial nerve paralysis. For this reason an obliterated external auditory meatus should be explored surgically and reconstructed (Smouha, Edelstein and Parisier, 1987). Three patients presented with massive temporal bone involvement and features of an intracranial space occupying lesion. The increased size of the temporal bone was usually postauricular often causing an anteroinferior protrusion of the auricle, but occasionally swellings of the preauricular and supra-auricular regions were present. Blockage of the eustachian tube leading to serous otitis media may occur. Rarely bony narrowing of the internal auditory meatus develops with progressive impairment of function of the VIIth and VIIIth cranial nerves.

Typically the serum calcium and phosphorus levels are normal, while the alkaline phosphatase level may be raised in the presence of an active lesion. If several bones are involved hyperparathyroidism must be excluded, although on occasions it appears that the two conditions may occur together. X-ray studies generally reveal an enlarged temporal bone associated with sclerosis, or a uniform 'ground glass' appearance (Figure 15.11). Areas of radiolucency and cortical thinning may occasionally be seen. The radiological appearance of the disease is a function of its

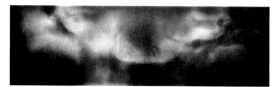

Figure 15.11 Fibrous dysplasia. Posteroanterior tomogram of 28-year-old man with a 1-year history of progressive hearing loss and recent painful otorrhoea. Typical ground-glass appearance of right petrous temporal bone. There is obliteration of the external auditory meatus, although the labyrinthine capsule appears unaffected. (Reproduced by kind permission of Mr Henry Grant)

histological structure. A predominance of osseous elements renders the lesion more opaque, while the mixture of fibrous and bony elements produces the 'ground glass' appearance (see Figure 2.66). The predominance of fibrous elements produces a radiolucent cyst-like picture. The high resolution CT scan features have been documented by Swartz and his colleagues (1985a) (Figure 15.12). Casselman *et al.* (1993) have decribed the MRI findings. Low to intermediate signal intensity is usually seen in the main part of the lesion on T1-and T2-weighted sequences. High clinical and pathological activity, however, correlates with high signal intensity on both spin-echo sequences and with strong gadolinium enhancement.

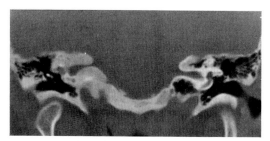

Figure 15.12 Fibrous dysplasia. High resolution CT scan showing narrowing of the internal auditory meatus

Treatment

At present there is no known conservative treatment for the control of fibrous dysplasia. Nevertheless, the prognosis is usually good and the decrease in disease activity at puberty is greater in the monostotic form. The presence of a lesion in the temporal bone does not in itself justify surgical intervention. However, more than one-half of the patients will probably undergo operative treatment. The main indication is external auditory meatus stenosis, while reduction of the unsightly local swelling for cosmetic reasons accounts for most of the other cases. The diseased bone

has characteristic macroscopic features. It is vascular, spongy and crumbly with a gritty consistency and can be readily removed by curettage. Half the cases reviewed by Nager, Kennedy and Kopstein (1982) underwent two or more operative procedures, but surgery was rarely curative. Management should therefore be conservative. Spontaneous decrease in disease activity may well help to reduce the recurrence rate. Radiotherapy appears to have a predisposing propensity to malignant generation of lesions in other sites (Schwartz and Alpert, 1964).

Osteopetrosis (marble bone disease)

Osteopetrosis is a rare inherited bone disorder which occurs as a benign dominant form, otherwise known as Albers-Schonberg disease, and a malignant recessive form. Pathologically there is a failure of resorption of cartilage and excessive formation of immature bone leading to thickening of the cortex and narrowing or obliteration of the medullary cavity. This may cause anaemia and a susceptibility to infection. Failure and impairment of bone maturation result in thick, dense and brittle bones (Figure 15.13). The skull may become extremely thick and when remodelling involves the cranial foramina, stenosis and compression of emergent nerves and vessels may occur. The optic, trigeminal, facial and auditory nerves are those most frequently affected (Myers and Stool, 1969; Hamersma, 1970). The hearing loss is usually conductive, but occasionally is mixed and is caused by impaired ossicular mobility by osteopetrotic bone (Jones and Mulcahy, 1968; Hamersma, 1970).

Otological features

Histological studies in established disease show that much of the bone tissue is expanded by dense lamellar bone, while the labyrinth and ossicles mainly consist of dense calcified cartilage (Milroy and Michaels, 1990b). Typically, pneumatization of the mastoids is absent. The internal auditory meatus may be narrowed, but the otic capsule remains unaffected (Myers and Stool, 1969; Hawke, Jahn and Bailey, 1981). A conductive hearing loss may be due to narrowing of the bony eustachian tube causing secondary chronic otitis media, in addition to bone deposition in the ossicles. The serum alkaline and acid phosphatase may be markedly elevated, while the urinary hydroxyproline levels are usually normal (Johnston *et al.*, 1968).

Most of the patients with malignant recessive disease die in early childhood and certainly none survive into their twenties. Elster and his colleagues (1992) have reviewed cranial imaging studies by conventional radiography, CT and MRI in 13 children. In

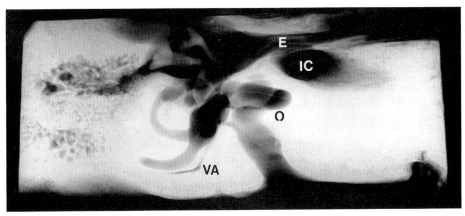

Figure 15.13 X-ray microslice of adult type osteopetrosis. The whole temporal bone is composed of dense bone. E = eustachian tube; IC = internal carotid artery; O = otic capsule; VA = vestibular aqueduct. (Reproduced by kind permission of Milroy and Michaels, 1990a and the Editor, *Journal of Laryngology and Otology*)

the majority, marked sclerosis and deposition of osteopetrotic bone was noted along the anterior occipitomastoid suture, and at the basioccipital-exoccipital and spheno-occipital synchondroses. Neurological deficits included blindness ($n = 11$), conductive hearing loss ($n = 11$), and facial nerve palsies ($n = 4$). Delayed myelination was seen with MR imaging in two of five retarded infants. Prominent extracerebral cerebrospinal fluid spaces were present over the frontal lobes in five of the eight developmentally normal patients, representing either subclinical parenchymal disease or a phenomenon related to discordant growth rates between the skull and brain.

In contrast, many patients with the benign autosomal dominant disease may be asymptomatic, the diagnosis only being made radiologically. Common symptoms are bone pain and fractures. Recent studies have suggested that two subgroups may be defined by imaging studies (Bollerslev, Grontved and Andersen, 1988). Type I osteopetrosis is characterized by a pronounced osteosclerosis of the skull and an enlarged and thickened cranial vault. In type II, osteosclerosis is most marked at the skull base. Interestingly all except one of the 14 patients studied had otoneurological manifestations, but these were primary complaints in only two cases. Trigeminal nerve involvement was only seen in type I, and a conductive hearing loss was also common in this group. In addition, tomography showed a significant narrowing of the internal auditory meatus ($P < 0.01$) compared to normal controls, but this feature was not present in type II. In contrast, facial nerve involvement, which is quite a frequent manifestation, was primarily found in type II. Recurrent facial palsy tends to result in progressive residual facial weakness with synkinesis and contracture. Clinical experience indicates that surgical intervention to alter the natural history of these recurrent facial palsies should include decompression of the proximal facial nerve in the fallopian canal by a middle fossa approach, as well as the more conventional transmastoid decompression of the horizontal and vertical segments (Benecke, 1993).

Neurofibromatosis

This is a common disorder of neural tissue which was described by von Recklinghausen in 1882. It is characterized by multiple areas of cutaneous pigmentation (café-au-lait spots), multiple naevi and neurofibromas of peripheral or cranial nerves. Within the cranial cavity, neurofibromas most often occur on the VIIIth nerve and are sometimes bilateral (type 2) (see Chapter 21). In addition, there is an increased incidence of gliomas and meningiomas, which may be multiple. The disease is familial with an autosomal dominant inheritance, although sporadic cases do occur (see Figure 2.59).

Bone lesions occur in about one-half of the cases (Hunt and Pugh, 1961; Nordin, 1973, Beighton, 1978). Common skeletal abnormalities include severe scoliosis, defects of the walls of the orbits, erosive defects caused by adjacent neurogenic tumours, apart from disorders of bone growth. The facial bones, mandible, occipital and temporal bones may be deformed and hypoplastic. Figure 15.14 shows the famous patient of Sir Frederick Treves, Joseph Merrick (alias the elephant man), who was treated at the London Hospital, and was commonly believed to be suffering from neurofibromatosis. It can be seen that he had marked narrowing of the right external auditory meatus resulting in a conductive hearing loss. There is no evidence, however, that one of his numerous misfortunes included vestibular schwannoma.

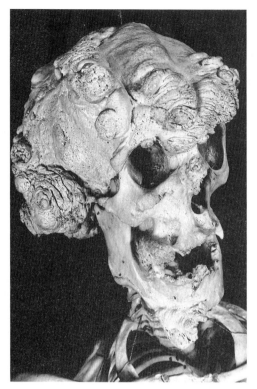

Figure 15.14 Neurofibromatosis. Oblique view of skull of Joseph Merrick (Reproduced from *Journal of Laryngology and Otology*, by kind permission of the Editor and Professor Sir Colin Berry, Royal London Hospital)

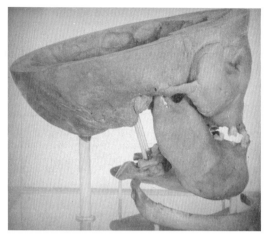

Figure 15.15 Hyperostosis corticalis generalisata. Lateral view of skull and rib. There is marked thickening and sclerosis of the bones of the calvarium, while both external auditory meatus are obliterated. The internal auditory meatus were similarly affected (Royal College of Surgeons Museum S.67.7). (Reproduced from *Journal of Laryngology and Otology* by kind permission of the Editor and the Medical Illustration Department, Royal College of Surgeons)

Genetic craniotabular hyperostoses

Hyperostosis corticalis generalisata (Van Buchem's disease)

This disease was first described by Van Buchem and his colleagues in 1955, who have since added further reports (Van Buchem *et al.*, 1962; Van Buchem, 1971). It is an autosomal recessive condition, in which normal stature but overgrowth of bone in the skull and skeleton are associated with facial palsy and conductive deafness.

There is osteosclerosis of the skull, mandible, clavicle and ribs and hyperplasia of the diaphyseal cortex of the long and short bones. The skull and mandible may enlarge from the age of 10 years onwards with thickening of the calvaria, skull base and clavicles (Figure 15.15). The facial paralysis may be unilateral or bilateral, and the gradually symmetrical hearing loss may be noted from the early teenage years. In some a sensorineural hearing loss and in others a mixed loss may occur. Optic nerve involvement is a late complication. The serum calcium and phosphorus remain normal, but the alkaline phosphatase is frequently raised by as much as 50–250%.

Sclerosteosis

This is an autosomal recessive condition in which skeletal overgrowth is associated with syndactyly and digital malformation; facial palsy and deafness are common complications and raised intracranial pressure may develop (Truswell, 1958).

The hearing loss may be bilateral, sensorineural, mixed, or conductive. Facial nerve paralysis is often unilateral in childhood, becoming bilateral in late adolescence. Dort, Pollak and Fisch (1990) have carried out a histopathological study of the dimensions of the fallopian canal using a new method of surface area measurement. They found narrowing in the labyrinthine, distal tympanic and mastoid segments of the facial nerve canal, and associated bony occlusion of the stylomastoid artery. They concluded that both ischaemia and bony compression are the underlying causes of recurrent facial palsy in this disease. As the labyrinthine segment is the most severely affected surgical decompression must include this portion of the fallopian canal. There is also decreased sensory function of the ophthalmic and maxillary divisions of the Vth cranial nerve, anosmia and chronic headache.

The alkaline phosphatase is markedly elevated in nearly all patients, although other biochemical skeletal indices are usually normal. Radiologically, the bones show increased density but abnormalities of bone modelling, if present, are of minor degree (Beighton, Crenin and Hamersma, 1976; Beighton, Durr and Hamersma, 1976).

Congenital hyperphosphatasia (osteoectasia)

This is a rare autosomal recessive condition with skeletal deformity developing in the second or third year of life. It is associated with dwarfing, fractures and blue sclerae. There is marked irregular thickening of the skull and enlargement of the calvaria. The external auditory meatus may become narrowed and there is a progressive mixed hearing loss which becomes evident from the fourth to the fourteenth year. Typically the hearing thresholds average about 70 dB. The serum alkaline and acid phosphatase levels are both consistently elevated.

Progressive diaphyseal dysplasia (Camurati-Engelmann's disease; osteopathia hyperostotica sclerositans multiplex infantilis)

This is an autosomal dominant condition principally involving the long bones, but the skull may be mildly affected. Generalized sclerosis of the base, similar to osteopetrosis, may be seen but in the vault of the skull fewer bones are involved and are less severely affected.

Sparkes and Graham (1972) have reported the case of a 26-year-old man with progressive hearing difficulty leading to total deafness on the right side associated with a facial paralysis. Bilateral decompression of the slit-like internal auditory meatus was carried out and some initial improvement was noted. Two cases who also underwent surgery have been described (Miyamoto, House and Brackmann, 1980). The first was a 26-year-old man who complained of bilateral hearing loss, right-sided facial paralysis and chronic unsteadiness. X-rays showed bilateral massive overgrowth of dense bone involving the petrous apex and mastoid bone. Both internal auditory meatus were partially obliterated by such bone. The second case was that of a 30-year-old woman with bilateral sensorineural hearing loss, occurring suddenly 14 months earlier on the right side and 9 months later on the left. Both cases were explored surgically by a middle cranial fossa approach, the first to improve the facial nerve function and the second to decompress the internal auditory meatus on the right side. Following surgery, the hearing of the second patient has remained stable and further X-rays did not show evidence of recompression.

One of the authors has recently managed a young female patient with bilateral progressive sensorineural hearing loss and vestibular dysfunction (Hellier and Brookes, 1996). In this case persistent dizziness and imbalance which was totally refractory to medical treatment was the overriding disability. It was associated with the localizing symptom of unilateral aural pressure. There was very marked narrowing of both internal auditory meatus (Figure 15.16) and surgical decompression was carried out via a retrosigmoid craniotomy to facilitate identification of the porus. Complete relief of vestibular symtoms was achieved, though some increased high frequency hearing loss resulted. The sclerotic bone in this disease is relatively avascular, and as one may expect no untoward technical difficulties were encountered at operation.

The genetic craniotabular dysplasias, craniofacial dysostoses and osteopathia striata are extremely rare conditions. They are usually only seen in infancy and are listed in Table 15.1 for completeness. The main clinical features of craniodiaphyseal dysplasia are somewhat similar to those described in Engelmann's disease, though facial distortion is typically more severe. Thus bony overgrowth results in a large head circumference and central nervous system dysfunction is frequently found due to mechanical compression, resulting in blindness, mental retardation, epilepsy or retarded growth. The VIIth and VIIIth cranial nerves are often involved. Himi *et al.* (1993) have recently described the temporal bone histopathology from a case of craniodiaphyseal dysplasia. Abnormal bone was not affecting the labyrinth directly, though the internal auditory meatus was elongated and narrowed to less than one-third of its normal diameter. They suggested that both direct mechanical neural compression or impaired vascular supply could well contribute to otovestibular dysfunction, and also to facial nerve compromise.

Dietary and metabolic disease

Osteomalacias (vitamin D deficiency)

Vitamin D deficiency has been recognized as an uncommon cause of bilateral sensorineural hearing loss only relatively recently (Brookes and Morrison, 1981; Brookes, 1983). It is a condition which occurs primarily in Asian immigrants and socioeconomically deprived populations. Since changing hospital appointments to a predominantly middle class practice in postgraduate hospitals without a metabolic medical unit on site, one of the authors (GBB) has only diagnosed and treated two new cases in the last 10 years.

Vitamin D refers to a group of steroids which, with parathyroid hormone, play an essential role in the regulation of calcium and bone metabolism. The main metabolic pathway is shown in Figure 15.17. Most is synthesized in the skin and, under normal circumstances, dietary requirements are minimal.

Rickets and osteomalacia are the juvenile and adult forms respectively of a group of disorders characterized by defective mineralization of bone and usually result from quantitative and qualitative impairment of vitamin D activity. A less common cause is hypophosphataemia, and secondary hyperparathyroidism is occasionally associated. A high incidence of osteomalacia has been recognized among Asian immi-

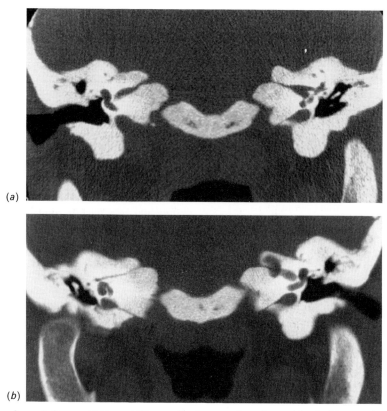

(a)

(b)

Figure 15.16 Engelmann's disease. (*a*) Coronal CT scan showing very dense bone of the skull base and marked narrowing of the internal auditory meatus. (*b*) Postoperative CT scan following retrosigmoid decompression of left internal auditory meatus

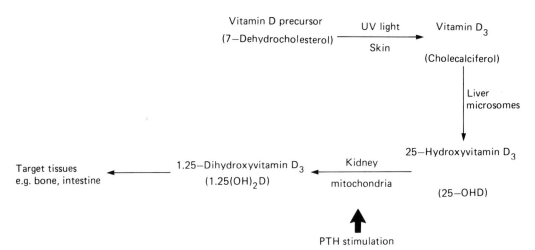

Figure 15.17 Main metabolic pathway of vitamin D. PTH = parathyroid hormone. (Reproduced by kind permission of the Editor, *Journal of Laryngology and Otology*)

grants living in the UK, due to a combination of dietary and genetic factors (British Medical Journal, 1976). In the classical deficiency state, the serum calcium and phosphate levels may be low, while the alkaline phosphatase is usually elevated. These biochemical parameters are often normal, however, due to compensatory metabolic mechanisms. Reduced mineralization may produce an altered trabecular bone pattern and pathological fractures on X-ray, but radiology in most early cases is normal, when the clinical condition is termed 'biochemical osteomalacia'. Serum assay of metabolic derivatives of vitamin D – 25-hydroxy vitamin D, the storage form, and 1,25-hydroxy vitamin D, the active form – are typically low in vitamin D deficient states including biochemical osteomalacia. However, the levels of these metabolites do not always show a close correlation.

Otological features

Brookes (1985a) has summarized the otological features and treatment results of 27 patients presenting to The London Hospital with deafness and low vitamin D levels. More than half were Asian immigrants and two-thirds reported associated tinnitus. Vestibular symptoms were infrequent. Nearly 50% had a progressive cochlear deafness. A characteristic trough-shaped pure-tone audiogram centred around 1–2 kHz frequencies was seen in two-thirds of these cases. Figure 15.18 is the audiogram of a 35-year-old Asian man at presentation. Three months later, when the diagnosis was established, his hearing had fallen to a mean level of 85 dB (Figure 15.19). Electrocochleography showed features of endolymphatic hydrops (Figure 15.20). Cochlear tomography demonstrated bilateral demineralization (Figure 15.21). However, this was only present in less than 15% of cases. All except one of the remaining patients in The London Hospital series had otosclerosis (see below).

The possible role of vitamin D in hearing impairment was subsequently investigated by Ikeda *et al.* (1989), who studied 28 patients with unexplained bilateral sensorineural hearing loss. They found a

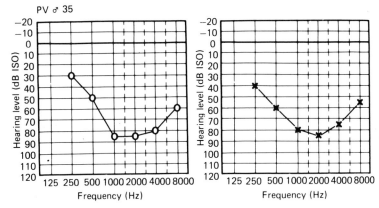

Figure 15.18 Vitamin D deficient deafness. Pure-tone audiogram of 35-year-old Asian man with a 2-year history of progressive hearing impairment and tinnitus (25-hydroxy vitamin D < 2.1 ng/ml). (Reproduced by kind permission of the Editor, *American Journal of Otology*)

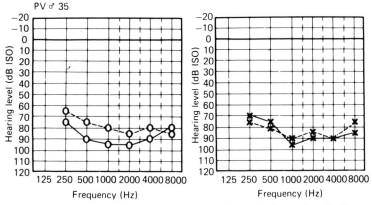

Figure 15.19 Pure-tone audiogram of same patient as in Figure 15.18, 3 months later, when the diagnosis of vitamin D deficient deafness was made. ——— = pretreatment threshold; – – – – = 2 months after treatment with calciferol. (Reproduced by kind permission of the Editor, *Journal of Laryngology and Otology*)

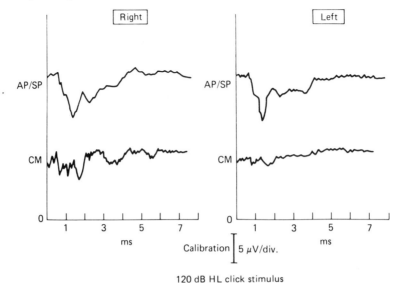

Figure 15.20 Vitamin D deficient deafness. Transtympanic electrocochleography showing large negative summating potentials (SPs) and small distorted cochlear microphonics (CMs). AP/SP = action potential/summating potential complex. (Reproduced by kind permission of the Editor, *Journal of Laryngology and Otology*)

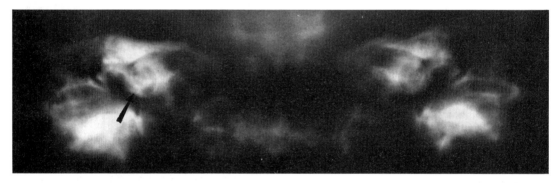

Figure 15.21 Vitamin D deficient deafness: cochlear polytomography. Bilateral demineralization is present. Arrow indicates obliteration of lumen of basal turn. (Reproduced by kind permission of the Editor, *Journal of Laryngology and Otology*)

significantly low 1,25-dihydroxyvitamin D_3 level in 23 cases, though 25-hydroxyvitamin D_3 levels were normal. Flock, Flock and Ulfendahl (1986) suggested that 1,25-dihydroxy vitamin D_3, the active metabolite, may regulate the intracellular calcium ion level in hair cells via a calcium binding protein, and affect the integrity of the membrane vessels in the cochlea. They concluded that a disturbance of such mechanisms could induce hair cell dysfunction and impaired microcirculation in the cochlea. On the other hand, Irwin (1986) screened 112 consecutive new patients with sensorineural hearing loss; though some had serum biochemical anomalies consistent with vitamin D deficiency, all vitamin D assays were normal. Perhaps this study merely emphasizes the low prevalence of this disorder in the UK Caucasian population.

Covell first reported the histopathological effects of

acute vitamin D deficiency in 1941. He studied a group of rats who were maintained on a vitamin D deficient diet for 3 weeks, followed by a vitamin replacement diet for 1 week. Pathological features were thus modified by various degrees of healing. Newly formed osteoid was found in the periosteal and endochondral layers of the otic capsule, together with slight degenerative changes in the cochlear nerve.

The effects of acute vitamin D deficiency alone on both cochlear function and morphology have been studied in the albino rat (Brookes, Lilly and Hawkins, 1983). A significant reduction in the amplitude of the brain-stem evoked responses and impaired mean hearing thresholds were seen in the vitamin D deficient animals, following a vitamin depleted diet for 10 weeks, compared with a control group. Preliminary morphological studies showed narrowing and, in some places, obliteration of the capillaries in the stria vascularis, features suggesting early strial atrophy. Ikeda *et al.* (1987a) conducted a similar study in rats, and found prolongation of the N1 latency with depression of the cochlear microphonic amplitude and elevation of the cochlear microphonic threshold. In a subsequent study in guinea-pigs the same group concluded that calcium ions are actively transported from perilymph, whereas the cacium ion concentration in perilymph is dependent on the serum concentration (Ikeda *et al.*, 1987b).

Treatment

Patients have been treated with replacement vitamin and mineral supplements, the dosage being dependent upon the degree of deficiency. Those with a 25-hydroxy vitamin D level of 5–10 ng/ml have received combined vitamin D and calcium tablets, two or three per day, to provide a dose of 1000–1500 units of vitamin D. Patients with levels less than 5 ng/ml have received treatment with the parent vitamin D_3 compound, calciferol, in doses of 3000–6000 units per day. Calcium and occasionally phosphate supplements have been added to this latter group if the patient's general diet was considered unsatisfactory. Careful biochemical monitoring is essential during replacement treatment because prolonged increases in plasma calcium and phosphate may lead to extra-skeletal calcification. Overall, the results have been generally disappointing, with a significant (greater than 10 dB) hearing improvement occurring in less than 15% of cases. Yamazaki *et al.* (1988), however, treated 12 patients with suspected abnormal bone metabolism as assessed by the novel technique of microdensitometry with an alternative active vitamin D preparation (1α-[OH]D_3) for 6–10 months and noted hearing improvement in six ears (four patients).

Vitamin D resistant rickets (hypophosphataemic)

Familial hypophosphataemic vitamin D resistant rickets is the commonest form of the genetically determined osteomalacias. It is due to a reduced renal tubular reabsorption capacity for phosphate and is most frequently transmitted as an X-linked dominant condition. Sporadic cases due to a new mutation are not uncommon. Davies, Kane and Valentine (1984) described the results of their survey of 16 families with the condition and found a high incidence of sensorineural hearing loss in 25 patients. General skeletal radiographs show osteosclerosis with an increase in bone density and a coarsened trabecular pattern (Davies and Stanbury, 1981).

Otological features

The petrous temporal bones in many cases also show a generalized increase in bone density (Figure 15.22) and, in some, narrowing of the internal auditory meatus was present (Figure 15.23). Similar radiological features were reported by Stamp and Baker (1976) who described two children from a first cousin marriage. The audiological features indicated a cochlear dysfunction but did not however support the original theoretical pathogenesis of hearing impairment suggested by Stamp and Baker, which was a retrocochlear loss due to pressure on the cochleovestibular nerve bundle in the narrowed internal auditory meatus. Nearly 75% of the cases were subsequently found to have typical features of endolymphatic hydrops on transtympanic electrocochleography (O'Malley *et al.*, 1985), while two displayed classical features of Menière's syndrome.

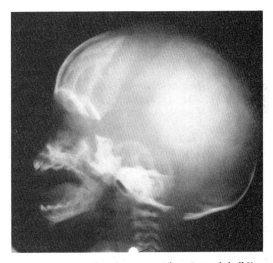

Figure 15.22 Hypophosphataemic rickets. Lateral skull X-ray showing demineralized cortical bone, but sclerotic temporal bone. (Reproduced by kind permission of the Institute of Orthopaedics and Dr D. J. Stoker)

The other main form of hypophosphataemic osteomalacia is recessive in type. Weir (1977) described two pairs of siblings who were known to suffer from this disorder. Three out of four developed some degree of sensorineural deafness, and all demonstrated the radiological finding of marked narrowing of the internal auditory meatus. In the X-linked hypophosphataemic variety, alkaline phosphatase levels return to normal on cessation of growth, but in the recessive form continued biochemical activity persists on attaining adult stature and maintenance therapy with vitamin D is necessary. Meister *et al.* (1986) conducted audiological tests in 19 subjects with hypophosphataemic bone disease. No hearing loss or significant auditory findings were noted among the children and

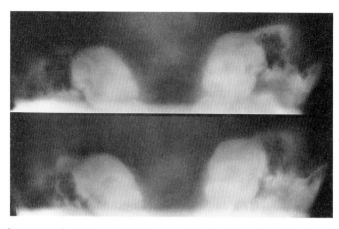

Figure 15.23 Hypophosphataemic rickets. Hypocycloidal tomography of a different case showing sclerotic bone involving the whole of the petrous pyramid with overall expansion. (Reproduced from *Journal of Laryngology and Otology*, by kind permission of the Editor and Dr G. A. S. Lloyd and Dr Peter Phelps)

young adults, and only one older patient had a cochlear loss for which an alternative cause could not be identified. They therefore concluded that auditory involvement in this condition will not develop until adulthood in treated patients.

Vitamin D intoxication

Cohen *et al.* (1979) reported a patient with pseudo-hyperparathyroidism who had continued to take calciferol 2.5 mg daily. Four years later a severe conductive hearing loss was present, and examination showed marked calcification of the tympanic membranes and cornea. Radiological investigation demonstrated extensive calcification of the kidneys and blood vessels, while the mastoids were cellular. Unfortunately the hearing loss was unchanged by treatment. One of the authors (GBB) has encountered a similar case. In 1972, a 4-year-old child, whose father was a serviceman stationed abroad, was eventually found to be suffering from a very rare growth disorder due to a primary growth hormone deficiency. The diagnosis of rickets had been made initially and calciferol treatment taken for more than 2 years. A bilateral hearing loss was present in addition to partial blindness and impaired growth. Calcification of the tympanic membranes and cornea was present, although the nature of the hearing loss could not be fully evaluated.

Osteoporosis

Most cases of osteoporosis are classified as idiopathic and typically affect the spine and long bones in the elderly. Pathologically there is a reduction in total bone mass due to loss of both the trabecular bone matrix with widening of the vascular channels and deficient mineralization. Radiologically there is rarefaction of bone, which is indistinguishable from osteomalacia. However, in this latter condition the histopathology is quite different because the bone matrix framework remains intact. Blood biochemistry is normal, although metabolic studies may show a negative nitrogen balance and evidence of calcium malabsorption.

Otological features

One of the very few accounts of the otological features associated with osteoporosis was reported by Henkin, Lifshitz and Larson (1972). They diagnosed a sensorineural deafness, significantly greater than their age related mean level, in five of seven patients with confirmed osteoporosis who presented with severe bone pain. The hearing loss commenced at the onset of symptoms of bone disease or soon after and was almost invariably bilateral and progressive. Temporal bone radiology showed increased sclerosis of the otic capsule in five cases.

The biochemistry is frequently normal and diagnosis may not be straightforward. Normal serum calcium, phosphate and alkaline phosphatase indices are also often seen in vitamin D undernutrition when clinical features of osteomalacia are also frequently absent and radiological bone changes are only found in the well established case. The association of osteoporosis and sensorineural loss clearly requires further investigation. The potential benefit of such studies for the hearing impaired population could be enormous. It is common knowledge that the body's positive calcium balance deteriorates with increasing age, particularly in postmenopausal women when plasma oestrogen levels are no longer maintained. It is quite possible therefore that this condition may well be an important contributory factor in the aetiology of presbyacusis, perhaps in association with relative vitamin D undernutrition which is also associated with increasing age. It is of great interest that the current treatment advocated for osteoporosis consists of a vitamin D metabolite, in conjunction with oestrogens in postmenopausal women. Calcium supplements are not considered necessary providing that the diet is satisfactory (Crilley *et al.*, 1981). The efficacy of such treatment on pre-existing hearing loss merits further study.

Hyperparathyroidism

This disorder may be primary, usually due to a parathyroid adenoma, or secondary, due to chronic renal disease. Occasionally it may be associated with osteomalacia. When the condition causes skeletal changes due to mobilization of phosphorus and calcium from bone, it is termed osteitis fibrosa cystica or von Recklinghausen's disease of bone. Plasma calcium levels are high and invariably diagnostic. Phosphate levels are often low, while elevation of the alkaline phosphatase, an index of osteoblastic activity, reflects bone involvement.

Otological features

The condition is only rarely encountered in otological practice. Rüedi (1968) described the temporal bone changes in two patients with osteitis fibrosa cystica, and Lindsay and Suga (1976) subsequently reported another. The histopathological features were very similar to those seen in Paget's disease. Morrison (1979) detailed the clinical features of one case; a 46-year-old man presenting with a 1-month history of a rapidly progressing hearing loss. Calcium deposits were observed beneath the tympanic membranes and a mixed hearing loss was found on pure-tone audiometry. The patient was lost to otological follow up, but terminal hypercalcinosis was subsequently diagnosed a few months later.

Acromegaly

Acromegaly is a chronic disease of middle life resulting from the action of excessive growth hormone usually caused by an eosinophil adenoma of the anterior pituitary gland. It occurs after fusion of the bony epiphyses and is characterized by enlargement of the bones, especially of the hands, feet, skull and mandible. The enlargement of bones is caused by deposition of new bone upon the surface of original cortex causing an increase in thickness but not in length. About 30% of patients develop overt diabetes mellitus.

Otological features

Richards (1968) investigated 15 patients. Five ears showed a marked conductive deafness, but otherwise the remainder developed a sensorineural loss which was substantially greater than in the 'normal' population, with the general tendency for the hearing loss to deteriorate with age. There was no relationship with the duration of the disease or the plasma growth hormone levels and hearing loss. Subsequently Doig and Gatehouse (1984) assessed the hearing in 56 patients with acromegaly requiring pituitary surgery and compared them with matched controls. They were unable to find any significant difference in hearing levels between the two groups nor any correlation with diabetes, growth hormone levels, blood pressure or other factors. In addition, no change in the hearing occurred after surgery to remove the tumour. In this series, three ears of the acromegalics showed evidence of otosclerosis compared with one in the control group.

Three cases of acromegaly with temporal bone involvement were reported by Graham and Brackman (1978). Radiology demonstrated massive thickening of the mastoid cortex and posterior bony canal wall with secondary lengthening of the bony external meatus. Some overgrowth diminishing the lumen also occurred. However, the internal auditory meatus, cochlea and vestibule appeared normal and the structure of the otic capsule including the facial nerve, remained in normal relationship.

Infective and granulomatous diseases
Syphilis

The effects of syphilis on the temporal bone are now seen very much less frequently in clinical practice. It is a disease which should, nonetheless, be suspected in any patient presenting with tinnitus and/or vertigo and/or sensorineural hearing impairment, particularly if fluctuant and of sudden onset. Prompt recognition and treatment may halt or possibly reverse the progressive audiovestibular symptoms, and prevent the development of serious systemic involvement in the tertiary stage, if this is not already present. These serious systemic features include cardiac and aortic involvement and parenchymatous neurosyphilis, manifested by general paralysis of the insane and tabes dorsalis. Both the congenital and acquired forms of syphilis can be complicated by inner ear disease.

The last half century has witnessed a dramatic decline in the number of reported new cases. Thus the incidence of new cases of congenital disease in the UK fell from 2439 in 1931 to 1223 cases in 1950 and 150 in 1974. In 1980, only eight new cases were diagnosed in children under 2 years of age (British Medical Journal, 1982). The universal antenatal serological screening programme in the UK has undoubtedly played an important part in the control of congenital syphilis; an untreated syphilitic mother has about a 50% chance of bearing a syphilitic child. Failure to eliminate this form of the disease altogether is probably due to the difficulty in administering antenatal care to some social groups. During the same period, the overall reported incidence of new cases of both congenital and acquired types fell from the post-war peak of nearly 28 000 cases per year to about 4500 cases in 1980. The prevalence in 1984 was 6.4 cases per 100 000 (British Medical Journal, 1986), but is now even lower due to the impact of AIDS on contemporary sexual practices. Currently well over 50% of syphilitic infections in men are reported to have been homosexually acquired. The male:female incidence is now about 4:1 and new cases of acquired syphilis are about 25 times more frequent than congenital ones.

Diagnosis

Of the established screening tests for syphilis, the Venereal Disease Research Laboratory (VDRL) slide test is probably still the one most commonly undertaken in clinical practice. Although the test is frequently negative in previously treated cases, and false positives may occur, it does give an indication of disease activity. It is invariably strongly positive in high dilution in early untreated cases and is usually accompanied by an elevated erythrocyte sedimentation rate.

More specific serological tests are now routinely employed, e.g. *Treponema pallidum* haemagglutination test (TPHA); *Treponema pallidum* immobilization test (TPI) and the fluorescent treponemal antibody absorption test (FTA-ABS). Of these the FTA-ABS is the most sensitive (Hughes and Rutherford, 1986). A positive result confirms previous syphilitic infection but does not reflect disease activity and stays positive even following adequate treatment. It is currently common practice to diagnose otosyphilis in any patient with inner ear symptoms of unknown cause and a positive FTA-ABS test result. However, a recent survey by Hoare *et al.* (1996) reported the results of a prospective study of syphilis serology in nearly 1800 new otolaryngological outpatients; 40 (2.2%) were positive. None had congenital or neurosyphilis, and as many had non-otological symptoms unrelated to their serological status as had cochleovestibular symptoms. Hughes and Rutherford (1986) have also highlighted the clinical dilemma caused by limitations in the predictive value of the serological tests for syphilis. A solution has recently been proposed by Birdsall, Baughn and Jenkins (1990), who advocated a new Western blot assay to eliminate the possibility of a false-positive result and to confirm whether the disease is active.

Examination of the cerebrospinal fluid in patients with syphilitic ear disease is desirable to look for possible evidence of central nervous system involvement which is more likely to be seen in the late acquired form. Typical cerebrospinal fluid abnormalities of neurosyphilis, apart from positive serological tests, include slightly raised globulin and IgG levels and a lymphocytosis. Such investigations and treatment are best coordinated by a venereologist, who will also need to examine possible contacts in cases of acquired syphilis. Gleich, Linstrom and Kimmelman (1992) found that the otovestibular symptoms of patients with syphilis and cerebrospinal fluid abnormalities invariably improved with high dose penicillin and steroid treatment.

General features

Congenital syphilis may be associated with other abnormalities outside the cochleovestibular systems. The ocular manifestations of interstitial keratitis and choroidoretinitis result in corneal opacity in about 90% of patients with otological symptoms. Such features may only be apparent on careful slit-lamp examination by an ophthalmologist but can be of diagnostic value. Hutchinsonian thickened wedge-shaped incisors which are occasionally notched are found in 20% of cases (Figure 15.24). The typical facies of frontal bossing of the skull due to periostitis of the cranial bones and saddle nose due to involvement and collapse of the nasal septal cartilage and bone are only present in about 10% of cases (Figure 15.25) (Morrison, 1975; Belal and Linthicum, 1980). Other features such as 'sabre tibia' are rare.

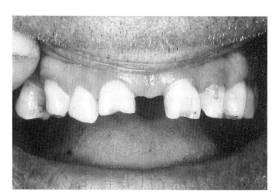

Figure 15.24 Congenital syphilis. Hutchinsonian teeth

Tabes dorsalis and general paralysis of the insane are manifestations of neurosyphilis and both are now rare. The neurological features include 'lightning' pains, early optic atrophy, Argyll Robertson pupils, bladder dysfunction and sensory loss from dorsal column involvement resulting in impaired vibration sense and joint disruption – Charcot's joints (Catterall, 1977). However, previous treatment which may have been inadequate often results in atypical features.

In late congenital and acquired disease, the main lesion is a rarefying gummatous osteitis of the temporal bone with secondary involvement of the membranous labyrinth (Mayer and Fraser, 1936; Goodhill, 1939; Schuknecht, 1974). All three layers of the otic capsule are involved in the osteitis, which is associated with underlying endarteritis and infiltration with chronic inflammatory cells and multinucleated giant cells (Figure 15.26). The inner ear features are dominated by endolymphatic hydrops and progressive degeneration of the neuroepithelial structures, particularly the cochlear neurons and organ of Corti, which may be severe (Figure 15.27; see also Figures 4.25 and 4.26).

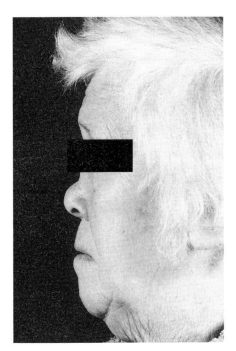

Figure 15.25 Congenital syphilis. Saddle nose and frontal bossing

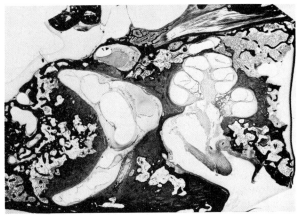

Figure 15.26 Late syphilitic osteitis. Horizontal section of left temporal bone of a 70-year-old woman with congenital syphilis and sensorineural deafness. There is erosion of all three layers of the otic capsule, and a gumma adjacent to the posterior semicircular canal. Severe hydrops of the cochlear and vestibular labyrinths is also seen. In the basal coil of the cochlea there is degeneration of the organ of Corti, atrophy of the stria vascularis and loss of the spiral ganglion. (Reproduced by kind permission of Professor H. F. Schuknecht)

A not infrequent clinical dilemma is posed by patients from the West Indies, Central America and Africa, who may display positive serological test results and similar clinical manifestations but who are suffering from yaws. This disorder is caused by a different spirochaete, *Treponema pertenue*, and typically is spread by direct contact among children. Old scarring from previously healed cutaneous ulcers is characteristically present on the lower legs. When these scars are absent, a patient from these countries should certainly be considered to be suffering from syphilis and treated accordingly.

Otological features

Histopathology

Two distinct types of histopathology are recognized. Treponemal labyrinthitis is the typical lesion in early congenital syphilis, and meningolabyrinthitis in the acute meningovascular phase of secondary and tertiary disease. In this latter form, the small blood vessels of the meninges show endarteritis obliterans. There is increased fibrosis of the meninges, with small areas of necrosis and a diffuse infiltration by plasma cells and lymphocytes. The VIIIth nerve may be involved in association with the infective basal meningitis, and the inflammatory process spreads from the spiral ganglion to the cochlear duct and membranous labyrinth (Goodhill, 1939).

It has long been held that the pathogenesis of the hydrops is probably by direct involvement of the endolymphatic duct which becomes obliterated. However, treponemal spirochaetes have been found in many different sites in humans with late syphilis following treatment, including the aqueous humour of the eye, cerebrospinal fluid, synovial fluid, temporal artery, lymph nodes and liver (Smith and Israel, 1967; Mack *et al.*, 1969). This continued presence of spirochaetes, in spite of apparently adequate previous antibiotic treatment, may well be a significant factor in the pathogenesis of the hearing loss (see below: Immunology and the temporal bone).

Early syphilis

Congenital syphilis is contracted by the developing fetus *in utero* as a consequence of acquired maternal

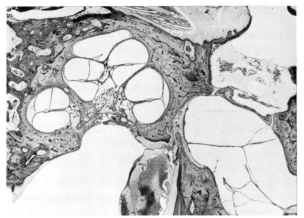

Figure 15.27 Late syphilitic osteitis. Horizontal section of the right temporal bone of a 43-year-old man with a 30-year history of progressive deafness. There is marked hydrops with degeneration of the organ of Corti, stria vascularis and cochlear neurons. (Reproduced by kind permission of Professor H. F. Schuknecht)

syphilis. The early infantile form is usually fatal due to multisystem involvement which dominates the features of otolabyrinthitis. As noted above, it is now exceedingly rare in the UK. Probably about 50% of cases develop bilateral hearing loss eventually. Earlier studies, e.g. Karmody and Schuknecht (1966) tended to underestimate the incidence because of the proportion of younger individuals who could be expected to develop symptoms later on.

Secondary syphilis is typically, although not exclusively, seen in adult homosexual men. The first symptoms last for a few weeks and include malaise, slight pyrexia, non-specific headaches, skin eruptions, pharyngitis and lymphadenopathy. They are relatively trivial and are hence frequently ignored by the patient until sudden hearing loss develops which is often bilateral. There may be some transient vestibular symptoms, which are frequently positional in character, and tinnitus. Ocular palsies and facial paralysis may occur as well in the acute meningovascular type of secondary disease. The sensorineural hearing loss preferentially affects the high frequencies; elevated stapedius reflex thresholds, possibly with reflex decay, are frequently present. Speech discrimination is often significantly worse than is suggested by pure-tone audiometry and the caloric responses are reduced. Increased latency and/or reduced wave V amplitude on brain stem evoked audiometry has been reported (Rosenhall, Löwhagen and Roupe, 1984). These audiovestibular symptoms may be partly reversible. If left untreated, the infection tends to run a benign course but the hearing loss remains.

Late syphilis

Late syphilis affects the temporal bone between 10 and 50 years after the primary infection. Once established, the untreated disease carries a poor prognosis with relentless progression to profound deafness, although fluctuations are common. There are some grounds, however, for optimism with antitreponemal agents and systemic steroids.

In general, the clinical features are similar in both the congenital and acquired forms of the disease, although the former is more common in women. It is often difficult to assign a patient to one of these groups, particularly since previous antibiotics have invariably been taken. The otological features in congenital cases can occur at any stage, but they are uncommon after middle age. In contrast, patients with late acquired disease are usually over 40 years of age. The hearing loss is typically symmetrical in congenital cases but more frequently unilateral in the acquired group, sometimes for many years. In about 20% the onset of aural symptoms is sudden and fluctuations are seen in 30%, particularly in the early stages (Hahn, Rosin and Haskins, 1962; Dawkins, Sharp and Morrison, 1968; Kerr, Smyth and Cinnamond, 1973). Apart from the fluctuation, there are other features which closely mirror the symptoms of Menière's disease and are a reflection of the underlying endolymphatic hydrops (Schuknecht, 1974). The early hearing loss is sensory in character with predominantly low or peaked patterns of pure-tone audiometry. Half the patients exhibit episodic attacks of vertigo which may be indistinguishable from those occurring in classical Menière's disease.

The results of transtympanic electrocochleography in a series of 18 cases of late syphilitic deafness have been described by Ramsden, Moffat and Gibson (1977). An enhanced negative summating potential was found in nearly 80% of ears tested in association with a small cochlear microphonic, both features indicating established endolymphatic hydrops. The summating potential characteristically affected the descending limb of the compound action potential. This feature, however, is not pathognomonic and in the authors' experience occurs relatively infrequently. Nagasaki *et al.* (1993) also found evidence of established hydrops on electrocochleography in a large proportion (56%) of patients with syphilitic labyrinthitis. Syphilitic hydrops tends to remain relentlessly active in the majority of cases, in contrast to idiopathic Menière's disease where only a relatively small proportion of patients have hydropic symptoms which are not self-limiting to some degree. Secondary neuronal degeneration associated with more profound degrees of hearing loss is therefore more frequent. The pattern of pure tone audiometry now becomes flattened or high tone in character. Alteration of the stapedius reflex to a retrocochlear pattern with elevated thresholds and decay is now evident in association with a relative greater impairment of speech discrimination.

Progressively severe peripheral vestibular damage leading to increasing imbalance and ataxia is also quite common. However, compensation for such a slowly developing deficit can significantly reduce the degree of disability, particularly in the younger patient, and may only come to light on formal vestibular assessment.

Two eponymous otological phenomena which are sometimes present in late congenital syphilitics are worthy of mention. Hennebert's (1911) sign consists of a transient positive fistula test without clinical evidence of middle ear disease (see Figure 5.3). Tullio's sign consists of transient vertigo and nystagmus following exposure to sudden high intensity sound. These phenomena are believed to be due to sound energy transmission through the stapes footplate on to the distended saccule, and are occasionally seen in other diseases associated with endolymphatic hydrops.

Treatment

Penicillin is still the most effective antibiotic for the treatment of syphilis. Its main bactericidal effect occurs when the organisms are dividing. This has been shown to take place much less rapidly in the late form of the disease, and hence the duration of treatment is as important as the maintenance of effective serum concentrations. In the presence of confirmed allergy, one of the cephalosporins is probably the second drug of choice.

The proven effective therapeutic regimen consists of 600 000 units of procaine penicillin by intramuscular injection daily for 21 days. This aqueous solution only has to be injected once a day and results in an effective serum level for 24 hours (Catterall, 1977). Oral probenecid 500 mg 6-hourly inhibits excretion of the drug and helps to raise tissue levels. This regimen has proved satisfactory for outpatient treatment (Dunlop, Al-Egaily and Houang, 1981). An alternative protocol which is probably as effective in patients who show good treatment compliance is high-dose ampicillin. A dosage of 1.5 g is prescribed four times daily for 4 weeks (Adams *et al.*, 1983). Unfortunately, there is no evidence that penicillin treatment alone prevents the progression of cochleovestibular manifestations.

There is now, however, considerable clinical evidence that systemic steroids alone can improve the hearing at least temporarily, in up to 50% of cases with late syphilitic deafness (Hahn, Rosin and Haskins, 1962; Karmody and Schuknecht, 1966; Morrison, 1969; Kerr, Smyth and Cinnamond, 1973) and suggests an immunological basis for at least part of the hearing loss. Steroids are also indicated to prevent the adverse effects of a possible Herxheimer reaction. This is a systemic phenomenon occurring within 2–12 hours of the first antitreponemal injection and is characterized by fever, followed by headache, malaise, flushing and sweating. The reaction lasts for a few hours and is often accompanied by worsening local tissue involvement and has been known to cause sudden increased hearing impairment. The reaction has been attributed to complement activation and to complex immunological reactions involving a hypersensitivity response to the disintegration products resulting from sudden destruction of large numbers of spirochaetes (Catterall, 1977).

Prednisolone 30 mg 8-hourly is therefore commenced prior to institution of antitreponemal treatment and continued for 4 weeks. Others have preferred to use ACTH (Kerr, Smyth and Cinnamond, 1973; Adams *et al.*, 1983). If there is no evidence of improvement in the auditory and vestibular symptoms by 6 weeks, it is discontinued. Improved hearing thresholds are more likely in patients with fluctuant symptoms and are an indication for longer term treatment on a maintenance dose of 2.5–5 mg daily. Unfortunately, any hearing gains often relapse on withdrawal of steroids which may well therefore need to be taken on a long-term basis to maintain improvement. Of course, prolonged steroid treatment has well recognized side-effects and the decisions to maintain steroids must be weighed carefully in each individual case. Discontinuation of steroids should be followed by a further course of antibiotics. Initial optimism about the successful outcome of treatment of late syphilis with penicillin and steroids has been tempered in recent years, although long-term results show that this regimen frequently prevents further hearing impairment and almost invariably preserves some hearing (Adams *et al.*, 1983; Chan, Adams, and Kerr, 1995).

Tuberculosis

Increasing numbers of patients with tuberculosis are currently presenting to various specialist departments in the UK, most often from among immigrant communities. Unfortunately it can no longer be considered a disease of the past. Although the infection primarily affects the middle ear, it may cause secondary involvement of the bony labyrinth.

Otological features

The possibility of tuberculous involvement is usually entertained by the presence of certain atypical features of chronic suppurative middle ear disease. Windle-Taylor and Bailey (1980) comprehensively reviewed a series of 22 patients with tuberculous ear disease who presented to The Royal National Throat, Nose and Ear Hospital, London, over a 30-year period and found one half to be under 20 years of age. None had a past history of pulmonary tuberculosis, although 18% had previously diagnosed disease at other sites. The middle ear features are dominated by the presence of florid, pale granulation tissue, which is often visible as a 'mass' behind the tympanic membrane (Figure 15.28). Occasionally, as in other granulomatous disorders, the tympanic membrane may be intact, but more often breakdown has occurred, characteristically resulting in multiple perforations. Coexistent secondary infection by other organisms is frequently found. Yaniv, Traub and Conradie (1986) subsequently reviewed a series of 24 cases of otological tuberculosis and reported similar findings.

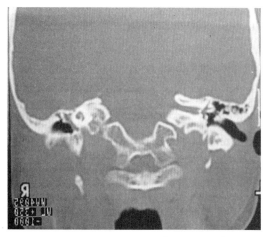

Figure 15.28 Tuberculosis otitis media. CT scan showing florid granulation tissue filling medial mesotympanum

Concomitant sensorineural hearing loss is encountered much more frequently than in 'conventional' chronic suppurative otitis media, and often results in a disproportionately large hearing loss. Windle-Taylor and Bailey (1980) did not detail the precise sensorineural hearing loss, but their data indicated that 60% had inner ear involvement, and in 25% this loss was total.

Treatment

Management obviously involves surgical excision and drainage of middle ear and mastoid disease in conjunction with antituberculous treatment. As in patients with syphilis, referral to a physician for general assessment, coordination of medical treatment and tracing of possible infective contacts is mandatory. Although there have been isolated reports of ototoxicity by rifampicin and ethambutol the risk is very considerably lower than following streptomycin therapy, which has therefore been largely discontinued. After the infection has been controlled by chemotherapy, any residual tympanic membrane defects can be managed successfully by conventional tympanoplastic surgical techniques (Ma, Tang and Chan, 1990).

Sarcoidosis

Sarcoidosis is a rare systemic granulomatous disease of unknown aetiology. Head and neck manifestations are uncommon and, when encountered in otolaryngological practice, the disease usually involves the parotid gland, facial nerve, nasal cavity and larynx. The nervous system is affected in only 5% of cases, although this rises to 50% if uveoparotid fever is present. The central nervous system lesion is presumed to be a granulomatous meningitis that directly infiltrates the cranial nerves or causes them to be compressed from involvement of adjacent intracranial structures. Any of the cranial nerves may be affected but the facial nerve is most frequently involved (see Chapter 24) while the VIIIth cranial nerve is fourth in order (Hybels and Rice, 1976). The disease has a higher prevalence among Blacks and Puerto Ricans in America.

The organs most frequently affected are the lymph nodes, lung, liver, spleen, skin and eyes, but any tissue may be involved and certain manifestations are known to be associated with particular HLA types. The course of the disease is usually chronic with minimal constitutional upset.

Serum angiotensin-converting enzyme (ACE) levels are raised in nearly two-thirds of cases of active sarcoidosis, but false positive elevation of this enzyme can occur. False positives, however, are extremely rare in the Kveim test. De Remee and Rohrbach (1980) noted that serum angiotensin-converting enzyme levels closely paralleled and occasionally antedated changes in clinical status in patients either undergoing spontaneous remission or being treated with steroids and suggested that enzyme determination should be of value in management. However, serum angiotensin-converting enzyme levels may also be raised in other conditions, such as Gaucher's disease and leprosy.

All patients with the disease should have assessment of their liver and renal function. The alkaline phosphatase is frequently raised and may be due to involvement of either liver or bone. Approximately 5–10% of patients with sarcoidosis have elevation of their serum calcium and this is thought to be due to hypersensitivity to vitamin D. There is hypoglobulinaemia in about 25% and this may also reflect disease activity. Electrophoresis of the serum proteins usually shows increased α-2 and γ globulins. The full blood count is frequently normal but the erythrocyte sedimentation rate may be raised in the active stages. It is a characteristic feature of sarcoidosis that infiltration of old scars often occurs and these may provide welcome biopsy material.

Otological features

Sarcoidosis involving the ear may be associated with other signs such as uveitis (80%), parotid swelling

(20%), facial nerve palsy (43%) and lymphadenopathy (55%). However, 40% of cases have shown no other neurological involvement, and isolated VIIIth nerve disease has also been reported (Souliere *et al.,* 1991).

The hearing loss may be sudden, fluctuating or progressive and the degree may vary from slight to severe to even total loss. It is usually bilateral although one side is frequently more affected than the other. Pure tone audiometry may show either a high or low frequency loss while caloric testing usually shows reduced or absent responses (Gristwood, 1958; Hooper and Holden, 1970; Kane, 1976). The pathogenesis of the hearing impairment is undecided. From the 50 or so recorded cases it would appear that the hearing loss is most probably sensorineural, but electrocochleography in two cases suggested the lesion may be retrocochlear with normal hair cell function (Majumdar and Crowther, 1983). One of the cases reported by Souliere *et al.* (1991) had a cerebellopontine angle granuloma that mimicked a vestibular schwannoma.

The temporal bones from a 32-year-old man, deaf for 5 years from central nervous system sarcoidosis, have been examined histologically (Babin, Liu and Ashenbrener, 1984). It was found that the acoustic, vestibular and facial nerves were involved in a striking perivascular lymphocytic infiltration resulting in myelin and axonal degeneration. The cochlear and labyrinthine neuroepithelium and stria vascularis had degenerated. Babin, Liu and Ashenbrener hypothesized that sensorineural deafness and vestibular dysfunction in sarcoidosis start as a reversible neuropathy; in some patients an ischaemia secondary to the vasculitis results in irreversible damage to the inner ear neuroepithelium.

Steroids remain the mainstay of treatment but their effectiveness is not assured, especially in those with a profound or total hearing loss. More recently immunosuppressive drugs have been used though because of the few cases treated their efficacy is as yet unproven.

Histiocytosis X

Histiocytosis X is a rare condition which is of clinical importance to the otolaryngologist because of the high incidence of head and neck involvement. Two recent large series reported head and neck lesions in 82% (DiNardo and Wetmore, 1989) and 73% (Irving, Broadbent and Jones, 1994) of cases.

Eosinophilic granuloma, Hand-Schüller-Christian disease and Letterer-Siwe disease were initially thought to be distinct clinical conditions. Major differences in the severity and prognosis of the disorders (see also Chapters 10 and 23) only served to reinforce the belief that they were separate entities. They are, however, now regarded as different parts of the same disease spectrum. Lichtenstein (1953) showed that the underlying pathological lesions were similar, and consisted of an inflammatory reticuloendotheliosis. He recognized all three as being of histiocyte origin, and suggested the term histiocytosis X, as the aetiology was unknown.

The condition is characterized by an accumulation of abnormal, though cytologically benign, histiocytes, together with lymphocytes and eosinophils, in various organs which normally contain elements of the reticuloendothelial system. These organs include the lung, skin, bone marrow, lymph nodes, thymus, liver, spleen and central nervous system. The Langerhans' cell, which is normally only only found in the dermis of the skin, has been identified as the characteristic cell. The contemporary term 'Langerhans' cell histiocytosis' is therefore now gaining widespread acceptance.

Langerhans' cells are characterized by the presence of pentilaminar cytoplasmic inclusion bodies seen on electron microscopy and called Birbeck granules. These are not always readily apparent, and immunohistochemical analysis may be necessary to confirm the diagnosis. The pathogenesis is most likely an underlying abnormality of immune regulation via lymphokines or other growth factors leading to faulty Langerhans' cell growth maturation and migration (Rabkin *et al.*, 1987).

The mildest form of histiocytosis X, which equates to the condition formerly known as eosinophilic granuloma, occurs typically in children and young adults, and there is a male predominance. It usually appears as a solitary osteolytic lesion in the long bones, skull including the temporal bone, ribs or vertebrae. The features of 19 cases recorded over a period of nearly 40 years at the Armed Forces Institute of Pathology Registry, Washington, DC, have been reviewed by Sweet, Kornblut and Hyams (1979). Although the tumour-like disorder is usually initially asymptomatic, growth progression in the temporal bone eventually may produce erosion of the mastoid cortex, tegmen, tympanic or sigmoid plates, and the bony labyrinth, leading to pain and local tenderness. Histopathology demonstrates sheets of benign histiocytes and scattered collections of small eosinophils. There may be areas of haemorrhage and necrosis with giant cells (Schuknecht, 1974). Treatment is by local curettage and steroids, and is invariably curative.

In its more severe form, which equates to the condition formerly termed Hand-Schüller-Christian disease, multiple lesions are present at diagnosis or develop within a few months. The onset is typically in childhood before 5 years of age, but has been reported in young adults. Skull lesions are quite common and may involve the temporal bone sometimes before other features are apparent (Tos, 1966). Destruction of the temporal bone may be asociated with secondary infection and otorrhoea. Lesions may occur in the scapulae, ribs and long bones, while infiltration may result in hepatosplenomegaly and lymphadenopathy. Systemic manifestations include pyrexia, anorexia, and recurrent upper respiratory tract infections. Perihylar infiltration may be evident on chest X-ray examination. This form is progressive and can be fatal in the young, although spontaneous regression may occur.

In the large series reported by Irving, Broadbent and Jones (1994), temporal bone lesions were found in 19% of children with histiocytosis X, and manifested as mastoid swelling, aural polyps or otorrhoea. The tympanic membrane and ossicles were frequently unaffected, which aids differentiation from infective mastoiditis. Sensorineural hearing loss was seen in 12%, due to otic capsule involvement which has been described previously (McCaffrey and McDonald, 1979; DeMarino *et al.*, 1985; Cunningham *et al.*, 1989) or as a result of surgical trauma. Middle ear surgery may predispose to inner ear involvement (Klimmelman, Nielsen and Snow, 1984), but in general the otic capsule is resistant to invasion by the disease. This group found that a conservative approach to treatment consisting mainly of local aural polypectomy with systemic steroids resulted in a more satisfactory outcome than their former policy of mastoidectomy with steroids ± radiotherapy.

In addition, 24% of children presented with involvement of the skin of the external auditory meatus, excluding those with underlying temporal bone disease. Widespread systemic disease was often associated, though most responded well to systemic treatment alone. This group has successfully used a 20% solution of mustine to treat otitis externa which is resistant to local steroid drops, provided the tympanic membrane is intact. They also recommended intralesional steroids (Depomedrone 40 mg) following local excision of aural polyps or bone curettage.

Autoimmune inner ear disease

The impact of immunological processes in inner ear disturbances has only become apparent relatively recently. Although there is already an abundance of contemporary experimental and clinical evidence demonstrating the many diverse ways in which these processes may affect cochleovestibular function, many fundamental questions remain unanswered. The umbrella term autoimmune inner ear disease has perhaps rather loosely been applied to all such disorders.

The concept was first postulated by Lehnhardt in 1958, on the basis of clinical observation in cases of recurrent bilateral sudden sensorineural hearing loss. McCabe, however, was the first to bring autoimmune inner ear disease to the attention of otologists in 1979. It is now becoming generally accepted as an uncommon, quite well defined, but poorly understood

entity. The term may well embrace several different clinical syndromes, which could explain why both cell-mediated and humoral-mediated pathways appear to be involved in the pathogenesis. It may occur as a primary autoimmune disorder confined to the inner ear, or may appear as an occasional local manifestation of a major systemic disease due to an underlying immune system defect (Tables 15.3 and 15.4).

Table 15.3 Otological 'immune' disorders

1 External ear
   a relapsing polychondritis
   b necrotizing external otitis
2 Tympanic membrane and middle ear
   a homograft tympanoplasty
   b tympanosclerosis
   c otosclerosis
   d chronic otitis media with effusion
   e chronic suppurative otitis media with cholesteatoma
3 'Autoimmune' inner ear disease
   a localized
   b systemic

(After Veldman *et al.*, 1984)

Table 15.4 Systemic 'immune' diseases which may develop otological involvement

1 Systemic lupus erythematosus
2 Vasculitis
   a hypersensitivity vasculitis
   b polyarteritis nodosa
   c Wegener's granulomatosis
   d temporal arteritis
   e Cogan's syndrome
   f Behçet's disease
3 Relapsing polychondritis
4 Polymyositis and dermatomyositis
5 Immunodeficiency diseases
   a T-cell deficiency
   b B-cell deficiency
   c disorders of phagocytosis
   d complement system disorders

(After Hughes, Barna and Calabrese, 1986)

Inner ear immunology

There is now substantial evidence that the inner ear possesses its own functioning host immune defence system. Lim and Silver first suggested in 1974 that the endolymphatic sac might be primarily involved in these processes on the basis of light and electron microscopic investigations. Subsequently Rask-Anderson and Stahle (1980) demonstrated interaction between macrophages and lymphocytes within the endolymphatic sac lumen, and also described the presence of a rich network of lymphatic capillaries and venules surrounding the sac and duct in guinea-pigs. They concluded from these studies that the endolymphatic sac could well be the main site in the inner ear for antigen processing activity, and could best be considered as analagous to a functioning lymph node. The hypothesis of an inner ear immune defence system primarily located in the endolymphatic sac was further supported by Arnold, Altermatt and Gebbers (1984), who observed free and tissue bound IgA and IgG immunoglobulins restricted to the endolymphatic sac region in human ears.

A number of animal studies have enabled models of the immunopathological effects on the inner ear to be documented. Beickert (1961) immunized guinea-pigs to inner ear antigen and produced lesions in the cochlea. Soon after, Terrayama and Sasaki (1968) replicated these results in a similar study, though they were unable to confirm the presence of anticochlear antibodies or inflammatory infiltration around local blood vessels due to technical limitations at this time. Yoo *et al.* (1983a,b) reported the induction of sensorineural hearing loss and endolymphatic hydrops in rats and guinea-pigs by stimulating autoimmunity to inner ear collagen. After sensitization with type II collagen, a booster dose was given before sacrifice. Histological examination showed ganglion cell degeneration, angiopathy, degeneration of the organ of Corti as well as hydrops. Pathological changes in the endolymphatic sac were not seen, and further immunohistochemical studies showed that type II collagen was localized in the endolymphatic duct. Two further groups have conducted similar studies, but were unable to replicate these findings. Soliman (1990) only found immunoglobulin deposition in the basilar membrane, perivascular region, as well as in other inner ear tissue, while Herdman *et al.* (1993) could not demonstrate functional hearing loss following systemic challenge with type II collagen. The cause of these discrepancies is uncertain.

Harris and Tomiyama (1987) described an animal model of autoimmune inner ear dysfunction following exposure to heterologous cochlear tissue. Guinea-pigs already previously immunized with fresh bovine cochlear antigen developed significant hearing impairment after further antigen administration compared to a control group. Anticochlear antibodies were detected in all animals in the experimental group, while one-third of the 38 ears tested had a marked hearing loss. Some animals only displayed unilateral changes, whereas others had varying degrees of bilateral inner ear damage. The authors pointed out the similarity of their findings with the clinical features of the syndrome of autoimmune sensorineural hearing loss in humans as described by McCabe (1981).

Harris (1983, 1984) conducted critically important studies which established how the normal inner ear immune defence mechanisms operated. He demonstrated that the inner ear reacted to antigenic challenge by mounting both a primary and secondary immune response. Thus direct sensitization of the perilymphatic compartment with antigen in non-sensitized guinea-pigs resulted in a low local perilymph antibody production and systemic immune response. However, when the animals had been initially immunized systemically, the introduction of a specific antigen into perilymph produced a very substantial increase in perilymph antibodies, which had declined towards pre-immunization values several weeks later.

In the secondary immune response, inner ear challenge with antigen in previously sensitized animals resulted in a significant increase in perilymph antibody levels after 2 weeks, whereas antibody titres in the non-immunized ear and CSF did not change. Further experiments showed that these phenomena were due to a local inner ear response and not due to increased vascular permeability or to a CSF antibody response. A limited infiltration of plasma cells and lymphocytes under the basilar membrane of the basal turn of the cochlea was invariably present histologically in animals exhibiting a primary inner ear immune response, though both sensory and neural elements of the membranous labyrinth were preserved. Subsequently Tomiyama and Harris (1986) confirmed that an intact endolymphatic sac was a prerequisite for these responses. They showed that experimental destruction of the endolymphatic duct resulted in a reduced perilymph antibody response to antigen challenge.

The secondary inner ear immune response following antigenic challenge of presensitized animals is an amplification of the primary responses. Histologically an even greater infiltration of plasma cells and lymphocytes occurred throughout the cochlea, endolymphatic sac lumen and perisaccular tissues. Perivascular cuffing was widespread and involved the posterior spiral modiolar veins. Woolf and Harris (1986) conducted electrophysiological auditory measurements in these animals and showed a progressive reduction in cochlear function. These various results have affirmed the central role which the endolymphatic sac plays in antigen processing and immune stimulation within the inner ear in addition to its absorptive function. The inner ear undoubtedly fulfils a protective role by neutralizing infective organisms within the cochlea, though secondary immune responses, as elsewhere, can have a marked deleterious effect.

Pathophysiology

Several specific types of immune response are currently recognized, and any of these may individually or in combination contribute to the development of autoimmune inner ear disease and cause adverse effects on inner ear function. The most useful classification of tissue-damaging hypersensitivity reactions between antigen and antibody is still that devised by Gell and Coombs (1968). They distinguished three types of initiating mechanisms involving humoral antibodies and a further type involving cell-mediated antibodies associated with delayed hypersensitivity reactions.

Type I

The type I reaction (anaphylactic) occurs as a result of free antigen interacting with cell-bound antibody in the tissues. Enzyme activation quickly causes the release of vasoactive substances from mast cells or basophils which increase capillary permeability, alter vascular tone and stimulate smooth muscle contraction. Many allergic reactions take place locally where the antibody is bound and do not necessarily induce a generalized anaphylactic response. Allergies, particularly associated with foods or chemicals, are believed to cause cochleovestibular disturbances (Boyles, 1984). Eliminating the offending antigen from the diet in conjunction with appropriate anti-allergic drug therapy may reverse a long-standing sensorineural loss (Clemis, 1974; Shambaugh, 1981). The authors have managed a few patients with Menière's syndrome and intolerance to dairy products in whom dietary management proved efficacious, but generally allergies do not appear to have a major impact in the pathogenesis of inner ear disorders.

Type II

This cytotoxic reaction occurs when free circulating antibody interacts with fixed antigen which already forms part of a cell surface or tissue membrane. Invariably this results in membrane change and, in the case of a cell, lysis and cell death. These processes involve complement fixation and activation. Immunofluorescent studies conducted by Arnold and Gebbers (1984) suggested that this mechanism is important in a number of immune-mediated inner ear disorders, on occasions in combination with delayed cell-mediated activity.

Type III

When both antigen and antibody are freely circulating, the resulting circulating immune complexes are still on occasions able to provoke a tissue response. Immune complexes are usually rapidly and harmlessly removed from the circulation by the phagocytic cells of the reticuloendothelial system. They can, however, become harmful if they are deposited in body tissues when complement activation enhances local inflammatory processes and cell damage. Immune complex reactions may be related to autoimmunity, or may also occur in response to exogenous antigens such as microorganisms and drugs.

Recognized clinical disorders relevant to otology which are probably mediated by immune complexes include systemic lupus erythematosus, polymyositis, and the various vasculitides. These are considered later.

The tissues involved depend on the size and specificity of the complexes. Biologically active complexes are of intermediate size and are poorly cleared from the circulation. They may become arrested on the endothelial lining of small blood vessels or in other tissues. There are specific receptors in some sites for the immune complexes or their breakdown products, and hence certain tissues may become preferentially involved to cause isolated organ or system disorders. Immune complex and complement activation in a vessel wall leads to a local inflammatory reaction, increased vascular permeability and permanent vessel damage. The stria vascularis vessels may be a possible location for immune complex deposition (Harada *et al.*, 1992), while the capillaries of the endolymphatic sac are another (Figure 15.29). The cochlear capillaries are non-fenestrated (Juhn and Rybar, 1981) and differ from the capillaries of the endolymphatic sac which are fenestrated (Lundquist, 1976) and arise from the external carotid system. The endolymphatic sac capillaries almost certainly have a filtration function and interference by antigen–antibody complexes may lead to inner ear fluid imbalance and secondary hydrops.

Syphilis is one specific disease in which the associated cochleovestibular features are believed to have an immunological basis, most probably due to immune complex deposition. Free circulating immune complexes have been identified in the serum of humans (Sølling *et al.*, 1978; Engel and Diezel, 1980) and animals (Baughn, Tung and Musher, 1980). Engel and Diezel (1980) found elevated circulating immune complexes in 41% of a series of 51 patients with early syphilis, and were able to prove that complexed antibodies were specifically anti-treponemal. Moreover, the complexes only decreased to levels within the normal range in about half of the cases following treatment. This indicates the persistence of viable organisms after treatment, and corroborates earlier reports of residual spirochaetes in various sites such as lymph nodes, aqueous humour and cerebrospinal fluid (Collart, Borel and Durel, 1964; Smith and Israel, 1967; Dunlop, King and Wilkinson, 1969; Mack *et al.*, 1969). One of the authors has suggested previously (Brookes, 1985b) that a persisting low-grade syphilitic infection causing continuous antigenic stimulation, may lead to continuous and excessive circulating immune complex production with secondary pathological changes including inner ear involvement.

The precise role of immune complexes in the pathogenesis of sensorineural hearing loss remains to be defined. The association was reported by Kanzaki and Ouchi (1981) and Stephens, Luxon and Hinch-

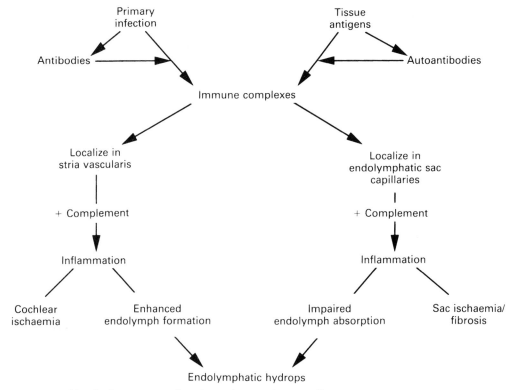

Figure 15.29 Possible role of immune complexes in autoimmune inner ear disease

cliffe (1982), and subsequently reviewed by one of the authors (Brookes, 1985b). Harada *et al.* (1992) reported significant hearing loss in three out of 22 patients with raised circulating immune complexes and renal failure, though tinnitus was present in all cases. Although circulating complexes may effect a final common pathophysiological pathway in a variety of cochleovestibular disorders, it is also possible that they are merely secondary epiphenomena resulting from local tissue damage.

Type IV

Cell-mediated delayed hypersensitivity reactions occur as a result of preliminary sensitization of T lymphocytes in the recirculating pool of immunologically competent cells. These subsequently become arrested and interact at the site of local concentration of antigen liberating chemotactic factors leading to infiltration of macrophages which cause tissue damage. Some tissue antigens are functionally sequestrated from the blood and reticuloendothelial system and do not produce an antibody response. However, a cell-mediated response may be induced following tissue damage, when the release of previously 'hidden' antigens results in a secondary immune response in similar tissues. Sympathetic ophthalmia

is a well known example of this type of disorder, when an immune-mediated ocular inflammation and progressive visual impairment follows a penetrating injury or surgery to the contralateral eye. Harris, Low and House (1985) postulated the likelihood of an analogous otological disorder which they termed 'sympathetic cochleolabyrinthitis'. They found a very small but consistent incidence of unexplained sensorineural hearing loss following previous translabyrinthine vestibular schwannoma surgery to the contralateral ear. As in sympathetic ophthalmia (Glynn and Holborrow, 1965) humoral antibodies causing immediate type II cytotoxic reactions can probably also occur. In other situations, an infective condition of the middle or inner ear may prime a cell-mediated otological immune response. Although the aetiology of autoimmunity is unknown, it has been suggested that involved tissues are either of ectodermal or endodermal origin and are recognized as 'foreign' by the immune system, which is mesodermal. The entire labyrinth is ectodermal in origin, and according to this theory is therefore a potential site for autoimmune activity.

Clinical features

McCabe (1979) described 18 patients, seen over a 10-year period, who presented with a similar clinical course and showed a uniform response to treatment. The main features consisted of progressive sensorineural hearing loss, often of sudden onset, fluctuant and bilateral, with associated aural pressure or fullness and variable tinnitus. Vestibular symptoms were frequently mild and transient but uncommonly acute and severe, while caloric tests showed reduced responses. Very occasionally disruption of soft tissue of the middle and external ear with facial paralysis was present. It was a disorder of young people in their 30s and 40s and characteristically the deafness progressed rapidly over weeks to months. On long-term follow up just under 20% went on to develop autoimmune diseases in other organ systems (McCabe, 1981). The lymphocyte inhibition test, in which the patients' own lymphocytes are challenged against inner ear antigen, was positive in about 25%. Treatment with steroids and cyclophosphamide either produced sustained hearing improvement or stabilization. The validity of the clinical concept of autoimmune deafness has been supported by others (Shea, 1982; Hughes *et al.*, 1983a, b), although soft tissue destruction and facial paralysis has only rarely been encountered.

Investigations

Unfortunately, there are no absolute diagnostic laboratory criteria, and often only a beneficial response to treatment has enabled a 'therapeutic' diagnosis to be made. Cell-mediated immunity may be assessed by the antigen-specific lymphocyte transformation test (Hughes *et al.*, 1983a) and immunofluorescence, as well as the lymphocyte migration inhibition test. However, a negative result does not necessarily exclude the diagnosis. The levels of serum immunoglobulins are probably of little relevance. Antigen-non-specific tests include assays of circulating immune complexes and complement, which may indicate enhanced immune activity perhaps due to a immune complex disorder if the levels are persistently elevated. A raised erythrocyte sedimentation rate may reflect systemic disease activity. Additional tests may be carried out to screen for rheumatoid factor and anti-DNA autoantibodies to various non-otological tissues, but these investigations are certainly less specific and their relevance uncertain.

Hughes and his colleagues have now treated more than 100 patients with a presumptive diagnosis of autoimmune inner ear disease (Hughes *et al.*, 1987; Hughes, 1991), and have long-term follow up in 47 cases. Table 15.5 lists the presenting diagnosis in the first 52 patients. Symptoms indistinguishable from Menière's syndrome were present in more than half the cases, while several cases of Dandy syndrome, or idiopathic bilateral labyrinthine failure, were seen. Although so-called 'antigen-specific' tests were used, Hughes acknowledged that these rely on crude inner ear preparations prepared from tissues removed during translabyrinthine surgery, so that the precise

antigens are not in fact known. Moreover, most of the inner ear tissue would normally be expected to consist of vestibular neuroepithelium, as the cochlear duct is not routinely removed in these procedures.

Table 15.5 Presenting diagnosis in 52 patients with autoimmune inner ear disease

Diagnosis	No.	Unilateral	Bilateral
Menière syndrome	27	8	19
Sensorineural hearing loss	15	2	13
Cogan's syndrome	7	1	66
Dandy syndrome	3	—	33

After Hughes *et al.*, 1987

Arnold, Pfaltz and Altermatt (1985) enjoyed less success with their own lymphocyte transformation test, and therefore elected to search for cross-reacting antibodies against inner ear structures using immunohistochemical methods with sections from healthy human temporal bones. They studied patients with bilateral inner ear disease of unknown aetiology and found antibodies against inner ear structures in more than half the cases. Antibodies bound preferentially to the cells of the stria vascularis in more than 75% while organ of Corti antibodies were found in less than 10%. Just over 40% of 12 patients with Menière's disease had antibodies exclusively to the stria vascularis. Arnold and co-workers concluded that their researches only justify the designation 'disease with autoimmune markers', as histopathological evidence of lymphocytic, plasma cell or macrophage infiltration in the temporal bones of patients with Menière's disease or progressive sensorineural hearing loss is still lacking. Furthermore, because the inner ear is able to produce those antibodies that are required locally via the endolymphatic sac, it may well not be possible to identify them in the circulation. This might explain why conventional clinical serum immunological parameters are negative in patients with presumed isolated autoimmune inner ear disease. In addition, the active stage of the disease may well be long past by the time temporal bone material becomes available for examination.

Harris and Sharp (1990) also found limitations in the lymphocyte transformation assay, and accordingly used the more specific Western blot technique to study inner ear reactivity. In this technique both cochlear and vestibular bovine membranous inner ear tissue were processed to form an antigen preparation which can then be electrophoresed onto a polyacrylamide gel for incubation with diluted test sera. The sera of animals in their guinea-pig model of experimental autoimmune sensorineural hearing loss, produced following immunizations with bovine inner ear tissue, all contained specific antibodies to inner ear antigens by this technique (Harris, 1987).

Subsequently, patients with rapidly progressive sensorineural hearing loss have been investigated by a similar blot assay. Thirty-five per cent showed similar autoantibodies to the sensitized animals to an antigen of 68 000 molecular weight. Two dimensional gel electrophoresis confirmed that both animals and patients reacted to identical components of inner ear antigen. One important problem concerns the purity of the test antigens. Yamanobe and Harris (1993) have recently studied various extraction procedures which use different solutions and detergents in an attempt to standardize antigen preparations. With their current technique, the potential contaminant bovine serum albumin can be removed in the water-soluble fractions, which will hopefully lead to more reproducible results.

Western blot techniques are complex and time consuming. They can be considered as a 'molecular dissection' and are probably more suited to research studies. The first author (GBB) has been involved in the application of a more straightforward screening test using an enzyme-linked immunoabsorbent assay (ELISA). This assay only requires very small amounts of antigen, perhaps less than one-tenth of that required for Western blotting. We have therefore been able to dissect the inner ear tissues from frozen human temporal bones and thus obtain more specific localization of antibodies. The test is relatively rapid, and many samples can be screened at a time, as opposed to the single assay technique in Western blot studies. Our preliminary results are highly promising though more normative data are required for standardization, while other workers have also reported successful applications with their own ELISA laboratory technique (Orozco *et al.*, 1990).

Genetic aspects

The discovery of associations between certain diseases and the major histocompatibility complex or human leucocyte antigen (HLA) locus represents one of the most important advances in clinical medicine in the last two decades. A number of striking associations of particular HLA haplotypes and diseases with a suspected or presumed autoimmune aetiology have been found. Certain haplotypes are known to be associated with susceptibility to disease, while others are associated with resistance. Correlations are invariably incomplete, however, probably largely reflecting a multifactorial pathogenesis. Other recognized factors in these disorders include the influence of other genes, or environmental factors such as trauma, bacterial or viral damage, drugs or toxins. Stress can also inhibit immune defences and lead to exacerbation of symptoms in autoimmune disease.

All chronic autoimmune diseases studied have shown a correlation with one or several of the HLA antigens compared with an appropriate control population. Indeed, failure to identify an association is very significant evidence against an autoimmune pathogenesis. An increased tendency for other autoimmune diseases should also be established in the same patient population, and in close family members. Immune disorders characteristically also display an hereditary predisposition, yet the familial distribution of cases is such that they do not follow classical mendelian laws.

Morrison and Xenellis (1987) studied the detailed medical history of 671 patients with the inner ear disorder Menière's disease and 689 controls. In the Menière's group, 10.3% had another autoimmune disorder compared with 4% of controls. In the Menière's group, 5.4% had a first degree relative with the Menière's disease, and a recognized autoimmune disorder was present in 9.7% of their relatives. In the control group, only 0.6% had a first degree relative with Menière's disease, and a recognized autoimmune disorder was present in 3.9% of their relatives. These differences were all highly significant.

Bowman and Nelson (1986) studied 39 patients with a clinical diagnosis of autoimmune inner ear disease, 28% of whom had other non-otological systemic autoimmune disease. They reported an increased frequency of the CW7 haplotype, which occurred in 51% of patients compared with 21% of 627 matched controls. A possible reduced frequency of DR4 was reported as well.

Xenellis *et al.* (1986) reported the results of an investigation of 41 patients with Menière's disease. Cases were selected with the intention of maximizing any possible association. There was therefore a very high incidence of bilateral involvement constituting nearly two-thirds of the cases. These patients were exclusively a tertiary referral population who were refractory to medical treatment and were severely disabled. The class I HLA allele CW7 was found in 75% of Menière's patients, a highly significant association ($P < 0.01$) when compared with controls. The frequencies of the HLA alleles A1 and B8 were also increased, but were not significant after corrections were made for the number of antigens tested. No association was found with class II DR3. In addition, no differences were found between males and females, or unilateral or bilateral cases.

The first author (GBB) has recently reported the results of a further collaborative HLA study in a more balanced and representative population of 60 Caucasian patients with Menière's disease (Brookes, Davey and Bachelor, 1992). The first 50 cases were seen consecutively, and included early, established and late stages of the disease activity spectrum. In the light of our findings a further 10 bilateral patients were added. There was an equal sex incidence, while the disorder was bilateral in 20 cases. Distinct differences were found between Menière's subjects with bilateral disease compared to unilateral cases. A highly significant ($P < 0.01$) positive correlation with the CW7 antigen was found in the bilateral group, and a highly significant ($P<0.01$) negative association with B12. In fact, B12 was never observed in the bilateral disease patients though the incidence in controls was 28%. In contrast, in the unilateral disease group there was only an association trend with CW7 ($P<0.1$), but a statistically highly significant ($P<0.01$) positive correlation with B12. The B12 antigen was identified in 43% of unilateral cases. The allele CW5 was also never found in the bilateral group though the numbers are insufficient to reach significance.

These three studies strongly support the contention that the class I allele CW7 is a genetic marker for susceptibility to the development of autoimmune inner ear disease. The last study suggested that the B12 antigen may well exert a protective influence, or alternatively its absence increases susceptibility, to the development of bilateral Ménière's disease. In the future early genetic screening may predict a population at risk of developing immune mediated inner ear disease, which could therefore have significant management implications.

Treatment

Many, but not all, patients respond to systemic steroids. Recommended regimens suggest enteric coated prednisolone 20 mg four times daily for 2 weeks before reducing to a maintainance dose of 5–10 mg on alternate days for 3–6 months in the face of continuing clinical improvement and lack of toxicity. In the authors' experience much lower dosages can sometimes lead to improvement and reduce unwanted side effects such as weight gain and dyspepsia. Hughes *et al.* (1990) found that 40% of their 47 patients who attended for long-term follow up improved with steroids, while stabilization was achieved in 40%. Twenty per cent continued to deteriorate.

Failure to respond to steroids may be an indication for immunosuppressive treatment with azathioprine or cyclophosphamide, but each case must be considered on its merits. Ethically it may be difficult to justify potentially hazadous immunosuppressive therapy in the absence of precise diagnostic criteria unless warranted by the severity of the clinical symptoms, usually marked bilateral hearing loss or rapid loss in an only hearing ear. Hughes *et al.* (1990) only treated less than 10% of their cases with cytotoxic therapy. The first author has, however, preferred to use the well established cytotoxic drug azathioprine (2 mg/kg body weight daily) at an early stage of active disease and when the diagnosis has been established. This has enabled steroid maintainance to be continued at a low alternate day dosage thereby avoiding long-term side effects. Figure 15.30 shows the efficacy of this combined regimen in a young man who presented with a short history of severe bilateral sensorineural hearing loss and positive inner ear autoantibodies.

Certain patients may show improvement with plasma exchange. This is an expensive therapeutic

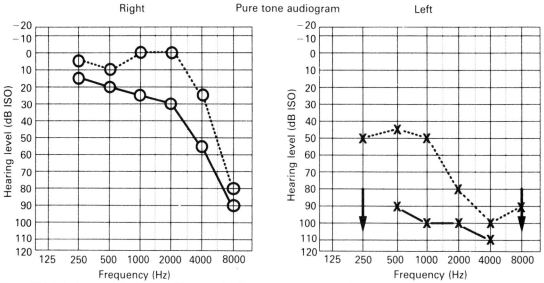

Figure 15.30 Audiometry of a 21-year-old man with bilateral autoimmune ear disease. He presented with sudden left hearing loss, distortion and vertigo 6 weeks previously, and a 10-day history of right hearing impairment and distortion. Solid line: pretreatent May 1989; broken line: post-treatment October 1989. His improved hearing has been maintained for more than 3 years on azathioprine and alternate-day low-dose steroids. (Reproduced by kind permission of the Editor, Kluwer Academic Publishers)

modality which is not widely available and whose beneficial effects are of a relatively temporary nature lasting, at the most, 3 months. It may, however, 'buy time' in the mangement of problem cases (Hamblin, Mufti and Bracewell, 1982; Brookes and Newland, 1986).

Connective tissue diseases

Certain systemic connective tissue diseases may affect the inner ear, in addition to many other organs and systems. The main pathological changes affect collagen, namely mucoid degeneration, fibrinoid necrosis and hyalinization. There is a significant female predominance, and many of the disorders often commence in young adults in their 20s and 30s. There is now considerable evidence that many are probably immunologically mediated disorders, largely on the basis of demonstrable autoantibodies. However, definite proof of an autoimmune aetiology is still lacking in most.

Conditions characterized by inflammation and necrosis of blood vessels constitute the hypersensitivity vasculitides. The varied features depend on the particular organs and blood vessel sites involved. There are several distinct types, though as this is a disease spectrum some overlap may occur. The pathogenesis is multifactorial, although in many instances the lesions are believed to be due to local tissue reaction to the deposition of immune complexes in vessel walls. Table 15.6 summarizes the main features found on investigation of the more important connective tissue and vasculitic disorders.

The systemic vasculitides were once considered to be quite rare. However, new laboratory tests notably for ANCA (antineutrophil cytoplasmic autoantibody) have led to an increased awareness of these diseases especially Wegener's granulomatosis. Scott and Watts (1994) recently studied a well defined unselected and stable population, and found an overall incidence of systemic vasculitis of 42/million, a figure some fourfold higher than previous estimates. There is also now less dependence on multiple tissue biopsy and/or angiography for diagnosis.

New classification criteria were proposed in 1990, based on the size of the dominant arteries and vessels involved (Hunder *et al.*, 1990), and these have been developed further (British Journal of Rheumatology, 1994.) Table 15.7 summarizes these criteria, though not all conditions are associated with secondary otological involvement. The new classification is particularly helpful in terms of management, because it appears that in general the response to treatment with systemic steroids, immunosuppressive drugs or alternative modalities varies with respect to the particular vessels affected (Table 15.8).

Disorders with small vessel and medium artery involvement are invariably associated with autoanti-

bodies directed against cytoplasmic components of neutrophils and monocytes, the so-called ANCA test. They carry a significant risk of renal involvement, but are most responsive to immunosuppression with cyclophosphamide. The ANCA serological marker has been divided into distinct cellular immunofluorescence staining patterns. The subtyping of ANCA into C-ANCA (cytoplasmic pattern) and P-ANCA (perinuclear pattern) has improved the test specificity. C-ANCA is highly specific for Wegener's granulomatosis (Nolle *et al.*, 1989). Schmitt, Csernok and Gross (1991) screened nearly 15 000 sera from 9000 patients and found that a classic ANCA was associated with Wegener's granulomatosis and closely related vasculitic disorders. In contrast a perinuclear pattern (P-ANCA) is a common finding in microscopic polyarteritis and may occur in about 10% of cases of rheumatoid arthritis. It is believed that these ANCA antibodies play an important role in pathogenesis, as ANCA-stimulated neutrophils and monocytes produce superoxide, degranulate and damage target cells *in vitro* (Ewert, Jennette and Falk, 1991).

Systemic lupus erythematosus

Systemic lupus erythematosus is a multisystem connective tissue disorder in which an autoimmune aetiology is most certain. Widespread immune complex deposition is present in many organs. Typically, lupus erythematosus cells (polymorphs with large engulfed basophilic material) are present and the serum antinuclear factor is positive. The erythrocyte sedimentation rate is very high and anaemia is frequently present. Although more than half the patients have central nervous system involvement, resulting in cranial neuropathies, otological features are very uncommon (Sheehy, 1981; Hamblin, Mufti and Bracewell, 1982; Bowman *et al.*, 1986; Caldarelli, Rejowski and Corey, 1986).

Otological features

Sudden sensorineural hearing loss which is usually bilateral is a common feature in reported cases. Hamblin, Mufti and Bracewell (1982) described a 42-year-old woman who developed sudden severe cochlear hearing loss 6 weeks after the onset of systemic symptoms. Prednisolone 40 mg daily resulted in general improvement but no hearing gain. Plasma exchange, however, effected immediate and complete restoration of hearing. A single plasma exchange was repeated at 6-monthly intervals to reverse the recurrent hearing loss which ensued. The dramatic response to plasma exchange infers a vascular mechanism, and it was suggested that circulating immune complexes could cause sludging in the stria vascularis. Kobayashi, Fujishiro and Sugiyama (1992) also described a patient who achieved dramatic hearing improvement after plasmapheresis.

Table 15.6 Laboratory results in main connective tissue disorders

Laboratory test	Normal population	Systemic lupus erythematosus	Cogan's syndrome	Wegener's granulomatosis	Polyarteritis nodosa
Full blood count (FBC) Haemoglobin		↓ normochromic normocytic	↓ in acute	↓ normochromic, normocytic	↓ normochromic, normocytic
White cell count		↓ lymphocytes	↑ lymphocytes ± eosinophils neutrophils monocytes (acute only)	↑ neutrophils	↑ neutrophils ± eosinophilia
Platelets		↓		↑	Normal
Erythrocyte sedimentation rate		↑	↑	↑	↑
Lupus erythematosus cells	Negative	Positive	Negative	Negative	May be positive
Coombs' test	Negative	May be positive	Negative	Negative	Negative
Antinuclear factor (ANF)	Low titres with increasing age	Positive – often high titre	Negative	Negative	May be positive in low titre
DNA-binding	Negative	Raised	Negative	Negative	Usually negative
Complement levels	C3 0.69–1.30 g/l C4 0.12–0.27 g/l	Low levels C3 may be high	Normal C3 and C4 may be raised acutely	Normal or raised	Normal or raised
Extractable nuclear antigen (ENA) (type RNP, S_m, P_o, La)	N	May be positive (S_m is most specific type)	Negative	Negative	Negative
C-reactive protein (CRP)	< 0.8 mg/dl	Only slightly raised unless infection present	Raised	Raised	Raised
Syphilis serology (RPR, TPHA)	Negative	RPR positive low titre TPHA negative	Negative	Negative	Negative

By kind permission of Jane Curley and Margaret Byron

Caldarelli, Rejowski and Corey (1986) reported a case in which the onset of bilateral profound sensorineural hearing loss associated with mild unsteadiness occurred over a period of 3 weeks. Systemic lupus erythematosus was diagnosed, but despite aggressive treatment with steroids and cyclophosphamide the profound deafness remained. The authors postulated that the pathogenesis was microinfarction of inner ear capillaries or arterioles, a mechanism responsible for CNS features. In the same year,

Bowman *et al.* (1986) reported their experience of nine patients with systemic lupus erythematosus and associated hearing loss. It is of interest that the diagnosis was made prior to the onset of otological symtoms in four patients. The same authors carried out a prospective study of 30 further systemic lupus erythematosus patients and found an 8% incidence of substantial previously unrecognized hearing loss without any other attributable cause, and strongly suspected a causal correlation. The hearing loss, how-

Table 15.7 Classification of systemic vasculitis

Dominant vessel involved	Primary	Secondary
Large arteries	Giant cell arteritis Takayasu's arteritis Isolated CNS angiitis	Aortitis associated with rheumatoid arthritis Infection (e.g. syphilis)
Medium arteries	Classical polyarteritis nodosa Kawasaki disease	Infection (e.g. hepatitis B)
Small vessels and medium arteries	Wegener's granulomatosis* Churg-Strauss syndrome* Microscopic polyangiitis*	Vasculitis secondary to rheumatoid arthritis, systemic lupus erythematosus and Sjögren's syndrome Drugs Infection (e.g. HIV)
Small vessels (leucocytoclastic)	Henoch-Schönlein purpura Essential mixed cryoglobulinaemia Cutaneous leucocytoclastic angiitis	Drugs Infection (e.g. hepatitis B, C)

*Diseases most commonly associated with ANCA (antineutrophil cytoplasmic autoantibody), a significant risk of renal involvement and which are most responsive to immunosuppression with cyclophosphamide. By kind permission the Editor, *British Journal of Rheumatology*

Table 15.8 Relationship between vessel size and treatment

Dominant vessel involved	Corticosteroids alone	Cyclophosphamide + corticosteroids	Others
Large arteries	+ + +	—	+
Medium arteries	+	+ +	+ +*
Small vessels and medium arteries	+	+ + +	—
Small vessels	+	—	+ +

* Includes plasmapheresis, antiviral therapy for hepatitis B-associated vasculitis and i.v. immunoglobulin for Kawasaki disease. By kind permission the Editor, *British Journal of Rheumatology*

ever, could not be correleated to age, sex, disease activity, organ system involvement, laboratory test abnormalities or duration of symptoms.

Cogan's syndrome

Cogan's syndrome is a rare condition in which a non-syphilitic interstitial keratitis is associated with fluctuant but aggressive cochleovestibular damage (Cogan, 1945). It usually affects young adults, and the ocular and otological symptoms commence suddenly and often simultaneously.

Otological features

McDonald, Vollertsen and Younge (1985) have reviewed the audiovestibular features and prognosis in 18 patients treated at the Mayo Clinic. The hearing loss is sensory in type and invariably bilateral. It progresses rapidly, though fluctuations may occur, and is associated with episodic vertigo, tinnitus and aural pressure, constituting a Menière's syndrome. Ultimately the deafness becomes profound and may be total. Vestibular assessment reveals significantly reduced or absent caloric responses. Central nervous system involvement is well recognized, and a recent report suggested that lower brain stem dysfunction may also cause reversible vestibuloauditory abnormalities (Benitez *et al.*, 1990). In contrast, the ophthalmic features consisting of irritation, lacrimation, photophobia and blurred vision typically progress more slowly. Patchy corneal infiltration is associated with neovascularization in the advanced stages.

There is now considerable evidence to support an autoimmune aetiology (McCabe, 1979; Hughes *et al.*, 1983b; Arnold and Gebbers, 1984; Brookes, 1985b).

Hughes *et al.* (1983b) studied two cases and found evidence of cell-mediated autoimmunity. One of the authors (Brookes, 1985b) studied two cases who were found to have very high levels of circulating immune complexes which fluctuated with disease activity as modified by treatment. Arnold and Gebbers (1984), using indirect immunofluorescent techniques, demonstrated IgG and IgA antibodies against human cornea and IgG antibodies against human inner ear tissue in the serum of a patient with Cogan's syndrome. These reactions were observed in the stria vascularis, Reissner's membrane, spiral ligament and dark cell areas. This study complements the main histopathological features in the temporal bone which include endolymphatic hydrops, degeneration of the organ of Corti and severe neuronal loss with infiltration of lymphocytes and plasmacytes in the region of the spiral ligament (Fisher and Hellstrom, 1961; Wolff and Bernard, 1965; Schuknecht and Nadol, 1994). Some cases of Cogan's syndrome are associated with systemic involvement consistent with polyarteritis nodosa and it has been suggested that the disorder may be a localized manifestation of this disorder.

Systemic steroids alone do not usually prevent the relentless progression towards severe cochleovestibular dysfunction. On the basis of the author's experience with two cases, immunosuppressive drugs are indicated at an early stage. The prognosis is so poor that there could be a place for intermittent plasma exchange therapy early in the natural history (Brookes, 1986).

Relapsing polychondritis

This disease entity was first described by Jaksch-Wartenhorst in 1923, and is characterized by an inflammatory reaction occurring in the cartilage of several different organs. Early features include tender swelling of the nasal septum and costal cartilages, perhaps associated with an underlying cough and dyspnoea from involvement of the larynx and trachea.

Otological features

The auricles are affected first in about 90% of cases (Ödkvist, 1970) resulting in pain, swelling and erythema. They are very tender on palpation and frequently associated with upper cervical lymphadenopathy. Chondritis of the cartilage of the eustachian tube may lead to serous otitis media, while involvement of the external auditory meatus may contribute to a conductive hearing loss. Sensorineural hearing impairment can occur independently or in conjunction with a conductive loss (Rabuzzi, 1970; Cody and Sones, 1971; Damiani and Levine, 1979). Cody and Sones (1971) found that 80% of patients had a sensory hearing loss which was usually bilateral and either of sudden onset or progressed over a period of a few weeks. Many had vestibular symptoms with

abnormalities on electronystagmography and caloric testing.

The condition has been considered an autoimmune disorder for some years mainly because of the efficacy of corticosteroids in reducing the inflammatory response. Cody and Sones reported some recovery of hearing in patients with early sensorineural involvement, although relapses tended to occur when drug therapy was discontinued or markedly reduced. Direct immunofluorescent examination of auricular cartilage obtained from patients with the disease, has demonstrated deposits of immunoglobulins and the C3 component of complement at the chondrofibrous junction (Valenzuela, 1980).

Wegener's granulomatosis

Wegener's granulomatosis is a discrete syndrome of necrotizing granulomatosis, vasculitis of the small arteries and veins of the upper and lower respiratory tract and kidney with less frequent involvement of other organs. There may be difficulties in differentiating this disorder from polyarteritis nodosa before the full complex develops. Patients will usually present with persistent epistaxis, and associated systemic features include weight loss, pyrexia, anaemia, leukocytosis and an elevated erythrocyte sedimentation rate. The average duration of untreated disease is about 6–9 months, and death is usually due to renal failure.

The C-ANCA immunofluorescent test, as described above, is now established as an important highly specific diagnostic tool. There is also good evidence that it correlates closely with disease activity, and hence is useful for monitoring response to treatment (Van der Woude *et al.* 1985; Egner and Chapel, 1990).

Otological features

Ear involvement occurs in 15–35% of cases and may be the only presenting feature (Blatt *et al.*, 1959; Kornblut *et al.*, 1980; Macias, Wackym and McCabe, 1993). Seromucinous otitis media is often present early in the course of the disease, and may result in frank otorrhoea (Karmody, 1978; Kornblut, Wolff and Fauci, 1982; McDonald and De Remee, 1983). On occasions the tympanic cavity becomes filled with granulomatous tissue containing giant cells, and may be associated with ossicular damage (Blatt and Lawrence, 1961; Friedmann and Bauer, 1973). Clinically, these patients still present as chronic middle ear effusions but, at myringotomy, there is usually excessive bleeding and a middle ear space cannot be readily identified through the granulation tissue. Figure 15.31 shows the audiometric features of a 56-year-old woman who presented to the first author with recurrent middle ear effusions prior to the develop-

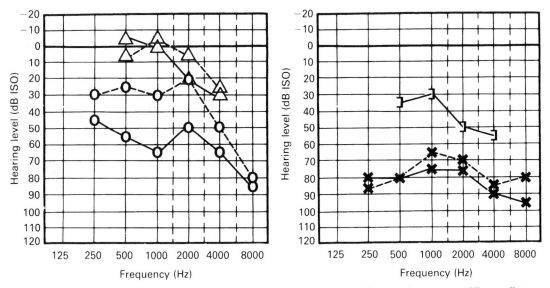

Figure 15.31 Wegener's granulomatosis. A 56-year-old woman with an 18-month history of recurrent middle ear effusions prior to the onset of multiple cranial nerve palsies due to central nervous system involvement. — = Baseline pure-tone audiometry; --- = thresholds following treatment with prednisolone 30 mg and cyclophosphamide 100 mg daily for 1 month. The improved right hearing threshold was maintained

ment of multiple cranial nerve palsies, and who responded to therapy.

Concomitant sensorineural hearing loss is uncommon (Blatt and Lawrence, 1961; Cody, 1971; McCaffrey *et al.*, 1980). McCaffrey and colleagues found evidence of inner ear involvement in 8% of 112 patients. In the case described by Blatt and Lawrence, direct spread of granulomatous tissue through the round window resulted in destruction of the membranous labyrinth (see Figure 4.35). Leone, Feghali and Linthicum (1984) described the temporal bone features in a patient who died of Wegener's granulomatosis. They found preferential involvement of the capillaries of the endolymphatic sac, but not those of the cochlea and suggested that a similar pathophysiology may well occur in other types of immune-complex mediated autoimmune disease, resulting in Menière-like symptoms. Although Wegener's granulomatosis has a sinister reputation, there is growing optimism for survival using combination regimens of steroids and cytotoxic immunosuppressant drugs. The long-term study of 85 patients by Fauci *et al.* (1985) showed that complete remissions can be achieved in more than 90% of cases.

Polyarteritis nodosa

Polyarteritis nodosa is a systemic necrotizing vasculitis of small and medium-sized arteries which demonstrates a 3:1 male to female predominance. There is frequently involvement of the renal, coronary, he-

patic and visceral circulations. A raised erythrocyte sedimentation rate, anaemia and leukocytosis are invariably present.

Otological features

Deafness is unusual but invariably involves the inner ear (Druss and Maybaum, 1934; McNeill, Berke and Reingold, 1952; Peitersen and Carlsen, 1966; Wing and Bulteau, 1967; Gussen, 1977; Lake-Bakaar and Gibbs, 1978; Jenkins, Pollak and Fisch, 1981). In rare instances it has been the presenting symptom. The onset is often sudden and typically bilateral and symmetrical (see Figure 17.3). Investigations show cochlear features which may be fluctuant. Occasionally, middle ear granulation tissue may be present causing a conductive component, though this feature is more typical of Wegener's granulomatosis. A pathological feature is involvement of arteries in the middle ear with an associated local tissue response. The other histopathological findings are described in Chapter 17. Significant hearing improvement following treatment with systemic steroids and in conjunction with the immunosuppressive drug chlorambucil has been reported (Peiterson and Carlsen, 1966; Wing and Bulteau, 1967).

Temporal arteritis

Pyrexia, bitemporal headaches and tender palpable thickening of the temporal arteries are the main features of this condition which occurs in older age groups. The underlying vasculitis is primarily confined to the extracranial arteries, which may undergo aneurysm formation, stenosis and even occlusion. Blindness occurs in about 30% of untreated cases due to involvement of the ophthalmic artery. Characteristically the erythrocyte sedimentation rate is extremely high and serum globulins are increased.

Otological features

Rapidly progressive hearing loss with vertigo has been described, presumably due to involvement of the internal auditory artery (Cody, 1971; Healy and Wilske, 1978). In the case reported by Cody, the cochleovestibular signs were partly reversible with systemic steroids.

Behçet's disease

Behçet's disease is a very uncommon chronic relapsing inflammatory disorder. The original classic symptom triad of uveitis and orogenital ulceration is now recognized as part of a multisystem vasculitic disorder which is very probably immunologically mediated. Lehner and Barnes (1986) have published a comprehensive review of the condition.

Otological features

Little attention has been given to otological aspects. Brama and Fainaru (1980) investigated 16 consecutive patients and found that 62% had features of inner ear involvement, which typically commenced about a decade after the initial manifestations of the disease. Elidan *et al.* (1991) studied 35 patients, and found that 80% showed some degree of hearing loss when compared to controls. Hearing loss is almost always bilateral and sensory in type, though only slowly progressive. It is frequently associated with vestibular symptoms. Elidan *et al.* (1991) studied the effects of the immunosuppressive drug cyclosporine A on audiological status. The hearing of five of the 28 Behçet's patients with at least a 1-year follow up showed improvement, while none deteriorated.

References

ADAIR-DIGHTON, C. A. (1912) Four generations of blue sclerotics. *Ophthalmoscope*, **10**, 188–189

ADAMS, D. A., KERR, A. G., SMYTH, G. L. and CINNAMOND, M. J. (1983) Congenital syphilitic deafness – a further review. *Journal of Laryngology and Otology*, **97**, 399–404

AEGERTER, E. E. and KIRKPATRICK, J. A. JR (1968) *Orthopedic Diseases*, 3rd edn. Philadelphia: Saunders. pp. 182–192

ALBRIGHT, F., BUTLER, A., HAMPTON, A. and SMITH, P. (1937) Syndrome characterised by osteitis fibrosa disseminata, areas of pigmentation and endocrine dysfunction, with precocious puberty in females. *New England Journal of Medicine*, **216**, 727–746

ARNOLD, W. and FRIEDMANN, I. (1988) Otosclerosis – an inflammatory disease of the otic capsule of viral aetiology? *Journal of Laryngology and Otology* **102**, 865–871

ARNOLD, W. and GEBBERS, J. O. (1984) Serum antibodies which bind to human cornea and inner ear tissues in a patient with Cogan's syndrome. *Laryngology, Rhinology and Otology*, **63/8**, 428–432

ARNOLD, W., ALTERMATT, H.-J. and GEBBERS, J.-O. (1984) Demonstration of immunoglobulins (IgA and IgG) in the human endolymphatic sac. *Laryngology, Rhinology and Otology*, **63**, 464–467

ARNOLD, W., PFALTZ, R. and ALTERMATT, H. J. (1985) Evidence of serum autoantibodies against inner ear tissues in the blood of patients with certain sensorineural hearing disorders. *Acta Otolaryngologica*, **99**, 437–444

BABIN, R. W., LIU, C. and ASHENBRENER, C. (1984) Histopathoplogy of neurosensory deafness in sarcoidosis. *Annals of Otology, Rhinology and Laryngology*, **93**, 389–393

BARKER, D. J. P., CHAMBERLAIN, A. T., GUYER, P. B. and CARDNER, M. J. (1980) Paget's disease of bone: the Lancashire focus. *British Medical Journal*, **280**, 1105–1107

BEICKERT, P. (1961) Zur Frage der Empfindungsschwerhörigkeit und Autoallergie. *Zeitschrift Laryngologie, Rhinologie und ihre Grenzgebiete*, **40**, 837–842

BEIGHTON, P. (1978) *Inherited Disorders of the Skeleton*. London: Churchill Livingstone

BEIGHTON, P., CRENIN, B. J. and HAMERSMA, H. (1976) The radiology of sclerosteosis. *British Journal of Radiology*, **49**, 393–397

BEIGHTON, P., DURR, L. and HAMERSMA, H. (1976) The clinical features of sclerosteosis. *Annals of Internal Medicine*, **84**, 934–937

BELAL, A. JR and LINTHICUM, F. M. JR (1980) Pathology of congenital syphilitic labyrinthitis. *American Journal of Otolaryngology*, **1**, 109–118

BENECKE, J. E. JR (1993) Facial nerve dysfunction in osteopetrosis. *Laryngoscope*, **103**, 494–497

BENITEZ, J. T., ARSENAULT M. A., LICHT, J. M., COHEN, S. D. and GREENBERG, R. V. (1990) Evidence of central vestibuloauditory dysfunction in atypical Cogan's syndrome: a case report. *American Journal of Otology*, **11**, 131–134

BIRDSALL, H. H., BAUGHN, R. E. and JENKINS, H. A. (1990) The diagnostic dilemma of otosyphilis. A new Western blot assay. *Archives of Otolaryngology – Head and Neck Surgery*, **116**, 617–621

BLAKELEY, B. W., HILGER, P. A., TAYLOR, S. and HILGER, J. (1986) Computed tomography in the diagnosis of cochlear otosclerosis. *Otolaryngology – Head and Neck Surgery*, **94**, 434–438

BLATT, I. and LAWRENCE, M. (1961) Otologic manifestations of fatal granulomatosis of respiratory tract: lethal midline granuloma – Wegener's granulomatosis. *Archives of Otolaryngology*, **73**, 639–643

BLATT, I., SELTZER, H., RUBIN, P., FURSTENBERG, A., MAXWELL, J. and SCHULL, W. (1959) Fatal granulomatosis of the respiratory tract (lethal midline granuloma – Wegener's granulomatosis). *Archives of Otolaryngology*, **70**, 707–711

BOLLERSLEV, J., GRONTVED, A. and ANDERSEN, P. E. JR (1988) Autosomal dominant osteopetrosis: an otoneurological investigation of the two radiological types. *Laryngoscope*, **98**, 411–413

BOUMANS, L. J. M. and POUBLON, R. M. L. (1991) The detrimental effect of aminohydroxypropylidene biphosphonate (APD) in otospongiosis. *European Archives of Oto-Rhino-Laryngology*, **248**, 218–221

BOWMAN, C. A. and NELSON, R. A. (1987) HLA antigens in autoimmune sensorineural hearing loss. *Laryngoscope*, **97**, 7–9

BOWMAN, C. A., LINTHICUM, F. H., NELSON, R. A., MIKAMI, K. and QUISMORIO, F. (1986) Sensorineural hearing loss associated with systemic lupus erythematosus. *Otolaryngology – Head and Neck Surgery*, **94**, 197–204

BOYLES, J. H. (1984) Allergy testing in otology. *American Journal of Otology*, **5**, 450–455

BRAMA, I. and FAINARU, M. (1980) Inner ear involvement in Behçet's disease. *Archives of Otolaryngology*, **106**, 215–217

BRETLAU, P., JORGENSEN, M. B. and JOHANSEN, H. (1970) Osteogenesis imperfecta. Light and electron microscopic studies of the stapes. *Acta Otolaryngologica*, **69**, 172–184

BRETLAU, P., CAUSSE, J., CAUSSE, J. B., HANSEN, H. J., JONSEN, N. J. and SALOMON, G. (1985) Otospongiosis and sodium fluoride. A blind experimental and clinical evaluation of the effect of sodium fluoride treatment in patients with otospongiosis. *Annals of Otology, Rhinology, and Laryngology*, **94**, 103–107

BRITISH MEDICAL JOURNAL (1976) Metabolic bone disease in Asians. **278**, 442–443

BRITISH MEDICAL JOURNAL (1982) Sexually transmitted disease surveillance in Britain – 1980. **284**, 124

BRITISH MEDICAL JOURNAL (1986) Sexually transmitted disease surveillance in Britain – 1984. **293**, 942–943

BRITISH JOURNAL OF RHEUMATOLOGY (1994) Editorial. Classification and epidemiology of systemic vasculitis. **33**, 897–900

BRONNER, F. (1973) Kinetic and cybernetic analysis of calcium metabolism. In: *Calcium and Phosphorus Metabolism*, edited by E. Irving. New York: Academic Press. pp. 149–186

BRONSON, E. (1917) On fragilitas ossium and its association with blue sclerotics and otosclerosis. *Edinburgh Medical Journal*, **18**, 240–274

BROOKES, G. B. (1983) Vitamin D deficiency – a new cause of cochlear deafness. *Journal of Laryngology and Otology*, **97**, 405–420

BROOKES, G. B. (1985a) Vitamin D deficiency and deafness: 1984 update. *American Journal of Otology*, **6**, 102–107

BROOKES, G. B. (1985b) Immune complex associated deafness: preliminary communication. *Journal of the Royal Society of Medicine*, **78**, 47–55

BROOKES, G. B. (1985c) Vitamin D deficiency and otosclerosis. *Otolaryngology – Head and Neck Surgery*, **93**, 313–321

BROOKES, G. B. (1986) Circulating immune complexes in Menière's disease. *Archives of Otolaryngology*, **112**, 536–540

BROOKES, G. B. and GRAHAM, M. D. (1984) Post-traumatic cholesteatoma of the external auditory canal. *Laryngoscope*, **94**, 667–670

BROOKES, G. B. and MORRISON, A. W. (1981) Vitamin D deficiency and deafness. *British Medical Journal*, **283**, 273–274

BROOKES, G. B. and NEWLAND, A. C. (1986) Plasma exchange in the treatment of immune-complex associated sensorineural deafness. *Journal of Laryngology and Otology*, **100**, 25–33

BROOKES, G. B., DAVEY, N. and BACHELOR, J. R. (1992) Is Menière's disease an autoimmune disorder? In: Otology

in the 90s – trends and perspectives. *Proceedings of the Politzer Society International Conference*, 76

BROOKES, G. B., LILLY, D. and HAWKINS, J. E. Jr (1983) The effects of acute vitamin D deficiency on cochlear function and morphology in the albino rat. Paper presented at the Research Forum of the *American Academy of Otolaryngology – Head and Neck Surgery*, Anaheim, California, Oct 23–27

BROOKES, G. B., PORTER, M. J. and PHELPS, P. D. (1992) CT densitometry of the cochlea in otosclerosis. *Clinical Otolaryngology*, **17**, 235–236

BROSNAN, M., BURNS, H., JAHN, A. F. and HAWKE, M. (1977) Surgery histopathology of the stapes in osteogenesis imperfecta tarda. *Archives of Otolaryngology*, **103**, 294–298

CALDARELLI, D. D., REJOWSKI, J. E. and COREY, J. P. (1986) Sensorineural hearing loss in lupus erythematosus. *American Journal of Otology*, **7**, 210–213

CANTRILL, J. A., BUCKLER, H. M. and ANDERSON, D. C. (1986) Low dose intravenous 3-amino-1-hydroxypropylidene-1, 1-biphosphonate (APD) for the treatment of Paget's disease of bone. *Annals of Rheumatic Diseases*, **45**, 1012–1018

CARRUTH, J. A. S., LUTMAN, M. E. and STEPHENS, S. D. G. (1978) An audiological investigation of osteogenesis imperfecta. *Journal of Laryngology and Otology*, **92**, 853–860

CASSELMAN, J. W., DE-JONGE, I., NEYT, L., DE-CLERCQ, C. and D'HONT, G. (1993) MRI in craniofacial fibrous dysplasia. *Neuroradiology*, **35**, 234–237

CATTERALL, R. D. (1977) Neurosyphilis. *British Journal of Hospital Medicine*, **17**, 585–604

CAUSSE, J., SHAMBAUGH, G. E. JR and CHEVANCE, L. G.. (1977) Cochlear otospongiosis: etiology, diagnosis and therapeutic implications. *Advances in Oto-Rhino-Laryngology*, **22**, 43–56

CAUSSE, J., CHEVANCE, L. G., BRETLAU, P., JORGENSEN, M. B., URIEL, J. and BERGES, J. (1977) Enzymatic concept of otospongiosis and cochlear otospongiosis. *Clinical Otolaryngology*, **2**, 23–32

CHAMBERS, T. J. and AZRIA, M. (1988) The effect of calcitonin on the osteoblast. Triangle. *Sandoz Journal of Medical Science*, **27**, 53–60

CHAN, C. C., GREEN, W. R., DE LA CRUZ, Z. and HILLIS, A. (1982) Ocular findings in osteogenesis imperfecta congenita. *Archives of Ophthalmology*, **100**, 1459–1463

CHAN, Y. M., ADAMS, D. A. and KERR, A. G. (1995) Syphilitic labyrinthitis – an update. *Journal of Laryngology and Otology*, **109**, 719–725

CHOLE, R. A. (1993) Differential osteoclast activation in endochondral and intramembranous bone. *Annals of Otology, Rhinology and Laryngology*, **102**, 616–619

CLEMIS, J. D. (1974) Cochleovestibular disorders and allergy. *Otolaryngologic Clinics of North America*, **7**, 757–780

CODY, D. T. (1971) *Rehabilitation for Sensorineural Hearing Loss.* **1**. *Clinical Otology – an international synopsis*, edited by M. Paparella, A Hohmann and J. C. V. Huff. St Louis: Mosby

CODY, D. T. R. and BAKER, H. L. (1978) Otosclerosis: vestibular symptoms and sensorineural hearing loss. *Annals of Otology, Rhinology and Laryngology*, **87**, 778–784

CODY, D. T. and SONES, D. A. (1971) Relapsing polychondritis: audiological manifestations. *Laryngoscope*, **81**, 1208–1222

COGAN, D. (1945) Syndrome of non-syphilitic interstitial keratitis and vestibuloauditory symptoms. *Archives of Ophthalmology*, **33**, 144–146

COHEN, H. N., FOGELMAN, I., BOYLE, I. T. and DOIG, J. A. (1979) Deafness due to hypervitaminosis D. *Lancet*, i, 985

COLLART, P., BOREL, C. J. and DUREL, P. (1964) Significance of spiral organisms found, after treatment, in late human and experimental syphilis. *British Journal of Venereal Disease*, 40, 81–89

COVELL, W. P. (1941) Pathologic changes in the peripheral auditory mechanisms due to avitaminosis (A, B complex, C, D, E). *Laryngoscope*, 50, 632–647

CRILLEY, R. G., HORSMAN, A., PEACOCK, M. and NORDIN, B. E. C. (1981) The vitamin D metabolites in the pathogenesis and management of osteoporosis. *Current Medical Research and Opinion*, 7, 337–344

CUNNINGHAM, M. J., CURTIN, H. D., JAFFE, R. and STOOL, S. E. (1989) Otologic manifestations of Langerhans' cell histiocytosis. *Archives of Otolaryngology – Head and Neck Surgery*, 115, 807–813

CZERNY, V. (1873) Eine lokale Malacie des Unterschenkels. *Wein Medizine Wochenschrift*, 23, 895

DAMIANI, J. M. and LEVINE, H. L. (1979) Relapsing polychondritis – report of ten cases. *Laryngoscope*, 89, 929–946

DAMSMA, H., DE GROOT, J. A., ZONNEVELD, F. W., VAN WAES, P. F. and HUIZING, E. H. (1984) CT of cochlear otosclerosis (otospongiosis). *Radiologic Clinics of North America*, 22, 37–43

DANDONA, P., GILL, D. S. and KHOKHER, M. A. (1989) Fluoride and osteoblasts. *Lancet*, i, 449–450

DAVIES, D. G. (1968) Paget's disease of the temporal bone. *Acta Otolaryngologica Supplementum*, 242, 1–47

DAVIES, D. G. (1970) The temporal bone in Paget's disease. *Journal of Laryngology and Otology*, 84, 553–560

DAVIES, M. and STANBURY, S. W. (1981) The rheumatic manifestations of metabolic bone disease. *Clinics in Rheumatic Diseases*, 7, 595–600

DAVIES, M., KANE, R. and VALENTINE, J. (1984) Impaired hearing in X-linked hypophosphataemic (vitamin D resistant) osteomalacia. *Annals of Internal Medicine*, 100, 230–232

DAWKINS, R. S., SHARP, M. and MORRISON, A. W. (1968) Steroid therapy in congenital syphilitic deafness. *Journal of Laryngology and Otology*, 82, 1095–1107

DE GROOT, J. A. M. and HUIZING, E. H. (1987) Computed tomography in otosclerosis and Menière's disease. *Acta Otolaryngologica*, Supplement 434, 1–94

DE GROOT, J. A. M., HUIZING, E. H., ZONNEVELD, F. W. and VELDMAN, J. E. (1987) New methods in studying the bony cochlear capsule in otosclerosis. In: *Immunobiology, Histophysiology, Tumour Immunology in Otorhinolaryngology, Proceedings 2nd International conference, Utrecht*, edited by J. E. Veldman. Amsterdam/Berkeley: Kugler Publications. pp. 193–200

DE MARINO, D. P., DUTCHER, P. O. JR, PARKINS, C. W. and HENGERER, A. S. (1985) Histiocytosis-X: otologic presentations. *International Journal of Pediatric Otorhinolaryngology*, 10, 91–100

DE REMEE, R. A. and ROHRBACH, M. S. (1980) Serum angiotension-converting enzymes in evaluating the clinical course of sarcoidosis. *Annals of Internal Medicine*, 92, 361–365

DETHERIDGE, F. M., GUYER, P. B. and BARKER, D. J. P. (1982) European distribution of Paget's disease of bone. *British Medical Journal*, 285, 1005–1008

DINARDO, L. J. and WETMORE, R. F. (1989) Head and neck manifestations of histiocytosis-X in children. *Laryngoscope*, 99, 721–724

DOIG, J. A. and GATEHOUSE, S. (1984) Hearing in acromegaly. *Journal of Laryngology and Otology*, 98, 1097–1011

DORT, J. C., POLLAK, A. and FISCH, U. (1990) The fallopian canal and facial nerve in sclerosteosis of the temporal bone: a histopathologic study. *American Journal of Otology*, 11, 320–325

DRUSS, J. B. and MAYBAUM, J. L. (1934) Periarteritis nodosa of the temporal bone. *Archives of Otolaryngology*, 19, 502–507

DU BOULAY, G. H. (1980) *Principles of X-ray Diagnosis of the Skull*. London: Butterworths

DUNLOP, E. M. C., AL-EGAILY, S. S. and HOUANG, E. T. (1981) Production of treponemicidal concentration of penicillin in cerebrospinal fluid. *British Medical Journal*, 283, 646

DUNLOP, E. M. C., KING, A. J. and WILKINSON, A. E. (1969) Study of late ocular syphilis. Demonstration of treponemes in aqueous humour and cerebrospinal fluid. 3. General and serological findings. *Transactions of the Ophthalmological Society*, 88, 275–294

EGNER, W. and CHAPEL, H. M. (1990) Titration of antibodies against neutrophil cytoplasmic antigens is useful in monitoring disease activity in systemic vasculitides. *Clinical and Experimental Immunology*, 82, 244–249

ELIDAN, J., LEVI, H., COHEN, E. and BENEZRA, D. (1991) Effect of cyclosporine A on the hearing loss in Behçet's disease. *Annals of Otology, Rhinology and Laryngology*, 101, 464–468

EL SAMMAA, M., LINTHICUM, F. H. Jr, HOUSE, H. P. and HOUSE, J. W. (1986) Calcitonin as treatment for hearing loss in Paget's disease. *American Journal of Otology*, 7, 241–243

ELSTER, A. D., THEROS, E. G., KEY, L. L. and CHEN, M. Y. (1992) Cranial imaging in autosomal recessive osteopetrosis. Part II. Skull and brain. *Radiology*, 183, 137–144

ENGEL, S. and DIEZEL, W. (1980) Persistent serum immune complexes in syphilis. *British Journal of Venereal Diseases*, 56, 221–222

EWERT, B. H., JENNETTE, C. J. and FALK, R. J. (1991) The pathogenic role of antineutrophil cytoplasmic autoantibodies. *American Journal of Kidney Diseases*, 18, 188–195

FAUCI, A. S., HAYNES, B. F., KATZ, P. and WOLFF, M. D. (1985) Wegener's granulomatosis: prospective clinical and therapeutic experience with 85 patients for 21 years. *Annals of Internal Medicine*, 98, 76–85

FISHER, E. R. and HELLSTROM, H. R. (1961) Cogan's syndrome and systemic vascular disease. *Archives of Pathology (Chicago)*, 72, 572–592

FLOCK, A., FLOCK, B. and ULFENDAHL, M. (1986) Mechanisms of movement in outer hair cells and a possible structural basis. *Archives of Otorhinolaryngology*, 243, 83–90

FORQUER, B. D., LINTHICUM, F. H and BENNETT, C. (1986) Sodium fluoride: effectiveness of treatment for cochlear otosclerosis. *American Journal of Otology*, 7, 121–125

FRIEDMANN, I. and BAUER, F. (1973) Wegener's granulomatosis causing deafness. *Journal of Laryngology and Otology*, 87, 449–464

GARRETSEN, T. J. and CREMERS, C. W. (1990) Ear surgery in osteogenesis imperfecta. Clinical findings and short-term and long-term results. *Archives of Otolaryngology*, 116, 317–323

GELL, P. G. H. and COOMBS, R. R. A. (1968) *Clinical Aspects of Immunology*, 2nd edn. Oxford: Blackwell Scientific Publications

GENNARI, C. and SENSINI, I. (1975) Diphosphonate therapy in deafness associated with Paget's disease. *British Medical Journal*, 1, 331–334

GLEICH, L. L., LINSTROM, C. J. and KIMMELMAN, C. P. (1992) Otosyphilis: a diagnostic and therapeutic dilemma. *Laryngoscope*, **102**, 1255–1260

GLYNN, L. E. and HOLBORROW, E. J. (1965) The eye. In: *Autoimmunity and Disease*. Oxford: Blackwell Scientific Publications. pp. 320–340

GOODHILL, V. (1939) Syphilis of the ear: a histopathological study. *Annals of Otology, Rhinology and Laryngology*, **48**, 676–706

GRAHAM, M. D. and BRACKMAN, D. E. (1978) Acromegaly and the temporal bone. *Journal of Laryngology and Otology*, **92**, 275–279

GRIMALDI, P. G. B., MOHAMEDALLY, S. A. and WOODHOUSE, N. J. Y. (1975) Deafness in Paget's disease: effect of salmon calcitonin treatment. *British Medical Journal*, **2**, 726

GRISTWOOD, R. E. (1958) Nerve deafness associated with sarcoidosis. *Journal of Laryngology and Otology*, **72**, 479–491

GUSSEN, R. (1977) Polyarteritis nodosa and deafness. A human temporal bone study. *Archives of Otorhinolaryngology*, **217**, 263–271

HAHN, R. D., ROSIN, P. and HASKINS, H. L. (1962) Treatment of syphilitic neural deafness with prednisone. *Journal of Chronic Diseases*, **15**, 395–409

HAMBLIN, T. J., MUFTI, G. J. and BRACEWELL, A. (1982) Severe deafness in SLE: its immediate relief by plasma exchange. *British Medical Journal*, **284**, 1374–1375

HAMERSMA, H. (1970) Osteopetrosis (marble bone disease) of the temporal bone. *Laryngoscope*, **80**, 1518–1539

HARADA, T., SANO, M., SAKAGAMI, M., OGINO, S. and MATSUNAGA, T. (1992) Mechanism of immune complex-mediated inner ear diseases. *Annals of Otology, Rhinology and Laryngology*, **101**, 72–77

HARCOURT, J. P., LENNOX, P., BROOKES, G. B. and PHELPS, P. D. (1996) CT screening for temporal bone diseases in bilateral sensorineural hearing loss. *Journal of Laryngology and Otology*, (In press)

HARNER, S. G., ROSE, D. E. and FACER, G. W. (1978) Paget's disease and hearing loss. *Otorhinolaryngology*, **86**, 869–874

HARRIS, J. P. (1983) Immunology of the inner ear: response of the inner ear to antigen challenge. *Otolaryngology – Head and Neck Surgery*, **91**, 17–23

HARRIS, J. P. (1984) Immunology of the inner ear: evidence of local antibody production. *Annals of Otology, Rhinology and Laryngology*, **93**, 157–162

HARRIS, J. P. (1987) Experimental autoimmune sensorineural hearing loss. *Laryngoscope*, **97**, 63–76

HARRIS, J. P. and SHARP, P. A. (1990) Inner ear autoantibodies in patients with rapidly progressive sensorineural hearing loss. *Laryngoscope*, **100**, 516–524

HARRIS, J. P. and TOMIYAMA, S. (1987) Experimental immune system of the inner ear. In: *Immunobiology, Histiophysiology and Tumour Immunology in Otolaryngology. Proceedings of the 2nd International Conference. Utrecht*, edited by J. E. Veldman. Amsterdam/Berkeley: Kugler Publications. pp. 113–121

HARRIS, J. P., LOW, N. C. and HOUSE, W. F. (1985) Contralateral hearing loss following inner ear injury: sympathetic cochlear-labyrinthitis? *American Journal of Otology*, **6**, 371–377

HARVEY, L. (1984) Viral aetiology of Paget's disease of bone: a review. *Journal of the Royal Society of Medicine*, **77**, 943–948

HAWKE, M., JAHN, A. F. and BAILEY, D. (1981) Osteopetrosis of the temporal bone. *Archives of Otolaryngology*, **107**, 278–282

HEALY, L. A. and WILSKE, K. R. (1978) *The Systemic Manifestations of Temporal Arteritis*. New York: Grune and Stratton

HELLIER, W. P. L. and BROOKES, G. B. (1996) Vestibular nerve dysfunction and decompression in Engelmann's disease. *Journal of Laryngology and Otology*, (in press)

HENKIN, R. I., LIFSCHITZ, M. D. and LARSON, A. L. (1972) Hearing loss in patients with osteoporosis and Paget's disease of bone. *American Journal of Medical Science*, **263**, 383–392

HENNEBERT, C. (1911) Un syndrome nouveau dans la labyrinthine heredo-syphilitique. *Clinique Bruxelles*, **25**, 545–550

HERDMAN, R. C. D., MORGAN, K., HOLT, P. J. L. and RAMSDEN, R. T. (1993) Type II collagen autoimmunity and Menière's disease. *Journal of Laryngology and Otology*, **107**, 994–998

HIMI, T., IGARASHI, M., KATAU, R. A. and ALFORD, B. R. (1993) Temporal bone findings in craniodiaphyseal dysplasia. *Auris Nasus Larynx (Tokyo)*, **20**, 255–261

HOARE, T. J., BROOKES, G. B., RIDGEWAY, G. L. and ROBINSON, A. J. (1996) The value of syphilis serology in otolaryngology practice. *Journal of Laryngology and Otology*, (in press)

HOOPER, R. and HOLDEN, H. (1970) Acoustic and vestibular problems in sarcoidosis. *Archives of Otolaryngology*, **92**, 385–391

HUGHES, G. B. (1991) Is surgery ever needed for immune inner ear disease? *Proceedings of Politzer Society International Conference on Reality in Ear Surgery and Otoneurosurgery*, Maastricht. p. 9

HUGHES, G. B. and RUTHERFORD, I. (1986) Predictive value of serologic tests for syphilis in otology. *Annals of Otology, Rhinology and Laryngology*, **95**, 250–259

HUGHES, G. B., BARNA, B. P. and CALABRESE, L. H. (1986) Immune mechanisms in auditory and vestibular disease. *Otolaryngology – Head and Neck Surgery, vol. 4, Ear and Skull Base*, edited by C. W. Cummings *et al.* St Louis: C. V. Mosby

HUGHES, G. B., KINNEY, S. E., BARNA, B. P. and CALABRESE, L. H. (1983a) Autoimmune reactivity in Menière's disease – a preliminary report. *Laryngoscope*, **93**, 1153–1154

HUGHES, G. B., KINNEY, S. E., BARNA, B. P., TOMSAK, R. I. and CALABRESE, L. H. (1983b) Autoimmune reactivity in Cogan's syndrome: a preliminary report. *Otolaryngology – Head and Neck Surgery*, **91**, 24–28

HUGHES, G. B., KINNEY, S. E., BARNA, B. P. and CALABRESE, L. H. (1987) Autoimmune inner ear disease: Five year review. In: *Immunobiology, Histopathology and Tumour Immunology in Otolaryngology. Proceedings of the 2nd International Conference, Utrecht*, edited by J. E. Veldman. Amsterdam/Berkeley: Kugler Publications. pp. 23–32

HUGHES, G. B., BARNA, B. P., KINNEY, S. E., CALABRESE, L. H., KOO, A. M., and NALEPA, N. J. (1990) Immune inner ear disease: 1990 report. *Proceedings of the XIV World Congress of Otorhinolaryngology, Head and Neck Surgery*, edited by T. Sacristan, J. J. Alvarez-Vicent, J. Bartual, F. Antoli-Candela and L. Rubio. Amsterdam: Kugler and Ghedini Publications. pp. 2855–2856

HUNDER, G. G., AREND, W. P., BLOCH, D. A., CALABRESE, L. H., FAUCI, A. S. and FRIES, J. F. *et al.* (1990) The American College of Rheumatology 1990 criteria for the classification of vasculitis: introduction. *Arthritis and Rheumatism*, **33**, 1065–1067

HUNT, J. C. and PUGH, D. G. (1961) Radiology of skeletal lesions in neurofibromatosis. *Radiology*, 76, 1–20

HYBELS, R. L. and RICE, D. H. (1976) Neuro-otologic manifestations of sarcoidosis. *Laryngoscope*, 86, 1873–1878

IKEDA, K., KUSAKARI, J., KOBAYASHI, T. and SAITO, Y. (1987a) The effect of vitamin D on the cochlear potentials and the perilymphatic ionized calcium concentration of rats. *Acta Otolaryngologica*, Supplement 435, 64–72

IKEDA, K., KUSAKARI, J., TAKASAKA, T. and SAITO, Y. (1987b) The calcium activity of cochlear endolymph of the guinea pig and the effect of inhibitors. *Hearing Research*, 26, 117–125

IKEDA, K., KOBAYASHI, T., ITOH, Z., KUSAKARI, J. and TAKASAKA, T. (1989) Evaluation of vitamin D metabolism in patients with bilateral sensorineural loss. *American Journal of Otology*, 10, 11–13

IRVING, R. M., BROADBENT, V. and JONES, N. S. (1994) Langerhans' cell histiocytosis in childhood: management of head and neck manifestations. *Laryngoscope*, 104, 64–70

IRWIN, J. (1986) Hearing loss and calciferol deficiency. *Journal of Laryngology and Otology*, 100, 1245–1249

JAKSCH-WARTENHORST, R. (1923) Polychondropathia. *Archives of Internal Medicine* (Vienna), 6, 93–97

JENKINS, H. A., POLLAK, A. M. and FISCH, U. (1981) Polyarteritis as a cause of sudden deafness. *American Journal of Otolaryngology*, 2, 99–107

JOHNSSON, L. G., HAWKINS, J. E. JR, ROUSSE, R. C. and LINTHICUM, F. H. Jr (1982) Cochlear and otoconial abnormalities in capsular otosclerosis and hydrops. *Annals of Otology, Rhinology and Laryngology*, 97 (suppl.), 3–15

JOHNSTON, C. C., LAVY, K., LORD, T., VELLIOS, F., MERRITT, R. D. and DEISS, W. P. (1968) Osteopetrosis. *Medicine (Baltimore)*, 47, 149–167

JUHN, S. K. and RYBAR, L. (1981) Nature of the blood-labyrinth barrier. In: *Ménière's disease: pathogenesis, diagnosis and treatment*, edited by K. H. Vosteen, H. F. Schuknecht, E. R. Pfaltz *et al.* New York: Thieme Verlag. pp. 59–67

KANE, K. (1976) Deafness in sarcoidosis. *Journal of Laryngology and Otology*, 90, 531–537

KANIS, J. A. and RUSSELL, R. G. G. (1981) Diphosphonates and Paget's disease of bone. *Metabolic Bone Disease Related Research*, 3, 4–5

KANZAKI, J. and OUCHI, T. (1981) Steroid-responsive bilateral sensorineural hearing loss and immune complexes. *Archives of Otolaryngology*, 230, 5–9

KARMODY, C. S. (1978) Wegener's granulomatosis: presentation as an otologic problem. *Otolaryngology – Head and Neck Surgery*, 86, 573–575

KARMODY, C. S. and SCHUKNECHT, H. F. (1966) Deafness in congenital syphilis. *Archives of Otolaryngology*, 83, 18–27

KASABACH, H. H. and GUTMAN, A. B. (1937) Osteoporosis circumscripta of the skull and Paget's disease. *American Journal of Roentgenology*, 37, 577–602

KENNEDY, D. W., HOFFER, M. E. and HOLLIDAY, M. (1993) The effects of etidronate disodium on progressive hearing loss from otosclerosis. *Otolaryngology – Head and Neck Surgery*, 109, 461–467

KERR, A. G., SMYTH, G. D. L. and CINNAMOND, M. J. (1973) Congenital syphilitic deafness. *Journal of Laryngology and Otology*, 87, 1–12

KHETARPAL, U. and SCHUKNECHT, H. F. (1990) In search of pathologic correlates for hearing loss and vertigo in Paget's disease. A clinical and histopathological study of 26 temporal bones. *Annals of Otology, Rhinology and Laryngology*, Suppl. 145, 1–16

KLIMMELMAN, C. P., NIELSEN, E. and SNOW, J. B. (1984) Histiocytosis X of the temporal bone. *Otolaryngology – Head and Neck Surgery*, 92, 588–590

KORNBLUT, A. D., WOLFF, S. M., DEFRIES, H. O. and FAUCI, A. S. (1980) Wegener's granulomatosis. *Laryngoscope*, 90, 1453–1465

KORNBLUT, A. D., WOLFF, S. M. and FAUCI, A. S. (1982) Ear disease in patients with Wegener's granulomatosis. *Laryngoscope*, 92, 713–717

KORNFIELD, M. (1967) Pathological changes in the stria vascularis in Paget's disease. *Practical Otorhinolaryngology*, 29, 406–432

KOSOY, J. and MADDOX, H. E., III (1971) Surgical findings in Van der Hoeve's syndrome. *Archives of Otolaryngology*, 93, 115–122

KOBAYASHI, S., FUJISHIRO, N. and SUGIYAMA, K. (1992) Systemic lupus erythematosus with sensorineural hearing loss and improvement after plasmapheresis using the double filtration method. *Internal Medicine*, 31, 778–781

LAKE-BAKAAR, G. and GIBBS, D. D. (1978) Polyarteritis nodosa presenting with bilateral nerve deafness. *Journal of the Royal Society of Medicine*, 71, 144–147

LANDO, M., HOOVER, L. A. and FINERMAN, G. (1988) Stabilisation of hearing loss in Paget's disease with calcium and etidronate. *Archives of Otolaryngology – Head and Neck Surgery*, 114, 891–894

LEHNER, T. and BARNES, C. G. (eds) (1986) *Recent Advances in Behçet's Disease*. Oxford: Royal Society of Medicine Services Ltd, University Press

LEHNHARDT, E. (1958) Plötzliche Hörstörungen auf beiden Sieten gleichseitig oder nacheinander aufgetreten. *Zeitschrift für Laryngologie Rhinologie*, 37, 1–16

LEONE, L. A., FEGHALI, J. G. and LINTHICUM, F. H. (1984) Endolymphatic sac: possible role in autoimmune sensorineural hearing loss. *Annals of Otology, Rhinology and Laryngology*, 93, 1984–1989

LEVENE, G. M., WRIGHT, D. J. M. and TURK, J. L. (1971) Cell-mediated immunity and lymphocyte transformation in syphilis. *Proceedings of the Royal Society of Medicine*, 64, 14–18

LICHTENSTEIN, L. (1953) Histiocytosis X: integration of eosinophilic granuloma of bone, Letterer-Siwe disease as related manifestations of a single nosologic entity. *Archives of Pathology*, 56, 84–102

LICHTENSTEIN, L. and JAFFE, H. L. (1942) Fibrous dysplasia of bone. *Archives of Pathology*, 33, 777–816

LIM, D. J. and SILVER, P. (1974) The endolymphatic duct system. A light and electron microscopic investigation. In: *Proceedings of the Barany Society Meeting, Los Angeles, 1974*, edited by J. Pulec. p. 390

LINDSAY, J. and LEHMAN, R. (1969) Histopathology of the temporal bone in advanced Paget's disease. *Laryngoscope*, 79, 213–227

LINDSAY, J. R. and SUGA, F. (1976) Sensorineural deafness due to osteitis fibrosa. *Archives of Otolaryngology*, 102, 37–42

LINTHICUM, F. H., HOUSE, H. P. and ALTHAUS, S. R. (1973) The effect of sodium fluoride on otosclerotic activity as determined by strontium-85. *Annals of Otology, Rhinology and Laryngology*, 82, 609–615

LLOYD, G. A. S., PHELPS, P. D. and DU BOULAY, G. H. (1980) High resolution computerised tomography of the petrous bone. *British Journal of Radiology*, 53, 631–641

LUNDQUIST, P.-G. (1976) Aspects of endolymphatic sac morphology and function. *Archives of Otorhinolaryngology,* **212,** 231–240

MA, K. H., TANG, P. S. O. and CHAN, K. W. (1990) Aural tuberculosis. *American Journal of Otology,* **11,** 174–177

MCCABE, B. F. (1979) Autoimmune sensorineural hearing loss. *Annals of Otology, Rhinology and Laryngology,* **88,** 585–589

MCCABE, B. F. (1981) Treatment of autoimmune inner ear disease. In: *Proceedings of the Sixth Shambaugh International Workshop on Otomicrosurgery and Third Shea Fluctuant Hearing Loss Symposium.* Huntsville: Strode. pp. 289–290

MCCAFFREY, T. V. and MCDONALD, T. J. (1979) Histiocytosis X of the ear and temporal bone: review of 22 cases. *Laryngoscope,* **89,** 1735–1742

MCCAFFREY, T. V., MCDONALD, T. J., FACER, G. W. and DE REMEE, R. A. (1980) Otologic manifestations of Wegener's granulomatosis. *Otolaryngology – Head and Neck Surgery,* **88,** 586–593

MCCUNE, D. J. (1936) Osteitis fibrosa cystica: the case of a nine year old girl who also exhibits precocious puberty, multiple pigmentation of the skin and hyperthyroidism. *American Journal of Diseases of Childhood,* **52,** 745–748

MCDONALD, T. J., VOLLERTSEN, R. S. and YOUNGE, B. R. (1985) Cogan's syndrome: audiovestibular involvement and prognosis in 18 patients. *Laryngoscope,* **95,** 650–654

MCDONALD, T. J. and DE REMEE, R. A. (1983) Wegener's granulomatosis. *Laryngoscope,* **93,** 220–231

MACIAS, J. D., WACKYM, P. A. and MCCABE, B. F. (1993) Early diagnosis of otologic Wegener's granulomatosis using the serologic marker C-ANCA. *Annals of Otology, Rhinology and Laryngology,* **102,** 337–341

MCKUSICK, V. (1972) Osteogenesis imperfecta. In: *Hereditary Disorders of Connective Tissue,* 3rd edn. St Louis: Mosby. pp. 33–48

MCNEIL, N. F., BERKE, M. and REINGOLD, I. M. (1952) Polyarteritis nodosa causing deafness in adults. *Annals of Internal Medicine,* **37,** 1253–1267

MACK, L. W. JR, SMITH, J. L., WALTER, E. K., MONTENEGRO, E. N. R. and NICOL, W. G. (1969) Temporal bone treponemes. *Archives of Otolaryngology,* **90,** 11–14

MAFEE, M. F., VALVASSOR, G. E., DEITCH, R. L., NOROUZI, P., HENRIKSON, G. C., CAPEK, V. *et al.* (1985) Use of CT in the evaluation of cochlear otosclerosis. *Radiology,* **156,** 703–708

MAJUMDAR, B. and CROWTHER, J. (1983) Hearing loss in sarcoidosis. *Journal of Laryngology and Otology,* **97,** 635–639

MAURER, H. (1967) Biochemical aspects of otosclerosis. *Archives of Otolaryngology,* **85,** 24–28

MAYER, O. and FRASER, J. (1936) Pathological changes in the ear in late congenital syphilis. *Journal of Laryngology and Otology,* **51,** 683 and 755

MEISTER, M., JOHNSON, A., POPELKA, G. R., KIM, G. S. and WHYTE, M. P. (1986) Audiologic findings in young patients with hypophosphatemic bone disease. *Annals of Otology, Rhinology and Laryngology,* **95,** 415–420

MILLS, B. G., SINGER, F. R., WEINER, L. P., SUFFIN, S. C., STABILE, E. and HOLST, P. (1984) Evidence for both respiratory syncytial virus and measles virus antigens in the osteoclasts of patients with Paget's disease of bone. *Clinical Orthopaedics,* **183,** 303–311

MILROY, C. M. and MICHAELS, L. (1990a) Pathology of the otic capsule. *Journal of Laryngology and Otology,* **104,** 83–90

MILROY, C. M. and MICHAELS, L. (1990b). Temporal bone pathology of adult-type osteopetrosis. *Archives of Otolaryngology – Head and Neck Surgery,* **116,** 79–84

MIRRA, J. M. (1987) Pathogenesis of Paget's disease based on viral etiology. *Clinical Orthopaedics and Related Research,* **217,** 162–170

MIYAMOTO, R. T., HOUSE, W. F. and BRACKMANN, D. E. (1980) Neurotologic manifestations of the osteopetroses. *Archives of Otolaryngology,* **106,** 210–214

MOFFATT, W. H., MORROW, J. D. and SIMPSON, N. (1977) Effects of calcitonin on deafness due to Paget's disease of bone. *British Medical Journal,* **2,** 485–487

MONSELL, E. M., CODY, D. D. and BONE, H. G. (1993) Measurement of regional bone mineral density: a new technique for the evaluation of the temporal bone. *American Journal of Otology,* **14,** 455–459

MONSELL, E. M., BONE, H. G., CODY, D. D., JACOBSON, G. P., NEWMAN, C. W., PATEL, S. C. *et al.* (1995) Hearing loss in Paget's disease of bone: evidence of auditory nerve integrity. *American Journal of Otology,* **16,** 27–33

MORRISON, A. W. (1967) Genetic factors in otosclerosis. *Annals of the Royal College of Surgeons,* **41,** 202–212

MORRISON, A. W. (1969) Management of severe deafness in adults. *Proceedings of the Royal Society of Medicine,* **62,** 959–965

MORRISON, A. W. (1975) *The Management of Sensorineural Deafness.* London: Butterworths

MORRISON, A. W. (1979) Disease of the otic capsule. In: *Scott-Brown's Diseases of the Ear, Nose and Throat,* 4th edn, edited by J. Ballantyne and J. Groves, vol. 2. London: Butterworths. pp. 465–498

MORRISON, A. W. and XENELLIS, J. (1987) Immunological aspects of Menière's disease. In: *Immunobiology, Histophysiology and Tumour Immunology in Otolaryngology. Proceedings of the 2nd International Academic Conference, Utrecht,* edited by J. E. Veldman. Amsterdam: Kugler Publications. pp. 9–14

MYERS, E. N. and STOOL, S. (1969) The temporal bone in osteopetrosis. *Archives of Otolaryngology,* **89,** 460–469

NAGASAKI, T., WATANABE, Y., ASO, S. and MIZUKOSHI, K. (1993) Electrocochleography in syphilitic hearing loss. *Acta Otolaryngologica, Supplement* 504, 68–73

NAGER, G. T. (1988) Osteogenesis imperfecta of the temporal bone and its relation to otosclerosis. *Annals of Otology, Rhinology and Laryngology,* **97,** 585–593

NAGER, G. T. (1993) Otosclerosis. In: *Pathology of the Ear and Temporal Bone.* Baltimore: Williams & Wilkins. pp. 943–1010

NAGER, G. T., KENNEDY, D. W. and KOPSTEIN, E. (1982) Fibrous dysplasia: a review of the disease and its manifestations in the temporal bone. *Annals of Otology, Rhinology and Laryngology, Supplement* 92, 1–52

NOLLE, B., SPECKS, U., LUDERMANN, J., ROHRBACH, M. S., DEREMEE, R. A. and GROSS, W. L. (1989) Anticytoplasmic autoantibodies; their immunodiagnostic value in Wegener's granulomatosis. *Annals of Internal Medicine,* **111,** 28–40

NORDIN, B. E. C. (1973) *Metabolic Bone and Stone Disease.* Edinburgh: Churchill Livingstone

ÖDKVIST, L. (1970) Relapsing polychondritis. *Acta Otolaryngologica,* **70,** 448–454

O'MALLEY, S., RAMSDEN, R. T., LATIF, A., KANE, R. and DAVIES, M. (1985) Electrocochleographic changes in the hearing loss associated with X-linked hypophosphataemic osteomalacia. *Acta Otolaryngologica,* **100,** 13–18

OROZCO, C. R., NIPARKO, J. P., RICHARDSON, B. C., DOLAND, D. F., PTOK, M. U. and ALTSCHULER, R. A. (1990) Experimental model of immune-mediated hearing loss using cross-species immunisation. *Laryngoscope*, **100**, 941–947

PAGET, J. (1877) On a form of chronic inflammation of bones (osteitis deformans). *Medico-Chirurgical Transactions*, **65**, 225–236

PARAHY, C. and LINTHICUM, F. H. Jr (1984) Otosclerosis and otospongiosis: clinical and histological comparisons. *Laryngoscope*, **94**, 508–512

PATTERSON, C. N. and STONE, H. B., III (1970) Stapedectomy in Van der Hoeve's syndrome. *Laryngoscope*, **80**, 544–558

PEDERSEN, U. (1984) Hearing loss in patients with osteogenesis imperfecta. A clinical and audiological study of 201 patients. *Scandinavian Audiology*, **13**, 67–74

PEDERSEN, U. (1985) Osteogenesis imperfecta. Clinical features, hearing loss and stapedectomy. *Acta Otolaryngologica Supplementum*, **415**, 1–36

PEDERSEN, U., CHARLES, P., HANSEN, H. H. and ELBROND, O. (1985) Lack of effects of human calcitonin in osteogenesis imperfecta. *Acta Orthopaedica Scandinavica*, **56**, 260–264

PEITERSEN, E. and CARLSEN, B. J. (1966) Hearing impairment as the initial sign of polyarteritis nodosa. *Acta Otolaryngologica*, **61**, 189–193

PETROVIC, A. and SHAMBAUGH, G. E. JR (1966) A study of the effects of fluoride on bone in laboratory animals and on otosclerotic bone in human subjects. *Archives of Otolaryngology*, **83**, 104–110

PETROVIC, A. G., STUTZMANN, J. J. and SHAMBAUGH, G. E. Jr (1985) Experimental studies on pathology and therapy of otospongiosis. *American Journal of Otology*, **6**, 43–50

PHELPS, P. D. and LLOYD, G. A. S. (1989) Otosclerosis and bone dysplasias. In: *Diagnostic Imaging of the Ear*, 2nd edn. London: Springer-Verlag. pp. 203–204

PRESTON, C. J., YATES, A. J. P., BENETON, M. N. C., RUSSELL, R. G. G., GRAY, R. E. S., SMITH, R. *et al.* (1986) Effective short-term treatment of Paget's disease with oral etidronate. *British Medical Journal*, **292**, 79–80

PRESTON, R. E., JOHNSSON, L. G., HILL, J. N. and SCHACHT, J. (1975) Incorporation of radioactive calcium into otolithic membranes and middle ear ossicles of the gerbil. *Acta Otolaryngologica*, **80**, 269–275

PROCKOP, D. J. (1992) Mutations in collagen genes as a cause of connective tissue disorders. *New England Journal of Medicine*, **326**, 540–546

PROOPS, D., BAYLEY, D. and HAWKE, M. (1985) Paget's disease and the temporal bone – a clinical and histopathological review of six temporal bones. *Journal of Otolaryngology*, **14**, 20–29

QUICK, C. A. (1975) Antigenic cause of hearing loss. *Otolaryngologic Clinics of North America*, **8**, 385–397

QUISLING, R. W., MOORE, G. R., JAHRSDOERFER, R. A. and CANTRELL, R. W. (1979) Osteogenesis imperfecta. A study of 160 family members. *Archives of Otolaryngology*, **105**, 207–211

RABKIN, M. S., WITTWER, C. T., KJELDSBERG, C. R. and PIEPKORN, M.W. (1987) Flow-cytometric DNA content of histiocytosis X (Langerhans cell histiocytosis). *American Journal of Pathology*, **131**, 283–289

RABUZZI, D. D. (1970) Relapsing polychondritis. *Archives of Otolaryngology*, **91**, 188–194

RAMSDEN, R. T., MOFFAT, D. A. and GIBSON, W. P. R. (1977) Transtympanic electrocochleography in patients with syphilis and hearing loss. *Annals of Otology, Rhinology and Laryngology*, **86**, 827–834

RASK-ANDERSON, H. and STAHLE, J. (1980) Immunodefence of the inner ear. *Acta Otolaryngologica*, **89**, 283–294

REBEL, A., BASLE, M., POUPLARD, A., KOUYOUMDJIAN, S., FILMON, R. and LEPATEZOUR, A. (1980) Viral antigens in osteoclasts from Paget's disease of bone. *Lancet*, ii, 344–346

REED, R. J. (1963) Fibrous dysplasia of bone. *Archives of Pathology*, **75**, 480–495

RICHARDS, S. (1968) Deafness in acromegaly. *Journal of Laryngology and Otology*, **82**, 1053–1065

RICHARDSON, A. C., TINLING, S. P. and CHOLE, R. A. (1993) Risedonate activity in the fetal and neonatal mouse. *Otolaryngology – Head and Neck Surgery*, **109**, 623–633

ROSENHALL, U., LÖWHAGEN, G. B. and ROUPE, G. (1984) Auditory function in early syphilis. *Journal of Laryngology and Otology*, **98**, 567–572

ROSS, M. D. (1979) Calcium ion uptake and exchange in otoconia. *Advances in Otorhinolaryngology*, **25**, 26–33

ROSS, U. H., LASZIG, R., BORNEMANN, H. and ULRICH, C. (1993) Osteogenesis imperfecta: clinical symptoms and update findings in computed tomography and tympano-cochlear scintigraphy. *Acta Otolaryngologica*, **113**, 620–624

RÜEDI, L. (1965) Histopathologic confirmation of labyrinthine otosclerosis. *Laryngoscope*, **75**, 1582–1609

RÜEDI, L. (1968) Are there cochlear shunts in Paget's and Recklinghausen's disease. *Acta Otolaryngologica*, **65**, 13–24

SCHMITT, W. H., CSERNOK, E. and GROSS, W. L. (1991) ANCA and infection. *Lancet*, i, 1416–1417

SCHRADER, M., POPPENDIECK, J. and PLESTER, D. (1987) Auto-immunological aspects of otosclerosis. *Proceedings of the 2nd International Academic Conference Utrecht*, edited by J. E. Veldman. Amsterdam Berkeley: Kugler Publications. pp. 433–443

SCHUKNECHT, H. F. (1974) *Pathology of the Ear*. Cambridge: Harvard University Press

SCHUKNECHT, H. F. (1978) Delayed endolymphatic hydrops. *Annals of Otology, Rhinology and Laryngology*, **87**, 743–748

SCHUKNECHT, H. F. (1983) Cochlear otosclerosis – an intractable absurdity. *Journal of Laryngology and Otology*, Suppl. 8, 81–83

SCHUKNECHT, H. F. and NADOL, J. B. (1994) Temporal bone pathology in a case of Cogan's syndrome. *Laryngoscope*, **104**, 1135–1142

SCHWARTZ, D. T. and ALPERT, M. (1964) The malignant transformation of fibrous dysplasia. *American Journal of Medical Science*, **247**, 35–54

SCOTT, D. G. I. and WATTS, R. A. (1994) Editorial. Classification and epidemiology of systemic vasculitis. *British Journal of Rheumatology*, **33**, 897–900

SHAI, F., BAKER, R. K. and WALLACH, S. (1971) The clinical and metabolic effects of calcitonin on Paget's disease of bone. *Journal of Clinical Investigation*, **50**, 1927–1940

SHAMBAUGH, G. E. JR (1981) Allergic causes for fluctuant hearing loss. *Proceedings of the Sixth Shambaugh and Third Shea International Workshop in Otology*. Huntsville: Strode

SHAMBAUGH, G. E. Jr and CAUSSE, J. (1974) Ten years experience with fluoride in otosclerotic (otospongiotic) patients. *Annals of Otology, Rhinology and Laryngology*, **83**, 635–645

SHAMBAUGH, G. E. Jr and SCOTT, A. (1964) Sodium fluoride for the arrest of otosclerosis. *Archives of Otolaryngology*, **80**, 263–270

SHEA, J. J. (1982) Autoimmune sensorineural hearing loss as an aggravating factor in Menière's disease. Paper presented to the *Barany Society*, Basel, Switzerland

SHEA, J. J. and POSTMA, D. S. (1982) Findings and long-term surgical results in the hearing loss of osteogenesis imperfecta. *Archives of Otolaryngology*, 108, 467–470

SHEEHY, J. L. (1981) Doctor's discussion. *American Journal of Otology*, 2, 405–407

SLY, W. S., HEWETT-EMMETT, D., WHYTE, M. P., LU, Y.-S. L. and TASIAN, R. E. (1983) Congenital carbonic anhydrase isoenzyme II deficiency and osteopetrosis. *Proceedings of the National Academy of Science (Washington)*, 80, 2752–2755

SMÄRS, G. (1961) *Osteogenesis imperfecta in Sweden*, translated by M. Marsden. Stockholm: Scandinavian University Books. pp. 1–240

SMITH, J. L. and ISRAEL, C. W. (1967) Spirochetes in the aqueous humour in seronegative ocular syphilis. Persistence after penicillin treatment. *Archives of Ophthalmology*, 77, 474–477

SMITH, R., FRANCIS, M. J. O. and HAUGHTON, G. R. (1983) *The Brittle Bone Syndrome: Osteogenesis Imperfecta*. London: Butterworths

SMOUHA, E. E., EDELSTEIN, D. R. and PARISIER, S. C. (1987) Fibrous dysplasia involving the temporal bone: report of three new cases. *American Journal of Otology*, 8, 103–107

SOLIMAN, A. M. (1990) Type II collagen induced inner ear disease: critical evaluation of the guinea pig model. *American Journal of Otology*, 11, 27–32

SØLLING, J., SØLLING, K., JACOBSEN, K. U., OLSEN, S. and FROM, L. (1978) Circulating immune complexes in syphilis. *Acta Dermato-Venereologica*, 58, 263–267

SOULIERE, C. R. JR, KAVA, C. R., BARRS, D. M. and BELL, A. F. (1991) Sudden hearing loss as the sole manifestation of neurosarcoidosis. *Otolaryngology – Head and Neck Surgery*, 105, 376–381

SPARKES, R. S. and GRAHAM, C. B. (1972) Camurati-Engelmann disease. Genetics and clinical manifestations with a review of the literature. *Journal of Medical Genetics*, 9, 73–85

SPARROW, N. J. and DUVAL, A. J. (1967) Hearing loss and Paget's disease. *Journal of Laryngology and Otology*, 81, 601–611

STAMP, T. C. B. and BAKER, L. R. I. (1976) Recessive hypophosphataemic rickets and possible aetiology of the vitamin D resistant syndrome. *Archives of Diseases in Childhood*, 51, 360–365

STEPHENS, S. D. G., LUXON, L. M. and HINCHCLIFFE, R. (1982) Immunological disorders and auditory lesions. *Audiology*, 21, 128–148

STEWART, E. J. and O'REILLY, B. F. (1989) A clinical and audiological investigation of osteogenesis imperfecta. *Clinical Otolaryngology*, 14, 509–514

STOLLER, F. M. (1982) The ear in osteogenesis imperfecta. *Laryngoscope*, 72, 855–869

SWARTZ, J. D., VANDERSLICE, R. B., KORSVIK, H., SALUK, P. H., POPKY, G. L., MARLOWE, F. I. et al. (1985a) High resolution computed tomography: part 6 craniofacial Paget's disease and fibrous dysplasia. *Otolaryngology – Head and Neck Surgery*, 7, 40–47

SWARTZ, J. D., MANDELL, D. W., BERMAN, S. E., WOLFSON, R., J., MARLOWE, F. I. and POPKY, G. L. (1985b) Cochlear otosclerosis (otospongiosis): CT analysis with audiometric correlation. *Radiology*, 155, 147–150

SWARTZ, J. D., MANDELL, D. W., WOLFSON, R. J. et al. (1985c) Fenestral and cochlear otosclerosis: CT evaluation. *American Journal of Otology*, 6, 476–481

SWEET, R. M., KORNBLUT, A. D. and HYAMS, V. J. (1979) Eosinophilic granuloma in the temporal bone. *Laryngoscope*, 89, 1545–1552

TERRAYAMA, Y. and SASAKI, Y. (1968) Studies on experimental allergic (isoimmune) labyrinthitis in guinea pigs. *Acta Otolaryngologica*, 58, 49–56

TOMIYAMA, S. and HARRIS, J. P. (1986) The endolymphatic sac: its importance in inner ear immune response. *Laryngoscope*, 96, 685–691

TOS, M. (1966) A survey of Hand-Schuller-Christian's disease in otolaryngology. *Acta Otolaryngologica*, 62, 217–228

TRUSWELL, A. S. (1958) Osteopetrosis with syndactyly. *Journal of Bone and Joint Surgery*, 408, 208–218

VALENZUELA, R. (1980) Relapsing polychondritis: immunomicroscopic findings in cartilage ear biopsy specimens. *Human Pathology*, 11, 19–26

VALVASSORI, G. E. and DOBBEN, G. D. (1985) CT densitometry of the cochlear capsule in otosclerosis. *American Journal of Neuroradiology*, 6, 661–667

VAN BUCHEM, F. S. P. (1971) Hyperostosis corticalis generalisata. *Acta Medica Scandinavica*, 189, 257–267

VAN BUCHEM, F. S. P., HADDERS, H. N., HANSEN, J. F. and WOLDRING, M. G. (1962) Hyperostosis corticalis generalisata. *American Journal of Medicine*, 33, 387–397

VAN DER HOEVE, J. and DE KLEYN, A. (1918) Blau sclera Knochenkrüchig-Keit und Schwerhorig-Keit. *Archives für Ophthalmologie*, 95, 81–93

VAN DER WOUDE, F. J., RASMUSSEN, N., LOBATTO, S., WIIK, A., PERMIN, H., VAN ES, L. A. et al. (1985) Autoantibodies against neutrophils and monocytes: tools for diagnosis and marker of disease activity in Wegener's granulomatosis. *Lancet*, i, 425–429

VAN TILBERG, W. (1972) Fibrous dysplasia. In: *Handbook of Clinical Neurology*, edited by P. J. Vinken and G. W. Bruyn. vol. 14. Amsterdam: North Holland Publishing. pp. 163–212

VELDMAN, J. E., ROORD, J. J., O'CONNOR, A. F. and SHEA, J. J. (1984) Autoimmunity and inner ear disorders: an immune-complex mediated sensorineural hearing loss. *Laryngoscope*, 94, 501–507

VON RECKLINGHAUSEN, F. D. (1882) *Uber die multiplen fibromen der Haut und ihre Beziehung zu den multiplen Neuromen*. Berlin: A. Hirschwald

WALKER, G. S., EVANSON, J. M., CANTY, D. P. and GIU, N. W. (1979) Effect of calcitonin on deafness due to Paget's disease of skull. *British Medical Journal*, 2, 364–365

WEIR, N. (1977) Sensorineural deafness associated with recessive hypophosphataemic rickets. *Journal of Laryngology and Otology*, 91, 717–722

WINDLE-TAYLOR, P. C. and BAILEY, C. M. (1980) Tuberculous otitis media: a series of 22 patients. *Laryngoscope*, 90, 1039–1044

WING, L. and BULTEAU, V. (1967) Deafness in Wegener's granulomatosis. *Journal of Otolaryngological Society of Australia*, 2, 91–92

WOLFF, D. and BERNARD (1965) The pathology of Cogan's syndrome causing profound deafness. *Annals of Otology, Rhinology and Laryngology*, 74, 507

WOODHOUSE, N. J. Y. (1973) Paget's disease and calcitonin therapy. *Ninth Symposium on Advanced Medicine*, edited by G. Walker. London: Pitman Medical

WOODHOUSE, N. J. Y. (1974) Clinical applications of calcitonin. *British Journal of Hospital Medicine*, 11, 677–684

WOOLF, N. K. and HARRIS, J. P. (1986) Cochlear pathophysiology associated with inner ear immune responses. *Acta Otolaryngologica*, **102**, 353–364

WULLSTEIN, N. (1960) Fundamentals and task of plastic surgery in operations for restriction of hearing. *Journal of Laryngology and Otology*, **73**, 515–526

XENELLIS, J., MORRISON, A. W., MCCLOWSKY, D. and FESTENSTEIN, H. (1986) HLA antigens in the pathogenesis of Menière's disease. *Journal of Laryngology and Otology*, **100**, 21–24

YAMANOBE, S. and HARRIS, J. P. (1993) Extraction of inner ear antigens for studies in inner ear autoimmunity. *Annals of Otology, Rhinology and Laryngology*, **102**, 22–27

YAMAZAKI, T., OGAWA, K., IMOTO, T., HAYASHI, N. and KOZAKI, H. (1988) Senile deafness and metabolic bone disease. *American Journal of Otology*, **9**, 376–382

YANIV, E., TRAUB, P. and CONRADIE, R. (1986) Middle ear tuberculosis – a series of 24 patients. *International Journal of Pediatric Otorhinolaryngology*, **12**, 59–63

YOO, T. J., STUART, J. M., CREMAR, M. A., OWNES, A. S. and KAWK, A. H. (1983a) Type II collagen-induced autoimmune sensorineural hearing loss and vestibular dysfunction in rats. *Annals of Otology, Rhinology and Laryngology*, **92**, 267–271

YOO, T. J., YAZAWA, Y., TMODA, K. and FLOYD, R. (1983b) Type II collagen-induced autoimmune endolymphatic hydrops in the guinea pig. *Science*, **222**, 65–67

16

Sensorineural hearing loss

J. E. T. Byrne and A. G. Kerr

Sensorineural hearing loss is considered in detail in the Adult Audiology volume. However any book on otology would be incomplete without some reference to the subject and the object of this chapter is to give a brief overview of the problem which, in terms of the number of patients seen, represents the greater part of the work load of the average otologist.

The clinician finds himself faced with a difficult diagnostic prospect each time he is confronted by a patient with sensorineural deafness. In this chapter an attempt is made to devise a practical approach to this problem in the everyday setting of the otolaryngology clinic.

Usually the patient has been aware of a hearing loss, but sometimes has not been until attention has been drawn to it, as for example, in pre-employment or some other routine medical examination. Not infrequently the remarks of family or friends will be the stimulus to seek an otological opinion, probably most often because of a tendency to turn up the volume of the television to the annoyance of the family.

Our aim is to devise a method which will chart a useful route through the symptoms and signs of sensorineural deafness towards the identification and management of the underlying pathology, a means by which the benefits of knowledge, experience and intuition, may be put to best use.

It is easy to slip into the habit of looking at an audiogram without enquiring about the nature of the underlying pathology. In many cases a diagnosis will prove elusive but consideration of the pathological basis of the audiogram should be routine practice. In some instances, the most important objective will be a negative one, that is to find out what is not wrong.

In the outpatient clinic

An initial long and detailed history may be wasteful of time and a brief general otological history is taken first. This is followed by clinical examination of the ear, including an assessment of the hearing by tuning fork tests. A pure tone audiogram is then carried out with the measurement of speech discrimination ability in each ear.

With the information gleaned from these initial steps, a more specifically directed history, examination and investigations may then be indicated.

History

Initially, enquiry is directed towards obtaining the patient's outline of his symptoms. When did he first notice hearing impairment? Was it of sudden or gradual onset? Is it unilateral or bilateral? Which ear does he consider to be the better? Is the hearing loss progressive, static or fluctuant? Is there or has there been otorrhoea? Were any incidents or specific circumstances associated with the onset of the deafness? How does the hearing loss affect him in his everyday life? Has he any tinnitus or vertigo?

Examination

A first requirement is the adequate visualization of both tympanic membranes. When the external auditory meatus is occluded by wax, hairs or debris, there may be a temptation to proceed with audiometry on the assumption that the bone conduction curve will at least give an idea of the severity of the sensorineural component of the deafness. This is not necessarily so. A small conductive component can convert a severe sensorineural deafness into an apparently profound deafness (Toner and Kerr, 1987). It is imperative that the ear canals are clear before carrying out audiometry. It is at this time that one ought to detect, and indicate to the audiology technician, an ear canal that may collapse under the pressure of the earphone.

An assessment of the overall ability to communicate will be made at this time and it is easy to eliminate any possibility of lipreading, by talking to the patient while cleaning out the ears and inspecting the tympanic membranes. Such an assessment is of importance both clinically and in medico-legal cases.

In clinical assessment of speech discrimination, it may be essential to mask the contralateral ear with the Bárány noise box. Routine use of tuning fork tests has been denigrated recently but we believe this to be an important clinical discipline.

Patients not infrequently have uncharacteristic difficulty when presented with choices. Allowance must be made for incorrect tuning fork responses occurring in patients who are unable to accept what to them is conflicting information from their senses, e.g. the lateralization to the deaf ear in conductive hearing loss. It may be helpful to use both the 256 Hz and 512 Hz tuning forks. In compensation cases, the responses to the tuning fork tests sometimes indicate a lack of cooperation, the knowledge of which is important when interpreting the audiogram.

Audiometry

Simple pure tone and speech audiometry (PBmax), with masking, have become the anchor of the clinical approach to sensorineural hearing losses. These routine measurements are generally very reliable, although constant vigilance should be maintained with regard to the possibility of spurious audiometric responses. The frequencies normally measured are 0.25, 0.5, 1, 2, 3, 4, and 8 kHz. In many situations it is desirable to include 6 kHz, as measurement of this frequency is required for certain pre-employment examinations including military service and also may be useful in cases of mild noise-induced hearing loss. Most otologists consider it practical to regard the lower limit of normal hearing to be 20 dB. Speech scores are measured, based on 25 phonetically balanced monosyllables, presented at approximately 40 dB above the average pure tone threshold for 0.5, 1 and 2 kHz (Kerr and Smyth, 1972). There is no necessity for the routine performance of the time-consuming speech discrimination curve.

Evaluation of the audiogram

In the absence of a conductive loss there will be three groups:

1 Bilateral hearing loss
2 Unilateral hearing loss
3 Those found to have apparently normal hearing.

In each group, it is important to consider two points:

1 Is the recorded pure tone loss consistent with the clinical assessment?
2 Is the speech discrimination score consistent with the clinical assessment?

In unilateral hearing loss, of course, with normal hearing in the other ear, there should be no difficulty in communicating in the normal clinic situation.

Bilateral sensorineural hearing loss

In bilateral sensorineural deafness, one should note whether the loss is symmetrical or nearly so, and how good or otherwise is the speech discrimination in each ear. In general clinical practice, the commonest cause of bilateral sensorineural deafness is presbyacusis. Schuknecht and Gacek (1993) have identified several types.

Sensory presbyacusis is due to loss of hair cells, possibly secondary to initial loss of supporting cells. This starts at the base of the cochlea and slowly progresses apically. Consequently the low frequencies are untouched initially with a steep fall off in hearing in the high frequencies. Speech discrimination in quiet surroundings remains good until the speech frequencies are affected.

Neural presbyacusis is due to loss of auditory neurons. The whole length of the spiral ganglion is affected, but the effect is more marked at the basal turn (see Figure 4.32). All the frequencies tend to be involved, but the higher frequencies are usually more affected. The prominent feature is a disproportionately severe loss of speech discrimination.

Atrophy of the stria vascularis gives a flat audiogram with good speech discrimination (see Figures 4.33 and 4.34). Although this is a degenerative condition it may also occur in younger people, and frequently affects other members of the family.

Inner ear 'conductive' deafness gives the well known ski-slope audiogram with only slightly impaired speech discrimination.

It is worth noting that the factors influencing speech discrimination scores are the severity of the loss for the speech frequencies, the angle of the audiometric curve, the presence or absence of recruitment and the number of available neurons in the auditory nerve.

Mixed presbyacusis is a combination of some or all of the foregoing types. Most audiograms will tend to be mixtures.

The term *indeterminate presbyacusis* has been applied by Schuknecht and Gacek (1993) to a group of cases that do not show light microscopic evidence of cochlear changes but clinically show as a bilateral symmetrical sensorineural hearing loss which progresses with age and without other obvious cause.

Industrial noise induced deafness is also common in many practices.

Before making a diagnosis of industrial noise-induced hearing loss, a careful work history should be taken. This should include some assessment of the noise exposure, its duration and probable levels. If the person has consistently to shout to communicate with colleagues close by, then there is a strong likelihood that the ambient noise is 90 dB(A) or above.

It is important that a diagnosis of noise-induced deafness should not be made simply on the patient's statement that his work is noisy. 'Noisy' is a relative term, but hair-cell damage does not usually occur in exposure to levels of less than 85–90 dB(A) for an average 40-hour week. A number of patients are likely to engage in litigation against their employers in respect of noise damage. A careful history is important and one must be circumspect in what one says lest a patient is induced to start on a spurious and potentially embittering claim.

Frequent mention is found in the recent literature to losses arising from the leisure activities of young people, including acoustic trauma from fireworks and noise damage from personal stereos, discos and rock concerts. However, as long as they are not also working in noisy environments, the risk to the audience is probably small because of the relative shortness of the periods of exposure. There is a definite risk for the performers, particularly if they engage in long practice sessions in small rooms.

Ototoxic hearing loss is usually bilateral and symmetrical. In those drugs which cause irreversible hair cell damage, the diagnosis usually becomes apparent from the history. However, in the reversible types, such as salicylate deafness, further enquiry may be necessary because some patients fail to admit to the consumption of aspirin or related drugs.

Salicylate deafness characteristically produces a 'flattish' hearing curve accompanied by good speech discrimination. It will usually reverse on withdrawal of the drug.

A *dish-shaped audiogram* is occasionally found, in which the curve exhibits a moderately severe loss for the middle frequencies and good hearing for the high and low frequencies. It is usually without obvious cause and is, by custom, attributed to heredity.

Asymmetrical bilateral hearing loss is often found following weapon firing, particularly one which is fired from the shoulder. The worse hearing is usually in the ear closer to the muzzle. Enquiry in these cases should be made into the type of weapons fired, e.g. high or low velocity, whether or not fired from the shoulder, the frequency of use and number of rounds. Other weapons such as anti-tank weapons, rocket launchers, and mortars should also be enquired about. A history of tinnitus or temporary threshold shift immediately after firing, may indicate ears at risk. When patients are asked about weapons they will sometimes forget to mention sporting weapons including shotguns. Members of shooting teams are particularly at risk. It is useful to remember that some earplugs or earmuffs may not provide adequate ear protection against high velocity weapons.

Asymmetry of high frequency loss may be associated with *head injury*. Indeed it is extremely unusual to find symmetrical high tone sensorineural loss from head trauma. Hearing loss is more probable in these cases if there is a history of unconsciousness following the injury. In general, the longer the period of unconsciousness, the greater the likelihood of a consequent hearing loss. Unconsciousness, bleeding or cerebrospinal fluid leak should be enquired about in deafness associated with head injury.

Hearing loss due to *explosion* is almost invariably asymmetrical. This effect results from the uneven nature of the blast pressure wave.

Hearing loss in late *Menière's disease* may be bilateral and non-fluctuant. Speech discrimination will, at that stage, usually be significantly reduced. Hearing loss associated with *congenital* or *late syphilis* is often bilateral and the speech discrimination tends to be reduced and to fluctuate.

Bilateral vestibular schwannomas (acoustic neuromas) are rare but must be kept in mind and the deafness may or may not be asymmetrical. Central neurofibromatosis (NF2) or a positive family history increase suspicion of this condition.

Each of the causes of unilateral deafness may, of course, occur either bilaterally, or in combination with each other, or with any of the causes of bilateral deafness, resulting in a bilateral sensorineural deafness which is usually asymmetrical.

Unilateral sensorineural hearing loss

Unilateral hearing loss is frequently of sudden onset. Trauma including head injury, acoustic accident, blast injury, and damage at surgery, will come to mind early in the consideration of unilateral hearing loss. There continue to be the sporadic cases of sudden hearing loss which are attributed to some interference with the cochlear blood supply, a viral infection, Reissner's membrane rupture, or a perilymph leak. Some cases may, with careful questioning, be found to be due to childhood mumps, half-forgotten head injury, or possible perinatal causes. A significant number of cases will be seen for which no cause can be determined.

It is in the unilateral group that one is most commonly placed in the position of excluding a vestibular schwannoma.

Recent developments point to the value of magnetic resonance imaging (MRI) with or without gadolinium in the early and secure diagnosis or exclusion of a vestibular schwannoma. Brain stem evoked responses (BSER), serial pure tone audiometry, and a CT scan may be considered valuable in the absence of MRI facilities. There are those who say that MRI must be performed in every patient with asymmetrical or unilateral hearing loss. The practicality of this will depend on local circumstances and hence it is important to make, where possible, an accurate diagnosis of the pathology so as to limit the number of cases in which expensive investigations are required.

Deafness with normal pure tone audiometry

About 5% of patients presenting at an otolaryngology clinic complain of difficulty in hearing against background noise despite normal pure tone audiograms and excellent speech discrimination. This has been given the title of obscure auditory disorder (OAD) by Saunders and Haggard (1989). It appears to be particularly common among patients such as teachers and social workers for whom communication is important in their employment.

Saunders and Haggard have devised a test package which detects psychoacoustic (impaired frequency resolution), cognitive/linguistic (low scores in a dichotic listening test), and personality (anxiety) factors. A patient questionnaire has shown a patient profile which includes difficulties in learning to read or write as a child, adult ear problems and tinnitus.

The major features of the early research into this syndrome have been confirmed by Higson, Haggard and Field (1994).

A diagnosis of neurosis in a patient should be made very reluctantly. Pressure on the central auditory pathways by a tumour has been known to cause severe reduction in speech discrimination in the presence of satisfactory or minimally reduced pure tone hearing loss. Demyelination (multiple sclerosis) affecting the auditory pathway may very occasionally be manifest by poor speech discrimination but a near-normal pure tone audiogram (Saunders and Haggard, 1993).

Fluctuating hearing loss

In taking a history of hearing loss it is important to ask specifically of the patient as to whether the hearing is fluctuant. Care must be taken in assessment of this symptom as occasionally the patient may be describing the variation in ability to hear in quiet and noisy surroundings.

Fluctuating hearing loss usually results from a small number of clear-cut pathological entities. The most common of these is a change in middle ear pressure resulting in minor degrees of conductive hearing loss.

The most common cause of fluctuation of inner ear function is endolymphatic hydrops which occurs in Menière's disease and syphilitic labyrinthitis. Perilymph fistula is a rare cause of fluctuating inner ear function.

In *Menière's disease*, the history of tinnitus and associated episodic rotatory vertigo will determine the 'true' Menière's case, but this leaves a number of cases of low frequency loss which may or may not have tinnitus or dizziness. These may be 'early' cases of Menière's disease. The disease is usually unilateral in the early stages and speech discrimination is generally well preserved until the later stages.

In *congenital* or *late syphilitic labyrinthitis*, the hearing loss fluctuates and the associated vertigo is episodic and rotatory in the early stages. In the later stages with destruction of vestibular function, it becomes constant and is described simply as unsteadiness. A history in early life of treatment, usually injections, for 'eye trouble' (interstitial keratitis), will suggest the diagnosis. Wassermann and Kahn tests will frequently be negative and the fluorescent treponemal antibody absorption (FTA Abs) test will be of most help. The loss is usually bilateral and asymmetrical. In established cases, speech discrimination tends to fluctuate more than the pure tone hearing.

It has been noted that HIV infection very markedly speeds up the development of luetic deafness in those patients who are in the latent stage of syphilis.

Perilymph fistula presents a difficult diagnostic problem and is discussed in Chapter 7.

Mixed sensorineural conductive hearing loss

Mixed sensorineural and conductive deafness presents a challenge to the physiological measurement technician and it is here that one most commonly encounters spurious audiometry. It is always important to ensure that the audiometric findings and clinical judgement are in agreement, especially if there is any question of surgery. A speech discrimination test (PBmax), with adequate masking of the other ear, will provide confirmation that the ear is serviceable or otherwise, and should not be overlooked.

The measurement of bone conduction is a rather artificial concept since it is not necessarily a true reflection of the function of the inner ear. It is well known that the middle ear makes a contribution to bone conduction and that correction of a middle ear conductive lesion causes an apparent improvement in inner ear function. The best known example is the Carhart notch in otosclerosis, but this may also be seen in chronic suppurative otitis media and secretory otitis media. The apparent inner ear hearing loss caused in this way may be to some extent reversible.

It has long been accepted that chronic suppurative

otitis media is often accompanied by sensorineural hearing loss related to the chronic suppurative otitis media but not due to the effect of conductive deafness on bone conduction. Toxins, it has been said, have damaged the inner ear. Walby, Barrera and Schuknecht (1983), in a clinical study of 87 patients with unilateral uncomplicated chronic otitis media, have confirmed that an abnormality of bone conduction does exist. However, in a study of 12 pairs of temporal bones with unilateral chronic otitis media, there was no evidence that the disease resulted in damage to the inner ear. They concluded that the sensorineural loss is due to altered mechanics of sound transmission.

There has been debate about the cause of the sensorineural deafness that is often seen with otosclerosis. Schuknecht (1993) has put forward good evidence that otosclerosis only rarely results in sensorineural loss in the absence of a conductive loss. He also has shown that there is no consistent histological explanation for the sensorineural loss found in ears with otosclerosis. However, all the other causes of sensorineural hearing loss also may occur in association with any of the conductive lesions. One cannot reasonably assume that inner ear function will necessarily improve with correction of the conductive component. Indeed, surgery carries the risk of trauma with an increase in the sensorineural deafness. In cases of industrial noise exposure, a concomitant conductive hearing loss may afford some protection to the inner ear. This is supported by unilateral cases of conductive hearing loss where inner ear function in the 'protected' ear is better than in the 'unprotected' one. However, not all investigators have confirmed this concept of protection for the inner ear by conductive deafness.

Suspected malingering or feigned 'hearing loss'

One must always be aware of the possibility of non-organic hearing loss. This, in the main, will arise in the litigant and less frequently is psychogenic. Public awareness of excessive noise as a cause of hearing loss has resulted in increased interest in civil action in this respect. The individual concerned may occasionally succumb to the temptation to exaggerate his hearing problems.

Suspicion will usually arise in the first few minutes of the interview with the patient. Not infrequently he will, in a rather obvious manner, fail to hear his name being called. In the initial stages of the interview each question may have to be repeated but will usually be heard the second time, despite the clinician keeping the volume of his voice at the same level. Later, as the interview comes to include questions which the patient feels are important to his case, such as enquiries designed to confirm the ab-

sence of other possible causes, he will tend to hear on the first occasion!

In psychogenic cases, suspicion may also arise when the patient appears to have a relative lack of concern about an apparently severe hearing loss.

At audiometry, attempts are made to exaggerate the severity of the loss. Suspicion of this will arise when the recorded hearing levels are inconsistent with his ability to hear the spoken word.

Sudden hearing loss

Sudden hearing loss presents a therapeutic dilemma. There are two schools of thought, broadly represented by nihilism and those who advocate simultaneous multiple drug therapy. The fact that early treatment appears to achieve better hearing need only mean that there is a high rate of spontaneous recovery and that the inclusion of early cases boosts the results! Controlled trials have failed to produce convincing evidence of success and often have produced conflicting conclusions.

If one considers the potential aetiological factors in sudden deafness, then certain treatments, for example steroids, could aggravate the problem they were intended to help; the deafness of viral labyrinthitis may be exacerbated by steroids. For those with a compulsion to prescribe active treatment there is little to be said against bed-rest accompanied by carbon dioxide inhalations in an effort to improve cochlear blood flow. In cases of acoustic incident a period of avoidance of noise exposure is advocated.

Immune sensorineural deafness

Interest continues in inner ear autoimmune disease as a cause of sensorineural hearing loss. There is no doubt that immune disorders can cause deafness which may reverse with immunosuppressive therapy. However, increasing numbers of alleged cases of immune sensorineural deafness are being reported. Many of these may be due to immune reactions but, so far, no clear pattern of clinical presentation has emerged and much more work will be required. It is said that the condition may be sudden in onset or slowly progressive and may be either unilateral or bilateral. It appears to be more common in middle-aged women and in patients with other autoimmune disease. There may also be associated fluctuation of hearing and vertigo. Tests including ESR, serum immunoglobulin assessment and C-reactive protein level, will be of some help. Specific antigen tests have been developed and are under evaluation. Meanwhile one must guard against spurious claims and poorly controlled trials of expensive but dubious treatment regimens.

General management

There is no doubt that demands and expectations with regard to hearing vary from person to person. The person with a hearing loss will, in the main, have five concerns:

1 How bad is the hearing loss?
2 Can it be reversed?
3 Will it be progressive?
4 How will it affect the future?
5 What can be done to help cope with the handicap?

The extent of the deafness should be clearly explained to the patient. He is frequently relieved to hear that he has not been imagining things and that his family have been justified in their complaints. The simple explanation that with a high tone loss one expects increased difficulties in noisy places is found by many patients to be reassuring.

The prognosis of the loss has then to be considered. Unfortunately, most sensorineural deafness is irreversible in our present knowledge, and this should be explained.

Treatment is obviously required for certain conditions such as a vestibular schwannoma or syphilitic deafness. Most cases cannot be improved. Indeed, although some may be static, most will progress slowly. Thus it has usually to be clearly explained that the loss will be permanent, but that any progression in the deterioration of hearing will be very gradual and that the patient will not become completely deaf.

Very occasionally young adults present with hearing problems where the prognosis will affect career choices. Care must be taken to avoid both the optimism that can leave him in a blind alley in middle life, and the pessimism that can put him there instantly. The question of the patient's future must be given serious consideration whether or not the matter is raised.

The Adult Audiology volume (Volume 2) contains chapters on rehabilitation and hearing aids in the management of sensorineural deafness. All that need be said here is that the main factors in success with a hearing aid are the ability to discriminate speech and the motivation to receive help from the aid. When both are poor the outlook is bleak. However, a positive approach from the otologist is of immense help. Constructive advice should be given on the selection and use of an aid, of avoiding if possible, attempting to communicate in noisy places and of the importance of non-auditory clues. Finally, it is reassuring for the patient to know that almost everyone with deafness experiences frustration with himself and irritation in his family.

References

HIGSON, J. H., HAGGARD, M. and FIELD, D. L. (1994) Validation parameters for assessing obscure auditory dysfunction-robustness of determinants of OAD status across samples and text methods. *British Journal of Audiology*, **28**, 27–39

KERR, A. G. and SMYTH, G. D. L. (1972) Routine speech discrimination tests. *Journal of Laryngology and Otology*, **86**, 33–41

SAUNDERS, G. H. and HAGGARD, M. P. (1989) The clinical assessment of obscure auditory dysfunction– 1. Auditory and psychological factors. *Ear and Hearing*, **10**, 200–208

SAUNDERS, G. H. and HAGGARD, M. P. (1993) The influence of personality-related factors upon consultation for two different 'marginal' organic pathologies with and without reports of auditory symptomatology. *Ear and Hearing*, **14**, 232–248

SCHUKNECHT, H. F. (1993) Disorders of bone. In: *Pathology of the Ear*, 2nd edn. Philadelphia: Lea and Febiger. p. 378.

SCHUKNECHT, H. F. and GACEK, R. R. (1993) Cochlear pathology in presbycusis. *Annals of Otology, Rhinology and Laryngology*, **102**, 1–16

TONER, J. G. and KERR, A. G. (1987) Severe sensorineural hearing loss presenting as profound deafness. *Journal of Laryngology and Otology*, **101**, 601–604

WALBY, A. P., BARRERA, A. and SCHUKNECHT, H. F. (1983) Cochlear pathology in chronic suppurative otitis media. *Annals of Otology, Rhinology and Laryngology*, **92**, (Suppl. 103), 3–19

17

Sudden and fluctuant sensorineural hearing loss

John B. Booth

Attention was first drawn to this subject by Citelli in 1926 but much more extensively by De Kleyn (1945) who reported three bilateral and 18 unilateral cases of 'sudden complete or partial loss of function of the octavus system in apparently normal persons'. There have been many contributions on the subject since including the first chapter in a textbook to be given over to it, which appeared in the fourth edition published in 1979.

The cause always remains the main challenge and must, therefore, be sought. Adopting an apathetic or nihilistic approach, because many cases improve spontaneously, will not lead to further understanding nor to the finding of new ways of treatment.

Many of the causes are in themselves extremely rare, not only in otological practice, but still more so to the general family practitioner. Many too, are associated with other symptoms which will initially, and quite rightly, command much greater attention even when the patient may have been admitted to hospital. These will often come within the specific causes listed in Table 17.1. It should be appreciated at the outset that much of what has been written on this subject contains two ingredients – the case report(s) followed by the theory of causation.

Sudden deafness has been reported in an increasing number of unlikely conditions; use of the relevant references will allow the reader with a particular problem to gain further help and information. Byl (1984) has reported a most helpful prospective study over 8 years of 2225 patients who presented with sudden deafness.

It is important to recognize that the classification given in Table 17.1 cannot be rigidly applied. Often two or more conditions may coexist in one patient, while some of the diseases listed may damage hearing at more than one anatomical level. The review of *specific causes* which follows must therefore seem

Table 17.1 Some causes of sudden or fluctuating sensorineural hearing loss

Cochlear
1 Inflammatory, e.g. bacterial, spirochaetal, viral
2 Traumatic
3 Vascular
4 Haematological, e.g. anaemia, embolism, coagulation disorders
5 Autoimmune disease/vasculitis
6 Endolymphatic hydrops, including Menière's disease
7 Metabolic disorders
8 Skeletal system – otic capsule
9 Ototoxicity
10 Miscellaneous (scleroderma, ulcerative colitis, sarcoidosis)

Retrocochlear and central nervous system
1 Meningitis, all forms
2 Multiple sclerosis
3 Friedreich's ataxia
4 Amyotrophic lateral sclerosis
5 Vogt-Koyanagi-Harada syndrome
6 Xeroderma pigmentosum
7 Tumours, e.g. vestibular schwannoma
8 Central deafness

Idiopathic

somewhat diffuse, and it must include some material which is also mentioned in Chapters 15, 16, 19 and 20.

Specific causes

Many of the cases reported seem to be isolated incidences. What can we learn from these widely varying aetiologies? In many the incidence is statistically no greater than chance, but in some the clinical and audiometric pattern, together with temporal bone findings, are of great importance. It should also be remembered that in several of the causes, hearing loss is but one manifestation of a systemic disease from which the patient may also have a generalized toxaemia, metabolic or other major disturbance. In some of these, the deafness occurs when the disease is at its height and is noticed only later when the patient's health improves sufficiently for him to be aware of his misfortune.

Cochlear causes

Inflammatory

Bacterial

Acute otitis media

While the vast majority of cases of acute otitis media never develop sudden deafness, a small proportion do and this may only become apparent in later life when it is noted that the child is turning the only hearing ear towards the sound source or the patient becomes aware of the fact that he cannot use the telephone on that side (Figure 17.1).

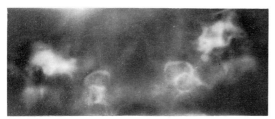

Figure 17.1 X-ray of a 9-year-old girl who suffered a single episode of acute otitis media (untreated with antibiotics) which led to total hearing and vestibular loss. The patient became aware of the hearing loss 2 months later but had no vertigo. Ossifying labyrinthitis is seen on the right side (half of the vestibule and semicircular canals) – left side of the illustration (Booth, 1984, by kind permission of the Editor, *The Physician*)

Typhoid fever

Escajadillo, Alatorre and Zarate (1982) have reported six cases of pathologically confirmed cochleovestibular lesions due to typhoid fever. The lesions occurred between the second and third weeks of the disease, and more often in females. In some of the patients the lesions were reversible. In all but one case the hearing loss was bilateral and slight to moderate in degree and when associated with reduced labyrinthine function on caloric testing, this was unilateral and occurred more often on the left side.

Brucellosis

Brucellosis is a zoonosis which humans contract either by direct contact with infected animals or ingestion of raw meat or unpasteurized milk from such animals. It is caused by one of three strains: *Brucella melitensis* (goats), *B. abortus* (cattle) or *B. suis* (hogs). Neurobrucellosis is an uncommon complication; most of such cases present to physicians with features of meningovascular or cranial nerve involvement. Although the vestibulocochlear nerve is one of the commonest cranial nerves to be involved it is a relatively late manifestation in the natural history of the disease.

Only relatively recently has involvement of the ear been appreciated (Elidan *et al.*, 1985) but there have been earlier reports in the Polish literature. Elidan *et al.* reported a case which showed progressive unilateral hearing loss but this did not start until nearly a year after the initial symptoms; the diagnosis was made 10 weeks after the patient presented when the blood culture was found to be positive for *B. melitensis*. The patient was a laboratory technician in the department of clinical microbiology. In a series of 15 patients with systemic brucellosis, in whom brucella meningitis was suspected clinically, in eight with abnormal CSF with a high brucella titre, the brain stem auditory evoked potentials were abnormal in all. In the seven with normal CSF, the evoked potentials were also normal (Yaqub *et al.*, 1992).

Thomas *et al.* (1993) reported a case in which isolated involvement of the VIIIth cranial nerve was the primary manifestation in neurobrucellosis. Serology showed *B. melitensis* and subsequent treatment with tetracycline and rifampicin failed to reverse the hearing loss.

Spirochaetes

Syphilis (see Chapters 4 and 15)

Either in the congenital or the acquired form, this all-invasive disease can cause sudden deafness. Karmody and Schuknecht (1966) reported congenital syphilis as a cause resulting in a profound and usually bilateral loss, especially in younger patients (see Figures 4.25 and 4.26). They also emphasized that the deafness is usually very sudden and may be partially asymmetrical, possibly with fluctuation.

In the milder case, the hearing loss may be more marked in the low and high frequencies rather than the more conventional flat pattern. It is frequently accompanied by poor speech discrimination. About 5% of patients with late syphilis of the temporal bone present with sudden deafness, while sudden deteriorations in one or both ears occur at later stages of the disease in a further 15%. Sudden bilateral loss in the patients with acquired disease is unusual (Morrison, 1975).

The otological symptoms of late congenital syphilis may be almost indistinguishable from those of Menière's disease. Black, Gibson and Capper (1982) described four cases of fluctuating hearing loss in West African and West Indian racial groups, two of which proved to be Menière's disease.

Lyme disease (*Borrelia burgdorferi*)

Lyme disease was first recognized, in 1975, in the town of Old Lyme, Connecticut, USA. In Great Britain, it is transmitted to man by the tick, *Ixodes dammini* and possibly other biting insects from reservoir infected mammals, particularly deer. Cattle, horses and smaller mammals may also harbour the disease. In the UK it is most common in the New Forest, Hampshire, where the disease is endemic, but it has been found in other areas of Britain, predominantly rural (O'Connell, 1995). A closely related borrelial spirochaetosis has also been identified in Europe, where the tick *I. ricinus* is the vector.

The infectious disease Lyme borreliosis is caused by the tick-borne *Borrelia burgdorferi* spirochaete. The dermatological signs of the disease have been known in Europe for nearly a century, although the causative agent was not known until recently. As in syphilis, neurological manifestations are common and may affect the cranial nerves. Antibody to the flagellin protein of Burgdorferi has been shown to bind to human nerve axons and neuroblastoma cell lines. Successful diagnosis rests on the recognition of a characteristic clinical picture and currently on serological tests. There are three main tests in use for the diagnosis at the moment: immunofluorescent assays (IFA), enzyme linked immunosorbent assays (ELISA) and immunoblots. Each of these tests has been plagued with problems of specificity and sensitivity; a patient suspected of having Lyme disease who is seronegative should have a second sample taken 4–6 weeks later (Curtin and Pennington, 1995) (Figure 17.2) (see Chapter 24).

Hanner *et al.* (1989) investigated the hearing impairment in patients with antibody production against *Borrelia burgdorferi* antigens. They studied 98 patients in 17% (17) of whom there was serological evidence of borreliosis. All but three of these had vertigo and three had a peripheral facial palsy. The hearing of five patients improved with treatment though all 17 were treated with intravenous benzylpenicillin. Two patients had a low frequency hearing loss of sudden onset; four patients had a sudden hearing loss in the high frequency area, one of whom also had a left-sided peripheral facial palsy and intense rotatory vertigo. The hearing of the latter patient returned to normal during treatment. Moscatello *et al.* (1991) investigated 256 patients in an area of New York state in which the disease was highly endemic. Bilateral hearing loss was noted in four patients, who described it as moderate, but no

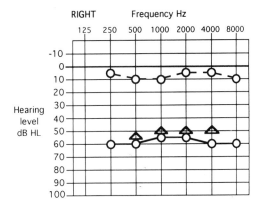

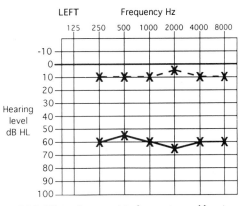

Figure 17.2 Bilateral, symmetrical sensorineural hearing loss in a 39-year-old woman; brain stem evoked response audiometry showed normal wave latency and morphology. The patient had previously been bitten on the legs in the New Forest. Serological tests for Lyme disease were negative. The patient was offered treatment for Lyme disease after further serum sampling and given a 2-week course of oral erythromycin followed by 3 weeks oral cefotaxime axetil 500 mg b.d. Three months after completion of the antibiotic therapy, the patient's hearing returned to normal. Serological tests for Lyme disease were weakly positive with a negative immunoblot test at the start of antibiotic therapy; positive immunoblot test 6 months after treatment confirming that she had had an infection with *Borrelia burgdorferi*. Illustration (audiogram) shows the air conduction thresholds in each ear before (continuous) and after treatment (interrupted lines)

patient underwent audiometry. All the patients were treated and reported resolution of their hearing losses after 10 days to 7 months. (Facial nerve palsy was seen in 12 patients.)

A late manifestation of Lyme borreliosis is acrodermatitis chronic atrophicans. Sandström *et al.* (1989) studied 26 patients with this condition and nine showed a pathological auditory brain stem response (four unilateral, five bilateral). The main pathological findings were: poor reproducibility of waves IV–V, or wave V, or increased latency of wave V. After antibiotic treatment, the auditory brain stem response was improved in eight out of the nine cases and in three it reverted to normal. It is of interest that the pure tone audiogram in all of these patients showed a sensorineural hearing loss of the presbyacusis type. The pure tone audiogram did not differentiate between those with normal and abnormal auditory brain stem responses. Speech audiometry (speech reception threshold and speech discrimination) was normal in all 26 patients. Impedance measurements (stapedial reflex thresholds and stapedial muscle reflex decay) were normal in all the patients except the two who could not be tested satisfactorily.

Richardson *et al.* (1994) investigated 100 consecutive patients who were undergoing investigations for asymmetrical hearing loss. They were a heterogeneous group, and included both subjects with sudden and gradual hearing losses of various patterns. Full serological testing for syphilis was performed, as this is known to give false-positive results in Lyme disease; all were negative for syphilis. Richardson *et al.* had questioned whether patients with an asymmetrical hearing loss should be routinely screened for Lyme disease but found only one patient who was positive; subsequent antibiotic treatment failed to bring about any improvement in her hearing.

Engervall, Carlsson-Nordlander and Bredberg (1990) investigated 82 patients with a facial palsy due to borreliosis. The aim of their study was to identify signs of central nervous system involvement by means of brain stem evoked response audiometry. None of the 82 patients was aware of any hearing loss but 10 had dysacusis. Sixteen of the 82 patients fulfilled the criteria for a diagnosis of borreliosis, 14 of whom underwent brain stem audiometry. Of these, the result was abnormal in five, though this reverted to normal in four patients between 4 and 24 months after the onset of the facial palsy. The brain stem evoked response abnormality mainly consisted of an abnormal amplitude of wave V, and abnormal test-retest reliability, and an unsatisfactory interpretability. The study showed that patients with a peripheral facial palsy due to borrelial infection often display signs of a brain stem lesion.

Rickettsiae

Typhus

Typhus exanthematicus of the louse-borne variety is caused by *Rickettsia prowazekii*. Rickettsiae are coccobacilli and are related to Gram-negative bacilli, having many features in common with viruses. The clinical picture may vary but so far as the otological signs are concerned, hearing loss is a serious, very early manifestation of the disease. A recent report on the temporal bone studies of five cases by Friedmann, Frohlich and Wright (1993) gives further details and is also referred to in Chapter 4 (see Figures 4.22, 4.23 and 4.24).

Mycoplasmas

Mycoplasma pneumoniae

While *Mycoplasma pneumoniae* is a common aetiological factor in a variety of respiratory diseases, involvement of the nervous system has only been observed in perhaps 5% of cases. Shanon *et al.* (1982) reported a girl with left-sided deafness, tinnitus and vertigo, whose investigations indicated a profound hearing loss with reduced labyrinthine activity following caloric stimulation. Brain stem evoked responses showed clear complexes but the transmission time was prolonged and the cochlear microphonic appeared to be abnormal. Three days after commencing treatment with doxycycline, the hearing on the affected side had virtually returned to normal and the discrimination had improved from 40 to 100%.

Nishioka *et al.* (1984) reported a girl who suffered from infection with *Mycoplasma pneumoniae* with primary atypical pneumonia, complicated first by meningitis followed by a mild bilateral acute otitis media with subsequent severe mixed hearing loss; the final outcome after the middle ear infection had settled, was that she was left with a bilateral high degree sensorineural hearing loss, more marked in the low and middle frequencies. Throughout the course of her serious illness she was treated with a variety of agents including minocycline and steroids. There was no impairment of any of the other cranial nerves and likewise no evidence of labyrinthine involvement.

Bullous myringitis

The possible pathology and clinical aspects of this condition have been discussed previously (see Chapters 3 and 7). Rarely, it may be associated with a sensorineural hearing loss, often of sudden onset. Merifield (1962) reported two cases. The first was a 22-year-old girl who developed a severe bilateral hearing loss, predominantly sensorineural, associated with tinnitus. The second case was a 31-year-old female with a unilateral, predominantly sensorineural loss, which returned to its probable earlier near normal level in just over 2 weeks. Wetmore and Abramson (1979) reported three cases, all unilateral (two male) with moderate to severe mixed hearing losses, although predominantly sensorineural, all of which were untreated and whose subsequent audiograms showed normal hearing.

A prospective study was reported by Hoffman and Shepsman (1983) on 15 patients with 21 ears diagnosed as bullous myringitis, seen over a 2-year period. Seven ears demonstrated a sensorineural hearing loss and seven a mixed loss. Recovery of hearing was complete in eight of the 14 ears.

An excellent review of the aetiology of this condition and the possible role of mycoplasmas was reported by Roberts (1980). He could find evidence of only one positive culture of *M. pneumoniae* and he stressed the considerable difficulties of obtaining un-contaminated specimens in this condition.

More recently, Hariri (1990) reported a prospective study of 18 patients studied over a 3-year period. Twenty ears were involved by bullous myringitis; pure tone audiograms and stapedial reflex thresholds were performed within 48 hours of referral. Seventeen ears were noted to have a significant hearing loss, six sensorineural and seven mixed (four conductive); recovery of the sensorineural loss was complete in 8 of the 13 cases. Four patients had a persistent high frequency sensorineural loss including one female who had a bilateral loss.

Chlamydia

The genus Chlamydia comprises two species – *C. trachomatis* and *C. psittaci*. The first is well known and causes a variety ocular and genital infections in man, the best known being trachoma. The second is less often encountered in man but causes several infections in animals, e.g. psittacosis, ornithosis. In recent years *C. psittaci* has been shown to cause endocarditis in man and is well recognized although infrequently as a cause of ocular infections.

Darougar *et al.* (1978) have reported a case with long-standing interstitial keratitis and uveitis associated with a marked otological syndrome and fatal cardiovascular lesions. The girl had a sudden bilateral hearing loss, tinnitus and imbalance. The deafness was initially moderate, sensorineural and symmetrical, with poor speech discrimination. Treatment with prednisolone failed to improve the hearing loss which fluctuated, but always relapsed leading ultimately to almost total loss. Later *C. psittaci* was isolated from the eye and the patient received two courses of doxycycline, which helped the keratouveitis, but otherwise after treatment, there was a definite increase in the intensity of the clinical signs and the number of recurrences.

Viral

Mumps

Hearing loss is uncommon, occurring in less than 0.1% of cases, but adolescents and adults are more likely to be affected. Most reported cases (80%) of sensorineural hearing loss are unilateral.

Bitnum, Rakover and Rosen (1986) reported a case of acute bilateral total deafness complicating mumps in 7-year-old girl. Brain stem evoked responses were completely absent bilaterally. They described three types of hearing loss with mumps: the commonest – insidious onset, unilateral, complete; the next most common – unilateral, partial and frequently undiagnosed at the time; the third, rare – bilateral and complete. Their patient also showed no recovery.

Murakami and Muzushima (1985) reported 53 cases seen over a 10-year period. The hearing loss in their patients was exclusively unilateral, profound or total and permanent, and more than 45% of the patients developed dysequilibrium of vestibular origin. As might be expected, two-thirds of the patients were under 10 years of age, with an equal sex ratio. They considered that the haematogenous infection 'theory' was the most valid, causing inflammatory changes in the stria vascularis of the cochlea, resulting in severe impairment of the endolymphatic system. They proposed 'viral endolymphatic labyrinthitis' as the possible pathogenesis of the deafness.

By an unusual combination of events, Westmore, Pickard and Stern (1979) were able to obtain a specimen of perilymph from a patient with mumps who had developed sudden deafness, which subsequently grew the mumps virus.

Several studies have now been published on sudden deafness and asymptomatic mumps making use of detection of the mumps IgM antibody to establish whether or not recent infection could have been the cause of the hearing loss (Nomura *et al.*, 1988; Koga *et al.*, 1988; Okamoto *et al.*, 1994). Patients with acute mumps deafness may occasionally have vestibular symptoms; Yamamoto, Watanabe and Mizukoshi (1993) in addition to carrying out caloric tests also used the galvanic body sway test (GBST), though only one of their four cases showed an abnormal result.

Hall and Richards (1987) examined the records of 33 children with profound unilateral sensorineural hearing loss of unknown origin. Fifteen gave a history of mumps in whom 12 contracted the infection between the last normal and first abnormal hearing test. They emphasized that the complications of mumps may arise, irrespective of the severity of infection and can occur even in the absence of parotitis.

There have been possible reports of a sensorineural deafness after measles, mumps, and rubella immunization. Of these, six children were reported whose deafness may be related to MMR immunization, or who may have received the Urabe strain of mumps vaccine. In this particular report (Stewart and Prabhu, 1993), the Jeryl Lynn strain was not implicated but both strains have previously been reported to cause deafness.

Measles (rubeola)

It has long been known that measles can cause inner ear deafness and estimates vary widely but in post-war years it seems to be between 5 and 10% of cases (see Figure 4.21). Measles is an important cause of acquired deafness. Before the introduction of rubeola vaccine, 3–10% of acquired deafness in children was secondary to measles.

Children with labyrinthine involvement usually develop abrupt bilateral hearing loss along with the measles rash. However, some children develop only unilateral deafness retaining normal hearing in the opposite ear. The characteristic audiogram is an asymmetric, bilateral hearing loss affecting hearing at higher more than lower frequencies which is usually permanent.

Hulbert *et al.* (1991) have reported a bilateral hearing loss after measles and rubella vaccination in a 27 year-old adult. Approximately 3 days afterwards she developed fever, headaches, tinnitus, dizziness, vomiting and unsteady gait; 22 days after vaccination she was aware of a progressive hearing loss. IgM but not IgG antibodies for rubella were found. A therapeutic trial of steroids and plasmapheresis failed to improve the patient's hearing. Kobayashi, Suzuki and Nomura (1994) reported a patient who developed mumps deafness in the left ear at the age of 26. Ten years later the patient had a rubella infection and a hearing loss in the opposite ear was noted 2 days after the disappearance of the macular rash. When tested 3 weeks later the patient had a mild ascending audiometric curve together with a marked loss at 4000 and 8000 Hz. Treatment with betamethasone for 14 days produced some hearing improvement on repeat pure tone audiometry.

Chickenpox (varicella)

Nervous system complications of chickenpox are relatively infrequent and include cerebellar ataxia, aseptic meningitis, acute transverse myelitis, chicken-pox-Reye syndrome and less commonly, aphasia, hemiplegia and VIIth cranial nerve palsy.

Bhandari and Steinman (1983) reported the case of a 14-month-old infant who developed bilateral sudden deafness. Brain stem auditory responses could not be evoked and there was no subsequent improvement.

Varicella zoster virus

Herpes zoster oticus is well known by all otologists, and sudden deafness with facial palsy forms part of the Ramsay Hunt syndrome. From a clinical standpoint, many patients afflicted by this virus present early because of their symptoms. In zoster deafness the site is sometimes neural, sometimes sensory but most often mixed (see Figures 4.19 and 4.20).

Treatment of this condition is now by oral acyclovir (9–2 hydroxyethoxy-methyl-guanine); this antiviral agent is a DNA nucleoside analogue which inhibits virus DNA replication, thus halting the cell cycle. Acyclovir is relatively insoluble in water and crystallizes in the renal tubules. As a result, it is essential to ascertain that the patient has good renal function throughout therapy.

Wilson (1986) reminds us that 19 out of the 60 patients reported by Ramsay Hunt had auditory symptoms. Wilson investigated the relationship between the herpes virus family to sudden hearing loss and found that herpes infections, in association with sudden viral hearing loss, occur as part of a multiple viral infection in 70% of instances. This feature is unique to herpes virus infections when compared to other neurotropic viral agents. The study also demonstrated the variables of viral hearing loss, such as degree of hearing loss, percentage of recovery, or the incidence of vertigo were unaffected by the presence of herpes virus infections. Hiraide *et al.* (1988) reported two cases of sudden progressive profound hearing loss associated with a Ramsay Hunt syndrome. In their first case, the unilateral hearing loss failed to recover with steroid hormone therapy; the second was treated by the antiviral drug vidarabine and also failed to recover.

Recently MR imaging in patients with Ramsay Hunt syndrome has shown enhancement, not only in the facial nerve but in the vestibular and cochlear nerves, particularly in those patients with vertigo and tinnitus. Kuo *et al.* (1995) have recently reported such a case showing discrete enhancement of the facial and vestibulocochlear nerves; while the facial nerve regained full function, the sensorineural hearing loss persisted. Downie *et al.* (1994) were able to demonstrate persistent enhancement beyond 6 weeks which had hitherto been thought to be the limit for such changes still to be demonstrable. Their case with labyrinthitis, sensorineural hearing loss and facial nerve palsy showed marked enhancement of inner ear structures 6 months after the onset of symptoms. They used axial and coronal T1-weighted images before and after contrast enhancement and they suggested that the fast spin echo high resolution imaging without enhancement, which is often used for screening patients with vestibular schwannoma, will probably miss the changes they found in the facial nerve and labyrinth in patients with Ramsay Hunt syndrome.

Koide *et al.* (1988) investigated 61 patients with sudden deafness who were seen within 7 days of onset. There was no significant difference in the incidence of positive tests for neutralizing antibodies to type 1 herpes simplex virus in the patients compared with the control. However, the proportion of subjects who were positive for antibody to type 2 herpes simplex virus was significantly higher than the patients in the control group. They felt that these results indicated there might be some relationship of herpes simplex virus to sudden deafness and that reactivation of a latent infection might play an important role in the aetiology of this disease.

Human spumaretrovirus (HSRV)

Pyykko *et al.* (1993) screened 1310 patients with various diseases in whom complement or other viral antibody assays were requested; only two patients were seropositive. However, in a group of 30 patients with sudden deafness, four had a positive antibody against HSRV.

The human spumaretrovirus is a recently characterized retrovirus which was originally isolated from patients with various neoplastic and degenerative diseases. Hitherto it has not been possible to identify HSRV as the causative agent of any specific disease. Experimental findings indicate that HSRV may be a neuropathic virus, similar to related retroviruses, the human immunodeficiency viruses and human T-cell leukaemia viruses. In two of the four cases associated with sudden deafness, the incidence was bilateral. Because of this unusually high proportion of positive results, the authors recommended further screening for this virus in sudden deafness.

Infectious mononucleosis

The nervous system may become involved in some 1% of cases of infectious mononucleosis. Schnell *et al.* (1966) reviewed 1285 patients seen at the Mayo Clinic over a 14-year period and reported one case who showed a temporary bilateral hearing loss on the fourteenth day, 7 days after admission; the audiogram showed a 60 dB hearing loss at 2000 Hz which gradually improved and was normal 1 year later.

Taylor and Parsons-Smith (1969) reported a patient who developed other cranial nerve signs; Petheram (1976) described a patient whose infection was characterized by a severe autoimmune haemolytic anaemia with autoantibody of anti-i specificity. Further cases have been documented by Gregg and Schaeffer (1964), Jaffe (1967) and more recently by Beg (1981). Site of lesion tests in these cases have indicated cochlear damage and in the two cases reported by Beg, brain stem evoked responses were normal as were caloric tests. Only the first and last cases mentioned have been bilateral and all but one have occurred in females! As also might be expected in this condition, the patients are young, only one being just over 30 years of age.

Lassa fever

Lassa fever is an acute, insidious arenavirus infection that is endemic in West Africa (Rybak, 1990). Cummins *et al.* (1990) in a most interesting paper described a prospective audiometric evaluation of 69 hospitalized febrile patients in Sierra Leone. There was a 29% incidence of sensorineural hearing loss in confirmed cases of Lassa fever, seven of which were bilateral. Sensorineural hearing loss was also present in 17.6% of 51 patients who had previously had Lassa fever. Many of the patients with severe disease were treated by a 10-day course of the intravenous antiviral agent Ribavarin. In all these 17 deaf patients the antibody to Lassa virus was present before the clinical onset of the hearing loss and their deafness occurred approximately 5–12 days after the fever had subsided. Eight patients showed significant recovery and at the final assessment, nine had a residual hearing deficit (six unilateral, three bilateral). There was no obvious association between the percentage of recovery and the severity of the initial hearing deficit. Antiviral therapy did not seem to reduce the severity of the deafness.

Liao, Byl and Adour (1992) investigated a series of 17 patients with Lassa fever. Data were available from 12 patients (20 ears) giving a bilateral incidence of 88%. The hearing loss was mild in seven ears but severe or profound in nine. They found the hearing recovery to be normal or complete in 10 ears, partial in five and there was no change or a worsening in the five remaining ears.

Human immunodeficiency virus (HIV) and acquired immunodeficiency syndrome (AIDS)

Infection by the human immunodeficiency virus may affect the external, middle and inner ear in addition to the condition on occasion producing vertigo and facial nerve involvement. The overall picture is well summarized by Lalwani and Sooy (1992). Representative cases of the various presentations were published by Linstrom *et al.* (1993). The human immunodeficiency virus is a retrovirus which has the enzyme reverse transcriptase which functions to transcribe viral RNA to DNA, which is then incorporated into the genetic make up of target cells. The HIV virus has been shown to be a lymphotropic virus, attacking principally T-helper cells, as well as a neurotropic virus. As a result, AIDS is characterized by an underlying suppression of cell-mediated response leading to the development of opportunistic infections and/or malignant tumours (Rarey, 1990).

In addition to the primary ear infection, secondary opportunistic infection is well recognized, the most common causative agent being *Toxoplasma*, others being *Pneumocystis carinii* and *Aspergillus*; cryptococcal meningitis may also occur (Breda *et al.*, 1988; Kohan, Rothstein and Cohen, 1988; Strauss and Fine, 1991; Hall and Farrior, 1993; Lyos *et al.*, 1993). Of course mycotic infections of the temporal bone did occur before AIDS and even in the non-immunocompromised patient, but were rare (McGill, 1978; Meyerhoff *et al.*, 1979). Some 35–55% of patients with AIDS have a past history of venereal disease including syphilis, though some people with AIDS may not live long enough to develop otosyphilis as it is a tertiary manifestation. The HIV virus may activate latent syphilis. It has also been noted that there is an increased incidence of otosyphilis and this appears to develop at an accelerated rate from the primary infection; it is thought that this may occur because of the profound defects in cell-mediated immunity (Johns, Tierney and Felsenstein, 1987; Hart *et al.*, 1989; Smith and Canalis, 1989).

In addition to the possible discharge from the external meatus and obvious hearing loss particularly due to conductive involvement, pain is frequently mentioned as one of the presenting symptoms. Auditory evoked responses had been investigated in patients infected with the human immunodeficiency virus in an attempt to ascertain early brain stem involvement (Figure 17.3). Isolated changes within the brain stem have been noted but Birchall *et al.* (1992) investigating 18 HIV-positive males in different CDC stages found one-third had abnormal brain stem evoked responses or pure tone audiometry. However, they could find no correlation with the T-cell subset and only a weak correlation with the pure tone audiometric average. Auditory and visual event-related potentials were investigated by Welkoborsky and Lowitzsch (1992) and Baldeweg *et al.* (1993).

Cases of sudden sensorineural hearing loss have been reported in HIV infection both as a presenting symptom (Timon and Walsh, 1989) and in a patient in whom the infection had already been diagnosed

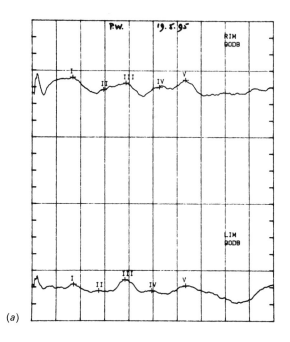

(a)

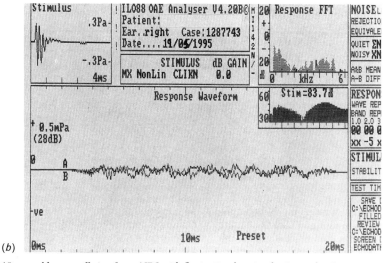

(b)

Figure 17.3 A 40-year old man suffering from AIDS with fluctuating hearing for 6 months. Pure-tone audiogram 16 days before showed a mild high tone sensorineural hearing loss. (*a*) Brain stem auditory evoked responses; (*b*) otoacoustic emissions

and with other symptoms evident (Real, Thomas and Gerwin, 1987). Grimaldi *et al.* (1993) reported a patient who presented with a febrile illness and who, 2 days later, suffered a sudden bilateral hearing loss. Patients with an appropriate background who experienced a sudden bilateral hearing loss must therefore now be considered candidates for infection with human immunodeficiency virus if no other obvious cause is apparent.

Primary central nervous system lymphoma and systemic lymphoma with central nervous system involvement constitute the majority of central nervous system tumours in the AIDS population. Kaposi's sarcoma metastatic to the central nervous system is less common but may also be associated with hearing loss (Lalwani and Sooy, 1992).

In recent years temporal bone reports of ears involved by AIDS have been reported. Michaels, Soucek and Liang (1994) reported on 49 bones from 25 patients, five with severe otitis media, 15 with low grade otitis media, two with labyrinthine cryptococcosis, one Kaposi's sarcoma with a deposit in the VIIIth nerve and six with cytomegalovirus in the inner and middle ear. Chandrasekhar, Siverls and Sekhar (1992) also reported histopathological and ultrastructural changes but noted that the organ of Corti was normal. Pappas *et al.* (1994) reported on the extracellular viral-like particles with morphological characteristics of HIV/1 identified in the tectorial membrane in three cases. Morris and Prasad (1990) noted that the HIV virus, which is known to be neurotropic as well as lymphotropic, has never yet been cultured from the VIIIth cranial nerve or from spiral ganglion cells.

Protozoa

Toxoplasmosis

Toxoplasmosis is an infectious disease caused by the protozoan, *Toxoplasma gondii*. The cat is the principal host and may excrete infectious oocysts. Infection in man occurs after ingestion of contaminated, undercooked meat or by contact with infected animals. The ingested parasites invade the epithelium of the intestine, multiply in the mesenteric lymph nodes and later spread haematogenously to other organs. The acquired infection is common. The most common clinical manifestation is lymphadenopathy which may be local or generalized. Infection of the central nervous system may occur but is uncommon in the immunocompetent patient. Hearing is rarely affected in acquired toxoplasmosis.

Katholm *et al.* (1991) reported a case of sudden deafness and a total loss of vestibular function first in the right ear and 3 months later also in the left. Treatment with sulphadiazine and pyrimethamine was successful in retrieving the hearing to such a degree that the patient was enabled to communicate by means of a body-worn hearing aid and lipreading.

Traumatic

Electricity

It is generally considered that individuals unlucky enough to be struck by lightning are either killed or suffer no untoward effects. While reports are few, lightning may affect the ears. Most incidents occur while the individuals are conversing on the telephone during a thunderstorm.

The most frequent damage is acoustic rupture of the tympanic membrane caused by the sonic shock wave emanating from the access of the lightning channel. This can occur whether the lightning strikes the person himself or the ground nearby. Burning of the skin surrounding the ear may be seen and an exit burn on the feet may also occur when the skin is wet. Although the perforation is usually unilateral, bilateral rupture has been reported. Redleaf and McCabe (1993) reported three cases of lightning injury to the tympanic membrane, one of which was bilateral. Analysis of their cases suggested that the mechanism of injury was direct conduction of electricity from the scalp to the soft tissues of the external auditory meatus to the tympanic membrane. They considered the conduits of the electrical surge to be the subcutaneous blood vessels, smaller being damaged more than larger vessels.

Recently Gordon *et al.* (1995) reported four cases of lightning injury to the tympanic membrane which they followed up for several months, before proceeding to myringoplasty closure. They emphasized the possibility of squamous epithelium being imploded leading to subsequent pearl formation. They also emphasized the possible poor hearing characteristics of such a perforation and possible reperforation after several months. Jones *et al.* (1991) reported four patients, the first of whom received bilateral oval window fistulae while the other three cases were in the same hunting party, all of whom were struck with different results. They commented upon the fact that in all the cases reported there had been no ossicular problems.

Sensorineural hearing loss may also occur and this too may be bilateral; the loss is usually transient but may last for a longer period, although it is seldom permanent. Bergstrom *et al.* (1974) reported the temporal bone pathology of one of their four cases who died 5 days after being struck.

In 1988, Youngs *et al.* reported the second temporal bone case of a patient who developed profound bilateral sensorineural hearing loss as a result of a lightning strike to the neck.

Cordless/portable telephones have also been found to pose a threat to hearing on a small number of occasions. These units have the ear receiver doubling as the ring or bell device. The output of the bell can be in the 140 dB range on the A scale. In those instances in which a permanent sensorineural hearing loss has been documented, the user was holding the telephone against the ear when the ringing occurred, and in three instances reported by Singleton *et al.* (1984) a loud extraneous crack was transmitted. Unlike regular cord-type telephones, these devices have no automatic gain control in the receiver unit. Singleton *et al.* (1984) reported 13 cases; five separate brands of cordless telephones were involved though one brand was involved in eight out of the 13 cases! They also reported a further 18 cases who had sufficient records and audiometric tests to be evaluated. The most severe hearing loss was found at 500 and 1000 Hz; at these two frequencies the mean pressure of the injured ear was poorer by 20 dB and 29 dB respectively. The ring in cordless telephones is a complex signal, characterized by a peak energy level of around 750 Hz (Orchik *et al.*, 1987).

Iatrogenic

Radiotherapy

Radiotherapy given to head and neck tumours, particularly those situated in the parotid and postnasal space, regularly involves its application to the ear and the organ of Corti. For many years it was considered that the cochlea was resistant to radiotherapeutic injury. This was strongly challenged first by Leach (1965) and later by Moretti (1976). Earlier work has been well summarized by Talmi, Finkelstein and Zohar (1989). They reviewed the seven papers published previously adding a single case of their own. More recently, Grau *et al.* (1991) reported on 22 patients whose hearing was tested, prior to irradiation for nasopharyngeal carcinoma, and again 7–84 months afterwards. They found a significant correlation between the total radiation dose to the inner ear and observed hearing impairment. Sensorineural hearing loss was most pronounced in the high frequencies with values of up to 35 dB (4 kHz) and 25 dB (2 kHz). The latent period for the complication appeared to be 12 months or more. The radiation dose was found to significantly influence the degree of hearing loss. The inner ears of six patients were not included in the treatment fields but the remaining 32 ears received 39–60 Gy; a significant correlation between the radiation dose and the level of sensorineural hearing loss was found in these patients. Four patients in the high dose group had severely abnormal auditory brain stem responses; two of these patients also had clinical signs of brain stem dysfunction and the hearing of these two patients was also severely affected. Schot *et al.* (1992) reported 30 patients who had been treated by surgery and radiotherapy for a parotid gland neoplasm (pleomorphic adenomas). Total doses less than 55 Gy seldom cause hearing loss in contrast to those above 65 Gy. Audiometry showed a significant increase in hearing loss in 1–2, 4–8 and 10–20 kHz ranges; the loss increased with frequency. Evans *et al.* (1988) reported on 45

patients after radiotherapy for unilateral parotid gland tumours who had been seen previously over a period of 18 years. Twenty attended for follow up review some 2–16 years later (mean 8 years). The total dose was 5500–6000 cGy over a 5–6 week period; the daily fractions were 200–220 cGy. The ipsilateral side received a full tumour dose while that on the contralateral was negligible. They found that a hearing loss was not detected in the irradiated ear when compared with the non-irradiated side of each patient. Chowdhury *et al.* (1988) carried out a prospective study of the effects of ventilation tubes on hearing after radiotherapy for carcinoma of the nasopharynx. From this, two small but interesting facts also emerged. The first was that tinnitus was frequently present and often distressing but in those without a ventilation tube, the tinnitus was significantly worse by the end of 6 months; conversely in those in whom a ventilation tube was inserted there was a marked and significant improvement in their tinnitus. The second fact was that there was a small increase of 3 dB in the average sensorineural threshold in the non-ventilated group after 6 months; this was not found in the ventilated group.

Gabriele *et al.* (1992) carried out a study on the vestibular apparatus disorders after external radiation therapy for head and neck carcinoma. Twenty-five patients had their vestibular function investigated by electronystagmography (ENG). The radiation dose administered to the vestibular system ranged from 2800 to 5120 cGy. Five patients suffered subjective vertigo or dizziness and three of these showed vestibular abnormalities on ENG. The patients were evaluated after the end of radiotherapy and at 3 and 6 months. At the first evaluation abnormal caloric responses were found in 12% and sinusoidal rotatory test abnormal responses in 4%. These figures increased to 36% and 20% respectively when re-evaluated at 6 months. They concluded that the vestibular disorders seemed to be related to the total radiation dose.

Smouha and Karmody (1995) emphasized the non-osteitic complications of therapeutic radiation on the temporal bone and described four cases as examples to show the soft tissue changes.

Radiotherapy to the postnasal space for carcinoma can also produce injury to the temporal lobe (Leung, Kreel and Tsao, 1992). In nine of the 60 patients examined by them the extent of the disease was such that one of the eye shields in the anterior portal had to be omitted to obtain adequate tumour coverage. This, and that the patients were treated with a hyperfractionation schedule giving 67.2 Gy in 42 fractions in 6 weeks were significant. No patient in their study had temporal lobe injury in the absence of these two factors. The earliest case of asymptomatic temporal lobe injury was found at 26.5 months after radiotherapy and the earlier symptomatic case at 28 months. All the symptomatic cases had well developed hypodense shadows in the white matter of the temporoparietal lobes associated with significant pressure effects such as midline shift.

Postoperative

Several cases of deafness following surgery have been reported. It seems most generally accepted that these are due to microembolism involving the cochlear division of the internal auditory artery.

Ness *et al.* (1993) carried out a prospective analysis of 1458 patients who underwent *aortocoronary bypass surgery* of whom 181 volunteers entered, and of these 145 patients completed the study. Acute or sudden sensorineural hearing loss within 2 weeks following the bypass surgery was not identified in any patient completing the study. It should not be forgotten that patients undergoing bypass surgery often have pre-existing and concurrent medical diseases which demand polypharmaceutical therapy. Preoperative sensorineural hearing loss of some type was present in 76.6% of the 145 patients who completed the study. The most frequent type of hearing loss was a high frequency sensorineural pattern. No patient had an immediate postoperative hearing change. Four patients actually showed objective improvement on postoperative testing. A subset of seven patients undergoing intraoperative brain stem evoked responses experienced increased absolute as well as intrapeak latency changes in waves I, II and V; the onset of these changes appeared to be related to hypothermia starting at 30°C. (All of these patients had essentially normal hearing.) Of the 145 patients, only four reported a subjective hearing loss after surgery and objective testing failed to confirm this. It is thought that new, smaller blood and pump filters of 60 μm, may prevent some of the possible microemboli causing central nervous system injury.

Perhaps it may be added as an interesting footnote that the effect of hypothermia upon the electrocochleogram and auditory evoked responses was investigated by Kusakari *et al.* (1984) in 10 children undergoing open heart surgery. The latencies of N1, waves III and V were prolonged. The summating potential was increased by hypothermia and never disappeared; on rewarming the summating potential appeared first, followed by N1, and finally waves III and V. Markand *et al.* (1987) reported 10 adult patients who underwent open heart surgery under induced hypothermia and had brain stem auditory evoked potentials recorded at 1–2 °C steps as the body temperature was lowered from 36° to 20 °C. Hypothermia produced increased latencies of waves I, III and IV. The latencies and, in particular latency I–IV, increased roughly 7% for each 1 °C drop; they doubled at a temperature around 26 °C. The amplitude rose with hypothermia to 27 °C but increased

linearly with further cooling. All components were present at temperatures above 23 °C but absent below 20 °C. With rewarming the change is reversed and the brain stem auditory evoked potentials returned to initial pre-hypothermia levels. Hypothermia produces several neurophysiological changes, the most prominent being the slowing of axonal conduction and depression of synaptic transmission due to impaired transmitter release. The effect on synaptic transmission appears to be more profound than on axonal conduction. The latency of the cochlear microphonic, which is a summated receptor potential, remains constant at a temperature as low as 18 °C, whereas the latency of N1 (compound cochlear nerve potential) of the electrocochleogram increases progressively with hypothermia. Conversely, raising the body temperature by 1°C in nine subjects significantly shortened the latency of wave V, while there were similar though less consistent changes in other waves (Bridger and Graham, 1985).

Anaesthesia

Much has been written in recent years about the effect caused by nitrous oxide on the middle ear pressure during general anaesthesia and as to whether the gas is given by inhalation or ventilation.

Patterson and Bartlett (1976) reported four cases of hearing impairment after anaesthesia, three receiving ear surgery and a fourth who underwent an orthopaedic operation but was already suspected of having a perilymph leak from a previous stapedectomy (which was subsequently confirmed at operation and closed). In all four, the hearing returned.

Davis, Moore and Lahiri (1979) reported the case of a patient who 1 year previously had undergone a successful left stapedectomy with complete closure of the air-bone gap and who subsequently underwent a hysterectomy operation. This was followed by a 20–25 dB conductive hearing loss which persisted thereafter.

Hearing loss after general anaesthesia has been reported on a small number of different occasions with widely differing procedures but it is almost always unilateral. Hochermann and Reimer (1987) reported a bilateral hearing loss following repair of a rectal prolapse under a 2-hour general anaesthetic; it was a low frequency loss, mainly sensorineural. A slight gradual spontaneous recovery was seen during the first 2 months but thereafter there was no further improvement. Journeaux *et al.* (1990) reported an interesting case of sudden hearing loss as a complication of a non-otological operation which occurred following a left adrenalectomy in a patient who had previously undergone bilateral stapedectomy operations for otosclerosis. The hearing loss occurred in the left ear on the sixth postoperative day; the right ear appeared to be unaffected.

Spinal anaesthesia

Transient hearing loss, occasionally associated with vestibular symptoms, has been reported on a few occasions following the use of water-soluble contrast media for lumbar myelography.

Panning, Mehler and Lehnhardt (1983) carried out a prospective study of 100 urological patients and found eight cases of transient hearing loss, in three of whom an audiogram was performed. A year later they found a further three cases. The results are identical: there was a hearing reduction of 10–40 dB in the low frequency range and usually both ears were affected. They commented that the hearing loss is transient, requires no therapy and is often overlooked. Two of the same authors (Panning and Lehnhardt, 1986) commented on the transient hearing loss after lumbar myelography with metrizamide. They thought that the delayed occurrence was explained by the indirect action of the contrast medium via systemic absorption. Panning and Lehnhardt thought that the more obvious explanation of the pathogenesis in the endolymphatic hydrops was due to the spinal fluid hypotension caused by the spinal puncture.

In 1986, Wang reported a case of sudden bilateral hearing loss after spinal anaesthesia. A 22 G needle had been inserted into the third lumbar interspace; the following day the patient noticed a bilateral hearing loss (10–45 dB within the low frequency range). The patient was treated with a low molecular weight Dextran and prednisolone for 3 days and the symptoms disappeared after 5 days and audiogram on the ninth postoperative day showed an improvement. At follow up 6 weeks later, the patient subjectively had no residual auditory deficit. This prompted the author to carry out further investigations publishing further papers in 1987 (Wang, Fog and Bove) in 1990 (Fog *et al.*) and 1992 (Sundberg, Wang and Fog). These investigations on patients undergoing spinal anaesthesia for transurethral resection of the prostate came to the conclusion that the shape of the tip of the needle seemed to be of some importance, i.e. the pencil-point design (Whitacre) was to be preferred to the standard design (Quincke), and the 26 was to be preferred to 22 gauge. Hearing loss was most noticed between 125 and 500 Hz. Earlier Vandam and Dripps (1956) had carried out a long-term follow up of patients who received 10 098 spinal anaesthetics. They had pointed out the incidence of headache was much less when needles of smaller diameter (24 as opposed to 22 gauge) were used. They found ocular difficulties in 0.4% and auditory difficulties in a similar proportion. 'Spinal' headache occurred in 11% and these were postural in nature, appearing in the assumption of the erect position and usually relieved by recumbancy. With few exceptions the hearing troubles were associated with typical postural headaches.

Lee and Peachman (1986) reported on a unilateral hearing loss in a patient undergoing elective caesarian section under spinal anaesthesia with a 25 gauge spinal needle who experienced a total left-sided hearing loss on the second postoperative day. This was still present on the fourth postoperative day and was associated with dizziness and nausea. They used a blood patch with 10 ml autologous blood injected into the epidural space at the site of the previous lumbar puncture. Shortly after the blood patch was performed the hearing began to improve and completely and permanently recovered about 1 hour later.

Hardy (1988) reported two cases of hearing loss following the implantation of an intrathecal catheter for the control of cancer pain. Withdrawal of fluid in his two cases was associated with a drop in hearing, on one occasion almost total, while if the volume of fluid withdrawn was replaced by 20 ml isotonic sodium chloride then the hearing improved in both patients. In the first patient this was only temporary and a few days later epidural blood patching was required which brought about a resolution of the hearing loss. More recently, Michel and Brusis (1992) published nine cases of hearing loss following myelography, lumbar puncture, and spinal anaesthesia. Hearing loss was seen in eight of the nine patients in the lower frequencies and on both sides in six. Recovery to normal hearing was noticed in six patients. They speculated that this rare complication only occurs in those with a wholly or partially patent cochlear aqueduct and occurs via the release of perilymph into the CSF. Hohmann, Lohmann and Schwager (1993) carried out auditory threshold and brain stem evoked potential studies on 50 patients before and after myelography. While significant functional disorders of the auditory pathway could be demonstrated, most of these were subclinical and only 12 patients showed slight subjective alterations. The changes in brain stem audiometry can be explained by changes in osmolality of the inner ear fluids which may lead to the development of temporary endolymphatic hydrops.

Sudden deafness after dental surgery

Farrell *et al.* (1991) reported four cases, all unilateral, seen over a 3-year period, in which one occurred bilateral extractions after a general anaesthetic. They occurred after 6 hours, 1, 3 and 7 days, were gradual in onset but all four remained permanently deaf. The duration of the procedures carried out is not stated.

Vascular

While vascular disease or its effects are frequently proposed as the principal cause of cochlear-type sudden hearing loss, the number of occasions when they have definitely been implicated is relatively few. Recent studies using casts have shown the vascular supply to the inner ear in great detail (Shatari, Hosoda and Kanzàki, 1994). It is therefore perhaps worth examining some of the conditions or factors which may be related.

Hypertension

An early study between sensorineural hearing loss and arterial hypertension by Hansen (1968) was uncontrolled and unconvincing. Drettner *et al.* (1975) looked at a series of cardiovascular risk factors including blood pressure and heart rate but could find no significant correlation between these and sensorineural hearing loss when assessing 1000 men aged fifty. Studies of the cochlear and vestibular arteries, as well as the labyrinthine arteries, showed that they remain patent at all ages (Fisch, Dobozi and Greig, 1972). No close relationship between the changes in the inner ear and the supplying vessels has been found, nor in patients dying of hypertensive disease. Similarly there is no evidence of atherosclerosis occurring in any of the smaller vessels supplying the ear.

Susmano and Rosenbush (1988) reported an investigation into hearing loss and ischaemic heart disease. They found that the probability of a patient with a hearing loss of unknown aetiology having ischaemic heart disease was eight times higher than in individuals with normal hearing. In the hearing loss groups, there were no significant differences in sex, hypertension, obesity or smoking.

A recent study by Gates *et al.* (1993) investigated the relationship of hearing in the elderly to the presence of cardiovascular disease and cardiovascular risk factors. They determined the hearing status in a cohort of 162 elderly men and women and compared this with their 30-year prevalence of cardiovascular disease. They found that the low frequency hearing was related to cardiovascular disease events in both sexes but more in women. Hypertension and systemic blood pressure were related to hearing thresholds in both sexes. The blood glucose level was related to the pure tone average in women and high density lipoprotein levels were inversely related to low frequency hearing thresholds, but only in women. There was a small but statistically significant association of cardiovascular disease and hearing status in the elderly that was greater for women than men and more in the lower than the higher frequencies.

Over the last 7–8 years a series of papers from a small number of centres has reported the work of a select group of distinguished investigators on cochlear blood flow comparing the different methods of radioactive microsphere measurements and laser Doppler (LD) flowmetry and the influence of various agents, both systemic and topical. These have shown the effect of haemodilution (Hultcrantz and Nuttal, 1987; Nuttal *et al.*, 1988), noise (Prazma *et al.*, 1988), breathing carbon dioxide, intravenous phenylephrine (Sillman *et al.*, 1988) and angiotensin II

(Kawakami *et al.*, 1989, 1991a), hydralazine, sodium nitroprusside, papavarine, nicotinic acid, verapamil and histamine (Ohlsen *et al.*, 1992).

As it will be appreciated the microsphere method can only be used in the experimental animal and it has therefore been investigations into the comparability of cochlear blood flow measured by laser Doppler flowmetry which is of the most interest in the hope that this might be possible clinically. Experiments in the guinea-pig have shown that the time-dependent flux change (wave form) was the same throughout a single cochlea but different between cochleae of the same animal (Ren, Nuttal and Miller, 1993). Flux motion could be limited by inhalation of pure oxygen or 5% CO_2 in oxygen. In experiments, also in the guinea-pig, Ohlsen *et al.* (1994) showed that laser Doppler flowmetry compared well with the microsphere surface method. As might be expected, the results indicate that the laser Doppler recording reflects the regional blood flow close to the probe but not the total cochlear blood flow. In their study they confirmed that nicotinic acid does not significantly increase cochlear blood flow and while they clearly demonstrated that sodium nitroprusside applied to the round window membrane did influence cochlear blood flow it would seem unlikely that this has clinical application in a patient in the light of our present knowledge!

It will be appreciated that the laser Doppler measures flux not flow. Because of the design of the laser Doppler flowmeter it is relatively insensitive to flow in large vessels. Miller *et al.* (1991) in their measurements on human cochlear blood flow suggested that the cochlear vasculature contributing to the LD measurement comprises principally if not exclusively the vessels of the lateral wall immediately beneath or under the probe tip. Nakashima *et al.* (1992) tried measuring cochlear blood flow with laser Doppler probe tips with optic fibre separations of 0.8, 0.9 and 1.0 mm with an outer diameter of 1.7 mm. Removal of the middle ear mucosa over the portion of the probe tip reduced the laser Doppler output from 50% to 80% of the previous level, demonstrating the blood flow of the middle ear mucosa should not be neglected. Even after the middle ear mucosa was removed, pulsatory movement of the laser output was still observed. The output from cochlear blood flow is considered to be detected from the lateral wall of the cochlea because laser light does not reach the central portion of the cochlea adequately. It is interesting to note that in both the experiments by Miller *et al.* (1991) and Nakashima *et al.* (1992) inhalation of carbogen (5% CO_2, 95% O_2) or even short periods with 10% CO_2 and 90% O_2 failed to produce any increase in cochlear blood flow!

The secondary effects of vascular obstruction to the inner ear in experimental animals are well known. Occlusion of the vertebral and basilar arteries has been reported in a single case associated with marked atherosclerotic changes in the vessel walls and an aneurysm of the left vertebral artery (Kitamura and Berreby, 1983). Ectasia of the basilar artery is a rare cause of sensorineural loss and this is usually unilateral and progressive, accompanied by vestibular symptoms and other neurological abnormalities. A study of seven patients with sudden unilateral partial vestibular loss has been described by Lindsay and Hemenway (1956). The findings in a 57-year-old man who had sudden onset of dizziness and unilateral deafness 2 months prior to death have been reported by Gussen (1976).

Belal (1980) reported on the pathology of vascular sensorineural hearing impairment. He examined the temporal bones of two patients with some sudden sensorineural hearing loss. He found the changes to be similar to those in the cochlea after it had been deprived of blood following surgical removal of an acoustic tumour resulting in severe degenerative changes that had progressed to total ossification of the cochlear spaces.

Sando, Ogawa and Jafek (1982) have reported the inner ear pathology including temporal bone findings following injury to the VIIIth cranial nerve and the labyrinthine artery. The first case, in which both the nerve and the artery were severed surgically revealed severe pathological changes in the cochlea including complete loss of the organ of Corti and moderate pathological changes in the fairly well-preserved vestibular end-organs. In the second case, in which the nerve only was sectioned but the artery preserved, the organ of Corti and vestibular end-organs appeared to be well preserved and normal. These findings suggest that the blood supply from the labyrinthine artery plays a major role in maintaining most of the structures in the inner ear except for the endolymphatic sac and that the vestibular end-organs are more resistant than the organ of Corti, to the effects of damage to the labyrinthine artery (see Figure 5.20).

There have been several recent reports using more modern diagnostic methods of assessing the blood flow through the vertebrobasilar system. Kikuchi *et al.* (1993) evaluating 102 patients with dizziness or vertigo who were 50 years of age or over, using magnetic resonance imaging, found slow blood flow in the vertebrobasilar system in 35%. They recommended that because MRI can detect both infarct in the hind-brain and slower blood flow in the vertebral and basilar arteries it should be used for evaluation of vascular disorders in older patients with vestibular symptoms. Mark *et al.* (1992) carried out MRI studies with gadolinium and showed cochlear enhancement on the side of the sudden hearing loss in all the patients. The vestibular enhancement correlated with both subjective and vestibular symptoms and objective measures of vestibular function by electronystagmography. They felt that labyrinthine enhancement in patients with auditory and vestibular symptoms was a new finding and indicative of labyrinthine

disease. Yamasoba *et al.* (1993a) have also carried out MRI studies and shown slow blood flow within the vertebrobasilar arteries in 57 patients with sudden deafness. They detected slow blood flow in 21% predominantly over the age of 50 years. A second MRI scan performed in five patients 2 months after the onset of symptoms showed recovery of blood flow. All 12 patients complained of vertigo. They emphasized in the discussion that the significance of the slow blood flow in sudden deafness is as yet unknown.

Biavati *et al.* (1994) reported a 68-year-old man who had a sudden hearing loss and an ipsilateral facial palsy. MRI demonstrated a lesion in the right inferior pons, suggestive of a postischaemic oedematous focus. Kano *et al.* (1994) performed MRI studies with contrast on 30 patients with unilateral sudden deafness. In seven of these, the cochlea and/or vestibule showed higher signal intensity on proton density and T2-weighted images on the diseased side. These findings suggest changes in the chemical composition of the perilymph and/or the endolymph since proton density and T2-weighted images reflect water content.

Takeuchi *et al.* (1994) have reported on the haemodynamic changes in the head and neck after ligation of the unilateral carotid artery using colour Doppler imaging. They performed the study more than 2 weeks after head and neck cancer surgery in eight patients who had undergone unilateral ligation of the external carotid artery and in three who had undergone unilateral ligation of a common carotid, internal and external carotid arteries. The main collateral pathway to the ligated external carotid artery region was the ipsilateral occipital artery through Richter's anastomosis from the vertebral artery.

Even with the advantage of laser Doppler flowmetry, the considerable anatomical variation in the branching of the cerebellar arteries in experimental animals such as the guinea-pig and the rat make experiments occluding various branches difficult in their interpretation and possible subsequent extrapolation to similar flow in man. Randolf, Haupt and Scheibe (1990) produced proximal obstruction of the basilar artery in the guinea-pig which led to a reduction in cochlear blood flow of between 10–25%. Inui *et al.* (1994) occluded the left anterior inferior cerebellar artery and using autoradiographic measurement of the regional brain stem blood flow showed a decrease in the ipsilateral vestibular nucleus of 31% and the cochlear nucleus of 47% compared with the same nuclei on the right. Using electrocochleography, the action potential disappeared completely after at least 7 minutes and the polarity of the summating potential changed from negative to positive but the cochlear microphonic did not disappear completely ante mortem. Experiments by Makino and Morimitsu (1994) examined the effect of occlusion of branches of the basilar artery on endocochlear DC potential and cochlear blood flow. From these it was clear that the anterior inferior cerebellar artery supplied blood to the cochlea in more or less all animals (guinea-pigs), although the reduction of the blood volume by its occlusion was not enough to decrease the endocochlear potential in some animals. When this vascular dysfunction occurred in the anterior inferior cerebellar artery of such animals, other branches of the basilar artery and/or posterior inferior cerebellar artery will play an important role to maintain cochlear circulation. Experiments in the guinea-pig by Suzuki, Nakashima and Yanagita (1993) investigated the effects of increased cerebrospinal fluid pressure on cochlear and cerebral blood flow. Cochlear blood flow was reduced by increased CSF pressure but the reduction was not persistent. Although inner ear pressure was elevated to the same level as CSF pressure, cochlear blood flow was not decreased by the pressure elevation as much as cerebral blood flow. Their results suggested the cochlear blood flow was relatively resistant to increases in CSF pressure.

Vertebrobasilar insufficiency is a clinical syndrome and should not be equated with a diagnosis (Hofferberth and Hirschberg, 1988). While vertigo is the most frequent accompaniment, hearing loss is relatively rare (Bruyn, 1988). According to consensus, the vertigo in vertebrobasilar insufficiency is the central vestibular type. However, Huang *et al.* (1993) have reported sudden bilateral hearing impairment in vertebrobasilar occlusive disease in seven out of a series of 503 patients with this problem. Watanabe *et al.* (1994) have reported two cases of sudden deafness from vertebrobasilar artery disease. The first was a 19-year-old man who had a right sudden hearing loss after a superselective embolization for the peripheral area of the right vertebral artery – operative procedure for removal of a right parietal temporal meningioma. The second was a 59-year-old woman who had an ipsilateral sudden hearing loss just after the accidental cutting of the left vertebral artery during the procedure of neurovascular decompression for facial spasms. Neither patient showed other signs of central nervous system disorder.

Grotemeyer (1990) investigated abnormal haemorheological parameters in vertebrobasilar insufficiency; 20% of these patients had no vascular risk factor. The distribution of haemorheological parameters was comparable to those in patients suffering from stroke or transient ischaemic attacks. Abnormal platelet reactivity was seen in 78%, plasma viscosity in 57%, fibrinogen in 23%, red blood cell aggregation in 13% and haematocrit in 11% of all cases. Fuse (1991) carried out auditory brain stem responses in two patients with vertebrobasilar ischaemia and found a decrease of the amplitude of all waves and a delay in wave latencies. The same author in an experimental study in the guinea-pig showed the changes in the auditory brain stem response reflected the degree of ischaemia in the auditory pathway but

noted that a non-responsive auditory brain stem response did not imply an irreversible ischaemic condition.

Brownson *et al.* (1986) reported two cases which may be of interest; following manipulation of the cervical spine a sudden unilateral sensorineural hearing loss was produced. The first case was of a 29-year-old woman who had her neck manipulated for a sprained shoulder, headaches and tension; immediately thereafter she had a moderately severe sensorineural hearing loss in the left ear with a speech discrimination of 16%. Aortic arch and cerebral angiograms revealed normal carotid arteries and a dominant right vertebral artery but the left vertebral artery had a 1 cm long focal high grade stenosis with a residual lumen of 1 mm width at the level of the second vertebral body. She was successfully treated with aspirin 600 mg and dipyridamole 100 mg t.d.s. for 1 month. Six weeks later her audiogram was almost normal. The second patient was a 45-year-old man with pain in the left shoulder and neck who was manipulated and who was immediately troubled by vertigo, nausea and vomiting and some diminution of vision. Further manipulation led to an immediate loss of hearing in the right ear with tinnitus. Angiography showed the caudal half of the basilar artery to be occluded, its cephalic portion filling through the posterior communicating artery. The hypoplastic right vertebral artery had a smooth tight diffuse stenosis with a lumen of less than 1 mm. The dominant left vertebral artery had luminal irregularities and stenoses at 20–30% of its diameter. Treatment was similar to the previous case; 6 months later the audiogram revealed only a slight improvement but there was a significant improvement in the speech discrimination score from 20 to 44%.

Rinehart *et al.* (1992) have reported the case of a 25-year-old man who presented with a left-sided hearing loss, tinnitus, vertigo and nausea of one day's duration. A profound sensorineural hearing loss was found but a CT scan showed no abnormality. Three months later, he presented with a 3-day history of a headache, vomiting and neck stiffness; the hearing loss was unchanged. A repeat CT scan and cerebral angiography revealed a 6–7 mm saccular aneurysm arising from a loop of the anterior inferior cerebellar artery at the porus acousticus. The patient's hearing loss was unchanged after surgical clipping of the aneurysm.

Buerger's disease (thromboangiitis obliterans cerebri)

Cerebral involvement in patients with Buerger's disease is rare; it has been estimated as less than 0.5%. Kirikae *et al.* (1962) have reported a single case. A moderate smoker, after developing intermittent claudication, noted a hearing loss on the same side. While an injection of vasodilator drugs improved the leg, there was no improvement in the hearing loss. Five years later the radial artery of the opposite side became slowly occluded over 2 months. At surgery, part of the artery was excised and the diagnosis was confirmed histologically. Seven months after the operation, the patient became suddenly deaf on the same side (that is the opposite side to the earlier loss). Both sides showed a sensorineural loss with absence of recruitment (see also Polyarteritis nodosa).

Hypercoagulation (thrombophilia)

In addition to the clinical syndromes with known haematological characteristics, a further, less well-defined group exists whose common feature can best be described as 'hypercoagulation'. The clinical diagnosis of hypercoagulation is characterized by recurring episodes of thrombosis and sometimes pulmonary embolism.

It is known that the stria vascularis has a slow blood flow in those with a high haematocrit value. It has therefore been suggested that stasis of blood flow and accelerated coagulation may be the twin interrelated factors responsible. There is no evidence of hypercoagulability in such patients except perhaps when their illness is at its most extreme.

Fibrinolytic activity and capacity were studied by Bomholt, Bak-Pedersen and Gormsen (1979) in a group of 18 patients with sudden sensorineural hearing loss and were found to be reduced in 12.

Noda *et al.* (1985) investigated 16 patients with vertigo (no mention is made of hearing loss or audiological tests) in whom no significant difference could be found in the fibrinogen or plasminogen content nor the fibrin-degradation product level and healthy adult controls. Similarly, no difference could be found in the alpha 2-macroglobulin content, alpha 1-antitrypsin or C1-inactivator content between the two groups. However, there was a significant difference in the antiplasmin activity and antithrombin activity and between the ADP- and collagen- induced platelet aggregations which were decreased in the patients with vertigo.

Vague *et al.* (1986) found significant correlations between body weight and plasma insulin, plasma insulin and triglyceride level and total cholesterol with age. They found plasma fibrinolytic activity did not correlate with the concentration of tissue-type plasminogen activator but there appeared to be a strong relationship between plasma insulin level and plasminogen activator inhibitor. They noted that several earlier studies in man had shown that obesity was associated with decreased fibrin activity and increased blood insulin levels. Lalanne *et al.* (1992) investigated 79 patients suffering from audiological disorders, mean age 61 years, for the possibility of haemostatic or rheological disorders. No statistical variation was observed in platelet count, packed cell volume, fibrinogen level or all other coagulation tests except TPI (thromboelastogram potential index).

Einer *et al.* (1994) investigated 32 consecutive patients with sudden sensorineural hearing loss to see if there was any apparent abnormality in their haemostatic mechanisms. Twenty-five showed some aberration of specific haemostasis parameters. Seven showed an increase in plasminogen 1 activator and increased plasminogen levels were most frequently observed among patients who were overweight. Seven of the oldest patients had an increase of D-dimers and most of these had a history of cardiovascular disease. From their results they considered that isolated aberrations in the haemostatic pathway did not seem to be of decisive importance for the pathogenesis of sudden hearing loss. It is of interest to add a study by Omori and Ikeda (1994) who investigated the possibility of intravascular hypercoagulability in patients with recent Bell's palsy. In their group of 84 patients, abnormally high levels of thrombin-antithrombin III complex (TAT) and alpha-II plasmin inhibitor-plasmin complex (PIC) were found. Values tended to be higher in patients seen within 3 days after the occurrence of the palsy compared with those seen 4 days or later. The severity of the facial nerve paralysis and its prognosis when compared with patients with high TAT and/or PIC levels did not show any significant difference. Patients with hypertension and/or diabetes, tended to have higher PIC levels than did their other patients.

Viscosity

Ischaemia is not only determined by vascular disease but also by blood viscosity and it has been suggested, particularly in patients with sudden deafness, that increased blood viscosity may play a role, but this has never been proven. Browning, Gatehouse and Lowe (1986) investigated the relationship between hearing threshold and blood viscosity, plasma viscosity, and haematocrit in 49 patients with idiopathic hearing loss. They established that hearing thresholds were unrelated to haematocrit or low shear blood viscosity but hearing impairment at high frequencies was directly related to high-shear blood viscosity and inversely related to plasma viscosity. The derived measure of red cell rigidity was significantly related to hearing thresholds at all frequencies. The significant negative relationship between plasma viscosity and pure tone hearing thresholds is perhaps contrary to expectations, but of even more interest is their finding that the greater the high shear blood viscosity, the poorer the sensorineural thresholds. High-shear blood viscosity, once corrected for the haematocrit and divided by plasma viscosity (relative viscosity), is a measure of red cell rigidity or lack of deformability under shear. It is unknown whether this lack of red-cell deformability is a primary or secondary phenomenon. Conversely, the high-shear viscosity values were all within the normal range and in conditions such as haemolytic anaemia, in which red cells are less deformable, there is no known association with hearing impairment. This situation is not dissimilar from the finding of fluctuating hearing in some patients with secondary hyperlipoproteinaemia, whereas so far hearing loss has never been reported in association with the primary condition.

In two further studies, Gatehouse *et al.* (1989) and Gatehouse and Lowe (1991) came to slightly different conclusions to their earlier report. In the 1989 contribution, they investigated a subset of 124 persons out of a total of 342, selected on a basis of likely sensorineural hearing loss. They found a significant relationship between whole blood viscosity and hearing level at all frequencies. In the 1991 report, Gatehouse and Lowe found strong correlations between whole blood viscosity of high shear rate and hearing thresholds of 250, 500, 1000 and 2000 Hz. At 4000 and 8000 Hz, the hearing threshold was related to red cell filterability. The data suggested a strong association between aspects of blood rheology and sensorineural hearing impairment, but in a more complex manner than had been suggested by their previous studies. The results imply that there are two processes associated with sensorineural hearing impairment, one of which can be considered due to bulk rheological properties, while the other appears more related to the properties of the individual red cells. The bulk properties are more important at lower frequencies, while the cellular properties are more influential at higher frequencies. Whole-blood filterability in sudden deafness was investigated by Ciuffetti *et al.* (1991). They found that the filterability of the red cells and whole blood were significantly impaired in those patients with sudden deafness. The impairment in red cell filterability was directly correlated with that in whole blood. No significant variations were observed in unfractionated leucocyte filterability or plasma viscosity. Hall, McGuigan and Rocks (1991) investigated red blood cell deformability in 12 patients with sudden sensorineural deafness; five patients had reduced deformability, including three out of four patients with a recent upper respiratory tract infection. Red cell deformability has a significant effect on blood flow in the peripheral circulation, particularly in small calibre vessels. Red cell deformability is an important determinant of whole blood viscosity, especially at high shear rates. One of the conditions by which it can be affected is diabetes mellitus.

A similar and more recent study by Ohinata *et al.* (1994) also investigated viscosity in patients with sudden deafness. In their 51 patients in the sudden deafness group, the blood and plasma viscosity were significantly higher than in the control group (70). The difference between the two groups was greater at the higher shear rates. During the course of treatment, blood and plasma viscosity decreased with the improvement of the hearing impairment. When the distribution of the average hearing level was 40–79 dB, a few of the recovery or good improvement and most of the fair improvement or no change patients belonged to the low viscosity group. Most of the patients of the flat type hearing impairment or a few patients with the high tone hearing impairment belong to the high viscosity group. (Blood and plasma viscosity were measured at three levels of shear rate: 75.22, 150.45 and 376.12/s^{-1} 37°C.)

Desloovere *et al.* (1991) have shown that patients with sudden hearing loss with a plasma viscosity > 1.7 (H$_2$O = 1) have a poorer prognosis. They also found evidence of superior treatment results with hydroxyethyl starch pentoxifylline infusions in patients with elevated plasma viscosity. Most patients were seen within 3 days. Following Dextran, plasma viscosity increased and the auditory improvement was significantly poorer than following hydroxyethyl starch when plasma viscosity fell.

Axial migration of the blood corpuscles is encountered in capillaries and arterioles with a diameter of < 100 μm. The corpuscular constituents of blood flow in the middle of the vessel surrounded by a plasma mantle. As a result blood viscosity in these small vessels approximates to plasma viscosity (the Fåhraeus-Lindqvist effect). Plasma viscosity depends primarily on the concentration of large molecular proteins. These include fibrinogen, α-2 macroglobulin and immunoglobulin M. The haematocrit is proportional to the log of whole blood viscosity. Determinations of fibrinogen concentration have not been found helpful in the management of sudden sensorineural hearing loss either as a causative factor or in treatment.

Haematological

Haemopoietic system

Anaemia, as such, has rarely been reported as being associated with deafness, sensorineural or otherwise. Morrison and Booth (1970) reported two patients with profound anaemia (haemoglobin levels of 6.2g/dl) associated with iron deficiency – both had a sudden bilateral total loss and neither showed any improvement following transfusion. A report from China by Sun *et al.* (1992) investigated 426 patients with idiopathic sudden hearing loss in a prospective study over a 14-year period. They found 42.5% of patients with haemoglobin concentrations less than 13.0 g/dl in men, 12.0 g/dl in women and 10.5 g/dl in children. The serum iron concentrations were also significantly lower than in the normal controls. Twenty-five patients (22.3%) with idiopathic sudden hearing loss who had either iron deficiency anaemia or had serum ferritin levels < 0.70 nm/l. Low concentrations of red cell basic ferritin and abnormal circadian variations in the serum iron level were also observed in the affected patients. Hearing improvement was still achieved in 53% of the patients whose treatment was started later than 3 months after the onset of hearing loss. It is interesting to note that the iron deficient cell is poorly deformable and can itself lead to a poor blood flow in small vessels; it may also lead to a considerable underestimation of the packed cell volume.

Morrison (1978) has reported a 58-year-old woman who awoke with sudden total bilateral deafness whose electrocochleogram confirmed that there was no action potential or cochlear microphonic on either side. She was found to have some megaloblastic change in the bone marrow and a plentiful supply of iron; she had a moderate anaemia due to folic acid deficiency. No recovery subsequently took place in the hearing.

Deafness may be associated with Fanconi's anaemia – constitutional aplastic anaemia (Harada *et al.*, 1980). Tinnitus has recently been reported as the presenting symptom in a case of pernicious anaemia, with normal hearing, which resolved with treatment (Cochran and Kosmicki, 1979). Aplastic anaemia in three patients who subsequently developed sudden sensorineural hearing loss has been reported by Ogawa and Kanzaki (1994). Their patients developed a sudden profound complete sensorineural hearing loss accompanied by tinnitus and severe vertigo. There was a marked drop in the platelet count prior to or just at the time of the acute episode of hearing loss. The prognosis for hearing recovery was poor in each patient.

Polycythaemia vera

In polycythaemia vera, the viscosity of the blood is increased five to eight times normal; the total red cell count becomes elevated by 20–50% and the total blood volume is increased to two to three times normal. These alterations affect the peripheral blood by causing engorgement of the capillaries, venules and arterioles with high viscosity, slowly circulating oxygen-deficient blood.

It had been indicated in an earlier report on two patients with a bilateral sensorineural hearing loss, that the hearing fluctuated in relation to the viscosity of the peripheral blood and that the level improved after phlebotomy (Davis and Nilo, 1965). However, Kenyon, Booth and Newland (unpublished data, 1984), in a small series of patients with this condition treated by large volume isovolaemic haemodilution and a separate group with Waldenstrom's macroglobulinaemia, treated by plasma exchange, showed that while the viscosity changed after 'treatment', there was no observable change or improvement either in the pure tone audiogram, or in the susceptance or conductance on otoadmittance measurements (220 and 660 Hz).

Cerebral blood flow in polycythaemia is significantly reduced.

Sickle-cell disease

While sickle-cell disease is not generally considered as a cause of deafness, it has been shown by Todd, Serjeant and Larson (1973) that sensorineural hearing loss of apparently gradual onset can occur. Until recently, this loss had only been reported in the homozygous disease (abnormal haemoglobin S–S disease). Both ends of the audiometric range may be affected but more often the higher tones. The sickling phenomena occur and crisis develops when certain intermolecular hydrophobic bonds form with subsequent polymerization. Any decrease in the Po_2 with associated hypoxaemia can initiate the process and the concomitant stasis, hyperviscosity, or acidosis significantly increases the likelihood of sickling. The end effect is tissue hypoxia. In the inner ear it is considered that the sickling and impaired blood flow in the cochlear venous system with secondary anoxia of the hair cells and stria vascularis are the most likely causes of the sensorineural hearing loss. Todd, Serjeant and Larson (1973) found a sensorineural loss in 22% of their 83 patients. They considered two possible pathological causes – anaemia and thrombosis. The haemoglobin level in SS disease was considered unlikely to reflect the oxygen carrying capacity since the decreased oxygen affinity of haemoglobin S allows greater oxygen release/gram haemoglobin than in haemoglobin A. Furthermore, the oxygen affinity is lower in cases with chronic anaemia.

The haemolytic process characteristic of sickle-cell disease is associated with an increase in bone-marrow activity. Active bone marrow is present in the petrous temporal bone in SS disease but Serjeant, Norman and Todd (1975) failed to find evidence that this caused any narrowing of the internal auditory meatus or compression of the VIIIth cranial nerve. In this condition the hearing loss may be gradually progressive, fluctuant or sudden in onset; in the last, partial or almost total recovery may occur (Morgenstein and Mannace, 1969; Urban, 1973; Orchik and Dunn, 1977). There is some dispute as to whether the number and frequency of the haemolytic crises may be a factor. Sensorineural hearing loss in patients with sickle cell disease may also be related to the increased susceptibility to bacterial meningitis. Neurological involvement is a common complication of sickle cell disease and vestibular dysfunction may occur.

Odetoyimbo and Adekile (1987), in their study on patients aged 6–15 years, reported that 58.3% of those who had sensorineural hearing loss had their first vaso-occlusive episode before the age of 1 year and more than 90% before the age of 5 years. They concluded therefore that the cochlear microvasculature in young infants was more susceptible to occlusion during sickle cell crises. Ajulo, Osiname and Myatt (1993) studied 52 patients with homozygous sickle cell disease but only seven (13.5%) were found to have sensorineural hearing loss at two or more frequencies. Hearing loss was unilateral in two and bilateral in five. There was no uniformity in the pattern of hearing loss affecting different frequencies in the relevant patients. Their results did not show any relationship between the incidence of hearing loss and age (age range 8–57 years). Gould *et al.* (1991) investigated 34 adults with sickle cell disease but could find no consistent audiometric pattern that was pathognomonic.

Morrison and Booth (1970) reported one case of bilateral deafness in sickle cell trait (haemoglobin S and C) which they presumed to be thrombotic. Tavin, Rubin and Camacho (1993) reported a case of sudden sensorineural hearing loss in haemoglobin SC disease. The abnormal haemoglobins S and C result from different substitutions of the sixth position of the beta chain of the haemoglobin molecule. Patients with haemoglobin SC disease may manifest the same symptoms as patients with sickle cell anaemia, although these symptoms occur less frequently. They reported a 43-year-old woman with sudden onset of decreased hearing in her right ear. On audiometry, a mild, sloping, sensorineural hearing loss was found with speech discrimination reduced to 48% on that side. Ten days later hearing in the same ear had diminished by an average 15 dB at each frequency but the speech discrimination reaching zero. She received two exchange transfusions of two units each. Post-transfusion haemoglobin electrophoresis showed values of S level of 18% and haemoglobin C of 22%; values when the pure tone and speech audiometry were repeated are not given. One year post-partial exchange transfusion showed pure tone speech thresholds of 20 dB and 96% discrimination. Brain stem auditory evoked responses 7 months after the initial presentation showed normal neural conduction. It should be noted that the patient subsequently became HIV positive and died of complications of that disease. It was presumed that she had developed this from HIV-infected blood either prior to the initial screening for the virus or from a donor with such recent acquisition that antibodies were not identifiable in the blood screening. Earlier Crawford *et al.* (1991) had investigated 75 adults with sickle cell disease and found that those with sickle cell C disease had the greatest incidence of hearing loss (9/13); those with Hb SB$^+$-thal also showed a high incidence of hearing loss (4/8) while those with Hb SB°-thal showed no association (0/4).

Sickle cell thalassaemia has been described in two out of a family of four sisters, another of whom had sickle cell trait and the fourth was normal. The two sisters with sickle cell thalassaemia showed symptoms of vertigo or hearing involvement, and vertigo after strenuous exercise. One sister with unilateral hearing loss subsequently developed a sudden, almost identical loss in the other ear, but unfortunately follow up was impossible (Marcus and Lee, 1976).

More recently, O'Keeffe and Maw (1991) reported a case of sudden total deafness in a patient with sickle cell thalassaemia. She developed bilateral otalgia on a holiday flight while cruising at high altitude and the following morning on waking had a bilateral partial deafness worse on the left side. On referral 1 month later, examination showed a marked sensorineural hearing loss on the left and a lesser loss on the right. The haemoglobin level was 7.9 g/dl, a drop of approximately 2 g/dl from the patient's normal level. Within 2 weeks there was almost no recordable hearing in the left ear and a falling curve on the right. Three weeks later there was no hearing in either ear whatsoever. One year later the patient remained completely deaf.

Thalassaemia

Onerci *et al.* (1994) carried out audiological and impedance measurements in 34 thalassaemic patients, 27 with thalassaemia major and seven intermedia. They noted the interesting finding that the majority of patients had an air-bone gap even though there was no negative middle ear pressure. In these patients, a high degree of static compliance and normal shaped, stiff amplitude normal pressure tympanograms were observed; in most acoustic reflexes could not be obtained.

Patients with thalassaemia require to be transfused to maintain their haemoglobin levels and in sickle cell disease regular exchange transfusion is used to maintain low HbS levels but in so doing there has been concern about the problem of iron overload. Conversely it has been known for quite a long time that there is the possibility of desferrioxamine (an iron chelating agent) causing ototoxicity and because of this there has been an obvious need to strike a balance between treatment and side effects.

Back in 1980, Cohen *et al.* investigated the vision and hearing during desferrioxamine (desferrioxamine) therapy. They investigated 52 regularly transfused/chelated patients, 51 of whom were symptom free but one developed a mild bilateral high frequency sensorineural hearing loss. It has also been noted that sensorineural hearing loss has occurred with unusual frequency in patients with primary haemochromatosis.

Olivieri *et al.* (1986) examined a series of 89 patients receiving nightly subcutaneous desferrioxamine infusions for transfusion-dependent thalassaemia major. Thirteen presented with visual loss or deafness, or both; examination revealed 27 more. The hearing loss was characteristically high frequency. Twenty-two patients had abnormal audiograms; with reduced dosage, reversal was complete in four, partial in one; those affected tended to be younger, have lower serum ferritin levels and self-administering higher doses of desferrioxamine per kilogram of body weight.

More recently, Porter *et al.* (1989) investigated risk factors in thalassaemic patients and attempted to produce guidelines for safer dosage. They studied 47 patients with thalassaemia; sensorineural hearing loss was only present in those who had previously received desferrioxamine (37, 30 in patients with thalassaemia major and seven with thalassaemia intermedia). Nine of the 37 patients who had received desferrioxamine had abnormal audiograms and displayed bilateral symmetrical high frequency sensorineural hearing loss in four of whom it was severe. Two patients developed tinnitus and one of these also had a vestibular neuropathy. Auditory brain stem responses in two patients with a severe hearing loss showed a normal result. Sensorineural hearing loss was only present in those patients who had received desferrioxamine but a clear trend was observed between the highest dose of the chelating agent received by each patient and the hearing loss. It was found that a low serum ferritin was also a risk factor. The younger patients with thalassaemia major showed the most severe sensorineural damage following use of the chelating agent. The authors went on to produce a therapeutic index in an attempt to produce a safe guideline for desferrioxamine administration.

Albera *et al.* (1988) carried out audiometric screening of 153 children aged 5–18 years affected by beta-thalassaemia treated with regular blood transfusions and iron overload chelation with desferrioxamine. Thirty-eight per cent showed a significant sensorineural hearing loss at high frequencies and the hearing loss was greater in the younger patients. It was also noted that the hearing loss appeared to be correlated with the mean and peak desferrioxamine doses administered and was higher in subjects with lower iron overload. Argiolu *et al.* (1991) reported 309 patients, aged 3–18 years, with thalassaemia major receiving desferrioxamine therapy. Until 1985 they had used a regimen of 40–100 mg/kg by subcutaneous infusion for 10–12 hours. In 1986, they had reduced it to 40–50 mg/kg per day. Of the 309 patients examined, 48 (15.5%) had sensorineural hearing impairment that was symptomatic in four.

The ability of the brain to biosynthesize ferritin in response to prolonged contact with haemoglobin iron was thought by Koeppen and Dentinger (1988) to be the most important factor in the pathogenesis of superficial siderosis. In a most interesting paper they note that the cerebellar cortex and VIIIth cranial nerves are especially susceptible to iron encrustation. They came to the conclusion that the severe damage of the VIIIth nerve in superficial siderosis was clearly related to the central nervous tissue in its substance. The transition from central to peripheral nervous system in the VIIIth nerve is located near the internal auditory meatus rather than near the brain stem as for most other cranial nerves, though they acknowledge this observation was by no means new. The VIIIth cranial nerves are as vulnerable to iron solutions as other central nervous system surfaces.

Parnes and Weaver (1992) reported on eight cases, seen over 30 years, of superficial siderosis of the central nervous system causing sensorineural hearing loss. Initially superficial siderosis was considered to be a form of haemochromatosis but was later diagnosed as a distinct entity. The condition is usually a result of repeated episodes of subarachnoid haemorrhage which can be derived from any source.

Bribitkin *et al.* (1994) have reported a case of superficial siderosis causing hearing loss and ataxia. The symptoms of the condition are caused by the deposition of haemosiderin in the central nervous system as a result of a current or persistent extravasation of blood into the cerebrospinal fluid. Clinically such patients present with cerebellar ataxia and progressive sensorineural hearing loss. Unfortunately, the signs and symptoms rarely indicate the site or cause of the bleeding. The diagnosis is confirmed by characteristic MRI findings (marginal hypointensity). The marked hypointensity is caused by the magnetic susceptibility effect of the iron of haemosiderin deposits in the pial and arachnoid membranes on the T2-weighted images. Lai *et al.* (1995) have also reported a case with bilateral progressive hearing loss over about 4 years accompanied by tinnitus and absent caloric responses (bilaterally) but good speech discrimination.

Waldenstrom's macroglobulinaemia

This condition, which tends to occur in elderly males, is characterized by retinal changes, an abnormal bleeding tendency from mucous membranes, generalized weakness and dyspnoea.

Waldenstrom's macroglobulinaemia is a primary plasma cell dyscrasia in which there is produced an excess of monoclonal macroglobulin of the IgM variety. This results in an increased blood viscosity which gives rise to circulatory disturbances caused by an increased resistance to blood flow. As a result the formation of complexes between macroglobulins and specific clotting factors, such as factor VIII, leads to a bleeding diathesis which is a feature of Waldenstrom's macroglobulinaemia and this is further complicated by interference of the macroglobulins with platelet function and a low platelet count due to bone marrow infiltration.

The condition is most often met in otolaryngological practice as a cause of epistaxis or bleeding from the gums, but a few cases of sudden deafness have been recorded, although vertigo may be the earliest symptom. Immediate diagnosis is essential if the patient is to be prevented from probable permanent bilateral deafness. The optic fundus must be examined and may reveal gross retinal haemorrhages or central vein thrombosis.

Keim and Sachs (1975) reported five patients, three

whom gave a history of periodic dizziness. They suggested that the cupulae may be altered by the macroglobulins affecting their ability to act as gravity receptors. The unique feature of the three cases with dysequilibrium was the episodic history of positional vertigo which historically resolved with their treatment for the macroglobulinaemia.

Feldman (1981) reported a single case of a 37-year-old man who suffered a sudden hearing loss and had been affected by Waldenstrom's macroglobulinaemia for 3 years. He stated that a complete recovery occurred but does not say how this was achieved. He also reported a sudden hearing loss in a patient with secondary porphyria and severe hepatosplenomegaly, leucopenia and thrombocytopenia.

Wells, Michaels and Wells (1977) reported four cases with otolaryngeal symptoms. A bleeding diathesis manifested itself as epistaxis in two cases. Hyperviscosity was thought to be the probable source of the hearing loss which occurred in all four, the characteristics of which were sudden onset, cochlear in type, bilateral, sequential involvement of the two sides and improvement of the disease with alkylating agents or plasmaphoresis. Histological examination of the temporal bone in one case showed disruption of the labyrinth by haemorrhage. The organ of Corti was totally destroyed and the stria vascularis could not be identified. The vestibular structures were similarly disrupted by haemorrhage and the saccule and utricle were unrecognizable.

Leukaemia

The first account of leukaemia of the inner ear was presented by Politzer in 1884; the patient experienced bilateral, severe deafness 1 year before death. The various forms of leukaemia may affect the ear but it is usually the middle ear that is involved. Otological complications occur almost invariably in those patients with the acute forms, particularly acute lymphocytic leukaemia. The changes seen in the temporal bone fall into three categories: leukaemic infiltration, haemorrhage, and infection (Paparella *et al.*, 1973).

Leukaemic infiltration may occur in the mucoperiosteum of the middle ear following the mucous membrane folds but this may extend on to the ossicles and the sheaths of the tendons of the intratympanic muscles. Infiltration into the bone marrow spaces of the petrous apex frequently occurs and also, to a lesser extent, within the ossicles. Infiltration into the inner ear is uncommon (Aikawa and Ohtani, 1991). Haemorrhage into the inner ear is also uncommon (see Figure 4.45).

Sudden deafness and/or vertigo is reported in acute leukaemia and seems to occur most often in the acute stem-cell type. As a general rule, the otological symptoms appear to be more associated with the degree of involvement. Nageris *et al.* (1993) reported

a single case later found to have chronic lymphocytic leukaemia. The patient presented with sudden hearing loss in the right ear with no other history except that 18 months before he had had a similar event on the left side for which he had received no investigation or treatment but it left him with some hearing loss on that side. When he experienced the sudden hearing loss on the right side he felt a further deterioration on the left. Combination chemotherapy including cyclophosphamide and prednisone was given and the hearing improved dramatically. After two cycles of treatment the hearing in the right ear returned to normal and that on the left showed an average improvement of 30 dB. The hearing subsequently remained unchanged for 4 years when the patient once again complained of bilateral sudden onset hearing deterioration. As previously there was an obvious increase in his B-CLL cells with the same morphology and immunophenotype. Three cycles of cyclic chemotherapy with prednisone and chlorambucil were given and the hearing improved quickly once again.

Haemorrhagic changes in the temporal bone are more frequently seen in patients with acute lymphocytic leukaemia than the other forms (Sando and Egami, 1977). Patients with acute leukaemia suffer a bone marrow failure with a resultant thrombocytopenia and other coagulation defects such as hypofibrinogenaemia may occur. Disseminated intravascular coagulation and secondary fibrinolysis may also occur.

Cryoglobulinaemia

Cryoglobulins are proteins which precipitate in the cold and redissolve on warming. They may occur in small amounts in systemic lupus erythematosus and other 'connective tissue' disorders and may be associated with multiple myeloma or macroglobulinaemia. Almost two-thirds are mixtures of IgG and IgM molecules, while a further one-quarter are G myeloma proteins and less than 10% are macroglobulins.

The characteristic clinical signs are purpura, arthralgia and a Raynaud-like phenomenon in the lower extremities. Patients with progressive sensorineural deafness, tinnitus and vestibular problems have been reported but neurological involvement is infrequent.

Autoimmune disease

Both humoral and cell-mediated immune abnormalities appear to be involved in the pathogenesis of sensorineural hearing disorders. The analysis of peripheral lymphocyte subsets is currently used to assess the immune status in a variety of diseases. Mayot *et al.* (1993) studied a group of 17 individuals with sudden deafness and 30 with progressive sensorineural hearing impairment. An autoimmune pattern was only observed in 30% of the patients but, in those with sudden deafness, a peculiar pattern appeared to stand out suggesting it to be a disorder involving different immune alterations more closely related to immune deficiency. Indeed the levels observed are strikingly low and suggestive of profound immune alterations. The decrease in LFA 1 + cells observed in their series has been reported before, both in viral immunodeficiency and in autoimmune disease. The incidence of antinuclear and antithyroid autoantibodies in the second group (progressive sensorineural hearing impairment) was similar to that reported by others in a different series of patients with sensorineural disorders. The low instance observed by Mayot and his colleagues in their group of sudden deafness contrasts with the normal population. This suggests that organ-specific rather than general dysimmunity develops in patients with sudden hearing loss. Mayot and colleagues found a severe depletion in CD3 + and CD4 + peripheral lymphocytes in their patients with sudden deafness and a marked decrease of CD8 + cells was observed in both groups. Patients with progressive sensorineural hearing impairment frequently had antinuclear and antithyroid antibodies while anticochlear antibodies were found in both groups (75 and 71%).

Audiovestibular manifestations are a common occurrence in several system non-organ-specific autoimmune diseases but may also present as an organ-specific autoimmune entity. The most common non-organ-specific autoimmune diseases that involve the inner ear are polyarteritis nodosa and Cogan's syndrome. Less commonly, the inner ear may be involved in relapsing polychondritis, Vogt-Koyanagi-Harada syndrome, giant cell arteritis, Takayasu's disease, hypersensitivity (small vessel involvement), sarcoidosis, and systemic lupus erythematosus.

Non-organ-specific autoimmune disease

Systemic lupus erythematosus

Systemic lupus erythematosus is a multisystem disease associated with high titres of circulating autoantibodies, most commonly the antinuclear factor and the antibody to double-stranded DNA. Joint and skin involvement are the most common presenting features (see Chapter 15).

In 1986, Caldarelli, Rejowski and Corey reported a case in which bilateral sensorineural hearing loss, initially on the right and 1 week later on the left, was the initial symptom in a patient with systemic lupus erythematosus. Investigation showed the patient to have an erythrocyte sedimentation rate of 125 mm/h, a positive antinuclear antibody titre and raised levels of C4 and C3. A temporal artery biopsy showed a small focus of chronic inflammatory cells around a small arteriole without active vasculitis of the temporal artery. Skin and muscle specimens showed a small focus of chronic perivascular infiltra-

tion in the muscle and a superficial perivascular lymphoid infiltrate in the skin. The biopsy of the skin showed immunofluorescence below the dermis, highly suggestive of systemic lupus erythematosus. Treatment with prednisone and a week later also with cyclophosphamide brought down the ESR (26 mm/h) but the audiogram 6 weeks and 1 year later after discharge showed no improvement in the hearing. In the same year, Bowman *et al.* (1986) investigated a possible association between hearing loss and systemic lupus erythematosus in a prospective study of 30 patients hospitalized for exacerbation of the disease. Twenty-nine were receiving immunosuppressive therapy at the time but they discovered an 8% incidence of substantial previously undetected hearing loss without attributable cause. Neuropsychiatric involvement is common in systemic lupus erythematosus but, in nearly half of the cases, indications are not present on examination. It was hoped therefore that brain stem evoked responses might be helpful in detecting CNS involvement. Borton *et al.* (1992) investigated 10 patients with systemic lupus erythematosus though with normal hearing; they were not statistically different from the controls in their brain stem evoked responses.

Central nervous system involvement in systemic lupus erythematosus is frequently occult and may be the presenting sign – when present it is a bad prognostic indicator. Fradis *et al.* (1989) performed brain stem evoked responses without and with increased click stimulus rates (10/s versus 55/s) in 15 patients and controls. With increased stimulus rate, subclinical involvement was demonstrated in patients with systemic lupus erythematosus; none had active signs of the disease and none had a history of central nervous system involvement. The interpeak latency differences at the more usual slower rate (10/s) showed no significant differences between the patients and the controls. Narula, Powell and Davis (1989) used psychoacoustical tuning curve measurements as a method to determine frequency-resolving ability in 20 patients with systemic lupus erythematosus but comparison with matched controls did not show significantly worse hearing in the patient group.

Vyse, Luxon and Walport (1994) reported two patients with acute audiovestibular failure with high titres of antiphospholipid antibodies one of whom had systemic lupus erythematosus. Hisashi *et al.* (1993) reported the case of an adolescent female with left lateral medullary syndrome and right internuclear ophthalmoplegia who was diagnosed as having systemic lupus erythematosus. Treatment with prednisolone markedly improved her symptoms but 2 years later she developed a sudden profound sensorineural hearing loss in the right ear. Her anticardiolipin antibody was positive. Anticardiolipin antibodies strongly correlate with episodes of recurrent venous or arterial thrombosis.

Systemic vasculitides

As has been mentioned in Chapter 15 the systemic vasculitides were generally considered to be rare, but investigation of the pathogenic mechanisms and new laboratory tests have led to an increased awareness. A suggested reclassification of systemic vasculitis according to the size of the dominant vessel and whether it is primarily or secondarily involved has been published (see Table 15.6; Scott and Watts, 1994). In addition to the introduction of the test for antineutrophil cytoplasmic autoantibody (ANCA) and the subtyping into c (cytoplasmic) and p (perinuclear) patterns, investigations have also taken place into circulating antiendothelial cell autoantibodies (AECA) (Frampton *et al.*, 1990). More recently it has been recognized that while proteinase 3 and myeloperoxidase are two of the major ANCA antigens, there remain a substantial number of serum samples which recognizes neither of these which are still positive to indirect immunofluorescence techniques. Zhao, Jones and Lockwood (1995) have investigated bactericidal/permeability-increasing protein (BPI) and found it to be an important antigen for antineutrophil cytoplasmic autoantibodies in vasculitis. BPI, a constituent of the azurophilic granules of neutrophils, is found only in cells of the myeloid series which directs its potent toxicity exclusively towards Gram-negative bacteria. The particular target cell specificity is attributable to the strong affinity of BPI for lipopolysaccharides. It seems likely therefore that further advances will be made in the diagnosis of this group of condition in the lifetime of this edition.

Cogan's syndrome

In 1945, Cogan reported four cases of non-syphilitic keratitis characterized by vestibular and auditory disorders. He noted that in syphilitic keratitis only 4% of the patients developed deafness, and that this did not occur until months or even years after the keratitis. He saw his first four cases all within 1 year and was impressed that while the corneal changes progressed relatively little, the vertigo became incapacitating but the deafness progressive and ultimately profound. Norton and Cogan reviewed the cases again in 1959. They confirmed the ocular signs of patchy, deep corneal infiltrates which tend to fluctuate in intensity and distribution, usually located in the periphery, and accompanied by deep corneal vascularization if they persist long enough. No evidence of syphilitic infection, by the tests then available, could be found. However, the sensorineural hearing loss is progressive, often sudden in onset, and always associated with tinnitus and vertigo. Very occasionally, the vestibular/auditory symptoms have preceded the eye changes but only by a few weeks or a month or so in all reported cases. More than three-quarters of the cases have occurred in patients under 30; two have been associated with pregnancy. Feldman (1981)

reminded us that the eye symptoms in Cogan's syndrome frequently cause lacrimation and the condition has therefore been characterized as the 'crying deafness'.

Haynes *et al.* (1980) carried out detailed investigations into 13 of Cogan's original series of 30 patients and also reviewed 111 patients from the literature. They again confirmed that while vestibular/auditory symptoms may appear before or after the onset of interstitial keratitis, they usually occur within 1–6 months of the onset of eye symptoms and progress to deafness over a period of 1–3 months. In their own series an elevated erythrocyte sedimentation rate was the most common abnormal laboratory finding (100%) followed by raised serum cryoglobulins (23%). Studies during flares of the disease showed C3 and C4 levels were normal and circulating immune complexes by the C1Q-binding assay failed to be demonstrated. Haynes *et al.* (1981) prospectively followed six patients with Cogan's syndrome who were treated within 4 weeks of the acute onset of the hearing loss. Within 1–2 weeks after the initiation of corticosteroid therapy, all six demonstrated improved hearing thresholds for pure tones and suprathreshold speech discrimination results which have since been maintained. No retrocochlear abnormalities were found in any patient. Hughes *et al.* (1981) reported cellular immune testing on two patients; lymphocyte migration inhibition tests on stimulation with inner ear membrane antigen were positive in both.

Majoor *et al.* (1992) reported two cases, the first of whom complained of bilateral hearing loss with tinnitus and fullness in the ears; an equilibrium loss without vertigo was noticed when he changed position. Audiometry showed a slightly sloping sensorineural hearing loss of 30 dB for the right ear and 40 dB for the left, while speech discrimination was found to be normal. Their second case initially showed vertigo, vegetative reactions, hearing loss and tinnitus the day after presenting with pain in the left eye together with redness and photophobia. Two weeks later an exacerbation of the condition occurred and audiometry then showed a flat sensorineural hearing loss of 90 dB for the right ear and a sloping sensorineural hearing loss of 50 dB for the left. Further investigations showed autoimmune reactivity against corneal antigens and in both cases the antibodies were found at the beginning or during an exacerbation of the disease. While the administration of high doses of corticosteroids caused the corneal antibodies to diminish the effect of such treatment on the audiovestibular systems was noted to be variable.

McDonald, Vollertsen and Younge (1985) reviewed their experience of 18 patients with Cogan's syndrome. Thirteen showed a typical presentation with audiovestibular symptoms quickly followed by the ocular findings. Five patients had an atypical presentation, two of whom had severe bilateral audiovestibular dysfunction 2 years before the onset of the classic ocular symptoms and signs. Reviewing 78 previously published cases, they noted that one-third of the patients had abdominal findings, most commonly gastrointestinal haemorrhage; one-quarter of the patients had cardiac involvement (aortic insufficiency was the most significant lesion) and there are several reports of such patients undergoing cardiac surgery. A number of patients are on record as developing systemic vasculitis in the course of their disease and in a few cases it has led to their death. A more extensive review of the same group of patients from the Mayo Clinic is reported by Vollertsen *et al.* (1986).

Morgan, Hochman and Weider (1984) reported two cases which presented with acute bilateral hearing loss and vestibular dysfunction. Slit-lamp examination confirmed initial interstitial keratitis. Cote *et al.* (1993) reported the case of a 41-year-old woman who gave a 1-week history of vertigo preceded by a viral upper respiratory tract infection. Audiometry then only showed a mild symmetric sensorineural hearing loss, but 7 days later she returned with a bilateral deafness coming on within a 24-hour period. Investigation showed the erythrocyte sedimentation rate (ESR) and the C-reactive protein (CRP) elevated to 112 mm/h and 2.6 mg/dl respectively. The authors pointed out that CRP is synthesized in the liver as an acute phase response after the onset of infection or inflammation and they found changes in the CRP corresponded well with the disease activity and steroid dose. The CRP rises soon after the onset of inflammation, undergoing an exponential increase within 4–6 hours. The decrease of CRP also correlated closely with remission of disease activity. They noted that in Cogan's syndrome typically, the hearing loss fluctuates, with periods of exacerbation and remission gradually resulting in profound hearing loss. Unlike the ophthalmological outcome, deafness will ensue in approximately 50% of patients despite adequate treatment.

Bicknell and Holland (1978) reported two patients in whom neurological problems were prominent and a review of 79 cases in the literature showed that more than one-half had involvement of the nervous system. Clinical syndromes of acute inferior cerebellar artery occlusion have also occurred on two occasions. It remains undecided whether Cogan's syndrome is a separate entity. Cases with systemic involvement tend to be labelled as polyarteritis nodosa.

Zeitouni, Tewfik and Schloss (1993) reported on a child aged 10 years, with a 10-year follow up but reminded us that the youngest patient to be diagnosed was only 2.5 years of age, though there are relatively few cases presenting in children. In their particular case the hearing worsened when prednisone was first given and only during the second month did it start to improve. The ears then appeared to be involved independently, the left improving while the right worsened and subsequently the reverse occurred!

Majoor, Albers and Casselman (1993) investigated five patients with Cogan's syndrome by a combined application of MR imaging and CT scanning. Their aim was to visualize the membranous labyrinth and correlate the pathology in Cogan's syndrome with the clinical findings. While one case was normal, in the remaining four there was narrowing or obliteration of parts of the vestibular labyrinth. In three they found aberrations in the cochlea consistent with the audiological data. They felt that the results of the radiological investigations were consistent with the hypothesis that the inner ear pathology in Cogan's syndrome is probably caused by an obstructive vasculitis.

Treatment with steroids remains the recommended treatment supplemented in the more progressive case by immunosuppressive drugs, e.g. azathioprine, cyclophosphamide, or chlorambucil. Plasma exchange has been successfully used on two occasions when other treatment has failed to halt the progress of the condition (Brookes and Newland, 1986). Serial audiometry in many cases has proved to be a satisfactory barometer for increasing or decreasing medication (McDonald, Vollertsen and Younge, 1985).

Recently, Schuknecht and Nadol (1994) have reported the temporal bone pathology in a case of Cogan's syndrome. This showed changes that were similar to those observed in other autoimmune disorders associated with audiovestibular dysfunction. They noted the following four pathological features which characterized autoimmune inner ear disease: acute labyrinthitis resulting in atrophy of inner ear tissues including the sense organs and their supporting structures; endolymphatic hydrops; focal and diffuse proliferation of fibrous tissue and bone; and retrograde neuronal degeneration. These pathological findings were noted to be consistent with an inflammatory (and possibly ischaemic) attack on the membranous labyrinth. Schuknecht and Nadol also compared the clinical manifestations and pathological findings of the four reported cases of polyarteritis nodosa, one of relapsing polychrondritis and four of Cogan's syndrome including their own case, together with a further case of inner ear autoimmune disease.

Relapsing polychondritis

Ocular inflammatory lesions, hearing loss, and dizziness are frequent manifestations of this condition. While the hearing loss may be secondary to a middle ear problem resulting from involvement of the eustachian tube cartilage, sensorineural deafness may also occur. In several of the reported cases the hearing loss has accompanied either an abrupt cessation of steroid therapy or a drastic reduction in the level of medication. Specialized audiometric tests show the loss to be of the cochlear type. The condition is dealt with more fully in Chapter 15.

In 1976, McAdam *et al.* carried out a prospective

study on 23 patients with well defined relapsing polychondritis and carried out a world literature review yielding a further 136 reported cases. Of the total 159 patients, 46 had audiovestibular damage but they felt this was an underestimate as often details of reported cases were lacking in some degree. From the frequencies of involvement, they produced a rank order of six diagnostic criteria with auricular chondritis in first (89%), nasal chondritis in third (72%) and audiovestibular involvement in sixth place. The last may be unilateral or bilateral and are usually sudden in onset. The vestibular symptoms typically decrease but the sensorineural hearing loss usually persists. Once all the vestibular involvement is present it is usually persistent rather than episodic. Damiani and Levine (1979) reported a series of 10 cases in whom cochlear vestibular damage and ocular inflammation were each seen in five.

Hoshino *et al.* (1978, 1980) have described a single case of a 56-year-old woman who suffered sudden deafness during the course of relapsing polychondritis. Audiometry showed a complete hearing loss in both ears and caloric testing did not elicit any responses. The patient was treated continuously with steroids which were supplemented over the last 6 years of her life with azathioprine before she died of gastrointestinal haemorrhage. They reported the temporal bone changes including scanning electron microscopy in this patient and described findings similar to those of viral deafness with endolymphatic labyrinthitis.

Albers, Majoor and Van der Gaag (1992) reported a case in which sudden deafness developed in both ears with tinnitus and vertigo. Circulating antibodies against corneal epithelium were determined by immunofluorescence before and after medical treatment.

Wegener's granulomatosis

While pathologically there may be difficulties in differentiating this from polyarteritis nodosa, clinically the two conditions are usually quite different in their presentation. Cases of polyarteritis nodosa seldom present to an otolaryngologist, while most will see Wegener's granulomatosis in their career and it will frequently present because of nasal symptoms. Similarly, while clinically it is different from lethal midline granuloma, pathologically these two · may also present problems; the latter is considered by some to be another variant of polyarteritis nodosa. Indeed, Wegener himself in 1939, stated that polyarteritis nodosa was a common finding in patients with lethal granulomas of the midline facial tisues (Wegener, 1990).

Wegener's granulomatosis has three principal components:

1 Necrotizing granulomatous lesions in the upper or lower respiratory tract or both
2 Generalized focal necrotizing vasculitis involving both arteries and veins, almost always present in the lungs and more or less widely disseminated in other sites
3 Glomerulonephritis, characterized by necrosis and thrombosis of loops or lobes of the capillary tuft, capsular adhesions, and evolution as a granulomatous lesion.

Wegener discovered the necrotizing granulomas in post-mortem tissue studies of three patients who had died of fulminant sepsis. The first of these, studied in 1934, showed 'involvement of the paranasal sinuses accompanied by a hearing loss'. Although the pathology predominantly involved the upper and lower respiratory tracts, a generalized vasculitis was also found, as well as evidence of end-stage glomerulonephritis. The disseminated vasculitis may involve both small arteries and veins and any organ system may be involved with granulomatous changes as disease progresses.

De Remee *et al.* (1976) reported a series of 50 patients over a 10-year period in which the ear was the most frequently involved site (37 patients), followed by the lung (35 patients) and kidney (23 patients). Karmody (1978) reported five patients seen over a 7-year period in which the ear was the presenting site. Illum and Thorling (1982) reported a series of 17 patients of whom 10 exhibited otological symptoms and in seven of whom it was the presenting sign.

In recent years there have been further reports. D'Cruz *et al.* (1989) published 22 cases in 15 of whom the ear was involved and the commonest presenting features were deafness in 13 and pain in 11 of these. Eight had a discharging ear, six serous otitis media and three otitis externa. Only 13 of the total group had an abnormal chest X-ray and seven showed impaired renal function. Kempf (1989) reported a series of 19 cases, in 16 of whom the early manifestations were limited to the ear and nose. Twenty-one of 26 ears presented with a low to moderate sensorineural hearing loss. One ear remained deaf after a sudden hearing loss in the early stage of the disease. On occasions it has been shown that it is possible to reverse the sensorineural hearing loss in Wegener's granulomatosis. Clements *et al.* (1989) reported two cases, both of which showed recovery but both required cyclophosphamide in addition to high dose prednisolone to bring this about.

Polyarteritis nodosa

Polyarteritis nodosa is a systemic vasculitis of unknown aetiology, involving mainly small and middle calibre arteries. The lesions are segmental with a predilection for the bifurcation of the vessels. The disease process spreads longitudinally along the arterioles and eventually involves accompanying venules. In the later stages, the vessels undergo fibrinoid necrosis, mainly in the media layer, with loss of elastic fibres in the elastic membrane of the arterial wall. In the classical form of polyarteritis, all three stages may occur simultaneously. Typically the distribution of the disease in the body spares the small vessels of the lung and spleen.

Deafness in this condition is itself unusual and only on rare occasions has it been the presenting symptom. The deafness is sensorineural. Lake-Bakaar and Gibbs (1978) reported a case with profound bilateral deafness and sudden tinnitus; electrocochleography pointed to an end-organ impairment. Before treatment, the patient's hearing improved to within normal limits (Figure 17.4).

Subsequently her polyarteritis nodosa was treated with prednisolone and there has been no recurrence of the deafness. Peiterson and Carlson (1966) reported a case, also with bilateral, and almost symmetrical, gradually deteriorating hearing loss. Subsequently the hearing fluctuated. After an interval of more than 6 months, polyarteritis nodosa seemed the most likely diagnosis and she was treated with prednisolone which brought about a considerable hearing improvement. The remaining reported cases totalled only approximately a dozen. The only common feature would seem to be that deafness is sensorineural and bilateral. In most of the earlier reports, minimal details are available. Later in the disease, or perhaps already present, other lesions of polyarteritis nodosa will be found in the body and it is by these that the diagnosis is made.

More recently, Rowe-Jones, Macallan and Sorooshian (1990) described a case of polyarteritis nodosa which presented with sudden bilateral cochlear-vestibular failure. Treatment with high dose prednisolone resulted in some improvement in her hearing; after she was re-admitted a fortnight later azathioprine was added to her treatment and a further improvement in her hearing and caloric response occurred on the right side.

It seems probable that the inner ear pathology is caused by obliterative vasculitis of the labyrinthine artery or its branches resulting in diffuse or focal areas of ischaemic necrosis. The inner ear changes therefore do not represent autoimmune disease in the sense that the immune system is reacting to proteins of the membranous labyrinth. The clinical features of suddenness of onset and profoundness of hearing loss are consistent with acute obstruction of the labyrinthine artery or the common cochlear artery (Schuknecht, 1991). In the same paper Schuknecht reported the case of organ-specific autoimmune inner ear disease in great detail. The pathological features that characterize the situation were the destruction of inner ear tissues including the sense organs, their supporting structures and eventually the membra-

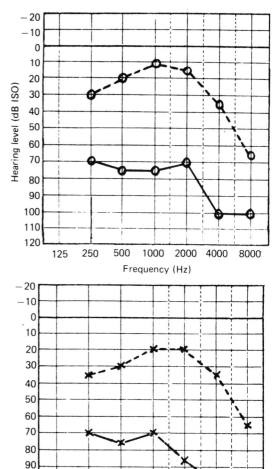

Figure 17.4 Audiograms of a 63-year-old woman who developed tinnitus and bilateral deafness with spontaneous return of hearing (right ○–○; left X–X; continuous line before; interrupted line after improvement). (Reproduced by kind permission of Dr D.D. Gibbs and Editor, *Journal of the Royal Society of Medicine*)

nous labyrinth; scattered infiltrates and free-floating aggregates of lymphocytes, plasma cells and macrophages; focal or diffuse proliferation of fibrous tissue and bone. Endolymphatic hydrops is a frequent but not a constant finding.

Yoon, Paparella and Schachern (1989) have also published a temporal bone histopathological study of 16 temporal bones from patients with systemic vasculitis: three with Wegener's granulomatosis, two with polyarteritis nodosa and three with systemic lupus erythematosus. In their patients the audiograms of only two ears demonstrated sensorineural hearing loss of sudden onset (one each) of polyarteritis nodosa and the other systemic lupus erythematosus; in five of the eight patients no audiometry was performed.

Giant cell arteritis (temporal arteritis)

In 1890, Jonathon Hutchinson mentioned a condition called arteritis obliterans which he believed was usually one of somewhat slow progress and not supposed to be accompanied by thrombosis. The condition to which he then wished to draw attention was one of rapid development and had as its principal feature thrombotic occlusion of the vessel implicated. He reported the case of an old man who was 'upwards of eighty years of age whom he was asked to see because of "streaks on his head" which were painful and prevented him wearing his hat.' The 'red streaks' proved, on examination, to be his temporal arteries which on both sides were found to be inflamed and swollen. He was of course describing the condition which we now know as temporal arteritis.

Inflammation of the vessels as in cranial arteritis may present to the otolaryngologist as headache, facial palsy, hearing loss, dysphagia, jaw claudication, lingual Raynaud's phenomenon, and tongue infarction. Sensorineural hearing loss with vertigo has been described (Sofferman, 1980).

Kinmont and McCallum (1965) described 18 cases of their own and examined the records of a further 42 patients. Of the total of 59, eight (13.3%) were affected by deafness. They noted that the ocular and aural complications, the most serious aspect of the disease, may occur within hours of the headache, or as long as 1 to 2 months subsequently. Cullen and Coleiro (1976) gave an excellent review of the ophthalmic complications of giant cell arteritis. They stressed that the erythrocyte sedimentation rate is of major significance in diagnosis but biopsy is necessary to prove or disprove the existence of temporal arteritis; however they make no mention of deafness. Malmvall and Bengtsson (1978) reported 68 patients with giant cell arteritis in whom a raised ESR was seen in all cases and an elevated platelet count in 24 patients. Reduced hearing capacity was demonstrated in five patients. They note the strong connection between giant cell arteritis and polymyalgia rheumatica.

Hall *et al.* (1983) followed up 134 residents from an area of Minnesota who had undergone temporal artery biopsy over a 15-year period for giant cell arteritis. Initial biopsies were positive in 46 and negative in 88. Over a median follow-up period of 70 months (range 1–192), only eight of the biopsy-negative patients had clinical courses which required long-term high-dose corticosteroid therapy. History of jaw pain, and abnormal temporal artery, or both were present in 78% of those with positive biopsies.

Sudden deafness complicating giant cell temporal arteritis has been reported on relatively few occasions.

Francis and Boddie (1982) reported a case which presented with acute hearing loss. Neurological examination revealed bilateral sensorineural deafness which deteriorated significantly over the subsequent 24 hours. The ESR was raised at 102 mm/h and the protein electrophoresis revealed a marked increase in alpha 1, alpha 2 and gamma globulin bands though the serum globulins were normal. Despite a negative temporal artery biopsy, a diagnosis of giant cell arteritis was made on clinical criteria and prednisolone therapy started at a dose of 80 mg daily. Within 24 hours the patient's headache had gone and his hearing had returned to normal. The case reported by Wolfovitz, Levy and Brook (1987) presented with bilateral sudden hearing loss during hospitalization! A trial of carbogen produced no improvement but prednisone, 40 mg daily, brought about a significant improvement in both ears.

Recently, McKennan *et al.* (1993) published a report of three patients with biopsy-proven giant cell arteritis who experienced significant auditory and vestibular symptoms. Two of the patients who presented with audiovestibular symptomatology died as a direct result of giant cell arteritis affecting the vertebral arteries. They emphasized the need for a high index of suspicion in elderly patients who present with acute onset of audiovestibular symptoms associated with giant cell arteritis. These symptoms can be a herald of brain stem infarction if giant cell arteritis is the underlying cause. Their first case was an 84-year-old woman who presented with a 5-day history of abrupt onset left-sided hearing loss, vertigo, and nausea. Two weeks before the onset of the hearing loss she had noticed blurring of vision in her left eye. Her initial audiogram showed a flat severe sensorineural hearing loss on the left side (pure tone average 65 dB) with a marked reduction in speech discrimination score (20%). Electronystagmography revealed completely absent caloric responses bilaterally. Her ESR was 45 mm/h and her temporal artery biopsy 2 days later showed classic giant cell arteritis. She needed to be admitted urgently because of a sudden change in her condition including a mild left motor neuron facial paralysis, right-sided ptosis and dysphagia due to a right Xth cranial neuropathy. MRI imaging with gadolinium revealed multiple sites of recent infarction of the brain stem and cerebellum. A flow void in the vertebral arteries was noticed indicative of vertebral artery occlusion. She was immediately commenced on prednisone but, in spite of a satisfactory response to steroid medication with a drop in her sedimentation rate to 15 mm/h within 9 days which enabled her to go home on prednisone 60 mg daily, she required to be readmitted 1 week later and died after a further week (Figure 17.5). Their second patient was an 85-year-old woman who again presented with acute onset of severe vertigo, nausea, vomiting and bilateral hearing loss. An audiogram demonstrated a flat bilaterally symmetric

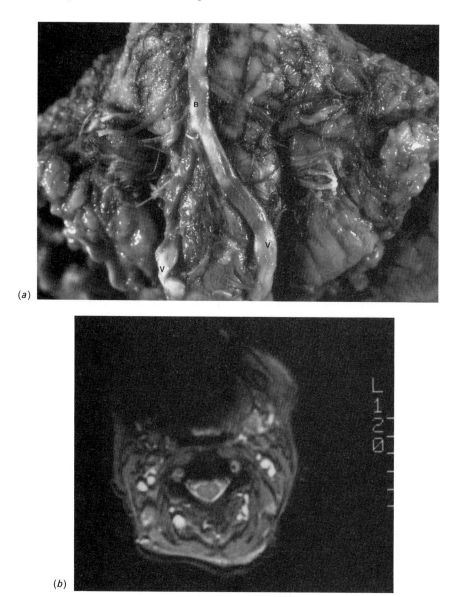

(a)

(b)

Figure 17.5 Giant cell arteritis (temporal arteritis). An 84-year-old woman presented with sudden unilateral sensorineural hearing loss and severe vertigo. Initial flat severe sensorineural hearing loss and vertigo could have been diagnosed as Menière's syndrome. Despite aggressive steroid treatment the patient still died as a result of underlying giant cell arteritis of the vertebral artery. (a) Illustration shows the ventral aspect of the brain stem showing thickening and tortuosity of the vertebral arteries (V) by the vasculitic process. The white plaques on the basilar artery (B) are due to atherosclerosis. The intracranial arteries were not affected by giant cell arteritis. (b) A flow void is seen in the vertebral arteries on MRI scan; these are seen as black holes rather than the normal white signal indicating arterial flow. The amorphous black region in the upper portion of the illustration is due to patient positioning. (Reproduced by kind permission of Dr Kevin X. McKennan and Editor, *The Laryngoscope*)

sensorineural hearing loss with a pure tone average of 40 dB in the right ear and 42 dB in the left. The following day she required to be admitted to hospital because of dysphagia, lethargy, dysarthria, ataxia and a mild left lower motor neuron facial paresis. She died before further investigations and treatment could be instituted. The third case was of a 79-year-old woman who was thought to have Menière's disease who presented with polymyalgia rheumatica and temporal headaches. Temporal artery biopsy was positive for giant cell arteritis and her ESR was 83 mm/h. Treatment with prednisone for 1 year successfully reduced her ESR to 7 mm/h. However, 21 months later she was again referred with the erroneous diagnosis of Menière's disease. Her ESR had climbed to 126 mm/h and she now had a right-sided severe sensorineural hearing loss which had developed over the preceding year. Auditory brain stem responses demonstrated very poor wave forms on the right and only wave IV and V could be identified. Her MRI scan and MR angiography were both normal. Audiograms during the last 7 months documented a fluctuating low tone sensorineural hearing loss in the right ear similar to that seen in classical Menière's syndrome. The authors emphasized that fluctuating Menière's symptoms can be a sign of vertebral artery ischaemia.

Kawasaki disease

Kawasaki disease is a self-limited acute vasculitis that affects predominantly medium-sized extraparenchymal muscular arteries. Coronary artery abnormalities occur in approximately 20% of untreated patients and are the major cause of morbidity. Neurological involvement however is rare. Cranial nerve palsy especially involving the VIIth nerve has been reported. The diagnostic criteria of Kawasaki disease are a fever lasting 5 days or more without any other explanation and at least four of the following criteria: bilateral conjunctival injection, change of the peripheral extremities including erythema of the palms or soles, oedema of the hands or feet (acute phase) or periungual desquamation (convalescent phase), mucus membrane changes, polymorphous rash, acute non-purulent cervical lymphadenopathy (with at least one lymph node 1.5 cm or greater in diameter). Sundel *et al.* (1990, 1992) prospectively evaluated the hearing of 40 consecutive patients with acute Kawasaki disease, 17 of whom were excluded from the analysis. Sixteen of the 23 children were found to have normal hearing but the seven others had results suggesting a transient hearing threshold shift of 10–25 dB, of whom six were re-tested at varying intervals and showed improvement over the ensuing 8 days to 4 months.

The mechanism of sensorineural hearing loss associated with acute Kawasaki disease remains to be determined. In their earlier report Sundel *et al.* (1990) examined five children and the sensorineural hearing losses varied in severity from mild to profound and were bilateral in four of the five patients. When the middle ear is involved then a conductive hearing loss may also be present. Auditory brain stem responses could only be carried out in three of the children because the severity of the hearing loss in the other two made this impossible. The results showed no indication of retrocochlear abnormality. Magnetic resonance imaging was carried out in two patients (those in whom auditory brain stem responses could not be obtained) and were found to be normal. Sundel *et al.* (1990) also examined seven patients who were being screened because of coronary artery aneurysms who were the most severely affected but no demonstrable hearing loss could be found. They felt this precluded a direct correlation between hearing loss and the intensity of the inflammation.

Takayasu's disease

Takayasu's disease, or aortitis syndrome, is named after a Japanese ophthalmologist who, in 1908, first described the ocular manifestation of the disease in a young female. The disease occurs predominantly in women. The classical clinical picture causes the absence of the pulse in the upper extremities due to the obstruction of the aortic arch branches. The syndrome is generally characterized by vasculitis of the large vessels; involvement of the small arteries has seldom been reported. No vasculitis has been observed in pathological examination of the temporal bones in cases of hearing loss associated with aortitis syndrome (Takayasu's disease).

Kanzaki, O-uchi and Tsuchihashi (1993) have reported a group of 17 patients with aortitis syndrome. Of these, seven had sensorineural hearing loss and in the remaining 10 there were no abnormalities observed on audiological tests. All but two were women. They also investigated a group of 42 patients with various autoimmune diseases, in 26 of whom there was a sensorineural hearing loss. In the latter group, rheumatoid arthritis was seen in 10 patients five of whom had a sudden onset hearing loss, systemic lupus erythematosus in 12 patients and again two had a sudden onset hearing loss, relapsing polychondritis in two out of three, dermatomyositis in one out of two and Burger's disease in one patient who had sudden onset hearing loss. They treated their patients with steroids (prednisolone) but also Sairei-to, a traditional herbal medicine which contains Shosaiko-to and Gorei-san. It is suggested that these may have glucocorticoid-like as well as antiallergic effects. None of the patients with systemic lupus erythematosus and sudden onset sensorineural hearing loss showed any improvement in hearing.

A single temporal bone report has been published on a patient with Takayasu's disease who died 5 years after complaining of a bilateral high tone sensorineural hearing loss. The temporal bones showed a marked loss of outer and inner hair cells and cochlear neurons (Nomura and Kitamura, 1979).

Behçet's disease

In recent years it has become recognized that Behçet's disease, previously thought of as an oculo-oral-genital syndrome, is a generalized vasculitis of small vessels affecting integument systems and other organs.

Histologically, this disease appears as perivascular infiltrates, small microhaemorrhages, subcortical white matter lesions and areas of fibrinoid degeneration. Auditory and vestibular lesions as part of the clinical manifestation of central nervous system involvement were first described by Alajouanine *et al.* (1961). Between 25 and 30% eventually develop neurological complications but only 5% present with such problems. Brama and Fainaru (1980) reported 16 patients, 10 of whom had sensorineural hearing loss, which was unilateral in one.

Gemignani *et al.* (1991) evaluated the problems of audiovestibular disturbances in Behçet's syndrome examining 20 consecutive patients and 20 control subjects which they had seen over the previous 3 years. Sensorineural hearing loss was found in 12 patients, in two of whom it had been of sudden onset. Two other patients showed a vestibular function deficit, and three others exhibited altered caloric test results. Two of the last group also revealed simultaneous bilateral auditory hearing losses. HLA typing showed the presence of the B51 antigen in 10 of the 14 patients with ear involvement, while only three of the six patients without ear involvement were positive. Berrettini *et al.* (1989) reported two cases of sudden deafness in Behçet's disease, the first bilateral though much worse in one ear and the second unilateral. More recently, Smith (1994) reported a case of unilateral hearing loss in a patient with known Behçet's disease and Tsunoda *et al.* (1994) reported simultaneous bilateral impairment of both vestibular and cochlear functions, in a patient with known Behçet's disease.

Endolymphatic hydrops

Hallberg (1956) thought that not more than 5% of all cases of sudden hearing loss eventually developed Menière's disease. He found only 57 such cases in his review of 1270 patients. Two cases of sudden hearing loss which showed endolymphatic hydrops at autopsy have now been reported (Takahara *et al.*, 1974; Sando *et al.*, 1977) (Figure 17.6). Menière's disease due to endolymphatic hydrops, as opposed to conditions producing a Menière-like disorder, displays a characteristic pattern (see also Chapter 19). It is well known that it may fail to oblige by producing its principal symptoms simultaneously and the fluctuant hearing associated with this condition has become a subject of particular interest.

In 1985, the Committee on Hearing and Equilibrium of the American Academy of Otololaryngology – Head and Neck Surgery decided to limit the diagnostic term, Menière's disease, to those cases with the full complement of classic symptoms resulting from endolymphatic hydrops. Thus cochlear and vestibular variants were excluded. Dornhoffer and Arenberg (1993) have described the use of electrocochleography to ascertain whether there may also be sub-

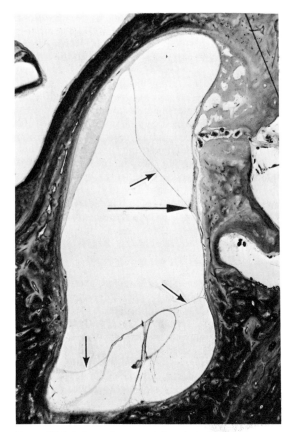

Figure 17.6 Left ear. Severe endolymphatic hydrops is seen at the extreme basal end of the cochlear duct (small arrows). Large arrow demonstrates collapsed ductus reuniens (× 23). (Reproduced by kind permission of Sando and Editor of *Annals of Otology, Rhinology and Laryngology*)

clinical cochlear involvement, in those who would previously have been diagnosed as vestibular Menière's disease; 73% (11/15) demonstrated findings consistent with endolymphatic hydrops.

Acute low tone sensorineural hearing loss without vertigo has been reported previously by Matsuoke *et al.* (1991) in 56 out of 106 cases of sudden deafness and 37 out of the total group developed vertigo within 2–24 months after steroid therapy (11/56 with low tone loss). More recently Yamasoba *et al.* (1993b, 1994) reported a series of 80 patients. Interestingly 74% (26/35) of those undergoing a glycerol test were positive. There was an abnormally increased negative SP/AP ratio in 63% (50/80). Hearing loss was improved within 3 months in 84% (67/80) of the patients. Of the 45 patients followed up for more than 3 years, 62% (28) showed no evidence of recurrence; 27% developed cochlear Menière's disease and 11% (5) developed classic Menière's disease.

In 1988, Kanzaki and Ogawa noted a possible association between vascular loops in the internal auditory meatus and sensorineural hearing loss; seven out of 23 presented with sudden hearing loss in a series of 61 cases found to have vascular loops (two out of 23 in the control group/healthy side). Transient low frequency retrocochlear hearing loss has also been reported in a small group of patients undergoing microvascular decompression for hemifacial spasm. All of them had excessively short perforating arteries surrounding the root entry zone of the VIIth and VIIIth cranial nerves (Fukuda, Nomura and Fukushima, 1991).

Of interest, is a recent paper by Rudd *et al.* (1993) of a patient with known Menière's disease initially on the left side who, some 10 years later, developed fluctuant hearing on the right side with normal investigations apart from transtympanic electrocochleography with glycerol dehydration, confirming probable Menière's disease on this side. The patient had noted that his right-sided hearing loss was of greatest severity when he had not eaten food for a prolonged period of time and his hearing returned to normal soon after eating. Serial pure tone audiometry and blood glucose levels at 30-minute intervals following the ingestion of 70 g of glucose confirmed the correlation. In 1979, Moffat, Booth and Morrison had found only three abnormal glucose tolerance curves (11%), none of which were hypoglycaemic, in a series of 27 patients with classical symptoms of Menière's disease. However, in the case reported by Rudd *et al.* (1993) there was no evidence of hypoglycaemia and a normal 5-hour glucose tolerance test.

Metabolic disorders

Renal failure

The analogy between the nephron and the organ of Corti is one which has become more frequent particularly with the increasing numbers of patients with renal failure who may be treated by haemodialysis or transplantation. It must be remembered that many of such patients have of necessity received ototoxic drugs, either to control their infection or to promote diuresis. Certain studies therefore, are not only of interest but helpful to the otologist, who is now more frequently involved with the management of such cases.

Yassin, Badry and Fatt-Hi (1970) found that the degree of hearing loss was directly related to the degree of hyponatraemia irrespective of the level of the blood urea. Urea by itself was non-toxic to the cochlear end-organs and the effects on the cochlear were greatly improved by correcting the renal failure and restoring the serum sodium. Eighty per cent of the cases with acute renal failure were improved by treatment, but only 52.4% of those with chronic forms.

Oda *et al.* (1974) have shown that in a study of 290 patients with chronic renal failure, 43 developed a significant hearing loss which could be attributed to the therapy of the kidney problem. None of the patients were complaining of hearing impairment before the kidney treatment was started. Five patients treated with less than 60 haemodialyses showed no subjective hearing loss; three who had received more than 260 haemodialyses and multiple transplants complained of hearing and vestibular difficulties. During haemodialysis frequent and intense osmotic changes occur. Johnson and Mathog (1976) noted fluctuations in hearing in a single dialysis period, but could find no correlation with corresponding changes in blood urea nitrogen, creatinine, Na, K, Ca, glucose, mean blood pressure level or weight.

Quick (1976), in a prospective study of a large series of patients receiving dialysis and/or transplantation, found that a hearing loss occurs quite frequently and while one factor might trigger off the loss, it was a combination effect of many factors, but this was not a simple addition of effects, more a potentiation. In his series, one in six had some form of hearing disorder. Six patients experienced sudden hearing loss and while a hypercoagulative state was evident in one patient, when the loss followed bilateral nephrectomy and splenectomy; there was no apparent cause in the others.

Kligerman *et al.* (1981), in a prospective study of 67 patients with chronic end-stage renal failure, noted a trend which appeared to suggest an association between haemodialysis and high frequency impairment, the degree of hearing loss did not vary with the length of treatment. Likewise, there was a striking similarity between the audiological findings obtained for all subjects with high frequency impairment, irrespective of medical treatment.

Hutchinson and Klodd (1982) assessed a series of 15 patients under the age of 60, suffering from chronic renal failure who were being treated by haemodialysis. They eliminated from their study any patient who was diabetic or in whom the cause of renal failure was considered to be congenital. Each patient was tested once when the effects of the renal failure were most severe and they were about to undergo dialysis. They were tested using pure tone audiometry, acoustic reflex thresholds and reflex decay tests, electronystagmography and brain stem auditory evoked responses. They concluded that when ototoxic drugs, noise exposure, diabetes, congenital nephritis, and age above 60 years are eliminated, that although individual abnormalities will occur, chronic renal failure does not in itself produce a clinically significant hearing loss; neither does it produce an abnormality of the peripheral or central vestibular function that is clinically significant; nor did it produce an abnormality within the brain stem that affects the auditory or vestibular brain stem function from the clinical standpoint.

A recent study by Gatland *et al.* (1991) investigated the prevalence of sensorineural hearing loss by pure tone audiometry in 66 patients with chronic renal failure and the threshold changes following haemodialysis in 31 patients. They found that the incidence of hearing loss was 41% in the low, 15% in the middle and 53% in the high ranges respectively. Of the 62 ears studied, 38% had a decrease in low frequency threshold after dialysis and 9% had an increase. They came to the conclusion that fluctuation of the low frequencies with dialysis was common. Where a sensorineural hearing loss was found they carried out additional tests (loudness discomfort levels and stapedial reflexes); these indicated the hearing loss to be of cochlear origin. Of their 66 patients, 51 were undergoing haemodialysis, seven continuous ambulant peritoneal dialysis, five were on diet alone and three underwent renal transplantation. There was a history of gentamicin administration in 20% and metabolic bone disease existed in 66%. The effect of the high and low frequency hearing losses produced a characteristic dome-shaped audiogram. Statistical analysis of the various parameters which they studied showed that age, derived plasma viscosity (from the globulin: albumin ratio) and gentamicin administration were significant factors in the aetiology of the high frequency loss. However, none of the parameters measured was significant in relation to the low frequency loss. They found no correlation between the fluctuation in hearing and weight change with dialysis.

Kusakari *et al.* (1992) carried out a long-term follow-up study on the hearing of patients treated by haemodialysis. They investigated 37 patients with observation periods of 4 years or longer; the average duration of the follow up study was 8 years 9 months (range 8 months – 11 years). Hearing tests were initially performed soon after the start of haemodialysis and every 3–12 months thereafter. Hearing corresponding to age was found in 43 ears whereas significant hearing loss was observed in 31 ears. The shape of the audiogram showed a high tone loss in the majority of cases and was bilateral and symmetrical in all except one case. They found two groups, the first in which the hearing deteriorated significantly in only three cases (five ears) during the period of observation, but in these the hearing had completely recovered in two ears, partially in one with no recovery in the remaining two. In the second group the hearing was already reduced at the first test and remained unchanged in all ears except for one case in which both ears exhibited further deterioration. In two of their 37 cases with an initial hearing loss the cause was due to acoustic trauma in one and streptomycin toxicity in another.

Alport's syndrome

Occasionally Alport's syndrome has been mentioned in relation to sudden hearing loss. Alport (1927) himself reported a relationship between nephritis and deafness and noted a familial occurrence. The aetiology of the hearing loss has never been clearly defined. Characteristically it varies in severity with the family, is slowly progressive and the high frequencies are those most severely affected. Myers and Tyler (1972) suggested that there may be as many as five variants – renal disease with organ of Corti damage, renal disease with spiral ganglion cochlear neuron loss, renal disease and deafness but no histological ear lesion, renal disease without deafness, and finally deafness without renal disease. Hearing loss with normal or only mild renal changes is especially typical of female members of affected families.

The commonest presenting signs are hypertension, proteinuria, and haematuria. Gubler *et al.* (1981) reported a series of 58 cases in one of whom, a boy, deafness was the presenting symptom. Some degree of hearing loss may be present by the time the renal lesion is diagnosed and in their series, 37 patients showed a hearing loss, in 22 of whom the defect was diagnosed by audiometry and in 15 there was an apparent hearing impairment. In eight of their patients the first audiogram was normal! The hearing loss is of the slowly progressive symmetrical sensorineural type which is often not significant until the second decade, appears to affect men much more than women, and is always bilateral. The rate of progression of the hearing loss is no greater in those receiving haemodialysis or showing hypertension. Three types of pure tone audiometric pattern have been described – trough-shaped, sloping and flat (Rintelmann, 1976). Gleeson (1984) noted unequal recruitment throughout the auditory range with a trend to it being greater in the middle frequencies, producing dynamic compression at 2 kHz. Speech reception thresholds are in agreement with pure tone averages and speech discrimination scores are consistent with the audiometric configuration. Brain stem auditory evoked responses were normal. Gleeson (1984) reported a series of 11 patients (from nine families) including seven with functioning transplants, one on regular haemodialysis, another on continuous ambulatory peritoneal dialysis and two (both female) still with functioning kidneys.

Arnold (1984) reported his own studies of four temporal bones from two patients with Alport's syndrome. These revealed a degeneration of the stria vascularis, a loss of cochlear neurons, atrophy of the spiral ligaments, or loss of hair cells (see Figure 4.10).

Alport's syndrome has also been reported in association with macrothrombopathic thrombocytopenia (Clare *et al.*, 1979). They followed a 20-year-old man from birth to autopsy in whom a kidney transplant had to be removed after signs of rejection at the age of 18 and thereafter he returned to haemodialysis. Audiometry prior to transplantation revealed a bilateral sensorineural hearing loss of 20 dB or less at 2000 Hz, a right hearing loss of 30 dB at 4000 Hz and of 50 dB in the left ear at 8000 Hz. Sadly when the patient died 2 years later there are abundant details of the pathology of the kidney and of platelet studies but only a single sentence comment about the changes in the cochlea: partial loss of the stria vascularis! Brodie *et al.* (1992) reported a kindred of hereditary macrothrombocytopaenia and progressive sensorineural hearing loss but none of the families had any evidence of renal dysfunction. Hearing impairment began in the third decade and progressed from severe to profound bilateral hearing loss by the fourth decade. The platelet disorder manifests itself in early childhood and persists lifelong, although it tends to remain subclinical. (The paper also contains a good discussion on Eckstein and Epstein's syndromes.)

Renal transplantation

Hearing improvement in sensorineural deafness has been reported in two papers. McDonald *et al.* (1978) have reported six cases with this syndrome who have undergone transplantation; of these one patient who received a cadaver kidney had a substantial improvement, the remainder (two received allograft kidneys from living, related donors) obtained stabilization of hearing (follow-up period 3 years).

Mitschke *et al.* (1977) reported audiometric studies on 13 patients before and after renal transplantation. During renal dialysis treatment there was a marked hearing loss for the higher frequencies between 2000 and 8000 Hz. The hearing capacity improved to normal after transplantation, the best results being obtained at 21.4 (8–42) months after surgery. There was a significant improvement in the hearing especially for the middle and high tone frequencies.

Quick (1976) reported a hearing loss in four patients after transplantation. Occasionally hearing loss was noted during transplantation and consideration was given as to whether this was due to the administration of frusemide (furosemide) but it was felt that the irrigation of the wound and peritoneal cavity prior to wound closure with neomycin was more likely; as a result this practice was discontinued.

Jordan *et al.* (1984) reported on seven patients with Alport's syndrome, four of whom underwent transplantation and three who were treated by dialysis; (as might be expected all those undergoing transplant had previously been on dialysis, three for 2 years and one for 3 months). One patient with a mild pre-transplant deficit had a slight improvement in hearing 2 years later; a second patient with a mild hearing loss had no change after 18 months; the patient with a severe deficit has not exhibited any change in the hearing 10 years after surgery and the patient with the moderate hearing loss showed significant deterioration 2 years after transplantation. Of the three patients with Alport's syndrome in the dialysis group, it was only a boy, who was diagnosed at the age of 4 years, had his first audiogram at the age of 11 and who commenced dialysis at the age of 20, whose hearing showed a mild loss over a 9-year period. The two other patients revealed a moderate hearing loss which was not progressive.

In the series reported by Gubler *et al.* (1981), three patients underwent transplantation of whom one was observed to have a hearing improvement (see also Duvall, Nelms and Williams, 1969). A single patient has been reported with unilateral sudden hearing loss which occurred in a renal transplant recipient on triple immunosuppressive treatment consisting of cyclosporin A, azathioprine and prednisolone (Arinsoy *et al.*, 1993). The hearing loss was attributed to a thromboembolic event due to the cyclosporin. One effect of the latter is to decrease vascular prostacyclin. Treatment with a variety of agents including dipyridamole and reduction in the cyclosporin dosage led to return of normal hearing.

So far, *liver transplantation* in children, which now has a one-year survival rate of over 70% using the immunosuppressive regimen of cyclosporin and prednisone, has not been associated with known inner ear problems, although middle ear effusion has been noted (Reilly *et al.*, 1984).

Renal tubular acidosis

In some patients with renal tubular acidosis there is an association with nerve deafness. This condition is one of disordered tubular function, characterized by a sustained metabolic acidosis and hyperchloraemia and an inappropriately high urinary pH. Classical renal tubular acidosis (type I) is a distal tubular defect, while type II is characterized by defective bicarbonate reabsorption in the proximal tubules. It is classical (type I) renal tubular acidosis which may be associated with deafness. While the condition may be sporadic there are many incidences of familial occurrence showing an autosomal dominant mode of transmission.

IgA nephropathy

IgA nephropathy is an immune complex glomerulonephritis. The disease is more common in men and occurs generally during the second or third decades of life. Ataya (1989) reported a case of a 25-year-old man who presented with a 2-day history of sudden deafness in one ear. He had been diagnosed 2 years previously with IgA nephropathy based on renal biopsy. He was treated by intravenous hydrocortisone followed by oral prednisolone. His hearing was monitored by daily audiometry and by the sixth day in hospital he had completely recovered from an 80 dB hearing loss throughout the frequencies to normal hearing on that side.

Diabetes mellitus

A relationship between diabetes and sensorineural hearing loss was first reported by Jordao in 1857.

Peripheral and central neuropathies are well known in diabetes mellitus and the vestibular neurons may also be affected. An excellent review by Taylor and Irwin (1978) endeavoured to put this into perspective and made the following points from their own initial survey and from the literature. The incidence of sensorineural hearing loss in diabetes will very largely depend on the limits of 'normality' and therein the statistical methodology. Second, nearly all the work has naturally been carried out in the group of diabetics most likely to be affected, that is those on insulin. They were careful to limit their upper age range to 50 years, thereby reducing the effect of presbyacusis. They noted that a diabetic with a family history had significantly better hearing thresholds than those without. They found that the diabetics, as a whole, were deafer particularly in the lower frequencies, than the controls and gradually approached each other in the middle range (1–4 kHz) and were similar at 8 kHz.

Friedman and Schulman (1975) studied 20 diabetic patients with peripheral neuropathy; 55% had a symmetrical hearing loss of the sensorineural type, involving at least one frequency, although none gave a history of hearing loss or ear disease. The hearing loss was unrelated to age, and the impairment was similar at low and high frequencies, with maximum deficiency between 750 and 2000 Hz.

Sieger *et al.* (1983) reported a study in children but found no statistically significant differences in auditory function between insulin-dependent diabetics and normal controls, between the diabetics in good or poor control, or between diabetics with or without neurological or vascular complications. Brain stem responses also showed no difference between the two groups.

A small group of patients suffering idiopathic sudden hearing loss was investigated by Wilson *et al.* (1982) to find out if there was a possible relationship to diabetes but no correlation could be found in the audiological pattern; a similar incidence of recovery was noticed in the two groups through the middle frequencies; however, the diabetic patients failed to recover as well in the high frequencies. Brain stem evoked responses also showed no abnormality and no evidence of retrocochlear dysfunction or pathology.

Mehra *et al.* (1985) investigated a series of 102 patients with diabetes and peripheral neuropathy to see if such patients were prone to dysfunction of the inner ear. Only 26 gave a history of hearing loss of mild degree, while 17 had tinnitus and 18 complained of vague giddiness. Investigations showed that one-half demonstrated some sensorineural hearing loss but when corrected for ageing, only 24 showed a mild loss (20–30 dB). Eleven out of 91 showed markedly diminished caloric responses but all of these were in the older age group and had long-standing diabetes. Brain stem auditory evoked responses were carried out in 20 diabetic patients and a matched group of normal controls; there was no difference in the latency of wave V and wave II, although waves III, IV and V were delayed in the diabetic patients.

Almost all studies on diabetic patients have been on those who are insulin-dependent. Piras *et al.* (1985) have reported a series of 30 diabetics of whom 27 were insulin-independent. Eight of the total group showed vascular lesions inherent to diabetics. They carried out auditory and vestibular studies both on the diabetic group and a similar number of normal controls and found that the influence of the disease was almost non-existent and the cochleovestibular response was similar in both groups.

Two centres in the UK (Nottingham and Cardiff) have combined in recent years. Gibbin and Davis (1981) investigated 50 diabetic subjects, 22 of whom were insulin-dependent, the remainder being managed by other regimens and 50 control subjects. No significant differences were found between the two groups on pure-tone audiometry or speech testing, nor between those who were insulin-dependent and those on different treatments.

Miller *et al.* (1983) from the same two centres investigated hearing loss in patients with diabetic retinopathy. They found that the hearing thresholds of patients with known diabetic retinopathy did not differ significantly from those of a control population. However, using a more subtle psychoacoustic test – filtered speech task – a definite difference in hearing acuity between the two groups was demonstrated.

Recent investigators have continued to find similar difficulties to their predecessors, some finding that there is no association between hearing loss and diabetes mellitus and others that there was quite definitely so depending at which sample you looked. Parving *et al.* (1990) investigated a group of long- and short-term insulin-dependent diabetics by a means of psychoacoustic testing and auditory brain stem responses. They tested those with and without diabetic microangiopathy. They could find no difference in the hearing threshold or discrimination scores between the two diabetic groups or between the diabetic patients and an age and sex-matched normal background population. Those with long-term insulin-dependent diabetes showed an auditory brain stem response abnormality in 40% which they thought indicated the presence of diabetic encephalopathy, whereas only 5% of those with short-term insulin-dependent diabetes showed an abnormal brain stem response. Virtaniemi *et al.* (1994a) studied a series of 53 patients with insulin-dependent diabetes mellitus and 42 randomly selected non-diabetic controls. They found that the hearing level tended to be worse in diabetic patients than in the controls but the difference was statistically different only in frequencies of 6000 Hz and 8000 Hz, a finding of several previous studies. Microvascular complications (retinopathy and nephropathy) and the duration of the diabetes was associated with elevated hearing thresholds. By contrast, poor metabolic control was not associated with increased hearing thresholds. Virtaniemi *et al.* concluded that the elevated sensorineural hearing threshold at the two highest frequencies tested were probably caused by the long duration of the diabetes and the microvascular complications associated with it. The same authors (Virtaniemi *et al.*, 1993) investigated auditory brain stem response latencies in insulin-dependent diabetics and compared their findings with a degree of metabolic control, microangiopathy, neuropathy, and the duration of diabetes. In this study all the subjects had normal hearing ability. The wave V latencies were longer in the diabetic patients. Their overall findings seem to indicate a central disturbance of the auditory pathway and the microvascular complications and the duration of the diabetes were associated with prolongation of auditory brain stem latencies. Poor metabolic control was only marginally associated with prolonged auditory brain stem latencies, but they felt that a causative role for diabetic neuropathy in the pathogenesis of prolonged auditory brain stem latencies remained unresolved. The same authors (Virtaniemi *et al.*, 1994b) also investigated the acoustic reflex response in patients with insulin-dependent diabetes mellitus. Patients with diabetes had longer acoustic reflex latencies and decreased amplitudes compared with those of the control subjects. The acoustic reflex amplitude showed a linear correlation with the amplitude of the tympanogram, whereas the acoustic reflex latency had no linear correlation with auditory brain stem latencies in the same subjects. The acoustic reflex responses in the diabetic patients was not associated with the duration of the diabetes, its metabolic control, microangiopathy or neuropathy. They felt the change was probably caused by stiffness in the middle ear system rather than disturbances in the brain stem.

Overall there is no doubt that perhaps the most interesting report is that by Wackym and Linthicum in 1986. They compared the audiometric and clinical histories together with the findings in the temporal bones of eight diabetic patients and 10 normal controls. Their group with diabetes mellitus had significantly more hearing loss than the controls and only patients with diabetes exhibited microangiopathy. In addition to examining the cochlea on both sides, they also examined the vestibular system including the endolymphatic sac. Patients with microangiopathic involvement of the endolymphatic sac had significantly greater hearing loss than those without such involvement and microangiopathy in the stria vascularis was highly significant in the diabetic group; however, they did not have a significant hearing loss! Diabetic patients with basilar membrane microangiopathy had significantly lower percentages of histologically normal hair cells and cells in the stria vascularis; they also had significantly greater hearing loss than diabetic patients without such changes. Their results indicated that the diabetics' sensorineural hearing loss resulted from microangiopathic involvement of the endolymphatic sac and/or basilar membrane vessels. Of their eight diabetic patients it is interesting to note that two were managed by oral hypoglycaemic agents, two were insulin-dependent and three were managed by diet alone; the diabetes was uncontrolled in one patient. Of the total group of eight diabetics and 10 controls, three were hypertensive (all diabetics) and retinopathy was present in two diabetics and neuropathy in three diabetics, but while it was absent in the controls, 11 of the total group were undocumented in both aspects. Interestingly only five diabetics had a hearing loss but this was significantly more than those in the controls. The diabetic group treated only by diet had the most severe hearing loss followed by the group taking oral hypoglycaemic agents; paradoxically the group receiving insulin and the uncontrolled diabetic showed the least hearing loss. From this study it is evident that other investigators should examine those on oral hypoglycaemic agents and those being treated by diet only as no significant clinical study of these groups appears to have been carried out.

Carmen *et al.*(1988, 1989) investigated 45 subjects undergoing a 5-hour glucose tolerance test and demonstrated a rising, progressively improving sensorineural hearing loss, i.e. from lower toward higher frequencies. Seven were found to have diabetes mellitus, five had impaired glucose tolerance and nine had a mild but non-diagnostic glucose intolerance – an overall total of 47%. No difference was found among any of the groups in terms of their ability to understand speech.

Phytanic acid storage disease (Refsum's disease)

Heredopathia atactica polyneuritiformis is a biochemically defined autosomal-recessive disease not a syndrome. The manifestations are characterized by pigmentary retinal degeneration (retinitis pigmentosa), chronic polyneuropathy, ataxia, and other cerebellar signs, and an increased CSF protein content with normal cell count. In most cases, anosmia, hearing loss of cochlear type, and cardiopathy have been present. Feldman (1981) reported a single case and Djupesland, Flottorp and Refsum (1983) reported two cases. By dietary measures (a low-phytanic-acid, low-phytol dietary treatment) there was no worsening of the hearing (see page 3/4/24).

Hyperlipoproteinaemia (hyperlipidaemia)

When considering this condition as a cause of fluctuating hearing loss, it is important to stress at the outset, the difference between primary and secondary hyperlipidaemia. There is a large number of conditions causing secondary hyperlipoproteinaemia, the most common of which are diabetes, alcoholism, chronic renal failure and gout. Pregnancy may also be a cause and oral contraceptives have been shown to elevate the plasma triglyceride in most subjects taking them. It is therefore essential to exclude these secondary causes, if not at the time of the original sampling, at least when the fasting lipids are being checked.

The next factor to be taken into account is the incidence of hyperlipoproteinaemia, not in populations elsewhere in the world, but in the same part of the same country and the normal value of the individual laboratory.

Booth (1977) investigated 44 patients with premature bilateral sensorineural hearing loss, without vertigo, and failed to find any incidence greater than in the local general population and no patient requiring treatment other than by a modification of the diet. Further cases have confirmed this finding and none so far has shown any significant improvement in hearing; conversely there has also been no progression apart from age-related changes.

Drettner *et al.* (1975) in a study of 1000, 50 year-old men investigated a number of cardiovascular risk factors to see if they might be of importance in the development of sensorineural hearing loss; no significant correlations were found. Included among the risk factors, which were studied, were serum cholesterol, serum triglycerides, uric acid and glucose tolerance. Spencer (1981) has carried out the largest series associating abnormal lipids and inner ear symptoms. Of his 1419 patients, 18.4% were classified as having type IIA or pure hypercholesterolaemia with normal triglycerides; 6.3% had type IIB primary hypercholesterolaemia associated with lesser hypertriglyceridaemia, while by far the largest part showed a type IV primary hypertriglyceridaemia with a lesser elevation of the cholesterol level. However, the incidence of obesity in these patients has varied from 72 to 100% depending upon the type of disorder and whether it was associated with an elevated glucose tolerance. In his patients, reversing their dietary habits by cutting out refined carbohydrates, reducing the intake of saturated fats and by increasing the amount of dietary fibre, avoidance of additional salt and sugar, and obtaining ideal body weight, he has reported improvements in hearing and has found similar therapy of value in treating patients with Menière's disease. Moffat, Booth and Morrison (1979) carried out detailed investigations including metabolic studies into 27 patients with Menière's disease, but found no increased abnormality on glucose tolerance testing, fasting serum cholesterol and triglyceride levels, or estimations of thyroid stimulating hormone. A similar evaluation was carried out by

Kinney (1980) in 134 patients showing a high correlation of abnormal carbohydrate metabolism (5-hour test) and hyperlipoproteinaemia.

Lowry and Isaacson (1978) examined the audiology records of 100 patients presenting with a 20 dB bilateral sensorineural hearing loss or greater. After a 14-hour fast and taking a history for the presence of diabetes, the height, weight and blood pressure were recorded. Lipoproteins were estimated and 12 patients with type IIA or IIB and eight patients with type IV abnormalities were found; they commented that such a finding was a lower proportion of patients with hyperlipoproteinaemia than in the general population. Jones and Davis (1992) investigated 279 men, aged 50–60 years, selected at random from those referred by general practitioners for lipid profiles. They found no relationship between the total cholesterol, low density lipoprotein or triglyceride measurements and hearing loss could be found at any frequency up to 14 kHz. The raised fasting glucose was associated with a higher hearing threshold at low frequencies; a raised ESR was associated with higher hearing threshold levels in mid-frequencies. The effect of high density lipoprotein level on hearing was highly dependent on the ESR. Ullrich, Aurbach and Drobik (1992) carried out a prospective study of hyperlipidaemia as a pathogenic factor in sudden hearing loss. They examined 25 patients with a first event of sudden hearing loss and nine with a repeated event of sudden deafness. Serum lipid patterns and atherogenic risk factors were the same in both groups and corresponded to lipid patterns in the average population. Histories of all the patients concerning smoking habits, alcohol and drug consumption, noise, stress and recent viral infections were documented. They noted that fibrinogen is assumed to be much more critical concerning blood rheology, but the plasma concentrations determined were within the normal range in all patients.

Ben-David *et al.* (1986) carried out a comparison of auditory brain stem evoked potentials in hyperlipidaemic and normolipaemic subjects. There were 25 hyperlipidaemic patients who were neurologically and audiologically asymptomatic and 20 normolipaemic controls. Auditory brain stem evoked potentials showed the effect of increasing stimulus rate to be significantly greater in hyperlipidaemic patients (click stimulus 10/s versus 55/s). There were 17 type IV, one type IIA and seven type IIB in the hyperlipidaemic group. There was no significant difference in the brain stem auditory evoked potentials at a stimulus rate of 10/s. It was considered that the highly significant difference with click stimuli at 55/s indicated subclinical impairment of brain stem function in hyperlipidaemic subjects. Strome, Topf and Vernick (1988) investigated the possibility of hyperlipidaemia being the cause of sensorineural hearing loss in children. They reported on this finding in three children, two aged 6 and one 9 years of age but they give no indication as to how many others were tested and found to be normal/negative.

Axelsson and Lindgren (1985) enquired about the possible relationship between hypercholesterolaemia and noise-induced hearing loss. They compared 75 50-year-old men with a high serum cholesterol level and 75 50-year-old men randomly selected from the same WHO material. The hearing was similar in both groups. They noted that noise was the most predominant factor influencing hearing at any specific frequency or combination of frequencies. There was a significant tendency for those with a high cholesterol level who suffered the most noise exposure to have a high frequency hearing loss; the tendency for the low cholesterol group was to have a high frequency hearing loss if excessively exposed to occupational noise.

Saadah (1993) reported on 31 patients seen over a 5-year period, mean age 58, in whom vestibular vertigo was associated with hyperlipidaemia and noted their response to antilipidaemic therapy. Complete resolution was finally achieved in 84% and it was noted that six of the 12 patients who stopped medication relapsed; three of these who resumed therapy responded satisfactorily again.

A cautionary reminder is given by Feher *et al.* (1992) emphasizing that in a group of 400 diabetic patients under their care, despite regularly supervised diabetes, including dietary advice, over one-quarter had a raised serum total cholesterol (> 6.5 mmol/l) while over one-quarter of the non-insulin-treated and one-eighth of the insulin-treated diabetic subjects had a high density lipoprotein-cholesterol less than < 0.9 mmol/l.

Hypothyroidism

Schuknecht (1974) found the literature up to that time unconvincing on the relationship between acquired idiopathic hypothyroidism and sensorineural hearing loss, although commented that clinicians seemed to have the impression that there probably was such an association. Post (1964) investigated 42 patients – seven with spontaneous primary hypothyroidism and 35 hypothyroid patients with treated carcinoma of the thyroid. He noted that slow mentation while hypothyroid may be interpreted by the patient as a subjective hearing loss. None of the patients with sensorineural loss attained entirely normal hearing when euthyroid. He was unable to demonstrate any specific correlation between age, degree of hypothyroidism and resulting deafness. He was also unable to determine the time required for patients to remain hypothyroid before experiencing a hearing loss. Stephens and Hinchcliffe (1968) found a significant correlation between the diagnosis of myxoedema, and fatigue or temporary threshold drift measured at 8000 Hz by the Carhart technique. Stephens (1970) later confirmed that this was not an

artefact relating to age, but a true finding. He suggested that the sensorineural lesion in myxoedema lies proximal to the hair cells. Meyerhoff (1976) reviewed the possible relationship between all forms of reduced thyroid function and hearing loss; under the heading 'non-genetic acquired' he reiterated the claims made up to that time, that is there was no definite association.

van't Hoff and Stuart (1979) reported an incidence of deafness of 85% in a consecutive series of 48 patients with myxoedema. The more severe the disease, the higher was the incidence of deafness; there was no difference between the effect on the high or low frequencies and in some cases the loss was unilateral. Testing after the patients became euthyroid showed improved hearing in 73% of ears. The percentage returning to normal (23%) showed no significant difference in the proportion of severe (20%) to mild myxoedema (26%). Repeat testing after becoming euthyroid, failed to show any further improvement. Age did not appear to be a factor in the cause of deafness in myxoedema. While severity of myxoedema was associated with a higher incidence of deafness, no other relationship could be found between severity in myxoedema and a variety of other neurophysiological measurements. van't Hoff and Stuart were in no doubt that the deafness was sensorineural.

Parving, Parving and Lyngsøe (1983) in a series of 15 patients with confirmed myxoedema, median age 76 years, demonstrated a bilateral symmetrical or nearly symmetrical sensorineural hearing loss in all patients before treatment. Treatment with L-thyroxine in this group of elderly patients showed no improvement in hearing sensitivity and the group demonstrated neither more nor less hearing loss than other hearing-impaired patients of the same age group.

Hall *et al.* (1985) reported a prospective study undertaken to compare the auditory acuity in hypothyroid patients and to assess the effect of thyroxine on these thresholds, for a mean period of 5.7 months (range 2–24 months). Auditory thresholds were reduced over all frequencies but the difference being significant only at 2000 and 4000 Hz. Speech discrimination was also significantly reduced in both ears. With thyroxine there was a small improvement in pure-tone thresholds and speech discrimination; this was only significant at 4000 Hz in both ears.

Himelfarb *et al.* (1981) attempted to correlate changes in the brain stem electric responses of patients with thyroid dysfunction (six hyperthyroid; six hypothyroid). A good correlation was observed between the brain stem conduction time and level of serum tetraiodothyronine (T4; thyroxine). In untreated hyperthyroidism, the brain stem conduction time was decreased and in some patients the brain stem electric response was characterized by high amplitude waves, sharp peaks and jittery contours becoming smoother in pattern and more well-defined after treatment (Figure 17.7).

In untreated hypothyroidism, the brain stem electric response was generally characterized by prolonged conduction time, diminished amplitudes, flattened peaks and poor synchronization; in the older patients the changes in wave pattern were more pronounced (Figure 17.8). Brain stem conduction time appears to be a sensitive index of the thyroxine-dependent cellular status in the neural pathways of the brain stem.

More recently, Anand *et al.* (1989) carried out auditory investigations in 20 patients with hypothyroidism. They were assessed before and after treatment with L-thyroxine, 3–7 months after becoming euthyroid (mean 3.7). Sixteen demonstrated a hearing loss: mild in five, moderate in 11; 12 sensorineural and four mixed. Special hearing tests revealed a cochlear type of hearing loss. Brain stem evoked responses showed prolonged, absolute latency of wave V and interpeak latencies I–III and I–V; the amplitude of waves I, II and V were reduced. Following treatment, a statistically significant improvement in the hearing thresholds was observed by pure tone audiometry, but brain stem evoked responses did not show signifi-

cant reversibility. Subjectively nine patients complained of diminished hearing acuity and three had tinnitus. Following treatment, 13 patients reported hearing improvement, the hearing thresholds improving by 5–10 dB in eight and by more than 10 dB in 12 at one or more frequencies, in one or both ears. Speech reception thresholds and speech discrimination scores were normal in all patients. Vanasse *et al.* (1989) investigated 15 adult hypothyroid patients by brain stem evoked responses before treatment and 17 also had pure tone audiometry. However, both tests were only repeated in five patients after treatment (2–22 months). They could find no significant changes in waves I, III, V latencies or in the I–V interval or in the I, III, V interpeak latencies. They commented on the different results achieved by themselves and Himelfarb *et al.* (1981), the latter authors measuring the brain stem conduction time from the peak of wave I to the peak of P4 (P4 being defined as the peak immediately following wave V and preceding wave VI).

Francois *et al.* (1993) investigated 11 congenital hypothyroid newborn babies; evoked otoacoustic emissions were present bilaterally in nine. Auditory brain stem responses in six newborns showed a prolonged wave I. When reassessed at 9–12 months of age after treatment, the auditory threshold was normal in nine and evoked otoacoustic emissions were present in at least one ear in all children. Four ears in two newborns could not be tested because the baby cried when the probe was inserted in the external ear canal. The authors found all waves on auditory brain stem responses to be clearly visible above the threshold in the congenitally hypothyroid newborn. Although there is a prolonged latency of wave I there was no modification of the I–IV interpeak latency. Earlier Hebert *et al.* (1986) using auditory brain stem response audiometry evaluated 34 congenital hypothyroid children receiving thyroid hormone therapy; their results suggested a significant incidence of auditory brain stem response abnormalities in treated hypothyroid children.

Parving *et al.* (1986) reported the audiological and temporal bone findings in myxoedema. They investigated 15 patients with confirmed myxoedema with a median age of 48 years before and after treatment with L-thyroxine. No improvement in hearing sensitivity could be demonstrated either in the younger patients (age 32–60 years) or in the older group (64–95 years). When compared to an age and sex-matched unscreened population, the myxoedematous patients did not demonstrate any different degree of hearing loss. Histological investigation of the temporal bones from an 83-year-old woman with myxoedema, however, showed no morphological changes or deposition of glycosaminoglycans, changes which were compatible with true age-related hearing loss. They concluded that those series which had previously indicated a hearing improvement after restoring

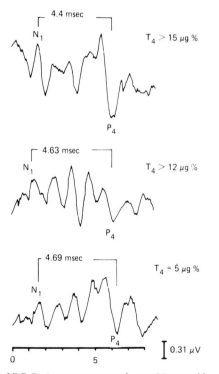

Figure 17.7 Brain stem responses from a 55-year-old woman with hyperthyroidism due to a toxic adenoma. Top tracing – recorded prior to onset of therapy. Middle trace – 5 weeks after receiving propylthiouracil and propranolol. Lower trace – shows normal response 6 weeks following hemithyroidectomy

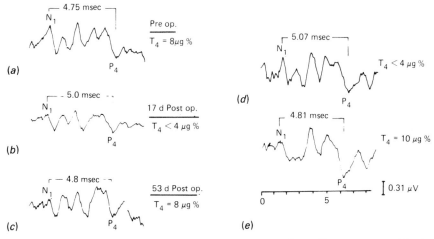

Figure 17.8 Brain stem responses from a 47-year-old man (*a*) prior to surgery for papillary carcinoma of the thyroid gland and squamous carcinoma of larynx; (*b*) trace 17 days after total thyroidectomy and laryngectomy; (*c*) trace 3 weeks after starting replacement therapy with L-thyroxine; (*d*) trace after patient had become clinically myxoedematous and failed to take thyroxine for past year; (*e*) trace 2 months after recommencing L-thyroxine. (Reproduced by kind permission of Himelfarb and Editor, *Journal of Laryngology and Otology*)

Skeletal system and otic capsule

the patients to a euthyroid state had been carried out on only a very limited number of patients and when the sample was larger no abnormal hearing levels could be found either before or after treatment in myxoedema.

Conditions under this heading are considered more fully in Chapter 15 but may rarely cause sudden cochlear hearing loss. Metastatic carcinoma may also occasionally occur in the ear producing such an effect and should not be overlooked (see Figure 5.43).

Johnson, Hawke and Berger (1984) reported a case of disseminated adenocarcinoma of the breast. The patient suffered sudden deafness with vertigo shortly before her death. The temporal bones revealed extensive perilymphatic haemorrhage as the probable cause of deafness; there were widespread deposits in the temporal bone. Pringle, Jefferis and Barrett (1993) reported a unilateral sudden sensorineural hearing loss caused by metastatic prostatic carcinoma. A patient has also been reported with multiple myeloma who, after a long remission, relapsed and developed a sudden and complete hearing loss in one ear followed 2 weeks later by that on the other side (Keay, 1988).

An osteoma of the internal auditory meatus is a rare finding and usually diagnosed only on CT scanning. Conversely an MRI scan of such a lesion shows no abnormality. Clerico, Jahn and Fontanella (1994) found only 12 cases in the world literature to which they added one of their own. In the majority of these there had been no histological report. Their own patient gave a 3-year history of occasional bouts of dizziness lasting a few seconds but vertigo became constant and violent in the few weeks prior to the referral, during which time she had also begun to notice decreased hearing and constant buzzing tinnitus in the affected ear. At operation, they found a loop of the anterior inferior cerebellar artery tethered between the two lobes of the bony mass which was abutting and compressing the vestibulocochlear nerve bundle. They concluded that the symptoms, when they occur, are presumably due to direct pressure on the bundle. Hearing loss which is unilateral and sensorineural, and vestibular abnormalities have been the most commonly reported symptoms. A case was reported by Singh, Annis and Todd (1992) producing a unilateral sensorineural hearing loss of sudden onset initially associated with slight dizzy spells. The latter settled spontaneously and, when investigated 2 years later, audiological tests confirmed sensorineural hearing loss with abnormal auditory adaptation indicating a retrocochlear hearing loss. A plain X-ray of the internal auditory meatus was normal. Brain stem evoked responses showed an increased interaural latency difference in wave V. A subsequent CT scan showed the internal auditory meatus to be of normal calibre but there was an osteoma arising from the posterior wall within the lateral part of the canal which occupied more than 50% of the anteroposterior diameter. This case was not one of those reported by Clerico, Jahn and Fontanella (1994).

Ototoxicity

This subject is discussed more fully in Chapter 20. It is well known that several types of medication, particularly certain groups of antibiotics, can cause sudden hearing loss, and likewise some diuretic agents. Less well known or expected are certain other agents.

Interferon

After seeing a single case of sudden sensorineural hearing loss during interferon therapy, Kanda *et al.* (1994) prospectively assessed the auditory function in 49 patients receiving interferon. Auditory disability (tinnitus, hearing loss or both) occurred in 22 patients (45%) during treatment with sensorineural hearing loss occurring in 18 (37%). The auditory disability often developed in the late stage of treatment and resolved in all patients within 7–14 days after discontinuation of interferon. The ototoxicity appeared to be dose related. All the patients receiving interferon alpha were affected at 8 kHz. In two patients receiving interferon beta, treatment had to be discontinued because of progressive sensorineural hearing loss. Interferon beta seems more ototoxic than interferon alpha but this may reflect a difference in administration.

Contraceptive pill

Oral contraception is in widespread use by women all over the world, but it seems that there are only a few reported cases of sudden deafness, all of which are presumed to be 'thrombotic', i.e. vascular. Sellars (1971) reported a case following the intramuscular injection of depoprogesterone (150 mg); the deafness developed in one ear, 7 days later together with tinnitus and vertigo. The woman became totally deaf with depressed labyrinthine function.

Gonzales, Istre and Rubin (1968) reported two cases, both considered to be cochlear losses in whom the labyrinthine caloric responses were reduced. The first developed a unilateral loss on norethindrone with mestranol and had partial recovery (after treatment) of the hearing loss which was thought to lie in the end-organ; the second, after taking Ortho-novum for 2 years.

Hanna (1986) reported a unilateral 90 dB loss in a patient who was taking a pill containing 500 μg norethisterone/35 μg ethinyl oestradiol. Next day there had been marked recovery at 500 Hz and 5 days after the event, her hearing had returned to normal. (She was treated with oral steroids and naftidrofuryl.) The patient was found to be allergic to Dextran 40.

Dickens and Graham (1993) have recently reported two cases of sagittal thrombosis. The first presented with sudden onset unilateral facial paralysis. The other with pressure/fullnes in one ear accompanied by nausea and vomiting together with left-sided tinnitus. The hearing of the first patient was normal though the stapedial reflexes were absent bilaterally; the hearing of the second was also normal but there

was a slight increase in the stapedial reflexes on the right side. The diagnosis in each case was made by MRI screening.

Dantrolene

Pace–Balzan and Ramsden (1988) reported a case of sudden bilateral sensorineural hearing loss in a 19-year-old Caucasian girl suffering from athetoid cerebral palsy who was known to have a normal hearing left ear and a long-standing, non-progressive sensorineural hearing loss on the right. She suffered from severe muscle spasms and dantrolene was added to her existing treatment of baclofen and diazepam at a starting dose of 25 mg daily. After 5 days the dose was increased to 50 mg daily. Within a few hours of taking the first dose at that level the patient became suddenly profoundly deaf. Pure tone audiometry 4 days after the event showed a sensorineural hearing loss of 70 dB in the left ear and virtually no measurable hearing in the right. In spite of treatment there was no improvement.

Mianserin

There have been reported cases of this drug causing tinnitus, but Marais (1991) reported a single case of a 22-year-old man in whom tinnitus began immediately after he was prescribed mianserin hydrochloride 20 mg twice daily for mild depression. The symptom became worse over the ensuing months and after 2 years he ceased taking the medication, though his tinnitus persisted at the same earlier level. Audiometry 3 years after the onset of the tinnitus showed bilateral, almost symmetrical high frequency sensorineural hearing loss.

Vaccination

Sudden deafness following vaccination has been reported; nine cases have been collected and analysed as a group (Mair and Elverland, 1977). The majority of these cases (eight) occurred following the administration of tetanus antitoxin but also one following tetanus toxoid. The deafness occurred from 2 days after the toxoid, up to 10 days. In all but three cases, the vaccine was given as a prophylaxis or re-vaccination, not as treatment. The sensorineural deafness appears to affect the cochlear nerve and only two cases have subsequently improved. Peripheral neuropathies following administration of antitetanus serum and tetanus toxoid are well documented. Hearing loss has also been reported following vaccination for whooping cough (including a booster), rabies injections, and possibly subsequent re-vaccination against smallpox. No case has been reported following diphtheria vaccination or oral polio immunization. These cases are presumed to be due to either a local hypersensitivity or antigen–antibody reaction and it is highly likely that many other cases have gone unnoticed or unreported.

Carbon monoxide intoxication

It will be a considerable surprise to most otolaryngologists to learn that probably more than 300 cases of hearing loss from carbon monoxide intoxication are on record. The gas, by its combination with haemoglobin to form carboxyhaemoglobin, may thereby deprive vital organs of oxygen. It is little wonder, therefore, that this may affect the inner ear, causing hearing loss, tinnitus, nystagmus and ataxia. The vestibular impairment is considered to be directly related to the duration of exposure, but there is argument as to whether the predominant lesion is central or peripheral. The intoxication may be chronic or acute. Chronic intoxication usually results in a permanent, symmetrical, high-frequency hearing loss. In one series, no less than 78% of 263 patients were affected and only 27% showed slight improvement (Lumio, 1948). Hearing returned to normal in 11%, only in cases having a slight deficiency. The hearing loss was unnoticed by the patients themselves and Lumio noted that hearing for speech and for whisper was seldom reduced.

Acute intoxication is much less common and hearing loss is quite unpredictable, though when it occurs, some improvement may be expected; it is usually bilateral and may be asymmetric. Morris (1969) reported a single case of bilateral sensorineural hearing loss following acute carbon monoxide poisoning. There was gradual improvement over the following 4 weeks. Baker and Lilly (1977) reported a case of fluctuating sensorineural hearing loss and acute carbon monoxide poisoning. They noted that while acute poisoning was said to cause diffuse haemorrhages in the brain stem and cerebrum, chronic poisoning often led to demyelination of the globus pallidus. At presentation audiometry showed a U-shaped audiogram which slowly improved over 7 months but maintained the basic shape throughout.

Miscellaneous

Ulcerative colitis

In a small number of patients an association between ulcerative colitis and sensorineural hearing loss usually bilateral and often sudden in onset has been reported; this may be associated with vestibular dysfunction (Summers and Harker, 1982; Weber, Jenkins and Coker, 1984; Hollanders, 1986). More recently a case in association with giant cell arteritis has been reported (Jacob *et al.*, 1990). Often the hearing loss has occurred at a time when the ulcerative colitis has been active and in each of the reported cases there has been a good response to treatment with steroids, sometimes supplemented by other immunosuppressive agents. The link between these conditions appears to be an immune complex vasculitis.

Scleroderma

Abou-Taleb and Linthicum (1987) reported a case including temporal bone pathology of a woman who in the last 2 years complained of slowly progressive hearing loss. Investigation showed a bilateral mixed hearing loss which was ultimately treated using cyclophosphamide. Three months later she claimed improvement in her hearing which was confirmed by closure of the air-bone gap and again in the sensorineural element on both sides.

Sarcoidosis

Neurological manifestations of sarcoidosis occur in 5% of affected patients. Of the cranial nerves, the VIIIth is the fourth most frequently involved. The central nervous system lesion is presumed to be a granulomatous meningitis that directly infiltrates the cranial nerves or causes them to be compressed from involvement of adjacent intracranial structures. Sensorineural hearing loss and vertigo usually occur in association with other neurological findings, but may be the only presenting complaint. Jahrsdoerfer *et al.* (1981) reported the case of a 35-year-old woman who experienced a form of tinnitus in her left ear while attending an outdoor concert. The following day she had a mild sensorineural hearing loss in the left ear which was slightly progressive over the next month. Two months later she returned complaining of a hearing problem in the right ear. A subsequent hearing test the following month continued to show a fluctuation of hearing in both ears, but additional investigations showed a raised serum calcium and hilar adenopathy on her chest X-ray. Examination of her eyes showed a granulomatous iritis consistent with sarcoidosis and biopsy of a pre-scalene lymph node showed a non-caseating granuloma. Subsequent treatment with prednisone led to an improvement in her hearing.

More recently, Souliere *et al.* (1991) reported two cases of neurosarcoidosis which presented with sudden onset sensorineural hearing loss as the only manifestation. One of these also had a cerebellopontine angle granuloma that mimicked a vestibular schwannoma. The first case presented with a total unilateral hearing loss and in subsequent investigations showed an absent ipsilateral caloric response. Radiological investigations showed a large non-enhancing mass filling the cerebellopontine angle with widening of the internal auditory meatus. The ESR was raised and likewise the angiotensin-converting enzyme (ACE) was elevated. Chest X-ray demonstrated bilateral perihilar adenopathy and biopsy of supraclavicular lymph nodes showed characteristic non-caseating granuloma. Subsequent treatment with prednisone led to complete resolution of the posterior fossa pathology but brain stem evoked responses which initially showed no response on the right side continued to demonstrate poor wave morphology and a prolonged though improved wave I–V latency. The second case showed a sudden onset asymmetrical bilateral hearing loss.

Recently, the first case of sarcoidosis affecting the middle ear has been reported (Tyndel *et al.*, 1994). This produced a mild conductive hearing loss and normal brain stem evoked responses. A pale, pink granular mass could be seen through the posterior part of the tympanic membrane and part was removed for biopsy revealing a non-caseating granuloma.

Retrocochlear (VIIIth nerve) and central nervous system

Meningitis

Leptomeningitis still causes a few cases of sudden deafness – it is typically bilateral, and total or subtotal. It may occur as a complication of acute otitis media, and is usually pneumococcal in origin. While this is a well-recognized complication of bacterial meningitis, sensorineural hearing loss in association with the less clinically obvious cryptococcal meningitis has been reported and has even been associated with sudden deafness (Maslan, Graham and Flood, 1985). A series of audiological examinations on five patients suffering from hearing loss following meningitis showed that extremely poor word discrimination scores as compared to pure tone audiograms were common in all five; acoustic reflex measurements showed absent reflexes when stimulating the better hearing ear (Harada *et al.* 1988).

Tuberculous meningitis may still rarely be encountered and the cranial nerves may be involved by the arachnoiditis and adhesions in spite of modern therapy; as in other bacterial forms of meningitis both the cochlear and vestibular nerves may be affected (McCabe, 1975) (see Figures 4.41 and 4.42).

Acute meningovascular syphilis still occurs and may present to the otologist.

Viral disease may also cause meningitis, although it is seldom the cause of sudden deafness.

Multiple sclerosis

Deafness in multiple sclerosis seems more likely to occur during the first 4 years of the presentation of the condition, but thereafter there is no relationship between the hearing loss and the duration of the disease. It has been estimated that some 3% of patients have a hearing problem but a higher percentage, perhaps 25%, are troubled by vertigo at some stage during the disease. The disparity between the pure tone result which may be good and speech discrimination scores which are often poor is well recognized.

Because by definition multiple sclerosis is a disease characterized by multiple areas of demyelination of the central nervous system, the clinical diagnosis depends on the demonstration of two or more lesions. For this reason, non-invasive techniques of investigation are of particular value. Included among these are auditory and vestibular tests particularly brain stem auditory evoked responses.

Cipparone *et al.* (1989) investigated the use of electronystagmography in 144 cases (116 definite and 28 possible) of multiple sclerosis. Pursuit movements and visual suppression tests were especially helpful being pathological in 56 and 58% of cases respectively; spontaneous and/or evoked nystagmus was present in 45%. Comparison between clinical and instrumental evidence of brain stem involvement indicated that 18% of the definite and 32% of possible cases of multiple sclerosis presented a negative clinical examination with positive instrumental findings.

Using a variety of tests, Jerger *et al.* (1986) examined 62 patients with definite multiple sclerosis. The acoustic reflex showed the highest identification rate (71%), followed by speech audiometry (55%), auditory brain stem responses (52%) and masking level difference (45%). A combination of abnormality on either acoustic reflex, auditory brain stem responses or speech audiometry yielded a 90% identification rate. Auditory brain stem responses showed some abnormality in one or both ears in only 52% of patients (Figure 17.9).

Wiegand and Poch (1988) investigated the acoustic reflex in normal controls, patients with sensorineural hearing loss and asymptomatic multiple sclerosis. The threshold, onset latency and rise time measurements were similar for all three groups. Unlike normal subjects, there is no increase in wave V amplitude on binaural stimulation in a large majority of patients with multiple sclerosis who have no hearing deficit. The first stage of bilateral innervation occurs at the level of the superior olivary complex. Binaural stimulation may be complete at this level, so that only the subsequent waves originating from the brain stem nuclei caudal to the superior olivary complex will result in increased amplitude on binaural stimulation. Prasher, Sainz and Gibson (1982) showed that the mean amplitude of wave V in patients with multiple sclerosis did not alter significantly when stimulation was changed from one ear to the other or even when both ears were stimulated simultaneously; the majority of their patients showed a decrease in amplitude on binaural stimulation. In patients with chronic disease, the amplitude of wave V was small and was not affected by changing from monaural to binaural stimulation. Their studies showed that the brain stem potentials in patients with multiple sclerosis who have no hearing deficit, did not increase in amplitude on binaural stimulation.

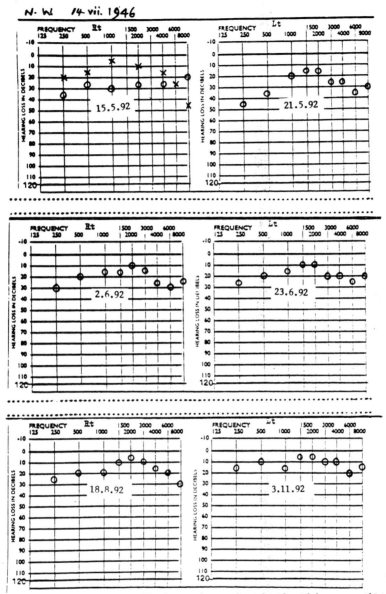

Figure 17.9 A 46-year-old man complaining of sudden hearing loss on the right side with known past history of multiple sclerosis. (*a*) Serial pure tone audiograms over a 6-month period show initially very little visible evidence of subjective hearing loss

There is no single characteristic pattern either in this or other series but prolongation of wave V latency appears to be the most consistent finding. By contrast Chiappa *et al.* (1980) reported brain stem auditory evoked responses in 202 patients with 'definite', 'probable', or 'possible' multiple sclerosis, but no patient presented with hearing difficulties. Only a few patients in their series had formal audiograms and all of these were normal. Using *monaural* stimulation, 68% had normal brain stem responses. In those showing abnormal responses, there was no signifi-

cant correlation between the multiple sclerosis classification and the abnormality in brain stem response. In the abnormal group, 13% had only interwave latency abnormalities, 55% had only wave V amplitude abnormalities, and 33% had abnormalities of both interwave latency and wave V amplitude.

Only relatively few patients are reported as developing acute hearing loss and two recent reports of such patients undergoing brain stem auditory evoked responses are of interest. Jabbari, Marsh and Gunderson (1982) reported two cases of acute unilateral

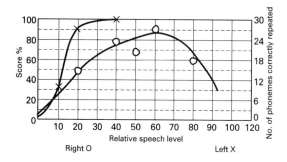

Figure 17.9 (*b*) Speech audiogram at presentation

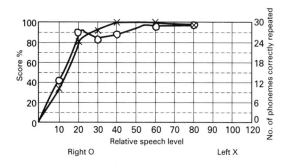

Figure 17.9 (*c*) Speech audiogram at presentation 6 months later showing return to normal

LEFT

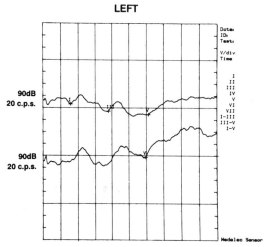

Figure 17.9 (*d*) Brain stem evoked responses (left) show waves I, III and V readily identifiable and absolute latencies within normal limits

LEFT   10 clicks per sec.

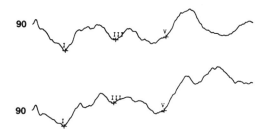

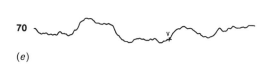

(*e*)

RIGHT

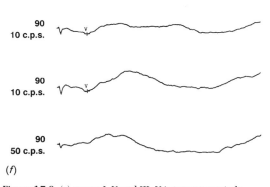

(*f*)

Figure 17.9 (*e*) waves I–V and III–V interwave periods indicate increased neural conduction time. (*f*) On the right side, only a poor wave form could be obtained and only wave I was identifiable at 90 and 100 dB HL indicating significantly impaired neural conduction

deafness whose responses showed an absence of waves II to IV in the first and the presence of only wave I in the second. Fischer *et al.* (1985) reported 12 patients with definite multiple sclerosis who experienced an acute hearing loss during a relapse of the demyelinating disease, in a series of 705 patients. Responses were recorded in all 12 patients, during the relapse with acute hearing loss in four and after the relapse with hearing loss in the remaining eight. During the relapse with hearing loss, brain stem electric response abnormalities were present in four, wave I being absent in two. Responses were also noted to improve substantially when recorded after the relapse in two of the three patients in whom such records were made. Brain stem electric response recordings were abnormal on the side of the earlier

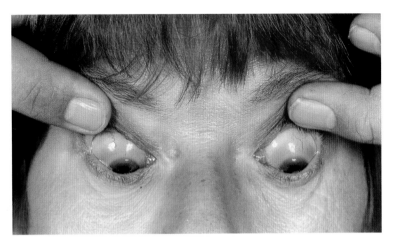

Plate 3/15/I Blue sclerae seen in a patient with osteogenesis imperfecta who underwent a successful stapedectomy, who also coincidentally had a family history of malignant hyperthermia.

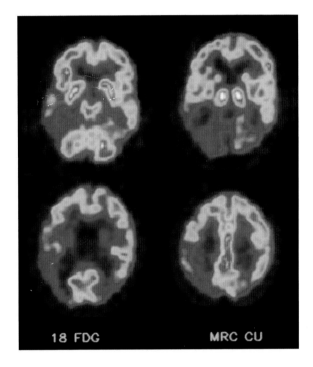

Plate 3/17/I Four slices from a positron emission tomogram showing cerebral glucose metabolism in a patient with probable Alzheimer's disease. A reduction (blue green) in the metabolism of the temporal and parietal regions is seen bilaterally

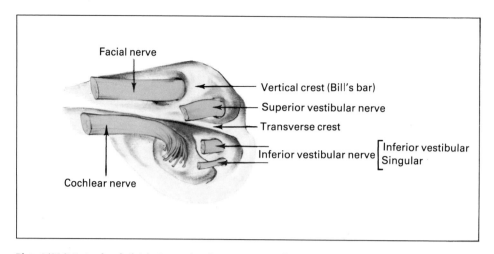

Plate 3/21/I Lateral end of right internal auditory meatus with normal neural structures

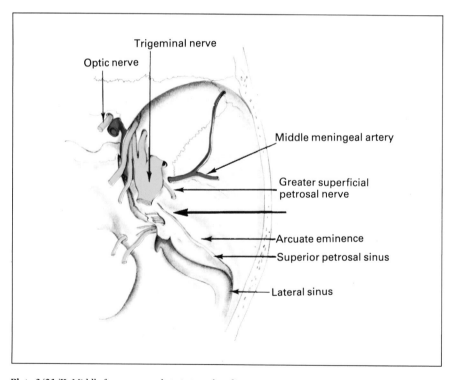

Plate 3/21/II Middle fossa approach to internal auditory meatus

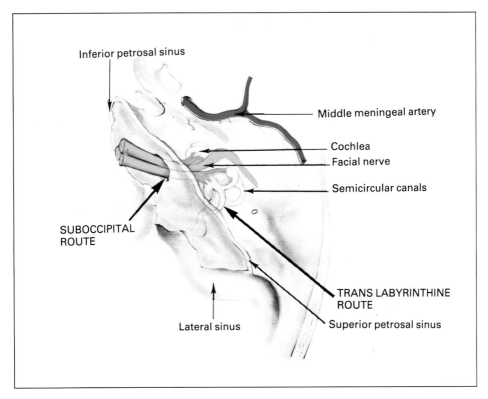

Plate 3/21/III The temporal bone seen from above to show the translabyrinthine and suboccipital transmeatal approaches

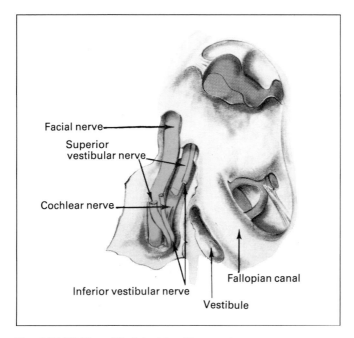

Plate 3/21/IV View of the internal auditory meatus as seen in the translabyrinthine approach

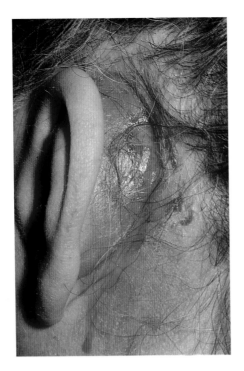

Plate 3/22/I Invasion of the retroauricular sulcus by cancer in the external auditory meatus

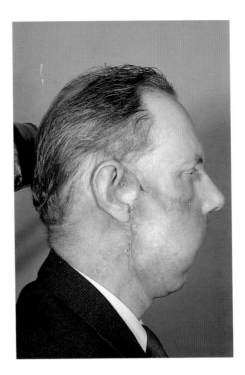

Plate 3/22/III Appearance of the patient after subtotal petrosectomy, the defect having been skin grafted

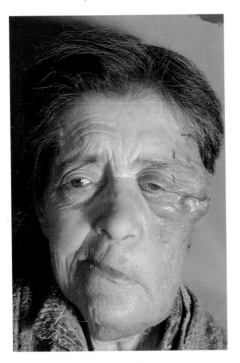

Plate 3/22/II Carcinoma of the middle ear invading the infratemporal fossa and causing a bulge in the temple and proptosis

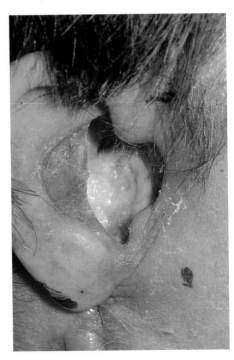

Plate 3/22/IV Patient with carcinoma of the ear treated surgically, following failed radiotherapy, and exhibiting osteoradionecrosis

hearing loss in five of the eight patients investigated after the relapse. Fisher *et al.* considered that the lesion causing unilateral hearing loss in multiple sclerosis could be situated in the cochlear nerve or close to its entry zone in the brain stem. In the classical case of a predominant, if not exclusive, central demyelination in multiple sclerosis, peak I remains present, well-shaped and of normal latency in most patients who have not experienced an acute episode of hearing loss in the course of their disease. Fishcher *et al.* reported an absence of wave I in only five cases in a series of 340 patients without a history of hearing loss. Arnold and Bender (1983) reported a case of particular interest in whom hearing tests were carried out over a 6-year period prior to the apparent development of multiple sclerosis. In spite of the subjective left-sided hearing loss, all the patient's investigations including specialized tests showed no abnormality. Brain stem auditory evoked responses using monaural stimulation showed that the latencies beyond wave II were delayed, particularly wave V. One month after the investigations, the patient was struck and killed by lightning. Histopathological examination of the brain stem showed extensive demyelination with specific sites of involvement in the superior olive, lateral lemniscus, and inferior colliculus.

Parving, Elberling and Smith (1981), using electrocochleography, showed prolonged action potential latencies and elevated thresholds at low intensity. At mid-intensities, there were significant deviations of action potential amplitudes. Hopf and Maurer (1983) examined a series of 71 consecutive patients suffering from clinically definite or clinically probable multiple sclerosis. Wave I, as measured by early auditory evoked potentials, showed delayed latency with or without reduced amplitude in 15 such patients and was interpreted as due to multiple sclerosis in eight. They concluded that the peripheral part of the acoustic nerve was involved in about 10% of multiple sclerosis patients.

Ferguson, Ramsden and Lythgoe (1985) sought to determine whether the combination of brain stem auditory evoked potentials and the blink reflex would yield a higher rate of abnormality than each test performed separately. In a series of 50 patients with multiple sclerosis (definite – 30, probable – 10, possible – 10) using monaural stimulation, they found that 64% had abnormal responses. The blink reflex was elicited using electrical stimulation to the supraorbital nerve. Fifty-two per cent had an abnormal blink reflex, but when the results were combined with the brain stem electric response, 76% were abnormal. In this series, symptomatic deafness was present in 20%.

Auditory temporal resolution has been examined in multiple sclerosis by Rappaport *et al.* (1994) and they gave a comprehensive review of the literature. They found that multiple sclerosis patients exhibited a temporal processing defect and that their patients' performances suggested a predominant role of forebrain pathways in mediating auditory temporal resolution.

Musiek *et al.* (1989) investigated 33 subjects with 'definite' multiple sclerosis using seven behavioural and electrophysiological measures; 40% of the subjects with normal peripheral hearing complained of hearing difficulties. They found the masking level difference to be the most useful test diagnostically. It is known for its sensitivity for testing low brain stem/pontine lesions. They found the auditory brain stem response to be abnormal in 61.5%; wave I was abnormal in five out of 26 (18%); wave III was absent in 25% of ears tested. Interwave latency measures I–III, III–V and I–V were not highly sensitive indices. Hendler, Squires and Emmerich (1990) assessed central auditory function in 15 patients with multiple sclerosis. They confirmed the demyelinating lesions can cause a deficit in temporal processing. Abnormal masking level differences were always accompanied by abnormal auditory brain stem responses and mid-latency responses; the subjects with abnormal masking level differences were more likely to have bilateral abnormalities in the auditory brain stem potentials. They also carried out MRI studies; MRI signals restricted to levels caudal to the lateral lemniscus did not have abnormal masking level differences (Figure 17.10).

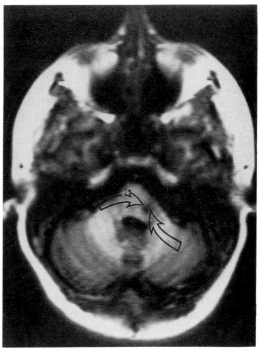

Figure 17.10 MR scan showing plaque of demyelination in the brain stem of a 29-year-old woman who experienced an episode of left-sided deafness and tinnitus. (Reproduced by kind permission of the Multiple Sclerosis Society's NMR Research Unit, National Hospital, London)

With the advent of MRI it has been possible to correlate electrophysiological abnormalities including brain stem evoked responses and this has totally changed the diagnostic picture. Barratt, Miller and Rudge (1988) published the report of one such patient who developed sequential hearing loss first on the right with recovery. MRI demonstrated lesions in the VIIIth nerve root entry zones which were thought to be responsible for the hearing loss; they carried out two scans with gadolinium enhancement 1 month apart. Antonelli *et al.* (1988) examined 32 patients with definite multiple sclerosis, 21 (65.5%) showed auditory brain stem response abnormalities in whom 13 proved positive on MRI studies; a further two patients (15/32, 46.8%) also showed demyelination plaques in the brain stem. Other reports with MRI imaging include those of Curé *et al.* (1990) and Gstoettner *et al.* (1993).

Sudden deafness as a presenting symptom has now been recorded on a number of occasions and it is likely this number will increase as MRI becomes a routine procedure. Cases have been recorded by Shea and Brackmann (1987), Franklin, Coker and Jenkins (1989), Furman, Durrant and Hirsch (1989), Schweitzer and Shepard (1989) and Drulović *et al.* (1993).

Multiple sclerosis has also been reported as the cause of sudden pontine 'deafness'. Drulović *et al.* (1994) reported two cases presenting with unilateral sensorineural hearing loss and tinnitus. Brain stem evoked responses showed only the first three waves in the first patient and only wave I in the second. MRI showed foci of demyelination in the pons in case one and on the border between the pons and medulla in case two. Pure tone audiometry showed recovery after 1 month in both patients and remained stable during 1 year; brain stem evoked responses however remained pathological after 1 month and again at 1 year. Morgenstern and Kau (1988) had reported six patients demonstrating the clinical features of pontine deafness. The latter is characterized by an interruption of the central auditory pathway cranial to the olive. They emphasized that the pathogenesis of pontine deafness is still unknown but that it should be taken into consideration in the diagnosis of sudden unilateral deafness. In one patient they carried out positron emission tomography (PET). Tabira *et al.* (1981) reported cortical deafness in a patient with multiple sclerosis. Complete recovery from total deafness was seen following stages of auditory agnosia and pure word deafness. A CT scan showed a transient low density area in the right parietotemporal region during the patient's second relapse. They pointed out that the most common cause of cortical deafness is cerebrovascular disease affecting both temporal lobes.

Friedreich's ataxia

In Friedreich's ataxia there is no relationship between the progressive clinical involvement and the degenerative changes affecting the peripheral nerves. Pelosi *et al.* (1984) investigated a series of 15 patients of whom only five had a hearing difficulty (three mild, one moderate and one severe). However brain stem electric responses were completely dissociated from the hearing disorder, being normal in one patient and abnormal in the remaining 12 investigated. Five showed severe abnormalities and there were mild to moderate abnormalities in the remaining seven, but wave I was present in all of this group (Figure 17.11). Patients without clinical acoustic disturbances showed abnormalities in brain stem response to the same degree or even greater than those who had a mild or moderate sensorineural hearing difficulty. However, the findings were significantly correlated with the level of clinical disability generally.

Visual evoked potentials showed abnormalities which corresponded to the severity of the clinical ophthalmological disturbance but were unrelated to the duration or severity of the clinical condition. Somatosensory evoked potentials showed findings which were also unrelated to either the duration or severity of the clinical conditions.

Jabbari *et al.* (1983) studied five children in an effort to find out the primary site of auditory dysfunction in classic Friedreich's ataxia; none of the children had any hearing complaints and all were tested soon after the onset of symptoms. The brain stem evoked potentials indicated dysfunction of the auditory system in the pontomesencephalic region. Acoustic reflex studies on two of the patients also suggested involvement of the brain stem auditory pathways. Wave I was retained in all patients and they thought it unlikely therefore that there was significant dysfunction of the spiral ganglia.

Ell, Prasher and Rudge (1984) reported on a group of 10 patients and noted that vestibular function and impaired hearing were common to most of the patients. Brain stem auditory evoked potentials were also abnormal in the majority. In their small series there was no obvious correlation between the type or severity of the neuro-otological abnormalities found and the duration of the disease. They commented on the high proportion of patients with vestibular and oculomotor abnormalities generally associated with cerebellar disease despite the absence of pathology at a gross level in that structure.

Amyotrophic lateral sclerosis (*van Laere's disease*)

Cristovao *et al.* (1985) have reported a family with this condition showing cochleovestibular involvement. This is an uncommon pattern of the disease and in the non-familial type such involvement has not been reported. The older two members of the family, aged 19 and 15 years, reported hearing loss as the first manifestation and on testing the eldest showed a severe bilateral sensorineural hearing loss

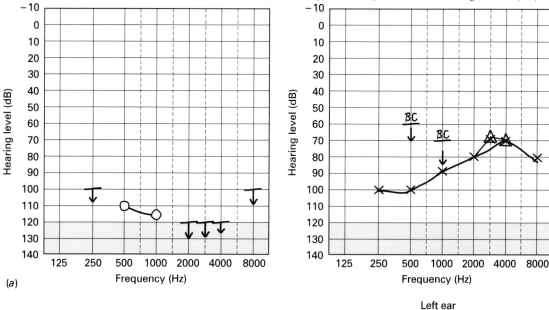

Figure 17.11 Friedreich's ataxia. (*a*) Pure tone audiogram from 10-year-old girl showing virtually absent hearing on the right and profound left-sided sensorineural hearing loss on the left. (*b*) Brain stem evoked responses only possible on the left side as only wave V was clearly visible and repeatable. (Mean latency 6.23 ms)

with very poor discrimination scores, pathological decay of the stapedius reflex bilaterally, asymmetry of the horizontal optokinetic nystagmus and bilateral absent responses in rotatory and caloric vestibular tests. The youngest member (aged 12) had no complaints and normal hearing but pathological decay of the stapedius reflex at one frequency in one ear was noted. Only the eldest member showed other neurological involvement which was severe by that time.

Vogt-Koyanagi-Harada syndrome

In 1926, Harada described what he believed to be a distinct entity comprising bilateral detachment of the retina, uveitis, mild meningeal irritation and 'dysacousia'. It is now generally considered that this 'disease' forms part of the now combined syndrome. Vogt in 1906, noted the association between bilateral uveitis, alopecia, vitiligo, poliosis (whitening of the hair) and 'dysacousia'. (Koyanagi described his variant in 1929 – this brought the vitiligo and the deafness together.) Most of the reported cases have occurred in people of pigmented race. The principal feature is the prolonged bilateral uveitis, causing blindness. The hearing loss develops at or near the time the blindness occurs; it is also usually bilateral, of varying degree, frequently associated with tinnitus and vertigo. The ear symptoms begin to improve after 1–3 weeks as the tinnitus and vertigo subside, gradually returning to normal. Vision often returns to normal in 2–6 months, but glaucoma and cataract may continue as complications. The vitiligo, poliosis and alopecia usually appear when the uveitis begins to improve. Rosen (1945) reported one case and reviewed those then in the literature – a total of 45; Maxwell has reported another (1963).

The percentage incidence of the various symptoms has been noted to differ between populations. Dysacousis is much more common in those cases presenting in Japan (70%) compared with those with the syndrome seen in the USA with only 17%, the same percentage as for tinnitus (Gilbert, Pollack and Pollack, 1994).

Xeroderma pigmentosum

Xeroderma pigmentosum is a rare autosomal recessive condition first described by Kaposi in 1874. Clinically the patients present with an abnormal sensitivity to sunlight, this is characterized by the appearance of a delayed yet marked erythema of skin exposed to ultraviolet light. Subsequently pigmented macules appear together with telangiectasia and skin atrophy and, in time, multiple cutaneous neoplasms develop. The condition is associated with abnormalities of excision and repair of DNA segments damaged by ultraviolet light. Complementation studies have shown seven different types of the condition, all of whom have an excision repair defect; there are still others known as xeroderma pigmentosum variants, in which no such defect is evident, but in whom synthesis of DNA is still abnormal with slow maturation of new DNA chains. Neurological abnormalities have also been described, particularly peripheral neuropathy and changes in the central nervous system may also occur. Deafness has also become recognized as being associated with this disease.

Longridge (1976) studied a pair of siblings and came to the conclusion that the disorder was central and not cochlear in origin. He based this opinion on absent stapedial reflexes, and absence of tone decay and a speech audiogram which he considered to be worse than would have been anticipated from the pure tone audiogram. More recently, Kenyon *et al.* (1985) reported three cases in whom detailed neuro-otological investigations had been carried out. These patients had widely differing ages (16, 46 and 57 years) and two showed a high and one a low tone recruiting hearing loss; brain stem auditory evoked responses obtained in one patient were completely normal and only mildly deranged in another, strongly suggesting the origin of the deafness to be more peripheral than the brain stem. Although the deafness was bilateral, in none of the patients was it entirely symmetrical. The vestibular pathways appear to be involved, but apparently to a lesser extent than the auditory ones and vestibulo-ocular reflex suppression is abnormal. The two older patients showed evidence of a mild supranuclear palsy that was only apparent on volitional movement.

Tumours

Vestibular schwannoma (acoustic neuroma)

It is interesting to note that Cushing in 1914 mentioned that two cases had sudden hearing loss as a manifestation of cerebellopontine angle tumour, but it was not described as the presenting symptom in the English literature until 1956 by Hallberg (see also Hallberg, Uihlein and Siekert, 1959). In addition, Edwards and Paterson (1951) mentioned five patients whose hearing loss was described as abrupt in their review of 157 cases. Higgs (1973) reported that 10% in his series of 44 patients presented with sudden deafness. Morrison (1975) showed that no less than 17% of his patients presented in this way. Pensak *et al.* (1985), in a retrospective analysis of 506 patients with surgically proven cerebellopontine angle lesions seen over a period of 14 years, found 77 (15.2%) who presented in this way (69 acoustic neuromas, seven meningiomas and one malignant cholesteatoma). They could find no characteristics which distinguished these cases from the remainder. Twenty-four were small lesions (up to 1.5 cm); 28 were medium-sized (1.6–2.9 cm) and 25 were large (3.0 cm or greater). The hearing patterns were in the same proportions as those for acoustic tumours generally; several had hearing losses which improved before they could be tested. Eleven had reasonably normal audiometric findings (tumour size 1–4.5 cm); the patient with the largest tumour (4.5 cm) had a pure tone threshold of 50 dB with 100% speech discrimination! Chow and Garcia (1985) reported a patient with sudden hearing loss whose hearing returned to normal 2 weeks later only to fall again 4 weeks later, with normal caloric responses and speech discrimination at that time of 24%, then recovering within 6 weeks to 76%. A CT scan showed a 1.5 cm mass and the patient refused surgical treatment.

In the 1960s it used to be said that a vestibular schwannoma had been excluded if there were normal caloric responses and that radiology of the internal auditory meatus with perhaps linear tomography showed no expansion. Everyone now accepts that both these statements may on occasion be untrue. However, in recent years, those without the most up-to-date radiological techniques being available to them, have often relied on auditory brain stem responses as a reliable method of screening for vestibular schwannoma. In 1989, Telian *et al.*, investigating a series of 120 vestibular schwannomas, found two patients with normal auditory brain stem responses. Every patient with a suspected vestibular schwannoma and/or sudden sensorineural hearing loss should undergo MRI with gadolinium enhancement wherever such facilities exist. Yanagihara and Asai

(1993) emphasized that even small tumours had the potential to produce sudden hearing loss (Figure 17.12). Moffat *et al.* (1994) examined their series of 284 patients with proven vestibular schwannoma and showed a 12% incidence of those presenting with sudden deafness. They noted that when present it was very likely to be the main presenting symptom and that this group presented some 8 months sooner than the non-sudden deafness patients. They also noted that while 16% of patients with vestibular schwannoma without sudden deafness presented with a dead ear, 29.5% of those presenting with sudden deafness already had a total hearing loss on that side. They felt that it was compression of the vasculature within the bony internal auditory meatus by a laterally arising tumour which may be the aetiological factor and may be more likely to occur than in tumours arising more medially. Cases of sudden sensorineural hearing loss responding to steroids should not escape complete investigation including an MRI scan (Suzuki *et al.*, 1987). Berenholz,

Eriksen and Hirsh (1992) reported a case in which sudden hearing loss in an only hearing ear which recovered to normal levels after steroid therapy on no less than four occasions; after the third episode, MRI was performed and this demonstrated a 1.5 cm mass in the right internal auditory meatus. The patient underwent middle cranial fossa decompression to allow expansion of the tumour without risk of the hearing loss associated with resection. The patient had a fifth episode of sudden hearing loss 3 months after the decompression which too resolved with steroid therapy. Rarely, a tumour may increase in size but the hearing loss remains the same (Van Leeuwen *et al.*, 1993).

Clemis, Mastricola and Schuler-Vogler (1982) reported three cases of sudden hearing loss postoperatively in the contralateral ear of patients with vestibular schwannoma. A further case (making a total of seven in the literature) has recently been reported by Walsh *et al.* (1994). The hearing in the contralateral ear can return but they found that this is less likely when the tumour is large, or a suboccipital approach has been used. In their own case, there was no return of hearing.

Sudden deafness has also been noted as the presenting symptom of a cerebellar tumour which was not localized strictly in the cerebellopontine angle. A CT scan showed an irregular density in the left cerebellar hemisphere displacing the fourth ventricle and subsequent surgery showed this to be a cerebellar desmoblastic medulloblastoma (Galvez *et al.*, 1994).

Transiently evoked otoacoustic emissions have been used to investigate both extrinsic and intrinsic brain stem lesions by Prasher, Ryan and Luxon (1994) together with the effect of contralateral suppression. Patients with hearing better than 30 dB were specifically chosen but at this stage the test remains in its infancy.

Metastases in the cerebellopontine angle

Secondary deposits may occur in the cerebellopontine angle from primary disease in the breast, bronchus and prostate.

Carcinomatous neuropathy

Peripheral neuropathy caused by malignant disease ranks second to the Guillain-Barré syndrome. Conversely, unexplained peripheral neuropathy should be the signal to search for malignant disease.

The highest incidence of this condition has been found in patients with carcinoma of the lung, ovary and stomach, and lowest in the rectum, cervix and uterus. Other malignant diseases may also have an associated involvement – progressive multifocal leucoencephalopathy is linked with Hodgkin's disease, lymphosarcoma and some other reticuloses. There is also an unusual form of encephalomyelitis nearly

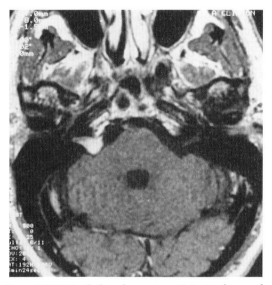

Figure 17.12 Vestibular schwannoma. Patient, when aged 45, developed high pitched tinnitus in the right ear followed 1 month later by total deafness on that side. The patient seen aged 64 has now developed a slight ticking sound in remaining left ear. A pure tone audiogram confirmed normal hearing on that side and total absence of hearing on the right. Brain stem evoked responses showed a normal result on the left and complete absence on the right. One month later the patient experienced short episodes of slight vertigo. Repeated episodes of minor 'floating/sailing' feeling occurred over a 6-month period. MRI scan shows small mass in the right cerebellopontine angle with enhancement after gadolinium. Further scans at intervals have shown a slight increase in size but no clinical increased disability. Hearing (left) remains normal

always associated with oat-cell bronchial carcinoma (*see* Figure 5.31).

No particular association with either branch of the VIIth nerve has so far been shown (Henson and Urich, 1982). Olson, Chernik and Posner (1974) carried out a clinical and pathological study in 50 patients over a 4-year period with infiltration of the leptomeninges by systemic cancer. They noted that neurological signs were more prominent than the patients' symptoms and, in 30, the clinical diagnosis was documented at autopsy. Acoustic and vestibular dysfunction occurred in 15 (30%) in 10 of whom there was deafness (four bilateral and six unilateral). Hearing loss has been reported in carcinomatous meningitis and five such cases have been seen in which the hearing loss was the presenting symptom (Alberts and Terrence, 1978).

There have been two case reports of sudden bilateral sensorineural loss occurring in association with meningeal carcinomatosis (Civantos, Choi and Applebaum, 1992; Houck and Murphy, 1992). In the first of these the complete bilateral hearing loss was the presenting sign of meningeal carcinomatosis and no other cranial nerves were involved; it occurred 3 weeks before death and the primary tumour was situated in the middle third of the oesophagus. Houck and Murphy (1992) reported the first case following carcinoma of the breast and, in addition to the sudden bilateral profound hearing loss, there was also bilateral absent vestibular function; the patient died 4 months later. These authors give a good review of meningeal carcinomatosis commenting that, of course, most diagnoses are made by lumbar puncture or at autopsy.

Central deafness

'Central' deafness may be unilateral or bilateral but it is the latter type that seems to yield the most helpful information so far. It should be stressed that cases are rare, autopsy reports are few and that there is no uniform pattern of hearing loss. However, certain features appear to give some diagnostic and investigative guide.

Jerger *et al.* (1969) and Jerger, Lovering and Wertz (1972) have reported two cases in great detail. Both were cases of bilateral temporal lobe damage, in men. Both experienced transient aphasia but no hearing problems after the first side (left) episode. Both reported severe hearing loss after the second (right) episode. In both, the presumed loss had essentially recovered within 3 months of the second episode; both showed marked inability to recognize either single words or sentences. However, there was one significant difference and that was in their ability to localize sound; in the younger case this was impaired but not in the older.

In the first (younger) patient, it was concluded

that he had experienced occlusion of the terminal branches of the middle cerebral artery on each side at different points in time, resulting in bilateral partial cerebral hemisphere infarction, maximal in the temporal lobes, and producing the clinical picture of cortical deafness. In the second case, at his second admission, angiography showed occlusion of the major middle cerebral trunk with anastomotic filling in a retrograde manner from the parieto-occipital branch of the right posterior cerebral artery. This patient had a third and final admission, 6 months later for acute cerebral infarction with right hemiplegia and aphasia; he died 1 week later of an acute myocardial infarct. Examination of the brain revealed bilateral and symmetrical areas of softening of the posterior segments of the superior temporal gyri, these were caused by cystic infarcts; the major arteries displayed moderate atherosclerosis but there was no evidence of embolism.

Earnest, Monroe and Yarnell (1977) reported a case of a man (left-handed) who subsequently had bilateral cerebral infarcts that caused a non-fluent aphasia, oral apraxia, and deafness and who, at the age of 27, had a mitral valve prosthesis fitted and received subsequent anticoagulation. They expressed the view that the cortical clinical syndrome of pure word deafness in many cases is probably a less severe form of cortical deafness and is due to less extensive bilateral temporal grey matter lesions. Strictly white matter lesions may produce cases of either syndrome.

Graham, Greenwood and Lecky (1980) carried out brain stem evoked responses (Figure 17.13*a*) on a 47-year-old woman (right-handed) who 3 years before had a mitral valve replacement. She was thought to have suffered three separate embolic lesions of cardiac origin, the first to the left temporal cortex producing dysphasia, the second, to the right occipital cortex, causing a left homonomous hemianopia and the third to the right temporal lobe, resulting in total deafness. The first and third events represent left and right middle cerebral artery embolism and the second, right posterior cerebral artery embolism. She also suffered a series of epileptic fits. A CT scan and isotope scan showed bilateral temporal infarction and a right occipital infarct (Figure 17.13*b*). Galvanic responses were negative. No cortical electrical response activity could be obtained but stapedius (acoustic) and postauricular myogenic responses were both present. A similar diagnosis to the other cases reported has been made, that is bilateral temporal lobe infarction of embolic origin. In addition to reporting their own case, Graham, Greenwood and Lecky (1980) gave an excellent review of the earlier literature and of the four cases published since 1969 making a total of 12 in all prior to their own study.

Tanaka *et al.* (1991) described two patients with severe persistent hearing loss caused by bilateral cerebral lesions which they examined using MRI and compared these lesions with those in two patients

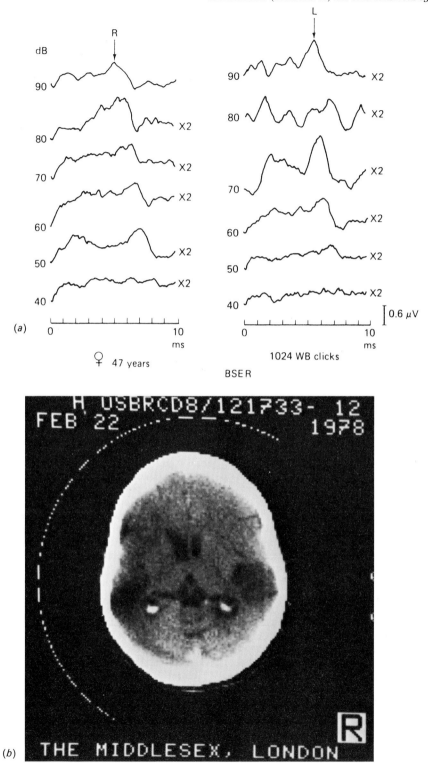

Figure 17.13 (*a*) Brain stem evoked response shows psychonormal responses with the usual five peaks and normal latencies, the fifth peak is shown by the arrow (case of central deafness). (Reproduced by kind permission of Dr C. J. Earl, Consultant Neurologist, Middlesex Hospital, Mr H. A. Beagley and Mr J. M. Graham, Nuffield Speech and Hearing Centre.) (*b*) CT scan with contrast (same patient as in (*a*)), showing bilateral opacities in the temporoparietal areas (Reproduced by kind permission of Dr C. J. Earl, Consultant Neurologist, Middlesex Hospital, Mr H. A. Beagley and Mr J. M. Graham, Nuffield Speech and Hearing Centre)

with only a mild hearing loss following extensive bilateral temporoparietal lesions. The extent of bilateral damage to the white matter adjacent to the posterior half of the putamen proved crucial in determining the severity of the hearing loss. The hearing loss was noted to be more severe when the white matter immediately central and lateral to the posterior half of the putamen was involved bilaterally. Such lesions appear to interrupt the projection fibres from the medial geniculate bodies to the auditory-related areas resulting in severe, persistent hearing loss. In addition to reporting these two groups of cases, they discussed the literature on word deafness in considerable detail which will be a particular help to those interested in this topic as many of the earlier papers were published in Japanese! Kido *et al.* (1994) published a case of cerebellar infarction which occurred producing VIIIth cranial nerve symptoms. MRI showed areas of infarction related to the anterior and posterior inferior cerebellar arteries on the right side. By the twelfth day, the hearing level and caloric response were significantly improved and by the fourteenth day the symptoms had disappeared. Auditory brain stem responses initially showed wave I but subsequent waves were unclear; a follow-up test is not reported. Two months after the initial illness, a right vertebral angiogram was performed, this showed the anterior inferior cerebellar artery diverging from the basilar artery and the posterior inferior arising from the anterior inferior cerebellar artery. There was an anastomosis between the occipital artery and the right vertebral artery. Ho *et al.* (1987) reported a 67-year-old woman who demonstrated intact peripheral and brain stem auditory evoked responses and who presented with sudden deafness secondary to sequential bilateral temporal lobe infarct. The hearing gradually returned but auditory agnosia persisted. Middle latency auditory evoked responses together with CT changes were analysed and suggested that the peak component of the middle latency response arises from Heschl's gyrus. Middle latency auditory evoked potentials have been examined in 19 patients with temporal lobe lesions by Shehata-Dieler *et al.* (1991).

Sudden cochlear hearing loss occurring successively or simultaneously in both ears was observed in four unrelated preschool children by Lenard *et al.* (1991). Three of the children also showed complete bilateral loss of vestibular function. All the patients had a mildly retarded motor development due to non-progressive muscular weakness. On MR imaging all patients showed multiple periventricular and subcortical white matter lesions. The children were aged 2–5 years and the almost identical symptoms and signs seemed to suggest a new disease entity.

An important short case report was published by Tobias *et al.* (1994) of a case of Creutzfeldt–Jakob disease presenting with cortical deafness. The patient,

a 65-year-old man, demonstrated bilateral hearing loss worse for speech than pure tones. Brain stem auditory evoked potentials showed waves III–V present on the right and wave III on the left. Cortical auditory evoked potentials showed normal wave forms bilaterally and normal absolute latencies of the N1 response. The patient died 2 weeks later and at autopsy the brain showed widespread subacute spongiform encephalopathy with vacuolation in the frontal, occipital and both temporal lobes. In the areas of severe spongiform change in the temporal lobes, there was extensive neuronal loss and there was active astrocytosis.

Lacunar syndromes

Lacunar cerebral infarcts are small, deep, ischaemic lesions (usually less than 20 mm diameter) localized in the area of cerebral perforant arteries. Clinical characteristics of a lacunar infarct are usually pure motor hemiparesis, pure sensory stroke, motor-sensory stroke, ataxic hemiparesis and dysarthria-clumsy hand. In general, dichotic listening tests have been used in the investigation of patients with large cortico–subcortical lesions. In these cases, the patients with auditory extinction had lesions encroaching upon the cochleocortical auditory pathways. Arboix *et al.* (1990) used the dichotic listening test to examine 28 patients with acute lacunar syndromes caused by small, deep, cerebrovascular lesions. Topographical studies showed that lesions in the external capsule and the anterior limb of the internal capsule in both hemispheres produced left ear extinction. They suggested the possibility that some of the auditory fibres travel through the external capsule, as well as the anterior limb of the internal capsule, before crossing the contralateral cerebral lobe.

Lacunar infarcts were reported in a patient who developed a thalamic syndrome with amnesia and dysphasia (Karni *et al.*, 1991). Some 3 months previously she had experienced sudden hearing loss, worse on the right, as the initial symptom of Cogan's syndrome and in spite of large doses of methylprednisolone, she became completely deaf on both sides. The authors could find only two cases of Cogan's syndrome complicated by strokes including one of Cogan's original patients.

Ghosh (1990) reported a case of 'central diplacusis' involving a lesion in the posterior thalamus resulting in diplacusis binauralis. He presumed the lesion to lie at the geniculate-collicula level. The patient had been diagnosed by the neurologist as having a thalamic syndrome, presumably resulting from infarction of the thalamogenicular branches of the posterior cerebral artery. The patient had slight impairment of hearing but no difficulty in day-to-day communication.

Cortical encephalitis

Diffuse cortical encephalitis causes an auditory aphasia when both temporal lobes are involved; the patients have normal pure-tone audiograms but no understanding of speech. The diagnosis is confirmed by EEG and the condition may develop over weeks or months with periods of fluctuation and acute episodes. Morrison (1975) reported three cases, all adult women, in all of whom the sudden hearing loss occurred relatively late in the disease but all made good recoveries after treatment with steroids followed by ACTH. However, one has continued to have occasional episodes of auditory aphasia.

Recently, it would appear that a new syndrome has been described which afflicts women in the third or fourth decade of life, is characterized by a subacute encephalopathy with sensorineural hearing loss and retinal artery branch occlusions, and shows no clinical or laboratory evidence of visceral lesions. It is associated with sclerosis of the media and adventitia of small pial and cortical vessels. Monteiro *et al.* (1985) have recorded two cases and reviewed the four reported previously. Hearing loss was present in all patients and was the first symptom in two and bilateral in all but one; tinnitus was described in three. Pure tone audiometry showed bilateral asymmetric sensorineural hearing loss with a preferential loss in the low and middle frequencies. Speech discrimination was poor in the ear on the more involved side. Brain stem auditory evoked responses were normal in the three patients tested. They felt it unlikely, therefore, that the deafness was of VIIIth nerve origin but was more attributable to cochlear damage. MRI was obtained in only one patient but this showed changes compatible with a small brain infarct in the white matter, as suspected clinically. Treatment with prednisone was given to all patients, but in three, progression of symptoms led to additional therapy with cyclophosphamide; it is noteworthy that none of the three patients receiving cyclophosphamide developed new symptoms. None of the patients had recurrence of symptoms after the disease subsided. However, treatment brought about no improvement in any of the six patients.

Alzheimer's disease

Alzheimer's disease is characterized by a pathological process with specific predilection for association with neocortex and medial temporal lobes. There is however an inconsistency in the post-mortem histopathological findings and the results of CT scanning during life. What is not clear is whether Alzheimer's disease is an age-dependent disease and thus intrinsic to ageing or whether it is age-related but not an inevitable part of the ageing process. Of the changes which occur, cerebral atrophy could reflect acceleration of the normal atrophy that occurs with age or indicate that those destined to develop Alzheimer's disease are born with smaller medial temporal lobes which then atrophy at the normal rate. Alternatively, the excessive atrophy could reflect some insult or catastrophic event that leads to fast degeneration of neurons in the medial temporal lobes.

Jobst *et al.* (1994) carried out yearly temporal lobe oriented CT scans and found that the average rate of atrophy of the medial temporal lobe in those with Alzheimer's disease was 15.1% per year compared with 1.5% in healthy ageing controls. They found that four patterns of atrophy could be discerned in patients with possible or probable dementia of the Alzheimer's type: little change in the medial temporal lobe thickness followed by rapid acceleration; rapid rate from the start that persisted (the commonest pattern); rapid rate at the start that levelled out; and no change. The findings of Jobst *et al.* (1994) were consistent with the overall view that the pathological signs of the disease are first manifest in the medial temporal lobe. However, it should be pointed out that atrophy of the medial temporal lobes is also found in other conditions, notably epilepsy and hypoxia, schizophrenia, and amnesia, so it is not unique to dementia of the Alzheimer's type. It has also been noted there is a reduced blood flow to the parietotemporal regions as demonstrated by single photon emission tomography and this was invariably associated with atrophy of the medial temporal lobe as shown by CT (Jobst *et al.*, 1992). In their group, 86% (44/51) of patients with dementia of the Alzheimer's type had a combination of medial temporal lobe atrophy and reduced parietotemporal blood flow. Of the 12 patients who died, 10 with a histological diagnosis of Alzheimer's disease all displayed the combination of CT evidence of atrophy of the medial temporal lobe with single photon emission tomography evidence of parietotemporal perfusion deficit (Jobst *et al.*, 1992).

Studies by Jagust *et al.* (1993) have suggested that the temporal lobe is the first neocortical brain region to be functionally affected by Alzheimer's disease. In their study the lowest metabolic rates in Alzheimer's disease patients were seen in the anterior temporal neocortex and the medial temporal cortex, but the same two regions were also the most hypometabolic in the controls. While glucose transport may be abnormal in Alzheimer's disease, the abnormality is not of sufficient magnitude to account for the metabolic disturbance seen which is more likely to be a consequence of reduction in neuronal number. Mounting evidence has suggested that synapse loss is the key determinant of dementia in Alzheimer's disease (Sheff and Price, 1993) (see Plate 3/17/I).

Baloyannis, Manolidis and Manolidis (1992) studied the acoustic cortex by light and electron microscopy in six post mortem cases of Alzheimer's disease. All the cases belonged to the early onset sub-type since all of them were under the age of 65. Compared with the normal controls they found serious morphological alterations in the acoustic cortex with regard to neurons, axons, dendrites and synapses as well as glial cells. They emphasize the morphological finding in their cases in particular the loss of the dendritic spines and the axionic collaterals as well as the dramatic abbreviation of the dendritic arborization. They felt that these changes might explain the profound deficit in verbal memory and language disturbance as the hallmarks in early cases of Alzheimer's disease.

Idiopathic
Pathogenesis

There have been two 'rival' theories as to the causation of the idiopathic case – *viral* and *vascular*. It has been known for a long time that certain viruses, e.g. mumps, measles, rubella, can cause sensorineural deafness, that the finding of a preceding 'viral' infection in many cases of sudden loss, varying in incidence from 30 to 40% according to the author, made the association of ideas, if not of facts, irresistible (e.g. van Dishoeck and Bierman, 1957). Conversely, the suddenness of onset made the analogy with similar events in the cardiovascular system equally attractive to the opposing school (e.g. Hallberg, 1956). As many of the cases occurred in patients over 40 years of age, the association looked even more tempting. Attempts have been made to reconcile these view points. The theory of *membrane breaks or ruptures* has also been put forward.

It is traditional in otology to try to match the clinical picture with the findings from the temporal bone laboratory, wherever possible. As in many other otological conditions, few patients die of their disease, so the interval between the event, in this case sudden deafness, and autopsy may be long, and reparative processes will have been at work. Alternatively, the end may come very rapidly from overwhelming disease, which in itself may complicate the histological picture. However, all this is familiar and expected by temporal bone experts (see Figures 4.18 and 4.19).

Membrane breaks

In an effort to understand the causation of sudden hearing loss, Simmons in 1968, considered the history and clinical findings in patients with this problem. He noted that all but two were under 45 years of age and that many could date their sudden onset to a particular day and time and he was struck by the association of a 'popping', 'clicking' preceding the hearing loss or of the sudden development of a marked roaring tinnitus. He also asked whether the patient's physical activity at the time could have caused any increase in the intrathoracic or intra-

cranial venous or cerebrospinal fluid pressure, or if more than a modest amount of alcohol had been drunk beforehand. He postulated that perhaps there was a disruption to the cochlear membranes which subsequently healed, in a similar manner to that in experimental animals exposed to intense sound. He reported a series of 15 patients and commented in this, and in a later paper discussing 56 patients (Simmons, 1973), that very few noticed vestibular symptoms at the time, but on questioning transient unsteady feelings were present in one third; a few were frankly vertiginous. He observed that untreated, there appeared to be an improvement in the hearing, sometimes quite suddenly, even after quite long intervals. He therefore advocated that nothing which would raise the pressure in the inner ear or might otherwise injure it further, e.g. high intensity audiometry, should occur in order to facilitate healing of the cochlear membranes.

Reports of three temporal bone studies have now been published, by Gussen (1981, 1983), showing cochlear membrane rupture in patients with sudden hearing loss. Gussen stressed the left-sided preponderance of such ruptures and the vulnerability of the ductus reuniens junction with the cochlea.

Koskas, Linthicum and House (1983) described membranous ruptures which they found only in patients with Menière's disease and occurred more frequently in Reissner's membrane than in the vestibular membrane.

Symptomatology

'Sudden hearing loss is a symptom in search of a diagnosis' (Simmons, 1973). It will be readily apparent that many of the causes of sudden hearing loss are in themselves rare. Many of them are discussed in other chapters. The preceding section is devoted to excluding the specific causes, thereby leaving the so-called 'idopathic' losses – still the largest single group and constituting the everyday case –' for treatment according to 'site-of-loss'.

For the purist, 'sudden' hearing loss means an instantaneous event; 'rapid' hearing loss means deafness occurring over a short period of time, for example hours. If the loss subsequently improves, either spontaneously or as a result of treatment, then some would label this 'fluctuant'! Terayama, Ishibe and Matsushima (1988) in a small series found that patients who had a rapidly progressing sensorineural hearing loss, i.e. from a few hours up to 3 days, had a relatively good prognosis but the recovery time was longer than in spontaneously healing sudden deafness. They also found that 32% (9/28) already had a hearing loss on the opposite side; one had experienced sudden deafness in the opposite ear which had remained unchanged for 8 years while in the other patients the cause of the hearing loss in the opposite ear was unknown. It should be appreciated that cases may present in any of these ways and the distinction between them from a diagnostic viewpoint is frequently somewhat artificial. It will become apparent that such divisions should not be interpreted too rigidly.

Veldman, Hanada and Meeuwsen (1993) reported a series of 76 patients with a hearing loss of greater than 30 dB in at least three frequencies and progressive over weeks to months, acute within hours or days (sudden deafness 31) or more slowly progressive over several months to years. Seventy-three per cent with rapidly progressive loss had cross-reacting antibodies (27, 45, 50, 68 kD); 65% of the group with sudden deafness also had cross-reacting antibodies (27, 45, 50, 80 kD). Spontaneous recovery occurred in approximately 50% of cases but only in those with a positive assay.

Age and sex distribution

In the 1220 cases reported by Shaia and Sheehy (1976), age at onset of the symptoms was as follows:

Under 30	13%
30–39	13%
40–49	21%
50–59	22%
60–69	18%
70 years +	13%

Three-quarters of the patients therefore were over the age of 40, but 1.4% dated the onset of their sudden hearing loss below the age of 10. Four per cent had a sudden bilateral loss, and one-half of these were simultaneous. Only one-quarter of the 1220 patients were seen within 1 month of onset. As all series show that the best results are obtained in those receiving their treatment within 15 days of onset, it will be immediately appreciated how vast is the wastage of untreated cases. In all series, the sex distribution is approximately equal at all age groups.

Bilateral simultaneous sudden hearing loss is fortunately rare and most quote an incidence of 4% or even less, but Mattucci and Bachoura (1982) in a series of 175 patients over a 10-year period, with an average age of 47 years, reported an incidence of 9.7%; vertigo was present in 26% and tinnitus in 52% of their series. At the other end of the scale Yanagita and Murahashi (1987) found 10 patients among their series of 997 cases who had been seen within 2 weeks of the onset of their bilateral sudden hearing loss. The average age in the incidence of vestibular symptoms was similar to those with unilateral deafness and the hearing recovery was much better in the ear which was less affected. No improvement was observed on the side with a total hearing loss. Those with bilateral sudden hearing loss or progressive hearing loss in young adult life should

be suspected as possible cases of HIV infection. In all age groups it is now appropriate to test for Lyme disease particularly in affected areas. In an older age group, vertebrobasilar occlusive disease may be a factor. Huang *et al.* (1993) reported sudden bilateral hearing loss with tinnitus and vertigo in seven out of a series of 503 patients; median age 61 years (range 46–71). Brain stem auditory evoked potentials were abnormal bilaterally in six of them with unilateral attenuation of the IV–V complex in the remaining patient.

Precipitating factors

Many published series state an incidence of a preceding viral infection in 30–40%.

Almost every virus has been reported or implicated as a causative factor in a proportion of these cases, but certain facts should be considered before such an aetiology is too readily accepted.

The viruses which have been suggested as causing sudden hearing loss may be divided into three groups. The first of these consists of viruses causing acute respiratory diseases such as influenza, parainfluenza and rhinoviruses. Such infections are very common. Adults suffer on average four to five respiratory infections a year, so that about one-third of any group of adults will give a history of a respiratory infection within the preceding 4 weeks. There is no confirmed evidence of a seasonal incidence as might be expected for the respiratory viruses and none following an epidemic such as might be expected after influenza. Although a high incidence might be expected in children because they sustain more infections than adults none such has been reported (Rowson, Hinchcliffe and Gamble, 1976).

The second group includes poliovirus, coxsackie virus, rubella, Epstein-Barr virus, adenovirus type 3 and herpes simplex virus. Following such infections, occasional cases of sudden hearing loss have been reported, but they are very uncommon. The third group comprises three viruses – mumps, measles and varicella zoster, all of which are known to produce sudden deafness.

Schuknecht and Donovan (1986) examined the temporal bone pathology in 12 ears with idiopathic sudden sensorineural hearing loss and found that the lesions present in these specimens and 10 others reported in the literature were similar to lesions occurring in known cases of viral cochleitis. Eight of the cases had been reported previously in two groups of four. Five of these eight cases showed evidence of upper respiratory tract infection at the time of onset of the hearing losses. The temporal bones showed atrophy of the organs of Corti, tectorial membranes and striae vasculares in varying combinations and severity. These changes were more like those occurring in labyrinthitis of known viral aetiology than in experimentally induced vascular lesions in animals.

Of the 12 temporal bones examined by Schuknecht and Donovan from the collection at the Massachusetts Eye and Ear Infirmary, the sudden hearing loss was unilateral in 10, while both ears were involved sequentially in one case with a time interval of 13 years. The hearing losses were permanent in 11, while one showed gradual and complete recovery over a time span of 11 days. Vertigo was severe in two cases, moderate in two, mild in three and absent in five. Six of the 12 cases occurred in association with upper respiratory tract infections. They also examined the significant pathological findings in 21 ears and 13 subjects available in the literature. Three of the reported temporal bone cases were of measles labyrinthitis, four of maternal rubella and three of herpes zoster oticus. None of the 12 cases reported by Schuknecht and Donovan showed fibrosis or ossification within the cochlea examined as might be expected as a result of arterial occlusion.

Kheterpal, Nadol and Glynn (1990) carried out a statistical comparison of 22 temporal bones from 18 patients with idiopathic sudden sensorineural hearing loss and post-viral labyrinthitis. They divided the bones into three groups on the basis of clinical data: idiopathic sudden sensorineural hearing loss but with no history of upper respiratory tract infection; idiopathic sudden sensorineural hearing loss with a history of upper respiratory tract infection preceding or concurrent with the hearing loss; and postnatal presumptive viral labyrinthitis with profound hearing loss following an attack of measles, mumps, or herpes zoster oticus. Statistically significant differences between groups one and two were only found on the loss of inner and outer hair cells and pillar cells. Wherever possible they examined the spiral ganglion cells in the opposite unaffected ear. Differences between total ganglion cell counts between 'unaffected and affected' ears of the same donor were small (groups one and two). However spiral ganglion counts in group three were markedly reduced from normal for age and contralateral ear. The authors suggested that perhaps idiopathic sudden sensorineural hearing loss is due to non-neurotropic viruses (e.g. adenovirus, influenza, parainfluenza virus, or rhinovirus). Neurotropism of cytopathic viruses like herpes, mumps and measles could account for severe neuronal atrophy seen in the third group.

Noise

Single episodes of noise leading to acute deafness have been reported, though they remain exceptional. Emmett (1994) reported simultaneous idiopathic sudden sensorineural hearing loss in identical twins listening to loud music at a rock concert – both had their right ears towards the wall of speakers. Both were followed up for 2 years; neither showed any improvement. Kellerhals (1991) has reported 58 bilat-eral and 17 unilateral cases of acute acoustic trauma which showed subsequent progression of more than 20 dB at least at one frequency.

Other symptoms

Many patients with sudden hearing loss can state the day, date and time that it occurred, or that they awoke with it. Others may recall severe physical effort at the time of onset. Nearly always it is a dramatic, well-remembered event. *Pain* or a feeling of pressure may be present in the affected ear, but so far no particular prognostic significance has been found to be attached to this.

Tinnitus occurs in approximately 80% of cases usually starting with, and alarmingly as, the deafness. In approximately 25% the tinnitus may precede the deafness by minutes or hours, very occasionally by some days. While tinnitus apparently does not affect the outcome, Danino *et al.* (1984) found it to be a favourable prognostic sign and felt that its presence seemed to indicate that cells were still functioning and therefore may recover. Tinnitus was present in 71% of the patients who recovered compared with 39% who did not.

Vertigo is commonest in those with a probable vascular aetiology. It carries a poorer prognosis for hearing recovery. Danino *et al.* agreed that vertigo was a bad prognostic factor (24% in the recovery and 54% in the non-recovery group), but not all reports agree with this (Noury and Katsarkas, 1989).

In the series of Shaia and Sheehy (1976), 60% of patients had no vestibular symptoms, 22% had them initially, and 18% persistently.

Vertigo of any duration associated with the hearing loss is an indication to investigate the patient very thoroughly, and the possibility of a vestibular schwannoma should never be overlooked.

Nakashima and Yanagita (1993) investigated 1313 patients with sudden deafness, 30% of whom had accompanying vertigo. The latter occurred frequently in patients with severe hearing loss in the high tones. Hearing recovery for these frequencies was worse in those with vertigo than in those without even when the initial hearing loss was the same. Kheterpal (1991) examined nine temporal bones of patients with sudden sensorineural hearing loss, of whom five ears had been affected by vertigo and four without. The differences between the vertiginous, non-vertiginous, and control (opposite) ears was not significant.

There is a series of reports of patients who, after developing sudden deafness, subsequently go on to develop episodic vertigo characteristic of endolymphatic hydrops. Wolfson and Leiberman (1975) recorded five such cases. The interval in their cases ranges from 6 to 10 years. After long observation, destruction labyrinthectomy was carried out with complete relief of the vertigo. Nadol, Weiss and Parker (1975) reported 12 cases, with vertigo developing from 1 to 68 years later! They found the long interval particularly puzzling. Few of the 12 had any coincidental vestibular symptoms at the time of onset of the sudden deafness. Again labyrinthectomy was curative. Both groups of authors question whether the cause could be Menière's disease.

Investigation of sudden or fluctuant sensorineural hearing loss may require:

Haematology

Haemoglobin, full blood count, erythrocyte sedimentation rate, prothrombin time, plasma viscosity, Paul Bunnell screening test and titre (Epstein-Barr virus)
Viral studies – repeat specimen will be required after 2–3 weeks to assess change in titre)
Syphilis serology (full – including fluorescent treponemal antibody-absorption (FTA-ABS) test and *Treponema pallidum* haemagglutination (TPHA) test)
Sickle-cell test (if appropriate and haemoglobin electrophoresis)
Fasting serum lipids (after 12–14 hours complete fast and 45 minutes total body rest; no stasis during blood withdrawal, i.e. no sphygmomanometer or other occluding cuff)
Glucose tolerance test
(serum electrolytes including urea, calcium, phosphorus, phosphate, uric acid, etc.)
Electrocardiogram
Radiology
Chest X-ray
Magnetic resonance imaging (with contrast)
CT scan (with contrast) if MRI unavailable
Audiometry
Pure tone audiogram
Acoustic impedance measurements including stapedius reflex thresholds and decay
Alternate binaural loudness balance (ABLB)
Speech audiometry loudness discomfort levels
Fistula test (electronystagmography + impedance) if appropriate
Brain stem auditory evoked response audiometry (Electrocochleography)
Promontory stimulation (if no hearing present)
Otoacoustic emissions
Lumbar puncture – for routine cerebrospinal fluid examination, serology, Lange curve and immunoglobulins (seldom now necessary unless multiple sclerosis suspected).

It must be remembered that when a patient with sudden hearing loss presents within the early stages, i.e. under 15 days, everyone carrying out investigations wants to help simultaneously. At the receiving end of this investigative enthusiasm and energy, lies a patient! Many of these investigations are time-consuming (e.g. glucose tolerance tests) and as they yield the least urgent information they should be left until last. Those conditions encompassed by the taking of blood on a rested, fasted patient can all be accomplished in a single venepuncture the morning after admission. Lumbar puncture if considered necessary (which is seldom now the case) should be left until last, as after this the patient may have much discomfort in the back and head. To follow this with any procedure requiring mobility, mental attention and cooperation or the maintenance of a prolonged position is cruel.

Audiometry

A patient with sudden hearing loss needs first the simplest tests, of pure tone thresholds, acoustic impedance measurements (except in cases of suspected oval or round window rupture or perilymph fistula); and stapedius (acoustic) reflex thresholds. Tests of longer duration can be more conveniently carried out later on. It should be remembered that tones above 85 dB can cause a temporary threshold shift even in the normal ear. In an already damaged cochlea, the possibility of further damage by test tones at high intensities is very real (Simmons, 1973).

From the simple pure-tone test, two most interesting prognostic factors have been reported (Mattox and Simmons, 1977). First, the less obvious, is the significance of the test frequency of 8 kHz, and the second is the shape of the audiogram. In their series they noted that all but one patient with an upward-sloping audiogram had complete or good recovery. Conversely all but two patients with a severe downward slope had a fair or poor recovery. Flat and less severe down-sloping patterns fell between the two extremes. Expressed in another way, if the threshold loss, going from the apex to the base of the cochlea was either improving or stable at 8 kHz, the prognosis for a good or complete recovery was 78%. If there was no hearing at 8 kHz, regardless of the hearing at other frequencies, the same prognosis was only 29%. Recovery was always better at the apex of the cochlea, than at the base. This seemed independent of the contour of the severity of the loss on the initial threshold audiogram. It should be remembered that these findings were noted on *untreated* patients.

In the series reported by Shaia and Sheehy (1976), 12% showed a low-tone loss, 32% a flat loss and 31% a high-tone loss. However, 25% showed a profound or total loss. It is this last group which deserves special mention and again they may be subdivided – first into those with a severe loss and second those with a total loss (Figure 17.14).

Audiometry in sudden hearing loss serves two purposes – first, to assess the day-to-day level of the loss by the level of the pure-tone threshold, and second to determine the site of the lesion. The site is of particular importance in determining the treatment. Many of the patients showing a retrocochlear pattern have the contour shown in Figure 17.14 and frequently they will be in the younger age group, that is below 40.

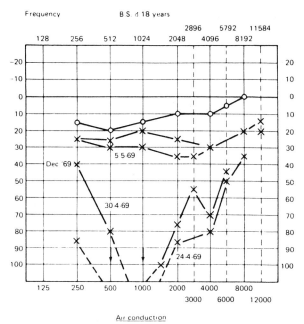

Figure 17.14 Retrocochlear lesion. The pure tone audiogram shows the low level of hearing in the left ear when first seen and the improvement after treatment at 1 week, at 2 weeks, and the final result at 8 months; ○–○ right, x–x left. (Reproduced by kind permission of Morrison and Booth and Editor, *British Journal of Hospital Medicine*)

Electrocochleography

Miyasaki and Kumagami (1988) emphasized the benefit of examining the cochlear microphonic by electrocochleography in patients with sudden deafness. They found that the detection threshold of the cochlear microphonic by electrocochleography, irrespective of the period after the onset of the hearing loss, seemed to be the most reliable tool in estimating the final level in the pure tone audiogram. Ikeda *et al.* (1987) carried out electrocochleography in 84 patients with sudden deafness. The difference of hearing threshold between the healthy and diseased ears was shown as a function of the difference of the N1 latency. The results of the patients were divided into three groups: the first group showed no change of the N1 latency despite the increase of the hearing threshold; the second exhibited a prolongation of N1 latency with the increase of the hearing threshold; and the third displayed no response of N1. The cause of the hearing loss was thought by the authors in the first group to be strial, postsynaptic or mild cochlear

damage and that in the second to be vascular, sensory or neural damage. In their series the first group showed a better prognosis than either of the other two.

In the group with a total loss, the primary audiometric tests will be of no avail in helping the worried clinician or patient, but electrocochleography has a useful part to play. Graham *et al.* (1978), used transtympanic electrocochleography to test 70 patients with sudden hearing loss. Of particular interest are the 24% where threshold audiometry was impossible. Of these 17 patients, a result was obtained indicating a retrocochlear pattern in seven. In the remaining 10 patients, neither a cochlear microphonic nor an action potential was found, suggesting a cochlear loss, with or without retrocochlear involvement. In two of these patients, the promonotry electrode was used to provide direct stimulation to the cochlea and this evoked a subjective sensation of sound, suggesting that the cochlar nerve was intact to some extent (Figure 17.15) (Graham and Hazell, 1977).

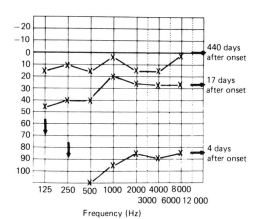

Figure 17.15 Serial audiograms in a man aged 61 years whose hearing completely recovered after sudden onset of nearly complete left-sided deafness. Electrocochleography, 5 days after the onset of the deafness, showed a large cochlear microphonic and no detectable action potential but promontory stimulation produced a sensation of sound. (Reproduced by kind permission of the Editor, *Journal of Laryngology and Otology*)

Otoacoustic emissions

The measurement of transient otoacoustic emissions evoked by a click stimulus is now a reliable technique for the qualitative detection of hearing impairment. Their use in patients with idiopathic sudden hearing loss has been thought by some authors to be helpful in predicting possible recovery. Tanaka, Suzuki and Inoue (1990) investigated otoacoustic emissions in 338 patients with sensorineural hearing loss including 286 with idiopathic sudden deafness. Three hundred and six patients with sudden deafness whose hearing losses were greater than 27 dB at the initial measurement were examined two or three times for otoacoustic emissions in the course of their treatment. Two hundred and six recovered to a greater or lesser degree from the hearing loss. They felt that the positive correlation between the interaural difference of audiometric threshold and the interaural difference of the otoacoustic emission threshold, resulting from the investigation of patients with sudden deafness suggested that the otoacoustic emission indicates the degree of impairment in the cochlea. Sakashita *et al.* (1991) showed that evoked otoacoustic emissions could be detected in about half of ears with sudden hearing loss and moreover the majority of these showed a good hearing prognosis in spite of the degree of hearing loss. Whereas in other conditions the test is not usually performed when the air conduction threshold exceeds 30 dB, the presence of such emissions in those with a greater hearing loss in sudden deafness does appear to be possible in some cases (Figure 17.16). The first to report this finding were Hinz and von Wedel (1984). Sakashita *et al.* stated that the emission thresholds did not show any correlation to the final hearing results. Hoth and Bönnhoff (1992) performed the test in 25 cases of sudden deafness and followed these during treatment. In some cases the transient otoacoustic emission parameters showed a recovery behaviour even if no improvement in hearing performance was observed on pure tone audiometry. Hattori, Niwa and Yanagita (1992) carried out transiently evoked otoacoustic emissions using click stimuli in 123 ears including 86 intact ears; 13 had sudden deafness but whose hearing had improved and six suffering from acoustic trauma with or without tinnitus. In the hearing improved cases with tinnitus in spite of a recovery of hearing thresholds to within normal levels, the detection thresholds of the emissions remained comparably high to that of intact ears. Truy *et al.* (1993) carried out a prospective study on 24 patients hospitalized with sudden idiopathic hearing loss. In addition to pure tone audiometry, transient evoked otoacoustic emissions were recorded and only those patients seen within 3 days of the onset of the hearing loss were included. The transient evoked otoacoustic emission amplitude at the first recording, i.e. at onset, was found to be correlated with improvement in pure tone threshold at a subsequent examination after a mean of 8.71 days at 2 kHz. However, they were unable to find any other correlation and expressed the view that the test did not form the basis of any prediction that could be clinically useful.

Vestibular tests

These have a particular place in those patients with sudden hearing loss which has been accompanied by

vertigo, but in most instances such tests can be deferred until all the necessary audiometric tests have been completed, and the patient's morale is beginning to improve. They are never urgent.

Electronystagmography is often helpful; it is of special benefit in diagnosing vertebrobasilar insufficiency or other possible vascular causes of positional nystagmus. It may be combined with impedance testing to demonstrate a possible perilymph fistula (see Chapter 14 on otosclerosis).

Radiology

If such facilities exist, then MR imaging with contrast is now obligatory in all patients with sudden hearing loss. This is not only to exclude a vestibular schwannoma, but it has recently been shown that in such patients changes within the cochlear vestibular and facial nerves together with the labyrinth may be demonstrated. T1-weighted images before and after contrast appear to be the most appropriate. The cause of enhancement is usually an infectious process, most often viral. However syphilitic and bacterial inner ear infections have also been reported as showing a similar effect. Recently, Mark and Fitzgerald (1993) reported six patients with sudden hearing loss with segmental enhancement of different areas of the cochlea on contrast-enhanced MR imaging; three of their patients were subsequently found on surgical exploration to have a perilymph fistula.

Management

Three unfavourable prognostic factors are known – the shape of the audiogram (especially the degree of involvement at 8 kHz), the severity of the hearing loss, and the presence of vertigo. It is also known that in the idiopathic case, there will be spontaneous improvement within 15 days in 50–60% of cases. However, failure to investigate patients will inevitably lead to a missed diagnosis and a missed opportunity for treatment.

Patients with a cochlear (sensory) loss should have a daily pure tone threshold audiogram under identical test conditions and ideally speech audiometry and discrimination scores should also be carried out on a daily basis. Those who fail to show spontaneous improvement under observation by the tenth or twelfth day should be offered treatment. On occasions, the pattern of hearing loss has been shown to change from neural to sensory as 'improvement' occurs.

Increasing cochlear blood flow
Vasodilators

There is little or no evidence that these are of proven value. The difference between the autoregulatory

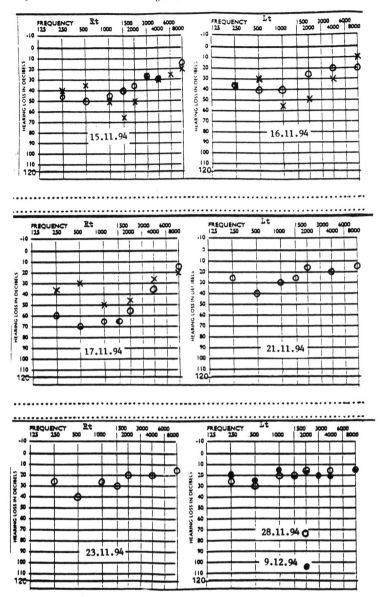

(a)

Figure 17.16 Patient when aged 48 went suddenly deaf in the left ear overnight and subsequent investigation including the CT scan showed no abnormality. The patient had left-sided tinnitus. Hearing on the left remained stable. The patient was seen 6 days after a possible viral infection affecting the nose and pharynx and feeling totally deaf on the right side with tinnitus. The patient was initially treated for a eustachian tube dysfunction. There was some subsequent spontaneous improvement in hearing before being seen. Audiometry confirmed the bilateral sensorineural hearing loss which was monitored at intervals. Investigations including an MRI scan were essentially normal apart from showing multiple high signal lesions within the white matter of both cerebral hemispheres more in keeping with ischaemic change. The patient's cardiac status was checked as he had undergone an angioplasty 7 years before. (a) Serial audiometry starting on sixth day after the incident (15 November) up to and including 9 December with restoration of hearing on the right side. Medication betahistine 16 mg t.d.s.

mechanisms in the circulation of the brain and of the inner ear have often been ignored; the cerebral circulation is practically unaffected by variations in the systemic blood pressure. Experimental work in animals (the cat) has shown that vasoconstrictor drugs

such as angiotensin produce, with some delay, a moderate increase in perilymphatic Po_2. Drugs inducing vasodilatation, such as histamine, are followed by the opposite effect. The changes observed in the perilymphatic Po_2 after injection of vasoactive drugs

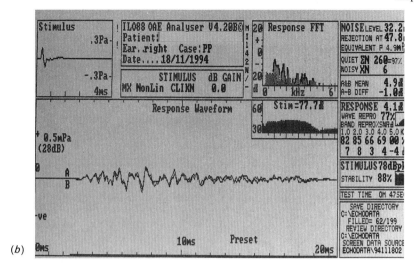

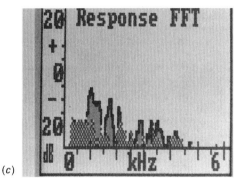

Figure 17.16 (*b*) and (*c*) Otoacoustic emissions (18 November)

indicate that there is a direct correlation between the systemic blood pressure and inner ear oxygenation. The evidence therefore implies that vasodilator drugs should be abandoned (Figure 17.17) (Yagi, Fisch and Murata, 1978). 'Cocktails' or 'shot gun' therapy have shown no worthhile benefit over more specific agents, or natural spontaneous recovery (Wilkins, Mattox and Lyles, 1987).

Laurikainen *et al.* (1993) reported work on betahistine-induced vascular effects in the rat cochlea. Betahistine has been widely used to treat cochlear disorders and the mechanism of its action is assumed to be based on its histamine-like effect on H1 receptors in the cochlear vasculature, leading to an increased cochlear blood flow. It has been shown that betahistine can strongly affect H3 heteroreceptors in the periphery via an autonomic ligand. Laurikainen *et al.*, using a laser Doppler flowmeter in 23 rats, concluded that betahistine affected the vascular conductivity in the cochlea in a dose-dependent fashion and that H1 receptors mediate the systemic and peripheral vascular effects of betahistine, whereas the cochlear effect involved cholinergic receptors.

Glycerol has been found to increase the cochlear and cerebral blood flow significantly after intravenous administration experimentally in the rabbit (Larsen, Angelborg and Hultcrantz, 1982).

Pentoxifylline/oxpentyfylline

Pentoxifylline is a phosphodiesterase inhibitor and haemorheological agent which has been found to increase oxygen delivery to ischaemic tissue. There are a number of studies suggesting that the intravenous use of this drug is helpful in the treatment of sudden sensorineural hearing loss of vascular origin but it is unavailable in the UK and the USA in the intravenous form. In a prospectively randomized trial conducted jointly in two clinics in two different countries on ·151 patients with sudden hearing loss, there was no difference between naftidrofuryl and pentoxifylline with respect of therapeutic success (Laskawi *et al.*, 1987); both were used in conjunction with low molecular weight Dextran and cortisone. Patients with concomitant vascular disease had less favourable treatment results than those who were otherwise

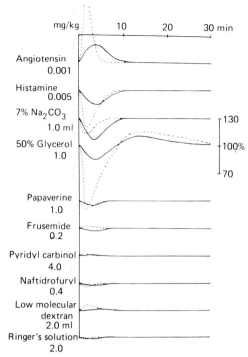

Figure 17.17 Average comparative response of the perilymphatic oxygen tension and systemic blood pressure following intravenous injection of various vasoactive drugs (in the cat). Only angiotensin induced a significant rise; histamine, 50% glycerol and 75% Na_2CO_3 caused a reduction; papaverine, frusemide, pyridylcarbinol, naftidrofuryl and low molecular weight Dextran had no significant effect on the perilymphatic oxygen. (Reproduced by kind permission of Professor Fisch and Editor, *Annals of Otology, Rhinology and Laryngology*)

healthy. (Naftidrofuryl is no longer available for intravenous use in the UK.) There is no evidence that when given by mouth, in common with all other oral vasodilating preparations, it has any value in increasing cochlear blood flow (Smith *et al.*, 1986).

Pentoxifylline has been observed to lower blood viscosity by altering red blood cell membrane flexibility; by increasing the latter it allows red blood cells to traverse capillaries more easily thereby increasing the oxygen delivery to ischaemic tissue. Given intravenously to guinea pigs (LaRouere *et al.*, 1992), it was found acutely to increase cochlear blood flow in a dose-dependent manner and this appeared to be strongly related to its rheological properties rather than as a vasodilator. The blood pressure was noted to decline in a similar manner and blood gas levels showed no significant difference between baseline and infusion levels (pH, Pco_2, Po_2 and HCO_3). Twenty minutes post-infusion the cochlear blood flow had returned to baseline values or below. Probst *et al.*

(1992) carried out a randomized double-blind placebo-control study of low molecular weight Dextran and pentoxifylline in acute acoustic trauma and sudden hearing loss. They treated 184 patients, because of sudden sensorineural hearing loss, by three different treatment regimens and there was no significant difference in respect of hearing recovery between the three groups; treatment with pentoxifylline was both by intravenous use and orally.

Calcium antagonists

The hope that a peripheral vasodilating drug whether given intravenously or orally might somehow increase cerebral circulation has so far proved totally fruitless. There is no indication that any of them are of the slightest value. However the 'calcium antagonists' have been shown to increase cerebral blood flow. In general, they prevent vascular smooth wall contraction induced by neurotransmitter and vasoconstrictor substances. The calcium antagonists also exhibit rheological properties by stabilizing the thrombocyte membrane. During ischaemia calcium antagonists counteract the depletion of the intracellular ATP-pool. It would seem therefore that they are a group of medicines which may have some application in the treatment of sudden sensorineural hearing loss of vascular cause. Class A calcium antagonists such as nifedipine, nimodipine, diltiazem and verapamil are of primary interest, while class B antagonists are less potent and less specific and include such drugs as cinnarizine and flunarizine.

Nimodipine is a 4-5-dihydropyridine calcium antagonist with selective spasmolytic and vasodilatory properties on cerebral vessels. Lenarz (1989) in a prospective randomized clinical study on 80 patients with idiopathic sudden hearing loss using parenteral treatment compared nimodipine with hydroxyethyl starch and naftidroduryl. There was no significant difference between the two groups, but there was a lower rate of side effects suggesting that nimodipine may have a possible future role.

Mann, Beck and Beck (1986) tried nifedipine given orally, 60 mg daily, and intravenous normal saline against intravenous oral naftidrofuryl and oral vitamins A and E, and zinc. They could find no significant difference between the two forms of treatment. Nimodipine was investigated both in guinea-pigs and rats by Jastreboff and Brennan (1988), in which the drug was given intraperitoneally. Subsequent levels in the perilymph were higher than those in the CSF suggesting that the drug enters the perilymph directly from the blood. Spontaneous activity of single cells recorded from the inferior colliculus and cerebellar vermis in the guinea-pigs before and after nimodipine injection revealed that while the activity of the inferior collicular cells increased significantly, the activity of cerebellar cells remained stable. Bobbin, Jastreboff and Fallon (1990) investigated the effect of perfusing the perilymph spaces of the guinea-pig cochlea with nimodipine and evaluating the cochlear potentials when stimulated by 10 kHz tone bursts. Their results supported the hypothesis that L-type calcium channels are directly involved in the operation of the organ of Corti. They speculated that L-type Ca^{2+} channels are integrally involved in generation of a negative summating potential and the decimation of the cochlear partition. In 1985, Theopold treated 30 patients with tinnitus, 12 of whom had shown sudden deafness and four with Menière's disease with almost universal benefit. A recent study by Davies, Knox and Donaldson (1994) reported some good responses in a smaller number of patients in the treatment of tinnitus and found a good correlation between the subjective and objective assessment of their responses. Coleman, Dengerink and Wright (1991) investigated the effects of intra-arterial infusion of hydroxyethyl starch and nimodipine in guinea-pigs. Given intra-arterially they found that nimodipine resulted in a pronounced increase in cochlear blood flow of 26% (compared with 12% for pentoxifylline).

Lassen, Hirsch and Kamerer (1995) reported on the use of nimodipine in the medical treatment of Menière's disease in 12 patients (30 mg b.d.) seen over a 27-month period who had failed first line treatment. Of these, seven showed the hearing to be improved or unchanged (58%) and eight (67%) had their vertigo controlled satisfactorily. Nimodipine (40 mg t.d.s. for 4 weeks) has been shown to produce a marked improvement compared with placebo in patients with vertebrobasilar insufficiency (Hirschberg and Hofferberth, 1988).

It is therefore a drug which seems to merit further trials in the treatment of sudden hearing loss.

Diatrizoate meglumine (Hypaque)

At the Fifth Shambaugh International Workshop, in March 1976, Morimitsu reported on the successful treatment of sudden hearing loss with diatrizoate meglumine after an initial case had stimulated his interest. A 1 ml test dose of intravenous Hypaque prior to vertebral angiography had produced a significant improvement in hearing in a patient who had sudden hearing loss of 40 days' duration. Subsequently, Morimitsu compared 39 patients treated within 2 weeks of the onset of the hearing loss who were treated with 10 ml Hypaque daily until maximum recovery was obtained. Later this treatment was incorporated with a regimen including inhalation of carbogen, intravenous histamine, dexamethasone, a diuretic and a low sodium diet by Emmett and Shea (1979). Interestingly they carried out electrocochleography studies in six patients treated with Hypaque and there was an immediate increase in the action potential (AP) and summating potential (SP) in four of the five patients and the fifth had an increase in the action potential

at 1 hour post-injection. This is perhaps not surprising when it is remembered that diatrizoate meglumine acts in a similar way to glycerol.

Ushisako and Morimitsu (1988) reported on their series of 47 patients treated with amidotrizoate. Twenty-four of 34 cases (71%) treated within 2 weeks showed either complete or marked recovery.

Huang et al. (1989) treated 142 patients with idiopathic sudden sensorineural hearing loss in three groups, although all received the vasodilator betahistine. All those in two of their groups were injected with 10 ml for a period of 5 days in hospital and subsequently on an outpatient basis up to a maximum of 30 doses. However, none of their three groups produced results which were consistently better than the spontaneous recovery rate of 65% reported by Mattox and Simmons (1977).

Most recently, Redleaf et al. (1995) treated 39 cases with a daily intravenous infusion of 40 ml of 66% diatrizoate meglumine (Hypaque 76) and 10 ml/kg of low molecular weight Dextran for 5–7 days. Sixty-four per cent showed hearing improvement while receiving treatment and 48% showed this after their first treatment dose. Those patients presenting early, i.e. before 7 days, showed the most marked improvement. Kano et al. (1994) reported the use of MR imaging in 30 cases of sudden unilateral hearing loss. They found that those who showed a higher signal intensity on proton density and T2-weighted images on the affected side responded less well to either amidotrizoate or steroid therapy; amidotrizoate seemed to be more effective in MRI negative cases of sudden deafness.

Low molecular weight Dextran (Rheomacrodex)

Among the aetiological factors proposed in sudden hearing loss is hypercoagulability of the blood. Low molecular weight Dextran by intravenous infusion has therefore been recommended. This preparation with a molecular weight of 40 000 is available as a 10% solution, either in 5% dextrose or in normal saline. No significant benefit has been demonstrated following its use (Kronenberg et al., 1992). It is contraindicated in patients with cardiac failure and bleeding disorders and has on rare occasions proven fatal (Zaytoun, Schuknecht and Farmer, 1983). Allergic reactions have also been recorded (Hanna, 1986).

Hydroxyethyl starch/ (Hetastarch-Hespan)

In those patients in which a vascular cause is considered the likely reason for sudden sensorineural hearing loss it has been assumed that a microcirculatory disturbance is involved either by vasospasm of the afferent blood vessels and or a sludging phenomenon in the region of the distal end-arteries of the cochlea. Such a disturbance results in the impairment of oxygen concentration of the perilymph thereby affecting the structure and metabolism of the hair cells. It is hoped therefore by treatment to bring about a reduction of the blood viscosity and flow resistance, a reduction in surface tension, and an influence on the glycogenolytic metabolism of the erythrocytes. It is thought to be ideal to do this by hypervolaemic haemodilution therapy with plasma substitutes choosing an agent which not only alters factors of the microcirculation such as packed cell volume and whole blood viscosity but also those important for the microcirculation, such as plasma viscosity and erythrocyte aggregation. Hydroxyethyl starch (10%) appears to fulfill these criteria ideally.

Hydroxyethyl starch (Hespan) is a 6% colloidal solution for plasma volume expansion. It is an artificial colloid derived from a waxy starch composed almost entirely of a myelopectin. The average molecular weight is 450000 and its colloidal properties approximate those of human albumin. It is given as a 6% colloidal solution in 0.9% sodium chloride. In common with all other plasma volume expanders it can produce dilutional effects on fibrinogen and prothrombin activity.

In the studies reported by Wilhelm *et al.* (1989) patients treated with Dextran 40 showed a significant deterioration in plasma viscosity and an increase in erythrocyte aggregation as well as a reduction in haematocrit. The reduction in haematocrit in the hydroxyethyl starch group was merely comparable with those of the Dextran group but the course of both plasma viscosity and erythrocyte aggregation differed significantly. There was no deterioration seen in either of these parameters but an improvement regarding tendency could be observed. They found the changes in these rheological parameters correlated with the clinical result and the mean increase in hearing in the speech range was significantly higher. Their treatment regimen was 2×500 ml 10% HES 200/0.5 i.v. transfused over a 4-hour period (to which they also added 400 mg naftidrofuryl).

Desloovere, Lörz and Klima (1989) and Desloovere (1989) reported the results using an infusion of hydroxyethyl starch 500 ml over a 4-hour period each day (including i.v. pentoxifylline); interestingly, patients with a systolic blood pressure above 130 mmHg performed better in the treatment group. The relative hearing improvement of patients with initial haematocrit value above 44 or haemoglobin value above 14 mg/dl, or both, was poorer in the control than in the treatment group. More recently Desloovere *et al.* (1991) have reported superior results with hydroxyethyl starch/pentoxifylline infusions in patients with an elevated plasma viscosity (> 1.7; $H_2O = 1$). Pilgramm (1991) in two independently conducted randomized clinical studies (sudden deafness; acute acoustic trauma) that in terms of hearing gain and the elimination of tinnitus, low molecular weight Dextran 40 and 6% hydroxyethyl starch did not produce any significant difference in therapy. Severe adverse reactions from hydroxyethyl starch are less common than with Dextran but generalized pruritus after an infusion is more frequent. The pruritus is assumed to be the result of HES deposition in the skin leading to release of non-histamine-related mediators; antihistamines are ineffective but capsaicin has been used with good effect (Szeimies *et al.*, 1994).

Inhalation of 5% carbon dioxide: 95% oxygen (carbogen)

It has been known for many years that carbon dioxide is a potent cerebral vasodilator, but for this to be achieved it is usual to use a mixture containing at least 10% CO_2 (Pollock *et al.*, 1974). Prazma showed, in guinea-pigs, that extreme hypercapnia caused an increase of the endocochlear potential; as the latter increased, so the cochlear microphonic decreased (Prazma, 1978; Prazma *et al.*, 1979) (see Figure 17.18). They concluded that the enzyme carbonic anhydrase may participate in the generation of the endocochlear potential. However, inhalations of 10% CO_2 in man may cause a dangerous increase in arterial blood pressure. Using inhalations of 5% CO_2 and 95% O_2 for a period of 20 minutes in a small series of patients with Menière's disease, the cochlear microphonic increased in some but there was no change in the summating potential and no obvious decrease in the width of the action potential (Booth, 1980).

Using the polarographic technique, Nagahara, Fisch and Yagi (1983) and Fisch (1983), measured the oxygen tension in human perilymph. Following the inhalation of carbogen (5% CO_2: 95% O_2) they demonstrated two different patterns of disturbed perilymphatic oxygenation; in sudden deafness and sudden cochleovestibular loss of inner ear function, there were low initial values but a normal response to inhalation, while patients with a slowly progressive sensorineural hearing loss showed normal initial values but a low response to carbogen (Figure 17.18). In a group of seven patients who presented with sudden deafness with or without vertigo but normal caloric responses, there was an initial value of perilymphatic oxygenation of 8.6 mmHg which rose after 13 minutes to an average of 14.8 mmHg (an increase of 175%). No significant correlation could be found between the hearing loss, or the initial value and maximal response to carbogen inhalation. Likewise there was no significant correlation between the initial value of oxygenation and the time interval between the onset of deafness and the measurement, i.e. the duration of the disease. In four patients with some cochleovestibular loss, the carbogen response started after 45 seconds and reached a maximum of 20.7 mmHg (an increase of 215%) 15 minutes after

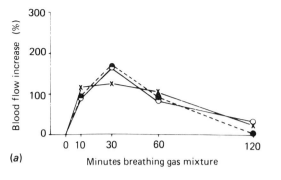

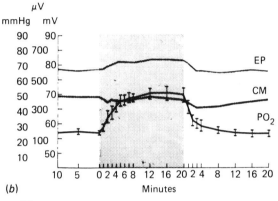

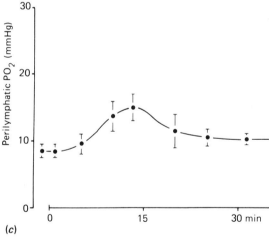

Figure 17.18 Mean blood flow changes in temporal bones. (a) Left and right with time; 5% CO_2–95% O_2, 14 dogs. x–x Brain; o–o temporal bone left (TBL); ●–● temporal bone right (TBR). (Reproduced by kind permission of authors and Editor, *Archives of Otolaryngology*). (b) Effects of ventilation with 5% CO_2–95% O_2 for 20 minutes (guinea-pig). Vertical bars represent the standard error of mean. CM, cochlear microphonic; EP, endolymphatic potential. (Reproduced by kind permission of Prazma and Editor, *Annals of Otology, Rhinology and Laryngology*). (c) Changes in perilymphatic oxygen tension by carbogen in seven patients with idiopathic sudden deafness (shown in x̄ ± s.d.) (Reproduced by kind permission of Professor Fisch and Editor, *Acta Otolaryngologica*)

the onset of inhalation. The mean initial values of perilymphatic oxygenation were below the normal range obtained in cats, and in otosclerotic patients. In patients with sudden cochleovestibular loss, a significant correlation was found between the initial value of perilymphatic oxygenation and the duration of the disease.

Fisch, Nagahara and Pollak (1984) have emphasized that the arterial Pco_2 has a stronger effect on the oxygenation of the perilymph than the arterial Po_2. Similarly hypoventilation induces an increase of the perilymphatic oxygen, while hyperventilation is followed by the opposite effect. Hypoventilation causes the arterial Po_2 to drop, while the Pco_2 increases. The combination of 5% CO_2 and 95% O_2 gives a fourfold increase in perilymphatic oxygen compared with pure oxygen alone or the inhalation of CO_2 in air. The recommended regimen, therefore, is the inhalation by mask of 95% O_2 and 5% CO_2 for 30 minutes eight times per day at intervals of one hour. Baghat and Shenoi (1982), using this regimen in four patients who were carefully monitored, achieved a good hearing improvement in three who received the treatment within a fortnight of the onset of deafness, but in the remaining patient, after an interval of 4 months, there was no change. It was originally Shea and Kitabchi (1971, 1973) who advocated inhalations of 5% CO_2 and 95% O_2 for 30 minutes four times a day, but this earlier work seems to have been largely overlooked.

Giger (1979) carried out a prospective randomized trial on 55 patients with sudden deafness treated by the inhalation of 95% O_2 and 5% CO_2, or intravenous infusion with papaverine and Dextran. Five days after treatment no significant difference could be found between the two therapies. However, audiometric results obtained 1 year later showed statistically better results for those who were managed by carbogen inhalations and he thought that this therapy may improve the spontaneous rate of recovery in sudden deafness. Grandis, Hirsch and Wagener (1993) used carbogen inhalations for 15 minutes every 2 hours while the patients were awake, together with other agents including steroids but failed to achieve results better than the 65% spontaneous recovery rate in their 41 patients.

Kawakami *et al.* (1991a) carried out experiments on guinea-pigs to test the feasibility of pulse oximetry to measure arterial O_2 saturation and its relationship to cochlear blood flow. They found that when the arterial oxygen saturation was measured in the foot pad by a pulse oximeter under respiratory conditions, the data showed a close correlation with the results of blood gas analysis. Their study demonstrated a slower reaction in the decrease of perilymphatic O_2 tension than of cochlear blood flow during stepwise induction of hypoventilation; under certain conditions of hyperventilation in which arterial O_2 saturation and perilymphatic oxygen tension increased gradually, cochlear blood flow was found to decrease. Experiments by the same authors (Kawakami *et al.*, 1991b), also on the guinea-pig, showed the cochlear blood flow generally parallels systemic blood pressure, indicating a close correlation. By contrast, perilymphatic oxygen tension was slower to increase and decrease. Kawakami *et al.* (1991c) also tested trimetaphan camsilate, a sulphonamide compound with ganglion blocking properties with an extremely short period of action. Its major therapeutic use has been to produce controlled hypotension for some surgical procedures during general anaesthesia or in the emergency treatment of hypertensive crises. They found that the cochlear blood flow and perilymphatic oxygen tension were found to be dose dependent (Kawakami *et al.*, 1991d). Experiments in the chinchilla by Ikeda and Morizono (1989) tested the effect of carbon dioxide upon the cochlear potentials and cochlear pH by flushing the gas into the tympanic bulla. Carbon dioxide did not affect the action potential threshold except for a slight decrease when 10% CO_2 was used. The endocochlear potential did not vary with carbon dioxide. However carbon dioxide gas mixture reduced the pH in perilymph significantly with both 5% and 10% CO_2. Carbon dioxide slightly but significantly decreased the endolymph pH.

More recently the inhalation of carbogen and the use of a peripheral vasodilator such as nicotinamide or pentoxifylline has been found to be effective as a non-toxic tumour radiosensitizer but is as yet unproven in every day clinical use (Rojas, Johns and Fiat, 1993). Hatch *et al.* (1991) investigated the effect of carbogen, carbon dioxide and oxygen on noise-induced hearing loss in guinea-pigs. Their results indicated that oxygen (i.e. cochlear-oxygenation) was a more important factor than CO_2 (i.e. a vasodilator) in protection of the cochlea for noise-induced damage.

Hyperbaric oxygenation

Reports so far from the few centres with such a facility appear encouraging, but no proper trial has yet been set up for the clinical treatment of patients with sudden deafness without the use of other agents. Where such a facility exists its use should certainly be considered and probably utilized.

Anticoagulants

There no longer seems any indication to give these unless indicated by the haematological investigations or other disease within the cardiovascular system. Heparin may be chosen in the initial stages and has an effect in reducing the serum lipid level and by stimulating lipoprotein lipase formation; it also binds with histamine.

Donaldson (1979) treated 23 patients with sudden unilateral sensorineural hearing loss with intra-venous heparin sodium within 1 week of the onset of the deafness. Complete or good recovery developed in a total of 70% but as he himself pointed out this is very similar to previous reported criteria of 66% spontaneous recovery.

Defibrinogenation therapy (Batroxobin)

A reduction in serum fibrinogen decreases blood viscosity. Four reports on the use of Batroxobin have been published from Osaka in Japan (Kubo *et al.*, 1988; Shiraishi, Kubo and Matsunaga, 1991; Kawakami *et al.*, 1992; Shiraishi *et al.*, 1993). Batroxobin is a thrombin-like enzyme (Gicopeptide).

Prostaglandins

Prostaglandin synthesis by the cochlea in the guinea-pig has been investigated by Escoubet *et al.* (1985) and Tran Ba Huy *et al.* (1987). Prostaglandins are synthesized by the vascular structures of the lateral wall of the inner ear (stria vascularis and spiral ligament). The main prostaglandins produced were PGI_2 (prostacyclin) PGF_{2alpha} and PGE_2; PGI_2 and PGF_{2alpha} were also found in the perilymph. Aspirin injected intraperitoneally decreased prostaglandin synthesis by the lateral wall and reduced the prostaglandin levels in the perilymph. (This effect was reversed after 3 days.) Arachidonic acid is metabolized to prostaglandins and to thromboxane by cyclo-oxygenase and to leukotrienes by lipo-oxygenase. Likewise treatment by aspirin which inhibits cyclo-oxygenase can cause disorders of the inner ear circulation. As to whether the depressive effect of aspirin upon the prostaglandin synthesis accounts for the drop in the microphonic and action potentials remains to be demonstrated. The administration of aspirin (or indomethacin) did not modify the basal endocochlear potential. The administration of PGI_2 reduced the endocochlear potential in three guinea-pigs but not in five others (Tran Ba Huy *et al.*, 1987). It should be noted that both of these sets of experiments were carried out *in vitro*. In the same experiments vasopressin and angiotensin II failed to stimulate prostaglandin synthesis. Nakashima, Kuno and Yanagita (1989) administered prostaglandin E_1 intravenously to 51 patients with sudden sensorineural hearing loss. The results are compared with those from 362 patients who had not received this type of treatment. They could find no significant difference in outcome between the two groups of patients.

In an earlier review of the prostaglandins in their effect on the body generally and in the ear, Booth (1982) predicted that when sodium prostacycline became commercially available it might prove to be a useful preparation for treating sudden sensorineural hearing loss. So far only a few reports have appeared on this subject. Olszewski *et al.* (1985) treated 22 patients with sudden unilateral sensorineural hearing loss with prostacycline. Ten of the patients were admitted within 7 days of the onset of the disease and the remainder within 8–24 days. Twelve (55%) achieved complete recovery, nine partial recovery and only one failed to show any improvement after 9 months of observation. Three of eight patients with total speech reception threshold and speech discrimination of score deafness experienced complete recovery, four showed partial recovery and one no return of hearing. Olszewski *et al.* (1990) treated 30 patients with sudden sensorineural hearing loss in a double blind test situation. In those receiving prostacycline 87% (15) were said to show a complete recovery. All of the patients had been deaf for at least 7 days before treatment was commenced (five 6-hour intravenous infusions at a dosage of 5 mg/kg per minute at 6-hourly intervals). Michel and Matthias (1991) treated 11 patients with a single infusion over 6 hours with prostacycline (10 mg/kg per minute). Eleven patients were treated and were initially given pentoxifylline 300 mg daily for 16 days. Subsequently they received the prostacycline and most cases showed a further hearing improvement (mean level 7.5 dB/frequency within 24 hours of the infusion). This improvement was subsequently maintained. Further trials of Epoprostenol (sodium prostacyclin) therefore seem worthwhile.

The drug has been used in severe Raynaud's disease with remarkable effect. Epoprostenol is a naturally occurring prostaglandin produced by the intima of blood vessels and is the most potent inhibitor of platelet aggregation known. Unlike many other prostaglandins it does not metabolize during passage through the pulmonary circulation. Epoprostenol is a potent vasodilator. It inhibits platelet aggregation by elevating platelet cyclic adenosine monophosphate. It reduces platelet procoagulant activity and the release of heparin neutralizing factor. The drug needs to be reconstituted with great care and given by a strict aseptic technique; the manufacturer's recommendations must be adhered to at all times.

Umemura *et al.* (1990, 1993) have reported on the effect of arachidonic acid on the circulation of the inner ear of the rat and the role of thromboxane A_2 respectively.

Indomethacin like aspirin and other non-steroidal anti-inflammatory drugs blocks the action of cyclooxygenase and is an inhibitor of prostaglandin synthesis. It was found by Arenberg and Goodfriend (1980) to block the effects of frusemide (furosemide) in two patients, whom they investigated with Menière's disease. It also blocked the concomitant rise in plasma renin level after frusemide (furosemide) administration. More recently, Michel and Matthias (1992) investigated 10 patients with Menière's disease to establish the effect of prostaglandin E_2 on their fluctuating hearing loss. Prostaglandin E_2 produced a transient hearing improvement comparable to the effects of the furosemide/frusemide test in the same patients.

Mori *et al.* (1990) investigated the effect of furosemide, canrenoate and aldosterone antagonists on the endocochlear potential and the endolymphatic sac potential in the guinea-pig. Furosemide produced no significant change in the latter but decreased the endocochlear potential to a negative level. Canrenoate produced no significant effect in the endocochlear potential but decreased the endolymphatic sac potential.

Steroid therapy

Treatment of a vascular cause by trying to improve the local circulation within the cochlea appears entirely reasonable, as has been outlined above. In all other branches of otology great stress is placed upon the tests designed to diagnose the site of the lesion. In our present state of knowledge therefore it appears illogical, having carried out such tests, to jettison the results in favour of a single treatment modality particularly when it involves the use of a group of potent drugs – steroids. It has been the experience of Morrison and Booth (1970), and remains so, that steroids are the treatment of choice when the loss is retrocochlear, and are the only effective treatment in the severe case of this type. It should be remembered that some two-thirds of cases with idiopathic sudden hearing loss may be expected to recover completely, or partially, particularly if the loss is moderate. Wilson, Byl and Laird (1980) and later Moskowitz, Lee and Smith (1984) carried out a double-blind clinical trial on the efficacy of steroids and concluded that they had a statistically significant effect on the recovery of hearing in patients with moderate hearing losses. However, in so doing, they assumed that a substantial proportion were of viral origin, but made no attempt to correlate this with the probable site of the lesion. It cannot be emphasized enough that such tests are required and may well need to be repeated as more hearing is recovered, thereby allowing more detailed testing (Kumar, Maudelonde and Mafee, 1986).

All forms of steroids have been used and selection should probably depend on personal experience. Patients receiving these drugs should be examined at regular intervals for side effects including checks on blood pressure, serum electrolytes and if appropriate, electrocardiography. For clinicians without an established or familiar scheme, enteric-coated prednisolone may be recommended, 60 mg on the first day in divided doses (every 6 hours), 50 mg on the second day, 40 mg daily for 3 days, 30 mg daily for 3 days and then the regimen may be tailed off, so that the patient ends medication after approximately 3 weeks. The complications of steroid therapy should never be overlooked; this has been well reviewed by Talar-Williams and Sneller (1994).

Bed rest

If there is the possibility of a membrane rupture, rest in bed may be indicated. Certainly, strenuous exertion should be avoided.

References

ABOU-TALEB, A. and LINTHICUM, F. H. (1987) Scleroderma and hearing loss (Histopathology of a case). *Journal of Laryngology and Otology*, 101, 656–662

AIKAWA, T. and OHTANI, I. (1991) Temporal bone findings in central nervous system leukemia. *American Journal of Otolaryngology*, 12, 320–325

AJULO, S. O., OSINAME, A. I. and MYATT, H. M. (1993) Sensorineural hearing loss in sickle cell anaemia – a United Kingdom study. *Journal of Laryngology and Otology*, 107, 790–794

ALAJOUANINE, T., CASTAIGNE, P., LHERMITTE, F., CAMBIER, J. and GAUTIER, J. C. (1961) La méningo-encéphalite de la maladie de Behçet. *Presse Medicale*, 69, 2579–2582

ALBERA, R., MORRA, B., LACILLA, M., BIANCO, L., GABUTTI, V. and PIGA, A. (1988) Hearing loss and desferrioxamine in homozygous beta-thalassemia. *Audiology*, 27, 207–214

ALBERS, F. W. J., MAJOOR, M. H. J. M. and VAN DER GAAG, R. (1992) Corneal autoimmunity in a patient with relapsing polychondritis. *European Archives of Otorhinolaryngology*, 249, 296–299

ALBERTS, M. C. and TERRENCE, C. F. (1978) Hearing loss in carcinomatous meningitis. *Journal of Laryngology and Otology*, 92, 233–241

ALPORT, A. C. (1927) Hereditary familial congenital haemorrhagic nephritis. *British Medical Journal*, 1, 504–506

ANAND, V. T., MANN, S. B., DASH, R. J. and MEHRA, Y. N. (1989) Auditory investigations in hypothyroidism. *Acta Otolaryngologica*, 108, 83–87

ANTONELLI, A. R., BONFIOLI, F., CAPPIELLO, J., PERETTI, G., ZANETTI, D. and CAPRA, R. (1988) Auditory evoked potentials test battery related to magnetic resonance imaging for multiple sclerosis. *Scandinavian Audiology*, Suppl. 30, 191–196

ARBOIX, A., JUNQUE, C., VENDRELL, P. and MARTI-VILALTA, J. L. (1990) Auditory ear extinction in lacunar syndromes. *Acta Neurologica Scandinavica*, 81, 507–511

ARENBERG, I. K. and GOODFRIEND, T. L. (1980) Indomethacin blocks acute audiologic effects of furosemide in Meniere's disease. *Archives of Otolaryngology*, 106, 383–386

ARGIOLU, F., DIANA, G., AVIGNONE, A. and CAO, A. (1991) Hearing impairment during deferoxamine therapy for thalassemia major. *Journal of Pediatrics*, 118, 826–827

ARINSOY, T., AKPOLAT, T., ATAMAN, M., ARIK, N., SUNGUR, C., YASAVAL, U. *et al.* (1993) Sudden hearing loss in a cyclosporin-treated renal transplantation patient. *Nephron*, 63, 116–117

ARNOLD, J. E. and BENDER, D. R. (1983) BSER abnormalities in a multiple sclerosis patient with normal peripheral hearing acuity. *American Journal of Otology*, 4, 235–237

ARNOLD, W. (1984) Inner ear and renal diseases. *Annals of Otology, Rhinology and Laryngology*, Suppl. 112, 119–124

ATAYA, N. L. (1989) Sensorineural deafness associated with IgA nephropathy. *Journal of Laryngology and Otology*, 103, 412

AXELSSON, A. and LINDGREN, F. (1985) Is there a relationship between hypercholesterolaemia and noise induced hearing loss. *Acta Otolaryngologica*, 100, 379–386

BAGHAT, M. S. and SHENOI, P. M. (1982) Sudden sensorineural hearing loss treated by carbon dioxide inhalation. *Journal of Laryngology and Otology*, 96, 73–81

BAKER, S. R. and LILLY, D. J. (1977) Hearing loss from acute carbon monoxide intoxication. *Annals of Otology, Rhinology and Laryngology*, 86, 323–328

BALDEWEG, T., GRUZELIER, J. H., CATALAN, J., PUGH, K., LOVETT, E., RICCIO, M. *et al.* (1993) Auditory and visual event-related potentials in a controlled investigation of HIV infection. *Electroencephalography and Clinical Neurophysiology*, 88, 356–368

BALOYANNIS, S. J., MANOLIDIS, S. L. and MANOLIDIS, L. S. (1992) The acoustic cortex in Alzheimer's disease. *Acta Otolaryngologica*, Supplement 494, 3–13

BARRATT, H. J., MILLER, D. and RUDGE, P. (1998) The site of the lesion causing deafness in multiple sclerosis. *Scandinavian Audiology*, 17, 67–71

BEG, J. A. (1981) Bilateral sensorineural hearing loss as a complication of infectious mononucleosis. *Archives of Otolaryngology*, 107, 620–622

BELAL, A. (1980) Pathology of vascular sensorineural hearing impairment. *Laryngoscope*, 90, 1831–1839

BEN-DAVID, Y., PRATT, H., LANDMAN, L., FRADIS, M., PODOSHIN, L. and YESHURIN, D. (1986) A comparison of auditory brain stem evoked potentials in hyperlipidemics and normolipemic subjects. *Laryngoscope*, 96, 186–189

BERENHOLZ, L. P., ERIKSEN, C. and HIRSH, F. A. (1992) Recovery from repeated sudden hearing loss in the presence of an acoustic neuroma. *Annals of Otology, Rhinology and Laryngology*, 101, 827–831

BERGSTROM, L. A., NEBLETT, I. M., SANDO, I., HEMENWAY, W. G. and HARRISON, C. D. (1974). The lightning damaged ear. *Archives of Otolaryngology*, 100, 117–121

BERRETTINI, S., BRUSCHINI, P., SELLARI-FRANCESCHINI, S., MITA, L., OLIVIERI, L. and GEMIGNANI, G. (1989) Sudden deafness and Behçet's disease. *Acta Otorhinolaryngologica Belgica*, 43, 221–229

BHANDARI, R. and STEINMAN, G. S. (1983) Sudden deafness in chickenpox: a case report. *Annals of Neurology*, 13, 347

BIAVATI, M. J., GROSS, J. D., WILSON, W. R. and DINA, T. S. (1994) Magnetic resonance imaging evidence of a focal pontine ischemia in sudden hearing loss and seventh nerve paralysis. *American Journal of Otology*, 15, 250–253

BICKNELL, J. M. and HOLLAND, J. V. (1978) Neurologic manifestations of Cogan's syndrome. *Neurology*, 28, 278–281

BIRCHALL, M. A., WRIGHT, R. G., FRENCH, P. D., COCKBAIN, Z. and SMITH, S. J. M. (1992) Auditory function in patients infected with the human immunodeficiency virus. *Clinical Otolaryngology*, 17, 117–121

BITNUM, S., RAKOVER, Y. and ROSEN, G. (1986) Acute bilateral total deafness complicating mumps. *Journal of Laryngology and Otology*, 100, 943–945

BLACK, R. J., GIBSON, W. P. R. and CAPPER, J. W. R. (1982) Fluctuating hearing loss in West African and West Indian racial groups: yaws, syphilis or Meniere's disease. *Journal of Laryngology and Otology*, 96, 847–855

BOBBIN, R. P., JASTREBOFF, P. J. and FALLON, M. (1990) Nimodipine, an L-channel Ca^2 antagonist, reverses the negative summating potential recorded from the guinea pig cochlea. *Hearing Research*, 46, 277–288

BOMHOLT, A., BAK-PEDERSEN, K. and GORMSEN, J. (1979) Fibrinolytic activity in patients with sudden sensorineural hearing loss. *Acta Otolaryngologica Supplementum*, **360**, 184–186

BOOTH, J. B. (1977) Hyperlipidaemia and deafness. *Proceedings of the Royal Society of Medicine*, **70**, 642–646

BOOTH, J. B. (1980) Menière's disease: the selection and assessment of patients for surgery using electrocochleography. *Annals of Royal College of Surgeons of England*, **62**, 415–425

BOOTH, J. B. (1982) Medical management of sensorineural hearing loss. *Journal of Laryngology and Otology*, **96**, 673–684, 773–795

BOOTH, J. B. (1984) Sudden deafness. *The Physician*, **2**, 467–469

BORTON, T. E., EBY, T. L., BALL, E. V., NOLEN, L. and BRADLEY, E. L. (1992) Stimulus repetition rate effect on the auditory brain stem response in systemic lupus erythematosus. *Laryngoscope*, **102**, 335–339

BOWMAN, C. A., LINTHICUM, F. H., NELSON, R. A., NIKAMI, K. and QUISMORIO, F. (1986) Sensorineural hearing loss associated with systemic lupus erythematosus. *Otolaryngology – Head and Neck Surgery*, **941**, 197–204

BRAMA, I. and FAINARU, M. (1980) Inner ear involvement in Behçets disease. *Archives of Otolaryngology*, **106**, 215–217

BREDA, S. D., HAMMERSCHLAG, P. E., GIGLIOTTI, F. and SCHINELLA, R. (1988) *Pneumocystis carinii* in the temporal bone as a primary manifestation of the acquired immunodeficiency syndrome. *Annals of Otology, Rhinology and Laryngology*, **97**, 427–431

BRIDGER, M. W. M. and GRAHAM, J. M. (1985) The influence of raised body temperature on auditory evoked brainstem responses. *Clinical Otolaryngology*, **10**, 195–199

BRODIE, H. A., CHOLE, R. A., GRIFFIN, G. C. and WHITE, J. G. (1992) Macrothrombocytopenia and progressive deafness: a new genetic syndrome. *American Journal of Otology*, **13**, 507–511

BROOKES, G. B. and NEWLAND, A. C. (1986) Plasma exchange in the treatment of immune complex-associated sensorineural deafness. *Journal of Laryngology and Otology*, **100**, 25–33

BROWNING, G. G., GATEHOUSE, S. and LOWE, G. D. O. (1986) Blood viscosity as a factor in sensorineural hearing impairment. *Lancet*, i, 121–123

BROWNSON, R. J., ZOLLINGER, W. K., MADEIRA, T. and FELL, D. (1986) Sudden sensorineural hearing loss following manipulation of the cervical spine. *Laryngoscope*, **96**, 166–170

BRUYN, G. W. (1988) Vertigo and vertebrobasilar insufficiency. *Acta Otolaryngologica* Supplement, 460, 128–134

BYL, F. M. (1984) Sudden hearing loss: eight years experience and suggested prognostic table. *Laryngoscope*, **94**, 647–661

CALDARELLI, D. D., REJOWSKI, J. E. and COREY, J. P. (1986) Sensorineural hearing loss in lupus erythematosus. *American Journal of Otology*, **7**, 210–213

CARMEN, R. E., SVIHOVEC, D., GOCKA, E. F., ERMSHAR, C. B., GAY, G. C., VANORE, J. F. *et al.* (1988) Audiometric configuration as a reflection of diabetes. *American Journal of Otology*, **9**, 327–333

CARMEN, R. E., SVIHOVEC, D. A., GOCKA, E. F., GAY, G. C. and HOUSE, L. R. (1989) Audiometric configuration as a reflection of low plasma glucose and diabetes. *American Journal of Otology*, **10**, 372–379

CHANDRASEKHAR, S. S., SIVERLS, V. and SEKHAR, H. K. (1992) Histopathologic and ultrastructural changes in the temporal bones of HIV-infected human adults. *American Journal of Otology*, **13**, 207–214

CHIAPPA, K. H., HARRISON, J. L., BROOKS, E. B. and YOUNG, R. R. (1980) Brainstem auditory evoked responses in 200 patients with multiple sclerosis. *Annals of Neurology*, **7**, 135–143

CHOW, J. M. and GARCIA, J. (1985) Acoustic neuroma presenting as sudden hearing loss. *American Journal of Otolaryngology*, **6**, 115–119

CHOWDHURY, C. R., HO, J. H. C., WRIGHT, A., TSAO, S. Y., AU, G. K. H. and TUNG, Y. (1988) Prospective study of the effects of ventilation tubes on hearing after radiotherapy for carcinoma of nasopharynx. *Annals of Otology, Rhinology and Laryngology*, **97**, 142–148

CIPPARRONE, L., FRATIGLIONI, L., SIRACUSA, G., AMATO, M. P., AMADUCCI, L., PAGNINI, P. *et al.* (1989) Electronystagmography in the diagnosis of multiple sclerosis. *Acta Neurologica Scandinavica*, **80**, 193–200

CITELLI, S. (1926) Surdité rapide par simple congestion cochleaire. *Oto-Rhino-Laryngologie Internationale*, **10**, 321–323

CIUFFETTI, G., SCARDAZZA, A., SERAFINI, G., LOMBARDINI, R., MANNARINO, E. and SIMONCELLI, C. (1991) Whole-blood filterability in sudden deafness. *Laryngoscope*, **101**, 65–67

CIVANTOS, F., CHOI, Y. S. and APPLEBAUM, E. L. (1992) Meningeal carcinomatosis producing bilateral sudden hearing loss: a case report. *American Journal of Otology*, **13**, 369–371

CLARE, N. M., MONTIEL, M. M., LIFSCHITZ, M. D. and BANNAYAN, G. A. (1979) Alport's syndrome associated with macrothrombopathic thrombocytopenia. *American Journal of Clinical Pathology*, **72**, 111–117

CLEMENTS, M. R., MISTRY, C. D., KEITH, A. O. and RAMSDEN, R. T. (1989) Recovery from sensorineural deafness in Wegener's granulomatosis. *Journal of Laryngology and Otology*, **103**, 515–518

CLEMIS, J. D., MASTRICOLA, P. G. and SCHULER-VOGLER, M. (1982) Sudden hearing loss in the contralateral ear in postoperative acoustic tumor: three case reports. *Laryngoscope*, **92**, 76–79

CLERICO, D. M., JAHN, A. F. and FONTANELLA, S. (1994) Osteoma of the internal auditory canal: case report and literature review. *Annals of Otology, Rhinology and Laryngology*, **103**, 619–623

COCHRAN, J. H. and KOSMICKI, P. W. (1979) Tinnitus as a presenting symptom in pernicious anemia. *Annals of Otology, Rhinology and Laryngology*, **88**, 297

COHEN, A., MARTIN, M., MIZANIN, J., KONKLE, D. F. and SCHWARTZ, E. (1980) Vision and hearing during deferoxamine therapy. *Journal of Pediatrics*, **117**, 326–330

COLEMAN, J. K. M., DENGERINK, H. A. and WRIGHT, J. W. (1991) Effects of hydroxyethyl starch, nimodipine, and propylene glycol on cochlear blood flow. *Otolaryngology – Head and Neck Surgery*, **105**, 840–844

COTE, D. N., MOLONY, T. B., WAXMAN, J. and PARSA, D. (1993) Cogan's syndrome manifesting as sudden bilateral deafness: diagnosis and management. *Southern Medical Journal*, **86**, 1056–1060

CRAWFORD, M. R., GOULD, H. J., SMITH, W. R., BECKFORD, N., GIBSON, W. R. and BOBO, L. (1991) Prevalence of hearing loss in adults with sickle cell disease. *Ear and Hearing*, **12**, 349–351

CRISTOVAO, C., ATHERINO, T., MATTOS, J. P. and ATHERINO, T. (1985) Cochleo-vestibular findings in the familial lateral amytrophic sclerosis (van Laere's disease). In: *New Dimen-*

sions in *Otorhinolaryngology – Head and Neck Surgery*, vol. 2, edited by E. Myers. Amsterdam: Excerpta Medica. pp. 239–240

CULLEN, J. F. and COLEIRO, J. A. (1976) Ophthalmic complications of giant cell arteritis. *Survey of Ophthalmology*, **20**, 247–260

CUMMINS, D., MCCORMICK, J. B., BENNETT, D., SAMBA, J. A., FARRER, B., MACHIN, S. J. *et al.* (1990) Acute sensorineural deafness in Lassa fever. *Journal of the American Medical Association*, **264**, 2093–2096

CURÉ, J. K., CROMWELL, L. D., CASE, J. L., JOHNSON, G. D. and MUSIEK, F. E. (1990) Auditory dysfunction caused by multiple sclerosis: detection with MR imaging. *American Journal of NeuroRadiology*, **11**, 817–820

CURTIN, S. M. and PENNINGTON, T. H. (1995) The diagnosis of Lyme disease. *Journal of the Royal Society of Medicine*, **88**, 248–250

CUSHING, H. W. (1917) *Tumors of the Nervus Acusticus and the Syndrome of the Cerebellopontile Angle*. Philadelphia: W. B. Saunders

DAMIANI, J. M. and LEVINE, H. L. (1979) Relapsing polychondritis – report of ten cases. *Laryngoscope*, **89**, 929–946

DANINO, J., JOACHIMS, H. Z., ELIACHAR, I., PODOSHIN, L., BEN-DAVID, Y. and FRADIS, M. (1984) Tinnitus as a presenting factor in sudden deafness. *American Journal of Otolaryngology*, **5**, 394–396

DAROUGAR, S., JOHN, A. C., VISWALINGAM, M., CORNELL, L. and JONES, B. R. (1978) Isolation of *Chlamydia psittaci* from a patient with interstitial keratitis associated with otological and cardiovascular lesions. *British Journal of Ophthalmology*, **62**, 709–714

DAVIES, E., KNOX E. and DONALDSON, I. (1994) The usefulness of nimodipine, an L-calcium channel antagonist, in the treatment of tinnitus. *British Journal of Audiology*, **28**, 125–129

DAVIS, E. C. and NILO, E. R. (1965) Hearing improvement induced by phlebotomy in polycythemia. *Laryngoscope*, **75**, 1847–1852

DAVIS, I., MOORE, J. R. M. and LAHIRI, S. K. (1979) Nitrous oxide and the middle ear. *Anaesthesia*, **34**, 147–151

D'CRUZ, D. P., BAGULEY, E., ASHERSON, R. A. and HUGHES, G. R. V. (1989) Ear, nose and throat symptoms in subacute Wegener's granulomatosis. *British Medical Journal*, **299**, 419–422

DEKKER, P. J. (1993) Wegener's granulomatosis: otological aspects. *Journal of Otolaryngology*, **22**, 364–367

DE KLEYN, A. (1945) Sudden complete or partial loss of function of the octavus-system in apparently normal persons. *Acta Otolaryngologica*, **32**, 407–429

DE REMEE, R. A., MCDONALD, T. J., HARRISON, E. G. and COLES, D. T. (1976) Wegener's granulomatosis. Anatomic correlates, a proposed classification. *Mayo Clinic Proceedings*, **51**, 777–781

DESLOOVERE, C. (1989) Sudden deafness therapy: hydroxyethylstarch-pentoxifylline versus normal saline in a double-blind study. In: *Sensorineural Hearing Loss and Equilibrium Disturbances*, edited by J. Helms. Stuttgart: Georg Thieme Verlag. pp. 41–43

DESLOOVERE, C., LÖRZ, M. and KLIMA, A. (1989) Sudden sensorineural hearing loss, influence of hemodynamical and hemorheological factors on spontaneous recovery and therapy results. *Acta Otorhinolaryngologica Belgica*, **43**, 31–37

DESLOOVERE, C., EHRLY, A. M., LÖRZ, M. and BETTINGER, R. (1991) Importance of plasma and blood viscosity in diag-

nosis and treatment of idiopathic sudden sensorineural hearing loss. *Otorhinolaryngologic Nova*, **1**, 210–215

DICKENS, J. R. E. and GRAHAM, S. S. (1993) Neurotologic presentation of sagittal sinus thromboses associated with oral contraceptive usage. *American Journal of Otology*, **14**, 544–547

DJUPESLAND, G., FLOTTORP, G. and REFSUM, S. (1983) Phytanic acid storage disease: hearing maintained after 15 years of dietary treatment. *Neurology*, **33**, 237–240

DONALDSON, J. A. (1979) Heparin therapy for sudden sensorineural hearing loss. *Archives of Otolaryngology*, **105**, 351–352

DORNHOFFER, J. L. and ARENBERG, I. K. (1993) Diagnosis of vestibular Meniere's disease with electrocochleography. *American Journal of Otology*, **14**, 161–164

DOWNIE, A. C., HOWLETT, D. C., KOEFMAN, R. J., BANERJEE, A. K. and TONGE, K. A. (1994) Prolonged contrast enhancement of the inner ear on magnetic resonance imaging in Ramsay Hunt syndrome. *British Journal of Radiology*, **67**, 819–821

DRETTNER, B., HEDSTRAND, H., KLOCKHOFF, I. and SVEDBERG, A. (1975) Cardiovascular risk factors and hearing loss. *Acta Otolaryngologica*, **79**, 366–371

DRULOVIĆ, B., RIBARIĆ-JANKES, K., KOSTIĆ, V. S. and STERNIĆ, N. (1993) Sudden hearing loss as the initial monosymptom of multiple sclerosis. *Neurology*, **43**, 2703–2705

DRULOVIĆ, B., RIBARIĆ-JANKES, K., KOSTIĆ, V. and STERNIĆ, N. (1994) Multiple sclerosis as the cause of sudden 'pontine' deafness. *Audiology*, **33**, 195–201

DUVALL, A. J., NELMS, C. R. and WILLIAMS, H. L. (1969) Necrotizing granuloma of the midline tissues following renal transplantation. *Transactions of American Academy of Ophthalmology and Otology*, **73**, 1187–1207

EARNEST, M. P., MONROE, M. A. and YARNELL, M. D. (1977) Cortical deafness: demonstration of the pathologic anatomy by CT scan. *Neurology*, **27**, 1172–1175

EDWARDS, C. H. and PATERSON, J. H. (1951) Review of symptoms and signs of acoustic neurofibromata. *Brain*, **74**, 144–190

EINER, H., TENGBORN, L., AXELSSON, A. and EDSTRÖM, S. (1994) Sudden sensorineural hearing loss and hemostatic mechanisms. *Archives of Otolaryngology – Head and Neck Surgery*, **120**, 536–540

ELIDAN, J., MICHEL, J., GAY, I. and SPRINGER, H. (1985) Ear involvement in human brucellosis. *Journal of Laryngology and Otology*, **99**, 289–291

ELL, J., PRASHER, D. and RUDGE, P. (1984) Neuro-otological abnormalities in Friedrich's ataxia. *Journal of Neurology, Neurosurgery and Psychiatry*, **47**, 26–32

EMMETT, J. R. (1994) Simultaneous idiopathic sudden sensorineural hearing loss in identical twins. *American Journal of Otology*, **15**, 247–249

EMMETT, J. R. and SHEA, J. J. (1979) Diatrozoate meglumine (Hypaque) treatment for sudden hearing loss. *Laryngoscope*, **89**, 1229–1238

ENGERVALL, K., CARLSSON-NORLANDER, B. and BREDBURG, G. (1990) Central nervous system involvement in patients with facial palsy due to borrelial infection. *Clinical Otolaryngology*, **15**, 537–544

ESCAJADILLO, J. R., ALATORRE, G. and ZARATE, A. (1982) Typhoid fever and cochleovestibular lesions. *Annals of Otology, Rhinology and Laryngology*, **91**, 220–224

ESCOUBET, B., AMSALLEM, P., FERRARY, E. and TRAN BA HUY, P. (1985) Prostaglandin synthesis by the cochlea of the guinea pig. Influence of aspirin, gentamicin and acoustic stimulation. *Prostaglandins*, 29, 589–599

EVANS, R. A., LIU, K. C., AZHAR, T. and SYMONDS, R. P. (1988) Assessment of permanent hearing improvement following radical megavoltage radiotherapy. *Journal of Laryngology and Otology*, 102, 588–589

FARRELL, R. W. R., PEMBERTON, M. N., PARKER, A. J. and BUFFIN, J. T. (1991) Sudden deafness after dental surgery. *British Medical Journal*, 303, 1034 (see also p. 1270)

FEHER, M. D., STEVENS, J., LANT, A. F. and MAYNE, P. D. (1992) Importance of routine measurement of HDL with total cholesterol in diabetic patients. *Journal of the Royal Society of Medicine*, 85, 8–11

FELDMAN, H. (1981) Sudden loss of cochlear and vestibular function. *Advances in Oto-Rhino-Laryngology*, 27, 40–69

FERGUSON, I. T., RAMSDEN, R. T. and LYTHGOE, M. (1985) Brain stem auditory evoked potentials and blink reflexes in multiple sclerosis. *Journal of Laryngology and Otology*, 99, 677–683

FISCH, U. (1983) Management of sudden deafness. *Otolaryngology – Head and Neck Surgery*, 91, 3–8

FISCH, U., DOBOZI, M. and GREIG, D. (1972) Degenerative changes of the arterial vessels of the internal auditory meatus during the process of aging. *Acta Otolaryngologica*, 73, 259–262

FISCH, U., NAGAHARA, K. and POLLACK, A. (1984) Sudden hearing loss: circulatory. *American Journal of Otology*, 5, 488–491

FISCHER, C., MAUGUIERE, F., IBANEZ, V., CONFAVREUX, C. and CHAZOT, G. (1985) The acute deafness of definite multiple sclerosis: BAEP patterns. *Electroencephalography and Clinical Neurophysiology*, 61, 7–15

FOG, J., WANG, L. P., SUNDBERG, A. and MUCCHIANO, C. (1990) Hearing loss after spinal anesthesia is related to needle size. *Anesthesia and Analgesia*, 70, 517–522

FRADIS, M., PODOSHIN, L., BEN-DAVID, J., STATTER, P., PRATT, H. and NAHIR, M. (1989) Brainstem auditory evoked potentials with increased stimulus rate in patients suffering from systemic lupus erythematosus. *Laryngoscope*, 99, 325–329

FRAMPTON, G., JAYNE, D. R. W., PERRY, G. J., LOCKWOOD, C. M. and CAMERON, J. S. (1990) Autoantibodies to endothelial cells and neutrophil cytoplasmic antigens in systemic vasculitis. *Clinical and Experimental Allergy*, 82, 227–232

FRANCIS, D. A. and BODDIE, H. G. (1982) Acute hearing loss in giant cell arteritis. *Postgraduate Medical Journal*, 58, 357–358

FRANCOIS, M., BENFILS, P., LEGER, J., AVAN, P., CZERNICHOW, P. and NARCY, P. (1993) Audiological assessment of eleven congenital hypothyroid infants before and after treatment. *Acta Otolaryngologica*, 113, 39–42

FRANKLIN, D. J., COKER, N. J. and JENKINS, H. A. (1989) Sudden sensorineural hearing loss as a presentation of multiple sclerosis. *Archives of Otolaryngology*, 115, 41–45

FRIEDMAN, I., FROHLICH, A. and WRIGHT, A. (1993) Epidemic typhus fever and hearing loss: a histological study. *Journal of Laryngology and Otology*, 107, 275–283

FRIEDMAN, S. A. and SCHULMAN, R. H. (1975) Hearing and diabetic neuropathy. *Archives of Internal Medecine*, 135, 573–576

FUKAYA, T., NOMURA, Y. and FUKUSHIMA, T. (1991) Transient retrocochlear low-frequency sensorineural hearing loss: a new clinical entity. *Laryngoscope*, 101, 643–647

FURMAN, J. M. R., DURRANT, J. D. and HIRSCH, W. L. (1989)

Eighth nerve signs in a case of multiple sclerosis. *American Journal of Otolaryngology*, 10, 376–381

FUSE, T. (1991) ABR findings in vertebrobasilar ischemia. *Acta Otolaryngologica*, 111, 485–490

GABRIELE, P., ORECCHIA, R., MAGNANO, M., ALBERA, R. and SANNAZZARI, G. L. (1992) Vestibular apparatus disorders after external radiation therapy for head and neck cancers. *Radiotherapy and Oncology*, 25, 25–30

GALVEZ, E. M., MESEGUER, D. H., ORTEGA, F. G. and MONDEJAR, J. M. (1994) Sudden deafness and cerebellar tumour. *Journal of Laryngology and Otology*, 108, 584–586

GATEHOUSE, S., GALLACHER, J. E. J., LOWE, G. D. O., YARNELL, J. W. G., HUTTON, R. D. and ISING, I. (1989) Blood viscosity and hearing levels in the Caerphilly collaborative heart disease study. *Archives of Otolaryngology*, 115, 1227–1230

GATEHOUSE, S. and LOWE, G. D. O. (1991) Whole blood viscosity and red cell filterability as factors in sensorineural hearing impairment in the elderly. *Acta Otolaryngologica*, Supplement 476, 37–43

GATES, G. A., COBB, J. L., D'AGOSTINO, R. B. and WOLF, P. A. (1993) The relation of hearing in the elderly to the presence of cardiovascular disease and cardiovascular risk factors. *Archives of Otolaryngology – Head and Neck Surgery*, 119, 156–161

GATLAND, D., TUCKER, B., CHALSTREY, S., KEENE, M. and BAKER, L. (1991) Hearing loss in chronic renal failure – hearing threshold changes following haemodialysis. *Journal of the Royal Society of Medicine*, 84, 587–589

GEMIGNANI, G., BERRETTINI, S., BRUSCHINI, P., SELLARI-FRANCESCHINI, S., FUSARI, P., PIRAGINE, F. *et al.* (1991) Hearing and vestibular disturbances in Behçet's syndrome. *Annals of Otology, Rhinology and Laryngology*, 100, 459–463

GHOSH, P. (1990) Central diplacusis. *European Archives of Otorhinolaryngology*, 247, 48–50

GIBBIN, K. P. and DAVIS, C. G. (1981) A hearing survey in diabetes mellitus. *Clinical Otolaryngology*, 6, 345–350

GIGER, H. L. (1979) Hörsturztherapie mit oxycarboninhalation. *HNO*, 27, 107–109

GILBERT, J. A., POLLACK, E. S. and POLLACK, C. V. (1994) Vogt-Koyanagi-Harada syndrome: case report and review. *Journal of Emergency Medicine*, 12, 615–619

GLEESON, M. J. (1984) Alport's syndrome: audiological manifestations and implications. *Journal of Laryngology and Otology*, 98, 449–465

GONZALES, G., ISTRE, C. and RUBIN, W. (1968) Labyrinthine catastrophe: is it the pill? *Journal of the Louisiana State Medical Society*, 120, 487–494

GORDON, M. A., SILVERSTEIN, H., WILCOX, T. O. and ROSENBERG, S. I. (1995) Lightning injury of the tympanic membrane. *American Journal of Otology*, 16, 373–376

GOULD, H. J., CRAWFORD, M. R., SMITH, W. R., BECKFORD, N., GIBSON, W. R., PETTIT, L. *et al.* (1991) Hearing disorders in sickle cell disease: cochlear and retrocochlear findings. *Ear and Hearing*, 12, 352–354

GRAHAM, J. M. and HAZELL, J. W. P. (1977) Electrical stimulation of the human cochlea using a transtympanic electrode. *British Journal of Audiology*, 11, 59–62

GRAHAM, J. M., GREENWOOD, R. and LECKY, B. (1980) Cortical deafness: a case report and review of the literature. *Journal of Neurological Sciences*, 48, 35–49

GRAHAM, J. M., RAMSDEN, R. T., MOFFAT, D. A. and GIBSON, W. P. R. (1978) Sudden sensorineural hearing loss: electrocochleographic findings in 70 patients. *Journal of Laryngology and Otology*, 92, 581–589

GRANDIS, J. R., HIRSCH, B. E. and WAGENER, M. M. (1993)

Treatment of idiopathic sudden sensorineural hearing loss. *American Journal of Otology*, **14**, 183–185

GRAU, C., MØLLER, K., OVERGAARD, M., OVERGAARD, J. and ELBROND, O. (1991) Sensori-neural hearing loss in patients treated with irradiation for nasopharyngeal carcinoma. *International Journal of Radiation, Oncology, Biology and Physics*, **21**, 723–728

GREGG, J. B. and SCHAEFFER, J. H. (1964) Unilateral inner ear deafness complicating infectious mononucleosis. *South Dakota Journal of Medicine*, **17**, 22–23

GRIMALDI, L. M., LUZI, L., MARTINO, G. V., FURLAN, R., NEMNI, R., ANTONELLI, A. *et al.* (1993) Bilateral eighth cranial nerve neuropathy in human immunodeficiency virus infection. *Journal of Neurology*, **240**, 363–366

GROTEMEYER, K-H. (1990) Abnormal hemorheological parameters in vertebrobasilar-insufficiency. *Acta Neurologica Scandinavica*, **81**, 529–532

GSTOETTNER, W., SWOBODA, H., MÜLLER, C. and BURIAN, M. (1993) Preclinical detection of initial vestibulocochlear abnormalities with multiple sclerosis. *European Archives of Otorhinolaryngology*, **250**, 40–43

GUBLER, M., LEVY, M., BROYER, M., NAIZOT, C., GONZALES, G., PERRIN, D. *et al.* (1981) Alport's syndrome: a report of 58 cases and review of the literature. *American Journal of Medicine*, **70**, 493–505

GUSSEN, R. (1976) Sudden deafness of vascular origin. A human temporal bone study. *Annals of Otology, Rhinology and Laryngology*, **85**, 94–100

GUSSEN, R. (1981) Sudden hearing loss associated with cochlear membrane rupture. *Archives of Otolaryngology*, **107**, 598–600

GUSSEN, R. (1983) Sudden deafness associated with bilateral Reissner's membrane ruptures. *American Journal of Otolaryngology*, **4**, 27–32

HALL, P. J. and FARRIOR, J. B. (1993) Aspergillus mastoiditis. *Otolaryngology – Head and Neck Surgery*, **108**, 167–170

HALL, R. and RICHARDS, H. (1987) Hearing loss due to mumps. *Archives of Diseases in Childhood*, **62**, 189–191

HALL, S., PERSELLIN, S., LIE, J. L., O'BRIEN, P. C., KURLAND, L. T. and HUNDER, G. G. (1983) The therapeutic impact of temporal artery biopsy. *Lancet*, ii, 1217–1220

HALL, S. J., MCGUIGAN, J. A. and ROCKS, M. J. (1991) Red blood cell deformability in sudden sensorineural deafness: another aetiology? *Clinical Otolaryngology*, **16**, 3–7

HALL, S. J., KERR, A. G., VARGHESE, M., PATTERSON, C. C. and MILLIKEN, T. G. (1985) Deafness in hypothyroidism. *Clinical Otolaryngology*, **10**, 292

HALLBERG, O. E. (1956) Sudden deafness of obscure origin. *Laryngoscope*, **66**, 1237–1267

HALLBERG, O. E., UIHLEIN, A. and SIEKERT, R. G. (1959) Sudden deafness due to cerebellopontine-angle tumor. *Archives of Otolaryngology*, **69**, 160–162

HANNA, G. S. (1986) Sudden deafness and the contraceptive pill. *Journal of Laryngology and Otology*, **100**, 701–706

HANNER, P., ROSENHALL, U., EDSTRÖM, S. and KAIJSER, B. (1989) Hearing impairment in patients with antibody production against *Borrelia burgdorferi* antigen. *Lancet*, i, 13–15

HANSEN, C. C. (1968) Perceptive hearing loss and arterial hypertension. *Archives of Otolaryngology*, **87**, 119–122

HARADA, T., SANDO, I., STOOL, S. E. and MYERS, E. N. (1980) Temporal bone histopathological features in Fanconi's anemia syndrome. *Archives of Otolaryngology*, **106**, 275–279

HARADA, T., SEMBA, T., SUZUKI, M., KIKUCHI, S. and MUROFUSHI, T. (1988) Audiological characteristics of hearing loss following meningitis. *Acta Otolaryngologica*, Supplement, **456**, 61–67

HARADA, Y. (1926) Beitrage zur klinischen Kenntniss von nichteitriger Choroiditis. *Acta Societatis Ophthalmologicae Japonicae*, **30**, 356–361

HARDY, P. A. J. (1988) Influence of spinal puncture and injection on VIIIth nerve function. *Journal of Laryngology and Otology*, **102**, 452

HARIRI, M. A. (1990) Sensorineural hearing loss in bullous myringitis. A prospective study of eighteen patients. *Clinical Otolaryngology*, **15**, 351–353

HART, C. W., COKELY, C. G., SCHUPBACH, J., DAL CANTO, M. C. and COPPLESON, L. W. (1989) Neurotologic findings of a patient with acquired immune deficiency syndrome. *Ear and Hearing*, **10**, 68–76

HATCH, M., TSAI, M., LA ROUERE, M. J., NUTTALL, A. L. and MILLER, J. M. (1991) The effects of carbogen, carbon dioxide, and oxygen on noise-induced hearing loss. *Hearing Research*, **56**, 265–272

HATTORI, T., NIWA, H. and YANAGITA, N. (1992) Transiently evoked otoacoustic emissions in ears with tinnitus after the recovery of acute hearing loss. *Auris, Nasus, Larynx (Tokyo)*, Supplement i, 575–580

HAYNES, B. F., KAISER-KUPFER, M. I., MASON, P. and FAUCI, A. S. (1980) Cogan syndrome: studies in thirteen patients, long-term follow-up, and a review of the literature. *Medicine*, **59**, 426–441

HAYNES, B. F., PIKUS, A., KAISER-KUPFER, M. and FAUCI, A. S. (1981) Successful treatment of sudden hearing loss in Cogan's syndrome with corticosteroids. *Arthritis and Rheumatism*, **24**, 501–503

HEBERT, R., LAUREAU, E., VANASSE, M., RICHARD, J. E., MORISSETTE, J., GLORIEUX, J. *et al.* (1986) Auditory brainstem response audiometry in congenitally hypothyroid children under early replacement therapy. *Paediatric Research*, **201**, 570–573

HENDLER, T., SQUIRES, N. K. and EMMERICH, D. S. (1990) Psychophysical measures of central auditory dysfunction in multiple sclerosis: neurophysiological and neuroanatomical correlates. *Ear and Hearing*, **11**, 403–416

HENSON, R. A. and URICH, H. (1982) Carcinomatous meningitis. In: *Cancer and the Nervous System*, ch. 4 Oxford: Blackwell Scientific Publications. pp. 100–119

HIGGS, W. A. (1973) Sudden deafness as the presenting symptom of acoustic neurinoma. *Archives of Otolaryngology*, **103**, 539–542

HIMELFARB, M. Z., LAKRETZ, T., GOLD, S. and SHANON, E. (1981) Auditory brain stem responses in thyroid dysfunction. *Journal of Laryngology and Otology*, **95**, 679–686

HINZ, M. and VON WEDEL, H. (1984) Otoakustiche emissionen bei patientien mit Hörsturz. *Archives of Otorhinolaryngology*, Supplement 11, 128–130

HIRAIDE, F., KAKOI, H., MIYOSHI, S. and MORITA, M. (1988) Acute profound deafness in Ramsay Hunt syndrome. Two case reports. *Acta Otolaryngologica*, Supplement 456, 49–54

HIRSCHBERG, M. and HOFFERBERTH, B. (1988) Calcium antagonists in an animal model of vertebrobasilar insufficiency. *Acta Otolaryngolohica*, Supplement 460, 61–65

HISASHI, K., KOMUNE, S., TAIRA, T., UEMURA, T., SADOSHIMA, S. and TSUDA, H. (1993) Anticardiolipin antibody-induced sudden profound sensorineural hearing loss. *American Journal of Otolaryngology*, **14**, 275–282

HO, K. J., KILENY, P., PACCIORETTI, D. and MCLEAN, D. R. (1987) Neurologic, audiologic and electrophysiologic sequelae of bilateral temporal lobe lesions. *Archives of Neurology*, **44**, 982–987

HOCHERMANN, M. and REIMER, A. (1987) Hearing loss after general anaesthesia. A case report and review of the literature. *Journal of Laryngology and Otology*, **101**, 1079–1082

HOFFERBERTH, B. and HIRSCHBERG, M. (1988) Treatment of vertebrobasilar insufficiency. *Acta Otolaryngologica*, Supplement 460, 154–159

HOFFMAN, R. A. and SHEPSMAN, D. A. (1983) Bullous myringitis and sudden hearing loss. *Laryngoscope*, **93**, 1544–1545

HOHMANN, D., LOHMANN, T. and HIRSCHBERG, M. (1988) Treatment of vertebrobasilar insufficiency. *Acta Otolaryngologica*, Suppl. 460, 154–159

HOHMANN, D., LOHMANN, T. and SCHWAGER, K. (1993) Effect of myelography on the curve of the auditory evoked early brain stem potentials. *Laryngorhinootologie*, **72**, 231–235

HOLLANDERS, D. (1986) Sensorineural deafness – a new complication of ulcerative colitis. *Postgraduate Medical Journal*, **62**, 753–755

HOPF, H. C. and MAURER, K. (1983) Wave I of early auditory evoked potentials in multiple sclerosis. *Electroencephalography and Clinical Neurophysiology*, **56**, 31–37

HOSHINO, T., ISHII, T., KODAMA, A. and KATO, I. (1980) Temporal bone finding in a case of sudden deafness and relapsing polychondritis. *Acta Otolaryngologica*, **90**, 257–261

HOSHINO, T., KATO, I., KODAMA, A. and SUZUKI, H. (1978) Sudden deafness in relapsing polychondritis. A scanning electron microscopy study. *Acta Oto-Laryngologica*, **86**, 418–427

HOTH, S. and BÖNNHOFF, S. (1992) Therapy induced changes in inner ear function as measured by oto-acoustic emissions. *European Archives of Otorhinolaryngology*, **249**, 411

HOUCK, J. R. and MURPHY, K. (1992) Sudden bilateral profound hearing loss resulting from meningeal carcinomatosis. *Otolaryngology – Head and Neck Surgery*, **106**, 92–97

HUANG, M. H., HUANG, C. C., RYU, S. J. and CHU, N. S. (1993) Sudden bilateral hearing impairment in vertebrobasilar occlusive disease. *Stroke*, **24**, 132–137

HUANG, T-S., CHAN, S-T., HO, T-L., SU, J-L. and LEE, F-P. (1989) Hypaque and steroids in the treatment of sudden sensorineural hearing loss. *Clinical Otolaryngology*, **14**, 45–51

HUGHES, G. B., KINNEY, S. E., BARNA, B. P., TOMSAK, R. L. and CALABRESE, L. H. (1981) Autoimmune reactivity in Cogan's syndrome: a preliminary report. *Otolaryngology – Head and Neck Surgery*, **91**, 24–32

HULBERT, T. V., LARSEN, R. A., DAVIS, C. L. and HOLTOM, P. D. (1991) Bilateral hearing loss after measles and rubella vaccination in an adult. *New England Journal of Medicine*, **325**, 134

HULTCRANTZ, E. and NUTTALL, A. L. (1987) Effect of hemodilution on cochlear blood flow measured by laser-doppler flowmetry. *American Journal of Otolaryngology*, **8**, 16–22

HUTCHINSON, J. (1889–1890) Diseases of the arteries. No. 1 On a peculiar form of thrombotic arteritis of the aged which is sometimes productive of gangrene. *Archives of Surgery*, **1**, 323–329

HUTCHINSON, J. C. and KLODD, D. A. (1982) Electrophysiological analysis of auditory function, vestibular and brain stem function in chronic renal failure. *Laryngoscope*, **92**, 833–843

IKEDA, K. and MORIZONO, T. (1989) Effects of carbon dioxide in the middle ear cavity upon the cochlear potentials and cochlear pH. *Acta Otolaryngologica*, **108**, 88–93

IKEDA, K., KUSAKARI, J., KOBAYASHI, T., INAMURA, N., SHIBUYA, M., TAKEYAMA, M. *et al.* (1987) Pathophysiology and prognosis of sudden deafness with special reference to the N1 latency. *ORL-Journal of Otorhinolaryngology and Related Specialties*, **49**, 234–241

ILLUM, P. and THORLING, K. (1982) Otologic manifestations of Wegener's granulomatosis. *Laryngoscope*, **92**, 801–804

INUI, H., MIYAHARA, H., NARIO, K. and MATSUNAGA, T. (1994) Autoradiographic measurement of regional brainstem blood flow: occlusion of the anterior inferior cerebellar artery. *European Archives of Otorhinolaryngology*, **251**, 233–237

JABBARI, B., MARSH, E. E. and GUNDERSON, C. H. (1982) The site of the lesion in acute deafness of multiple sclerosis – contribution of the brain stem auditory evoked potential test. *Clinical Electroencephalography*, **13**, 241–244

JABBARI, B., SCHWARTZ, D. M., MACNEIL, D. M. and COKER, S. B. (1983) Early abnormalities of brainstem auditory evoked potentials in Friedreich's ataxia: evidence of primary brainstem dysfunction. *Neurology*, **33**, 1071–1074

JACOB, A., LEDINGHAM, J. G., KERR, A. I. G. and FORD, M. J. (1990) Ulcerative colitis and giant cell arteritis associated with sensorineural deafness. *Journal of Laryngology and Otology*, **104**, 889–890

JAFFE, B. F. (1967) Sudden deafness: an otologic emergency. *Archives of Otolaryngology*, **86**, 55–60

JAGUST, W. J., EBERLING, J. L., RICHARDSON, B. S., REED, B. R., BAKER, M. G., NORDAHL, T. E. *et al.* (1993) The cortical topography of temporal lobe hypometabolism in early Alzheimer's disease. *Brain Research*, **629**, 189–198

JAHRSDOERFER, R. A., THOMPSON, E. G., JOHNS, M. M. E. and CANTRELL, R. W. (1981) Sarcoidosis and fluctuating hearing loss. *Annals of Otology, Rhinology and Laryngology*, **90**, 161–163

JASTREBOFF, P. J. and BRENNAN, J. F. (1988) Specific effect of nimodipine on the auditory system. *Annals of the New York Academy of Science*, **522**, 716–718

JERGER, J., LOVERING, L. and WERTZ, M. (1972) Auditory disorder following bilateral temporal lobe insult: report of a case. *Journal of Speech and Hearing Disorders*, **37**, 523–535

JERGER, J., WEIKERS, N. J., SHARBROUGH, F. W. and JERGER, S. (1969) Bilateral lesions of the temporal lobe: a case study. *Acta Otolaryngologica Supplementum*, **258**

JERGER, J. F., OLIVER, R. A., CHMIEL, R. A. and RIVERA, V. M. (1986) Patterns of auditory abnormality in multiple sclerosis. *Audiology*, **25**, 193–209

JOBST, K. A., SMITH, A. D., BARKER, C. S., WEAR, A., KING, E. M., SMITH, A. *et al.* (1992) Association of atrophy of the medial temporal lobe with reduced blood flow in the posterior parietotemporal cortex in patients with a clinical and pathological diagnosis of Alzheimer's disease. *Journal of Neurology, Neurosurgery and Psychiatry*, **55**, 190–194

JOBST, K. A., SMITH, A. D., SZATMARI, M., ESIRI, M. M., JASKOWSKI, A. HINDLEY, N. *et al.* (1994) Rapidly progressing atrophy of medial temporal lobe in Alzheimer's disease. *Lancet*, **343**, 829–830

JOHNS, D. R., TIERNEY, M. and FELSENSTEIN, D. (1987) Alteration in the natural history of neurosyphilis by concurrent infection with the human immunodeficiency virus. *New England Journal of Medicine*, **316**, 1569–1572

JOHNSON, A., HAWKE, M. and BERGER, G. (1984) Sudden deafness and vertigo due to inner ear hemorrhage – a temporal bone case report. *Journal of Otolaryngology*, **13**, 201–207

JOHNSON, D. W. and MATHOG, R. H. (1976) Hearing function and chronic renal failure. *Annals of Otology, Rhinology and Laryngology*, **85**, 43–49

JONES, D. T., OGREN, F. P., ROH, L. H. and MOORE, G. F. (1991) Lightning and its effect on the auditory system. *Laryngoscope*, **101**, 830–834

JONES, N. S. and DAVIS, A. (1992) Hyperlipidaemia and hearing loss: a true association? *Clinical Otolaryngology*, **17**, 463

JORDAN, B., NOWLIN, J., REMMERS, A., SARLES, H., FLYE, M. H. and FISH, J. (1984) Renal transplantation and hearing loss in Alport's syndrome. *Transplantation*, **38**, 308–309

JORDAO, A. M. D. (1857) Considération sur un cas du diabète. *Union médicale, Paris*, **11**, 446

JOURNEAUX, S. F., MASTER, B., GREENHALGH, R. M. and BULL, T. R. Sudden sensorineural hearing loss as a complication of non-otologic surgery. *Journal of Laryngology and Otology*, **104**, 711–712

KANDA, Y., SHIGENO, K., KINOSHITA, N., NAKAO, K., YANO, K. and MATSUO, H. (1994) Sudden hearing loss associated with interferon. *Lancet*, **343**, 1134–1135

KANO, K., TONO, T., USHISAKO, Y., MORIMITSU, T., SUZUKI, Y. and KADAMA, T. (1994) Magnetic resonance imaging in patients with sudden deafness. *Acta Otolaryngologica*, Supplement 514, 32–36

KANZAKI, J. and OGAWA, K. (1988) Internal auditory canal vascular loops and sensorineural hearing loss. *Acta Otolaryngologica*, Supplement 447, 88–93.

KANZAKI, T., O-UCHI, T. and TSUCHIHASHI, N. (1993) Steroid-responsive sensorineural hearing loss combination therapy with prednisolone and Sarei-to. *ORL – Journal of Otorhinolaryngology and Related Specialties*, **55**, 24–29

KAPOSI, M. (1874) Xeroderma parchment skin. In: *On Diseases of the Skin*, vol. 3, edited by F. von Hebra and M. Kaposi. London: New Sydenham Society. pp. 252–258

KARMODY, C. S. (1978) Wegener's granulomatosis: presentation as an otologic problem. *Transactions of the American Academy of Ophthalmology and Otology*, **86**, 573–584

KARMODY, C. S. and SCHUKNECHT, H. F. (1966) Deafness in congenital syphilis. *Archives of Otolaryngology*, **83**, 18–27

KARNI, A., SADEH, M., BLATT, I. and GOLDHAMMER, Y. (1991) Cogan's syndrome complicated by lacunar brain infarcts. *Journal of Neurology, Neurosurgery and Psychiatry*, **54**, 169–171

KATHOLM, M., JOHNSEN, N. J., SIIM, C. and WILLUMSEN, L. (1991) Bilateral sudden deafness and acute acquired toxoplasmosis. *Journal of Laryngology and Otology*, **105**, 115–118

KAWAKAMI, M., MAKIMOTO, K., NAKAJIMA, T. and TAKAHASHI, H. (1989) Observations of cochlear blood flow dynamics using the laser doppler flowmeter. *European Archives of Otorhinolaryngology*, **246**, 147–150

KAWAKAMI, M., MAKIMOTO, K., NOI, O. and TAKAHASHI, H. (1991a) Feasibility of pulse oxymetry to measure arterial O_2 saturation in studies on cochlear blood circulation. *Acta Otolaryngologica*, **111**, 908–916

KAWAKAMI, M., MAKIMOTO, K., NOI, O. and TAKAHASHI, H. (1991b) Relationship between cochlear blood flow and perilymphatic oxygen tension. *European Archives of Otorhinolaryngology*, **248**, 465–470

KAWAKAMI, M., MAKIMOTO, K., FUKUSE, S. and TAKAHASHI, H. (1991c) Effects of a depressor on cochlear blood flow and

perilymphatic oxygen tension. *Acta Otolaryngologica*, **111**, 743–749

KAWAKAMI, M., MAKIMOTO, K., FUKUSE, S. and TAKAHASHI, M. (1991d) Autoregulation of cochlear blood flow. *European Archives of Otorhinolaryngology*, **248**, 471–474

KAWAKAMI, M., MAKIMOTO, K., YAMAMOTO, H. and TAKAHASHI, H. (1992) The effect of batroxobin on cochlear blood flow. *Acta Otolaryngologica*, **112**, 991–997

KEAY, D. (1988) Total bilateral hearing loss as a complication of myeloma. *Journal of Laryngology and Otology*, **102**, 357–358

KEIM, R. J. and SACHS, G. B. (1975) Positional nystagmus in association with macroglobulinemia. *Annals of Otology, Rhinology and Laryngology*, **84**, 223–227

KELLERHALS, B. (1991) Progressive hearing loss after single exposure to acute acoustic trauma. *European Archives of Otorhinolaryngology*, **248**, 289–242

KEMPF, H-G. (1989) Ear involvement in Wegener's granulomatosis. *Clinical Otolaryngology*, **14**, 451–456

KENYON, G. S., BOOTH, J. B., PRASHER, D. K. and RUDGE, P. (1985) Neuro-otological abnormalities in xeroderma pigmentosum with particular reference to deafness. *Brain*, **108**, 771–784

KHETERPAL, U. (1991) Investigation into the cause of vertigo in sudden sensorineural hearing loss. *Otolaryngology – Head and Neck Surgery*, **105**, 360–371

KHETERPAL, U., NADOL, J. B. and GLYNN, R. J. (1990) Idiopathic sudden sensorineural hearing loss and post viral labyrinthitis: a statistical comparison of temporal bone findings. *Annals of Otology, Rhinology and Laryngology*, **99**, 969–976

KIDO, T., SEKITANI, T., OKINAKA, Y., TAHARA, T. and HARA, H. (1994) A case of cerebellar infarction occurred with the 8th cranial nerve symptoms. *Auris, Nasus, Larynx (Tokyo)*, **21**, 111–117

KIKUCHI, S., KAGA, K., YAMASOBA, T., HIGO, R., O'UCHI, T. and TOKUMARU, A. (1993) Slow blood flow of the vertebrobasilar system in patients with dizziness and vertigo. *Acta Otolaryngologica*, **113**, 257–260

KINMONT, P. D. C. and MCCALLUM, D. E. (1965) The aetiology, pathology and course of giant-cell arteritis. The possible role of light sensitivity. *British Journal of Dermatology*, **77**, 193–202

KINNEY, S. E. (1980) The metabolic evaluation in Ménière's disease. *Otolaryngology – Head and Neck Surgery*, **88**, 594–598

KIRIKAE, I., NOMURA, Y., SHITARA, T. and KOBAYASHI, T. (1962) Sudden deafness due to Buerger's disease. *Archives of Otolaryngology*, **75**, 502–505

KITAMURA, K. and BERREBY, M. (1983) Temporal bone histopathology associated with occlusion of vertebrobasilar arteries. *Annals of Otology, Rhinology and Laryngology*, **92**, 33–38

KLIGERMAN, A. B., SOLANGI, K. B., VENTRY, I. M., GOODMAN, A. I. and WESELEY, S. A. (1981) Hearing impairment associated with chronic renal failure. *Laryngoscope*, **91**, 583–591

KOBAYASHI, H., SUZUKI, A. and NOMURA, Y. (1994) Unilateral hearing loss following rubella infection in an adult. *Acta Otolaryngologica*, Supplement 514, 49–51

KOEPPEN, A. H. and DENTINGER, M. P. (1988) Brain hemosiderin and superficial siderosis of the central nervous system. *Journal of Neuropathology and Experimental Neurology*, **47**, 249–270

KOGA, K., KAWASHIRO, N., NAKAYAMA, T. and MAKINO, S.

(1988) Immunological study on association between mumps and infantile unilateral deafness. *Acta Otolaryngologica* Suppl. 456, 55–60

KOHAN, D., ROTHSTEIN, S. G. and COHEN, N. L. (1988) Otologic disease in patients with acquired immunodeficiency syndrome. *Annals of Otology, Rhinology and Laryngology*, 97, 636–640

KOIDE, J., YANAGITA, N., HONDO, R. and KURATA, T. (1988) Serological and clinical study of herpes simplex virus infection in patients with sudden deafness, *Acta Otolaryngologica*, Supplement 456, 21–26

KOSKAS, H. J., LINTHICUM, F. H. and HOUSE, W. F. (1983) Membranous ruptures in Menière's disease: existence, location and incidence. *Otolaryngology – Head and Neck Surgery*, 91, 61–67

KOYANAGI, Y. (1929) Dysakusis, Alopecia und Poliosis bei schwerer Uveitis nicht traumatischen Urspurngs. *Klinische Monatsblätter für Augenheilkunde*, 82, 194–211

KRONENEBERG, J., ALMAGOR, M., BENDET, E. and KUSHNIR, D. (1992) Vasoactive therapy verus placebo in the treatment of sudden hearing loss: a double-blind clinical study. *Laryngoscope*, 102, 65–68

KUBO, T., MATSUNAGA, T., ASAI, H., KAWAMOTO, K., KUSAKARI, J., NOMURA, Y. *et al.* (1988) Efficacy of defrinogenation and steroid therapies on sudden deafness. *Archives of Otolaryngology*, 114, 649–652

KUMAR, A., MAUDELONDE, C. and MAFEE, M. (1986) Unilateral sensorineural hearing loss: an analysis of 200 consecutive cases. *Laryngoscope*, 96, 14–18

KUO, M., DRAGO, P. C., PROOPS, D. W. and CHAVDA, S. V. (1995) Early diagnosis and treatment of Ramsay Hunt syndrome: the role of magnetic resonance imaging. *Journal of Laryngology and Otology*, 109, 777–780

KUSAKARI, J., INAMURA, N., SAKURAI, T. and KAWAMOTO, K. (1984) Effect of hypothermia upon electrocochleogram and auditory evoked brainstem response. *Tohuku Journal of Experimental Medicine*, 143, 351–359

KUSAKARI, J., HARA, A., TAKEYAMA, M., SUZUKI, S. and IGARI, T. (1992) The hearing of the patients treated with hemodialysis: a long term follow-up study. *Auris, Nasus, Larynx (Tokyo)*, 19, 105–113

LAI, M.-T., OHMICHI, T., YUEN, K., EGUSA, K. YORIZANE, S. and MASUDA, Y. (1995) Superficial siderosis of the central nervous system: a case with an unruptured intracranial aneurysm. *Journal of Laryngology and Otology*, 109, 549–552

LAKE-BAKAAR, G. and GIBBS, D. D. (1978) Polyarteritis nodosa presenting with bilateral nerve deafness. *Journal of the Royal Society of Medicine*, 71, 144–147

LALANNE, M. C., DOUTREMEPUICH, C., BOJ, F., TRAISSAC, L. and QUICHAUD, F. (1992) Some hemostatic and hemorrheological disorders in auditory and vestibular impairments. *Thrombosis Research*, 66, 787–791

LALWANI, A. K. and SOOY, C. D. (1992) Otologic and neurotologic manifestations of acquired immunodeficiency syndrome. *Otolaryngologic Clinics of North America*, 25, 1183–1197

LAROUERE, M. J., SILLMAN, J. S., TSAI, M. T. and NUTTALL, A. L. (1992) The effect of pentoxifylline on cochlear blood flow. *Otolaryngology – Head and Neck Surgery*, 106, 87–91

LARSEN, H. C., ANGELBORG, C. and HULTCRANTZ, E. (1982) The effect of glycerol on cochlear blood flow. *Oto-Rhino-Laryngology and its Borderlands*, 44, 101–107

LASKAWI, R., SCHRADER, B., SCHRODER, M., POSER, R. and VON-DER-BRELIE, R. (1987) Therapy of sudden deafness—

naftidrofuryl (Dusodril) and pentoxifylline (Trental) compared. *Laryngologie, Rhinologie, Otologie (Stuttgart)*, 661, 242–245

LASSEN, L. F., HIRSCH, B. E. and KAMERER, D. B. (1995) Use of nimodipine in the medical treatment of Meniere's disease: preliminary clinical experience. Presented to American Society of Neurootology (May 1995)

LAURIKAINEN, E. A., MILLER, J. M., QUIRK, W. S., KALLINEN, J., REN, T., NUTTALL, N. L. *et al.* (1993) Betahistine-induced vascular effects in the rat cochlea. *American Journal of Otology*, 14, 24–30

LEACH, W. (1965) Irradiation of the ear. *Journal of Laryngology and Otology*, 79, 870–880

LEE, C. M. and PEACHMAN, F. A. (1986) Unilateral hearing loss after spinal anesthesia treated with epidural blood patch. *Anesthesia and Analgesia*, 65, 312

LENARD, H. G., VOIT, T., LAMPRECHT, A., KAHN, T., NEUEN-JACOB, E. and RUITENBEEK, W. (1992) Sudden loss of hearing and vestibular function, muscular weakness, and multiple white matter lesions in preschool children. *Neuropediatrics*, 23, 221–224

LENARZ, T. (1989) Treatment of sudden deafness with the calcium antagonist nimodipine. Results of a comparative study. *Laryngorhinootologie*, 68, 634–637

LEUNG, S. F., KREEL, L. and TSAO, S. Y. (1992) Asymptomatic temporal lobe injury after radiotherapy for nasopharyngeal carcinoma: incidence and determinants. *British Journal of Radiology*, 65, 710–714

LIAO, B. S., BYL, F. M. and ADOUR, K. K. (1992) Audiometric comparison of Lassa fever hearing loss and idiopathic sudden hearing loss: evidence for a viral cause. *Otolaryngology – Head and Neck Surgery*, 106, 226–229

LINDSAY, J. R. and HEMENWAY, W. G. (1956) Postural vertigo due to unilateral sudden partial loss of vestibular function. *Annals of Otology, Rhinology and Laryngology*, 65, 692–706

LINSTROM, C. J., PINCUS, R. L., LEAUITT, E. B. and URBINA, M. C. (1993) Otologic neurotologic manifestations of HIV-related disease. *Otolaryngology – Head and Neck Surgery*, 108, 680–687

LONGRIDGE, N. S. (1976) Audiological assessment of deafness associated xeroderma pigmentosa. *Journal of Laryngology and Otology*, 90, 539–551

LOWRY, L. D. and ISAACSON, S. R. (1978) Study of 100 patients with bilateral sensorineural hearing loss for lipid abnormalities. *Annals of Otology, Rhinology and Laryngology*, 87, 404–408

LUMIO, J. S. (1948) Hearing deficiencies caused by carbon monoxide (generator gas). *Acta Otolaryngologica*, Supplement 71, 11–112

LYOS, A. T., MALPICA, A., ESTRADA, R., KATZ, C. D. and JENKINS, H. A. (1993) Invasive aspergillosis of the temporal bone: an unusual manifestation of acquired immunodeficiency syndrome. *American Journal of Otolaryngology*, 14, 444–448

MCADAM, L. P., O'HANLAN, M. A., BLUESTONE, R. and PEARSON, C. M. (1976) Relapsing polychondritis. *Medicine*, 55, 193–215

MCCABE, B. F. (1975) Diseases of the end organ and vestibular nerve. In: *The Vestibular System*, edited by R. F. Naunton. New York: Academic Press. p. 299

MCDONALD, T. J., VOLLERTSEN, R. S. and YOUNGE, B. R. (1985) Cogan's syndrome: audiovestibular involvement and prognosis in 18 patients. *Laryngoscope*, 95, 650–654

MCDONALD, T. J., ZINCKE, H., ANDERSON, C. F. and OTT, N. T.

(1978) Reversal of deafness after renal transplantation in Alport's syndrome. *Laryngoscope*, **88**, 38–42

MCGILL, T. J. (1978) Mycotic infection of the temporal bone. *Archives of Otolaryngology*, **104**, 140–144

MCKENNAN, K. X., NIELSEN, S. L., WATSON, C. and WIESNER, K. (1993) Meniere's syndrome: an atypical presentation of giant cell arteritis (temporal arteritis). *Laryngoscope*, **103**, 1103–1107

MAIR, I. W. S. and ELVERLAND, H. H. (1977) Sudden deafness and vaccination. *Journal of Laryngology and Otology*, **91**, 323–329

MAJOOR, M. H. J. M., ALBERS, F. W. J., VAN DER GAAG, R., GMELIG-MEYLING, F. and HUIZING, E. H. (1992) Corneal autoimmunity in Cogan's syndrome. Report of two cases. *Annals of Otology, Rhinology and Laryngology*, **101**, 679–684

MAJOOR, M. H. J. M., ALBERS, F. W. J. and CASSELMAN, J. W. (1993) Clinical relevance of magnetic resonance imaging and computed tomography in Cogan's syndrome. *Acta Otolaryngologica*, **113**, 625–631

MAKINO, K. and MORIMITSU, T. (1994) Effects of arterial occlusion on endocochlear DC potential and cochlear blood flow in guinea pigs. *Auris, Nasus, Larynx (Tokyo)*, **21**, 75–83

MALMVALL, B. E. and BENGTSSON, B. A. (1978) Giant cell arteritis. *Scandinavian Journal of Rheumatology*, **7**, 154–158

MANN, W., BECK, C. and BECK, C. (1986) Calcium antagonists in the treatment of sudden deafness. *Archives of Otorhinolaryngology*, **243**, 170–173

MARAIS, I. (1991) Cochleotoxicity due to mianserin hydrochloride. *Journal of Laryngology and Otology*, **105**, 475–476

MARCUS, R. E. and LEE, Y. M. (1976) Inner ear disorders in a family with sickle cell thalassemia. *Archives of Otolaryngology*, **102**, 703–705

MARK, A. S. and FITZGERALD, D. (1993) Segmental enhancement of the cochlea on contrasrt-enhanced MR: correlation with the frequency of hearing loss and possible sign of perilymphatic fistula and autoimmune labyrinthitis. *American Journal of Neuroradiology*, **14**, 991–996

MARK, A. S., SELTZER, S., NELSON-DRAKE, J., CHAPMAN, J. C., FITZGERALD, D. C. and GULYA, A. J. (1992) Labyrinthine enhancement on gadolinium-enhanced magnetic resonance imaging in sudden deafness and vertigo. Correlation with audiologic and electronystagmography studies. *Annals of Otology, Rhinology and Laryngology*, **101**, 459–464

MARKAND, O. N., LEE, B. I., WARREN, C., STOELTING, R. K., KING, R. D., BROWN, J. W. *et al.* (1987) Effects of hypothermia on brain stem auditory evoked potentials in humans. *Annals of Neurology*, **22**, 507–513

MASLAN, M. J., GRAHAM, M. D. and FLOOD, L. M. (1985) Cryptococcal meningitis: presentation as sudden deafness. *American Journal of Otology*, **6**, 435–437

MATSUOKA, I., KURATA, K., KAZAMA, N., NAKAMURA, T., SUGIMARU, T. and SATOH, M. (1991) The beginning of Menière's disease. *Acta Otolaryngologica*, Supplement 481, 505–509

MATTOX, D. E. and SIMMONS, F. B. (1977) Natural history of sudden sensorineural hearing loss. *Annals of Otology, Rhinology and Laryngology*, **86**, 463–480

MATTUCCI, K. F. and BACHOURA, L. (1982) Sudden hearing loss: ten years' experience. *Bulletin of the New York Academy of Medicine*, **58**, 464–470

MAXWELL, O. N. (1963) Hearing loss in uveitis. *Archives of Otolaryngology*, **78**, 138–142

MAYOT, D., BENE, M. C., DRON, K., PERRIN, C. and FAURE, G. C. (1993) Immunologic alterations in patients with sensorineural hearing disorders. *Clinical Immunology and Immunopathology*, **68**, 41–45

MEHRA, Y. N., SHARMA, Y. K., MANN, S. B. S. and DASH, R. J. (1985) Inner ear function in diabetes mellitus with peripheral neuropathies. In: *New Dimensions in Otorhinolaryngology – Head and Neck Surgery*, vol. 2, edited by E. Myers. Amsterdam: Excepta Medica. pp. 794–795

MERIFIELD, D. O. (1962) Hemorrhagic bullous myringitis: its relation to perceptive deafness. *Annals of Otology, Rhinology and Laryngology*, **71**, 124–133

MEYERHOFF, W. L. (1976) The thyroid and audition. *Laryngoscope*, **86**, 483–489

MEYERHOFF, W. L., PAPARELLA, M. M., ODA, M. and SHEA, D. (1979) Mycotic infections of the inner ear. *Laryngoscope*, **89**, 1725–1734

MICHAELS, L., SOUCEK, S. and LIANG, J. (1994) The ear in the acquired immunodeficiency syndrome: 1. Temporal bone histopathologic study. *American Journal of Otology*, **15**, 515–522

MICHEL, O. and BRUSIS, T. (1992) Hearing loss as a sequel of lumbar puncture. *Annals of Otology, Rhinology and Laryngology*, **101**, 390–394

MICHEL, O. and MATTHIAS, R. (1991) Probational treatment of sudden deafness with prostacyclin: a pilot study. *Auris, Nasus, Larynx (Tokyo)*, **18**, 115–123

MICHEL, O. and MATTHIAS, R. (1992) Effects of prostaglandin E_2 on the fluctuating hearing loss in Ménière's disease. *Aurus, Nasus, Larynx (Tokyo)*, **19**, 7–16

MILLER, J. J., BECK, L., DAVIS, A., JONES, D. E. and THOMAS, A. B. (1983) Hearing loss in patients with diabetic retinopathy. *American Journal of Otolaryngology*, **4**, 342–346

MILLER, J. M., BREDBERG, G., GRENMAN, R., SUONPÄÄ, J., LINDSTROM, B. and DIDIER, A. (1991) Measurement of human cochlear blood flow. *Annals of Otology, Rhinology and Laryngology*, **100**, 44–53

MITSCHKE, H., SCHMIDT, P., ZAZGORNIK, J., KOPSA, H. and PILS, P. (1977) Effect of renal transplantation on uremic deafness: a long-term study. *Audiology*, **16**, 530–534

MIYAZAKI, M. and KUMAGAMI, H. (1988) Prognostic estimation of sudden deafness by cochlear microphonics of electrocochleography. *ORL-Journal of Otorhinolaryngology and Related Specialties*, **50**, 371–376

MOFFAT, D. A., BAGULEY, D. M., VON BLUMENTHAL, H., IRVING, R. M. and HARDY, D. G. (1994) Sudden deafness in vestibular schwannoma. *Journal of Laryngology and Otology*, **108**, 116–119

MOFFAT, D. A., BOOTH, J. B. and MORRISON, A. W. (1979) Metabolic investigations in Ménière's disease. *Journal of Laryngology and Otology*, **93**, 545–561

MONTEIRO, M. L. R., SWANSON, R. A., COPPETO, J. R., CUNEO, R. A., DE ARMOND, S. J. and PRUSINER, S. B. (1985) A microangiopathic syndrome of encephalopathy, hearing loss, and retinal arteriolar occlusions. *Neurology*, **35**, 1113–1121

MORETTI, J. A. (1976) Sensorineural hearing loss following radiotherapy to the nasopharynx. *Laryngoscope*, **86**, 598–602

MORGAN, G. J., HOCHMAN, R. and WEIDER, D. J. (1984) Cogan's syndrome: acute vestibular and auditory dysfunction with interstitial keratitis. *American Journal of Otolaryngology*, **5**, 258–261

MORGENSTEIN, K. M. and MANNACE, E. D. (1969) Temporal bone histopathology in sickle cell disease. *Laryngoscope*, 79, 2172–2180

MORGENSTERN, C. and KAU, R. (1988) Pontine deafness – a new disease picture? *Laryngologie, Rhinologie, Otologie (Stuttgart)*, 67, 621–623

MORI, N., UOZUMI, N., YURA, K. and SAKAI, S. (1990) The difference in endocochlear and endolymphatic sac d.c. potentials in response to furosemide and canrenoate as diuretics. *European Archives of Otorhinolaryngology*, 247, 371–373

MORIMITSU, T. (1977) New theory and therapy of sudden deafness. Proceedings of the Fifth International Shambaugh Workshop on Middle Ear Microsurgery and Fluctuant Hearing Loss, edited by G. E. Shambaugh and J. J. Shea. Huntsville: Strode. pp. 412–421

MORRIS, M. S. and PRASAD, S. (1990) Otologic disease in the acquired immunodeficiency syndrome. *Ear, Nose and Throat Journal*, 69, 451–453

MORRIS, T. M. O. (1969) Deafness following acute carbon monoxide poisoning. *Journal of Laryngology and Otology*, 83, 1219–1225

MORRISON, A. W. (1975) *Management of Sensorineural Deafness*. London and Boston: Butterworths

MORRISON, A. W. (1978) Acute deafness. *British Journal of Hospital Medicine*, 19, 237–249

MORRISON, A. W. and BOOTH, J. B. (1970) Sudden deafness – an otological emergency. *British Journal of Hospital Medicine*, 4, 287–298

MOSCATELLO, A. L., WORDEN, D. L., NADELMAN, R. B., WORMSER, G. and LUCENTE, F. (1991) Otolaryngologic aspects of Lyme disease. *Laryngoscope*, 101, 592–595

MOSKOWITZ, D., LEE, K. J. and SMITH, H. W. (1984) Steroid use in idiopathic sudden sorienenural hearing loss. *Laryngoscope*, 94, 664–666

MURAKAMI, Y. and MUZUSHIMA, N. (1985) Deafness following mumps: the possible pathogenesis and incidence of deafness. In: *New Dimensions in Otorhinolaryngology – Head and Neck Surgery*, vol. 2, edited by E. Myers. Amsterdam: Excerpta Medica. pp. 1031–1032

MUSIEK, F. E., GOLLEGLY, K. M., KIBBE, K. S. and REEVES, A. G. (1989) Electrophysiologic and behavioral auditory findings in multiple sclerosis. *American Journal of Otology*, 10, 343–350

MYERS, G. J. and TYLER, H. R. (1972) The etiology of deafness in Alport's syndrome. *Archives of Otolaryngology*, 96, 333–340

NADOL, J. B., WEISS, A. D. and PARKER, S. W. (1975) Vertigo of delayed onset after sudden deafness. *Annals of Otology, Rhinology and Laryngology*, 84, 841–846

NAGAHARA, K., FISCH, U. and YAGI, N. (1983) Perilymph oxygenation in sudden and progressive sensorineural hearing loss. *Acta Otolaryngologica*, 96, 57–68

NAGERIS, B., OR, R., HARDAN, I. and POLLIACK, A. (1993) Sudden onset of deafness as a presenting manifestation of chronic lymphocytic leukaemia. *Leukaemia-Lymphoma*, 9, 269–271

NAKASHIMA, T. and YANAGITA, N. (1993) Outcome of sudden deafness with and without vertigo. *Laryngoscope*, 103, 1145–1149

NAKASHIMA, T., KUNO, K. and YANAGITA, N. (1989) Evaluation of prostaglandin E_1 therapy for sudden deafness. *Laryngoscope*, 99, 542–546

NAKASHIMA, T., SUZUKI, T., MORISAKI, H. and YANAGITA, N. (1992) Measurement of cochlear blood flow in sudden deafness. *Laryngoscope*, 102, 1308–1310

NARULA, A. A., POWELL, R. J. and DAVIS, A. (1989) Frequency-resolving ability in systemic lupus erythematosus. *British Journal of Audiology*, 23, 69–72

NESS, J. A., STANKIEWICZ, J. A., KANIFF, T., PIFARRE, R. and ALLEGRETTI, J. (1993) Sensorineural hearing loss associated with aortocoronary bypass surgery: a prospective study. *Laryngoscope*, 103, 589–593

NISHIOKA, K., FUJIMOTO, M., DATE, R., MASUDA, Y., HIRAMOTO, K. and TANAKA, T. (1984) Bilateral sensorineural deafness associated with *Mycoplasma pneumoniae* infection: the first case report. *Hiroshima Journal of Medical Sciences*, 33, 585–589

NODA, Y., URA, M., NAKAMURA, M. and KOSUGI, T. (1985) Hemostatic study in patients with vertigo and the effect of antiplatelet drug. In: *New Dimensions in Otorhinolaryngology – Head and Neck Surgery*, vol. 2, edited by E. Myers. Amsterdam: Excerpta Medica. pp. 301–303

NOMURA, Y. and KITAMURA, K. (1979) Abrupt (sharp cut) type sensorineural hearing loss – a human temporal bone study. *Auris, Nasus, Larynx (Tokyo)*, 6, 13–21

NOMURA, Y., HARADA, T., SAKATA, H. and SUGIURA, A. (1988) Sudden deafness and asymptomatic mumps. *Acta Otolaryngologica* Supplement 456, 9–11

NORTON, E. W. D. and COGAN, D. G. (1959) Syndrome of non-syphilitic interstitial keratitis and vestibuloauditory symptoms. *Archives of Ophthalmology*, 61, 695–697

NOURY, K. A. and KATSARKAS, A. (1989) Sudden unilateral sensorineural hearing loss: a syndrome or a symptom. *Journal of Otolaryngology*, 18, 274–278

NUTTALL, A. L., HULTCRANTZ, E., LARSEN, H-C. and ANGELBORG, C. (1988) Cochlear blood flow increases after systemic hemodilution: comparison of simultaneous laser doppler flowmetry and radioactive microsphere measurements. *Hearing Research*, 34, 215–224

O'CONNELL, S. (1995) Lyme disease in the United Kingdom. *British Medical Journal*, 310, 303–308

ODA, M., PRECIADO, M. C., QUICK, C. A. and PAPARELLA, M. M. (1974) Labyrinthine pathology of chronic renal failure patients treated with haemodialysis and kidney transplantation. *Laryngoscope*, 84, 1489–1506

ODETOYINBO, O. and ADEKILE, A. (1987) Sensorineural hearing loss in children with sickle cell anemia. *Annals of Otology, Rhinology and Laryngology*, 96, 258–260

OGAWA, K. and KANZAKI, J. (1994) Aplastic anemia and sudden sensorineural hearing loss. *Acta Otolaryngologica*, Supplement 514, 85–88

OHINATA, Y., MAKIMOTO, K., KAWAKAMI, M., HAGINOMORI, S. I., ARAKI, M. and TAKAHASHI, H. (1994) Blood viscosity and plasma viscosity in patients with sudden deafness. *Acta Otolaryngologica*, 114, 601–607

OHLSEN, K. A., DIDIER, A., BALDWIN, D., MILLER, J. M., NUTTALL, A. L. and HULTCRANTZ, E. (1992) Cochlear blood flow in response to dilating agents. *Hearing Research*, 58, 19–25

OHLSEN, A., HULTCRANTZ, E., LARSEN, H. C. and ANGELBORG, C. (1994) The cochlear blood flow: a comparison between the laser doppler and the microsphere methods. *Acta Otolaryngologica*, 114, 4–10

OKAMOTO, M., SHITARA, T., NAKAYAMA, M., TAKAMIYA, H., NISHIYAMA, K., ONO, Y. *et al.* (1994) Sudden deafness accompanied by asymptomatic mumps. *Acta Otolaryngologica* Supplement 514, 45–48

O'KEEFE, L. J. and MAW, A. R. (1991) Sudden total deafness in sickle cell disease. *Journal of Laryngology and Otology*, 105, 653–655

OLIVIERI, N. F., BUNCIC, J. R., CHEW, E., GALLANT, T.,

HARRISON, R. V., KEENAN, N. et al. (1986) Visual and auditory neurotoxicity in patients receiving subcutaneous deferoxamine infusions. *New England Journal of Medicine*, **314**, 869–873

OLSON, M. E., CHERNIK, N. L. and POSNER, J. B. (1974) Infiltration of the leptomeninges by systemic cancer. A clinical and pathologic study. *Archives of Neurology*, **30**, 122–137

OLSZEWSKI, E., SEKULA, J., KOSTKA–TRABKA, E., GRODZINSKA, K., BASISTA, M., KEDZIOR, K. et al. (1985) Prostacyclin in the treatment of sudden deafness. *Prostacyclin – Clinical Trials*, 77–82

OLSZEWSKI, E., KOSTKA-TRABKA, E., RERON, E., GRODZINSKI, L. TUREK, J., DEMBINSKA-KIEC, A. et al. (1990) Administration of prostacyclin in sudden deafness. Evaluation with the double blind method. *Otolaryngologie Polki*, **44**, 62–65

OMORI, H. and IKEDA, M. (1994) Intravascular hypercoagulability in patients with recent Bell's palsy. *European Archives of Otorhinolaryngology*, **251**, 278–282

ÖNERCI, M., ASLAN, S., GÜMRÜK, F., AKSOY, S., BELGIN, E., OZCELIK, T. et al. (1994) Audiologic and impedancemetric findings within thalassaemic patients. *International Journal of Pediatric Otorhinolaryngology*, **28**, 167–172

ORCHIK, D. J. and DUNN, J. W. (1977) Sickle cell anemia and sudden deafness. *Archives of Otolaryngology*, **103**, 369–370

ORCHIK, D. J., SCHMAIER, D. R., SHEA, J. J., EMMETT, J. R., MORETZ, W. H. and SHEA, J. J. (1987) Sensorineural hearing loss in cordless telephone injury. *Otolaryngology – Head and Neck Surgery*, **96**, 30–33

PACE–BALZAN, A. and RAMSDEN, R. T. (1988) Sudden bilateral sensorineural hearing loss during treatment with dantrolene sodium (Dantrium). *Journal of Laryngology and Otology*, **102**, 57–58

PANNING, B. and LEHNHARDT, E. (1986) Letter. *Laryngoscope*, **96**, 1303

PANNING, B., MEHLER, D. and LEHNHARDT, E. (1983) Transient low-frequency hypoacousia after spinal anaesthesia. *Lancet*, ii, 582

PAPARELLA, M. M., BERLINGER, N. T., ODA, M. and EL FIKY, F. (1973) Otological manifestations of leukemia. *Laryngoscope*, **83**, 1510–1526

PAPPAS, D. G., SEKHAR, H. K. C., LIM, J. and HILLMANN, D. E. (1994) Ultrastructural findings in the cochlea of AIDS cases. *American Journal of Otology*, **15**, 456–465

PARNES, S. M. and WEAVER, S. A. (1992) Superficial siderosis of the central nervous system: a neglected cause of sensorineural hearing loss. *Otolaryngology – Head and Neck Surgery*, **107**, 69–77

PARVING, A., ELBERLING, C. and SMITH, T. (1981) Auditory electrophysiology: findings in multiple sclerosis. *Audiology*, **20**, 123–142

PARVING, A., ELBERLING, C., BALLE, V., PARBO, J., DEJGAARD, A. and PARVING, H. H. (1990) Hearing disorders in patients with insulin-dependent diabetes mellitus. *Audiology*, **29**, 113–121

PARVING, A., OSTRI, B., HANSEN, J. M., BRETLAU, P. and PARVING, H-H. (1986) Audiological and temporal bone findings in myxedema. *Annals of Otology, Rhinology and Laryngology*, **95**, 278–283

PARVING, A., PARVING, H-H. and LYNGSØE, J. (1983) Hearing sensitivity in patients with myxoedema before and after treatment with L-thyroxine. *Acta Otolaryngologica*, **95**, 315–321

PATTERSON, M. E. and BARTLETT, P. C. (1976) Hearing impairment caused by intratympanic pressure changes during general anaesthesia. *Laryngoscope*, **86**, 399–404

PEITERSON, E. and CARLSON, B. H. (1966) Hearing impairment as the initial sign of polyarteritis nodosa. *Acta Otolaryngologica*, **61**, 189–195

PELOSI, L., FELS, A., PETRILLO, A., SENATORE, R., RUSSO, G., LONEGREN, K., CALACE, P. et al. (1984) Friedreich's ataxia: clinical involvement and evoked potentials. *Acta Neurologica Scandinavica*, **70**, 360–368

PENSAK, M. L., GLASSCOCK, M. E., JACKSON, C. G., JOSEY, A. F. and GULYA, A. J. (1985) Sudden hearing loss and cerebellopontine angle tumors. *Laryngoscope*, **95**, 1188–1193

PETHERAM, I. S. (1976) Severe haemolysis and unilateral sensorineural deafness in infectious mononucleosis. *Practitioner*, **217**, 945–948

PILGRAMM, M. (1991) Hemodilution therapy of acute inner ear damage. *Acta Medica Austriaca*, **18** (Supplement 1), 60–62

PIRAS, A. G., OLIVEIRA, E., LOCKHART, P., BRANDI, P., GUAITA, H. E. and SAHAGUN, N. B. (1985) Diabetes mellitus and cochleovestibular disturbance. In: *New Dimensions in Otorhinolaryngology – Head and Neck Surgery*, vol. 2, edited by E. Myers. Amsterdam: Excerpta Medica. pp. 933–934

POLITZER, A. (1884) *see* Politzer, A. (1902) *A Textbook of Diseases of the Ear*, 4th edn, translated and edited by M. J. Ballin and C. L. Heller, London

POLLOCK, R. A., JACKSON, R. T., CLAIRMONT, A. A. and NICHOLSON, W. L. (1974) Carbon dioxide as an otic vasodilator. *Archives of Otolaryngology*, **100**, 309–313

PORTER, J. B., JASWON, M. S., HUEHNS, E. R., EAST, C. A. and HAZELL, J. W. P. (1989) Desferrioxamine ototoxicity: evaluation of risk factors in thalassaemic patients and guidelines for safe dosage. *British Journal of Haematology*, **73**, 403–409

POST, J. T. (1964) Hypothyroid deafness. *Laryngoscope*, **74**, 221–232

PRASHER, D., RYAN, S. and LUXON, L. (1994) Contralateral suppression of transiently evoked otoacoustic emissions and neuro-otology. *British Journal of Audiology*, **28**, 247–254

PRASHER, D. K., SAINZ, M. and GIBSON, W. P. R. (1982) Binaural voltage summation of brainstem auditory evoked potentials: an adjunct to the diagnostic criteria for multiple sclerosis. *Annals of Neurology*, **11**, 86–91

PRAZMA, J. (1978) Carbonic anhydrase in the generation of cochlear potentials. *American Journal of Physiology*, **235**, F317–320

PRAZMA, J., FISCHER, N. D., BIGGERS, W. P. and ASCHER, D. (1979) Variation of endocochlear PO_2 and cochlear potential by breathing carbon dioxide. *Annals of Otology, Rhinology and Laryngology*, **88**, 222–227

PRAZMA, J., SMALLEY, W. E., COVINGTON, S. and PILLSBURY, H. C. (1988) Cochlear blood flow. The effect of six hours of noise exposure. *Archives of Otolaryngology – Head and Neck Surgery*, **114**, 657–660

PRIBITKIN, E. A., RONDINELLA, L., ROSENBERG, S. I. and YOUSEM, D. M. (1994) Superficial siderosis of the central nervous system: an underdiagnosed cause of sensorineural hearing loss and ataxia. *American Journal of Otology*, **15**, 415–418

PRINGLE, M. B., JEFFERIS, A. F. and BARRETT, G. S. (1993) Sensorineural hearing loss caused by metastatic prostatic carcinoma: a case report. *Journal of Laryngology and Otology*, **107**, 933–934

PROBST, R., TSCHOPP, K., LÜDIN, E., KELLERHALS, B., PODVINEC, M. and PFALTZ, C. R. (1992) A randomized, double-blind, placebo-controlled study of dextran/pentoxifylline in acute acoustic trauma and sudden hearing loss. *Acta Otolaryngologica*, 112, 435–443

PYYKKO, I., VESANEN, M., ASIKAINEN, K., KOSKINIEMI, M., AIRAKSINEN, L. and VAHERI, A. (1993) Human spumaretrovirus in the etiology of sudden hearing loss. *Acta Otolaryngologica*, 113, 109–112

QUICK, C. A. (1976) Hearing loss in patients with dialysis and renal transplants. *Transactions of the American Academy of Ophthalmology and Otology*, 105, 838–843

RABUZZI, D. D. (1970) Relapsing polychondritis. *Archives of Otolaryngology*, 91, 188–194

RANDOLF, H-B., HAUPT, H. and SCHEIBE, F. (1990) Cochlear blood flow following temporary occlusion of the cerebellar arteries. *European Archives of Otorhinolaryngology*, 247, 226–228

RAPPAPORT, J. M., GULLIVER, J. M., PHILLIPS, D. P., VAN DORPE, R. A., MAXNER, C. E. and BHAN, V. (1994) Auditory temporal resolution in multiple sclerosis. *Journal of Otolaryngology*, 23, 307–323

RAREY, K. E. (1990) Otologic pathophysiology in patients with human immunodeficiency virus. *American Journal of Otolaryngology*, 11, 366–369

REAL, R., THOMAS, M. and GERWIN, J. M. (1987) Sudden hearing loss and acquired immunodeficiency syndrome. *Otolaryngology – Head and Neck Surgery*, 97, 409–412

REDLEAF, M. I. and MCCABE, B. F. (1993) Lightning injury of the tympanic membrane. *Annals of Otology, Rhinology and Laryngology*, 102, 867–869

REDLEAF, M. I., BAUER, C. A., GANTZ, B. J., HOFFMAN, H. T. and MCCABE, B. F. (1995) Diatrizoate and dextran treatment of sudden sensorineural hearing loss. *American Journal of Otology*, 16, 295–303

REILLY, J. S., CASSELBRANT, M. L., STOOL, S. E. and BLUESTONE, C. D. (1984) Liver transplants in children: importance for the laryngologist. *Annals of Otology, Rhinology and Laryngology*, 93, 494–497

REN, T-Y., NUTTALL, A. L. and MILLER, J. M. (1993) Provoked flux motion of cochlear blood flow measured with laser doppler flowmetry in guinea pig. *Acta Otolaryngologica*, 113, 609–614

RICHARDSON, H., BIRCHALL, J. P., HILL, J. and MCMASTER, T. (1994) Should we routinely screen for Lyme disease in patients with asymmetrical hearing loss? *British Journal of Audiology*, 28, 59–61

RINEHART, R., HARRE, R. G., ROSKI, R. A. and DOLAN, K. D. (1992) Aneurysm of the anterior inferior cerebellar artery producing hearing loss. *Annals of Otology, Rhinology and Laryngology*, 101, 705–706

RINTELMANN, W. F. (1976) Auditory manifestations of Alport's disease syndrome. *Transactions of the American Academy of Ophthalmology and Otology*, 82, 375–387

ROBERTS, D. B. (1980) The etiology of bullous myringitis and the role of mycoplasmas in ear disease: a review. *Pediatrics*, 65, 761–766

ROJAS, A. M., JOHNS, H. and FIAT, P. R. (1993) Should carbogen and nicotinamide be given throughout the full course of fractionated radiotherapy regimens. *International Journal of Radiation, Oncology, Biology and Physics*, 27, 1101–1105

ROSEN, E. (1945) Uveitis, with poliosis, vitiligo and alopecia and dysacousia (Vogt-Koyanagi syndrome). *Archives of Ophthalmology*, 33, 281–292

ROWE-JONES, J. M., MACALLAN, D. C. and SOROOSHIAN, M. (1990) Polyarteritis nodosa presenting as bilateral onset cochleo-vestibular failure in a young woman. *Journal of Laryngology and Otology*, 104, 562–564

ROWSON, K. E. K., HINCHCLIFFE, R. and GAMBLE, D. R. (1976) The role of viruses in acute auditory failure. *British Journal of Audiology*, 10, 107–109

RUDD, M. J., HARRIES, M. L. I., LYNCH, C. A. and MOFFAT, D. A. (1993) Hearing loss fluctuating with blood sugar levels in Meniére's disease. *Journal of Laryngology and Otology*, 107, 620–622

RYBAK, L. P. (1990) Deafness associated with Lassa fever. *Journal of the American Medical Association*, 264, 2119

SAADAH, H. A. (1993) Vestibular vertigo associated with hyperlipidemia: response to antilipidemic therapy. *Archives of Internal Medicine*, 153, 1848–1849

SAKASHITA, T., MINOWA, Y., HACHIKAWA, K., KUBO, T. and NAKAI, Y. (1991) Evoked otoacoustic emissions from ears with idiopathic sudden deafness. *Acta Otolaryngologica*, Supplement 486, 66–72

SANDO, I. and EGAMI, T. (1977) Inner ear hemorrhage and endolymphatic hydrops in a leukemic patient with sudden hearing loss. *Annals of Otology, Rhinology and Laryngology*, 86, 518–524

SANDO, I., HARADA, T., LEHR, A. and SOBEL, J. H. (1977) Sudden deafness: histopathologic correlation in temporal bone. *Annals of Otology, Rhinology and Laryngology*, 86, 269–279

SANDO, I., OGAWA, A. and JAFEK, B. W. (1982) Inner ear pathology following injury to the eighth cranial nerve and the labyrinthine artery. *Annals of Otology, Rhinology and Laryngology*, 91, 136–141

SANDSTRÖM, M., BREDBERG, G., ÅSBRINK, E., HOVMARK, A. and HOLMKVIST, C. (1989) Brainstem response audiometry in chronic Lyme borreliosis. *Scandinavian Audiology*, 18, 205–210

SCHEFF, S. W. and PRICE, D. A. (1993) Synapse loss in the temporal lobe in Alzheimer's disease. *Annals of Neurology*, 33, 190–199

SCHNELL, R. G., DYCK, P. J., BOWIE, E. J. W., KLASS, D. W. and TASWELL, H. T. (1966) Infectious mononucleosis: neurologic and EEG findings. *Medicine*, 45, 51–63

SCHOT, L. J., HILGERS, F. J. M., KEUS, R. B., SCHOUWENBURG, R. F. and DRESCHRER, W. A. (1992) Late effects of radiotherapy on hearing. *European Archives of Otorhinolaryngology*, 249, 305–308

SCHUKNECHT, H. F. (1974) *Pathology of the Ear*. Cambridge, Mass: Havard University Press

SCHUKNECHT, H. F. (1991) Ear pathology in autoimmune disease. Bearing of Basic Research on Clinical Otolaryngology, edited by C. R. Pfaltz, W. Arnold and O. Kleinsasser. *Advances in Otorhinolaryngology*, 46, 50–70.

SCHUKNECHT, H. F. and DONOVAN, E. D. (1986) The pathology of idiopathic sudden sensorineural hearing loss. *Archives of Otorhinolaryngology*, 243, 1–15

SCHUKNECHT, H. F. and NADOL, J. B. (1994) Temporal bone pathology in a case of Cogan's syndrome. *Laryngoscope*, 104, 1135–1142

SCHWEITZER, V. G. and SHEPARD, N. (1989) Sudden hearing loss: an uncommon manifestation of multiple sclerosis. *Otolaryngology – Head and Neck Surgery*, 100, 327–332

SCOTT, D. G. I. and WATTS, R. A. (1994) Classification and epidemiology of systemic vasculitis. *British Journal of Rheumatology*, 33, 897–900

SELLARS, S. K. (1971) Acute deafness associated with depo-progesterone. *Journal of Laryngology and Otology*, 85, 281–282

SERJEANT, G. R., NORMAN, W. and TODD, G. B. (1975) The internal auditory canal and sensorineural hearing loss in homozygous sickle cell disease. *Journal of Laryngology and Otology*, **89**, 453–455

SHAIA, F. T. and SHEEHY, J. L. (1976) Sudden sensorineural hearing impairment: a report of 1220 cases. *Laryngoscope*, **86**, 389–398

SHANON, E., REDIANU, C., ZIKK, D. and EYLAN, E. (1982) Sudden deafness due to infection by *Mycoplasma pneumoniae*. *Annals of Otology, Rhinology and Laryngology*, **91**, 163–165

SHATARI, T., HOSODA, Y. and KANZAKI, J. (1994) Study on the vasculature of the internal auditory artery in humans by casts. *Acta Otolaryngologica*, Supplement 514, 101–107

SHEA, J. J. III and BRACKMANN, D. E. (1987) Multiple sclerosis manifesting as sudden hearing loss. *Otolaryngology – Head and Neck Surgery*, **97**, 335–338

SHEA, J. J. and KITABCHI, A. E. (1971) Management of fluctuant hearing loss. *Journal of Tennessee Medical Association*, **64**, 862–869

SHEA, J. J. and KITABCHI, A. E. (1973) Management of fluctuant hearing loss. *Archives of Otolaryngology*, **97**, 118–124

SHEHATA-DIELER, W., SHIMIZU, H., SOLIMAN, S. M. and TUSA, R. J. (1991) Middle latency auditory evoked potentials in temporal lobe disorders. *Ear and Hearing*, **12**, 377–388

SHIRAISHI, T., KUBO, T. and MATSUNAGA, T. (1991) Chronological study of recovery of sudden deafness treated with defibrinogenation and steroid therapies. *Acta Otolaryngologica*, **111**, 867–871

SHIRAISHI, T., KUBO, T., OKUMURA, S., NARAMURA, H., NISHIMURA, M., OKUSA, M. *et al.* (1993) Hearing recovery in sudden deafness patients using a modified defibrinogenation therapy. *Acta Otolaryngologica*, Supplement 501, 46–50

SIEGER, A., SKINNER, M. W., WHITE, N. H. and SPECTOR, G. J. (1983) Auditory function in children with diabetes mellitus. *Annals of Otology, Rhinology and Laryngology*, **93**, 237–241

SILLMAN, J. S., LAROUERRE, M. J., NUTTALL, A. L., LAWRENCE, M. and MILLER, J. M. (1988) Recent advances in cochlear blood flow measurements. *Annals of Otology, Rhinology and Laryngology*, **97**, 1–8

SIMMONS, F. B. (1968) Theory of membrane breaks in sudden hearing loss. *Archives of Otolaryngology*, **88**, 68–74

SIMMONS, F. B. (1973) Sudden idiopathic sensori-neural hearing loss: some observations. *Laryngoscope*, **83**, 1221–1227

SINGH, V., ANNIS, J. A. D. and TODD, G. B. (1992) Osteoma of the internal auditory canal presenting with sudden unilateral hearing loss. *Journal of Laryngology and Otology*, **106**, 905–907

SINGLETON, G. T., WHITAKER, D. L., KEIM, R. J. and KEMKER, F. J. (1984) Cordless telephones: a threat to hearing. *Annals of Otology, Rhinology and Laryngology*, **93**, 565–568

SMITH, L. N. (1994) Unilateral sensorineural hearing loss in Behçet's disease. *American Journal of Otolaryngology*, **15**, 286–288

SMITH, M. E. and CANALIS, R. F. (1989) Otologic manifestations of AIDS: the otosyphilis connection. *Laryngoscope*, **99**, 365–372

SMITH, P. V., WALLER, E. S., DOLUISIO, J. T., BAUZA, M. T., PURI, S. K. and LASSMAN, H. B. (1986) Pharmacokinetics of orally administered pentoxifylline in human. *Journal of Pharmacological Science*, **75**, 47–52

SMOUHA, E. E. and KARMODY, Y. S. (1995) Non-osteitic complications of therapeutic radiation to the temporal bone. *American Journal of Otology*, **16**, 83–87

SOFFERMAN, R. A. (1980) Cranial arteritis in otolaryngology. *Annals of Otology, Rhinology and Laryngology*, **89**, 215–219

SOULIERE, C. R., KAVA, C. R., BARRS, D. M. and BELL, A. F. (1991) Sudden hearing loss as the sole manifestation of neurosarcoidosis. *Otolaryngology – Head and Neck Surgery*, **105**, 376–381

SPENCER, J. T. (1981) Hyperlipoproteinaemia, hyperinsulinism, and Menière's disease. *Southern Medical Journal*, **74**, 1194–1200

STEPHENS, S. D. G. (1970) Temporary threshold shift in myxoedema. *Journal of Laryngology and Otology*, **84**, 317–321

STEPHENS, S. D. G. and HINCHCLIFFE, R. (1968) Studies on temporary threshold drift. *International Audiology*, **7**, 267–279

STEWART, B. J. A. and PRABHU, P. U. (1993) Reports of sensorineural deafness after measles, mumps and rubella immunisation. *Archives of Diseases in Childhood*, **69**, 153–54

STRAUSS, M. and FINE, E. (1991) Aspergillus otomastoiditis in acquired immunodeficiency syndrome. *American Journal of Otology*, **12**, 49–53

STROME, M., TOPF, P. and VERNICK, D. M. (1988) Hyperlipidemia in association with childhood sensorineural hearing loss. *Laryngoscope*, **98**, 165–169

SUMMERS, R. W. and HARKER, L. (1982) Ulcerative colitis and sensorineural hearing loss: is there a relationship? *Journal of Clinical Gastroenterology*, **4**, 251–252

SUN, A. H., WANG, Z. M., XIAO, S. Z., LI, Z. J., DING, J. C., LI, J. Y. *et al.* (1992) Idiopathic sudden hearing loss and disturbance of iron metabolism. A clinical survey of 426 cases. *ORL – Journal of Otorhinolaryngology and Related Specialties*, **54**, 66–70

SUNDBERG, A., WANG, L. P. and FOG, J. (1992) Influence on hearing of 22G Whitacre and 22G Quincke needles. *Anaesthesia*, **47**, 981–983

SUNDEL, R. P., NEWBURGER, J. W., MCCILL, T., CLEVELAND, S. S., MILLER, W. M., BERRY, B. *et al.* (1990) Sensorineural hearing loss associated with Kawasaki disease. *Journal of Pediatrics*, **117**, 371–377

SUNDEL, R. P., CLEVELAND, S. S., BEISER, A. S., NEWBURGER, J. W., MCGILL, T., BAKER, A. L. *et al.* (1992) Audiology profiles of children with Kawasaki disease. *American Journal of Otology*, **13**, 512–515

SUSMANO, A. and ROSENBUSH, S. W. (1988) Hearing loss and ischemic heart disease. *American Journal of Otology*, **9**, 403–408

SUZUKI, M., SAKAI, T., HIRAKAWA, K., OYA, T., YAJIN, K., HARADA, Y. *et al.* (1987) Acoustic neuroma presenting with sudden and fluctuating hearing loss – A case report. *Auris, Nasus, Larynx (Tokyo)*, **14**, 165–170

SUZUKI, T., NAKASHIMA, T. and YANAGITA, N. (1993) Effects of increased cerebrospinal fluid pressure on cochlear and cerebral blood flow. *European Archives of Otorhinolaryngology*, **250**, 332–336

SZEIMIES, R. M., STOLZ, W., WLOTZKE, U., KORTING, H. C. and LANDTHALER, M. (1994) Successful treatment of hydroxyethyl starch-induced pruritus with topical capsaicin. *British Journal of Dermatology*, **131**, 380–382

TABIRA, T., TSUJI, S., NAGASHIMA, T., NAKAJIMA, T. and KUROIWA, Y. (1981) Cortical deafness in multiple sclerosis. *Journal of Neurology, Neurosurgery and Psychiatry*, **44**, 433–436

TAKAHARA, S., SAITO, R., KONISHI, S. and IGARASHI, M. (1974) Idiopathic endolymphatic hydrops with history of sudden deafness. *Journal of Otolaryngology of Japan*, **77**, 959–969

TAKAYASU, M. (1908) A case with peculiar changes of the central retinal vessels. *Acta Societas Ophthalmologica Japonica*, **12**, 554–555

TAKEUCHI, Y., NUMATA, T., KONNO, A., SUZUKI, H., HINO, T. and KANEKO, T. (1994) Hemodynamic changes in the head and neck after ligation of the unilateral carotid arteries: a study using color doppler imaging. *Annals of Otology, Rhinology and Laryngology*, **103**, 41–45

TALAR-WILLIAMS, C. and SNELLER, M. C. (1994) Complications of corticosteroid therapy. *European Archives of Otorhinolaryngology*, **251**, 131–136

TALMI, Y. P., FINKELSTEIN, Y. and ZOHAR, Y. (1989) Post irradiation hearing loss. *Audiology*, **28**, 121–126

TANAKA, Y., SUZUKI, M. and INOUE, T. (1990) Evoked otoacoustic emissions in sensorineural hearing impairment: its clinical implications. *Ear and Hearing*, **11**, 134–143

TANAKA, Y., KAMO, T., YOSHIDA, M. and YAMADORI, A. (1991) 'So-called' cortical deafness. *Brain*, **114**, 2385–2401

TAVIN, M. E., RUBIN, J. S. and CAMACHO, F. J. (1993) Sudden sensorineural hearing loss in haemoglobin SC disease. *Journal of Laryngology and Otology*, **107**, 831–833

TAYLOR, I. G. and IRWIN, J. (1978) Some audiological aspects of diabetes mellitus. *Journal of Laryngology and Otology*, **92**, 99–113

TAYLOR, L. and PARSONS–SMITH, G. (1969) Infectious mononucleosis, deafness and facial paralysis. *Journal of Laryngology and Otology*, **83**, 613–616

TELIAN, S.A., KILENY, P. R., NIPARKO, J. K., KEMINK, J. L. and GRAHAM, J. M. (1989) Normal auditory brainstem response in patients with acoustic neuroma. *Laryngoscope*, **99**, 10–14

TERAYAMA, Y., ISHIBE, Y. and MATSUSHIMA, J. (1988) Rapidly progressive sensorineural hearing loss (rapid deafness). *Acta Otolaryngologica*, Supplement **456**, 43–48

THEOPOLD, H.-M. (1985) Nimodipin (Bay e 9736) ein neues therapiekonzept bei innenohrerkrankungen? *Laryngologie, Rhinologie, Otologie*, **64**, 609–613

THOMAS, R., KAMESWARAN, M., MURUGAN, V. and OKAFOR, B. C. (1993) Sensorineural hearing loss in neurobrucellosis. *Journal of Laryngology and Otology*, **107**, 1034–1036

TIMON, C. I. and WALSH, M. A. (1989) Sudden sensorineural hearing loss as a presentation of HIV infection. *Journal of Laryngology and Otology*, **103**, 1071–1072

TOBIAS, E., MANN, C., BONE, I., DE SILVA, R. and IRONSIDE, J. (1994) A case of Creutzfeldt–Jakob disease presenting with cortical deafness. *Journal of Neurology, Neurosurgery and Psychiatry*, **57**, 872–873

TODD, G. B., SERJEANT, G. R. and LARSON, M. R. (1973) Sensorineural hearing loss in Jamaicans with SS disease. *Acta Otolaryngologica*, **76**, 268–272

TRAN BA HUY, P., FERRARY, E., ESCOUBET, B. and STERKERS, O. (1987) Strial prostaglandins and leukotrienes. *Acta Otolaryngologica*, **103**, 558–566

TRUY, E., VEUILLET, E., COLLET, L. and MORGON, A. (1993) Characteristics of transient otoacoustic emissions in patients with sudden idiopathic hearing loss. *British Journal of Audiology*, **27**, 379–385

TSUNODA, I., KANNO, H., WATANABE, M., SHIMOJI, S., HIRAYAMA, K., SUMITA, H. *et al.* (1994) Acute simultaneous bilateral vestibulocochlear impairment in neuro-Behçet's disease: a case report. *Auris, Nasus, Larynx (Tokyo)*, **211**, 243–247

TYNDEL, F. J., DAVIDSON, G. S., BIRMAN, H., MODZELEWSKI, Z. A. and ACKER, J. J. (1994) Sarcoidosis of the middle ear. *Chest*, **105**, 1582–1583

ULLRICH, D., AURBACH, G. and DROBIK, C. (1992) A prospective study of hyperlipidemia as a pathogenic factor in sudden hearing loss. *European Archives of Otorhinolaryngology*, **249**, 273–276

UMEMURA, K., ASAI, Y., UEMATSU, T. and NAKASHIMA, M. (1993) Role of thromboxane A_2 in a microcirculation disorder of the rat inner ear. *European Archives of Otorhinolaryngology*, **250**, 342–344

UMEMURA, K., TAKIGUCHI, Y., NAKASHIMA, M. and NOZUE, M. (1990) Effect of arachidonic acid on the inner ear blood flow measured with a laser doppler flowmeter. *Annals of Otology, Rhinology and Laryngology*, **99**, 491–495

URBAN, G. E. (1973) Reversible sensori-neural hearing loss associated with sickle cell crisis. *Laryngoscope*, **83**, 633–638

USHISAKO, Y. and MORIMITSU, T. (1988) Studies on amidotrizoate therapy in sudden deafness (1978–1987). *Acta Otolaryngologica*, Supplement **456**, 37–42

VAGUE, P., VAGUE, J. V., AILLAUD, M. F., BADIER, C., VIARD, R., ALESSI, M. C. *et al.* (1986) Correlation between blood fibrinolytic activity, plasminogen activator inhibitor level, plasma insulin level, and related body weight in normal and obese subjects. *Metabolism*, **35**, 250–253

VANASSE, M., FISCHER, C., BERTHEZÈNE, F., ROUX, Y., VOLMAN, G. and MORNEX, R. (1989) Normal brainstem auditory evoked potentials in adult hypothyroidism. *Laryngoscope*, **99**, 302–306

VANDAM, L. D. and DRIPPS, R. D. (1956) Long-term follow-up of patients who received 10,098 spinal anesthetics. *Journal of the American Medical Association*, **1**, 586–591

VAN DISHOECK, H. A. E. and BIERMAN, Th. A. (1957) Sudden perceptive deafness and viral infection. *Annals of Otology, Rhinology and Laryngology*, **66**, 963–980

VAN LEEUWEN, J. P. P. M., CREMERS, C. W. R. J., THIJSSEN, H. O. M. and MEYER, H. E. (1993) Unchanged unilateral hearing loss and ipsilateral growth of an acoustic neuroma from 1 to 4 cm. *Journal of Laryngology and Otology*, **107**, 230–232

VAN'T HOFF, W. and STUART, D. W. (1979) Deafness in myxoedema. *Quarterly Journal of Medicine*, **48**, 361–367

VELDMAN, J. E., HANADA, T. and MEEUWSEN, F. (1993) Diagnostic and therapeutic dilemmas in rapidly progressive sensorineural hearing loss and sudden deafness. *Acta Otolaryngologica*, **113**, 303–306

VIRTANIEMI, J., LAAKSO, M., KÄRJÄ, J., NUUTINEN, J. and KARJALAINEN, S. (1993) Auditory brainstem latencies in type I (insulin-dependent) diabetic patients. *American Journal of Otolaryngology*, **14**, 413–418

VIRTANIEMI, J., LAAKSO, M., NUUTINEN, J., KARJALAINEN, S. and VARTIAINEN, E. (1994a) Acoustic-reflex responses in patients with insulin-dependent diabetes mellitus. *American Journal of Otolaryngology*, **15**, 109–113

VIRTANIEMI, J., LAAKSO, M., NUUTINEN, J., KARJALAINEN, S. and VARTIAINEN, E. (1994b) Hearing thresholds in insulin-dependent diabetic patients. *Journal of Laryngology and Otology*, **15**, 109–113

VOGT, A. (1906) Frühzeitiges Ergranen der Zilien und Bemerkungen über den sogenannten plötzlichen Eintritt dieser Veränderung. *Klinische Monatsblätter für Augenheilkunde*, **45**, 228–242

VOLLERTSEN, R. S., MCDONALD, T. J., YOUNGE, B. R., BANKS, P.

M., STANSON, A. W. and ILSTRUP, D. M. (1986) Cogan's syndrome: 18 cases and review of the literature. *Mayo Clinic Proceedings*, **611**, 344–361

VYSE, T., LUXON, L. M. and WALPORT, M. J. (1994) Audiovestibular manifestations of the antiphospholipid syndrome. *Journal of Laryngology and Otology*, **108**, 57–59

WACKYM, P. A. and LINTHICUM, F. H. (1986) Diabetes mellitus and hearing loss: clinical and histopathologic relationships. *American Journal of Otology*, **71**, 176–182

WALSH, R. M., MURTY, G. E., PUNT, J. A. G. and O'DONOGHUE, G. M. (1994) Sudden contralateral deafness following cerebellopontine angle tumor surgery. *American Journal of Otology*, **15**, 244–246

WANG, L. P. (1986) Sudden bilateral hearing loss after spinal anaesthesia. *Acta Anaesthesiologica Scandinavica* **30**, 412–413

WANG, L. P., FOG, J. and BOVE, M. (1987) Transient hearing loss following spinal anaesthesia. *Anaesthesia*, **42**, 1258–1263

WATANABE, Y., OHI, H., SHOJAKU, H. and MIZUKOSHI, K. (1994) Sudden deafness from vertebrobasilar artery disorder. *American Journal of Otology*, **15**, 423–426

WEBER, R. S., JENKINS, H. A. and COKER, N. J. (1984) Sensorineural hearing loss associated with ulcerative colitis. *Archives of Otolaryngology*, **110**, 810–812

WEGENER, F. (1936) Über generalisierte septische Gefässerkrankungen. *Verhandlungen der Deutschen Pathologischen Gesellschaft*, **29**, 202–209

WEGENER, F. (1939) Über eine eigenartige rhinogene granulomatose mit besonderer Beteiligung des arteriensystems und der nieren. *Beitrage zür Pathologischen Anatomie und zür Allgemeinen Pathologie*, **109**, 36–68

WEGENER, F. (1990) Wegener's granulomatosis. *European Archives of Otorhinolaryngology*, **247**, 133–142

WELKOBORSKY, H. J. and LOWITZSCH, K (1992) Auditory brain stem responses in patients with human immunotropic virus infection of different stages. *Ear and Hearing*, **13**, 55–57

WELLS, M., MICHAELS, L. and WELLS, D. G. (1977) Otolaryngological disturbances in Waldenstrom's macroglobulinaemia. *Clinical Otolaryngology*, **2**, 327–338

WESTMORE, G. A., PICKARD, B. H. and STERN, H. (1979) Isolation of mumps virus from the inner ear after sudden deafness. *British Medical Journal*, **1**, 14–15

WETMORE, S. J. and ABRAMSON, M. (1979) Bullous myringitis with sensorineural hearing loss. *Otolaryngology – Head and Neck Surgery*, **87**, 66–70

WIEGAND, D. A. and POCH, N. E. (1988) The acoustic reflex in patients with asymptomatic multiple sclerosis. *American Journal of Otolaryngology*, **9**, 210–216

WILHELM, H. J., JUNG, F., KIESEWETTER, H. and RECHTENWALD, C. (1989) Sudden deafness therapy: HES 200/0.5 10% versus dextran 40 in a double-blind study. In: *Sensorineural Hearing Loss and Equilibrium Disturbances*, edited by J. Helms. Stuttgart: Georg Thieme Verlag. pp. 36–40

WILKINS, S. A., MATTOX, D. E. and LYLES, A. (1987) Evaluation of a 'shotgun' regimen for sudden hearing loss. *Otolaryngology – Head and Neck Surgery*, **97**, 474–480

WILSON, W. R. (1986) The relationship of the herpes virus family to sudden hearing loss: a prospective clinical study and literature review. *Laryngoscope*, **96**, 870–877

WILSON, W. R., BYL, F. M. and LAIRD, N. (1980) The efficacy of steroids in the treatment of idiopathic sudden hearing loss. *Archives of Otolaryngology*, **106**, 772–776

WILSON, W. R., LAIRD, N., SOELDNER, J. S., MOO-YOUNG, G., KAVESHI, D. A. and MACMEEL, J. W. (1982) The relationship of idiopathic sudden hearing loss to diabetes mellitus. *Laryngoscope*, **92**, 155–160

WOLFOVITZE, E., LEVY, Y. and BROOK, J. G. (1987) Sudden deafness in a patient with temporal arteritis. *Journal of Rheumatology*, **14**, 384–385

WOLFSON, R. J. and LEIBERMAN, A. (1975) Unilateral deafness with subsequent vertigo. *Laryngoscope*, **85**, 1762–1766

YAGI, N., FISCH, U. and MURATA, K. (1978) Perilymphatic oxygen tension and vasoactive drugs. *Annals of Otology, Rhinology and Laryngology*, **87**, 364–370

YAMAMOTO, M., WATANABE, Y. and MIZUKOSHI, K. (1993) Neurotological findings in patients with acute mumps deafness. *Acta Otolaryngologica*, Supplement 504, 94–97

YAMASOBA, T., KIKUCHI, S., HIGO, R., O'UCHI, T. and TOKUMARU, A. (1993a) Sudden sensorineural hearing loss associated with slow blood flow of the vertebrobasilar system. *Annals of Otology, Rhinology and Laryngology*, **102**, 873–877

YAMASOBA, T., SUGASAWA, M., KIKUCHI, S., YAGI, M. and HARADA, T. (1993b) An electrocochleographic study of acute low tone sensorineural hearing loss. *European Archives of Otorhinolaryngology*, **250**, 418–422

YAMASOBA, T., KIKUCHI, S., SUGASAWA, M., YAGI, M. and HARADA, T. (1994) Acute low-tone sensorineural hearing loss without vertigo. *Archives of Otolaryngology*, **120**, 532–535

YANAGIHARA, N. and ASAI, M. (1993) Sudden hearing loss induced by acoustic neuroma: significance of small tumours. *Laryngoscope*, **103**, 308–311

YANAGITA, N. and MURAHASHI, K. (1987) Bilateral simultaneous sudden deafness. *Archives of Otorhinolaryngology*, **244**, 7–10

YAQUB, B. A., KABIRAJ, M. M., SHAMENA, A., AL-BUNYAN, M., DAIF, A. and TAHAN, A. (1962) Diagnostic role of brain-stem auditory evoked potentials in neurobrucellosis. *Electroencephalography and Clinical Neurophysiology*, **84**, 549–552

YASSIN, A., BADRY, A. and FATT-HI, A. (1970) The relationship between electrolyte balance and cochlear disturbances in cases of renal failure. *Journal of Laryngology and Otology*, **84**, 429–435

YOON, T. H., PAPARELLA, M. and SCHACHERN P. A. (1989) Systemic vasculitis; a temporal bone histopathologic study. *Laryngoscope*, **99**, 600–609

YOUNGS, R., DECK, J., KWOK, P. and HAWKE, M. (1988) Severe sensorineural hearing loss caused by lightning. *Archives of Otolaryngology – Head and Neck Surgery*, **114**, 1184–1187

ZAYTOUN, G. M., SCHUKNECHT, H. F. and FARMER, H. S. (1983) Fatality following the use of low molecular weight dextran in the treatment of sudden deafness. *Advances in Oto-Rhino-Laryngology*, **31**, 240–246

ZEITOUNI, A. G., TEWFIK, T. L. and SCHLOSS, M. (1993) Cogan's syndrome: a review of otologic management and 10-year follow-up of a pediatric case. *Journal of Otolaryngology*, **22**, 337–340

ZHAO, M. H., JONES, S. J. and LOCKWOOD, C. M. (1995) Bactericidal/permeability-increasing protein (BPI) is an important antigen for antineutrophil autoantibodies (ANCA) in vasculitis. *Clinical and Experimental Immunology*, **99**, 49–56

18

Vertigo

A. G. Kerr and J. G. Toner

Vestibular disorders have been considered in depth in Volume 2. However, every day the otolaryngologist is actively involved in the management of patients with vestibular problems and this volume would be incomplete without a chapter on vertigo. This chapter differs from those in Volume 2 in that it takes a more practical, day-to-day look at the problem, omitting much of the detail.

Vertigo tends to be a subject which depresses both patient and doctor. Generally, the patient has difficulty in describing his symptoms and, in the time he has available, the doctor may have difficulty in grasping the picture that the patient is trying to convey.

The patient often feels foolish and thinks that the doctor may be secretly smiling at his naivety in producing these bizarre complaints. On the other hand, the doctor, in approaching this difficult symptom complex, may have a haphazard system, or none at all, and try to make a diagnosis with inadequate information.

Unfortunately, when the conscientious doctor turns to the standard textbooks he may find that he does not get much help. This is not because the information is not available. There are many excellent and comprehensive books on this subject. The problem is that, with few exceptions, the textbooks tend to start with the diagnosis and then give the clinical features. For example, having made a diagnosis of dizziness secondary to vestibulotoxic drugs, there is little difficulty in finding a description of this condition and its management. However, if one starts with the symptoms, but not the diagnosis, it may be necessary to read through most of the textbook to find the appropriate section.

There is only one straightforward way of overcoming this difficulty. That is to start with the detailed symptoms and work backwards through the differential diagnosis to the identification of the underlying problem.

Despite the bizarre histories which one frequently obtains from patients complaining of vertigo, there are certain characteristic patterns. Many of these are consistent with a specific underlying pathology and, obviously, this pathology should be considered in the management of the patient.

Definition of vertigo

The definitions of vertigo which have been given are often as bizarre as the histories given by the patient. Although the Latin root of the word implies a sensation of turning, in general clinical usage of this term a sensation of spinning or turning need not necessarily be implied. Probably the most effective definition is 'a subjective sense of imbalance'. If this contains a sensation of spinning then one can add the adjective 'rotatory' when describing the symptom.

Types of vertigo

The diagnosis of the underlying cause of vertigo is usually made on the basis of the history. Subsequent examination and investigations are normally used to confirm the diagnosis and it is likely that, in 80% of cases, if one does not have an idea of the diagnosis at the end of the history, one is unlikely to have it at the end of the examination and investigations.

Basically, vertigo can be described in one of two ways; either it is rotatory or it is not. If it is rotatory, patients usually have little difficulty in saying so. Where there is no obvious sense of rotation patients have more difficulty in giving a good description. They use various terms but, in essence, the complaint is that they are unsteady. Many will have associated symptoms such as deafness, tinnitus, nausea or vomiting.

Generally speaking, each of the two groups (rotatory or unsteady) can be further subdivided into those where the symptom is episodic and those where it is more or less continuous. When it is episodic it may be very short-lived, i.e. less than a minute, or very much longer, such as hours or days. Consequently, the vast majority of patients with vertigo can be classified as in Table 18.1. It would be naive to expect every patient to fit neatly into any classification but, remarkably, most do. Broadly speaking, each group has a basic underlying pathological correlate which is discussed later in the chapter.

Table 18.1 Classification of vertigo

Rotation
1 Episodic
   a seconds
   b hours

2 Prolonged
   weeks

Unsteadiness
1 Episodic
   a seconds
   b hours to days

2 Prolonged
   weeks to months

A certain degree of licence has been taken in that 15 minutes are equivalent to hours

History

Certain precautions must be observed when taking a history. The first is to ensure that the story given by the patient starts at the onset of the complaint. There is a tendency in any condition which has been going on for some years, for the patient to start the history somewhere other than at the beginning. It is important to establish when the patient was last perfectly steady.

The doctor must control the history-taking. It is through this that he develops a picture of the condition. If he does not have a systematic way of covering all aspects he will get an incomplete picture. If left to their own devices, patients rarely give the complete story because they will emphasize the aspects which have impressed them most. For example, the periods of freedom from vertigo are almost as important as the periods with vertigo, but most patients do not talk about these without prompting.

When seeking a description of the symptoms the patients may need some guidance. One must be care-ful about leading questions, but many patients find it impossible to describe symptoms without help. It is necessary to know the speed of both onset and resolution.

Throughout the history one must ensure that both the patient and the doctor are on the same mental wavelength. For example, many patients will say that they are dizzy 'all the time' when they mean 'frequently', but some are, in truth, dizzy 'all the time'. One can ensure that one has an accurate history by asking the same question in two different ways and confirming that consistent answers come back. If not, one must identify where the misunderstanding has arisen and resolve it.

Finally, the patient may well try to interpret the symptoms himself and the doctor must check that both he and the patient are using the same interpretation.

By and large, the history is best taken chronologically with specific details being sought of the first and of a typical recent attack.

Details must be sought of associated symptoms such as deafness, tinnitus, nausea, vomiting, diplopia, blurring of vision, paraesthesia of the face, headaches, sudden falling and loss of consciousness.

Examination

In an ideal world, every patient complaining of vertigo would have a detailed neurological examination. Clearly, this is not possible in the average busy otolaryngological outpatient department. Even in vertigo clinics, which are desirable in all sizeable units, this is difficult. However, it is usually possible, within a few minutes, to identify those patients who require a detailed neurological examination.

Following a routine ear, nose and throat examination it is usually possible to make a rapid assessment of cranial nerves III to XII, of cerebellar function and the ability to perform balance tests. It is extremely unusual that the need for a detailed neurological assessment will be overlooked if these are all normal and the history does not point to a central lesion. Although olfactory and ophthalmic symptoms may occur in association with vestibular problems, routine examination of these systems is not required unless some aspect of the history points to them. However, every patient with vertigo should be examined for nystagmus (see below, section on nystagmus). During this examination cranial nerves III, IV and VI will automatically be checked. If there is direction changing or vertical nystagmus, a neurological lesion is usually present and a detailed neurological examination is required. Usually a test of the corneal reflex is sufficient for the assessment of the Vth cranial nerve. Weakness of the VIIth cranial nerve will often become apparent simply by looking at the patient while taking the history. A slower blink on the affected side is usually obvious. Very minor weakness of the facial nerve can be detected by the inability of the patient to bury the eyelashes in tight closing of the eyes.

The auditory part of the VIIIth cranial nerve will be tested during the routine examination and subsequent audiogram. The IXth and Xth cranial nerves can be rapidly checked by the gag reflex, the XIth by shrugging the shoulders and, theoretically, the XIIth by having the patient protrude the tongue. Unilateral atrophy of the tongue is a much more reliable sign but apparent only when the paralysis is of long standing. Involvement of the XIIth cranial nerve is uncommon in vertiginous problems which is fortunate as early lesions of this cranial nerve are difficult to detect.

The assessment of balance should have begun when the patient walked into the room. If he walked in steadily there will be no further need to check his walking. A positive Romberg test usually means considerable impairment of function. An extended or tandem Romberg test is more refined. In this the patient is asked to stand in a heel to toe position, first with the eyes open and then closed. One-leg standing, with eyes open or closed, gives a further clarification of balance. In the elderly the significance of these more difficult tests lies often in the exclusion of serious disease when they are performed well.

Nystagmus

Nystagmus is a disturbance of ocular posture, characterized by a more or less rhythmical oscillation of the eyes. The speed of the eye movements may be the same in both directions or may be quicker in one than the other. There is little or no interval between consecutive movements, which may be horizontal, vertical or rotatory.

The posture of the eyes, and consequently the nystagmus, depends on two sets of afferent impulses – visual and vestibular. The visual impulses are concerned with regulation of the position of the eyes in relation to the object of visual interest. It is by means of the vestibular impulses that the position of the eyes is regulated in relation to the position and movements of the head and the remainder of the body. Eye posture is coordinated by a central mechanism that receives these afferent impulses and controls the efferent impulses to the ocular muscles. Nystagmus may result from any lesion involving these afferent pathways, their central connections or, less frequently, the efferent pathways.

There are two broad categories of nystagmus depending upon the appearance of the movements. Pendular nystagmus is characterized by ocular oscillations that are approximately equal in velocity in both directions. These are almost always horizontal. There may be a jerk component on extreme lateral gaze. Phasic, or jerk, nystagmus is characterized by rhyth-

mic oscillations in which the movement in one direction is significantly faster than in the other. Although the slow movement is the pathological one, the fast, or corrective, movement is used to denote the direction of the nystagmus. The position in which the nystagmus is least marked is called the null point.

Examination for nystagmus

Nystagmus found at examination may be either spontaneous or induced.

Spontaneous nystagmus is said to be present when there are rhythmical eye movements on forward gaze. Induced nystagmus is said to be present when rhythmical movements are brought about by some specific test. There is an intermediate nystagmus, or gaze nystagmus, which is demonstrated by altering the gaze to the right or left, or up or down. For the purposes of this discussion intermediate or gaze nystagmus will be considered under the heading of spontaneous nystagmus.

When examining the nystagmus it is essential that the patient is in good light. The object at which the patient is asked to look must be within a comfortable range. Ideally, it should be at infinity but a few feet away will suffice, so that excessive accommodation is not required. Care must be taken that, on looking laterally, the nose does not impinge on the field of vision and on looking upwards, that the object remains comfortably in view. Otherwise, searching or nystagmoid movements may be mistakenly interpreted as nystagmus.

Causes of spontaneous nystagmus

Labyrinthine

Labyrinthine nystagmus, which is phasic, has four main characteristics. It is usually associated with a sensation of vertigo, is always unidirectional, is more marked when looking in the direction of the fast phase, and it is enhanced by removal of fixation by eye closure, Frenzel's glasses or darkness. Following a labyrinthine destructive lesion, the nystagmus decreases with time and clinically has usually disappeared entirely within 4 weeks. However, even then it may still be detected by removal of visual fixation.

Mechanism of vestibular nystagmus

In the normal subject, the tone of the extraocular muscles is to some extent controlled by the vestibular nuclei. The vestibular nuclei tend to drive the eyes to the opposite side. Hence, the vestibular nuclei on the right side influence the left lateral and the right medial rectus muscles, moving the eyes to the left side. Normal ocular posture is maintained by a correct balance between the vestibular nuclei on the two sides.

If there is an abnormality of function of the vestibular nuclei on one side there will be a change in the tone in the corresponding muscles. Consequently, stimulation of the vestibular nuclei on one side will result in movement of the eyes to the opposite side. Unilateral inhibition of the vestibular nuclei will result in movement of the eyes towards that side. The effect is to move the eyes from the point of visual interest. There is then a correcting movement to restore the eyes to the original position. This repeated deviation of the eyes, and repeated correction, is nystagmus.

A destructive lesion involving the right labyrinth, and hence the right vestibular nuclei, will result in slow deviation of the eyes to the right side with the quick correcting movement being to the left side resulting in so-called left beating nystagmus.

In describing unidirectional phasic nystagmus one should state not only the direction, but also the degree. First degree nystagmus is said to be present when phasic eye movements are detected only when looking in the direction of the quick phase. Second degree nystagmus is present when the phasic movements are also seen on looking straight ahead, and third degree even when looking in the direction away from the nystagmus.

The logical nature of this is easy to understand when one considers a specific example. A major lesion resulting in reduced function in the right vestibular nuclei will cause grossly reduced tone in the left lateral and right medial rectus muscles. Consequently, the opposing recti muscles which move the eyes to the right will, in comparison, be so hyperactive that there is a drift of the eyes to the right, even when already looking to the right side. As the disproportion between the two groups of vestibular nuclei diminishes as a result of central nervous system compensation, the nystagmus will slowly reduce to second degree, then first degree, and finally nystagmus only when fixation is removed.

Alexander's law states that, in general, if vestibular nystagmus is present it can be enhanced by moving the eyes in the direction of the fast phase and diminished by moving the eyes in the direction away from the fast phase.

Central nervous system lesions

Nystagmus due to central nervous system lesions presents in a multitude of different forms, some of which are not clearly understood. However, most neurological lesions causing nystagmus produce a bidirectional (direction changing) form. Labyrinthine lesions never do this. Similarly, it has been said that labyrinthine lesions never produce a vertical nystagmus which is therefore always indicative of a central lesion. This is a good general rule but it is not quite

true as excitation of the posterior canal crista, as in benign paroxysmal positional vertigo may cause an upbeat nystagmus, and transection of the posterior ampullary nerve may cause a downbeat nystagmus (Gacek, 1991).

Unidirectional nystagmus which is diminished by removal of fixation or which does not vary in amplitude or velocity in different directions of gaze, is almost certainly of central origin.

Textbooks of neurology and ophthalmology describe rare and bizarre forms of nystagmus, e.g. monocular, involving only one eye, or see-saw, where one eye moves up and the other down. In these and in other central types of nystagmus, most otolaryngologists will wish to seek the opinion of a neurologist!

Toxic

Many drugs including alcohol, barbiturates, tranquillizers and anticonvulsants are potential causes of nystagmus. It is likely that, in most instances, the effects of the drug are on the central nervous system. Indeed, it has been suggested that drugs are the most common cause of vertical nystagmus. However, the positional nystagmus which is associated with alcohol, may well be peripheral in its action. Positional alcoholic nystagmus has two phases, in opposite directions. The first phase occurs shortly after the ingestion of alcohol and passes off after a few hours. The second phase occurs about 8 hours later. It has been suggested that the nystagmus is due to partial replacement by alcohol of water-containing components of the semicircular canal ampullae, followed by later metabolism, each phase resulting in abnormal but opposite impulses.

Ocular

Any lesion affecting the macula, especially where peripheral vision is still maintained, may result in nystagmus which is usually pendular. This may occur in amblyopia. In the past, miners' nystagmus also fell into this category although it has been suggested that neurosis played a part in maintaining the disorder.

Central nervous system lesions affecting the ocular pathways may also result in ocular nystagmus.

Congenital

Congenital nystagmus, which is often familial, is usually horizontal and pendular although it may be phasic (jerk). The null point is close to the position of forward gaze. Unlike that in any other condition, horizontal nystagmus continues even when the eyes are turned upwards. Closure of the eyes results in a marked reduction in the nystagmus but the effects of darkness, with eyes open, are variable and in some instances the nystagmus increases.

In the everyday life of the otolaryngologist, the diagnosis is usually verified by the patient confirming that the nystagmus has been present since as long as he can remember.

Causes of induced nystagmus

Nystagmus may be induced by clinical testing or by certain investigations. The most common clinical test inducing nystagmus is the positional test (Dix-Hallpike manoeuvre). This is useful in diagnosing positional vertigo and differentiating between the common benign paroxysmal positional type and the uncommon positional vertigo of central origin (Table 18.2).

In the fistula test, nystagmus is induced by altering the pressure in the external auditory meatus, producing both nystagmus and a sensation of dizziness. The Tullio phenomenon is a variation of this cause of nystagmus and is induced by acoustic stimuli of high intensity.

Induced nystagmus in clinical investigation is produced by the optokinetic drum, pendulum tracking and caloric and rotational tests.

Oscillopsia is the term which describes the illusion of motion of the environment caused by inadequacy of the vestibular-ocular reflex. During head and body movements images are held steady on the retina by the vestibular-ocular reflex. Patients with reduced peripheral vestibular function or acquired nystagmus often suffer from oscillopsia, those with congenital nystagmus seldom have this problem. One test for oscillopsia involves testing the patient's visual acuity with a Snellen eye chart with the head still, and then during passive high frequency head movements produced by the examiner. A reduction of more than two lines is to be regarded as significant. As oscillopsia is caused by unilateral or bilateral vestibular hypofunction, no treatment is available.

Investigations

The only investigation that is required routinely is an audiogram. By and large, if an air conduction audiogram is normal, no further audiometric tests need be done. However, it is the authors' routine to do an air and bone conduction audiogram and, in addition, a simple speech discrimination assessment (PBmax). There is a danger of over investigation of patients with vertigo, by multiple biochemical screening tests, in an attempt to compensate for ignorance.

Electronystagmography and caloric testing are not routine. Indeed, there are many who claim that the caloric test is of no practical value. The authors disagree with this conclusion but feel that it does not need to be carried out in the majority of vertiginous patients and especially *not* in the elderly.

Radiological investigations and blood examinations are not required routinely. However, in the light of the clinical features, it may be desirable to exclude a vestibular schwannoma or syphilis. The advent of gadolinium-enhanced magnetic resonance imaging has provided access to some additional information on the exact site of the lesion in some cases of vertigo. Enhancement of the vestibular apparatus has been noted on T1-weighted images in some cases, though in practical terms this imaging technique has not altered clinical management apart from enabling retrocochlear lesions to be excluded.

Recently, quantification of the balancing responses

Table 18.2 Comparison of the positional nystagmus of benign paroxysmal vertigo (BPPV) with that of certain lesions of the central nervous system (CNS)

	BPPV	*CNS*
Latent period	A few seconds	Nil
Distress	Present; may be severe with patient clutching at couch or examiner	Nil
Direction of nystagmus	This is usually rotatory and is anticlockwise with the right ear down and clockwise with the left ear down. (When the nystagmus is horizontal it is towards the undermost ear)	Variable
Duration of nystagmus	Less than 30 seconds	Persists while position maintained
On sitting up again	Similar events with nystagmus in opposite direction	Nystagmus stops
Fatiguability	Nystagmus and dizziness stop with repeated testing	Nystagmus persists with repeated testing

Table 18.3 Suggested pathological correlates for the different types of vertigo

Rotation
1 Episodic
  a seconds: short-lived stimulation or depression of the labyrinth
  b hours: metabolic or physiological failure of the labyrinth or central connections
2 Prolonged
  weeks: destructive lesion of the labyrinth or central connections

Unsteadiness
1 Episodic
  a seconds: physiological overload of the vestibular system
  b hours to days: temporary impairment of the central connections or decompensation of the vestibular system
2 Prolonged
  weeks to months: vestibular inadequacy

to induced sways has become possible with force plates. This procedure, called *dynamic posturography*, is being increasingly used in the diagnosis and rehabilitation of those with chronic balance disorders.

Pathological correlates

Table 18.3 shows the suggested pathological correlates for the different types of vertigo.

Rotatory

Short-lived stimulation or depression of the labyrinth

Episodic rotatory vertigo, lasting for only seconds, would be expected from short-lived depression or stimulation of one of the labyrinths or its central connections. The main causes of such vertigo are benign paroxysmal positional vertigo, labyrinthine fistula, the caloric effect and alternobaric vertigo (Table 18.4). Also included in this group, although not in such pure form, are the post-concussional syndrome, vertebrobasilar insufficiency, cervical vertigo and the Coriolis phenomenon which results from stimulation of another pair of semicircular canals while the first pair is still being stimulated.

Table 18.4 Short-lived episodic rotatory vertigo

Benign paroxysmal positional vertigo
Labyrinthine fistula
Caloric effect
Alternobaric vertigo
Post-concussional syndrome
Vertebrobasilar insufficiency
Cervical vertigo
Coriolis phenomenon

These short-lived episodic types of vertigo can recur frequently, many times each day, depending on the frequency of the stimulus.

Metabolic failure of the labyrinth

The episodic types of vertigo lasting from a few minutes to less than 24 hours, are due to a physiological or metabolic failure of the labyrinth (Table 18.5). They include Menière's disease, syphilitic labyrinthitis and other types of endolymphatic hydrops of immediate or delayed onset. Also included in this group are decompensation of a previously compensated lesion and the dizziness which may occur in the first 24 hours after middle ear surgery.

Metabolic failure and recovery can recur frequently but not as often as the short-lived attacks.

Table 18.5 Metabolic failure

Menière's disease
Syphilitic labyrinthitis
Delayed endolymphatic hydrops
Decompensation of previous vestibular lesion
Following middle ear surgery

Destructive lesions

Prolonged rotatory vertigo, lasting for more than 24 hours and usually for less than 3–4 weeks, can be expected when there is some destruction of the labyrinth or the central connections (Table 18.6). This is a large disparate group where the clinical picture is of severe incapacitating rotatory vertigo associated with nausea and vomiting.

Table 18.6 Destructive lesions

Vestibular neuronitis
Trauma
    head injury
    ear surgery
    labyrinthectomy
    vestibular neurectomy
Labyrinthitis
    bacterial
    viral
Vascular lesions
Metastatic deposits in cerebellopontine angle

Vestibular neuronitis, bacterial or viral labyrinthitis and vascular lesions of the inner ear fall into this group (see Figure 5.30). Traumatic lesions, either accidental as in head injury or inexpert ear surgery, or planned as in labyrinthectomy or vestibular neurectomy, are also included in this group. A rare but definite clinical entity is metastatic malignant disease in the cerebellopontine angle, from lesions in the breast, kidney, lung and prostate gland (see Figure 5.43).

In many cases of naturally occurring destructive lesions the damage is incomplete and therefore similar vertiginous episodes may recur. A destructive lesion cannot recur if it is complete. The central neurological compensation which follows such lesions may, however, break down in the future as a result of stress or some intercurrent illness.

Unsteadiness

In those patients with unsteadiness, the picture is usually not quite so clear-cut. However, it still bears some attempt at pathological classification.

Physiological overload

The unsteadiness that lasts for only seconds can be due to a physiological overload of the vestibular or central processing systems (Table 18.7). The central processor deals with impulses, not only from the labyrinth, but also from the visual and proprioceptive systems. If the central processing system is overloaded, imbalance will be experienced. This may occur for any one of three reasons. First, there may be excessive input, as can happen in a normal person with very rapid movements. Second, it may occur as a result of abnormal input, especially from the visual apparatus. Third, it may result from minor inadequacies in the visual, proprioceptive or labyrinthine systems, when the central processor cannot keep pace with all the signals that are arriving, so that short-lived unsteadiness occurs.

Table 18.7 Physiological overload of central processor

Rapid movement
Abnormal input – especially visual
Minor inadequacies
    visual
    vestibular
    proprioceptive

In young people, this is seen in the later stages of recovery from the post-concussional syndrome or benign paroxysmal positional vertigo. It may also be seen in those who have compensated for a destructive labyrinthine lesion. It is probably seen most often in the elderly, in such activities as rising quickly to the feet or turning rapidly. The dizziness is usually only momentary.

By its nature, this short-lived unsteadiness can occur many times each day.

Temporary impairment or decompensation

The unsteadiness which lasts from hours to days may be due to temporary impairment of the central vestibular connections or decompensation of the vestibular system (Table 18.8). Drugs are a common cause of the temporary impairment. They may be self-inflicted as in drug overdose or alcohol. They may be iatrogenic where drugs such as tranquillizers or anticonvulsants are used which, even in normal therapeutic dosage, can cause unsteadiness. Travel sickness also produces unsteadiness and is included in this category.

Table 18.8 Temporary impairment or decompensation

Drugs
    self-inflicted
    iatrogenic
Travel sickness
Perilymph fistula
Active chronic suppurative otitis media
Decompensation of pre-existing lesion
Hyperventilation
Functional

It is difficult to categorize the dizziness due to perilymph fistula, but it can reasonably be inserted here, even though the unsteadiness may persist for weeks or months. Similarly, the unsteadiness sometimes seen in active chronic suppurative otitis media, which resolves with control of the infection, can also be included here. When it is prolonged it falls into the next category.

The unsteadiness due to stress, both in normal subjects and in those where decompensation of a pre-existing lesion occurs, can also be included. This may be precipitated by hyperventilation.

Vestibular inadequacy

Prolonged unsteadiness, lasting for weeks or months, is usually due to vestibular inadequacy (Table 18.9). This is most often seen in the elderly. It may also be seen in the group who continue to take the offending drugs, usually unaware that they are the cause of any unsteadiness. Vestibulotoxic drugs such as gentamicin or streptomycin, which cause permanent damage to the labyrinth also produce this problem.

Table 18.9 Vestibular inadequacy

The elderly
Drugs
    metabolic effect, e.g. anticonvulsants
    destructive effect, e.g. gentamicin
Central nervous system lesions
'Floating females'
Toxic products from chronic middle ear infections

There are many central nervous system lesions producing chronic vestibular inadequacy but, usually, these are accompanied by other neurological symptoms or signs which indicate the nature of the problem and point to the site of the lesion. Large unilateral or smaller bilateral vestibular schwannomas fall into this group.

There is a large group of patients whose dizziness is thought to be psychogenic and who have in the past been categorized somewhat unsympathetically as 'floating females'. These patients need not necessarily be female! On examination and caloric testing they are normal so that they are not, technically, suffering from any identifiable vestibular inadequacy. However, the unsteadiness may persist for months. Remarkably, this rarely interferes with everyday activities.

Head trauma

Head trauma causes such a diversity of vertigo that it is an aetiological factor in many of the tables. The six different causes of vertigo following head trauma are listed in Table 18.10.

Table 18.10 Vertigo following head injury

Post-concussional syndrome
Benign paroxysmal positional vertigo
Destructive labyrinthine lesion
Perilymph fistula
Delayed endolymphatic hydrops
Functional

The principles of treatment

One of the persisting difficulties in assessing any treatment plan for vertigo is the lack of a simple, reliable and repeatable objective means of assessing the degree of handicap. There have been several attempts at producing vertigo scales and handicap inventories but these have proven either too cumbersome or not sufficiently reproducible for routine clinical use.

In the management of vertigo there are certain basic principles which can be applied to most conditions. Once enumerated they appear to be basic common sense, but then that applies to much of medicine.

Treat or eliminate the cause

Treating or eliminating the cause is a perfectly obvious way of dealing with any problem. Unfortunately, many of the causes of vertigo are either untreatable with our present knowledge or irreversible by the time the patient presents and consequently this mode of management is not always applicable.

Suppress the vestibular system

In labyrinthine vertigo, the sensation of dizziness is due to a disproportion between the activity in the two sets of vestibular nuclei. In an acute labyrinthine destructive lesion, the more or less equal and opposite activity in the vestibular nuclei is lost. In an effort to correct this, the cerebellum imposes an attempt at a shut down of electrical activity in the vestibular nuclei, the so-called 'cerebellar clamp'. This reduces the disproportion between the two sides. This can be augmented by the use of labyrinthine sedative drugs including cinnarazine, cyclizine, dimenhydrinate and prochlorperazine. These drugs are of particular value in acute situations, including travel sickness, not only reducing dizziness but also exercising an antiemetic effect. Diazepam also is a potent labyrinthine sedative drug and has, in addition, anxiolytic properties.

Two notes of caution need to be sounded. First, these drugs may not only delay central compensation but can make it incomplete and therefore they should be used for only a few days and certainly no longer than a week when there is a destructive lesion. Second, in dizziness due to vestibular inadequacy, as in the elderly, these labyrinthine sedative drugs will simply increase the unsteadiness.

Suppress the patient's emotional reaction

Vertigo is a most distressing symptom, especially if it is accompanied by vomiting and is occurring in a random and unpredictable manner. There are few patients who do not develop some emotional reaction to severe, episodic labyrinthine vertigo. This may result in aggravation of the symptoms as it may disturb even further the dysequilibrium between the two sets of vestibular nuclei.

These patients need strong reassurance both about the nature of their dizziness and the prognosis. In addition, a short period of suppression of the emotional reaction with a mild tranquillizer may be desirable. However, it is important to be alert to the possibility that the central effects of tranquillizers, especially in high dosage, can aggravate the dizziness.

Wait for compensation

Nature has a marvellous way of compensating for any imbalance, not least in the activity of the vestibular nuclei. In the early stages there is the 'cerebellar clamping' of the activity of the vestibular nuclei. In time, spontaneous activity is generated in the affected vestibular nuclei with gradual restoration of comfortable balance. Thus, following a labyrinthectomy in a young person, the simple passage of time may result in a return of balance function which is normal for most everyday activities. In peripheral lesions, time tends to be on our side. Unfortunately, this is not so common with the dizziness due to lesions of the central nervous system. In many instances the process of compensation can be accelerated by the performance of Cawthorne-Cooksey exercises (see Chapter 12, Appendix 12.1).

Eliminate the offending labyrinth

Although nature can compensate readily for the complete loss of function of a labyrinth, it may have some difficulty in compensating for incomplete loss and will have considerable difficulty in compensating for fluctuating loss. Labyrinthectomy, or vestibular nerve section, may be the treatment of choice in any condition where labyrinthine function is fluctuating or where nature has failed to compensate, despite the passage of an adequate length of time. Unfortunately, labyrinthectomy always, and vestibular nerve section occasionally, results in loss of all auditory function in the affected ear.

Acceptance of the problem

There are some conditions where, despite the application of the appropriate methods of management outlined above, there is persisting imbalance. It is desirable that the physician should understand the prognosis and, where appropriate, explain to the patient that some degree of imbalance will have to be accepted. With the explanation, appropriate aids should be recommended. A walking stick is the first and most obvious but it is often overlooked. Very often this is all that is required to restore the patient's confidence and enable the resumption of reasonably normal everyday activity. In severe cases a walking frame and strategically placed hand rails will be needed.

Surgery for vertigo

It is only occasionally that surgery has any part to play in the management of vertigo. Most conditions where surgery is indicated have been discussed elsewhere in this volume.

In Menière's disease, surgery may be seen as first, correcting the underlying problem, e.g. saccus decompression or cervical sympathectomy; second, having a metabolic or even non-specific effect, e.g. saccus decompression or 'cortical mastoidectomy'; or third, ablating all vestibular function in an offending labyrinth, such as vestibular neurectomy or labyrinthectomy.

The management of labyrinthine fistulae is discussed in the section on chronic suppurative otitis media (see Chapter 12). Active chronic suppurative otitis media may be associated with vague imbalance, even in the absence of a labyrinthine fistula. It is possibly due to the absorption of toxins or an enhanced caloric effect. Although the mechanism is obscure, the alleviation of the unsteadiness is often dramatic when the infection is dealt with by either open or closed cavity techniques.

When a labyrinthectomy is carried out in the presence of an open cavity, there may be persisting imbalance, thought to be due to stimulation of vestibular nerve endings. Subsequent vestibular nerve section may be necessary to control this unsteadiness.

Any incomplete destructive lesion of the labyrinth may be followed by persistent vertigo. In some cases this may be due to delayed endolymphatic hydrops. A complete drill-out (bony) labyrinthectomy, or even a vestibular nerve section, may be required.

Perilymph fistulae are discussed in Chapter 7.

The surgery of benign paroxysmal positional vertigo deserves special mention as this is not considered elsewhere. This condition tends to be self-limiting and is only rarely sufficiently severe to warrant surgery. Spontaneous resolution may be enhanced by several recently described manoeuvres which are described in Volume 2, Chapter 22.

Initial reports suggest that these may be simple and effective forms of management which will hasten resolution in many cases. However, in the small proportion of patients whose daily life has become crippled by dizziness, or whose symptoms have persisted for some years, surgery may be indicated.

Gacek first described section of the posterior ampullary nerve for this condition and recently has reported on the results of over a hundred cases (Gacek, 1991). In this difficult procedure, the posterior ampullary, or singular nerve, is exposed via the middle ear. The bone overhanging the round window membrane is removed. Drilling of the bone inferior to the round window membrane will expose the nerve at a depth of 1–2 mm. The nerve is divided with a hook and the canal sealed with absorbable gelatin sponge. Unfortunately in a small proportion of patients the nerve is inaccessible under the basal turn of the cochlea.

The main risk of this procedure is sensorineural hearing loss, which occurs in about 10% of patients. There is also the risk of opening into the labyrinth, causing persistent unsteadiness. Very infrequently, a cerebrospinal fluid leak may occur from the singular canal. This is a difficult procedure which is only rarely indicated, but, in experienced and competent hands, produces excellent results.

A technically less demanding procedure has recently been advocated by Parnes and McClure (1990). This procedure involves a transmastoid approach to the posterior semicircular canal. The canal is blue-lined and then curetted to produce a 2–3 mm fenestration leaving the membranous labyrinth intact; occlusion of the posterior semicircular canal is performed with bone paté. This technique should be within the competence of most experienced otologists, and initial reports suggest excellent control of the positional vertigo with reduced risk to hearing and the facial nerve.

References

GACEK, R. R. (1991) Singular neurectomy update. Review of 102 cases. *Laryngoscope*, **101**, 855–862

PARNES, L. S. and MCCLURE, J. A. (1990) Posterior semicircular canal occlusion for intractible benign paroxysmal positional vertigo. *Annals of Otology, Rhinology and Laryngology*, **99**, 330–334

19

Menière's disease

David A. Moffat and Robert H. Ballagh

Menière's disease has fascinated generations of physicians who have struggled to understand and explain the various features of this entity. Even Menière himself could not have anticipated that the disease which bears his name would prove to be so enigmatic. The world literature on Menière's disease has become vast, and continues to grow (Dickins and Graham, 1990). Over 3000 citations for Menière's disease have been added to the *Index Medicus* in the past three decades. Despite this, controversy exists in almost every aspect of this disease. The study of 'Menierology' (Torok, 1983) must therefore involve a healthy scepticism, and requires the student of the subject to separate what is fact from what is purely conjecture. The amount of proven scientific knowledge is embarassingly small, and many questions remain unanswered. This has resulted in widely varying views within the specialty regarding the nature of this disease, its pathophysiology and its precise diagnosis and treatment.

History

In 1861, Dr Prosper Menière (Figure 19.1) described a series of similarly afflicted patients in a series of six articles (1861a,b,c,d,e,f). An excellent English translation of these papers exists (Atkinson, 1961) and provides an interesting insight into the man and the medical philosophy of the time. Earlier, in 1848, Menière had been the translator of a book on diseases of the ear by Kramer in which the account of the patient whose temporal bone he later reported can be read. A condition characterized by recurrent episodes of vertigo, hearing loss, and tinnitus of sudden onset is described. These symptoms had previously been ascribed to a condition called 'apoplectic cerebral congestion' (Trousseau, 1861), a form of threatened

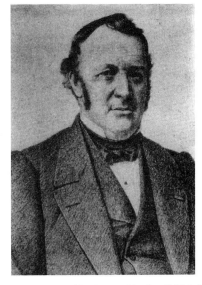

Figure 19.1 Portrait of Dr Prosper Menière (1799–1862)

or actual intracranial haemorrhage and a condition which was treated by bleeding, leeching and purging. Menière was aware of experimental work performed on the inner ear by Flourens in 1842. In a study designed to look at the effect of destruction of the hearing apparatus on the behaviour of birds, the horizontal semicircular canals of pigeons were sectioned. The birds were then noted to have strong rhythmic movements of the head and neck, unusual eye movements, and they were unable to fly. It was concluded that the inner ear contained an apparatus involved in controlling body equilibrium. Menière was the first to suggest that the symptom complex he was seeing in his patients was due to a disturbance of the inner ear, a suggestion which has led to the lasting association of his name with the disorder and his recognition as one of the great pioneers of nineteenth century otology.

Even the correct spelling of his name has evoked controversy. The man himself signed all his correspondence and papers 'Meniere', and this is the preferred spelling of most current authors (Atkinson, 1961; Colman, 1987). Curiously, after his death, his family published his memoirs with the spelling 'Ménière', and used the same name to decorate his tomb in Paris, a situation which has led to the use of this alternative spelling in the medical literature ever since. It may be that the family were not unduly concerned about the exact spelling since the name Meniere on the outside of the family grave in the Montmartre cemetery in Paris does not have any accents!

In 1927, Guild produced the first description of the longitudinal flow of endolymph, accurately identifying the stria vascularis as the principal source of endolymph and the endolymphatic sac as the site of endolymphatic 'outflow'. One year prior to this, following a fascinating series of experiments on the elasmobranch fishes, Dr Georges Portmann published a paper documenting the first endolymphatic sac drainage operation for the treatment of vertigo. His studies of patients with Menière's triad of symptoms led him to believe that the entity was due to intralabyrinthine hypertension, a form of 'auricular glaucoma', and he reported improvement in symptoms following his drainage operation (Portmann, 1926, 1927a,b). In 1928, Dandy described his successful experience in treating Menière's disease in nine patients by sectioning the VIIIth cranial nerve, an operation first suggested and performed for this indication by Parry in 1904.

Endolymphatic hydrops, the principal pathological feature of Menière's disease, was first described by Hallpike and Cairns in 1938. They demonstrated the increased volume of endolymph in the scala media in two patients afflicted by this disorder. The first opportunity to visualize the pathology was provided by the death, from postoperative complications, of both patients shortly after VIIIth nerve section procedures intended to treat the symptoms of Menière's disease. In the same year Yamakawa (Yamakawa, 1938; Yamakawa and Naito, 1954) independently described this pathological entity. The finding of endolymphatic hydrops was confirmed in subsequent examinations by Hallpike and Wright (1940), Lindsay (1942), Altmann and Fowler (1943), and Brunner (1948). In 1952, Tasaki and Fernandez caused cochlear paralysis by instilling artificial endolymph into the perilymph-containing part of the inner ear, a result which would lead to the addition of the membrane rupture theory to the explanation of the pathophysiology of Menière's disease.

Kimura and Schuknecht produced the first consist-

ent and reproducible animal model of endolymphatic hydrops in 1965 by obliterating the endolymphatic duct and sac of the guinea-pig. In repeating and confirming this original observation, Kimura (1967) discovered that he could induce membranous hydrops following a variety of traumatic insults to the endolymphatic duct and sac, but unfortunately none of the animals developed any signs of vestibular dysfunction after 14 months' observation. A true animal model of Menière's disease itself has thus proved elusive, a situation which continues to frustrate research into this disease.

In studying the history of this disorder, it is interesting to consider that some famous historical figures may have suffered its symptoms, even before the disease was formally described. A review of the papers and personal descriptions of Vincent Van Gogh have recently led some to suggest that he suffered from this condition (Arenberg *et al.*, 1991). It is thought that the severe symptoms of uncontrolled Menière's disease caused his psychological turmoil and finally, his famous episode of auricular amputation.

Definitions of terms in Menière's disease

The lack of clear definitions and uniformity in Menière's disease has led to misunderstanding and confusion in the past. As a result, in 1972, the American Academy of Ophthalmology and Otolaryngology Committee on Equilibrium defined Menière's disease as follows: 'a disease of the membranous inner ear characterized by deafness, vertigo, and usually tinnitus, which has as its pathologic correlate hydropic distension of the endolymphatic system' (Alford, 1972). The additional symptom of aural fullness is often added to the current definition. Except for a few refinements, little has changed in the classical description of Menière's disease since his original report. Owing to its long-standing clinical usage, the designation 'Menière's disease' has achieved a time-honoured place in the medical nomenclature. However, ambiguities in the use of the term have arisen, particularly as it is sometimes used in diagnosis as an umbrella term for symptoms of vertigo (Balkany, Pillsbury and Arenberg, 1980).

Confusion about whether to describe the disorder as a 'disease' or a 'syndrome' has resulted from a lack of understanding of the causation of the symptom complex. The term 'Menière's syndrome' implies that this group of symptoms occurs together but is the result of diverse aetiologies. This term has been abandoned in favour of the term 'Menière's disease' for simplicity and uniformity (Williams, 1968; Alford, 1972). The expression 'endolymphatic hydrops' is often employed but is unacceptable because although it is the chief histopathological finding in Menière's disease, it is present in other diseases. Pfalz and Thomsen (1986) quite correctly cautioned against using this term to define the disorder because the cause and effect relationship between endolymphatic hydrops and the clinical findings remains unclear. The term 'secondary endolymphatic hydrops' is now used to describe this pathological feature when it is caused by another disease such as syphilis.

Variations in the clinical presentation of patients with some but not all of the features of Menière's disease has resulted in the definition of subtypes of the disorder. 'Atypical Menière's disease' is a term which has been suggested to describe patients who complain of some but not all of the classical symptoms of the triad (Schessel and Nedzelski, 1993). The terms 'cochlear' and 'vestibular' Menière's disease are terms which have been introduced in the past to describe patients who complain of auditory or vestibular symptoms only (Alford, 1972; Pfalz and Thomsen, 1986). The former is thought to relate to endolymphatic hydrops of the pars inferior and the latter to hydrops confined to the pars superior. It has been suggested by the Hearing and Equilibrium Committee of the American Academy of Otolaryngology – Head and Neck Surgery that these terms be discarded for simplicity (Pearson and Brackmann, 1985). The terms 'atypical Menière's disease' and 'recurrent vestibulopathy' are suggested as preferable because they more appropriately describe the clinical and pathophysiological nature of these two disorders (Wallace and Barber, 1983; Schessel and Nedzelski, 1993).

Two additional variants of Menière's disease are recognized and thought to be due to endolymphatic hydrops. 'Lermoyez syndrome' is a term describing characteristic sudden sensorineural hearing loss which improves during or immediately after the attack of vertigo (Lermoyez, 1919). 'Tumarkin's otolithic catastrophe' or 'drop attack Menière's disease' is a variant which features abrupt falling attacks of brief duration without loss of consciousness (Tumarkin, 1936; Baloh, Jacobson and Winder, 1990).

Incidence

The estimates of the incidence of Menière's disease in the world literature vary significantly. In Great Britain, Cawthorne and Hewlett (1954) reported an incidence of 1 per 636 persons per year, or 157 per 100 000 population. Harrison and Naftalin (1968) reported an incidence in the UK of 0.1%, or 100 per 100 000. In Sweden, in a study examining hospital discharge and outpatient data on a population of over two million, the incidence of Menière's disease was found to be 46 per 100 000 (Stahle, Stahle and Arenberg, 1978). In France, Michel, Fouillet and Trovero (1977) have indicated an incidence of only 7.5 per 100 000. In Japan, the incidence of Menière's disease appears to have increased dramatically since the Second World War (Watanabe, 1981). In Africa, the diagnosis of Menière's disease is uncommon, de-spite the fact that vertigo is a common presenting complaint (Watanabe, 1983). Estimates of the prevalence of Menière's disease are even more difficult to obtain than incidence figures. In view of its nature as a non-lethal non-communicable disease, inadequate public health records exist in most countries. Based on the Swedish study, however, conservative estimates and data indicate that Menière's disease is at least four times more common than clinical otosclerosis (Arenberg *et al.*, 1980). Clinically, Menière's disease is responsible for 10% of visits to a busy dizziness unit in a tertiary referral centre (Nedzelski, Barber, and McIlmoyl, 1986).

A *racial variation* has been suggested in the past, but in a large survey, Kitahara, Futaki and Nakano (1971) concluded that the incidence is the same in Caucasians and Blacks, and that the frequency of associated symptoms such as nausea and headache is the same for American whites as for Japanese patients. Menière's disease is rare in the south western American Indian population (Pfalz and Thomsen, 1986).

A *sexual preponderance* in Menière's disease has been suggested by the work of some authors. In Sweden, Stahle, Stahle and Arenberg (1978) found a female preponderance in a ratio of 3:2. In Japan, a 3:2 male preponderance in a data survey from 1934 to 1960 disappeared when the survey was more rigorously repeated in 1981 by Watanabe. Balkany, Pillsbury and Arenberg (1980) found no sexual preponderance, nor did Paparella (1985). The right and left ears are affected with equal frequency.

A *familial tendency* has been described in Menière's disease, with a positive family history in up to 20% (Paparella, 1985). Birgerson, Gustavson and Stahle (1987) found that 14% of affected patients had a first order relative with the disorder, including a family with three generations of Menière's disease and another with an aberration in chromosome 7. It is generally felt that, while genetic transmission may play a role in Menière's disease, transmission is variable and inheritance is multifactorial (Paparella, 1985).

The *age at onset* of symptoms is extremely variable. Menière's disease in children under the age of 10 years is rare, with the youngest case described in a four year old. The disease begins in most patients before the age of 60 years (Thomas and Harrison, 1971; Greven and Oosterveld, 1975; Stahle, Stahle and Arenberg 1978) with a noticeable peak in incidence in the fifth and sixth decades of life (Oosterveld, 1980).

The *frequency of bilateral Menière's disease* ranges from 2 to 78% in the literature (Balkany, Sizes and Arenberg, 1980; Green, Blum and Harner, 1991). The difficulties that may give rise to this wide range are the lack of consensus about the diagnostic criteria and the length of time Menière's disease patients should be followed up for the development of contralateral disease. In the largest study, a British survey of 610 patients with Menière's disease followed for at least 5 years found that the incidence of bilateral disease was 31.8% (Thomas and Harrison, 1971). Rosenberg *et al.* (1991) found that 72% of patients who developed bilateral Menière's disease did so within 5 years of diagnosis in the first ear. Interestingly they found that the incidence of bilateral Menière's disease was 17% in medically treated patients and significantly lower at 5.9% (P < 0.01) in surgically treated patients. Friberg, Stahle and Svedberg (1984) reported an incidence of 47% in 34 patients who were followed for 20 years, and showed a relationship between incidence and follow-up observation time. Kitahara (1991) found a 9% incidence in the first year of follow up and 41% when the patients had been observed for more than 20 years. It is now generally agreed that the incidence of bilateral disease increases continuously over time (Paparella and Griebie, 1984; Stahle 1991). Subclinical Menière's disease may exist in the second ear long before the development of overt symptoms (Moffat *et al.*, 1992). Greven and Oosterveld (1975) found 10% of 292 patients had developed classical Menière's disease in the second ear, but that 73% of the patients in this group had signs of hearing disturbance in the second ear, such as sensorineural hearing loss, recruitment, or tinnitus. Paparella and Griebie (1984) studied 360 patients the same way and obtained numbers of 32% and 78.6% respectively. More compelling are recent results using transtympanic electrocochleography, the only proven investigation that can demonstrate objectively the presence of endolymphatic hydrops. Electrophysiological evidence of hydrops was seen in 35% of second ears in a population of 40 patients with unilateral clinical Menière's disease (Moffat *et al.*, 1992). The early recognition of incipient Menière's disease in the asymptomatic contralateral ear of a patient with known unilateral disease has profound implications for patient management and follow up. The high frequency of bilateral disease dictates that, when considering therapeutic options, every attempt should be made to conserve hearing.

Pathophysiology

Menière's disease appears to be one member of a group of disorders of the inner ear linked by the common pathophysiological condition of endolymphatic hydrops (Hallpike and Cairns, 1938; Altmann and Kornfeld, 1965; Antoli-Candela, 1976; Schuknecht and Igarashi, 1986). Endolymphatic hydrops is thought to be a pathological condition that is the end result of a variety of insults to the inner ear, and may be subdivided into symptomatic and asymptomatic forms. This was further subclassified by Schuknecht and Gulya in 1983 (Table 19.1). The

Table 19.1 Classification of endolymphatic hydrops

Symptomatic	Asymptomatic
Embryopathic	Embryopathic
Acquired	Acquired
postinflammatory	postinflammatory
post-traumatic	post-traumatic
Idiopathic	Idiopathic

From Schuknecht and Gulya, 1983

symptomatic form is characterized by the classical triad of fluctuating sensorineural hearing loss, episodic vertigo and, usually, tinnitus and the asymptomatic form is clinically silent (Rauch, Merchant and Tuedinger, 1989). The acute attacks of the symptomatic form are superimposed on a gradual progressive reduction in the auditory and vestibular functions of the affected ear over time.

Endolymphatic hydrops is a physical distortion in the membranous labyrinth. Since the original report of endolymphatic hydrops by Hallpike and Cairns (1938) and Yamakawa (1938), 134 temporal bone cases have been reported (Paparella, 1985). Cochlear hydrops was seen in all cases and saccular hydrops was seen in most. Utricular hydrops was uncommon. Endolymphatic hydrops therefore was observed most consistently in the pars inferior (Altmann and Kornfeld, 1965; Schuknecht and Igarashi, 1986; Okuno and Sando, 1987) and could be identified by the typical bowing of Reissner's membrane and distension of the saccule (Schuknecht, 1974) (Figure 19.2). Enlargement of the endolymphatic space clearly occurred at the expense of the perilymphatic space (Antoli-Candela, 1976; Klis, Buijs and Smoorenburg, 1990). The degree of endolymphatic space expansion was variable. The endolymphatic space bulged in the region of the helicotrema in half of the cases, while the saccule bulged against the footplate in 60% of

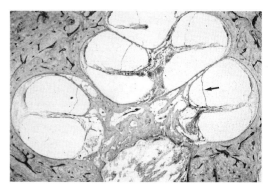

Figure 19.2 Histopathology of endolymphatic hydrops demonstrating gross distension of Reissner's membrane (black arrow)

the cases reviewed by Paparella (1985) and into a semicircular canal (usually the horizontal semicircular canal) in about one-third of cases. Fibrous adhesions can form between the saccule and the undersurface of the stapedial footplate (Issa *et al.*, 1983). This contact may explain Hennebert's sign, which is subjective vertigo and tonic eye deviation and nystagmus observed during a pressure-induced excursion of the footplate (Nadol, 1977). It may also explain the 'Tullio phenomenon' which is experienced by some Menière's patients, namely a subjective imbalance and nystagmus observed in response to loud, low frequency noise exposure (Tullio, 1938; Ishizaki *et al.*, 1991) (Figure 19.3).

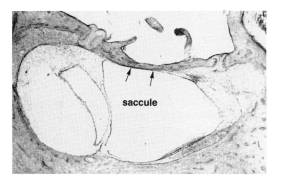

Figure 19.3 Marked hydrops of the saccule. Saccular wall has attached to footplate of the stapes (arrows). (From Nomura *et al.*, Modality of endolymphatic hydrops, Figure 4, In: *Menière's Disease. Proceedings of the Second International Symposium*, 1988, edited by J. B. Nadol. Amsterdam: Kugler & Ghedini Publications. Reproduced with kind permission)

Changes in the pars superior (utricle and semicircular canals) are observed less frequently and are less dramatic, and more likely to be seen in cases of longstanding Menière's disease. Utricular dilatation and herniation into the crus commune has been observed (Lindsay, 1942), as well as ampullary distortion and displacement of the cupula from the ampullary wall (Antoli-Candela, 1976; Rizvi, 1986).

Interestingly, despite the progressive decline in auditory and vestibular function witnessed in these patients over the years, there is relative sparing of hair cells and the first order neurons in this disease. Only in the most severe cases will these structures show damage and a depletion in numbers (Schuknecht and Igarashi, 1986; Schuknecht, Suzuka and Zimmerman,1990) (Figure 19.4).

Endolymph is derived predominantly from the stria vascularis; the planum semilunatum and dark vestibular cells contribute a small amount. Endolymph may also be produced from perilymph across the labyrinthine membranes (Paparella, 1985). The circulation of endolymph is both radial and longitudinal (Lawrence, 1980) (Figure 19.5). The *longitudinal pattern* starts with the production of endolymph in the stria vascularis of the cochlea, circulation via the scala media occurs through the ductus reuniens to the saccular duct, where it proceeds into the vestibular labyrinth. Elimination of endolymph occurs via circulation through the vestibular aqueduct and on to the endolymphatic sac, where it is absorbed. *Radial flow* results from the production of endolymph in the dark vestibular cells and planum semilunatum with local absorption. The evidence strongly suggests that both longitudinal (slow process) and radial (rapid process)

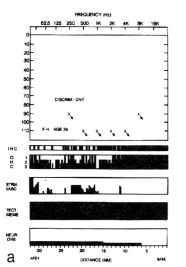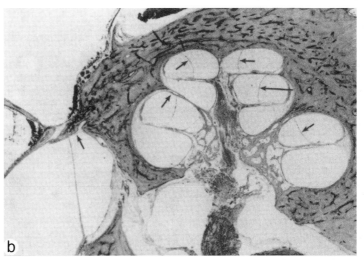

Figure 19.4 (*a*) Audiogram and cytocochleogram. There is near-total loss of hair cells in the basal half and about 50% loss in the apical half of the cochlea. Tectorial membrane is totally non-functional. (*b*) Moderately severe hydrops of cochlear duct and saccule (arrows). (Reproduced with kind permission of Professor Schuknecht)

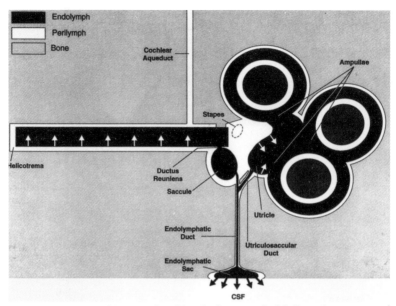

Figure 19.5 Schematic representation of the normal cochlear fluid spaces. The labelling of structures such as the utricle and saccule is by an arrow to the endolymphatic part of these strucures. The rectangular structure at the left represents the cochlea. The white arrows indicate where endolymph is thought to be secreted based on the presence of dark cells. The black arrows indicate where endolymph is thought to be resorbed. Abnormalities in endolymph formation or absorption would lead to endolymphatic hydrops which would be represented by distension of the black spaces in this figure. (Reproduced from Kiang, N. Y. S., 1989, An auditory physiologist's view of Menière's syndrome. In: *Second International Symposium on Menière's Disease*, edited by J. B. Nadol. Amsterdam: Kugler & Ghedini. pp. 13–24, with kind permission)

circulations are concurrently operational and subject to both hydrostatic and osmotic pressure gradients.

Endolymphatic hydrops occurs through the accumulation of endolymph, either through its overproduction (Henriksson, Gleissner and Johansson, 1986) or through its inadequate absorption. The prevalent theory is that the fundamental problem is one of longitudinal flow, specifically endolymphatic malabsorption, with the site of this dysfunction being the endolymphatic sac or duct (Schuknecht, 1968; Paparella, 1985). This concept is supported by several studies in which endolymphatic hydrops has been induced by injury and disruption of the endolymphatic sac in guinea-pigs, rabbits and cats. The successful mechanisms of this injury include mechanical means (Kimura and Schuknecht, 1965; Beal, 1968; Horner, Erre and Cazals, 1989), chemical cauterization (Yazawa, Shea and Kitahara, 1985), viral inoculation and infection (Fukuda, Keithley and Harris, 1988), or by an immunologically induced inflammatory response (Yoo, 1984; Sawada *et al.*, 1987; Tomiyama, 1992). Despite this, the hydrops which is histologically identified in these animal models has not resulted in the clinical presentation of the symptoms of Menière's disease experienced in humans.

Even in the normal ear there are enormous variations in the surgical anatomy of the endolymphatic sac (Friberg *et al.*, 1988) (Figure 19.6). Studies in humans with endolymphatic hydrops have revealed

hypoplasia of the vestibular aqueduct (Sando and Ikeda, 1984), narrowing of the endolymphatic duct (Yuen and Schuknecht, 1972; Ikeda and Sando, 1984), perisaccular fibrosis (Altmann and Fowler, 1943), loss of epithelial integrity and atrophy of the sac (Arenberg, Marovitz and Shambaugh, 1970), and positive immunofluorescent staining for immunoglobulins of the sac wall (Yazawa and Kitahara, 1989). Temporal bone studies of otosclerosis have implicated bony narrowing of the vestibular aqueduct and duct obstruction in explaining the coexistence of otosclerosis and endolymphatic hydrops (Sismanis, Hughes and Abedi, 1986; Franklin, Pollak and Fisch, 1990; Yoon, Paparella and Schachern, 1990). The wall of the endolymphatic sac in Menière's disease has been shown to have significantly fewer and smaller blood vessels than normal controls, suggesting a microvascular contribution to the pathogenesis of the disorder (Ikeda and Sando, 1985). When the lumen of the endolymphatic sac is studied in patients with Menière's disease, stainable proteinaceous material can be seen (Takumida, Bagger-Sjoback and Rask-Anderson, 1989; Friberg *et al.*, 1988) (Figure 19.7). Other authors have found this secretion to have the staining characteristics of a glycoprotein and have suggested that the endolymphatic duct may function as an organ of merocrine secretion as well as endolymph absorption (Wackym *et al.*, 1990; Rask-Anderson *et al.*, 1991). Wackym (1995) has

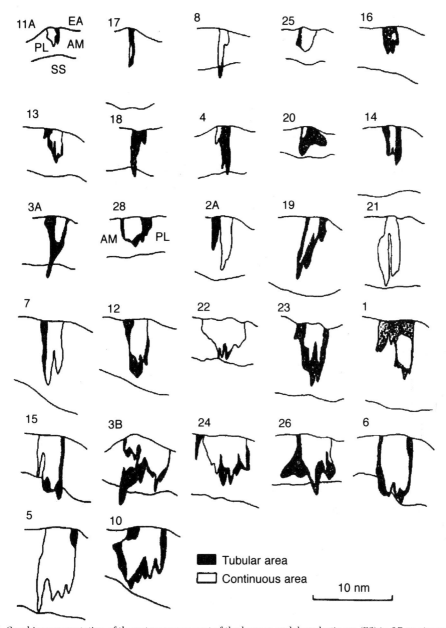

Figure 19.6 Graphic representation of the extraosseous part of the human endolymphatic sac (ES) in 27 specimens. White area represents part of the ES with open continuous lumen; dotted area, the area with interrupted (tabular) lumen. Specimens are arranged in order of increasing area. EA indicates external aperture; SS, sigmoid sinus; PL, posterolateral aspect of ES; AM, anteromedial aspect of ES. (Reproduced from Friberg *et al.*, 1988, Variations in surgical anatomy of the endolymphatic sac. *Archives of Otolaryngology–Head and Neck Surgery*, **114**, 389–394, with kind permission)

recently suggested three possible pathophysiological mechanisms to account for the histopathological changes in Menière's disease; fibrosis of the endolymphatic sac and vestibular epithelia, altered glycoprotein metabolism and inner ear viral infection. Tightly adherent dura in the region of the endolymphatic sac

has been seen at the time of revision endolymphatic sac surgery, and this is thought greatly to increase local sac pressure and resistance to endolymph flow, supporting the malabsorption theory (Paparella and Sajjadi, 1987a).

Blockage of the duct and hypoplasia of the sac,

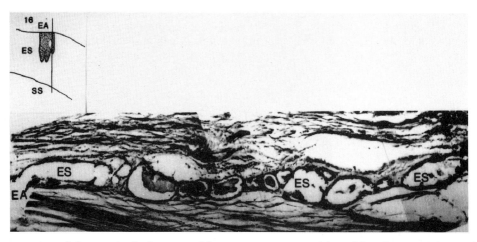

Figure 19.7 Composite light micrograph of a section of the extraosseous portion of the endolymphatic sac (ES) towards the extreme anteromedial end. The lumen is tubular and the tubules are filled with densely staining material (haematoxylin-eosin × 70). The vertical line on the small drawing indicates the location of the section. EA, the external aperture; SS, sigmoid sinus. (Reproduced from Friberg *et al.*, 1988, Variations in surgical anatomy of the endolymphatic sac. *Archives of Otolaryngology – Head and Neck Surgery*, **114**, 389–394, with kind permission)

however, are not seen in all cases of Menière's disease, and it therefore seems likely that other mechanisms may play a role in the development of endolymphatic hydrops. Stahle and Wilbrand (1983) described a lack of periaqueductal pneumatization, with its concomitant effect on the angulation of the vestibular aqueduct within the inner ear, lack of pneumatization medial to the arcuate eminence, a short vestibular aqueduct with a narrow external aperture and a reduction in the overall size of the mastoid air cell system as the characteristic features of the temporal bones of patients with Menière's disease which they studied. Sando and Ikeda (1985) also noted the poor mastoid pneumatization, although others have been unable to verify this finding (Arnhold-Schneider, 1990). Paparella *et al.* (1989) noted a significant anterior and medial displacement of the lateral sinus and consequent reduction in the size of Trautmann's triangle in patients with Menière's disease. They hypothesized that long-term endolymphatic malabsorption is related to a developmental abnormality of the endolymphatic duct and sac in association with hypogenesis of Trautmann's triangle. Impeded local venous drainage, such as one might see in a displaced lateral venous sinus, may result in a disruption of hydrodynamic forces in the labyrinth and endolymphatic hydrops (Gussen, 1982).

Endolymphatic hydrops may be due to a pathological lesion of the dark cells. Masutani, Takahashi and Sando (1992) found abnormalities in dark cell morphology and density in patients with Menière's disease which were not present in normal controls.

Endolymphatic hydrops alone is probably not the whole explanation for Menière's disease and its related symptoms. In a review of 1200 temporal bones,

Paparella (1984b) found endolymphatic hydrops in 310, but could only find a convincing history of Menière's disease in 22 patients and 26 bones. Rauch, Merchant and Thedinger (1989) found hydrops in 26 of 125 cases reviewed, and of these, only 13 had clinical Menière's disease and six had clinical histories incompatible with a diagnosis of Menière's disease. It must be assumed, therefore, that something occurs in concert with the hydrops to bring on the clinical symptoms of the disease. Ruptures occurring in the hydropic membranous labyrinth may be this pathophysiological factor (Lawrence and McCabe, 1959; Schuknecht, 1963, 1968; Schuknecht and Igarashi, 1986; Koskas, Linthicum and House, 1983; Kimura, 1984) (Figure 19.8). Since their discovery in the temporal bones of patients with Menière's disease, ruptures have been described in almost every part of the membranous labyrinth. Ruptures are seen significantly more in the temporal bones of patients with Menière's disease than in those with asymptomatic endolymphatic hydrops (Sperling *et al.*, 1993). Repair of tears has been observed in animal models (Lawrence and McCabe, 1959; Kimura and Schuknecht, 1975) and fibrous tissue proliferation seen within the vestibules of humans with Menière's disease may represent healing of these breaks (Schuknecht and Igarashi, 1986).

The presence of these ruptures has led to the theory that Menière's attacks are due to sudden mixing of the endolymph and perilymph, and disruption of the normal electrochemical activity of the end organ (Brown, McClure and Downar-Zapolski, 1988). When the boundaries of the fluid compartments were studied anatomically, chemically and electrophysiologically, it was shown that the sensory organs and the first order neurons of the auditory and vestibular

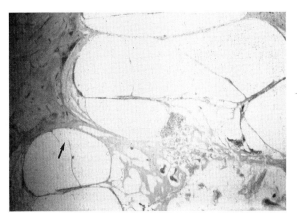

Figure 19.8 Histological section of the cochlea demonstrating endolymphatic hydrops and ruptures of Reissner's membrane (black arrow)

systems are located in the perilymphatic compartment (Schuknecht and Igarashi, 1986). Potassium concentration in the endolymph is high, about 140 mmol/l, a level toxic to neural tissue, whereas the low levels present in the perilymph are ideal for neural conductivity. A rupture in the membranous labyrinth would allow the leakage of this neurotoxic endolymph into the perilymph, resulting in a sustained depolarization and inactivation of the hair cells and neurons of the VIIIth nerve. The subsequent healing of the membrane rupture and the return of the endolymph/perilymph barrier would result in the return of normal inner ear function and the resolution of the symptoms of the Menière's attack (Dohlman, 1977). Chronic repeated exposure of the delicate neural elements of the inner ear to endolymph contamination would result in the progressive irreversible deterioration in auditory and vestibular function seen over the long term.

The histopathological discovery of membrane ruptures and their repair is compelling evidence for this theory and moreover, Tasaki and Fernandez (1952) found that perfusion of the perilymphatic compartment of the cochlea with a solution of potassium blocked the cochlear microphonic responses and action potentials. This would explain the difficulty in recording these responses when transtympanic electrocochleography is carried out in a patient during an acute attack. A similar acute, intense, reversible paralysis of vestibular function was shown when the perilymphatic space was perfused with artificial endolymph (Dohlman and Johnson 1965; Silverstein, 1970). Other groups have detected changes in the composition of endolymph after several weeks of experimentally-induced endolymphatic hydrops, suggesting that hydrops itself may cause pathological permeability of the endolymph–perilymph barrier (Jahnke, 1981; Sziklai *et al.*, 1989).

Despite all of this evidence, the theory remains controversial, however, as some authors believe that membrane ruptures occur rarely and constitute catastrophic events in the inner ear (Tonndorf, 1968, 1986; Thomsen and Bretlau, 1986). A belief held by some is that high endolymphatic pressure alone can produce the Menière's symptom complex. Animal work by Andrews, Bohmer and Hoffman (1991) has looked at the pressure measurements of endolymph and perilymph in normal and hydropic ears and found that endolymph pressures in hydrops are elevated compared with normal endolymph and perilymph pressures. The cochlear damage and hearing loss of Menière's disease can be reproduced by manipulating and increasing endolymphatic pressure alone (Simmons and Mongeon, 1967). Tonndorf (1975, 1983) has suggested that the mechanical distortion and increased tension in the membranes of the inner ear caused by high endolymphatic pressures can explain all the clinical symptoms and findings of Menière's disease, an idea also supported by Fraysse, Alonso and House (1980) after a comprehensive temporal bone study. Paparella (1985) has pointed out that the saccule blocks and fills the vestibule, and that a break in the membrane of the cochlea may not therefore result in contamination of the perilymph of the pars superior. He has reasoned that multiple membrane ruptures would therefore be necessary to produce the classical symptoms of Menière's disease, an unlikely event which is not supported by existing temporal bone studies. He has proposed that the observed ruptures actually alleviate the symptoms of a Menière's attack, a theory supported by the fact that many patients enjoy relief from the attack when the aural pressure subsides.

Aetiology of Menière's disease

The cause of Menière's disease remains unknown. Recent research has incriminated various hypo- and hyper-metabolic states as well as allergy and personality type in the causation of the disease. This has again brought to light the unanswered question of whether Menière's disease is a disease in its own right or simply a symptom complex. Mygind and Dederding (1932) stated that 'Menière's disease is not a disease *sui generis*, but a typical reaction of a predisposed labyrinth to an almost infinite series of exo- and endo-genic influences, which have, however, this in common, that they express themselves throughout the vessels, especially the capillaries'. Many modern otologists concur with this view, believing that metabolic factors can produce endolymphatic hydrops and that, when all of these entities have been discovered, Menière's disease will cease to exist.

The alternative viewpoint held by the present authors is that abnormal metabolic states, infection, allergy, and autoimmunity which have been well documented and are known to produce symptoms and pathological inner ear changes similar to Menière's disease exist separately from the disease *per se*. It is thought that Menière's disease is indeed a disease *sui generis* and that these other disorders should be regarded as constituting a group of diseases associated with 'secondary endolymphatic hydrops' and should not be called Menière's disease (Moffat, Booth and Morrison, 1979). Table 19.2 lists the aetiological factors felt to be involved in Menière's disease and those which result in secondary endolymphatic hydrops.

Table 19.2 Aetiological factors in Menière's disease and 'secondary endolymphatic hydrops'

Menière's disease

1   Genetic
2   Anatomical
3   Traumatic
4   Viral infection
5   Allergy
6   Autoimmunity
7   Psychosomatic and personality features

'Secondary endolymphatic hydrops'

1   Developmental insult
2   Abnormal metabolic and endocrine states
3   Syphilis
4   Chronic otitis media
5   Viral infection
6   Autoimmunity
7   Otosclerosis
8   Abnormal fluid balance
9   Leukaemia

Aetiological factors in Menière's disease

Genetic

There have been several reports of familial Menière's disease dating from Brown in 1941. The observation of a familial tendency has been described in 14–20% of patients with Menière's disease (Paparella, 1985; Birgerson, Gustavson and Stahle, 1987) and has resulted in the search for a locus of genetic aberration to explain the disorder. Oliveira and Braga (1992) described a family with a father, three daughters, and one son afflicted with typical Menière's disease and paroxysmal headaches, a pedigree which suggests an autosomal dominant transmission of the disease in some familial cases. The association, in both sporadic and familial cases, of Menière's disease and partial HLA class I haplotypes (Xenellis *et al.*, 1986) points to a possible locus lying between the HLA-C and HLA-A loci on the short arm of chromosome 6. It is likely that the predisposition to familial Menière's disease is attributable to a mutation on

chromosome 6, which has been designated M1 (Morrison *et al.*, 1994). Others have specified the HLA-DRB1*1602 subtype of the HLA-DR2 locus in Menière's disease (Koyama *et al.*, 1993).

Anatomical

Anatomical causes of Menière's disease have been suggested. A small vestibular aqueduct has been proposed as a cause of the disorder, and some radiological studies of the temporal bones of patients with Menière's disease support this hypothesis (Clemis and Valvassori, 1968). A significant reduction of the volume of the rugose portion of the endolymphatic sac has been detected with computer-aided graphic reconstruction (Antunez *et al.*, 1980; Bagger-Sjoback *et al.*, 1990) (Figures 19.9 and 19.10). The histopathological studies, however, have not supported these radiological observations (Yuen and Schuknecht, 1972; Sackett, Kozarek and Arenberg, 1980). High-resolution magnetic resonance imaging of the inner ear has resulted in good visualization of the structures of the membranous labyrinth (Tanioka *et al.*, 1992; Suchato, Vejvechaneyom and Charoensuwan, 1993). Considerable difficulty was experienced in visualizing the endolymphatic duct and sac in ears affected by Menière's disease, whereas these structures were more easily seen in the normal hearing ears, leading to the suggestion that these structures are smaller in ears with Menière's disease (Tanioka *et al.*, 1992).

Traumatic

An association has been noted between Menière's disease and trauma, either physical or acoustic (Paparella and Mancini, 1983). The chronological sequence of events in certain cases suggests that trauma may have had a role to play in the genesis of Menière's-related symptoms. Trauma may produce biochemical dysfunction in the cells of the membranous labyrinth, or it may simply cause the release of debris into the endolymph which could then obstruct the endolymphatic duct and sac.

Viral infection

Damage to the endolymphatic sac and duct by viral infection has been proposed as an aetiological mechanism in Menière's disease (Schuknecht, 1986). Neurotropic viruses have been considered the most likely offenders. Viruses have been implicated as aetiological agents in a number of clinical conditions related to the temporal bone. These include Bell's palsy, vestibular neuronitis, and benign positional vertigo, and suspicion exists that they may play a role across the spectrum of idiopathic disorders of inner ear function (Bance and Rutka, 1990). Recent work in Sweden has found a higher antibody reactivity to herpes simplex virus type I polypeptides in patients with

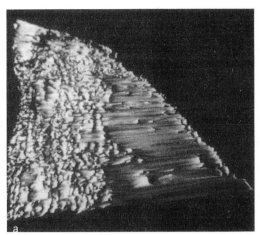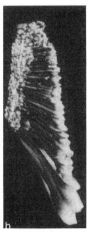

Figure 19.9 Computer-aided reconstruction of the microscopic anatomy of the pars canalicularis of an endolymphatic sac in a patient with Menière's disease. The highlighted mass of small canaliculi at the anterior edge is the rough pars canalicularis. The unhighlighted portion is the smooth pars canalicularis. (Reproduced from Galey, 1988, Quantative evaluation of the structure of the endolymphatic sac. In: *Second International Symposium on Menière's Disease*, edited by J. B. Nadol. Amsterdam: Kugler & Ghedini. pp. 105–111, with kind permission)

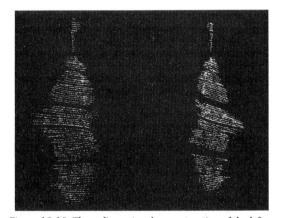

Figure 19.10 Three-dimensional reconstruction of the left human endolymphatic duct and sac. For technical reasons the angle at the isthmus was straightened out. The external aperture of the vestibular aqueduct was situated just above the second partition of the specimen. Left: anterolateral view (× 7). Right: Lateral view (× 7). (Reproduced from Bagger-Sjöback, 1990, Three-dimensional anatomy of the human endolymphatic sac. *Archives of Otolaryngology - Head and Neck Surgery*, **116**, 345–349, with kind permission)

Menière's disease, as well as discovering herpes simplex viral DNA in the endolymphatic sac tissue of two patients (Bergstrom *et al.*, 1992). A significant association has been detected between Menière's disease and circulating levels of the group-specific protein of enterovirus, VP1, implicating this virus in the disorder (Morrison *et al.*, 1994). VP1 was found to be present in more patients with active disease and the absence of the protein correlated with remission,

suggesting that disease activity may mirror periods of active viral infection.

Allergy

Allergy is a proposed aetiological factor in Menière's disease (Duke, 1923; Powers and House, 1969; Endicott and Stucker, 1977). The presence of allergy was the most common association with Menière's disease in a study of 120 patients by Pulec (1972). In another study, 81% of patients with Menière's disease had a history of childhood allergy, and 87% had significant symptoms of a systemic disorder suggesting allergy at the time of assessment. Both food and inhalant allergy were implicated. Relief of Menière's symptoms occurred in 62% of patients treated with immunotherapy by Derebery and Valenzuela (1992) but in only 32% of the patients treated by Shaver (1975). Duke (1923) put his original patient on a diet free of all fruits, vegetables and nuts and this led to a remission of the disease. Despite this clinical evidence, failure to document the diagnostic changes in IgE and IgE antibody that are normally seen in allergic disorders has cast doubt on allergy as a true aetiological factor in Menière's disease (Stahle, Deutschl and Johansson, 1974).

Autoimmunity

Autoimmunity as a causative factor has been seriously considered in Menière's disease. Numerous immunological abnormalities have been noted in these patients. The endolymphatic sac has been shown to contain immunoglobulins and lymphocytes, and is thought to be capable of generating a humoral or cellular immune response (Harris, 1989). Immuno-globulins have been seen deposited in the walls and luminal fluid of the endolymphatic sacs of Menière's patients (Brookes, 1986; Futaki, Semba and Kudo, 1988; Yazawa and Kitahara, 1989; Dorn-hoffer *et al.*, 1993). Severe immunological abnormalities, as measured by erythrocyte sedimentation rate (ESR), serum immunoglobulin levels, complement assays, and autoantibodies, were present in 16% of people with bilateral Menière's disease (Suzuki and Kitahara, 1992) and in many patients with unilateral disease (Evans *et al.*, 1988). Elevated levels of circulating immune complexes have been detected in the serum of Menière's patients (Brookes, 1986; Morrison, 1986; Hsu, Zhu and Zhao, 1990; Derebery *et al.*, 1991), suggesting that circulating immune complexes may be involved in the pathogenesis of the disease, either as a direct cause of damage or as a by-product of an underlying autoimmune abnormality.

Antibodies directed against the mesenchymal elements of the normal inner ear have also been discovered in this patient population (Arnold, Pfalz and Altermatt, 1985). Antibodies directed against type II collagen have been found in the serum of Menière's patients (Yoo *et al.*, 1982; Tomoda *et al.*, 1993). Autoimmune reactivity against type II collagen is a proposed aetiological mechanism for otosclerosis, and animals in whom an immune reaction to type II collagen is induced develop auditory and vestibular dysfunction, endolymphatic hydrops and lesions resembling otosclerotic foci (Yoo, 1984).

Psychosomatic and personality features

A basic disorder of personality occurring in Menière's disease was described by Fowler and Zeckel in 1952 and emotion as a precipitating factor was reported by Hinchcliffe (1967a). The personality profile of patients with Menière's disease was investigated by Hinchcliffe (1967b) using the Minnesota Multiphasic Personality Inventory. An increased prevalence of psychosomatic type personality profiles in people with Menière's disease compared with a control population was found. In 1975, Stephens evaluated the personality of patients with Menière's disease using the Eysenck Personality Inventory and the Middlesex Hospital Questionnaire. The most notable finding was an elevated obsessionality score. Czubalski, Bochenek and Zawisza (1976) found psychic stresses experienced in childhood and overt neurosis to be more common in patients with Menière's disease. Psychological factors occurring in Menière's disease have also been described by Crary and Wexler (1977), Barber (1983) and Eagger *et al.* (1992). Patients with inner ear disorders as a group were found to have significantly higher objective scores of psychiatric morbidity than healthy patients and than patients afflicted with other physical disorders (Berrios *et al.*, 1988). No discernible organic cerebral impairment

has been discovered in Menière's patients which would explain this association (Crary, Wexler and Riley, 1976). A psychosomatic aetiology has even been suggested for Menière's disease (Watson *et al.*, 1967), but subsequent reports tended to show that the psychological features seen in these patients are due to the presence of the physical disease (Crary and Wexler, 1977). Psychiatric morbidity has been shown to increase along with an increase in vestibular symptoms (Eagger *et al.*, 1992).

Aetiological factors in 'secondary endolymphatic hydrops'

Developmental insult

Developmental causes of symptomatic endolymphatic hydrops fall under the heading 'embryopathic symptomatic endolymphatic hydrops' (see Table 19.1). Mondini dysplasia can exhibit endolymphatic hydrops, which is thought to be due to dysplasia of the endolymphatic sac (Schuknecht and Gulya, 1983).

Abnormal metabolic and endocrine states

Certain abnormal metabolic and endocrine states produce the pathological inner ear changes of 'secondary endolymphatic hydrops' and symptoms similar to Menière's disease (Moffat, Booth and Morrison, 1979; Morrison and Booth, 1988). Both hypo- and hyperglycaemia have been associated with inner ear dysfunction and hearing may fluctuate with blood glucose levels (Rudd *et al.*, 1993). An abnormal 5-hour oral glucose tolerance test may be elicited in up to 30% of patients with Menière's triad of symptoms (Powers, 1972). The relationship between diabetes mellitus and sensorineural hearing loss and vestibular dysfunction has been known for some time and the histopathological changes in the temporal bone have been clearly documented (Moffat, Booth and Morrison, 1981). Similarly, a relationship exists between hypoglycaemia and vestibular complaints (Currier, 1969). Weille (1967) reported that 42% of a series of 19 patients with Menière's disease were suffering from reactive hypoglycaemia compared with only 15% in a control group. Mendelsohn and Roderique (1972) demonstrated that induced hypoglycaemia resulted in a decrease in the potassium concentration of the endolymph and a rise in endolymphatic sodium, changes that resemble the cationic changes demonstrated in other studies of Menière's disease. Hyperlipoproteinaemia has been proposed as an aetiological factor in Menière's triad of symptoms by Spencer (1975) and Booth (1977). It was found that 42% of a group of patients with this clinical picture of inner ear disease had a clearly defined hyperlipoproteinaemia (Spencer, 1973).

A number of endocrinological associations have been made with Menière's disease. An aetiological role of hypothyroidism has been proposed by Poulsen (1966) who found that 12% of patients with Menière's disease were hypothyroid. Hypothyroidism alone is associated with a higher than average incidence of hearing impairment (Bhatia *et al.*, 1977). A statistical relationship has also been reported between Menière's disease and adrenal pituitary insufficiency and lowered adrenocortical reserve (Powers, 1972; Pulec, 1972). Menière's disease has been reported in a set of twins with nephrogenic diabetes insipidus, suggesting an association with this disorder as well as posing interesting questions about the role of antidiuretic hormone in fluid and electrolyte regulation in the inner ear (Comacchio *et al.*, 1992). Andrews, Ator and Honrubia (1992) identified a subgroup of women patients with Menière's disease whose symptoms correlated with the premenstrual period, or late luteal phase of the menstrual cycle, indicating that sex hormones and their effect on compartmental fluid redistribution within the body may play a role in some. As with so many secondary disorders, the symptoms of vestibuloauditory dysfunction often improve when these other aetiological factors are treated. Moffat, Booth and Morrison (1979, 1981) have shown that the incidence of abnormal metabolic and endocrine states in a group of 50 patients with Menière's disease was no greater than in the general population lending support to the argument that Menière's disease is a disease *sui generis*. There is therefore good evidence to suggest that patients with Menière's triad of symptoms should undergo a programme of metabolic screening to rule out metabolic and endocrine abnormalities (Powers, 1978; Moffat, Booth and Morrison, 1981).

Syphilis

Syphilis is a known cause of endolymphatic hydrops and the Menière's triad of symptoms, and it is therefore part of the group of disorders of 'secondary endolymphatic hydrops'. Up to 7% of patients presenting with fluctuant sensorineural hearing loss, episodic vertigo and tinnitus have congenital or acquired syphilis (Pulec, 1972). Schuknecht has studied the temporal bones of syphilitics and found endolymphatic hydrops in association with syphilitic osteitis of the otic capsule (Schuknecht, 1974) and it has also been found with syphilitic endolymphatic duct obstruction (Linthicum and El-Rahman, 1987). It has been suggested that the inner ear's reaction to this local inflammation is the progressive over-accumulation of endolymph, the subsequent rupture of membranes and long-term degeneration of the membranous labyrinth.

The diagnosis and treatment of luetic endolymphatic hydrops has been reviewed by Amenta *et al.* (1992) and the long-term outcome of the hearing by Chan, Adams and Kerr (1995).

Chronic otitis media

The clinical observation of patients with fluctuant sensorineural hearing loss occurring with or following chronic otitis media led to the hypothesis that endolymphatic hydrops can be caused by chronic otitis media (Paparella, deSousa and Mancini, 1983). Endolymphatic hydrops has been observed in the temporal bones of animals with otitis media (Kimura, 1982). A correlation has also been observed in human temporal bone studies. Paparella *et al.* (1979) found that out of a set of 109 temporal bones demonstrating endolymphatic hydrops, 75 also had evidence of otitis media. The effect of otitis media on the inner ear may be through the influence of infectious products, toxins and associated enzymes migrating through the round window membrane into the fluids of the inner ear, or through the effects of osteitis from mastoiditis on the development and blood supply of the endolymphatic sac (Paparella, deSousa and Mancini, 1983). The presence of middle ear bacterial endotoxin has been shown to cause a potent inflammatory response in the inner ear leading to sensory cell degeneration and endolymphatic hydrops in an animal model (Kawauchi, Lim and DeMaria, 1989).

Viral infection

The temporal bones of patients with the clinical entity 'delayed endolymphatic hydrops', or hydrops developing in an ear many years after an unexplained deafness, resemble those known to have suffered a measles or mumps labyrinthitis (Schuknecht, 1978; Schuknecht, Suzuka and Zimmermann, 1990). This suggests that endolymphatic hydrops may occur as a delayed sequela of inner ear damage sustained during an attack of subclinical viral labyrinthitis occurring much earlier in life. Contralateral delayed endolymphatic hydrops was first described by Schuknecht in 1978 and a recent report by Harris and Aframian (1994) has suggested that this is an autoimmune event directed against the remaining inner ear.

Autoimmunity

Cogan (1945, 1949) described a syndrome characterized by interstitial keratitis, vestibular and auditory dysfunction, and non-reactive serological tests for syphilis. More recent studies confirmed the autoimmune aetiology of this condition, which occurs via a cell-mediated autoimmune inflammatory response (Hughes *et al.*, 1983a; Peeters *et al.*, 1986). Subsequent cellular and humoral tests of patients with bilateral Menière's disease suggested that at least some cases have an autoimmune aetiology (Hughes *et al.*, 1983b). The diagnosis of 'autoimmune sensorineural hearing loss' has been proposed to explain bilateral, asymmetrical, progressive sensorineural hearing loss, with or without dizziness, tinnitus or aural pressure (McCabe, 1979). This disorder is related to endolymphatic hydrops, and possibly represents part of a spectrum of autoimmune inner ear diseases (Hughes *et al.*, 1988a). The fact that symptoms improve with steroid and electrophoresis therapy in many patients with Menière's disease supports the autoimmune hypothesis (Futaki, Semba and Kudo, 1988; Hughes *et al.*, 1988b). It has been suggested that autoimmune endolymphatic hydrops be considered in middle-aged women with other pre-existing systemic autoimmune disorders such as rheumatoid arthritis (Hughes *et al.*, 1988b).

Otosclerosis

Patients with otosclerosis may occasionally develop auditory and vestibular symptoms similar to those seen in Menière's disease. This relationship is well documented in the clinical and experimental literature (Black *et al.*, 1969; Liston *et al.*, 1984; Paparella, Mancini and Liston, 1984; Sismanis, Hughes and Abedi, 1986; Franklin, Pollak and Fisch, 1990; Yoon, Paparella and Schachern, 1990) and has resulted in the introduction of the term 'otosclerotic inner ear syndrome' (McCabe, 1966; Ghorayeb and Linthicum, 1978). The cause of this association may be the physical impingement of otosclerotic bone on the vestibular aqueduct or in the biochemical alteration of the perilymph and endolymph (Paparella, Mancini and Liston, 1984).

Abnormal fluid balance

Haemodialysis has been reported to precipitate endolymphatic hydrops in the contralateral ear of a patient with known Menière's disease (Moffat, Cumberworth and Baguley, 1990). This was thought to be due to the sudden changes in plasma osmolality brought on by haemodialysis affecting a predisposed inner ear.

Other possible aetiologies

Leukaemia is reported to have an association with endolymphatic hydrops (Sando and Egami, 1977), although a causal relationship remains in doubt. An association between Shy-Drager syndrome and Menière's disease has been noted (Hinton, Ramsden and Saeed, 1993), supporting the idea that Menière's disease may be due to a breakdown in normal autonomic nervous system function. An association has also been observed between Menière's disease and temporal arteritis in three patients (McKennan *et al.*, 1993) (see Figure 17.5).

Clinical manifestations

The typical presenting history of Menière's disease is of episodic attacks of rotatory vertigo (96.2%), with tinnitus (91.1%) and ipsilateral hearing loss (87.7%) (Paparella and Mancini, 1985). Aural pressure, or fullness, in the affected ear or on both sides is a common complaint (74.1%). The attacks of vertigo may be preceded by an aura consisting of aural fullness, increasing tinnitus, and hearing loss and lasting 15–60 minutes (Stahle and Klockhoff, 1986). On the other hand, they may be associated with little or no warning, and may even suddenly wake a patient from a deep sleep (Barber, 1983). The length of the attacks is variable, with most episodes lasting 2–3 hours (Oosterveld, 1980). Ten per cent of patients with Menière's disease report episodes lasting less than 30 minutes, while a small number of patients have more prolonged attacks. Attacks lasting longer than 24 hours may represent two or more attacks occuring in series with continuing symptoms, but a history of more prolonged episodes than this is considered inconsistent with the diagnosis of Menière's disease (Stahle and Klockhoff, 1986). The clinical rule-of-thumb that attacks of vertigo in Menière's disease last '24 minutes to 24 hours' is valid for the majority of cases. The frequency of attacks is similarly variable, with some severe cases suffering attacks on a daily basis or more, while other patients suffer clusters of attacks, and still others have long quiescent periods which may last years (Paparella and Mancini, 1985).

Episodic vertigo

Episodic vertigo associated with vegetative signs such as nausea and vomiting is the most distressing and disabling symptom of Menière's disease and the one for which most patients seek medical attention (Barber, 1983; Paparella, 1984a). The first attacks begin in otherwise healthy patients with normal equilibrium. The vertigo begins suddenly, with a severe spinning sensation, and is accompanied by pallor, diaphoresis, nausea, diarrhoea and vomiting. The vertigo is often most severe at the beginning of the attack. Head movement exacerbates the symptoms, as is seen with most acute peripheral vestibular lesions. During the attack, the patient has a normal level of consciousness and orientation and suffers no focal neurological symptoms, such as diplopia, dysarthria, paraesthesia, or muscular weakness. The nystagmus associated with acute vertigo may cause visual blurring (Paparella, 1984a).

Over the following minutes to hours, the symptoms gradually subside, and the patient often falls asleep. Following the attack, patients often feel entirely normal. Some patients complain of dysequilibrium, light-headedness, or motion intolerance, and this is most common in the first 24 hours (Barber, 1983). The severity of different acute attacks may vary.

A variation of this pattern is seen in the condition described by Lermoyez (1919). The vertiginous episode is preceded by increasing tinnitus and hearing loss, but unlike the classic condition, the hearing loss and tinnitus dramatically resolve during or shortly after the onset of dizziness (Schmidt and Schoonhaven, 1989). An explanation of the pathophysiology of this disorder is lacking.

Another variation of Menière's disease relating to vestibular symptoms is 'Tumarkin's crisis' or drop attacks (Tumarkin, 1936; Barber, 1983). Sudden unexplained falls without vertigo or loss of consciousness are suffered by about 2% of patients with Menière's disease. Patients describe a sensation of being pushed, or thrown to the ground, or a sudden illusion of movement of the environment, Tumarkin felt that this was to do with acute dysfunction in the otolithic organs. Sudden changes in the output of gravity reference information from the saccule and utricle results in an inappropriate postural adjustment via the vestibulospinal tract (Odkvist and Bergenius, 1988; Baloh, Jacobson and Winder, 1990). The majority of these episodes remit spontaneously, although the Menière's disease often continues (Baloh, Jacobson and Winder, 1990).

Another variant of Menière's disease has recently been proposed by Meyerhoff (1989), the 'abnormal oculovestibular response'. He described a series of nine patients, each of whom had an abnormal oculovestibular response. These patients experienced vertigo with its attentive vegetative symptoms of nausea, vomiting, and diaphoresis when exposed to optokinetic stimuli, such as riding in a car or train. Most of them had the symptoms of aural fullness, tinnitus, and fluctuating sensorineural hearing loss, and seven of them had abnormal electronystagmography.

An association has been noted between Menière's disease and benign paroxysmal positional vertigo (Barber, 1983; Baloh, Honrubia and Jacobsen, 1987). A complaint of positional vertigo between attacks was found in 85.9% of patients with Menière's disease (Paparella, 1984a). Unlike the definitive spells of vertigo, these attacks are short-lived, lasting seconds only, and are provoked by certain head movements. Patients may present to the clinician with a classical history of Menière's disease and have the classical benign paroxysmal positional vertigo finding of rotatory nystagmus on Dix-Hallpike testing. In Canada, Parnes and Price-Jones (1993) have suggested that the aetiology of the majority of cases of benign paroxysmal positional vertigo may be free-floating particles in the posterior semicircular canal, and that repositioning of these particles into the utricle results in resolution of the vertigo in 68% of cases. In Menière's disease, these particles may be generated by coalescence and concretion of the endolymphatic glycoproteins or inflammatory products seen in temporal bone studies (Wackym *et al.*, 1990; Rask-Anderson *et al.*, 1991) or they may be otoconia dislodged by metabolic or degenerative changes occurring in the sensory organs of the vestibule.

Acute attacks of Menière's disease are rarely observed by the physician, but if they are, a horizontal nystagmus is the classical physical finding. The direction of the nystagmus varies over the time course of the attack. The initial direction of the nystagmus is the subject of some controversy because of the difficulties experienced in trying to observe this. Bance *et al.* (1991) reported a patient who suffered an attack while undergoing electronystagmography. A 'near-instantaneous' recording in the caloric test position captured a nystagmus beating toward the affected ear, a so-called 'irritative nystagmus', for 20 seconds. A very short time into the attack, the nystagmus is observed to beat towards the healthy ear, a so-called 'paralytic nystagmus' (McClure, Copp and Lyett, 1981). Hours into the attack, as the auditory and vestibular symptoms subside, nystagmus is seen to reverse again, beating toward the affected ear, the so-called 'recovery nystagmus' (Brown, McClure and Downar-Zapolski, 1988; McClure, Copp and Lyett, 1981). Recovery nystagmus may be horizontal or rotatory, necessitating inspection of the patient's eye movements to observe this phenomenon, because rotatory nystagmus may not appear on an ENG (Parnes and McClure, 1990). While Stahle and Klockhoff (1986) cautioned against using the direction of the nystagmus to determine which ear is causing the patient's symptoms, others have shown that, with careful evaluation, recovery nystagmus can be an important localizing sign (Parnes and McClure, 1990).

The membrane rupture theory is thought to be supported by these observations of changing nystagmus (Bance *et al.*, 1991). Soon after a membrane rupture, rising perilymphatic potassium would initially have an excitatory effect in the first order vestibular neurons (i.e. an increased spontaneous activity), resulting in an irritative nystagmus. Quickly thereafter, as the concentration of potassium increased, a blockade of action potentials would occur, resulting in the paralytic nystagmus seen within minutes of the onset of the attack. The recovery nystagmus may be the result of vestibular adaptation (McClure, Copp and Lyett, 1981).

The natural history of Menière's disease is poorly depicted in the literature, because few studies have been performed on large numbers of patients over a long period. There are, however, several studies that indicate the average outcome of persistent disease. Generally, the pattern of vertigo in Menière's disease is a gradual increase in the frequency of attacks over a period of years until a maximum is reached, followed by a decreasing frequency as the disease runs its course and irreversible damage occurs to the inner ear (Paparella, 1984a). Silverstein, Smouha and Jones (1989) found that in 57% of patients with Menière's disease the vertigo resolved after only 2 years without therapy, while in 71%, complete control of vertigo occurred after 8.3 years. Friberg, Stahle and Svedberg (1984) noted that the mean frequency of attacks was six to 11 per year for the first 20 years and only three or four per year after 20 years. The average reduction in caloric response is approximately 50% over the long term (Stahle, 1976). It has been suggested that predictions can be made about the course of the vestibular symptoms of Menière's disease based on the characteristics of the progressive hearing loss (Sakurai, Yamane and Nakai, 1991). Shea (1993a) has recently proposed a five-stage classification of Menière's disease based on the clinical presentation, which he stated mirrors the natural progression of classical Menière's disease for most of his patients. In stage I, the patient has solely cochlear symptoms, stages II–IV feature progressively more cochlear and vestibular symptoms, and stage V represents end-stage Menière's disease.

Sensorineural hearing loss

Sensorineural hearing loss is a cardinal feature of Menière's disease. The hearing loss is typically fluctuant and progressive. Hearing may fluctuate significantly over the course of the illness, particularly in the first year or two (Schuknecht, 1963; Paparella, 1984a). During the acute spell, auditory acuity is always decreased and may remain so for some time after the vertigo has subsided. Early in the disease, the characteristic pattern is one of a low frequency, fluctuant hearing loss. A second early pattern is one of low frequency hearing loss occurring in concert with a high frequency hearing loss, resulting in an 'inverted V' shape in the audiogram centred at 2 kHz (Barber, 1983). Other audiometric configurations such as U-shaped or downward sloping hearing loss are described less frequently (Oosterveld, 1980). The hearing loss tends to flatten with time and variability decreases. Profound deafness is the end-point only rarely in the progression of Menière's disease (Stahle, 1976). Friberg, Stahle and Svedberg (1984) noted that the average pure tone hearing loss over the long term is 50 dB and average speech discrimination drops to 53%. It has been suggested that predictions can be made regarding the progression of hearing loss and the final hearing result, based on a study of the changes in hearing in the first 3 years (Sakurai, Yamane and Nakai, 1991).

The clinical evaluation of a patient suspected of having Menière's disease should include tuning fork assessment. This should confirm the presence of a sensorineural hearing loss, although a false-negative Rinne test may be present in the rare patient with a severe unilateral sensorineural hearing loss and Bárány noise box masking of the contralateral ear should always be employed.

The decrease in hearing acuity is typical of the cochlear type of sensorineural hearing loss (Paparella, 1984a). Distortion of sounds occurs during attacks and may occur between them. Most patients experience 'dysacusis', in which sounds are perceived to have an abnormally tinny nature, during the course of their disease (Stahle and Klockhoff, 1986). 'Diplacusis' is a complaint in 43.6% of patients with Menière's disease (Paparella, 1984a). The same sound frequently is perceived as a different pitch in the two ears (diplacusis binauralis dysharmonica), with the affected ear usually perceiving a higher pitch. Loudness intolerance due to recruitment is another common feature, present in 56%. Recruitment, defined as oversensitivity to suprathreshold acoustic stimuli, is considered to be a manifestation of hair cell injury and is absent in lesions of the auditory nerve (Schuknecht, 1963).

Tinnitus

Tinnitus in Menière's disease is also variable in character. It may be the first symptom of the disorder and it may begin with the first attack. It is always present during a spell if a patient is able to listen for it, and it is often present between attacks (Paparella, 1984a). Tinnitus may be continuous or intermittent, and it is non-pulsatile. Although little objective information is available when evaluating tinnitus, certain generalizations have been made. The pitch of the tinnitus tends to correspond to the region of most severe hearing loss, and its severity may be loosely related to the severity of the hearing loss (Paparella, 1984a). Early in the disease, tinnitus becomes loud when the hearing is reduced and then becomes softer as the hearing improves. Later, the tinnitus is constant and more distracting between attacks. This may result in tinnitus being the patient's primary complaint in the late stages of Menière's disease, especially in bilateral disease (Barber, 1983).

Aural fullness

Aural fullness is an interesting symptom of Menière's disease. Most of the time, the pressure sensation is limited to the ear, but some patients may consistently feel pressure elsewhere in the head and neck with attacks (Paparella, 1984a).

Somatopsychic effects

Just as psychosomatic elements may play a part in the aetiology of this condition, the somatopsychic effects of the vertigo are equally important and effects such as secondary agoraphobia produced by frightening vertigo may occur, particularly in the elderly.

Due to the variability that is so much a part of this disorder, the classical clinical manifestations of Menière's disease are not always present. Kitahara *et al.* (1984) found that 50% of patients presented with vestibular and auditory complaints together, while 19% had vertigo only, and 26% had hearing loss only. Wilmot (1974) realized this and suggested eight positive and eight negative criteria to aid a more accurate diagnosis of Menière's disease.

Variations in the clinical presentation of patients with some but not all features of Menière's disease have resulted in the definition of subtypes of the disorder. The disorder previously called 'cochlear Menière's disease' or 'Menière's disease without vertigo' is characterized solely by fluctuating and progressive sensorinerual hearing loss with all the audiometric tests typical of Menière's disease (Williams, Hortorn and Day, 1947). The term 'atypical Menière's disease' is now favoured. Longitudinal follow up of these patients has revealed that up to 80% go on to develop classical Menière's disease (Kitahara *et al.*, 1984) and then the qualifying 'atypical' is dropped. The disorder known as 'vestibular Menière's disease' or 'Menière's disease without deafness' is characterized solely by the definitive spells of vertigo. Interestingly, only 20% of these patients go on to develop the auditory symptoms of classical Menière's disease (Paparella and Mancini, 1985) and there is no pathological correlation for this variant (Kitahara *et al.*, 1984). This has led some authors to suggest that the majority of these patients do not actually have Menière's disease and has led to the introduction of the term 'recurrent vestibulopathy' for this disorder (LeLiever and Barber, 1981).

Another variation in the classical pattern of Menière's disease is that of delayed endolymphatic hydrops. This disorder is defined as recurrent attacks of rotatory vertigo in an ear that has been previously deafened. It was first described by Nadol, Weiss and Parker (1975) and has subsequently been well investigated (LeLiever and Barber, 1980; Hicks and Wright, 1988). Schuknecht (1978) elaborated further on this entity by classifying it into an ipsilateral form, in which the vertigo arises in the same ear as the hearing loss, and a contralateral form, in which fluctuant hearing loss and/or vertigo occurs in the opposite ear. The aetiology of the original hearing loss does not appear to have an affect on the development of delayed endolymphatic hydrops, although there is much support for a viral aetiology of the disorder itself (Schuknecht, Suzuka and Zimmermann, 1990). One report implicated heavy noise exposure in the development of delayed endolymphatic hydrops in a group of professional soldiers (Ylikoski, 1988). This distinctive entity typically affects young adults, with the mean age at clinical presentation of 32 years in one study (LeLiever and Barber, 1980). The latency between the onset of deafness and the onset of vertigo is from 1 to 68 years, with an average of 23–28 years (Nadol, Weiss and Parker, 1975; LeLiever and Barber, 1980).

Differential diagnosis

In the event of a monosymptomatic onset, or if the full triad of symptoms is not manifest from the outset, difficulties may be encountered in establishing a diagnosis. This is particularly true when the initial symptoms are vestibular in nature. Usually within several months, other features will arise which will clarify the clinical picture and make the diagnosis of Menière's disease, but a good knowledge of the differential diagnosis is essential if the clinician is to avoid missing another pathology or an associated illness. The history is the most important aspect of diagnosis in Menière's disease, and other causes of inner ear symptoms may be ruled out by taking a meticulous, detailed history and carrying out a careful and complete otoneurological examination. Detailed descriptions of the disease entities can be found in other chapters, but a diagnostic framework is provided. Stahle and Klockhoff (1986) divided the differential diagnosis of Menière's disease into: conditions with vertigo without auditory symptoms; conditions with auditory symptoms without vertigo; and conditions with a combination of auditory symptoms and vertigo.

Conditions with vertigo without auditory symptoms

Conditions with vertigo without auditory symptoms include vestibular neuronitis and benign paroxysmal positional vertigo. *Vestibular neuronitis* is a condition characterized by a change in the vestibular output of one inner ear, resulting in severe vertigo. The patient is generally very ill initially and the vertigo and vegetative symptoms subside over 24–48 hours, the time taken for central compensation to occur. Milder attacks of vertigo may persist for up to 2 months, rarely for as long as 6 months. If compensation is incomplete, the patient may complain of transitory dysequilibrium exacerbated by fast head movements and this may persist indefinitely. Patients may be more prone to travel sickness and motion intolerance than they were in the past. ENG reveals a reduced caloric response on the affected side and a paralytic nystagmus. Repeated attacks of vertigo are very uncommon. The length of the attack and the lack of auditory symptoms or aural fullness are the features which distinguish this disorder from Menière's disease (see Figure 5.30).

Benign paroxysmal positional vertigo is evoked by changes in head position. An attack is usually triggered when the patient lies back on the affected side, rolls over onto that side, sits up quickly, or tilts the head back while looking up. A latent period of some seconds after the head movement is followed by severe vertigo, which usually lasts less than 1 minute. Dix-Hallpike testing is positive when a rotatory nystagmus is induced with the affected ear dependent, a response which is fatiguable. The positive Dix-Hallpike test can be abolished in the majority of patients by the correct and careful application of the particle repositioning manoeuvre, which will abolish the positional vertigo (Parnes and Price-Jones, 1993).

Conditions with auditory symptoms without vertigo

Conditions with auditory symptoms without vertigo include those which result in sudden hearing loss and vestibular schwannoma. *Sudden deafness* is distinguished from the initial stages of Menière's disease by the fact that the hearing loss develops more quickly, usually across the frequency spectrum. Aural fullness is usually absent, although discomfort in the ear may be a feature, depending on the aetiology.

Vestibular schwannomas (acoustic neuromas) usually present with a progressive sensorineural hearing loss and often tinnitus. Sudden hearing loss is the presenting symptom in 12% of patients with vestibular schwannoma (Moffat, Irving and Hardy, 1994) and it tends not to recover. Rotatory vertigo is unusual in vestibular schwannoma, and most patients complain of dysequilibrium. The pure tone audiogram demonstrates a high frequency loss in 42% of patients with vestibular schwannoma and in only 2% of a series of 284 tumours was there a low frequency loss similar to Menière's disease (Moffat, Irving and Hardy, 1994). The absence of recruitment, very poor discrimination, and absent stapedial reflexes or marked stapedial reflex decay may be present and helps the clinician differentiate a vestibular schwannoma from Menière's disease. Despite this, it may be very difficult to differentiate between these two conditions, particularly since 2% of patients with a vestibular schwannoma present with the classical Menière's triad of symptoms including rotatory vertigo. Secondary endolymphatic hydrops can occur in patients with vestibular schwannoma perhaps relating to the high CSF protein present in some cases. All patients should have the diagnosis of a vestibular schwannoma excluded by MRI with gadolinium-DTPA enhancement.

Conditions with a combination of auditory symptoms and vertigo

Conditions with a combination of auditory symptoms and vertigo include Cogan's syndrome, craniocervical dysplasia, vertebrobasilar insufficiency and the non-specific cochleovestibulopathies. *Cogan's syndrome* has been discussed above, and can be diagnosed by ophthalmological assessment looking for interstitial keratitis. *Cranioverteberal junction abnormalities*, also known as craniocervical dysplasia or basilar impression, is a combination of congenital or acquired bony, vascular and neural malformations resulting in pressure on the brain stem and symptoms which may resemble those of Menière's disease (Harker, 1989). The most common of these is a high odontoid process with protrusion into the foramen magnum, a diagnosis which can be made radiologically (see Figure 2.67). These patients will often have other malformations or disease processes, such as rheumatoid arthritis, which will increase clinical suspicion. *Vertebrobasilar*

insufficiency is characterized by transient vertigo or dysequilibrium following certain head movements. Auditory symptoms are unusual, but other focal neurological symptoms may occur. *Migraine* is another cause of the symptom of vertigo, presenting most commonly in adolescents and in post-menopausal women (Harker, 1989). Basilar migraine may present in a similar way to Menière's disease (Olsson, 1991). The category of *non-specific cochleovestibulopathies* is meant to include those patients presenting with a progressive, non-fluctuating, usually unilateral hearing loss, attacks of vertigo and/or dysequilibrium, and an abnormal ENG. Numerous aetiological mechanisms can result in these symptoms. The absence of fluctuation and low frequency hearing loss may point to this diagnosis, but transtympanic electrocochleography is often necessary to exclude established endolymphatic hydrops.

Investigations

Assessment of cochlear function

Standard audiological assessment

Evaluation by means of pure tone audiometry is very important in the diagnosis of Menière's disease. The classical sequential pattern of the hearing loss has been previously described. As a whole, patients with Menière's disease will most often demonstrate a flat audiogram (42%), followed by a peaked pattern (32%), a downward sloping pattern (19%), and a rising pattern (7%) (Meyerhoff, Paparella and Gudbrandsson, 1981). Most patients have good air and bone thresholds at 2000 Hz. In patients with a predominantly low frequency hearing loss, the hearing acuity for consonant sounds may be so good that there is no complaint of hearing loss. Serial audiometry over time may demonstrate fluctuation in the degree of sensorineural hearing loss. Fluctuations are most often seen in the frequency range 250–1000 Hz, usually with an average amplitude of 20–30 dB (Stahle and Klockhoff, 1986) (see Figure 5.29).

Special audiometric tests can indicate whether the sensorineural hearing loss is a cochlear or hair-cell related disease. Recruitment can be elicited by tests of the alternate binaural loudness balance in unilateral disease or the loudness discomfort level and the short increment sensitivity index in unilateral or bilateral disease (Hood, 1983). Fowler's alternate loudness balance test will indicate complete recruitment and the stapedius reflex thresholds are often found at a normal level (Stahle and Klockhoff, 1986). Tone decay and acoustic reflex decay tests will usually fall between the values seen in normal patients and patients with a vestibular schwannoma, although in patients with Menière's disease whose hearing loss exceeds 60 dB there may be a mixture of 'retrocochlear' findings in these tests which may make them unreliable (Stahle and Klockhoff, 1986).

Speech discrimination scores are widely variable, but tend to resemble closely the pure tone average in most patients. Poor speech discrimination out of keeping with the degree of pure tone loss should arouse suspicion of a retrocochlear lesion (Penrod, 1985). The pheomenon known as 'rollover', a marked decrease in discrimination performance at high presentation levels, is seen in retrocochlear lesions and is unusual in purely cochlear lesions (Bess, Josey and Humes, 1979).

Evoked response audiometry

Evoked response audiometry has proved to be instrumental in the diagnosis of Menière's disease (Moffat, 1987a). It is a means of determining the electrical activity occurring in the cochlea and central auditory pathways in response to sound stimuli. Electrocochleography evaluates the evoked potential activity of the cochlea and VIIIth nerve, while brain stem evoked response audiometry gives information about the transmission of electrical stimulation through the brain stem nuclei. Together, these modalities form the backbone of modern neuro-otological audiological diagnosis by distinguishing abnormalities of the end organ from retrocochlear lesions, and in determining whether end organ dysfunction is due to endolymphatic hydrops. Electrocochleography is the best existing objective test for Menière's disease, and it has provided considerable insight into the pathophysiology of the condition.

The term *electrocochleography* refers to the measurement of electrical events generated either within the cochlea or by primary afferent neurons. This includes the cochlear microphonic potential and summating potential from the cochlea, and the whole nerve or compound action potential from the cochlear division of the VIIIth nerve. The advent of electronic averaging techniques revolutionized evoked response audiometry and made it possible to obtain recordings of these potentials from several sites, including the tympanic membrane, external auditory meatus, ear lobe, mastoid, and scalp. Large amplitude potentials are needed to monitor the small changes in inner ear electrical activity, and the changes in inner ear physiology that occur in response to drugs, surgery and dehydrating agents.

Transtympanic electrocochleography

The most satisfactory potentials, in terms of amplitude, are obtained from the middle ear promontory near the round window niche or via a silver ball electrode placed on the round window membrane. This method involves the placement of a thin, Teflon coated 0.3 mm diameter stainless steel needle elec-

trode through the tympanic membrane, which has been anaesthetized using iontophoresis (Ramsden, Gibson and Moffat, 1977) or by EMLA cream (Figure 19.11).

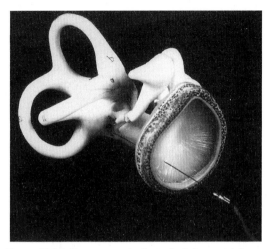

Figure 19.11 Transtympanic electrode, 0.3 mm stainless steel and Teflon coated, *in situ* resting on the promontory close to the round window niche

Sound stimuli are produced from a loudspeaker in earphones and may be clicks, usually with a centre frequency of 3 kHz, or tone pips, which are frequency specific sine waves. Tone bursts are diagnostically more useful than clicks in Menière's disease because low frequency stimuli can be used (Gibson and Rose, 1993). Low noise binaural amplifiers are required with a high input impedance and a high common mode rejection. The shape of the action potential/summating potential complex can be altered by changing the bandwidth of the high and low pass filters. A high-pass filter of 3.2 Hz and a low-pass filter of 3.2 kHz are satisfactory for most recordings. An averaging computer is used to average out the background electrical activity and produce the clear electrophysiological potentials. The test environment should be properly soundproofed and electrically screened.

The *cochlear microphonic potential* (Figure 19.12): sound energy is transduced in the inner ear from a mechanical vibration of the basilar membrane into an electrical waveform by the hair cells. This alternating current potential is an electrical image of the sound stimulus, and represents the sum of the microphonics from many individual hair cells produced by different phases of the travelling wave. Most of the cochlear microphonic potential is produced by outer hair cells within the first few millimetres of the basal turn of the cochlea (Moffat, 1987a).

The *summating potential* (see Figure 19.12) is a

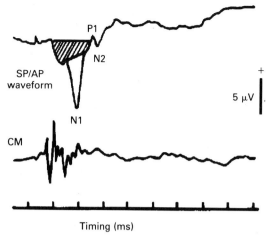

Timing (ms)

Figure 19.12 Normal summating potential/action potential (SP/AP) complex. Normal cochlear microphonic (CM). (Reproduced from Moffat, 1987a, Electrocochleography. In: *Handbook of Neurotological Diagnosis*, edited by J.W. House and A. F. O'Connor. New York: Marcel Dekker. Ch. 5, p. 107)

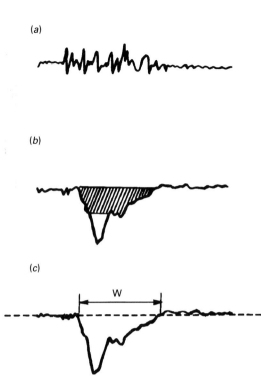

Figure 19.13 Typical transtympanic electrocochleographic recordings in Menière's disease. (*a*) Small distorted cochlear microphonic (CM). (*b*) Widened action potential/summating potential (AP/SP) waveform due to enhanced negative SP. (*c*) W, width of AP/SP waveform in milliseconds from the onset of the N1 to the point of return to the baseline. (Reproduced from Moffat, 1987a, Electrocochleography. In: *Handbook of Neurotological Diagnosis*, edited by J. W. House and A. F. O'Connor. New York: Marcel Dekker. Ch. 5, p. 126)

potential of short latency (0.3 ms) and is usually only present at high stimulus intensities. It is characterized by a DC shift in the baseline of the response, generally in a negative direction, and occurs for the duration of the stimulus. The summating potential is a complex, multicomponent response representing the sum of various electrical events occurring within the cochlea.

The *evoked action potential* (see Figure 19.12) is a compound action potential representing the synchronous firing of multiple cochlear neurons derived mainly from the basal turn of the cochlea. A click stimulus, owing to its faster rise time, will stimulate more of the basilar membrane than frequency-specific tone bursts, and alteration in the intensity of the stimulus affects the amplitude, latency and configuration of the action potential.

In Menière's disease, the most common findings on electrocochleography are an increased summating potential/action potential ratio, a widened summating potential/action potential complex, and a small distorted cochlear microphonic potential (Figure 19.13) (Gibson, Moffat and Ramsden, 1977). In some cases, marked 'after ringing' (sinusoidal wave) of the cochlear microphonic potential is seen, but its significance is unknown. These changes in the electrocochleographic potentials have also been seen in an experimental animal model of endolymphatic hydrops (Klis, Buijs and Smoorenburg, 1990; Ximing, Yuqing and Musan, 1990). The observed electrical findings are explained by the mechanical deformations seen in cochlear endolymphatic hydrops. Whitfield and Ross

(1965) showed that a major component of the summating potential was derived from an asymmetry in the vibration-induced deflection of the basilar membrane. In normal ears, at high stimulus intensities, the basilar membrane vibrates more upwards towards the scala media than downwards generating a negative summating potential. Endolymphatic hydrops accentuates this asymmetry by stretching and stiffening the basilar membrane, limiting its downward vibration. The mechanical deformation of the basilar membrane is greatest at its basal end, where it is most compliant due to its physical properties, and this is the region where the majority of the summating potential is being generated. The normal up-going asymmetry is enhanced, leading to a negative summating potential of increased amplitude and width and an increase in the summating potential/action potential ratio (Figure 19.14).

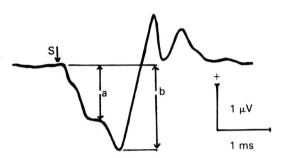

Figure 19.14 Enhanced negative summating potential (SP) producing a notch on the descending limb of the action potential (AP). The SP to AP ratio is a/b on the diagram. a = SP amplitude, b = AP amplitude; S = stimulus onset. Band pass filters 250 Hz to 3.2 kHz, 100 μsec click at 110 dB HL. (Reproduced from Ramsden, Moffat and Gibson, 1977, with permission from *Annals of Otology, Rhinology and Laryngology*)

A summating potential/action potential ratio of up to 1:3 is within the normal range, and a higher ratio is suggestive of hydrops. The more exact figure of summating potential/action potential ratio of 29% has been provided by Gibson, Prasher and Kilkenny (1983) as a dividing line between sensory damage and Menière's disease. When the amplitudes are easily identified and measurable, the summating potential/action potential ratio is a very efficient diagnostic measure, with 62% of patients with Menière's disease patients demonstrating abnormal ratios in one study (Goin, Staller and Asher, 1982). The summating potential can be difficult to measure, however, because of the problem of separating it from the action potential on the trace. In Menière's disease, enhancement of the negative summating potential will widen the summating potential/action potential complex, and the width of the complex is directly proportional to the size of the negative summating potential (Moffat, 1987a). The normal width of the summating potential/action potential complex is 1.2–1.8 ms and widening of greater than 2 ms is usually significant. Measurement of the summating potential/action potential ratio can sometimes give misleading information, particularly when the responses are poor or if the patient's hearing threshold is close to the maximum stimulus intensity. Widening of the summating potential/action potential complex is still a very useful measure of the degree of endolymphatic hydrops. It

should be noted that during an attack, it may be difficult to record an action potential at all and the cochlear microphonic potential may be very distorted, due to the profound electrophysiological disruption of the acute episode.

In 1966, Klockhoff and Lindblom reported that dehydration of patients with Menière's disease using parenteral glycerol produces significant improvement in hearing thresholds, particularly in cases where the hearing loss is still fluctuant. This finding is supported by research using an animal model of endolymphatic hydrops looking at the effect of glycerol on hearing (Magluilo *et al.*, 1993). These findings were supported by further studies, in which improvements in speech discrimination scores with glycerol were also noted (Arenberg *et al.*, 1974; Snyder, 1974). Glycerol is a trivalent alcohol (1, 2, 3 propanetriol) and, when given in high doses, it is incompletely metabolized and acts as an osmotic diuretic. The osmotic effect of the glycerol is thought to reduce the endolymphatic hydrops and intralabyrinthine pressure, resulting in more symmetrical basilar membrane vibration (Juhn, Prado and Pearce, 1976). Changes visualized in the endolymphatic sac following glycerol administration support the theory that glycerol reduces endolymphatic pressures (Rask-Anderson *et al.*, 1989). Another theory is that improvements in cochlear blood flow induced by the osmotic agent are responsible, and significant improvements have been documented in an animal model (Baldwin *et al.*, 1992).

Continuous transtympanic electrocochleographic recording during glycerol dehydration in patients with Menière's disease was first carried out by Moffat *et al.* (1978); 63% of these patients demonstrated a significant decrease in the width of the summating potential within 2 hours of oral glycerol administration (Figure 19.15). Electrocochleography was found to be more sensitive than subjective audiometric tests in detecting glycerol-induced changes in the cochlea. A change in the summating potential/action potential ratio of 15% is thought to be significant (Arenberg, Gibson and Bohlen, 1989). Using tone bursts, the best glycerol-induced improvements in summating potential are seen in the low frequency range (Daumann *et al.*, 1988). The use of dehydrating or osmotic agents in concert with electrocochleography in the investigation of Menière's disease has become a part of most standard current protocols. Some clinicians feel that the glycerol should be administered intravenously, as the characteristic diagnostic electrocochleographic changes are seen less reliably following oral glycerol ingestion (Aso, Watanabe and Mizukoshi, 1991). Similar electrocochleographic results occur following the intravenous administration of 200 ml of 10% glycerol solution as 500 ml of the same solution (Aso *et al.*, 1993).

The side effects of glycerol administration include headache, nausea, and drowsiness, but these are rarely severe enough to cause the patient to request

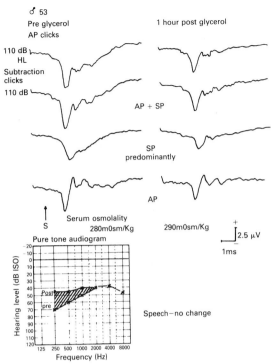

♂ 53
Pre glycerol
AP clicks

1 hour post glycerol

110 dB
HL
Subtraction
clicks
110 dB

AP + SP

SP
predominantly

AP

S ↑ Serum osmolality
280m0sm/Kg

290m0sm/Kg

+ ⌐2.5 μV

1ms

Pure tone audiogram

Post
Pre

Speech—no change

Figure 19.15 Transtympanic electrocochleography during glycerol dehydration. A reduction in the amplitude of the negative summating potential (SP) restores the action potential/summating potential (AP/SP) complex to a more normal width. The low frequency pure tone threshold has improved significantly. (Reproduced from Moffat *et al.*, 1978, with the kind permission of *Acta Otolaryngologica*)

termination of the diagnostic procedure (Morrison, Moffat and O'Connor, 1980). Fewer side effects are experienced with intravenous administration of the agent (Aso *et al.*, 1993).

Other agents used include frusemide (furosemide), a diuretic which induces a rapid diuresis by depressing the reabsorption of water and sodium chloride in the loop of Henle, and urea, a mild osmotic diuretic (Angelborg, Klockhoff and Stahle, 1977). Similar effects on the audiogram and electrocochleogram are seen with both agents as with glycerol. Less marked improvements in the audiogram have been seen with intravenous administration of the osmotic agents mannitol, Macrodex, and Rheomacrodex (Babighian, 1976). The success of these tests in reversing the subjective and objective clinical findings of Menière's disease has led to the introduction of diuretics as therapy for the disorder, now a firmly entrenched therapeutic modality (Klockhoff and Lindblom, 1967; Klockhoff, Lindblom and Stahle, 1974).

Acetazolamide, a carbonic anhydrase inhibitor, has been used to increase the cochlear endolymphatic hydrops, a sort of 'reverse glycerol test' (Brookes, Morrison and Booth, 1982). Documentation of deterioration in pure tone thresholds and in speech discrimination scores, as well as a significant increase in the enhancement of the negative summating potential following acetazolamide administration supports a diagnosis of Menière's disease. Despite greater patient acceptance and fewer side effects than glycerol dehydration, any test that increases the pathological changes within the cochlea, however briefly, may be open to criticism.

In patients suspected of having Menière's disease, it is therefore possible to determine the existence of endolymphatic hydrops by examining the electrocochleographic potentials and their changes with dehydration. It has been shown that, the more certain the diagnosis of Menière's disease is clinically, the greater the likelihood of finding an enhanced negative summating potential (Gibson, Moffat and Ramsden, 1977). Electrocochleography may confirm the diagnosis of Menière's disease when it is in the prevertiginous stage, and is useful in identifying incipient disease in the second ear in patients with documented unilateral disease (Moffat *et al.*, 1992). Electrocochleography is most likely to be positive when the patient is experiencing one or more of the classical symptoms of Menière's disease, particularly aural fullness (Ferraro, Arenberg and Hassanein, 1985). It is important to realize that other conditions producing secondary endolymphatic hydrops, such as syphilis, will exhibit these characteristic electrocochleographic findings (Ramsden, Moffat and Gibson, 1977), although in syphilis, the action potential/summating potential complex is more likely to be W-shaped with an enhanced negative summating potential notch confined to the descending limb of N1. Electrocochleographic studies of patients with 'vestibular Menière's disease', or 'recurrent vestibulopathy', demonstrate endolymphatic hydrops in 73% of cases, fuelling the debate about whether or not this is a disease entity separate from Menière's disease (Dornhoffer and Arenberg, 1993).

The degree of hydrops and the electrophysiological changes in the ear will vary and it is therefore not surprising that the variation in the amplitude of the summating potential can be related to the clinical status of the patient with Menière's disease (Figure 19.16) (Moffat, 1979; Kumagami, Nishida and Baba, 1982). In the early stages of the disease, with complete recovery of auditory function between acute attacks, the summating potential/action potential waveform is often completely normal (Moffat, 1979; Ferraro, Best and Arenberg, 1983). This may explain the frustration some authors have experienced in using the summating potential/action potential waveform alone when using electrocochleography to diagnose Menière's disease (Campbell, Harker and Abbas,

1992). Perhaps, not surprisingly, the likelihood of obtaining a positive electrocochleogram in patients with Menière's disease is strongly related to the degree of hearing loss (Orchik, Shea and Ge, 1993). As the disease becomes established, the enhanced negative summating potential is more consistently recorded between attacks, implying that the hydrops is a more permanent pathological feature. An elevated summating potential/action potential ratio can be found in up to 83.7% of Menière's ears, with a false positive rate as low as 12% (Orchik, Shea and Ge, 1993), making transtympanic electrocochleography generally accepted as a valuable clinical tool (Shea, 1993b).

Preoperative electrocochleography is thus of value in selecting patients for surgery (Booth, 1980) and of some prognostic value in patients undergoing conservative surgery. Those with a normal summating potential/action potential complex do significantly better after endolymphatic sac surgery (Morrison, Moffat and O'Connor, 1980), which might imply the patient is at an early stage in the natural history of the disease, when the inner ear returns to normal between attacks.

Another exciting potential application of electrocochleography may be its use in monitoring the electrophysiological changes occurring in the cochlea and VIIIth nerve in Menière's disease in response to various therapeutic modalities and to surgery. Electrocochleography has also been used with some success to monitor antigenic challenges in patients whose Menière's disease is thought to be due to allergy (Viscomi and Bojrab, 1992). During infusion of the vasodilating agent naftidrofuryl, an increase in the amplitude of the cochlear microphonic potential and decrease in the negativity of the summating potential was seen in some patients, providing support for the use of vasodilators in the therapy of Menière's disease (Gibson, Ramsden and Moffat, 1977). Intraoperative electrocochleography has been used to monitor the progress of endolymphatic sac surgery, and it is claimed that over half the ears demonstrated improvement in the summating potential/action potential ratio during the actual procedure (Arenberg *et al.*, 1993). Those who employ intraoperative monitoring conclude that it provides strong evidence that endolymphatic sac surgery alters the inner ear physiology in a significant number of ears with endolymphatic

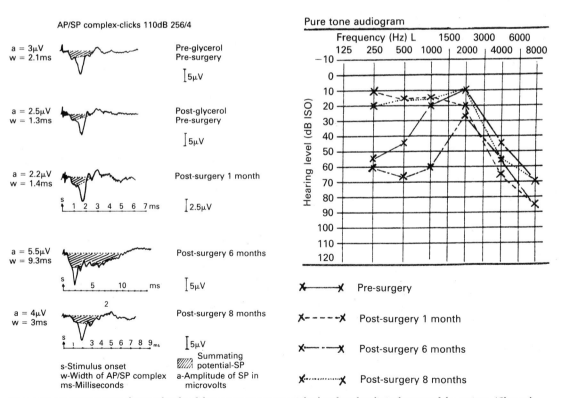

Figure 19.16 Variation in the amplitude of the summating potential related to the clinical status of the patient. (Glycerol dehydration, saccus endolymphaticus/mastoid shunt surgery and the clinical stage of the disease.) (Reproduced from Moffat, 1979, with the kind permission of the *British Journal of Audiology*)

hydrops (Gibson, 1991). It should be pointed out, however, that meaningful changes in the electrocochleographic recording during surgery may be difficult to interpret at the present time.

Glycerol dehydration has also been shown to have an effect on the inner ear impedance and, in a small way, on impedance as measured at the tympanic membrane. Hall (1978), using an impedance bridge with a probe tone of 220 Hz, reported reduced compliance in patients who complained of fullness or pressure in the ear at the time of testing. Morrison, Moffat and O'Connor (1980) reported changes in otoadmittance following glycerol dehyration, and the change was in proportion to the improvement seen in low tone hearing loss on the pure tone audiogram. Paradoxically, when the hearing improves after dehydration, there is an increased resistance to the flow of sound energy through the inner ear, or decreased inner ear conductance (Morrison, 1986). Brookes, Morrison and Richard (1984) confirmed these findings in a larger series of patients and found that glycerol induced significant maximum conductance changes in 53.4% of hydropic ears, while subjective audiometric threshold shifts were seen in only 23.2%. The same group went on to demonstrate that significant changes in maxiumum conductance could be demonstrated in 40.7% of the asymptomatic contralateral ears in patients with Menière's disease (Brookes, Morrison and Richard, 1985).

Audiological techniques under investigation

Auditory brain stem evoked responses are useful in the investigation of patients with asymmetrical sensorineural hearing loss in excluding the wave latency prolongation associated with retrocochlear lesions. Recently, Thornton, Farrell and Haacke (1991) have proposed a test for Menière's disease which uses the auditory brain stem evoked responses as a non-invasive monitor of the mechanical state of the cochlea. The test is based upon the theory that endolymphatic hydrops and increased pressure in the scala media result in increased stiffness of the basilar membrane and increased speed of the travelling wave. It involves the measurement of a properly masked auditory brain stem evoked response prior to and following glycerol administration. A positive test includes the finding of reduced latency of wave V in the hydropic ear, followed by prolongation of the wave V latency after glycerol infusion, with a progressive increase in the latency again as the glycerol is excreted. Preliminary efforts have been met with some success, indicating the technique may show promise as a future non-invasive test for endolymphatic hydrops and as a means of monitoring the response to medical therapy or surgery. It should be noted, however, that a recent report (Munro, Smith and Thornton, 1995) examined the difficulties experienced in implementing the auditory brain stem evoked response travelling

wave velocity (delta V) technique with two commercially available systems and this test, theoretically exciting as it is, may not fulfil its early diagnostic promise.

Otoacoustic emissions have been examined in patients with Menière's disease. Transiently evoked otoacoustic emissions obtained from patients with Menière's disease demonstrate features which are atypical compared with normal hearing ears or from ears with sensorineural hearing loss due to other aetiologies (Harris and Probst, 1992). In patients with a mean hearing loss of less than 30 dB, the measurement of otoacoustic emissions may reveal a hearing improvement of as little as 5 dB following glycerol dehydration, leading some to suggest that this non-invasive test be employed in patients suspected of having early Menière's disease (Uziel and Bonfils, 1993). The lack of a consistent abnormal pattern in the otoacoustic emissions of patients with Menière's disease, however, and the inability to test patients with anything more than a mild hearing loss, makes this technique less attractive than electrocochleography.

Lowering the ambient pressure has been reported to have a positive effect on the symptoms and objective audiometric findings of Menière's disease (Larsen and Angelborg, 1991). While this has led to the introduction of pressure chamber treatment of Menière's disease (Tjernstrom, 1980), the usefulness of this phenomenon as a test of Menière's disease is limited by the bulky and expensive equipment needed to perform it.

Assessment of vestibular function

The assessment of vestibular labyrinthine function is an integral part of a complete investigative protocol in Menière's disease. This evaluation may be useful in assessing disease localization, and may give insight into the related balance disorders these patients may suffer.

The most common observation in the vestibular investigation is hypoactivity of the vestibulo-ocular reflex upon caloric stimulation of the involved labyrinth. In 1942, Cawthorne, Fitzgerald and Hallpike clearly showed that as many as 94% of patients with Menière's disease had abnormal reactions to the caloric test. Evaluation of the reaction is usually based on the maximum speed of the slow phase of the generated nystagmus, although other measurements can be made (Stahle and Klockhoff, 1986). A slow phase velocity difference of 20% is considered significant (Cawthorne, Fitzgerald and Hallpike, 1942; Black and Kitch, 1980). Meyerhoff. Paparella and Gudbrandsson (1981) found that 65% of 211 patients with Menière's disease demonstrated a canal paresis, although the caloric response was normal in 21%. The caloric response decreases over the duration of the disease, with the greatest fluctuation seen earlier in Menière's disease (Stahle and Klockhoff, 1986). The monothermal differential caloric test allows a differentiation between vestibular recruitment and decruitment and may therefore be helpful in excluding an VIIIth nerve or brain stem disorder (Kumar, 1981). Galvanic stimulation of the vestibular system can similarly differentiate between Menière's disease and retrolabyrinthine disorders, but it is technically difficult to perform (Black and Kitch, 1980).

A directional preponderance is present in 13–36% of these patients, and has been reported to be, on the whole, just as often away from the diseased ear as towards it (Stahle and Klockhoff, 1986). Therefore, while directional preponderance constitutes a good indication of vestibular dysfunction, its use in localizing the affected side is limited.

Futaki, Kitahara and Morimoto (1975) developed the frusemide, (furosemide) test to measure changes in the caloric response following administration of the diuretic, a sort of 'vestibular glycerol test'. Significant improvements (defined as greater than 9.4% pre-furosemide slow phase velocity) were seen in as many as 80% of ears affected by Menière's disease (Futaki, Kitahara and Morimoto, 1975) and up to 89% of patients with delayed endolymphatic hydrops (Futaki *et al.*, 1984). A variation on the same theme, called the 'frusemide (furosemide) VOR test' measures changes in the slow phase velocity generated during harmonic sinusoidal rotation with eyes closed (Kobayashi *et al.*, 1989). Sensitivities of 54% and 67% were obtained for Menière's disease and delayed endolymphatic hydrops respectively. A comparison of the frusemide (furosemide) test with electrocochleography/glycerol dehydration suggested a much higher sensitivity of the frusemide (furosemide) test (Futaki, Kitahara and Morimoto, 1977), but a lack of enthusiasm for the test is probably because of its low specificity for Menière's disease. The combination of the frusemide (furosemide) VOR test and electrocochleography with glycerol dehydration is recommended for detecting endolymphatic hydrops in the vestibular and cochlear systems (Ito *et al.*, 1993).

Rotational chair testing has been used to evaluate patients with Menière's disease in several studies, but a wide variety of response and failure to develop a diagnostic pattern of the vestibular dysfunction have limited its usefulness (Black and Kitch, 1980). Similar confusion has plagued tests of optokinetic function (Stahle and Klockhoff, 1986) and ocular counter-rolling (Black and Kitch, 1980).

Clinical evaluations of the vestibulospinal reflex arch are included in the neuro-otological examination, but are rather insensitive in detecting subtle abnormalities in Menière's disease. In one study, gait and stepping tests were abnormal in 28% of the patients and the Romberg test was positive in only 12.8% (Hulshof and Baarsma, 1981). The Unterberger stepping test is more useful than the Romberg test. In Menière's disease, the clinician may see a directional preponderance but, in the patient who is grossly unsteady, a vestibular schwannoma should be suspected and ruled out. Vestibulospinal testing by dynamic posturography, however, shows the greatest promise in the clinical vestibular evaluation in Menière's disease. Posturography proved to be more sensitive than caloric responses and rotational testing in a busy vestibular laboratory, with 71% of those afflicted with Menière's disease showing abnormal results (Black and Kitch, 1980). Posturography also carried the lowest false positive rate, of just 5%. Posturography has proved to be of value in assessing the effects of therapy in Menière's disease (Black, 1982).

In 1977, Nadol found that a positive Hennebert's sign was found in 30% of Menière's affected ears. The required stimulus was negative pressure applied to the external auditory meatus, and the elicited response was horizontal nystagmus in 92% of cases. Others have found that changes in the pressure of the external auditory meatus can affect vestibulospinal function, causing deviation in the stepping or standing position or head deviation toward the opposite side (Naito *et al.*, 1989). Indeed, even stapes movement due to an electrically induced stapedial reflex has been shown adversely to affect body sway as measured by posturography, a technical means of reproducing what is essentially the Hennebert sign (Watanabe *et al.*, 1989). This phenomenon is probably due to the close proximity between the stapedial footplate and saccule following the saccular dilatation of endolymphatic hydrops. This finding is a medical curiosity and is not specific for Menière's disease.

Metabolic and other screening tests

Patients should be put through a protocol of investigations to exclude all of these causes of 'secondary endolymphatic hydrops' before making the diagnosis of pure or classical Menière's disease (Table 19.3). It is the firm belief of the current authors that many

Table 19.3 Investigative protocol for causes of secondary endolymphatic hydrops

Full blood count (FBC)
Erythrocyte sedimentation rate (ESR)
Urea, electrolytes
Venereal disease research laboratory test (VDRL)
Treponema pallidum haemagglutination antibody (TPHA)
Random serum glucose (fasting glucose)
Glucose tolerance test (GTT)
Cholesterol, triglycerides (fasting lipid profile)
Thyroid function tests
Immunological assays, autoantibody screening

clinical studies of Menière's disease have been blighted and made invalid by the fact that the patients included have not been put through a comprehensive series of investigations to exclude patients with 'secondary endolymphatic hydrops' and that the cohort of patients studied are not all 'pure' Menière's disease.

Treatment

The precise aetiology of Menière's disease remains obscure and it is therefore not surprising that no cure for the disorder exists. At present, almost every medical treatment and a bewildering array of surgical procedures have been tried without universal success. There is no single therapy for Menière's disease embraced by the majority of doctors who are experts in its management. There is a vast, often contradictory literature on the subject. No known therapeutic modality has been scientifically and statistically proven to alter significantly the course of the disease. In 1977, Torok published a paper demonstrating that all treatments, medical and surgical, reported significant improvement in the symptoms of Menière's disease in 60–80% of cases and therapeutic failures occurred in 10–20%. These figures remain accurate,

according to more recent longitudinal studies (Green, Blum and Harner, 1991). This suggests either a significant placebo effect or a natural history which results in spontaneous resolution of symptoms. Silverstein, Smouha and Jones (1989) shed further light on this issue when reporting that, in patients refusing any treatment, 57% had complete resolution of vertigo at 2 years, 71% at 8.3 years. Most recent papers on therapy for Menière's disease have poor or absent controls, and fail to demonstrate a significant difference between the therapy and placebo (Ruckenstein, Rutka and Hawke, 1991).

Difficulty exists in quantifying the effect of the various treatments for Menière's disease because of its broad clinical variability. A significant advance in the science of Menière's treatment has been the development of fixed criteria for the evaluation of therapy and the reporting of therapeutic results. These were devised by the American Academy of Otolaryngology's (AAO–HNS) Subcommittee on Hearing and Equilibrium and their Measurements (Alford, 1972; Pearson and Brackmann, 1985). The most recent formula, generated in 1985, provides criteria for hearing changes and disability, and offers a numerical score to quantify changes in vertigo spells (Table 19.4). Most current studies of therapy for Menière's

Table 19.4 Summary of the American Academy of Otolaryngology – Head and Neck Surgery Subcommittee on Hearing and Equilibrium criteria for evaluating Menière's disease therapy

A Vertigo

Requires 6 months of pre-treatment observation and 24 months post-treatment follow up

1   Vertigo control − numerical value =

$$\text{Vertigo control} = \frac{\text{Average number of spells per month post-treatment (24 months)} \times 100}{\text{Average number of spells per month pre-treatment (6 months)}}$$

Numerical value	Verbal score
= 0	Complete control
= 1–40	Substantial control
= 41–80	Limited control
= 81–120	Insignificant control
= > 120	Patient worse

2   Disability status

    0 = No disability
    1 = Mild disability: mild unsteadiness/dizziness that precludes working in a hazardous environment
    2 = Moderate disability: unsteadiness/dizziness that results in necessity for a sedentary occupation
    3 = Severe disability: symptoms exclude gainful employment

B Hearing

Pure tone average (PTA) = Average threshold over 0.5, 1, 2, 3 kHz

Pre-treatment audiogram = worst PTA and speech discrimination (SD) over the 6 months prior to therapy

Post-treatment audiogram = worst PTA and SD over 24 months post-treatment

Unchanged	+/− 10 dB PTA or +/− 15% SD
Improved	> 10 dB PTA decrease or 15% SD increase
Worse	< 10 dB PTA increase or 15% SD decrease

From Pearson and Brackmann, 1985

disease include an analysis of data pertaining to both the 1972 and 1985 scoring methods (Moffat, 1994). A further revision is currently in preparation (see addendum). Current therapy is largely aimed at alleviating vertigo, which is the most troublesome symptom of Menière's disease and, except in long-standing bilateral disease where hearing loss may be severe, is the single most important symptom producing a profound effect on the quality of the patient's life.

Medical treatment

In the treatment of Menière's disease, it is of paramount importance that a good doctor–patient relationship be established. After the initial attack, the patient is often very apprehensive and requires considerable support and reassurance. An explanation of the nature of the disease and the fact that it is not life threatening, is often very encouraging to these anxious people, who may initially imagine they have a brain tumour or are experiencing strokes. A discussion of long-term expectations is important, and it should be stated that although there is no cure, modern treatment can usually dramatically improve the quality of life by controlling the vertigo (Blair, 1984). Psychological support is possibly the most important aspect of medical treatment for this chronic disorder (Weit, Kazan and Shambaugh, 1981; Berrios *et al.*, 1988).

Symptomatic relief during acute episodes

The acute vertigo suffered during an attack of Menière's disease is due to a sudden asymmetry in vestibular input to the central nervous system. 'Vestibular suppressants' are a group of drugs which have a well established record of controlling attacks of vertigo and associated vegetative symptoms. These drugs all have variable anticholinergic, antiemetic and sedative properties. They include phenothiazines, such as prochlorperazine and perphenazine, antihistamines, such as cinnarizine, cyclizine, dimenhydrinate, promethazine hydrochloride and meclizine hydrochloride, and benzodiazepines, such as lorazepam and diazepam (Weit, Kazan and Shambaugh, 1981; Beck, 1986a; Pyykko *et al.*, 1988; Birchall, 1991). The benzodiazepines reduce activity in the vestibular nuclei, and probably relieve anxiety associated with the attack as well. Transdermal scopolamine hydrobromide, an anticholinergic agent which crosses the blood–brain barrier, has also recently been added successfully to the medical armamentarium of Menière's disease (Babin, Balkany and Fee, 1984). Astemizole, a new antihistamine which apparently does not cross the blood-brain barrier, has been shown in a preliminary study substantially to reduce symptoms in patients with unilateral Menière's disease (Turner and Jackson, 1989).

Prophylaxis between acute episodes

The medical therapies aimed at prophylaxis and prevention of vertigo in Menière's disease are based on concepts about the pathophysiology of the disorder (Beck, 1986a). Salt restriction, diuretic therapy, and hyperosmolar dehydration are aimed at reducing endolymphatic accumulation. Vasodilators are given in the belief that Menière's disease is the result of strial ischaemia or endolymphatic sac hypoperfusion. Steroids and immunological therapy are aimed at the possible causes of the disorder generated by the immune system.

In 1934, Furstenberg, Lashmet and Lathrop noted the 'salt sensitivity' of many patients with Menière's disease. Diuretics and dietary salt restriction are now believed by many otolaryngologists to be the mainstays of medical therapy (Jackson, Glasscock and Davis, 1981; Santos *et al.*, 1993). The perceived goal of this therapy is the reduction of endolymph volume and pressure, either by fluid removal or reduction in production. Substantial relief of symptoms has been reported in several studies, with vertigo control occurring in up to 79% and hearing stabilization in 69% (Klockhoff and Lindblom, 1967; Klockhoff, Lindblom and Stahle, 1974; Santos *et al.*, 1993). Success has been reported with the use of hydrochlorothiazide (Klockhoff and Lindblom, 1967), chlorthalidone (Klockhoff, Lindblom and Stahle, 1974), acetazolamide (Shinkawa and Kimura, 1986; Corvera and Corvera, 1989), and Dyazide (Van Deelen and Huizing, 1986). Many of these studies, however, have been criticized for poor design and control, leading some authors to question whether diuretics are truly better than placebo or the natural history of the disorder (Ruckenstein, Rutka and Hawke, 1991). The best designed diuretic study to date, a cross-over placebo-controlled study of Dyazide (a combination of hydrochlorothiazide and triamterene) showed a statistically favourable effect on vestibular complaints, but no effect on hearing loss or tinnitus (Van Deelen and Huizing, 1986). Most authors agree that, especially with regard to hearing loss, diuretics do not halt the progression of the disease (Horner *et al.*, 1989).

Carbonic anhydrase inhibitors, such as acetazolamide, were initially recommended because of the presence of carbonic anhydrase in the endolymph-producing dark cells and stria vascularis. Their use, however, has not been shown to be clinically superior to other diuretics (Shinkawa and Kimura, 1986; Corvera and Corvera, 1989) and the fact that the immediate effect of acetazolamide is to increase hydrops and hearing loss indicates that caution should be exercised when using this medication (Brookes, Morrison and Booth, 1982). Brookes and Booth reported the results of a pilot study in 1984 which concluded that oral acetazolamide had no place in the treatment of Menière's disease.

The cerebrally effective calcium antagonist, flunarizine, has been evaluated in patients with Menière's disease by means of a vestibular index and a positive therapeutic effect has been reported (Haid, 1988).

The use of vasodilators in Menière's disease is also widespread (Beck, 1986a). Betahistine dihydrochloride (Serc), an oral preparation of a histamine precursor, has received the most attention and use (Fischer, 1991). Early studies have been criticized because of small sample sizes, poor controls, and lack of long term follow up (Hommes, 1970; Wilmot and Menon, 1976). Two recent large, well designed and controlled studies contradict each other in their findings regarding the use of betahistine in Menière's disease. One study showed a benefit of the use of betahistine, both in terms of vertigo relief and cochlear symptoms (Fraysse *et al.*, 1991); the study did not use the 1985 AAO-HNS criteria to evaluate the response to the drug. The better designed study by Schmidt and Huizing (1992) shows no advantage of betahistine over placebo in a double-blind, randomized, crossover, placebo-controlled trial of 35 patients over 33 weeks. Recent reports of an improvement in 80% of patients with Menière's disease treated with betahistine have led some to suggest it is the most effective drug in maintenance therapy of the disorder (Aantaa, 1991). As with diuretic therapy, however, no benefit in long-term hearing loss is seen with betahistine, and the disease continues to progress despite symptom relief (Weintraub *et al.*, 1976).

Other vasodilators used in the treatment of Menière's disease include papaverine, isoxsuprine, nylidrin, dipyridamole, amyl nitrite, nitroglycerin, nicotinic acid, carbon dioxide and thymoxamine (Pollock *et al.*, 1974; Young, 1978; Glasscock *et al.*, 1984; Beck, 1986a). Adenosine triphosphate, whose effects on the inner ear are thought to include improvement of the microcirculation, has been shown in a large, well controlled, double-blind trial to be more effective than betahistine in the treatment of Menière's disease (Mizukoshi *et al.*, 1988). Other methods of attempting an improvement in inner ear blood flow and oxygenation in Menière's disease include the use of low molecular weight Dextran infusion and inhalation of a 5% CO_2/95% O_2 mixture (carbogen) (Shea and Kitabchi, 1973; Glasscock *et al.*, 1984).

Confusion about the use of vasodilators begins with theoretical concerns regarding the proposed pathophysiology of Menière's disease. If this disorder is due to ischaemia of the stria vascularis and dark cells, it seems logical to some authors that increasing blood flow to these organs, which produce endolymph, should actually make hydrops worse (Blair, 1984; Ruckenstein, Rutka and Hawke, 1991). One trial showed that betahistine relieved the vertigo suffered by patients with a variety of peripheral vestibular disorders, including Menière's disease, indicating

that relief of vertigo may not be due to resolution of endolymphatic hydrops at all but via another mechanism (Oosterveld, 1984). It also seems odd, in the case of betahistine, to treat patients with histamine in a disease that is also relieved by systemic antihistamines. Despite these objections, the literature does offer some qualified support for the use of betahistine for the control of vertigo in Menière's disease (Ruckenstein, Rutka and Hawke, 1991).

Recent evidence that Menière's disease may have an autoimmune aetiology has led some authors to use therapeutic modalities aimed at the immune system. Hughes *et al.* (1983b, 1988a) advocated the use of steroids, cytotoxic drugs and/or lymphocytoplasmaphoresis in patients suspected to have an immune aetiology to their Menière's disease, while Futaki, Semba and Kudo (1988) have administered immunoglobulin G with methyl B12 in the same patient group.

Other therapies have been proposed for the treatment of Menière's disease. Holistic treatment using acupuncture and herbal preparations have been employed (Eichner, Kampik and Gleditch, 1986). Long-term relief of the vertigo of Menière's disease using hypobaric pressure chamber therapy has also been described (Tjernstrom, 1986). The problem of scientifically studying these techniques is magnified by their previous empirical application and poor description of the techniques themselves.

One must not forget that part of the medical therapy for Menière's disease involves treatment of the less troubling symptoms of hearing loss and tinnitus. Hearing loss is generally rehabilitated through the use of hearing aids, although recruitment and impaired speech discrimination may make this difficult. Tinnitus may be treated with reassurance or with masking. Tinnitus clinics and self-help groups can be very helpful and reassuring to some patients. The tinnitus associated with Menière's disease is usually easily masked by a low level of many different external sounds, and the use of hearing aids and tinnitus maskers can usually provide an acceptable level of relief for the tinnitus of Menière's disease (Vernon, Johnson and Schleuning, 1980).

While inattention to aural auditory rehabiliation is rarely an issue, few centres concentrate on vestibular rehabilitation of patients with inner ear disorders. Vestibular rehabilitation programmes have recently been developed which integrate the diagnostic, clinical and audiological investigation with a comprehensive assessment of the balance system and the patient's general state of fitness (Shepard, Telian and Smith-Wheelock, 1990). A programme of specific exercises is then designed for the patient by the medical and physiotherapy team, the goal of which is improved central compensation for vestibular asymmetry and improved attention to non-vestibular balance clues. While vestibular rehabilitation is not tremendously helpful for patients with rapidly changing vestibular outputs, such as a patient suffering frequent vertiginous episodes, it is helpful for patients with relatively static vestibular function, such as a patient with end-stage Menière's disease or a patient who has undergone a procedure which involved partial or total vestibular ablation. In Menière's disease, vestibular rehabilitation is very helpful for patients with poorly compensated unilateral vestibular hypofunction and for patients with bilateral vestibular hypofunction (Telian *et al.*, 1990).

Surgical treatment

Surgical treatment of Menière's disease is reserved for the 10–20% of patients who fail conservative medical management (Torok, 1977; Brown, 1983). As with medical therapy, no surgical cure has been devised for Menière's disease. Clearly, labyrinthectomy will eradicate the patient's symptoms, but the cost is total ablation of auditory and vestibular function. There is still great controversy surrounding the various surgical procedures advocated in Menière's disease. Scientific papers containing passionate diatribes claiming the superiority of one procedure over the rest abound in the literature. Increased fervour and foment has been stirred up by the emergence of several studies of sham operations claiming to show that equally good results can be achieved in this way.

A study of the history of surgery for Menière's disease makes interesting reading. Perhaps it is not surprising that, in view of the diverse aetiological factors that have been implicated, a constellation of fascinating and sometimes bizarre procedures has been advocated, some, but not all, with a rational basis in the light of our current knowledge. In 1877, Gowers reported that blistering behind the ear afforded very marked relief of the vertigo. Babinski, in 1903, first proposed the therapeutic effects of lumbar puncture as a treatment for Menière's disease, a practice which conferred only temporary benefit and required repetition to be effective. In the same year (1903) Crockett reported the removal of the stapes in two cases of auditory vertigo, but most authors consider that the first effective definitive surgical procedure was reported in 1904. Lake (1904) and Milligan (1905) independently described labyrinthectomy for aural vertigo. Lake described a transmastoid approach, opening the lateral semicircular canal to gain access to the vestibule. The ampullae were opened, the vestibule curetted, stapes removed and the cavity filled with iodoform emulsion. Milligan carried out a radical mastoidectomy, drilled out all three semicircular canals and curetted the resulting cavity which was then packed with dry gauze. Also in 1904, R. H. Parry performed the first intracranial VIIIth nerve section for Menière's disease via a middle fossa approach. In 1907, T. W. Parry advocated the use of a 'seton', a thread or tape placed in a subcutaneous tract fashioned in these cases over the nape of the neck on the side of the affected ear. Parry also suggested hypnosis as a treatment for Menière's disease. Other procedures, such as stapedectomy and cervical sympathectomy (Passe and Seymour, 1948), have been described, used for a time and abandoned as generations of surgeons have sought to relieve their patients with Menière's disease (McKee *et al.*, 1991) (Table 19.5).

The operations for Menière's disease may be divided into those that preserve auditory function and those that do not. Within the hearing preservation group are procedures which preserve vestibular function and those which ablate it.

Procedures involving hearing preservation and vestibular preservation

The operations described in this group are those procedures which attempt to reverse endolymphatic hydrops and restore normal endolymph volume and pressure. These include the endolymphatic sac decompression procedures and the Cody (1973) and Fick (1964) cochleosacculotomies.

Procedures on the endolymphatic sac

In 1926, Portmann performed the first surgery on the saccus endolymphaticus after having conducted research in comparative and human anatomy and pathology of the endolymphatic sac. His interesting series of experiments on the lateral line organ of elasmobranch fishes make fascinating reading. It is interesting to note that this occurred 12 years before Hallpike and Cairns (1938) discovered that endolymphatic hydrops was the pathological correlate of Menière's disease. Despite the many modifications in technique that have been described in the intervening years, little has changed in terms of the overall objective of the surgery. All forms of this operation seek either to decompress or open the endolymphatic sac and increase the drainage or resorption of endolymph, so as to reduce or eliminate endolymphatic hydrops and its clinical sequelae. Whether, in fact, this occurs through the decompression itself, or by passive diffusion of endolymph, osmotic pull, or alteration of blood supply following manipulation of the endolymphatic sac is a question which remains unanswered (Alford, Cohn and Igarashi, 1977; Paparella and Sajjadi, 1987a,b).

Portmann's operation simply opened the sac (Portmann, 1987), but drainage through the medial wall of the sac creating an endolymphatic-subarachnoid fistula was advocated by Naito (1962) and used subsequently by many authors (Glasscock *et al.*, 1989). Shambaugh (1968) advocated a wide decompression of the saccus by removing the bone overlying

Table 19.5   A concise history of surgical therapy for Menière's disease

1877	Gowers reported the results of blistering the skin behind the affected ear
1903	Babinski uses repeated lumbar punctures
1903	Crockett performs stapedectomy for Menière's disease
1904	Lake describes labyrinthectomy
1904	R. H. Parry performs the first VIIIth cranial nerve section
1905	Milligan describes labyrinthectomy
1907	T. W. Parry employs a subcutaneous thread in the nape of the neck
1912	Bárány operates to 'break down posterior fossa adhesions'
1920	Ballance injects absolute ethanol into the labyrinth
1926	Portmann performs the first endolymphatic sac drainage operation
1928	Dandy recommends posterior fossa VIIIth nerve section
1932	McKenzie performs the first selective section of the vestibular nerve
1943	Cawthorne advocates membranous labyrinthectomy via lateral semicircular canal
1948	Lempert describes the transmeatal approach to labyrinthectomy
1948	Passe and Seymour employ sympathectomy for Menière's disease
1957	Cawthorne describes the stapedectomy approach to labyrinthectomy
1957	Schuknecht describes intratympanic streptomycin
1958	Fick and Cody describe separate 'tack' procedures
1960	Angell-James employs inner ear ultrasonic stimulation
1960	Several authors use cryotherapy to the inner ear for Menière's disease
1966	Tumarkin advocates grommet insertion for Menière's disease
1970	Arslan applies crystallized salt to the round window as osmotic therapy
1978	Beck describes the use of intratympanic gentamicin for this disorder
1986	Janetta describes fossa microvascular decompression

(After McKee *et al.*, 1991)

it and the adjacent posterior fossa dura. In 1966, Shea described the use of a Teflon film, inserted into an opening in the endolymphatic sac to keep it patent and allow continuing drainage of endolymph into the mastoid cavity. Various prosthetic materials of silicone or Teflon in the form of sheets or tubes have since been inserted into the saccus (Morrison, 1979; Booth, 1980; Glasscock *et al.*, 1984; Arenberg, 1987; Kitahara *et al.*, 1987) as have autologous items like vein grafts (Futaki and Nomura, 1989). Valves have been developed for the same purpose, including the one-way valve used by Arenberg (1987) and the tubed capillary sponge introduced by Austin, Pfalz and Altermatt (1984; Huang and Lin, 1989a). No studies conclusively demonstrate the superiority of one technique over the others (Ruckenstein, Rutka and Hawke, 1991) and it is hard to believe that drainage of the saccus endolymphaticus is achieved in such a low volume, low pressure system. Even if drainage did occur initially it is highly likely that fibrinous occlusion occurs in the fullness of time. Proponents of the operation say that it works by producing surgical trauma and increases blood flow as a result. Others think that surgery may damage the saccus. Indeed, Gibson (personal communication, 1994), believing that endolymphatic sac surgery works by damaging the sac and speeding up the progression of the disease, is now attempting sac ablation rapidly to create 'end stage' disease. This may quickly reduce the severity of the vertigo, but

will increase the sensorineural deafness and is open to the same criticism as the acetazolamide test. His results will be awaited with interest.

All of these methods have been advocated and the literature is punctuated by scattered papers with results that are often confusing and conflicting, based on widely different sets of criteria for reporting success rates (Moffat, 1994). The quoted results of all the procedures described are quite similar. In those studies using the uniform objective guidelines provided by the AAO-HNS in 1985 (see Table 19.4), approximately 50–80% of patients reported complete resolution of vertigo, with another 12–25% reporting substantial relief of vertigo for at least 2 years after the operation (Brackmann and Nissen, 1987; Paparella and Sajjadi, 1987a; Luetje, 1988; Monsell and Wiet, 1988; Huang and Lin, 1989a; Moffat, 1994). In these studies, hearing improvement or stabilization occurred in 60–70% and improvement in tinnitus in 40–60%. While these numbers may not differ appreciably from those quoted for the majority of Menière's disease treatments (Torok, 1977), the fact that these patients have failed medical management indicates that patients with more severe or persistent Menière's disease make up this group in the first place. A 50–80% success rate in this patient population is therefore a respectable result, particularly since the surgery carries a low morbidity. Success has also been experienced in revision sac surgery for recurrent symptoms (Paparella and Sajjadi, 1987a; Huang and

Lin, 1989b), endolymphatic saccotomy for endolymphatic hydrops caused by syphilis (Paparella, Kim and Shea, 1980), and in hydrops associated with chronic otitis media (Huang and Lin, 1991). Complications of this surgery are low and consist primarily of severe postoperative hearing loss, which occurs in 1–2% of cases (Arenberg, 1987; Brackmann and Nissen, 1987; Paparella and Sajjadi, 1987a). Other complications related to the mastoidectomy, such as facial nerve injury and wound infection, and to the peridural manipulations, such as CSF leak and meningitis, have been reported.

Even more so than in other areas of the study of Menière's disease, controversy rages over the effectiveness of the endolymphatic sac decompression and drainage procedures. Behind this furore, there is serious scientific debate over the technique, and many questions have been raised. Foremost in generating and perpetuating this controversy is the 'sham study,' performed by Thomsen *et al.* (1981). In a double-blind, placebo-controlled study, the authors performed a simple mastoidectomy with or without endolymphatic sac drainage. Results were identical for the two operations, with improvement in 73% of patients receiving an endolymphatic shunt and in 80% of patients who had a simple mastoidectomy only, and these results have not changed during longer term subsequent follow up (Bretlau *et al.*, 1984; Thomsen *et al.*, 1986). The study has been criticized for its design and statistics, and a subsequent re-analysis by Pillsbury *et al.* (1983) using the 1972 AAOO criteria concluded that 87% of endolymphatic sac surgery patients improved while only 47% improved in the placebo surgery group. From a statistical point of view, the small sample size renders the study virtually useless. Owing to ethical considerations, it is unlikely that this study will ever be repeated, and therefore controversy surrounding its results will probably always exist. Although the results of the sham study do not necessarily discredit the merit of endolymphatic sac surgery, it will have forced investigators to consider whether the relief of vertigo is due to the intended pathophysiological effect on the inner ear or whether other factors in common with the placebo operation are important (Thomsen *et al.*, 1995).

When comparing a group of patients who underwent endolymphatic sac surgery to a group of patients who chose no therapy over an 8.7 year period, Silverstein, Smouha and Jones (1989) found that endolymphatic sac surgery did not cause a significant difference in the reported relief of vertigo. Glasscock *et al.* (1989) reported complete control of vertigo in 65% of patients at 3 years, which decreased to 50% at 10 years. They subsequently abandoned the endolymphatic sac operation for the vestibular nerve section. This trend of waning success over several years of follow up has been noted in a review of several other current papers on sac surgery (Ruckenstein,

Rutka and Hawke, 1991). This has led to the opinion of some authors that endolymphatic sac surgery does not provide adequate long-term control of vertigo as compared with other surgical methods. Despite the questions regarding endolymphatic sac surgery, the fact remains that many patients have benefitted significantly from it and avoided bigger and more complicated procedures, and it therefore continues to be the initial surgical procedure of choice in many major centres (Brackmann, 1990; Moffat, 1994).

The other advantage of endolymphatic sac procedures is that, since hearing and vestibular neuroepithelium are preserved, the technique is particularly suitable for patients with bilateral disease. Therapeutic destruction of the vestibular neuroepithelium in these patients may trade rotatory vertigo for failed vestibular compensation, as well as the possibility of increased hearing loss.

Procedures on other ear structures

The other surgical procedures which attempt to preserve hearing and vestibular function include grommet insertion, middle ear osmotic therapy and the various forms of fistulization of the cochlea and/or saccule.

In 1966, Tumarkin proposed that endolymphatic hydrops could be secondary to negative middle ear pressure acting at the round window. He therefore advocated the insertion of a grommet in the tympanic membrane to equalize atmospheric and middle ear pressures. However, no association between Menière's disease and eustachian tube dysfunction has been established and despite the lack of scientific rationale some otologists still practise this.

Given the fact that Menière's disease is associated with endolymphatic hydrops, some authors have used osmotic agents to attempt to reduce this inner ear fluid imbalance. In 1970, Arslan applied crystallized salt to the round window with some success. Morrison and Morrison (1989) reported a new technique of hyperosmolar perfusion of the scala tympani using mannitol, calling this procedure 'cochlear dialysis'. Vertigo was substantially or completely controlled in 63% of their patients, and hearing losses occurred in 27%.

The Fick and Cody tack procedures were similarly designed to create a fistula in the saccule via the oval window, in the hope of decompressing endolymphatic hydrops (Fick, 1964; Cody, 1973; Cody and McDonald, 1983). The Fick procedure accomplished this through direct manipulation of the saccule with a pick via the oval window, and the Cody procedure involved the insertion of a sharp, 1.5 mm tack through the membranous attachments of the stapes footplate. These techniques have largely been abandoned because of their inconsistent results and their high incidence of hearing loss (Brackmann, 1990). Schuknecht (1982a) first described the round window cochleosacculotomy procedure after observing that a fracture of the osseous spiral lamina led to a permanent fistula. This procedure was reported to control vertigo in 70% of patients, although the long-term results of others have been disappointing (Giddings *et al.*, 1991). Significant hearing loss occurs frequently, in as many as 80% of patients, and those who continue to use this procedure consider it a destructive one and reserve it for use in elderly patients with good vestibular function and poor preoperative hearing (Brackmann, 1990). Given this high incidence of hearing loss, these procedures should probably be considered under the category of 'vestibular conservation – hearing ablation'.

Procedures involving hearing preservation and vestibular ablation

This category of surgical procedures for Menière's disease includes operations which disrupt the flow of sensory input from the vestibular end organ to the brain. This is done by the selective chemical ablation of the vestibular end organ itself or by the disruption of the vestibular component of the VIIIth nerve.

Procedures involving ablation of the VIIIth nerve

The first VIIIth nerve division for persistent 'aural vertigo' was performed by R. H. Parry in 1904. Frazier also reported this procedure in 1912. In 1928, Dandy successfully treated nine patients with Menière's disease by sectioning the VIIIth cranial nerve by the suboccipital approach. He went on to perfect and popularize the procedure, performing over 400 such operations for this indication in the following 13 years, with complete success in terms of symptom relief in all but a very few (Dandy, 1941). While Dandy advocated lysis of the vestibular nerves and up to three quarters of the cochlear nerve, McKenzie (1936) was the first selectively to section the vestibular component alone, and he showed that vertigo could be controlled with good preservation of hearing in the majority of patients with good preoperative hearing. Barber and Ireland (1952) reported an 83% rate of complete relief from vertigo following the performance of 117 of these selective operations.

This operation was overshadowed for some time by the total osseous labyrinthectomy, partly because of the greater ease of the latter procedure for the otologist and partly because of the potentially much greater side effects of the intracranial procedure. A revival of enthusiasm for the vestibular nerve section occurred following the description by House in 1961 of exposure of the internal auditory meatus through the middle cranial fossa. He advocated this operation over the labyrinthectomy because he felt that residual hearing preservation should be attempted as often as possible in a disease which, it was emerging, had a significant incidence of bilaterality in the long term. The great strength of this procedure is the ease with which the vestibular nerves can be differentiated from the cochlear and facial nerves in the lateral internal auditory meatus, allowing greater accuracy of the nerve section and decreasing the likelihood of injury to hearing and facial movement. House continued to section the nerve medial to Scarpa's ganglion, as this was felt to reduce the likelihood of any regeneration or neuroma formation. This operation has seen much use and success in the past three decades, with Smyth, Kerr and Gordon (1976), Glasscock *et al.* (1984) and Fisch (1984), all reporting a 94% success rate in relieving vertigo. However, even in Los Angeles, the birthplace of the operation, reluctance to use the middle fossa approach emerged in the late 1970s and early 1980s, especially in elderly patients. This was because of the increased difficulty of elevating the middle fossa dura experienced in older patients and in the poor tolerance older patients have of temporal lobe retraction (Brackmann, 1983). Fisch (1984) proposed a variation on the middle fossa approach called the 'transtemporal supralabyrinthine' approach. This involves removal of the root of the zygoma and roof of the epitympanum, in addition to as much bone as possible from above the labyrinth itself, allowing better visualization of the internal auditory meatus from a lateral approach and minimizing the degree of temporal lobe retraction necessary to perform the procedure.

It is interesting to note that, although this is categorized as a hearing conservation procedure, hearing losses due to surgery occur in 8–58% of the patients, with the average in large series being about 45% (Glasscock *et al.*, 1989a; Moffat *et al.*, 1991; Nguyen *et al.*, 1992). Also, although hearing is reported to stabilize or improve postoperatively in 51–83% of patients (Brackmann, 1990), actual long-term hearing results are in keeping with the natural history of the disease (Glasscock, Johnson and Poe, 1989a). Changes in tinnitus are unpredictable, but improvements occur in up to 50% (Brackmann, 1990). Complications of the middle fossa procedure included a 3–7% incidence of transient or delayed facial palsy, a 3–6% incidence of total hearing loss, and a variable but uncommon incidence of meningitis, haematoma, CSF leak and temporal lobe epilepsy (Fisch, 1984; Moffat, 1988; Brackmann, 1990).

Selective incomplete supralabyrinthine transtemporal vestibular neurectomy in the internal auditory meatus has been described by Bohmer and Fisch (1995). Intentional preservation of parts of the inferior vestibular nerve has been practised for better hearing preservation. Patients with bilateral vestibular neurectomy had preserved horizontal vestibulo-ocular reflexes in response to high angular accelerations with gain enhancement over time. A torsional down-beating spontaneous nystagmus and an important tilt of the subjective vertical were observed when the remaining VIIIth nerve was sectioned after homolateral incomplete supralabyrinthine vestibular neurectomy. These findings suggest that a reorganization of vestibular reflexes may occur after incomplete neurectomy if afferents of the inferior vestibular branch are partially spared. The vestibular function after incomplete supralabyrinthine vestibular neurectomy does not affect the postoperative control of vertiginous attacks and may have positive effects in case of deterioration of the contralateral inner ear.

As an alternative to the middle fossa approach, Silverstein, Norrell and Haberkamp reintroduced a form of the suboccipital vestibular nerve section in 1987. This involves the sectioning of the superior vestibular and posterior ampullary nerves via the retrosigmoid approach after removal of some bone from the posterior aspect of the internal auditory meatus, although many surgeons now do not remove the posterior lip of the meatus. Its advantages were the familiarity of this dissection to the otologist, good exposure of the VIIth and VIIIth cranial nerves and less risk of injury to the facial nerve, labyrinth and temporal lobe.

This procedure was found to alter significantly the natural history of Menière's disease, where endolymphatic sac surgery had failed to meet the statistical threshold (Silverstein, Smouha and Jones, 1989). After some modifications in technique, including the use of the presigmoid-retrolabyrinthine and retrosigmoid routes to the vestibular nerve, success rates in terms of vertigo relief are identical to the middle fossa approach (Silverstein, Norrell and Rosenberg, 1990). This success rate has been verified in other large series of retrolabyrinthine vestibular nerve sections for Menière's disease, and is identical for presigmoid, retrosigmoid and combined approaches (Kemink and Hoff, 1986; Glasscock *et al.*, 1991; Nguyen *et al.*, 1992). In Cambridge, all patients who have undergone the posterior fossa vestibular neurectomy reported marked improvement in vertigo symptoms (Moffat *et al.*, 1991). Postoperatively, 98% of patients report that they consider the operation worthwhile, prompting some authors to offer this as the first line of surgical therapy (Glasscock *et al.*, 1991).

Stabilization or improvement in hearing was reduced in 55–88% of patients (Kemink and Hoff, 1986; Silverstein, Norrell and Rosenberg, 1990; Glasscock *et al.*, 1991). Long-term postoperative hearing results are not available but, as with the middle fossa procedure, deterioration with time and progression of the disease would be anticipated. Tinnitus results are more variable with 31–36% reporting improvement and 7–15% reporting worsening of their tinnitus.

The complications vary somewhat from those seen following middle fossa nerve sections. While facial nerve injury remains a potential problem, it is rare with this procedure (Brackmann, 1990). A CSF leak rate of 5%, a meningitis rate of 1–3%, a wound infection rate of up to 20% (Silverstein, Norrell and Haberkamp, 1987), and a 9% incidence of severe postoperative headache (Silverstein, Norrel and Rosenberg, 1990) have been reported. This last complication can be the most miserable in the long term, with up to 27% of these patients reporting continuing headache requiring medication 2 years following surgery (Silverstein, Norrel and Rosenberg, 1990). Although this postoperative headache may relate to drilling the posterior lip of the internal auditory meatus, it may still occur as occipital neuralgia in those cases where the nerve is sectioned in the posterior fossa and no bone is removed from the internal auditory meatus. Prevention of this may be possible by not dividing the upper cervical muscles and by interposing fat between the dura and pericranium to prevent dural adhesions.

Interestingly, most patients report continuing aural fullness following vestibular nerve section, confirming that the disease remains active in the end organ but the labyrinth has been effectively denervated (Moffat *et al.*, 1991). Many patients still have the premonitory symptoms without the vertigo and know when they would have had an attack. This also seems to indicate that the sensory input that is decoded by the central nervous sytem as aural fullness must be carried from the labyrinth by a non-vestibular nerve, the cochlear nerve being the most likely.

Attention should be paid to pre- and postoperative vestibular and postural function tests. The patterns of vestibular function following vestibular nerve section are widely variable, and failure of central compensation may occur (Cass, Kartush and Graham, 1992). Vestibular rehabilitation should be considered in patients troubled by continuing postoperative dysequilibrium, and it may be a useful adjunct in the routine early postoperative care of these people in helping to facilitate and speed central compensation.

Bilateral vestibular neurectomy has been advocated for some patients with bilateral Menière's disease (Bohmer and Fisch, 1993). These patients suffer dysequilibrium and oscillopsia due to the bilateral loss of vestibular input, especially at higher levels of angular acceleration of the head, but they are reported to compensate well through the use of 'extra-vestibular' balance cues.

Procedures involving chemical ablation of the vestibular end organ

The ototoxicity associated with aminoglycoside antibiotics has long been recognized (Moffat, 1987b). Within this class of drugs, there exists a spectrum of cochlear and vestibular toxicity, with neomycin and kanamycin being known for their high cochlear toxicity, and gentamicin and streptomycin for their vestibular toxicity. These latter drugs have been used by otolaryngologists topically, in the middle ear or applied to the inner ear via a labyrinthotomy, and systemically to control the symptoms of Menière's disease.

Schuknecht (1956) was the first to use intratympanic streptomycin to cause a chemical ablation of vestibular function for Menière's disease, and succeeded in curing 63% of patients of their vertigo. All these patients, however, also suffered a profound hearing loss and Schuknecht abandoned the method. Lange (1976) subsequently used streptomycin in conjunction with ozothin, a substance which was felt selectively to protect the sensory epithelium of the cochlea, and this was met with somewhat better hearing results. Most reports on intratympanic aminoglycoside administration since that time have focused on the use of gentamicin. Between the years 1968 and 1978, Beck used low dose intratympanic gentamicin alone on 39 patients with Menière's disease and reported a 95% rate of improvement in the vertigo and a 15% incidence of hearing deterioration (Beck and Schmidt, 1978). These rates did not change in his subsequent report on a total of 118 patients (Beck, 1986b), and his method of administration became the standard and was used in several centres.

Nedzelski has popularized this technique in Canada (Nedzelski, Bryce and Pfleiderer, 1992). Indications for the treatment are active unilateral Menière's disease with frequent disabling attacks of vertigo which have not responded to conservative medical management. Contraindications include a pre-existing tympanic membrane perforation, active inflammation of the middle ear, allergy to aminoglycosides, impaired renal function, high risk of poor post-procedural central nervous system compensation, and Menière's disease in an only hearing ear. A T-tube is inserted in the tympanic membrane and is attached to a tubal apparatus. This tube is attached to the external ear to prevent movement. A solution containing 26.4 mg/ml of gentamicin is instilled at a volume of about 0.8 ml into the middle ear. The patient lies on the contralateral side for 20 minutes in such a way as to cause pooling of the solution over the round and oval windows. This treatment is repeated three times daily for 4 days, for a total of 12 doses or 208 mg. Treatment is terminated prematurely if nystagmus is observed, if the patient complains of unsteadiness associated with a deterioration of tandem gait, or if a significant deterioration of hearing occurs (a change of 10 dB or greater at three consecutive frequencies) (Nedzelski et al., 1992). Using this regimen Nedzelski, Bryce and Pfleiderer (1992) reported a 100% rate of vertigo relief as judged by the 1985 AAO-HNS criteria, with 89% declaring themselves cured. Caloric excitability was diminished or ablated in 89%.

In Nedzelski's series of patients, hearing improved in 30%, remained unchanged in 43%, and worsened in 27% (Nedzelski et al., 1993). There is a 10% risk of total deafness with this protocol which has remained unchanged as the technique has evolved, and retreatment using the same protocol does not seem to be associated with an increased risk to hearing.

Interestingly, subjective dizziness and objective caloric changes began to occur after the last dose of gentamicin in most patients, and the ablative process occurred gradually over the 2 weeks which followed the therapy. This indicates that the effect on the vestibular sensory organ is delayed (Magnusson et al., 1991), either because of slow transport of the drug into the inner ear or because of the slow accumulation of the drug in the target cells which reaches a critical ablative threshold over time. The chief route of transport between the middle and inner ears is thought to be the round window membrane. The target cells appear to be the endolymph-producing dark cells and the sensory epithelium (Monsell, Cass and Rybak, 1993). This may explain the results of several investigators who obtained poorer hearing results using daily instillations of intratympanic gentamicin or until signs of cochlear and vestibular loss were evident (Odkvist, Bergholtz and Lundgren, 1984; Odkvist, 1988; Laitakari, 1990). 'Overdosing' with too much of this aminoglycoside may actually have a more deleterious effect on the cochlea than on the vestibule (Bagger-Sjöback, Bergenius and Lundberg, 1990). Another interesting point is that the aminoglycoside-induced vestibular ablation may be partially reversible. An irritative spontaneous nystagmus has been seen in some patients during the early post-treatment period, and this may represent a recovery phenomenon resulting from the temporary reversible ototoxic effect in the treated ear (Parnes and Riddell, 1993).

In the presence of this delayed effect, some workers hypothesized that it may make pharmacodynamic sense to alter the Nedzelski protocol (Magnusson and Padoan, 1991; Parnes and Toth, personal communication, 1994). Extremely low dose therapy has been proposed by Magnusson and Padoan (1991) and Inoue et al. (1994) in the hope of optimizing the ratio of vestibular to cochlear damage, but scientific evidence in support of this proposal is still being collected. By prolonging the interval between gentamicin doses to several days or a week, more precise vestibular ablation can be undertaken and earlier detection of hearing loss can occur at a lower total gentamicin dose. Whether such alterations bear fruit in terms of the incidence of profound sensorineural hearing loss, or whether the vestibular ablative effect is negatively altered, remain the subject of an ongoing study (Parnes and Toth, personal communication, 1994).

When compared with vestibular neurectomy, the current most effective hearing conservation operation, topical gentamicin is equally effective in relieving vertigo (Nedzelski, Bryce and Pfleiderer, 1992). If the caloric response is only partially reduced and the patient continues to have symptoms, further treatments can be tailored and titrated to reduce vestibular function until symptomatic relief is achieved (Nedzelski *et al.*, 1993). Such revisions following a failed vestibular neurectomy, while uncommon, are difficult technically, require another intracranial procedure with its attendant risks, and may require the surgeon to sacrifice a good portion of the cochlear nerve to divide residual vestibular fibres which may intermingle there. Also, a therapy aimed at ablation of dark cell function is more theoretically attractive than nerve section, as it may be closer to the pathophysiological source of endolymphatic hydrops and Menière's disease. Whether this will result in improvements in the long-term hearing in the affected ear, or in the emergence of disease in the contralateral ear, remains to be seen following longitudinal study of these patients. The risk of hearing loss is similar to or even less than that seen in most series of vestibular neurectomies. Vestibular neurectomy is a major intracranial operation with a previously documented morbidity. In contrast, intratympanic gentamicin instillation is a technically simple operation for all otolaryngologists, requires little or no time in hospital, and has much less morbidity. Otologists should therefore give careful consideration to intratympanic aminoglycoside use as an alternative to vestibular neurectomy in the treatment of Menière's disease.

Another application of aminoglycoside ototoxicity is the application of aminoglycoside preparations directly into the perilymphatic space via an opening created in the horizontal semicircular canal. First described by Shea (1988), perfusion of the inner ear with 100 μg of streptomycin, followed by intramuscular injections of 1 μg of streptomycin daily, was associated with relief of vertigo in 78% and hearing loss in 38% of patients. Animal experiments using this technique with streptomycin demonstrated reasonable vestibular ablation, but substantial dose-related cochlear damage (Norris *et al.*, 1988). An instilled dose of 125 μg of this drug is recommended following successful dose-response animal research by the same group (Norris *et al.*, 1990). Subsequent studies by several authors indicated that, while this method has some merit as a vestibular ablation technique, the incidence of hearing loss as a result of the surgery can be as high as 68%, with a 57% rate of severe to profound loss (Amedee, Norris and Risey, 1991; Monsell and Shelton, 1991). As many as 17% of patients will require another secondary procedure to control vertigo, provoking some proponents of the technique to abandon it. Given the greater simplicity and the smaller risk to hearing complications of transtympanic aminoglycoside therapy, persistence with aminoglycoside perfusion of the inner ear seems regressive. Shea, however, following success with 166 streptomycin perfusions, continued to promote the technique and its future modifications as 'the ultimate answer to Menière's disease' (Shea, 1990).

The final application of the vestibular toxicity of streptomycin is its parenteral use in bilateral Menière's disease. The objectives of treatment of patients with bilateral disease are the reduction or elimination of vertigo with maximal hearing preservation. When streptomycin is administered parenterally, it causes bilateral peripheral vestibular ablation while leaving the cochlea undamaged and the hearing largely unchanged (Hanson, 1951; Graybiel *et al.*, 1967). This is thought to be mainly due to damage to the sensory cells of the vestibule (Kimura *et al.*, 1991). Given its effects in both inner ears, its use is inappropriate in unilateral disease (Glasscock, Johnson and Poe, 1989b). In the past, high doses of up to 39 g over 2.5 weeks were recommended to abolish completely the ice water caloric response (Wilson and Schuknecht, 1980). We now realize, however, that complete abolition of bilateral vestibular function is unnecessary to control vestigo in Menière's disease, and that some residual vestibular function is beneficial to the patient and helps in reducing ataxia and oscillopsia (Dix and Morales-Garcia, 1972; Silverstein *et al.*, 1984). Titrated doses of parenteral streptomycin, in amounts up to 20 g and with monitoring of vestibular function during therapy, is now the preferred method (Graham, Sataloff and Kemink, 1984; Langman, Kemink and Graham, 1990). Patients with recurrent vertigo following this therapy can always be considered for a further, smaller dose to reduce symptoms.

Procedures involving non-chemical ablation of the vestibular end organ

The application of ultrasonic irradiation to the labyrinth has been advocated as a surgical method to ablate vestibular function while preserving hearing. Ultrasonic energy was applied to the inner ear either by placing the source on the thinned out capsule of the horizontal semicircular canal or on the round window (Kossof, Wadsworth and Dudley, 1967; Angell-James, 1969). This was associated with a measurable irritative nystagmus for the first half hour, then a period without nystagmus, followed by a paralytic nystagmus (Altmann and Hager, 1968). This cycle of eye movements could repeat itself with recovery, and therapy was concluded when no further irritative nystagmus was seen, indicating total or subtotal vestibular ablation. The initial effects were encouraging but the longer term results have been disappointing, with many patients suffering continuing or recurrent vertigo (Moffat, 1988). Vertigo is diminished in 75% of lateral canal procedures and only 25% of round window procedures. Animal studies failed to show significant morphological alteration in the inner ear due to ultrasound (Peron *et al.*, 1983).

Cryosurgery is a similar attempt to injure selectively the vestibular end organ while preserving hearing. Wolfson (1984) reported on his technique, which involved the transmastoid application of a cryoprobe cooled to −160°C to the lateral semicircular canal for three cycles of 2 minutes each. Seventy-three per cent of 215 patients had their vertigo controlled by this procedure at the 1 year follow-up visit. A similar success rate of 71% of 69 patients was reported by Horowitz, Flood and Hampal (1989). Hearing is reportedly unaffected by this therapy. The serious complication of delayed facial paralysis, however, which occurs in 5–8% of these procedures makes this procedure less desirable than most of the other conservative operations. As with ultrasonic therapy, a high rate of recurrent vertigo has caused all but a few to abandon this modality (Brackmann, 1990).

Procedures involving hearing and vestibular ablation

Patients with Menière's disease and poor, non-serviceable hearing may be considered for a destructive procedure. Total and irreversible destruction of the sensory cells of the inner ear should be associated with complete relief of the vertigo of Menière's disease. This destruction is called a labyrinthectomy, and has taken three basic forms.

The first technique, the 'transcanal labyrinthectomy', is a limited exposure technique in which the labyrinth is approached via the external auditory canal and opened. Neuroepithelium is destroyed by mechanical means, through hooking and removing or dessicating (Brackmann, 1990), or by chemical means with high concentrations of aminoglycoside antibiotics or crystals of sodium chloride (Colletti, Fiorino and Sittoni, 1989). While this technique is simple and has been shown to relieve the vertigo of Menière's disease in over 90% of cases (Schuknecht, 1956), a disturbing number of patients develop recurrent symptoms. Brown (1983) reported that patients who underwent transcanal labyrinthectomy were three times more likely to require revision surgery for recurrent vertigo than those who had undergone a transmastoid labyrinthectomy. This is thought to be due to incomplete removal and destruction of inner ear neuroepithelium. This procedure is therefore either not performed or is reserved for patients with other medical problems which contraindicate any more extensive surgery (Brackmann, 1990). A variation of the transcanal labyrinthectomy was described by Silverstein in 1976, in which the lateral internal auditory meatus is exposed through the oval window via a permeatal approach. This technique has similarly been largely abandoned because of poor exposure of the contents of the internal auditory meatus (Brackmann, 1990).

The second technique is the transmastoid labyrinthectomy. This involves the removal of the osseous and membranous portions of the vestibular labyrinth via a cortical mastoidectomy (Graham and Colton, 1980). It is important to remove the neuroepithelium of the ampulla of the posterior semicircular canal so that no troublesome neuroepithelial remnants are left to return to function and cause recurrent symptoms. This is a well-established procedure with minimal complications. Current indications for this procedure are a pure tone average of greater than 60 dB and speech discrimination scores of less than 50% (Graham and Kemink, 1984). Barring incomplete central compensation for the vestibular loss, almost all patients report complete relief of vertigo from this procedure alone (Schuknecht, 1982b).

Translabyrinthine vestibular neurectomy has been described as the gold standard for control of vertigo in resistant Menière's disease (Glasscock, 1973; Brackmann, 1990). However, most authors now feel that the nerve section has no advantage over transmastoid labyrinthectomy alone, and that the potential intracranial complications can be avoided by performing a labyrinthectomy alone (Schuknecht, 1982b). Animal studies have shown that osseous labyrinthectomy is associated with progressive, steady atrophy of the vestibular nerve with no tendency to post-traumatic neuroma formation (Schuknecht, 1982b). We therefore reserve this operation for those rare patients with non-serviceable hearing who present with persisting Menière's attacks following osseous labyrinthectomy. These are usually people who have undergone a transcanal labyrinthectomy, in whom neuroepithelium remains in the labyrinth and may retain some function.

With the increasing recognition of the bilateral nature of Menière's disease, some authors have questioned the continuing use of labyrinthectomy, with its concomitant complete hearing loss, in any of its forms (Schessel and Nedzelski, 1993). When promontory stimulation testing is performed on patients who have undergone osseous labyrinthectomy, threshold, discomfort levels and dynamic ranges were found to be comparable with patients successfully implanted with Nucleus 22 channel cochlear implants (Ramsden and Timms, 1991). This exciting result suggests that cochlear implantation might be possible in a labyrinthectomized ear.

Conclusions

The study of Menière's disease and its treatment continues to evoke mixed emotions in the modern otologist. The initial excitement of the early description of the condition gave way to expectancy when the pathology of endolymphatic hydrops was first described and the discovery of the precise aetiology seemed so close at hand. The initial enthusiasm which greeted the supersedence of destructive labyrinthectomy by conservative surgery on the endolymphatic sac, a procedure which seemed so logical in the light of current knowledge, was replaced by intense frustration that the cause of the disease remained elusive. The fact that surgical therapies have not lived up to expectations has fostered cynicism and sham operations. The birth of otoneurosurgery brought with it ingenious methods of sectioning the vestibular nerve but the might of major intracranial operations and their attendant risk has tempered the hand of the clinician, who, while relentlessly continuing the search for the aetiology, has sagely focused on the less risky vestibular ablation afforded by the ototoxic effects of the aminoglycoside antibiotics.

While continuing the research into this enigmatic disease, it is paramount that scientific, carefully planned and controlled trials are carried out comparing medical therapy and surgery and critically analysing the effect of treatment in relation to the natural history of the disease. Scientific papers should define what is meant by 'Menière's disease', excluding secondary endolymphatic hydrops and heterogeneity within the group by meticulously assessing patients by means of a comprehensive protocol of investigations to obtain a much more homogeneous group. This will facilitate valid comparison of studies from different centres. Only if like patients are compared with like will the results of medical treatment and surgery be meaningful. The results must be analysed according to accepted and laid down criteria as has been established by the Equilibrium Committee of the American Academy of Otolaryngology, Head and Neck Surgery. In this way, international uniformity of patient selection and analysis of results can be achieved.

Addendum

1995 – American Academy of Otolaryngology – Head and Neck Surgery

Committee on Hearing and Equilibrium guidelines for the diagnosis and evaluation of therapy in Menière's disease (*Otolaryngology – Head and Neck Surgery* (1995), *113*, 181–185)

Definition of Menière's disease

For reporting purposes Menière's disease is a clinical disorder defined as the idiopathic syndrome of endolymphatic hydrops. This syndrome is defined as the presence of the following: recurrent, spontaneous episodic vertigo; hearing loss; aural fullness; and tinnitus. Either tinnitus or aural fullness (or both) must be present on the affected side to make the diagnosis for reporting purposes under these guidelines.

Vertigo

The definitive spell of Menière's disease is spontaneous rotational vertigo lasting at least 20 minutes (commonly several hours), is often prostrating, and is accompanied by dysequilibrium, which may last for days. It is usually accompanied by nausea and commonly by vomiting or retching. Consciousness is not lost. During the definitive episode, horizontal or horizontal rotatory nystagmus is always present. This type of vertigo is termed *episodic vertigo of the Menière type*. Although vertiginous episodes of variable duration and character may occur in patients with Menière's disease, at least two definitive episodes of 20 minutes or longer must occur to permit the diagnosis of definite Menière's disease.

Hearing loss

Sensorineural hearing loss must be documented audiometrically in the treated ear on at least one occasion to permit the diagnosis of Menière's disease. Diagnostic hearing loss may take any of the following forms:

1   The average (arithmetical mean) of hearing thresholds at 0.25, 0.5 and 1 kHz is 15 dB or more higher than the average of 1, 2 and 3 kHz.
2   In unilateral cases, the average of threshold values at 0.5, 1, 2 and 3 kHz is 20 dB or more poorer in the ear in question than on the opposite side.
3   In bilateral cases, the average of threshold values at 0.5, 1, 2 and 3 kHz is greater than 25 dB in the studied ear.
4   In the judgement of the investigator, the patient's hearing loss meets reasonable audiometric criteria for hearing loss characteristic of Menière's disease. The rationale for using this criterion should be stated and justified for each case.

Although hearing usually fluctuates early in Menière's disease, fluctuation is not universally present and is not essential to the diagnosis, provided that hearing loss is documented at some time, as above. The determination of hearing change should be based on the four-tone average (arithmetical mean) of thresholds at 0.5, 1, 2 and 3 kHz. A change of 10 dB or more or a change in word recognition score (speech discrimination) of 15 percentage points or more is considered clinically significant. In case the pure tone average and word recognition scores change in opposite directions, the pure tone average will determine the overall nature of the change for reporting purposes. The four tone average of 0.5, 1, 2 and 3 kHz has been adopted because this average takes into account the importance of high frequencies in normal hearing. This four tone average is consistent with the 1985 version of the guidelines and the Academy's formula for calculating hearing handicap.

Tinnitus and aural fullness

These are difficult to quantify independent of results for hearing and control of vertigo. Investigators are free to create and validate scales for tinnitus, fullness and other measures.

Other diagnostic considerations

Conditions producing all or part of *Menière's triad of symptoms* but not true Menière's disease should be excluded. These have been described in detail in this chapter and in Chapter 17.

Diagnostic scale

Certain Menière's disease

- Definite Menière's disease, plus histopathological confirmation.

Definite Menière's disease

- Two or more definitive spontaneous episodes of vertigo 20 minutes or longer.
- Audiometrically documented hearing loss on at least one occasion.
- Tinnitus or aural fullness in the teated ear.
- Other causes excluded.

Probable Menière's disease

- One definitive episode of vertigo
- Audiometrically documented hearing loss on at least one occasion.
- Tinnitus or aural fullness in the treated ear
- Other causes excluded.

Possible Menière's disease

- Episodic vertigo of the Menière's type without documented hearing loss, or
- Sensorineural hearing loss, fluctuating or fixed, with dysequilibrium but without definitive episodes.
- Other causes excluded.

Only patients in the definite or certain categories should be reported as having Menière's disease.

Staging

A staging system based solely on hearing has been devised. It is not implied that all patients will progress through a series of stages in sequence.

Staging of definite and certain Menière's disease

Stage	Four tone average (dB)
1	≤ 25
2	26–40
3	41–70
4	> 70

Staging is based on the four-tone avarage of the pure tone thresholds at 0.5, 1, 2 and 3 kHz of the worst audiogram during the interval 6 months before treatment. This is the same audiogram that is used as the baseline evaluation to determine hearing outcome from treatment. Staging should be applied only to cases of definite or certain Menière's disease. Once a stage has been established for a given patient and a given course of treatment, the stage of disease for that patient does not change for reporting purposes even if hearing does change after treatment.

Functional impairment and disability

To help assess the effects of episodic vertigo on daily activities, a six-point functional level scale has been introduced which better reflects disability than the 1985 guidelines.

Functional level scale

Regarding my current state of *overall* function, *not just during attacks* (check the ONE that best applies):

1   My dizziness has no effect on my activities at all.
2   When I am dizzy I have to stop what I am doing for a while, but it soon passes and I can resume activities. I continue to work, drive and engage in any activity I choose without restriction. I have not changed any plans or activities to accommodate my dizziness.
3   When I am dizzy I have to stop what I am doing for a while, but it does pass and I can resume activities. I continue to work, drive and engage in most activities I choose, but I have had to change some plans and make some allowance for my dizziness.
4   I am able to work, drive, travel, take care of a family or engage in most essential activities, but I must exert a great deal of effort to do so. I must constantly make adjustments in my activities and budget my energies. I am barely making it.
5   I am unable to work, drive or take care of a family, I am unable to do most of the active things which I used to. Even essential activities must be limited. I am disabled.
6   I have been disabled for 1 year or longer and/or receive compensation (money) because of my dizziness or balance problem.

It is suggested that clinicians review the choices of disability level with each patient and allow the patient to make the final selection.

The raw data of the functional level scale should be reported for each patient at each time interval recorded (baseline, 2 years, etc.). The treatment outcome regarding disability should also be expressed as improved, unchanged or worse for each patient.

Vertigo control

Numerical value	Class
0	A (Complete control of definitive spells)
1 to 40	B
41 to 80	C
81 to 120	D
> 120	E
Secondary treatment initiated due to disability from vertigo	F

Numerical value = $(X/Y) \times 100$, rounded to the nearest whole number, where X is the average number of definitive spells per month for the 6 months 18 to 24 months after therapy and Y is the average number of definitive spells per month for the 6 months before therapy.

Reporting results of treatment

To make comparisons among studies and to facilitate meta-analysis, the Committee believes that the frequency of definitive attacks for the period 6 months before treatment should be compared with the interval occurring between 18 and 24 months after treatment. In this manner, the two intervals are of the same duration, and the elapsed time after treatment is standardized. Hearing comparisons should be made with the worst audiogram of each of the two 6-month intervals. Characterization of the treatment response for an individual patient should not be made until the patient has been observed for 24 months after treatment.

The worst pre-operative audiogram for 6 months before treatment should be compared with the worst post-operative audiogram between 18 and 24 months after treatment. Investigators are encouraged to report results 4 years after treatment (frequency of definitive spells and worst audiogram 42 to 48 months after treatment). Publication of extensive data in tabulatory form is recommended to facilitate meta-analyses.

References

AANTAA, E. (1991) Treatment of acute vestibular vertigo. *Acta Otolaryngologica Supplementum,* **479,** 44–47

ALFORD, B. R. (1972) Menière's disease: criteria for diagnosis and evaluation of therapy for reporting. Report of subcommittee on equilibrium and its measurement. *Transactions of the American Academy of Ophthalmology and Otolaryngology,* **76,** 1462–1464

ALFORD, B. R., COHN, A. M. and IGARASHI, M. (1977) Current status of surgical decompression and drainage procedures upon the endolymphatic system. *Annals of Otology, Rhinology and Laryngology,* **86,** 683–687

ALTMANN, F. and FOWLER, E. P. (1943) Histological findings in Menière's symptom complex. *Annals of Otology, Rhinology and Laryngology,* **52,** 52–80

ALTMANN, F. and HAGER, E. (1968) Ultrasonic treatment for Menière's disease. *Otolaryngologic Clinics of North America,* **1,** 575–586

ALTMANN, F. and KORNFELD, M. (1965) Histological studies of Menière's disease. *Annals of Otology, Rhinology and Laryngology,* **74,** 915–943

AMEDEE, R. G., NORRIS, C. H. and RISEY, J. A. (1991) Selective chemical vestibulectomy: preliminary results with human application. *Otolaryngology – Head and Neck Surgery,* **105,** 107–112

AMENTA, C. A. DAYAL, V. S., FLAHERTY, J. AND WEIL, R. J. (1992) Luetic endolymphatic hydrops: diagnosis and treatment. *American Journal of Otology,* **13,** 516–524

ANDREWS, J. C., ATOR, G. A. and HONRUBIA, V. (1992) The exacerbation of symptoms in Menière's disease during the premenstrual period. *Archives of Otolaryngology – Head and Neck Surgery,* **118,** 74–78

ANDREWS, J. C., BOHMER, A. and HOFFMAN, L. F. (1991) The measurement and manipulation of intralabyrinthine pressure in experimental endolymphatic hydrops. *Laryngoscope,* **101,** 661–668

ANGELBORG, C., KLOCKHOFF, I. and STAHLE, J. (1977) Urea and hearing in patients with Menière's disease. *Scandinavian Audiology,* **6,** 143–146

ANGELL-JAMES, J. (1969) Menière's disease: treatment with ultrasound. *Journal of Laryngology and Otology,* **83,** 771–785

ANTOLI-CANDELA, F. (1976) The histopathology of Menière's disease. *Acta Otolaryngologica Supplementum,* **340,** 5–42

ANTUNEZ, J. C. M., GALEY, F. R., LINTHICUM, F. H. and MCCANN, G. D. (1980) Computer-aided and graphic reconstruction of the human endolymphatic duct and sac. *Annals of Otology, Rhinology and Laryngology,* **89** (Supplement 76), 23–32

ARENBERG, I. K. (1987) Results of endolymphatic sac to mastoid shunt surgery for Menière's disease refractory to medical therapy. *American Journal of Otology,* **8,** 335–344

ARENBERG, I. K., GIBSON, W. P. R. and BOHLEN, H. K. H. (1989) Improvements in audiometric and electrophysiologic parameters following nondestructive inner ear surgery utilizing a valved shunt for hydrops and Menière's disease. In: *Proceedings of the Second International Symposium on Menière's Disease: Pathogenesis, Pathophysiology, Diagnosis and Treatment,* edited by J. B. Nadol. Amsterdam: Kugler Publications. pp. 545–562

ARENBERG, I. K., MAROVITZ, W. P. and SHAMBAUGH, G. E. (1970) The role of the endolymphatic sac in the pathogenesis of endolymphatic hydrops in man. *Acta Otolaryngologica Supplementum,* **275,** 1–49

ARENBERG, I. K., BALKANY, T. J., GOLDMAN, G. and PILLSBURY, R. C. (1980) The incidence and prevalence of Menière's disease – a statistical analysis of limits. *Otolaryngologic Clinics of North America,* **13,** 597–601

ARENBERG, I. K., COUNTRYMAN, L. L., BERNSTEIN, L. H. and SHAMBAUGH, G. E. JR (1991) Vincent's violent vertigo. An analysis of the original diagnosis of epilepsy vs. current diagnosis of Menière's disease. *Acta Otolaryngologica Supplementum*, **485**, 84–103

ARENBERG, I. K., KOBAYASHI, H., OBERT, A. D. and GIBSON, W. P. R. (1993) Intraoperative electrocochleography of endolymphatic hydrops surgery using clicks and tone bursts. *Acta Otolaryngologica Supplementum*, **504**, 58–67

ARENBERG, I.K., STROUD, M. H., SPECTOR, G. J. and CARVER, W. F. (1974) The salt loading provocative glycerol test for the early diagnosis of auditory endolymphatic hydrops (Menière's disease). *Revue de Laryngologie*, **95**, 709–719

ARNHOLD-SCHNEIDER, M. (1990) Degree of pneumatization of the temporal bone and Menière's disease: Are they related? *American Journal of Otolaryngology*, **11**, 33–36

ARNOLD, W., PFALZ, R. and ALTERMATT, H. (1985) Evidence of serum antibodies against inner ear tissues in the blood of patients with certain sensorineural hearing disorders. *Acta Otolaryngologica*, **99**, 437–444

ARSLAN, M. (1970) Choice of surgical procedure in Menière's disease. Proposal for a new osmotic 'induction' method. *Journal of Laryngology and Otology*, **84**, 131–147

ASO, S., WATANABE, Y. and MIZUKOSHI, K. (1991) A clinical study of electrocochleography in Menière's disease. *Acta Otolaryngologica*, **111**, 44–52

ASO, S., KIMURA, H., TAKEDA, S., MIZUKOSHI, K. and WATANABE, Y. (1993) The intravenously administered glycerol test. *Acta Otolaryngologica Supplementum*, **504**, 51–54

ATKINSON, M. (1961) Menière's original papers: reprinted with an English translation together with commentaries and biographical sketch. *Acta Otolaryngologica Supplementum*, **162**, 1–78

AUSTIN, W., PFALZ, R. and ALTERMATT, H. (1984) Endolymphatic fistulization. *Annals of Otology, Rhinology and Laryngology*, **93**, 534–539

BABIN, R. W., BALKANY, T. J. and FEE, W. E. (1984) Transdermal scopolamine in the treatment of acute vertigo. *Annals of Otology, Rhinology, and Laryngology*, **93**, 25–27

BABIGHIAN, G. (1976) Audiological findings following intravenous administration of hypertonic solutions in cases of long-standing Menière's disease. *Minerva Otorinolaringologica*, **26**, 83–87

BABINSKI, J. (1903) Du traitement des affections auriculaires par la ponction lombaire. *Bulletin et Memoirs du Societé Medicale*, **3**, 450–458

BAGGER-SJÖBACK, D., BERGENIUS, J. and LUNDBERG, A. M. (1990) Inner ear effects of topical gentamicin treatment in patients with Menière's disease. *American Journal of Otology*, **11**, 406–410

BAGGER-SJÖBACK, D., JANSSON, B., FRIBERG, U. and RASK-ANDERSON, H. (1990) Three-dimensional anatomy of the human endolymphatic sac. *Archives of Otolaryngology – Head and Neck Surgery*, **116**, 345–349

BALDWIN, D. L., OHLSEN, K. A., MILLER, J. M. and NUTTALL, A. L. (1992) Cochlear blood flow and microvascular resistance changes in response to hypertonic glycerol, urea, and mannitol infusions. *Annals of Otology, Rhinology and Laryngology*, **101**, 168–175

BALKANY, T. J., PILLSBURY, H. C. and ARENBERG, I. K. (1980) Defining and quantifying Menière's disease. *Otolaryngologic Clinics of North America*, **13**, 589–595

BALKANY, T. J., SIZES, B. and ARENBERG, I. (1980) Bilateral aspects of Menière's disease; an underestimated clinical entity. *Otolaryngologic Clinics of North America*, **13**, 603–609

BALOH, R., HONRUBIA, V. and JACOBSEN, K. (1987) Benign positional vertigo: clinical and oculographic features in 240 cases. *Neurology*, **37**, 371

BALOH, R. W., JACOBSON, K. and WINDER, T. (1990) Drop attacks in Menière's syndrome. *Annals of Neurology*, **28**, 384–387

BANCE, M. and RUTKA, J. (1990) Speculation into the aetiological role of viruses in the development of Bell's palsy and disorders of inner ear dysfunction: a case history and review of the literature. *Journal of Otolaryngology*, **19**, 46–49

BANCE, M., MAI, M., TOMLINSON, D. and RUTKA, J. (1991) The changing direction of nystagmus in acute Menière's disease: pathophysiological implications. *Laryngoscope*, **101**, 197–201

BARBER, H. O. (1983) Menière's disease: symptomatology. In: *Menière's Disease: A Comprehensive Appraisal* edited by W. J. Oosterveld. New York: John Wiley. pp. 25–34

BARBER, H. O. and IRELAND, P. E. (1952) Surgical treatment of hydrops of the labyrinth: the clinical results following differential section of the VIIIth nerve. *Laryngoscope*, **62**, 566–576

BEAL, D. D. (1968) Effect of endolymphatic sac ablation in the rabbit and cat. *Acta Otolaryngologica*, **66**, 333–346

BECK, C. (1986a) Medical treatment. In: *Controversial Aspects of Menière's Disease*, edited by C. R. Pfalz. New York: George Thieme. pp. 88–95

BECK, C. (1986b) Intratympanic gentamicin for treatment of Menière's disease. *Keio Journal of Medicine*, **35**, 36–41

BECK, C. and SCHMIDT, C. L. (1978) 10 years experience with intratympanically applied streptomycin (gentamicin) in the therapy of morbus Menière. *Archives of Otorhinolaryngology*, **221**, 149–152

BERGSTROM, T., EDSTROM, S., TJELLSTRÖM, A. and VAHLNE, A. (1992) Menière's disease and antibody reactivity to herpes simplex virus type 1 polypeptides. *American Journal of Otolaryngology*, **13**, 295–300

BERRIOS, G. E., RYLEY, J. P., GARVEY, T. P. N. and MOFFAT, D. A. (1988) Psychiatric morbidity in subjects with inner ear disease. *Clinical Otolaryngology*, **13**, 259–266

BESS, F. H., JOSEY, A. F. and HUMES, L. E. (1979) Performance intensity functions in cochlear and eighth nerve disorders. *American Journal of Otology*, **1**, 27–31

BHATIA, P. L., GUPTA, O. P., AGRAWAL, M. K. and MISHR, S. K. (1977) Audiological and vestibular function tests in hypothyroidism. *Laryngoscope*, **87**, 2082–2089

BIRCHALL, J. (1991) Therapeutic options in Menière's disease. *Prescriber*, **31**, 33–39

BIRGERSON, L., GUSTAVSON, K. and STAHLE, J. (1987) Familial Menière's disease: a genetic investigation. *American Journal of Otology*, **8**, 323–326

BLACK, F. O. (1982) Vestibular function assessment in patients with Menière's disease: the vestibulospinal system. *Laryngoscope*, **92**, 1419–1436

BLACK, F.O. and KITCH, R. (1980) A review of vestibular test results in Menière's disease. *Otolaryngologic Clinics of North America*, **13**, 631–642

BLACK, F. O., SANDO, I., HILDYARD, V. H. and HEMENWAY, W. G. (1969) Bilateral multiple otosclerotic foci and endolymphatic hydrops: histopathological case report. *Annals of Otology, Rhinology and Laryngology*, **78**, 1062–1073

BLAIR, R. L. (1984) Medical management of vestibular dysfunction. *Otolaryngologic Clinics of North America*, **17**, 679–684

BOHMER, A. and FISCH, U. (1993) Bilateral vestibular neurectomy for treatment of vertigo. *Otolaryngology – Head and Neck Surgery*, **109**, 101–107

BOHMER, A. and FISCH, U. (1995) Clinical pathophysiology of vestibular neurectomy. *Otolaryngology – Head and Neck Surgery*, **112**, 183–188

BOOTH, J. B. (1977) Hyperlipidaemia and deafness: a preliminary survey. *Proceedings of the Royal Society of Medicine*, **70**, 642–646

BOOTH, J. B. (1980) Menière's disease: the selection and assessment of patients for surgery using electrocochleography. *Annals of the Royal College of Surgeons of England*, **62**, 415–425

BRACKMANN, D. E. (1983) Menière's disease: surgical treatment. In: *Menière's Disease: A Comprehensive Appraisal*, edited by W. J. Oosterveld. New York: John Wiley. pp. 91–108

BRACKMANN, D. E. (1990) Surgical treatment of vertigo. *Journal of Laryngology and Otology*, **104**, 849–859

BRACKMANN, D. E. and NISSEN, R. L. (1987) Menière's disease: results of treatment with the endolymphatic subarachnoid shunt compared with the endolymphatic mastoid shunt. *American Journal of Otology*, **8**, 275–282

BRETLAU, P., THOMSEN, J., TOS, M. and JOHNSEN, N. J. (1984) Placebo effect in surgery for Menière's disease: a three year follow-up study of patients in a double blind placebo controlled study on endolymphatic sac shunt surgery. *American Journal of Otology*, **5**, 558–561

BROOKES, G. B. (1986) Circulating immune complexes in Menière's disease. *Archives of Otolaryngology – Head and Neck Surgery*, **112**, 536–540

BROOKES, G. B. and BOOTH, J. B. (1984) Oral acetazolamide in Menière's disease. *Journal of Laryngology and Otology*, **98**, 1087–1095

BROOKES, G. B., MORRISON, A. W. and BOOTH, J. B. (1982) Acetazolamide in Menière's disease: evaluation of a new diagnostic test for reversible endolymphatic hydrops. *Otolaryngology – Head and Neck Surgery*, **90**, 358–366

BROOKES, G. B., MORRISON, A. W. and RICHARD, R. (1984) Otoadmittance changes following glycerol dehydration in Menière's disease. *Acta Otolaryngologica*, **98**, 30–41

BROOKES, G. B., MORRISON, A. W. and RICHARD, R. (1985) Unilateral Menière's disease: is the contralateral ear normal? *American Journal of Otology*, **6**, 495–499

BROWN, D. H., MCCLURE, J. A. and DOWNAR-ZAPOLSKI, Z. (1988) The membrane rupture theory of Menière's disease – is it valid? *Laryngoscope*, **98**, 599–601

BROWN, J. S. (1983) A ten year statistical follow-up of 245 consecutive cases of endolymphatic shunt and decompression and 328 cases of labyrinthectomy. *Laryngoscope*, **93**, 1419–1424

BROWN, M. R. (1941) Menière's syndrome. *Archives of Neurological Psychiatry*, **46**, 561–565

BRUNNER, H. (1948) Menière's disease. *Journal of Laryngology and Otology*, **62**, 627–638

CAMPBELL, K. C. M., HARKER, L. A. and ABBAS, P. J. (1992) Interpretation of electrocochleography in Menière's disease and normal subjects. *Annals of Otology, Rhinology and Laryngology*, **101**, 496–500

CASS, S. P., KARTUSH, J. M. and GRAHAM, M. D. (1992) Patterns of vestibular function following vestibular nerve section. *Laryngoscope*, **102**, 388–394

CAWTHORNE, T. and HEWLETT, A. B. (1954) Menière's disease. *Proceedings of the Royal Society of Medicine*, **47**, 663–670

CAWTHORNE, T. E., FITZGERALD, G. and HALLPIKE, C. S. (1942) Studies in human vestibular function. III Observations on the clinical features of Menière's disease: with special reference to the results of the caloric tests. *Brain*, **65**, 161–180

CHAN, Y. M., ADAMS, D. A. and KERR, A. G. (1995) Syphilitic labyrinthitis – an update. *Journal of Laryngology and Otology*, **109**, 719–725

CLEMIS, J. D. and VALVASSORI, G. E. (1968) Recent radiographic and clinical observations on the vestibular aqueduct. *Otolaryngologic Clinics of North America*, **1**, 339–346

CODY, D. T. (1973) The tack operation. *Archives of Otolaryngology*, **97**, 109–111

CODY, D. T. and MCDONALD, T. J. (1983) Tack operation for idiopathic endolymphatic hydrops: an update. *Laryngoscope*, **93**, 1416–1418

COGAN, D. G. (1945) Syndrome of non-syphilitic interstitial keratitis and vestibuloauditory symptoms. *Archives of Ophthalmology*, **33**, 144–149

COGAN, D. G. (1949) Nonsyphilitic interstitial keratitis with vestibuloauditory symptoms: report of four additional cases. *Archives of Ophthalmology*, **42**, 42–49

COLLETTI, V., FIORINO, F. G. and SITTONI, V. (1989) NaCl deposition in the vestibule: a simple, safe and effective method of cochleovesibular deafferentation. *American Journal of Otology*, **10**, 451–455

COLMAN, B. H. (1987) Menière's disease. In: *Scott-Brown's Otolaryngology*, 5th edn, edited by A.G. Kerr, vol. 3 *Otology*, edited by J. B. Booth. London: Butterworths. pp. 444–464

COMACCHIO, F., BOGGIAN, O., POLETTO, E., BEGHI, A., MARTINI, A. and RAMPAZZO, A. (1992) Menière's disease in congenital nephrogenic diabetes insipidus: report of two twins. *American Journal of Otology*, **13**, 477–481

CORVERA, J. and CORVERA, G. (1989) Long-term effect of acetazolamide and chlorthalidone on hearing loss of Menière's disease. *American Journal of Otology*, **10**, 142–145

CRARY, W. G. and WEXLER, M. (1977) Menière's disease: a psychosomatic disorder? *Psychological Reports (Monograph supplement)*, **41**, 603–645

CRARY, W. G., WEXLER, M. and RILEY, M. A. (1976) Menière's disease and cerebral impairment. *Archives of Otolaryngology*, **102**, 368–370

CROCKETT, E. A. (1903) The removal of the stapes for the relief of auditory vertigo. *Annals of Otology, Rhinology and Laryngology*, **12**, 67–72

CURRIER, W. D. (1969) Dizziness related to hypoglycemia: the role of adrenal steroids and nutrition. *Laryngoscope*, **79**, 18–35

CZUBALSKI, W., BOCHENEK, W. and ZAWISZA, E. (1976) Psychological stress and personality in Menière's disorder. *Journal of Psychosomatic Research*, **20**, 187–191

DANDY, W. E. (1928) Menière's disease: its diagnosis and a method of treatment. *Archives of Surgery*, **16**, 1127–1152

DANDY, W. E. (1941) The surgical treatment of Menière's disease. *Surgery, Gynecology and Obstetrics*, **72**, 421–425

DAUMANN, R., ARAN, J. M., CHARLET DE SAUVAGE, R. and PORTMANN, M. (1988) Clinical significance of the summating potential in Menière's disease. *American Journal of Otology*, **9**, 31–38

DEREBERY, M. J., RAO, V. S., SIGLOCK, T. J., LINTHICUM, F. H. and NELSON, R. A. (1991) Menière's disease: an immune complex-mediated illness? *Laryngoscope*, **101**, 225–229

DEREBERY, M. J. and VALENZUELA, S. (1992) Menière's syndrome and allergy. *Otolaryngologic Clinics of North America*, **25**, 213–224

DICKINS, J. R. E. and GRAHAM, S. S. (1990) Menière's disease – 1983–1989. *American Journal of Otology*, **11**, 51–65

DIX, M. R. and MORALES-GARCIA, C. (1972) Modern concepts in the management of Menière's disease. *British Journal of Hospital Medicine*, 623–625

DOHLMAN, G. F. (1977) Experiments on the mechanism of Menière's attacks. *Journal of Otolaryngology*, **6**, 135–156

DOHLMANN, G. F. and JOHNSON, W. H. (1965) Experiments on the mechanism of Menière's attack. *Proceedings of the Canadian Otolaryngology Society*, **19**, 73

DORNHOFFER, J. L. and ARENBERG, I. K. (1993) Diagnosis of vestibular Menière's disease with electrocochleography. *American Journal of Otology*, **14**, 161–164

DORNHOFFER, J. L., WANER, M., ARENBERG, I. K. and MONTAGUE, D. (1993) Immunoperoxidase study of the endolymphatic sac in Menière's disease. *Laryngoscope*, **103**, 1027–1034

DUKE, W. W. (1923) Menière's syndrome caused by allergy. *Journal of the American Medical Association*, **81**, 2179–2181

EAGGER, S., LUXON, L. M., DAVIES, R. A., COELHO, A. and RON, M. A. (1992) Psychiatric morbidity in patients with peripheral vestibular disorder: a clincial and neuro-otological study. *Journal of Neurology, Neurosurgery and Psychiatry*, **55**, 383–387

EICHNER, H., KAMPIK G. and GLEDITCH, J. (1986) Treatment of Menière's disease by natural remedies. In: *Controversial Aspects of Menière's Disease*, edited by C. R. Pfalz. New York: George Thieme. pp. 99–103

ENDICOTT, J. N. and STUCKER, F. J. (1977) Allergy in Menière's disease related fluctuating hearing loss preliminary findings in a double-blind crossover clinical study. *Laryngoscope*, **87**, 1650–1657

EVANS, K. L., BALDWIN, D. L., BAINBRIDGE, D. and MORRISON, A. W. (1988) Immune status in patients with Menière's disease. *Archives of Otorhinolaryngology*, **245**, 287–292

FERRARO, J. A., BEST, L. G. and ARENBERG, I. K. (1983) The use of electrocochleography in the diagnosis of endolymphatic hydrops. *Otolaryngologic Clinics of North America*, **16**, 69–82

FERRARO, J. A., ARENBERG, I. K. and HASSANEIN, R. S. (1985) Electrocochleography and symptoms of inner ear dysfunction. *Archives of Otolaryngology*, **111**, 71–74

FICK, I. A. (1964) Decompression of the labyrinth: a new surgical procedure for Menière's disease. *Archives of Otolaryngology*, **79**, 447–458

FISCH, U. (1984) Vestibular nerve section for Menière's disease. *American Journal of Otology*, **5**, 543–545

FISCHER, A. J. (1991) Histamine in the treatment of vertigo. *Acta Otolaryngologica Supplementum*, **479**, 24–28

FLOURENS, P. (1842) *Recherches experimental sur les proprietes et les fonctions du system nerveux dans les animaux vertebres*, 2nd edn. Paris: Balliere

FOWLER, E. P. Jr, and ZECKEL, A. (1952) Psychosomatic aspects of Menière's disease. *Journal of the American Medical Association*, **148**, 1265–1269

FRANKLIN, D. J., POLLAK, A. and FISCH, U. (1990) Menière's symptoms resulting from bilateral otosclerotic occlusion of the endolymphatic duct: an analysis of the causal relationship between otosclerosis and Menière's disease. *American Journal of Otology*, **11**, 135–140

FRAYSSE, B., ALONSO, A. and HOUSE, W. (1980) Menière's disease and endolymphatic hydrops: clinical-histopathological correlations. *Annals of Otology, Rhinology and Laryngology*, **89** (Supplement 76), 2–22

FRAYSSE, B., BEBEAR, J. P., DUBREUIL, C., BERGES, C. and DAUMAN, R. (1991) Betahistine hydrochloride versus flunarizine. A double-blind study on recurrent vertigo with or without cochlear syndrome typical of Menière's disease. *Acta Otolaryngologica Supplementum*, **490**, 1–10

FRAZIER, C. H. (1912) Intracranial division of the auditory nerve for persistent aural vertigo. *Surgery, Gynecology and Obstetrics*, **15**, 524–529

FRIBERG, U., STAHLE, J. and SVEDBERG, A. (1984) The natural course of Menière's disease. *Acta Otolaryngologica Supplementum*, **406**, 72–77

FRIBERG, U., JANSSON, B., RASK-ANDERSEN, H. and BAGGER-SJÖBACK, D. (1988) Variations in surgical anatomy of the endolymphatic sac. *Archives of Otolaryngology – Head and Neck Surgery*, **114**, 389–394

FUKUDA, S., KEITHLEY, E. M. and HARRIS, J. P. (1988) The development of endolymphatic hydrops following CMV inoculation of the endolymphatic sac. *Laryngoscope*, **98**, 439–443

FURSTENBURG, A. C., LASHMET, F. H. and LATHROP, F. (1934) Menière's symptom complex: medical treatment. *Annals of Otology, Rhinology and Laryngology*, **43**, 1035–1046 Reproduced 1992. **101**, 20–31

FUTAKI, T. and NOMURA, Y. (1989) The surgical procedures and evaluation of two modifications of endolymphatic sac surgery: the epidural shunt and vein graft drainage. *Acta Otolaryngologica Supplementum*, **468**, 117–127

FUTAKI, T., KITAHARA, M. and MORIMOTO, M. (1975) The furosemide test for Menière's disease. *Acta Otolaryngologica*, **79**, 419–424

FUTAKI, T., KITAHARA, M. and MORIMOTO, M. (1977) A comparison of the furosemide and glycerol tests for Menière's disease. *Acta Otolaryngologica*, **83**, 272–278

FUTAKI, T., SEMBA, T. and KUDO, Y. (1988) Treatment of hydropic patients by immunoglobulin with methyl B12. *American Journal of Otology*, **9**, 131–135

FUTAKI, T., YAMANE, M., KAWABATA, I. and NOMURA, Y. (1984) Detection of delayed endolymphatic hydrops by the furosemide test. *Acta Otolaryngologica*, **406**, 37–41

GHORAYEB, B. Y. and LINTHICUM, F. H. (1978) Otosclerotic inner ear syndrome. *Annals of Otology, Rhinology and Laryngology*, **87**, 85–90

GIBSON, W. P. R. (1991) The use of intraoperative electrocochleography in Menière's surgery. *Acta Otolaryngologica Supplementum*, **485**, 65–73

GIBSON, W. P. R. and ROSE, E. (1993) The use of tone burst electrocochleography in the diagnosis of Menière's disease. In: *Menière's Disease – Pathogenesis, Pathophysiology, Diagnosis and Treatment. Proceedings of the Third International Symposium. Rome, Italy, October 20–23, 1993*, edited by M. Barbara and R. Filipo. Amsterdam/New York: Kugler Publications. pp. 1–4.

GIBSON, W. P. R., MOFFAT, D. A. and RAMSDEN, R. T. (1977) Clinical electrocochleography in the diagnosis and management of Menière's disorder. *Audiology*, **16**, 389–401

GIBSON, W. P. R., PRASHER, D. K. and KILKENNY, G. P. G. (1983) Diagnostic significance of transtympanic electrocochleography in Menière's disease. *Annals of Otology, Rhinology and Laryngology*, **92**, 155–159

GIBSON, W. P. R., RAMSDEN, R. T. and MOFFAT, D. A. (1977) The immediate effects of naftidrofuryl on the human electrocochleogram in Menière's disorder. *Journal of Laryngology and Otology*, **91**, 679–696

GIDDINGS, N., SHELTON, C., O'LEARY, M. J. and BRACKMANN, D. E. (1991) Cochleosacculotomy revisited: long-term results poorer than expected. *Archives of Otolaryngology – Head and Neck Surgery*, 117, 1150–1152

GLASSCOCK, M. E. (1973) Vestibular nerve section: middle fossa and translabyrinthine. *Archives of Otolaryngology*, 97, 112–114

GLASSCOCK, M. E., JOHNSON, G. D. and POE, D. S. (1989a) Long-term hearing results following middle fossa vestibular nerve section. *Otolaryngology – Head and Neck Surgery*, 100, 35–40

GLASSCOCK, M. E., JOHNSON, G. D. and POE, D. S. (1989b) Streptomycin in Menière's disease: a case requiring multiple treatments. *Otolaryngology – Head and Neck Surgery*, 100, 237–241

GLASSCOCK, M. E., GULYA, A. J., PENSAK, M. L. and BLACK, J. N. JR (1984) Medical and surgical management of Menière's disease. *American Journal of Otology*, 5, 536–542

GLASSCOCK, M. E., JACKSON, C. G., POE, D. S. and JOHNSON, G. D. (1989) What I think of sac surgery in 1989. *American Journal of Otology*, 10, 230–233

GLASSCOCK, M. E., THEDINGER, B. A., CUEVA, R. A. and JACKSON, C. G. (1991) An analysis of retrolabyrinthine vs. retrosigmoid vestibular nerve section. *Otolaryngology – Head and Neck Surgery*, 104, 88–95

GOIN, D. W., STALLER, S. J. and ASHER, D. L. (1982) Summating potential in Menière's disease. *Laryngoscope*, 92, 1383–1389

GOWERS, W. R. (1877) The diagnosis and treatment of auditory nerve vertigo. *British Medical Journal*, 1, 287–289, 418–420, 477–478

GRAHAM, M. D. and COLTON, J. J. (1980) Transmastoid labyrinthectomy indications. Technique and early postoperative results. *Laryngoscope*, 90, 1253–1262

GRAHAM, M. D. and KEMINK, J. L. (1984) Transmastoid labyrinthectomy: surgical managment of vertigo in the nonserviceable hearing ear: five year experience. *American Journal of Otology*, 5, 295–299

GRAHAM, M., SATALOFF, R. T. and KEMINK, J. L. (1984) Titration streptomycin therapy for bilateral Menière's disease: a preliminary report. *Otolaryngology – Head and Neck Surgery*, 92, 440–447

GRAYBIEL, A., SCHUKNECHT, H. F., FREGLY, A. R., MILLER, E. F. and MCLEOD, M. E. (1967) Streptomycin in Menière's disease: long-term follow-up. *Archives of Otolaryngology*, 85, 156–170

GREEN, J. D., BLUM, D. J. and HARNER, S. G. (1991) Longitudinal follow up of patients with Menière's disease. *Otolaryngology – Head and Neck Surgery*, 104, 783–788

GREVEN, A. J. and OOSTERVELD, W. J. (1975) The contralateral ear in Menière's disease: a survery of 292 patients. *Archives of Otolaryngology*, 101, 608–612

GUILD, S. (1927) The circulation of the endolymph. *American Journal of Anatomy*, 39, 5781

GUSSEN, R. (1982) Vascular mechanism in Menière's disease. *Archives of Otolaryngology*, 108, 544–549

HAID, T. (1988) Evaluation of flunarizine in patients with Menière's disease. *Acta Otolaryngologica Supplementum*, 460, 149–153

HALL, C. M. (1978) Maximum compliance and Menière's disease. *Laryngoscope*, 88, 1521–1517

HALLPIKE, C. and CAIRNS, H. (1938) Observations on the pathology of Menière's syndrome. *Journal of Laryngology and Otology*, 53, 625–655

HALLPIKE, C. S. and WRIGHT, A. J. (1940) On the histological changes in the temporal bones of a case of Menière's

disease. *Journal of Laryngology and Otology*, 55, 59–65. Reproduced 94, 805–844

HANSON, H. V. (1951) The treatment of endolymphatic hydrops (Menière's disease) with streptomycin. *Annals of Otology*, 60, 676–691

HARKER, L. A. (1989) Differential diagnosis in Menière's disease. In: *Proceedings of the Second International Symposium on Menière's Disease: Pathogenesis, Pathophysiology, Diagnosis and Treatment*, edited by J. B Nadol. Amsterdam: Kugler Publications. pp. 29–36

HARRIS, F. P. and PROBST, R. (1992) Transiently evoked otoacoustic emissions in patients with Menière's disease. *Acta Otolaryngologica*, 112, 36–44

HARRIS, J. P. (1989) Autoimmunity of the inner ear. *American Journal of Otology*, 10, 193–195

HARRIS, J. P. and AFRAMIAN, D. (1994) Role of autoimmunity in contralateral delayed endolymphatic hydrops. *American Journal of Otology*, 15, 710–716

HARRISON, M. S. and NAFTALIN, L. (1968) *Menière's Disease. Mechanism and Management*. Springfield: Charles C. Thomas

HENRIKSSON, N. G., GLEISSNER, L. and JOHANSSON, G. (1986) Experimental pressure variations in the membranous labyrinth of the frog. *Acta Otolaryngologica*, 61, 281–286

HICKS, G. W. and WRIGHT, W. J. (1988) Delayed endolymphatic hydrops: a review of 15 cases. *Laryngoscope*, 98, 840–845

HINCHCLIFFE, R. (1967a) Emotion as a precipitating factor in Menière's disease. *Journal of Laryngology and Otology*, 81, 471–475

HINCHCLIFFE, R. (1967b) Personality profile in Menière's disease. *Journal of Laryngology and Otology*, 81, 477–481

HINTON, A. E., RAMSDEN, R. T. and SAEED, S. (1993) Shy-Drager syndrome presenting as Menière's disease. *American Journal of Otology*, 14, 407–408

HOMMES, O. R. (1970) A study of the efficacy of betahistine in Menière's syndrome. *Acta Otolaryngologica*, 305, 70–79

HOOD, J. D. (1983) Audiology. In: *Menière's disease: A Comprehensive Appraisal*, edited by W. J. Oosterveld. New York: John Wiley. pp. 35–53

HORNER, K. C., ERRE, J. P. and CAZALS, Y. (1989) Asymmetry of evoked rotatory nystagmus in the guinea pig after experimental induction of endolymphatic hydrops. *Acta Otolaryngologica Supplementum* 468, 65–69

HORNER, K. C., AUROUSSEAU, C., ERRE, J. P. and CAZALS, Y. (1989) Long-term treatment with chlorthalidone reduces experimental hydrops but does not prevent hearing loss. *Acta Otolaryngologica*, 108, 175–183

HOROWITZ, M., FLOOD, L. M. and HAMPAL, S. (1989) Cryosurgical treatment of endolymphatic hydrops. *Journal of Laryngology and Otology*, 103, 481–484

HOUSE, W. F. (1961) Surgical exposure of the internal auditory canal and its contents through the middle cranial fossa. *Laryngoscope*, 71, 1363–1385

HSU, L., ZHU, X. and ZHAO, Y. (1990) Immunoglobulin E and circulating immune complexes in endolymphatic hydrops. *Annals of Otology, Rhinology and Laryngology*, 99, 535–538

HUANG, T. and LIN, C. (1989a) Austin endolymph dispursement shunt surgery for Menière's disease. *Acta Otolaryngologica Supplementum*, 468, 99–103

HUANG, T. and LIN, C. (1989b) Revision endolymphatic sac surgery for recurrent Menière's disease. *Acta Otolaryngologica Supplementum*, 485, 131–144

HUANG, T. S. and LIN, C. C. (1991) Surgical treatment of

chronic otitis media and Menière's syndrome. *Laryngoscope*, **101**, 900–904

HUGHES, G. B., BARNA, B. P., KINNEY, S. E., CALABRESE, L. H., HAMID, M. A. and NALEPA, N. J. (1988a) Autoimmune endolymphatic hydrops: five year review. *Otolaryngology – Head and Neck Surgery*, **98**, 221–225

HUGHES, G. B., BARNA, B. P., KINNEY, S. E., CALABRESE, L. H. and NALEPA, N. J. (1988b) Clinical diagnosis of immune inner-ear disease. *Laryngoscope*, **98**, 251–253

HUGHES, G. B., KINNEY, S. E., BARNA, B. P., TOMSAK, R. L. and CALABRESE, L. H. (1983a) Autoimmune reactivity in Cogan's syndrome: a preliminary report. *Otolaryngology – Head and Neck Surgery*, **91**, 24–32

HUGHES, G. B., KINNEY, S. E., BARNA, B. P., TOMSAK, R. L. and CALABRESE, L. H. (1983b) Autoimmune reactivity in Menière's disease: a preliminary report. *Laryngoscope*, **93**, 410–417

HULSHOF, J. H. and BAARSMA, E. A. (1981) Follow-up vestibular examination in Menière's disease. *Acta Otolaryngologica*, **92**, 397–401

IKEDA, I. and SANDO, I. (1984) Endolymphatic duct and sac in patients with Menière's disease: a temporal bone histopathological study. *Annals of Otology, Rhinology and Laryngology*, **93**, 540–546

IKEDA, M. and SANDO, I. (1985) Vascularity of endolymphatic sac in Menière's disease: a histopathological study. *Annals of Otology, Rhinology and Laryngology*, **94** (Supplement 118), 6–10

INOUE, H., UCHI, Y., NOGAMI, K. and UEMURA, T. (1994) Low dose intratympanic gentamicin treatment in Menière's disease. *European Archives of Otorhinolaryngology*, **251** (suppl. 1), S12–S14

ISHIZAKI, H., PYYKKO, I., AALTO, H. and STARCK, J. (1991) The Tullio phenomenon in patients with Menière's disease as revealed with posturography. *Acta Otolaryngologica Supplementum*, **481**, 593–595

ISSA, T. K., BAHGAT, M. A., LINTHICUM, F. H. and HOUSE, H. P. (1983) The effect of stapedectomy on hearing of patients with otosclerosis and Menière's disease. *American Journal of Otology*, **4**, 323–326

ITO, M., WATANABE, Y., SHOJAKU, H., KOBAYASHI, H., ASO, S. and MIZUKOSHI, K. (1993) Furosemide VOR test for the detection of endolymphatic hydrops. *Acta Otolaryngologica Supplementum*, **504**, 55–57

JACKSON, C. G., GLASSCOCK, M. E. and DAVIS, W. E. (1981) Medical management of Menière's disease. *Annals of Otology, Rhinology and Laryngology*, **90**, 142–147

JAHNKE, K. (1981) Permeability barriers of the inner ear in respect to the Menière's attack. In: *Menière's Disease: Pathogenesis, Diagnosis and Treatment*, edited by K. H. Vosteen. Stuttgart: George Thieme. pp. 67–74

JUHN, S. K., PRADO, S. and PEARCE, J. (1976) Osmolality changes in perilymph after systemic administration of glycerin. *Archives of Otolaryngology*, **102**, 683–685

KAWAUCHI, H., LIM, D. J. and DEMARIA, T. F. (1989) Role of middle ear endotoxin in inner ear inflammatory response and hydrops. Long-term study. In: *Proceedings of the Second International Symposium on Menière's Disease: Pathogenesis, Pathophysiology, Diagnosis and Treatment*, edited by J. B. Nadol. Amsterdam. Kugler Publications. pp. 113–124

KEMINK, J. L. and HOFF, J. (1986) Retrolabyrinthine vestibular nerve section: analysis of results. *Laryngoscope*, **96**, 33–36

KIMURA, R. S. (1967) Experimental blockage of the endolymphatic duct and sac and its effect on the inner ear of the guinea pig: a study on endolymphatic hydrops. *Annals of Otology, Rhinology and Laryngology*, **76**, 664–687

KIMURA, R. S. (1982) Animal models of endolymphatic hydrops. *American Journal of Otology*, **3**, 447–451

KIMURA, R. S. (1984) Fistulae in the membranous labyrinth. *Annals of Otology, Rhinology and Laryngology*, **93** (Supplement 112), 36–43

KIMURA, R. S. and SCHUKNECHT, H. F. (1965) Membranous hydrops in the inner ear of the guinea pig after obliteration of the endolymphatic sac. *Practica Otorhinolaryngologica*, **27**, 343–354

KIMURA, R. S., and SCHUKNECHT, H. F. (1975) Effect of fistulae on endolymphatic hydrops. *Annals of Otology, Rhinology and Laryngology*, **84**, 271–286

KIMURA, R. S., LEE, K. S., NYE, C. L. and TREHEY, J. A. (1991) Effects of systemic and lateral canal administration of aminoglycosides on normal and hydropic inner ears. *Acta Otolaryngologica*, **111**, 1021–1030

KITAHARA, M. (1991) Bilateral aspects of Menière's disease. Menière's disease with bilateral fluctuant hearing loss. *Acta Otolaryngologica Supplementum*, **485**, 74–77

KITAHARA, M., FUTAKI, T. and NAKANO, K. (1971) Ethnic aspects of Menière's disease. *Equilibrium Research Supplement*, **1**

KITAHARA, M., KITAJIMA, K., YAZAWA, Y. and UCHIDA, K. (1987) Endolymphatic sac surgery for Menière's disease: eighteen years' experience with the Kitahara sac operation. *American Journal of Otology*, **8**, 283–286

KITAHARA, M., TAKEDA, T., YAZAWA, Y., MATSUBARA, H. and KITANO, H. (1984) Pathophysiology of Menière's disease and its subvarieties. *Acta Otolaryngologica*, **406**, 52–55

KLIS, S. F. L., BUIJS, J. and SMOORENBURG, G. F. (1990) Quantification of the relation between electrophysiologic and morphologic changes in experimental endolymphatic hydrops. *Annals of Otology, Rhinology and Laryngology*, **99**, 566–570

KLOCKHOFF, I. and LINDBLOM, U. (1966) Endolymphatic hydrops revealed by the glycerol test. Preliminary report. *Acta Otolaryngologica*, **61**, 459–462

KLOCKHOFF, I. and LINDBLOM, U. (1967) Menière's disease and hydrochlorothiazide – a critical analysis of symptoms and therapeutic effects. *Acta Otolaryngologica*, **63**, 347–365

KLOCKHOFF, I., LINDBLOM, U. and STAHLE, J. (1974) Diuretic treatment of Menière's disease. *Archives of Otolaryngology*, **100**, 262–265

KOBAYASHI, H., ITO, M., MUZUKOSHI, K., WATANABE, Y., OHASHI, N. and SHOJAKU, H. (1989) The furosemide VOR test for Menière's disease: a preliminary report. *Acta Otolaryngologica Supplementum*, **468**, 81–85

KOSKAS, H. J., LINTHICUM, F. H. and HOUSE, W. F. (1983) Membranous rupture in Menière's disease: existence, location, and incidence. *Otolaryngology – Head and Neck Surgery*, **91**, 61–67

KOSSOFF, G., WADSWORTH, J. R. and DUDLEY, P. F. (1967) The round window ultrasonic technique for treatment of Menière's disease. *Archives of Otolaryngology*, **86**, 535–542

KOYAMA, S., MITSUSHI, Y., BIBEE, K., WATANABE, I. and TERASAKI, P. I. (1993) HLA associations with Menière's disease. *Acta Otolaryngologica*, **113**, 575–578

KRAMER, G. (1848) *Traite des maladies de l'oreille*. Paris: Germer Bailliere, Libraire-Editeur pp. 397–399

KUMAGAMI, H., NISHIDA, H. and BABA, M. (1982) Electrocochleographic study in Menière's disease. *Archives of Otolaryngology*, **108**, 284–288

KUMAR, A. (1981) Diagnostic advantages of the Torok monothermal differential caloric test. *Laryngoscope*, **91**, 1679–1694

LAITAKARI, K. (1990) Intratympanic gentamicin in severe Menière's disease. *Clinical Otolaryngology*, **15**, 545–548

LAKE, R. (1904) Removal of the semicircular canals in a case of unilateral aural vertigo. *Lancet*, i, 1567–1568

LANGE, G. (1976) Ototoxische antibiotika in der behandlung des morbus Menière. *Therapiewoche*, **26**, 3366–3372

LANGMAN, A. W., KEMINK, J. L. and GRAHAM, M. D. (1990) Titration streptomycin therapy for bilateral Menière's disease. Follow-up report. *Annals of Otology, Rhinology and Laryngology*, **99**, 923–926

LARSEN, H. C. and ANGELBORG, C. (1991) Low-pressure chamber test in Menière's disease. *Acta Otolaryngologica Supplementum*, **481**, 474–476

LAWRENCE, M. (1980) The flow of endolymph – a unified concept. *Otolaryngologic Clinics of North America*, **13**, 577–583

LAWRENCE, M. and MCCABE, B. F. (1959) Inner ear mechanics and deafness: special considerations of Menière's syndrome. *Journal of the American Medical Association*, **171**, 1927–1932

LELIEVER, W. C. and BARBER, H. O. (1980) Delayed endolymphatic hydrops. *Journal of Otolaryngology*, **9**, 375–380

LELIEVER, W. C. and BARBER, H. O. (1981) Recurrent vestibulopathy. *Laryngoscope*, **91**, 1–6

LERMOYEZ, M. (1919) Le vertige qui fait entendre (angiospasme labyrinthique). *Presse Medicale*, **27**, 1–3

LINDSAY, J. R. (1942) Labyrinthine dropsy and Menière's disease. *Archives of Otolaryngology*, **35**, 853–867

LINTHICUM, F. H. and EL-RAHMAN, A. G. (1987) Hydrops due to syphilitic endolymphatic duct obliteration. *Laryngoscope*, **97**, 568–574

LISTON, S. L., PAPARELLA, M. M., MANCINI, F. and ANDERSON, J. H. (1984) Otosclerosis and endolymphatic hydrops. *Laryngoscope*, **94**, 1003–1007

LUETJE, C. M. (1988) A critical comparison of results of endolymphatic subarachnoid shunt and endolymphatic sac incision operations. *American Journal of Otology*, **9**, 95–101

MCCABE, B. F. (1966) Otosclerosis and vertigo. *Transactions of the Pacific Coast Otoophthalmological Society*, **47**, 37–42

MCCABE, B. F. (1979) Autoimmune sensorineural hearing loss. *Annals of Otology, Rhinology and Laryngology*, **88**, 585–589

MCCLURE, J. A., COPP, J. C. and LYETT, P. (1981) Recovery nystagmus in Menière's disease. *Laryngoscope*, **91**, 1727–1737

MCKEE, G. J., KERR, A. G., TONER, J. G. and SMYTH, G. D. L. (1991) Surgical control of vertigo in Menière's disease. *Clinical Otolaryngology*, **16**, 216–227

MCKENNAN, K. X., NIELSEN, S. L., WATSON, C. and WIESNER, K. (1993) Menière's syndrome: an atypical presentation of giant cell arteritis (temporal arteritis). *Laryngoscope*, **103**, 1103–1107

MCKENZIE, K. G. (1936) Intracranial division of the vestibular portion of the auditory nerve for Menière's disease. *Canadian Medical Association Journal*, **34**, 369–381

MAGLIULO, G., VINGOLO, G. M., PETTI, R. and CRISTOFARI, P. (1993) Experimental endolymphatic hydrops and glycerol. Electrophysiologic study. *Annals of Otology, Rhinology and Laryngology*, **102**, 596–599

MAGNUSSON, M. and PADOAN, S. (1991) Delayed onset of ototoxic effects of gentamicin in treatment of Menière's disease. Rationale for extremely low dose therapy. *Acta Otolaryngologica*, **111**, 671–676

MAGNUSSON, M., PADOAN, S., KARLBERG, M. and JOHANSSON, R. (1991) Delayed onset of ototoxic effects of gentamicin in treatment of Menière's disease. *Acta Otolaryngologica Supplementum*, **481**, 610–612

MASUTANI, H., TAKAHASHI, H. and SANDO, I. (1992) Dark cell pathology in Menière's disease. *Acta Otolaryngologica*, **112**, 479–485

MENDELSOHN, M. and RODERIQUE, J. (1972) Cationic changes in endolymph during hypoglycemia. *Laryngoscope*, **82**, 1533–1540

MENIÈRE, M. P. (1861a) Sur une forme de surdité grave dependant d'une lésion de l'oreille interne. *Gazette Medicale de Paris*, **16**, 29

MENIÈRE, M. P. (1861b) Académie de Médicine: congestions cérébrales apoplectiformes: M. Trousseau. Discussion: MM. Bouillaud, Piorry, Tardieu, Durand-Fardel. *Gazette Medicale de Paris*, **16**, 55–57

MENIÈRE, M. P. (1861c) Maladies de l'oreille interne offrant les symptômes de la congestion cérébrale apoplectiforme. *Gazette Medicale de Paris*, **16**, 88–89

MENIÈRE, M. P. (1861d) Nouveaux documents relatifs aux lesions de l'oreille interne caractérisés par des symptômes de congestion cérébrale apoplectiforme. *Gazette Medicale de Paris*, **16**, 239–240

MENIÈRE, M. P. (1861e) Observations de maladies de l'oreille interne caractérisés par des symptomes de la congestion cérébrale apoplectiforme. *Gazette Medicale de Paris*, **16**, 379–380

MENIÈRE, M. P. (1861f) Memoire sur des lesions de l'oreille interne donnant lieu des symptômes de congestion cérébrale apoplectiforme. *Gazette Medicale de Paris*, **16**, 597–601

MEYERHOFF, W. L. (1989) Abnormal oculo-vestibular response. A newly described variant of Menière's disease. In: *Proceedings of the Second International Symposium on Menière's Disease: Pathogenesis, Pathophysiology, Diagnosis and Treatment*, edited by J. B. Nadol. Amsterdam: Kugler Publications. pp. 25–28

MEYERHOFF, W. L., PAPARELLA, M. M. and GUDBRANDSSON, F. K. (1981) Clinical evaluation of Menière's disease. *Laryngoscope*, **91**, 1663–1668

MICHEL, J., FOUILLET, J. and TROVERO, A. (1977) Recherches concernant l'evolution spontane de 135 cass de la maladie de Menière. *Annales d'Otolaryngologie (Paris)*, **78**, 377–385

MILLIGAN, W. (1905) Menière's disease – a clinical and experimental enquiry. *Journal of Laryngology and Otology*, **20**, 105–109

MIZUKOSHI, K., WATANABE, I., MATSUNAGA, T., HINOKI, M., KOMATSUZAKI, A., TAKAYASU, S. *et al.* (1988) Clinical evaluation of medical treatment for Menière's disease, using a double-blind controlled study. *American Journal of Otology*, **9**, 418–422

MOFFAT, D. A. (1979) Transtympanic electrocochleography in Menière's disease: variation in the amplitude of the summating potential related to clinical status. *British Journal of Audiology*, **13**, 149–152

MOFFAT, D. A. (1987a) Electrocochleography. In: *Handbook of Neurotological Diagnosis*, edited by J. W. House and A. F. O'Connor. New York: Marcel Dekker Inc. pp. 105–139

MOFFAT, D. A. (1987b) Ototoxicity. In: *Scott-Brown's Otolaryngology*, 5th edn. edited by A. G. Kerr, Vol. 3 *Otology*, edited by J. B. Booth. London: Butterworths. pp. 465–499

MOFFAT, D. A. (1988) The surgery of vertigo. *Practitioner*, **232**, 1322–1324

MOFFAT, D. A. (1994) Endolymphatic sac surgery: analysis of 100 operations. *Clinical Otolaryngology*, **19**, 261–266

MOFFAT, D. A., BOOTH, J. B. and MORRISON, A. W. (1979) Metabolic invesitigations in Menière's disease. Preliminary findings. *Journal of Laryngology and Otology*, **93**, 545–561

MOFFAT, D. A., BOOTH, J. B. and MORRISON, A. W. (1981) Metabolic investigations in Menière's disease. *Journal of Laryngology and Otology*, **95**, 905–913

MOFFAT, D. A., CUMBERWORTH, V. L. and BAGULEY, D. M. (1990) Endolymphatic hydrops precipitated by hemodialysis. *Journal of Laryngology and Otology*, **104**, 641–642

MOFFAT, D. A., IRVING, R. M. and HARDY, D. G. (1994) Sudden deafness in acoustic neuroma. *Journal of Laryngology and Otology*, **108**, 116–119

MOFFAT, D. A., BAGULEY, D. M., HARRIES, M. L., ATLAS, M. D. and LYNCH, C. A. (1992) Bilateral electrocochleographic findings in unilateral Menière's disease. *Otolaryngology – Head and Neck Surgery*, **107**, 370–373

MOFFAT, D. A., GIBSON, W. R. P., RAMSDEN, R. T., MORRISON, A. W. and BOOTH, J. B. (1978) Transtympanic electrocochleography during glycerol dehydration. *Acta Otolaryngologica*, **85**, 158–166

MOFFAT, D. A., TONER, J. G., BAGULEY, D. M. and HARDY, D. G. (1991) Posterior fossa vestibular neurectomy. *Journal of Laryngology and Otology*, **105**, 1002–1003

MONSELL, E. M. and SHELTON, C. (1991) Labyrintotomy with streptomycin infusion: early results of a multicenter study. *American Journal of Otology*, **13**, 416–422

MONSELL, E. M. and WIET, R. J. (1988) Endolymphatic sac surgery: methods of study and results. *American Journal of Otology*, **9**, 396–402

MONSELL, E. M., CASS, S. P. and RYBAK, L. P. (1993) Therapeutic use of aminoglycosides in Menière's disease. *Otolaryngologic Clinics of North America*, **26**, 737–746

MORRISON, A. W. (1979) Menière's disease saccus surgery technique. *Revue de Laryngologie*, **100**, 327–329

MORRISON, A. W. (1986) Predictive tests for Menière's disease. *American Journal of Otology*, **7**, 5–10

MORRISON, A. and BOOTH, J. (1988) Systemic disease and otology. In: *Otologic Medicine and Surgery*, edited by P. Alberti and R. Ruben. New York: Churchill Livingstone. pp. 287–298

MORRISON, A. W. and MORRISON, G. A. (1989) Cochlear dialysis for Menière's disease: an update. *American Journal of Otology*, **10**, 148–149

MORRISON, A. W., MOFFAT, D. A. and O'CONNOR, A. F. (1980) Clinical usefulness of electrocochleography in Menière's disease: an analysis of dehydrating agents. *Otolaryngologic Clinics of North America*, **13**, 703–721

MORRISON, A. W., MOWBRAY, J. F., WILLIAMSON, R., SHEEKA, S., SODHA, N. and KOSKINEN, N. (1994) On genetic and environmental factors in Menière's disease. *American Journal of Otology*, **15**, 35–39

MUNRO, K. J., SMITH, R. and THORNTON, A. R. D. (1995) Difficulties experienced in implementing the ABR travelling wave velocity (Delta V) technique with two commercially available systems. *British Journal of Audioogy*, **29**, 23–29

MYGIND, S. H. and DEDERDING, D. (1932) Significance of water metabolism in general pathology as demonstrated by experiments on ear. *Acta Otolaryngologica*, **17**, 424–466

NADOL, J. B. (1977) Positive Hennebert's sign in Menière's disease. *Archives of Otolaryngology*, **103**, 524–530

NADOL, J. B., WEISS, A. D. and PARKER, S. W. (1975) Vertigo of delayed onset after sudden deafness. *Annals of Otology, Rhinology and Laryngology*, **84**, 841–846

NAITO, T. (1962) Notre experience de l'operation de G. Portmann (Ouverture du sac endolymphatique dans le maladie de Menière). *Revue de Laryngologie*, **83**, 643–645

NAITO, T., TABAYASHI, N., ITO, J., YAGI, N. and HONJO, I. (1989) Influence of external auditory canal pressure on head movement of patients with Menière's disease. In: *Proceedings of the Second International Symposium on Menière's Disease: Pathogenesis Pathophysiology, Diagnosis and Treatment*, edited by J. B. Nadol. Amsterdam: Kugler Publications. pp. 385–390

NEDZELSKI, J. M., BARBER, H. O. and MCILMOYL, L. (1986) Diagnosis in a dizziness unit. *Journal of Otolaryngology*, **15**, 101–104

NEDZELSKI, J. M., BRYCE, G. E. and PFLEIDERER, A. G. (1992) Treatment of Menière's disease with topical gentamicin: a preliminary report. *Journal of Otolaryngology*, **21**, 95–101

NEDZELSKI, J. M., SCHESSEL, D. A., BRYCE, G. E. and PFLEIDERER, A. G. (1992) Chemical labyrinthectomy: local application of gentamicin for the treatment of unilateral Menière's disease. *American Journal of Otology*, **13**, 18–22

NEDZELSKI, J. M., CHIONG, C. M., FRADET, D., SCHESSEL, D. A., BRYCE, G. E. and PFLEIDERER, A. G. (1993) Intratympanic gentamicin instillation as treatment of unilateral Menière's disease: an update of an ongoing study. *American Journal of Otology*, **14**, 278–282

NGUYEN, C. D., BRACKMANN, D. E., CRANE, R. T., LINTHICUM, F. H. Jr and HITSELBERGER, W. E. (1992) Retrolabyrinthine vestibular nerve section: evaluation of technical modification in 143 cases. *American Journal of Otology*, **13**, 328–332

NORRIS, C. H., SAWATSKY, S. L., BROCATO, G. D. and TABB, H. G. (1988) Application of streptomycin to the lateral semicircular canal. *Transactions of the American Otology Society*, **75**, 84–88

NORRIS, C. H., AMEDEE, R. G., RISEY, J. A. and SHEA, J. J. (1990) Selective chemical vestibulectomy. *American Journal of Otology*, **11**, 395–400

ODKVIST, L. M. (1988) Middle ear ototoxic treatment for inner ear disease. *Acta Otolaryngologica Supplementum*, **457**, 83–86

ODKVIST, L. M. and BERGENIUS, J. (1988) Drop attacks in Menière's disease. *Acta Otolaryngologica Supplementum*, **455**, 82–85

ODKVIST, L. M., BERGHOLTZ, L. M. and LUNDGREN, A. (1984) Topical gentamicin treatment for disabling Menière's disease. *Acta Otolaryngologica Supplementum*, **412**, 74–76

OKUNO, T. and SANDO, I. (1987) Localization, frequency, and severity of endolymphatic hydrops and pathology of the labyrinthine membrane in Menière's disease. *Annals of Otology, Rhinology and Laryngology*, **96**, 438–445

OLIVEIRA, C. A. and BRAGA, A. M. (1992) Menière's syndrome inherited as an autoosomal dominant trait. *Annals of Otology, Rhinology and Laryngology*, **101**, 590–594

OLSSON, J. E. (1991) Neurotologic findings in basilar migraine. *Laryngoscope*, **101**, Supplement 52, 1–41

OOSTERVELD, W. J. (1980) Menière's disease: signs and symptoms. *Journal of Laryngology and Otology*, **94**, 885–894

OOSTERVELD, W. J. (1984) Betahistine dihydrochloride in the treatment of vertigo of peripheral origin. *Journal of Laryngology and Otology*, **98**, 37–41

ORCHIK, D. J., SHEA, J. J. and GE, X. (1993) Transtympanic electrocochleography in Menière's disease using clicks and tone-bursts. *American Journal of Otology*, **14**, 290–294

PAPARELLA, M. M. (1984a) Pathogenesis of Menière's disease and Menière's syndrome. *Acta Otolaryngologica Supplementum*, **406**, 10–25

PAPARELLA, M. M. (1984b) Pathology of Menière's disease. *Annals of Otology, Rhinology and Laryngology*, **93** (Supplement 112), 31–35

PAPARELLA, M. M. (1985) The cause (multifactorial inheritance) and pathogenesis (endolymphatic malabsorption) of Menière's disease and its symptoms (mechanical and chemical). *Acta Otolaryngologica*, **99**, 445–451

PAPARELLA, M. M. and GRIEBIE, M. S. (1984) Bilaterality of Menière's disease. *Acta Otolaryngologica*, **97**, 233–237

PAPARELLA, M. M. and MANCINI, F. (1983) Trauma and Menière's syndrome. *Laryngoscope*, **93**, 1004–1012

PAPARELLA, M. M. and MANCINI, F. (1985) Vestibular Menière's disease. *Otolaryngology – Head and Neck Surgery*, **93**, 148–151

PAPARELLA, M. M. and SAJJADI, H. (1987a) Endolymphatic sac enhancement: principles of diagnosis and treatment. *American Journal of Otology*, **8**, 294–300

PAPARELLA, M. M. and SAJJADI, H. (1987b) Endolymphatic sac revision for recurrent Menière's disease. *American Journal of Otology*, **9**, 441–447

PAPARELLA, M. M., DESOUSA, L. C. and MANCINI, F. (1983) Menière's syndrome and otitis media. *Laryngoscope*, **93**, 1408–1415

PAPARELLA, M. M., KIM, C. and SHEA, D. A. (1980) Sac decompression for refractory luetic vertigo. *Acta Otolaryngologica*, **89**, 541–546

PAPARELLA, M. M., MANCINI, F. and LISTON, S. L. (1984) Otosclerosis and Menière's syndrome: diagnosis and treatment. *Laryngoscope*, **94**, 1414–1417

PAPARELLA, M. M., GOYCOOLEA, M. V., MEYERHOFF, W. L. and SHEA, D. (1979) Endolymphatic hydrops and otitis media. *Laryngoscope*, **81**, 43–54

PAPARELLA, M. M., SAJJADI, H., DACOSTA, S. S., YOON, T. H. and LE, C. T. (1989) The significance of the lateral sinus and Trautmann's triangle in Menière's disease. In: *Proceedings of the Second International Symposium on Menière's Disease: Pathogenesis, Pathophysiology, Diagnosis and Treatment*, edited by J. B. Nadol. Amsterdam: Kugler Publications. pp. 139–146

PARNES, L. S. and MCCLURE, J. A. (1990) Rotatory recovery nystagmus: an important localizing sign in endolymphatic hydrops. *Journal of Otolaryngology*, **19**, 96–99

PARNES, L. S. and PRICE-JONES, R. G. (1993) Particle repositioning maneuver for benign positional vertigo. *Annals of Otology, Rhinology and Laryngology*, **102**, 325–331

PARNES, L. S. and RIDDELL, D. (1993) Irritative spontaneous nystagmus following intratympanic gentamicin for Menière's disease. *Laryngoscope*, **103**, 745–749

PARRY, R. H. (1904) A case of tinnitus and vertigo treated by division of the auditory nerve. *Journal of Laryngology and Otology*, **19**, 402–406. Reproduced 1991, **105**, 1099–1100

PARRY, T. W. (1907) On the treatment of Menière's disease and Menière's symptoms. *British Medical Journal*, **2**, 83

PASSE, E. R. G. and SEYMOUR, J. S. (1948) Menière's syndrome: successful treatment by surgery on the sympathetic. *British Medical Journal*, **2**, 812–816

PEARSON, B. W. and BRACKMANN, D. E. (1985) Committee on hearing and equilibrium guidelines for reporting treatment results in Menière's disease. *Otolaryngology – Head and Neck Surgery*, **93**, 579–581

PEETERS, G. J., CREMERS, C. W., PINCKERS, A. J. and HOEFNAGELS, W. H. L. (1986) Atypical Cogan's syndrome: an autoimmune disease? *Annals of Otology, Rhinology and Laryngology*, **95**, 173–175

PENROD, J. P. (1985) Speech discrimination testing. In: *Handbook of Clinical Audiology*, edited by J. Katz. Baltimore: Williams & Wilkins. pp. 235–258

PERON, D. L., KITAMURA, K., CARNIOL, P. J. and SCHUKNECHT, H. F. (1983) Clinical and experimental results with focused ultrasound. *Laryngoscope*, **93**, 1217–1221

PFALZ, C. R. and THOMSEN, J. (1986) Symptomatology and definition of Menière's disease. In: *Controversial Aspects of Menière's Disease*, edited by C. R. Pfalz. New York, George Thieme. pp. 2–7

PILLSBURY, H. C., ARENBERG, I. K., FERRARO, J. and ACKLEY, R. S. (1983) Endolymphatic sac surgery. The Danish Sham study: an alternative analysis. *Otolaryngologic Clinics of North America*, **16**, 123–127

POLLOCK, R. A., JACKSON, R. T., CLAIRMONT, A. A. and NICHOLSON, L. (1974) Carbon dioxide as an otic vasodilator. *Archives of Otolaryngology*, **100**, 309–313

PORTMANN, G. (1926) Le traitement chirurgical des vertiges par l'overture du sac endolymphatique. *Presse Medicale*, **104**, 1635–1637

PORTMANN, G. (1927a) Vertigo surgical treatment by opening the saccus endolymphaticus. *Archives of Otolaryngology*, **6**, 309–319

PORTMANN, G. (1927b) The saccus endolymphaticus and an operation for draining the same for the relief of vertigo. *Journal of Laryngology and Otology*, **42**, 809–917. Reproduced **105**, 1109–1113

PORTMANN, M. (1987) The Portmann procedure after sixty years. *American Journal of Otology*, **8**, 271–274

POULSEN, H. (1966) Thyrotropic and thyroid control of the inner ear with special reference to myxoedema and Menière's disease. In: *Hormones and Connective Tissue*, edited by G. Ashboe-Hanson. Baltimore: Williams and Wilkins. p. 239

POWERS, W. H. (1972) Metabolic aspects of Menière's disease. *Laryngoscope*, **82**, 1716–1725

POWERS, W. H. (1978) Metabolic aspects of Menière's disease. *Laryngoscope*, **88**, 122–129

POWERS, W. H. and HOUSE, W. F. (1969) The dizzy patient – Allergic aspect. *Laryngoscope*, **79**, 1330–1338

PULEC, J. L. (1972) Menière's disease: results of a two and one-half year study of aetiology, natural history and results of treatment. *Laryngoscope*, **82**, 1703–1715

PYYKKO, I., MAGNUSSON, M., SCHALEN, L. and ENBOM, H. (1988) Pharmacological treatment of vertigo. *Acta Otolaryngologica Supplementum*, **455**, 77–81

RAMSDEN, R. T. and TIMMS, M. S. (1991) Promontory stimulation following labyrinthectomy. *Journal of Laryngology and Otology*, **105**, 729–731

RAMSDEN, R. T., GIBSON, W. P. R. and MOFFAT, D. A. (1977) Anaesthesia of the tympanic membrane using iontophoresis. *Journal of Laryngology and Otology*, **91**, 779–785

RAMSDEN, R. T., MOFFAT, D. A. and GIBSON, W. P. R. (1977) Transtympanic electrocochleography in patients with syphilis and hearing loss. *Annals of Otology, Rhinology, and Laryngology*, **86**, 827–834

RASK-ANDERSON, H., FRIBERG, U., ERWALL, C. and JANSSON, B. (1989) Effects of hyperosmolar substances on the endolymphatic sac. *Acta Otolaryngologica Supplementum*, **468**, 49–52

RASK-ANDERSON, H., DANCKWARDT-LILLIESTROM, N., LINTHICUM, F.H. and HOUSE, W. F. (1991) Ultrastructural evidence of a merocrine secretion in the human endolymphatic sac. *Annals of Otology, Rhinology and Laryngology*, **100**, 148–156

RAUCH, S. D., MERCHANT, S. N. and THEDINGER, B. A. (1989) Menière's syndrome and endolymphatic hydrops: a double blind temporal bone study. *Annals of Otology, Rhinology and Laryngology*, **98**, 873–883

RIZVI, S. S. (1986) Investigations into the cause of canal paresis in Menière's disease. *Laryngoscope*, **96**, 1258–1271

ROSENBERG, S., SILVERSTEIN, H., FLANZER, J. and WATANABE, H. (1991) Bilateral Menière's disease in surgical versus non-surgical patients. *American Journal of Otology*, **12**, 336–340

RUCKENSTEIN, M. J., RUTKA, J. A. and HAWKE, M. (1991) The treatment of Menière's disease: Torok revisited. *Laryngoscope*, **101**, 211–218

RUDD, M. J., HARRIES, M. L., LYNCH, C. A. and MOFFAT, D. A. (1993) Hearing loss fluctuating with blood sugar levels in Menière's disease. *Journal of Laryngology and Otology*, **107**, 620–622

SACKETT, J. F., KOZAREK, J. A. and ARENBERG, I. K. (1980) The clinical significance of tomographic visualization of the vestibular aqueduct. *Otolaryngologic Clinics of North America*, **13**, 657–664

SAKURAI, T., YAMANE, H. and NAKAI, Y. (1991) Some aspects of hearing change in Menière's patients. *Acta Otolaryngologica Supplementum*, **486**, 92–98

SANDO, I and EGAMI, T. (1977) Inner ear hemorrhage and endolymphatic hydrops in a leukemic patient with sudden hearing loss. *Annals of Otology, Rhinology and Laryngology*, **86**, 518–524

SANDO, I. and IKEDA, M. (1984) The vestibular aqueduct in patients with Menière's disease: a temporal bone histopathological investigation. *Acta Otolaryngologica*, **97**, 558–570

SANDO, I. and IKEDA, M. (1985) Pneumatization and thickness of the petrous bone in patients with Menière's disease: a histopathologicalal study. *Annals of Otology, Rhinology and Laryngology*, **94** (Supplement 118), 2–5

SANTOS, P. M., HALL, R. A., SNYDER, J. M., HUGHES, L. F. and DOBIE, R. A. (1993) Diuretic and diet effect on Menière's disease evaluated by the 1985 Committee on Hearing and Equilibrium guidelines. *Otolaryngology – Head and Neck Surgery*, **109**, 680–689

SAWADA, I., KITAHARA, M., KITAJIMA, K. and YAZAWA, Y. (1987) Induction of experimental endolymphatic hydrops by immunologic techniques. *American Journal of Otology*, **8**, 330–334

SCHESSEL, D. A. and NEDZELSKI, J. M. (1993) Menière's disease and other peripheral vestibular disorders. In: *Otolaryngology, Head and Neck Surgery*, 2nd edn, edited by C. W. Cummings. St Louis: Mosby. pp. 3152–3176

SCHMIDT, R. H. and HUIZING, E. H. (1992) The clinical drug trial in Menière's disease with emphasis on the effect of betahistine SR. *Acta Otolaryngologica Supplementum*, **497**, 1–189

SCHMIDT, R. H. and SCHOONHAVEN, R. (1989) Lermoyez's syndrome: a follow-up study in 12 patients. *Acta Otolaryngologica*, **107**, 467–473

SCHUKNECHT, H. F. (1956) Ablation therapy for relief of Menière's disease. *Laryngoscope*, **66**, 859–870

SCHUKNECHT, H. F. (1963) Menière's disease: a correlation of symptomatology and pathology. *Laryngoscope*, **73**, 651–665

SCHUKNECHT, H.F. (1968) Pathology of Menière's disease. *Otolaryngologic Clinics of North America*, **1**, 331–337

SCHUKNECHT, H.F. (1974) *Pathology of the Ear*, Boston: Harvard University

SCHUKNECHT, H.F. (1978) Delayed endolymphatic hydrops. *Annals of Otology, Rhinology and Laryngology*, **87**, 743–748

SCHUKNECHT, H.F. (1982a) Cochleosacculotomy for Menière's disease: theory, technique and results. *Laryngoscope*, **92**, 853–858

SCHUKNECHT, H.F. (1982b) Behaviour of the vestibular nerve following labyrinthectomy. *Annals of Otology, Rhinology and Laryngology*, **91**, 16–32

SCHUKNECHT, H.F. (1986) Endolymphatic hydrops: can it be controlled? *Annals of Otology, Rhinology and Laryngology*, **95**, 36–39

SCHUKNECHT, H. F. and GULYA, A. J. (1983) Endolymphatic hydrops: an overview and classification. *Annals of Otology, Rhinology and Laryngology* **106** (suppl.), 1–20

SCHUKNECHT, H. F. and IGARASHI, M. (1986) Pathophysiology of Menière's disease. In: *Controversial Aspects of Menière's Disease*, edited by C. R. Pfalz. New York: George Thieme. pp. 46–54

SCHUKNECHT, H. F., SUZUKA, Y. and ZIMMERMANN, C. (1990) Delayed endolymphatic hydrops and its relationship to Menière's disease. *Annals of Otology, Rhinology and Laryngology*, **99**, 843–853

SHAMBAUGH, G. E. (1968) Decompression of the endolymphatic sac for hydrops. *Otolaryngologic Clinics of North America*, **1**, 607–611

SHAVER, E. F. (1975) Allergic management of Menière disease. *Archives of Otolaryngology*, **101**, 96–99

SHEA, J. J. (1966) Teflon film drainage of the endolymphatic sac. *Archives of Otolaryngology*, **83**, 40–43

SHEA, J. J. (1988) Perfusion of the inner ear with streptomycin. *Transactions of the American Otology Society*, **75**, 89

SHEA, J. J. (1990) Streptomycin perfusion of the labyrinth. *Acta Otolaryngologica Supplementum*, **485**, 123–130

SHEA, J. J. (1993a) Classification of Menière's disease. *American Journal of Otology*, **14**, 224–229

SHEA, J. J. (1993b) Interpretation of electrocochleography in Menière's disease and normal subjects. *Annals of Otology, Rhinology and Laryngology*, **102**, 77

SHEA, J. J. and KITABCHI, A. E. (1973) Management of fluctuant hearing loss. *Archives of Otolaryngology*, **97**, 118–124

SHEPARD, N. T., TELIAN, S. A. and SMITH-WHEELOCK, M. (1990) Habituation and balance retraining therapy: a retrospective review. *Neurologic Clinics of North America*, **8**, 459–475

SHINKAWA, H. and KIMURA, R. S. (1986) Effects of diuretic on endolymphatic hydrops. *Acta Otolaryngologica*, **101**, 43–52

SILVERSTEIN, H. (1970) The effects of perfusing the perilymphatic space with artificial endolymph. *Annals of Otology, Rhinology and Laryngology*, **79**, 754–765

SILVERSTEIN, H. (1976) Transmeatal labyrinthectomy with and without cochleovestibular neurectomy. *Laryngoscope*, **86**, 1777–1791

SILVERSTEIN, H., NORRELL, H. and HABERKAMP, T. (1987) A comparison of retrosigmoid IAC, retrolabyrinthine, and middle fossa vestibular neurectomy for treatment of vertigo. *Laryngoscope*, **97**, 165–173

SILVERSTEIN, H., NORRELL, H. and ROSENBERG, S. (1990) The resurrection of vestibular neurectomy: a 10 year experience with 115 cases. *Journal of Neurosurgery*, **72**, 533–539

SILVERSTEIN, H., SMOUHA, E. and JONES, R. (1989) Natural history vs. surgery for Menière's disease. *Otolaryngology – Head and Neck Surgery*, **100**, 6–16

SILVERSTEIN, H., HYMAN, S. M., FELDBAUM, J. and SILVERSTEIN, D. (1984) Use of streptomycin sulfate in the treatment of Menière's disease. *Otolaryngology – Head and Neck Surgery*, **92**, 229–232

SIMMONS, F. B. and MONGEON, C. J. (1967) Endolymphatic duct pressure produces cochlear damage. *Archives of Otolaryngology*, **85**, 39–46

SISMANIS, A., HUGHES, G. B. and ABEDI, E. (1986) Coexisting otosclerosis and Menière's disease: a diagnostic and therapeutic dilemma. *Laryngoscope*, **96**, 9–13

SMYTH, G. D. L., KERR, A. G. and GORDON, D. S. (1976) Vestibular nerve section for Menière's disease. *Journal of Laryngology and Otology*, **90**, 823–831

SNYDER, J. M. (1974) Extensive use of a diagnostic test for Menière's disease. *Archives of Otolaryngology*, **100**, 360–365

SPENCER, J. T. (1973) Hyperlipoproteinemias in the aetiology of inner ear disease. *Laryngoscope*, **83**, 639–678

SPENCER, J. T. (1975) Hyperlipoproteinemia and inner ear disease. *Otolaryngologic Clinics of North America*, **8**, 483–492

SPERLING, N. M., PAPARELLA, M. M., YOON, T. H. and ZELTERMAN, D. (1993) Symptomatic versus asymptomatic endolymphatic hydrops: a histopathological comparison. *Laryngoscope*, **103**, 277–285

STAHLE, J. (1976) Advanced Menière's disease: a study of 356 severely disabled patients. *Acta Otolaryngologica*, **81**, 113–119

STAHLE, J. (1991) Long term progression of Menière's disease. *Acta Otolaryngologica Supplementum*, **485**, 78–83

STAHLE, J. and KLOCKHOFF, I. (1986) Diagnostic procedures, differential diagnosis and general conclusions. In: *Controversial Aspects of Menière's Disease*, edited by C. R. Pfalz. New York: George Thieme. pp. 71–86

STAHLE, J. and WILBRAND, H. F. (1983) The temporal bone in patients with Menière's disease. *Acta Otolaryngologica*, **95**, 81–94

STAHLE, J., DEUTSCHL, H. and JOHANSSON, S. G. O. (1974) Menière's disease and allergy: with special reference to immunoglobulin E and IgE antibody (reagin) in serum. *International Journal of Equilibrium Research*, **4**, 22–27

STAHLE, J., STAHLE, C. and ARENBERG, K. (1978) Incidence of Menière's disease. *Archives of Otolaryngology*, **104**, 99–102

STEPHENS, S. D. G. (1975) Personality tests in Menière's disorder. *Journal of Laryngology and Otology*, **89**, 479–490

SUCHATO, C., VEJVECHANEYOM, W. and CHAROENSUWAN, P. (1993) MR imaging in a patient with Menière's disease. *American Journal of Roentgenology*, **161**, 1263–1264

SUZUKI, M. and KITAHARA, M. (1992) Immunologic abnormality in Menière's disease. *Otolaryngology – Head and Neck Surgery*, **107**, 57–62

SZIKLAI, J., HOMER, K. C., FERRARY, E., STERKERS, O. and AMIEL, C. (1989) Electrochemical composition of the cochlear fluids in early experimental hydrops. *Acta Otolaryngologica*, **107**, 371–374

TAKUMIDA, M., BAGGER-SJÖBACK, D. and RASK-ANDERSON, H. (1989) The effects of glycerol on vestibular function and the endolymphatic sac after pre-treatment with colchicine. *Acta Otolaryngologica Supplementum*, **468**, 59–63

TANIOKA, H., ZUSHO, H., MACHIDA, T., SASAKI, Y. and SHIRAKAWA, T. (1992) High-resolution MR imaging of the inner ear: findings in Menière's disease. *European Journal of Radiology*, **15**, 83–88

TASAKI, I. and FERNANDEZ, C. (1952) Modification of cochlear microphonics and action potentials by KCl solution and by direct currents. *Journal of Neurophysiology*, **15**, 497–512

TELIAN, S. A., SHEPARD, N. T., SMITH-WHEELOCK, M. and KEMINK, J. L. (1990) Habituation therapy for chronic vestibular dysfunction: preliminary results. *Otolaryngology – Head and Neck Surgery*, **103**, 89–95

THOMAS, K. and HARRISON, M. S. (1971) Long term follow-up of 610 cases of Menière's disease. *Proceedings of the Royal Society of Medicine*, **64**, 853–856

THOMSEN, J. and BRETLAU, P. (1986) General conclusions. In: *Controversial Aspects of Menière's Disease*, edited by C. R. Pfalz. New York: George Thieme. pp. 120–136

THOMSEN, J., BRETLAU, P., TOS, M. and JOHNSEN, N. J. (1981) Placebo effect in surgery for Menière's disease, a double-blind, placebo-controlled study on endolymphatic sac shunt surgery. *Archives of Otolaryngology*, **107**, 271–277

THOMSEN, J., BRETLAU, P., TOS, M. and JOHNSEN, N. J. (1986) Endolymphatic sac-mastoid shunt surgery: a nonspecific treatment modality? *Annals of Otology, Rhinology and Laryngology*, **95**, 32–35

THOMSEN, J., KERR, A. G., BRETLAU, P., OLSSON, J. and TOS, M. (1995) Endolymphatic sac surgery: why we don't do it. *Clinical Otolaryngology*, (in press)

THORNTON, A. R., FARRELL, G. and HAACKE, N. P. (1991) A non-invasive, objective test of endolymphatic hydrops. *Acta Otolaryngologica Supplementum*, **479**, 35–43

TJERNSTRÖM, O. (1980) Current status of pressure chamber treatment. *Otolaryngologic Clinics of North America*, **13**, 723–729

TJERNSTRÖM, O. (1986) Pressure chamber treatment. In: *Controversial Aspects of Menière's Disease*, edited by C. R. Pfalz. New York: George Thieme. pp. 96–98

TOMODA, K., SUZUKA, Y., IWAI, H., YAMASHITA, T. and KUMAZAWA, T. (1993) Menière's disease and autoimmunity: clinical study and survery. *Acta Otolaryngologica Supplementum*, **500**, 31–34

TOMIYAMA, S. (1992) Development of endolymphatic hydrops following immune response in the endolymphatic sac of the guinea pig. *Acta Otolaryngologica*, **112**, 470–478

TONNDORF, J. (1968) Pathophysiology of the hearing loss in Menière's disease. *Otolaryngologic Clinics of North America*, **1**, 375–388

TONNDORF, J. (1975) Mechanical causes of fluctuant hearing loss. *Otolaryngoloic Clinics of North America*, **8**, 303–311

TONNDORF, J. (1983) Vestibular signs and symptoms in Menière's disorder: mechanical considerations. *Acta Otolaryngologica*, **95**, 421–430

TONNDORF, J. (1986) Physiologic aspects. In: *Controversial Aspects of Menière's Disease*, edited by C. R. Pfalz. New York: George Thieme. pp. 34–45

TOROK, N. (1977) Old and new in Menière's disease. *Laryngoscope*, **87**, 1870–1877

TOROK, N. (1983) Prosper Menière, a pioneer in otology of the 19th century. In: *Menière's Disease: A Comprehensive Appraisal*, edited by W. J. Oosterveld. New York, John Wiley & Sons. pp. 1–7

TROUSSEAU, A. (1861) De la congestion cerebrale apoplectiforme, dans ses rapports avec epilepsie. *Gazette Medicale de Paris*, **16**, 51–52

TULLIO, P. (1938) Demonstration des methodes pour la stimulation acoustique des caneaux semicirculaires. *Acta Otolaryngologica*, **26**, 267–273

TUMARKIN, A. (1936) The otolithic catastrophe: a new syndrome. *British Medical Journal (Clinical Research)*, **2**, 175–177

TUMARKIN, A. (1966) Thoughts on the treatment of labyrinthopathy. *Journal of Laryngology and Otology*, **80**, 1041–1053

TURNER, J. S. and JACKSON, R. T. (1989) Astemizole use in Menière's patients with intractable vertigo. In: *Proceedings of the Second International Symposium on Menière's Disease: Pathogenesis, Pathophysiology, Diagnosis and Treatment*, edited by J. B. Nadol. Amsterdam: Kugler Publications. pp. 459–461

UZIEL, A. and BONFILS, P. (1993) Assessment of endolymphatic cochlear hydrops by means of evoked acoustic emissions. In: *Proceedings of the Second International Symposium on Menière's Disease: Pathogenesis, Pathophysiology, Diagnosis and Treatment*, edited by J. B. Nadol. Amsterdam: Kugler Publications. pp. 379–383

VAN DEELEN, G. W. and HUIZING, E. H. (1986) The use of a diuretic (Dyazide) in the treatment of Menière's disease. *Otorhinolaryngology*, **48**, 287–292

VERNON, J., JOHNSON, R. and SCHLEUNING, A. (1980) The characteristics and natural history of tinnitus in Menière's disease. *Otolaryngologic Clinics of North America*, **13**, 611–619

VISCOMI, G. J. and BOJRAB, D. I. (1992) Use of electrocochleography to monitor antigenic challenge in Menière's disease. *Otolaryngology – Head and Neck Surgery*, **107**, 733–737

WACKYM, P. A. (1995) Histopathologic findings in Menière's disease. *Otolaryngology – Head and Neck Surgery*, **112**, 90–100

WACKYM, P. A., LINTHICUM, F. H., WARD, P. H., HOUSE, W. F., MICEVYCH. P. E. and BAGGER-SJÖBACK, D. (1990) Re-evaluation of the role of the human endolymphatic sac on Menière's disease. *Otolaryngology – Head and Neck Surgery*, **102**, 732–744

WALLACE, I. R. and BARBER, H. O. (1983) Recurrent vestibulopathy. *Journal of Otolaryngology*, **12**, 61–63

WATANABE, I. (1981) Menière's disease in males and females. *Acta Otolaryngologica*, **91**, 511–514

WATANABE, I. (1983) Incidence of Menière's disease, including some other epidemiological data. In: *Menière's Disease: A Comprehensive Appraisal*, edited by W. J. Oosterveld. New York. John Wiley & Sons. p. 16

WATANABE, I., OKUNO, H., MASUDA, Y., ISHIDA, H., NIIZEKI, Y. and OKUBO, J. (1989) Studies on electrically induced stapedius reflex in cases of Menière's disease. In: *Proceedings of the Second International Symposium on Menière's Disease: Pathogenesis Pathophysiology, Diagnosis and Treatment*, edited by J. B. Nadol. Amsterdam: Kugler Publications. pp. 391–398

WATSON, C. G., BARNES, C. M., DONALDSON, J. A. and KLETT, W. G. (1967) Psychosomatic aspects of Menière's disease. *Archives of Otolaryngology*, **86**, 491–549

WEILLE, F. L. (1967) Hypoglycemia in Menière's disease. *Archives of Otolaryngology*, **87**, 129–131

WEINTRAUB, J., ARENBERG, I. K., SPECTOR, G. J. and STROUD, M. H. (1976) The efficacy of 'conservative' medical regimens on the rate of hearing losses in Menière's syndrome: a retrospective computerized statistical analysis. *Laryngoscope*, **86**, 1391–1396

WEIT, R. J., KAZAN, R. and SHAMBAUGH, G. E. (1981) An holistic approach to Menière's disease: medical and surgical management. *Laryngoscope*, **91**, 1647–1656

WHITFIELD, I. C. and ROSS, H. F. (1965) Cochlear-microphonic and summating potentials and the outputs of individual hair-cell generators. *Journal of the Acoustic Society of America*, **38**, 126–131

WILLIAMS, H., HORTORN, B. and DAY, L. (1947) Endolymphatic hydrops without vertigo. *Transactions of the American Otological Society*, **35**, 116

WILLIAMS, H. L. (1968) Definition of terms in Menière's disease. *Otolaryngologic Clinics of North America*, **1**, 267–271

WILMOT, T. J. (1974) Vestibular analysis in Menière's disease. *Journal of Laryngology and Otology*, **88**, 295–306

WILMOT, T. J. and MENON, G. N. (1976) Betahistine in Menière's disease. *Journal of Laryngology and Otology*, **90**, 833–840

WILSON, W. and SCHUKNECHT, H. (1980) Update on the use of streptomycin therapy for Menière's disease. *American Journal of Otology*, **2**, 108–111

WOLFSON, R. J. (1984) Labyrinthine cryosurgery for Menière's disease – present status. *Otolaryngology – Head and Neck Surgery*, **92**, 221–224

XENELLIS, J., MORRISON, A. W., MCCLOWSKY, D. and FESTENSTEIN, H. (1986) HLA antigens in the pathogenesis of Menière's disease. *Journal of Laryngology and Otology*, **100**, 21–24

XIMING, J., YUQING, G. and MUSAN, H. (1990) Electrocochleography in an experimental animal model of acute endolymphatic hydrops. *Acta Otolaryngologica*, **110**, 334–341

YAMAKAWA, K. (1938) Uber pathologische Veraenderung bei einem Ménière-kranken. *Japanese Journal of Otology, Tokyo*, **44**, 2310

YAMAKAWA, K. and NAITO, T. (1954) The modification of Portmann's operation for Menière's disease (Yamakawa–Naito's operation) *Medical Journal of Osaka University*, **5**, 167–175

YAZAWA, T. and KITAHARA, M. (1989) Immunofluorescent study of the endolymphaic sac in Menière's disease. *Acta Otolaryngologica Supplementum*, **468**, 71–76

YAZAWA, T., SHEA, J. J. and KITAHARA, M. (1985) Endolymphatic hydrops in guinea pig after cauterizing the sac with silver nitrate. *Archives of Otolaryngology*, **111**, 301–304

YLIKOSKI, J. (1988) Delayed endolymphatic hydrops syndrome after heavy exposure to impulse noise. *American Journal of Otology*, **9**, 282–285

YOO, T. J. (1984) Etiopathogenesis of Menière's disease: a hypothesis. *Annals of Otology, Rhinology and Laryngology*, **93** (suppl. 113), 6–12

YOO, T. J., STUART, J. M., KANG, A. H., TOWNES, A. S., TOMODA, K. and DIXIT, S. (1982) Type II autoimmunity in otosclerosis and Menière's disease. *Science*, **217**, 1153–1155

YOON, T. H., PAPARELLA, M. M. and SCHACHERN, P. A. (1990) Otosclerosis involving the vestibular aqueduct and Menière's disease. *Otolaryngology – Head and Neck Surgery*, **103**, 107–112

YOUNG, J. R. (1978) Retrospective assessment of thymoxamine (opilon) in the treatment of Menière's disease. *Journal of International Medical Research*, **6**, 166–168

YUEN, S. S. and SCHUKNECHT, H. F. (1972) Vestibular aqueduct and endolymphatic duct in Menière's disease. *Archives of Otolaryngology*, **96**, 553–555

20

Ototoxicity

A. Wright, A. Forge and B. Kotecha

The inner ear is prone to damage caused by various external factors such as noise, drugs and infections. In this chapter only damage to the inner ear secondary to drugs will be considered.

Hawkins (1976) defined ototoxicity as: 'the tendency of certain therapeutic agents and other chemical substances to cause functional impairment and cellular degeneration of the tissues of the inner ear, and especially of the end-organs and neurons of the cochlear and vestibular divisions of the eighth cranial nerve'. The sensitivity of the inner ear to the toxic effects of various therapeutic agents has been recognized for centuries. For an excellent historical review the reader is referred to Hawkins (1976) and Stephens (1982).

This chapter is divided into two sections: clinical ototoxicity and research methods for evaluation of ototoxicity.

Clinical ototoxicity

Many drugs have been blamed for the hearing loss, tinnitus and dysequilibrium that can arise during the course of treatment for illness. This blame is not always justified since the patient's illness itself can frequently be associated with auditory and vestibular symptoms. The use of ear drops containing ototoxic aminoglycoside antibiotics in patients with discharging ears and a perforated tympanic membrane is a case in point. Is it the drug or is it the disease that causes the severe sensorineural hearing loss that sometimes occurs?

In patients who are systemically ill, the presence of infected emboli, renal failure, hypoxia, dehydration and many other factors, could all cause a hearing loss or, at the very least, potentiate the effects of potential, or actual, ototoxic drugs.

This dilemma is made more difficult to resolve when the practical problems of testing the hearing and balance in sick patients in ward settings are realized. Without pre-illness or pretreatment audiometry it may be impossible to tell whether small hearing losses were already in existence given the widespread incidence of hearing loss in the general population. Thus, many studies on the incidence of drug-induced hearing loss are quite meaningless when there are neither control groups nor a pretreatment hearing assessment. A more detailed study addressing this problem will be described in the subsection on aminoglycoside toxicity.

Some drugs also appear to have central effects, delaying brain stem auditory impulses or altering higher central processing so that patients complain of hearing loss which in turn is wrongly ascribed to an ototoxic action. For example, acute and chronic treatment with imipramine has no effect on brain stem auditory evoked potentials but chronic treatment delays the large negative wave at 17 ms (N17) of the middle latency auditory evoked potentials. This change can be enhanced by 5-hydroxytryptophan which by itself causes an increased latency of N17 and also delays the later waves of the brain stem auditory evoked potentials in the rat (Rowen, O'Connor and Anwyl, 1988).

More centrally, carbamazepine appears to dampen cortical responses to sound with an increased latency of N1 on cortical auditory evoked potential testing in healthy adults (Rockstroh *et al.*, 1988). This effect may relate to the altered hearing that is sometimes noted in patients taking this drug.

Despite these general reservations about using the label 'ototoxic' rather freely, it is clear that several classes of drugs do damage the inner ear. The effects can be seen either in the auditory or vestibular components or in both and can be transient or permanent, depending on the site of damage. The warning signs are tinnitus, hearing loss or dysequilibrium.

Tinnitus

This symptom often represents the initial manifestation of changes in the cochlea. The mechanism of the production of the tinnitus is unclear and probably differs among the various classes of ototoxic agents. With the salicylates and their derivatives it is possible that a direct neural element is involved. With the aminoglycosides changes in the outer hair cells, without cell death, may alter the cochlear micromechanics and induce the symptom. Alternatively, or additionally, the slight changes in hearing may alter central processing so that to 'hear' sound above the internal background noise of the cochlea which is not usually appreciated, the central 'gain' is increased to the extent that the background is now detected.

Whatever the mechanism, the tinnitus is frequently high frequency at onset, often continuous and usually of a relatively pure tone (at least with the aminoglycosides). Many patients with progressive damage notice a lowering of the pitch of the tinnitus presumably as the damaged area becomes more extensive within the cochlea. Some drugs can cause a crashing wide band noise and this is especially common when the loop diuretics are given by rapid intravenous bolus injection.

Hearing loss

The classic pattern of aminoglycoside damage is said to be an initial high frequency loss that subsequently extends to include the speech frequencies with severe effects on hearing. The initial losses may go relatively unnoticed by the patient and since there seems to be a progression of the loss, at least for a short while after treatment with the aminoglycosides, the onset of noticeable loss may not be detected by the prescribing doctor.

Following withdrawal of the aminoglycosides there may be long-term recovery of some auditory function. This is the exception rather than the rule and may be related to a general improvement in health rather than specific recovery in the cochlea. Nevertheless, there does seem to be a group where specific recovery occurs and whether this arises because of spontaneous recovery of partially damaged hair cells (much as occurs in noise-induced temporary threshold shift) or because of regeneration and replacement of terminally damaged hair cells, is a matter for speculation at present. Hair cell regeneration is discussed later in the chapter.

Compared to the aminoglycosides the loop diuretics can cause an immediate loss noticed by the patient and involving frequencies across the audiogram. Fortunately this nearly always recovers. Similarly, the rare cases of hearing loss associated with use of erythromycin (one of the macrolide antibiotics) also tends to be a 'flat' sensorineural loss that usually recovers.

Dysequilibrium

When vestibulotoxic drugs are given systemically, both ears are usually affected symmetrically. Therefore, vertigo (defined here as an illusion of movement) is particularly uncommon and nystagmus rare, unless some other unilateral or central event has occurred. The patients are unsteady with a global reduction in vestibular function and need to hold on to safe objects for stability. In profound losses they may not be able to move out of bed in the initial phases since the rapid labyrinthine responses to movement are missing and they have not yet adapted to using only vision and proprioception. Darkness or poor vision makes the symptoms worse and indeed the occasional patient is completely disabled. Caloric tests show a bilaterally diminished or absent response and rotating chair tests confirm this with no vestibular evoked ocular responses as opposed to optokinetic nystagmus which is intact.

An additional symptom has earned itself the intriguing name 'bobbing oscillopsia'. Here the fast labyrinthine responses to head movement are inadequate to correct eye position which, therefore, lags behind head movement so that the surroundings, in turn, appear to continue to move for a short while. This symptom, which is also particularly distressing, is noticed most when travelling on bumpy roads hence the name. It also occurs on turning the head when the surroundings appear to continue to rotate. By definition, this is vertigo and if the history of ototoxic drug administration is not available may cause some diagnostic confusion.

Clinical aspects of specific drugs

Many drugs are known to be toxic to the inner ear. The most significant compounds, both from the point of view of clinical incidence of ototoxicity, and also because of the extent to which they have been studied experimentally, are the aminoglycoside antibiotics, cisplatin, the salicylates, quinine, the loop diuretics, and erythromycin. Only these compounds will be discussed further. These drugs may cause damage to either the auditory and/or the vestibular system. However, as exemplified by the aminoglycosides, which will be discussed in detail, a predilection for either the cochlea or the vestibular organs is often characteristic of a particular drug. The UK Adverse Reaction Register data for drug-induced ototoxicity has been analysed over the period from 1964 to 1984 (Griffin, 1988). The most commonly reported drug-induced cochleotoxicity was found to be secondary to salicylates.

The aminoglycosides

Following a period of research directed towards obtaining antimicrobial agents from various soil microorganisms, Waksman and his associates in 1944 isolated streptomycin from *Actinomycoses griseus*, later termed *Streptomyces griseus* (Schatz, Bugie and Waksman, 1944). The antibiotic was found to have activity against *Mycobacterium tuberculosis* (Waksman, Bugie and Schatz, 1944) and so was soon evaluated for use in the treatment of clinical tuberculosis after it had been found to be effective in an animal model (Feldman and Hinshaw, 1944). The first report of its use in humans (Hinshaw and Feldman, 1945) mentioned the unexpected finding that of the 34 patients treated, one developed a transient deafness, and three had disturbances of balance. Although the authors tentatively ascribed the symptoms to a selective neurotoxic effect on the VIIIth cranial nerve, they could not exclude the possibility that the tuberculosis itself caused the symptoms.

Other reports of deafness in association with streptomycin treatment soon appeared in the literature (Brown and Hinshaw, 1946; Fowler and Seligman, 1947; Farrington *et al.*, 1947). An assessment of the case reports in these three papers alone casts considerable doubt on the idea that the symptoms of 'otic toxicity' – a term used by Fowler and Seligman – were caused by streptomycin *per se*.

Fowler and Seligman assessed 81 American servicemen directly, and included another group of about 80, members of which were referred to the authors if tinnitus or impaired hearing developed during long-term streptomycin treatment. Only one patient had severe hearing loss, documented by audiometry, that improved with time and was thought by the authors to be caused by streptomycin. However, the report of this case stated that the patient had similar symptoms some 9 years previously when he started antisyphilitic treatment, and that a fluctuating hearing loss had occurred in the intervening period. It would seem likely that the fluctuating hearing loss was secondary to late syphilis, as this is a well-recognized symptom of that disease.

This difficulty in assessing whether the prolonged use of streptomycin does in fact result in deafness in humans has been painstakingly reviewed by Walby and Kerr (1982). From 1945 to 1980, 55 publications were found that suggested streptomycin as a cause of deafness in 558 patients. After carefully pruning out the cases of deafness that were probably caused by other medical conditions, by other drug combinations, or that had been improperly assessed, only 271 cases remained. Of these, 24 had a deafness that caused a handicap. Seven of the 24 had coincidental renal disease, so the authors concluded that after 35 years' use only 17 patients could be identified who had developed 'a handicapping deafness with no obvious contributing factor other than streptomycin

sulphate', and thought that this was less than general opinion might have expected. A number of genuine cases must have been lost by the authors' rigorous selection criteria, but in spite of this there are surprisingly few unequivocal cases.

All the aminoglycosides consist of two or more amino-sugars joined in a glycosidic linkage to a hexose nucleus. This hexose nucleus (an aminocyclitol) is streptidine in streptomycin and dihydrostreptomycin, and 2 deoxy-streptamine in all the other aminoglycosides. The aminocyclitol is in a terminal position in the streptomycins while it is central in all the other aminoglycosides (Figures 20.1 and 20.2).

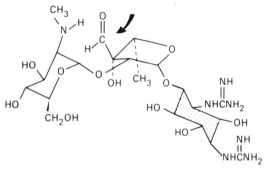

Figure 20.1 The structure of streptomycin. The shaded ring is the terminal aminocyclitol – streptidine. The heavy arrow indicates the site of reduction of the side chain -CHO to - CH_2OH during the formation of dihydrostreptomycin

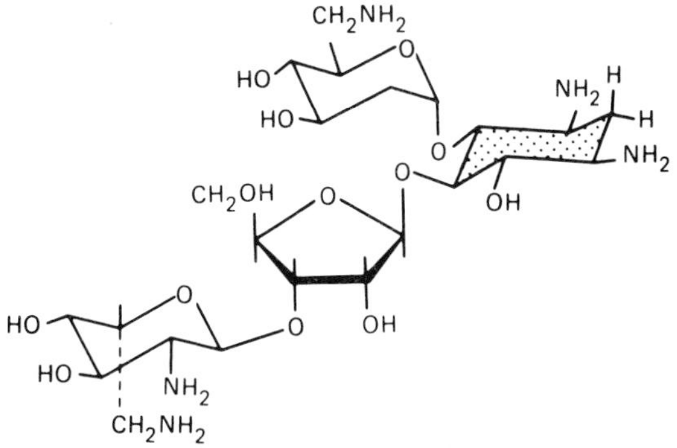

Figure 20.2 The structure of neomycin B. The shaded ring is the aminocyclitol 2,deoxy-streptamine, which is in a central position and this feature is typical of all the newer aminoglycosides. In the kanamycin group the four carbon ring next to the 2,deoxy-streptamine is absent and this structure is the core of all the newer aminoglycosides

The structure of kanamycin forms the basis of the deoxy-streptamine aminoglycosides currently in clinical use.

The gentamicins, the next group to be introduced clinically in the late 1960s, were unique in that they were the first aminoglycoside to be isolated from a source other than *Streptomyces*, in this case *Micro-*

monospora purpurea and *echinospora*, hence the difference in the spelling of the terminal micin (Weinstein *et al.*, 1963). The structure was similar to that of kanamycin except that the 6-position sugar was 3 methylamino, 3 deoxy, 4C methyl beta L-arabinose (garosamine) instead of 3 amino, 3 deoxy D-glucose (kanosamine). A whole family of different gentamicins exists, each with slight differences in the side groups attached to the sugar backbone, but the marketed product contains a mixture of gentamicin C1, C1a, and C2.

Tobramycin, the next major successful aminoglycoside, was one of several components of a complex of aminoglycosides, termed nebramycin, produced by *Streptomyces tenebranus* (Higgins and Kastners, 1967). It differs from kanamycin A in only two ways; by having an amino group at the 2′ position, and by not having a hydroxyl at the 3′ position, thereby making it much more resistant to bacterial degradation (Nagabushan, Miller and Weinstein, 1982).

A second family of aminoglycosides, the sisomicins, were isolated from *Micromonospora* again by Weinstein and co-workers in 1970. Sisomicin has a spectrum of activity similar to that of gentamicin, but is more potent. Sisomicin differs from gentamicin C1a by having one less proton at C′4 and therefore a C′4–C′5 double bond, and by having the epimer of -CHNH$_2$ at C′5.

As knowledge of the structural activity relationships increased, semisynthetic aminoglycosides were developed in a rational attempt to overcome the problems of bacterial resistance. Amikacin was the first successful derivative of kanamycin described by Kawaguchi *et al.* in 1972. This has a 4 amino, 2 hydroxy butyl chain attached to the N1 position of the 2 deoxy-streptamine moiety of kanamycin, and proved to be active against most of the kanamycin resistant organisms.

Subsequently the 1-N ethyl derivative of sisomicin (netilmicin) was produced and found to have, as predicted, a broader spectrum of antibiotic activity, by being resistant to a number of the bacterial enzymes that inactivated the parent sisomicin (Wright, 1976).

Continued clinical and commercial pressure to produce broad-spectrum antibiotics especially active against the Gram-negative organisms, and resistant to inactivation by bacterial enzymes has resulted in the production of large numbers of new aminoglycosides, some of which will surely enter the clinical field.

With neomycin, the oto- and nephrotoxic potential was realized early on in its use so that the drug was generally restricted to topical and oral administration. There are reports of parenteral administration that occurred accidentally (Lowry, May and Pastore, 1973), or when other aminoglycosides were not available (Lindsay, Proctor and Work, 1960) and which resulted in symptomatic deafness. One case, unsupported by audiometry, is reported in each of these papers. Both patients died, one in renal failure, the other from bacterial endocarditis. Leach (1962) had audiometry available and detected two low and two high frequency hearing losses in four seriously ill patients undergoing neomycin therapy. There was a latency of onset and a slow progression of the hearing loss in his cases.

The topical application of neomycin in burns and wound irrigation brought forth reports of associated deafness (Sugarbaker, Sabath and Morgan, 1974; Little and Lynn, 1975; Masur, Whelton and Whelton, 1976; Bamford and Jones, 1978). These papers each reported a small number of patients, all of whom were either in severe renal failure, or had other biochemical abnormalities. The anuric patients became profoundly deaf, while Bamford and Jones' six children developed a progressive deafness that in five cases did not develop until some months after cessation of treatment. In two of the five the deafness did not start until 16 and 26 months after, and this extremely long delay must cast some doubt on their inclusion.

Neomycin, which was not considered to be absorbed by the gut, was administered orally to patients with cirrhosis in the hope of sterilizing the bowel to prevent or ameliorate hepatic coma or pre-coma. Last and Sherlock (1960) reported one of their 27 patients, thus treated, who developed a high frequency, sensorineural hearing loss following two episodes of hepatic pre-coma and who had neomycin detectable in the blood. The belief that neomycin could be absorbed through the gut wall in the seriously ill was confirmed by Berk and Chalmers (1970) and Ward and Routhwaite (1978) who made similar reports of deafness following oral administration.

The lack of pretreatment audiometry in these patients is not really surprising as most were seriously ill or too young to be tested. The rigorous audiometric studies carried out during trials with streptomycin and dihydrostreptomycin, when patients with pulmonary tuberculosis were fit enough to be tested, were unfortunately only performed infrequently with the newer aminoglycosides, thereby invalidating much of the data on hearing loss because of the lack of knowledge of the pretreatment hearing level. This is especially important because of the level of hearing loss in the general population. The early reports of the Medical Research Council's study (Browning and Davis, 1983) on the characterization of the hearing of the adult British population suggested that 9% of those in the age band 31 to 50 years have a mean sensorineural loss greater than 25 dB in their poorer hearing ear (averaged at 0.5, 1, 2 and 4 kHz). This figure rises to 23% for the age band 51 to 70 years. Although this level of hearing loss is slightly higher than that found in the earlier studies of Hinchcliffe (1959) and Ward *et al.* (1977) the scope and organization of the Medical Research Council survey makes these results the most reliable to date. However, large studies without baseline audiometry continued to be published as newer aminoglycosides became available.

With kanamycin, for example, Finegold (1966) found that 17 of his 106 parenterally treated patients had a 'hearing loss'. Thirteen had a high frequency audiometric change without any subjective loss, and four had a low frequency, 'conversation' loss. It is not clear whether pretreatment audiometry was performed. Kreis (1966) reviewing 22 European papers dealing with 1121 kanamycin-treated patients, found a wide range in the incidence of audiometric hearing loss (0 to 82%) and a wide range in the frequencies affected. Again it is not clear whether pretreatment audiometry was performed.

With tobramycin, Neu and Bendush (1976) reviewed 3506 patients whose charts had been made available to the parent drug company. They distinguished quite clearly between a symptomatic hearing loss and an audiometric loss. An audiometric loss had to be greater than 15 dB to be included. They were able to assess a group of 23 patients with adequate audiometry, who complained of hearing loss following treatment. Four had this confirmed by their audiometric findings. Three of the four had a preceding high frequency loss at 6 and 12 kHz, that increased during and persisted after cessation of treatment. These three were aged 52, 60 and 70 years. The fourth was 22 years old, had received concomitant gentamicin, and had a 'slight' low frequency loss after treatment which resolved spontaneously. A separate group of 99 patients with good pre- and post-treatment audiometry could also be assessed. None of these complained of any hearing loss and 49 had no audiometric change. Of the rest 17 had audiometric losses, 24 had gains and 9 had both losses and gains at various frequencies.

With gentamicin, an early report from Meyers (1972) on patients with renal failure who had been treated with this drug, described how one out of 40 developed a documented flat hearing loss (45 dB at 250 and 500 Hz, 35 dB at 1 kHz, 30 dB at 2 and 4 kHz, 35 dB at 8 kHz) in one ear associated with severe vestibular failure. This single case had also received high doses of bumetanide. A low frequency loss was also detected by Smith *et al.* (1977), who classified toxicity by a fall in the hearing level of greater than 10 dB at any frequency and found two patients with a mean loss of 20 dB at 250 Hz and 22.5 dB at 500 Hz, out of 30 who had had serial audiograms. Cox (1976), however, found no losses occurring when gentamicin was given for urinary tract infections in 29 patients who also had serial audiometry. This same negative finding occurred in healthy volunteers given 80 mg of intravenous gentamicin and then tested audiometrically at one hour, one week and one month (Dobbs and Mawer, 1976). Tjernstrom *et al.* (1973) found that vestibular function was more likely to become abnormal following gentamicin if there was a preceding hearing loss, but failed to find any cases where the hearing had deteriorated in their group of 45 patients.

With the newer antibiotics more extensive prospective trials have been undertaken. Amikacin is well documented and it appears that although most of the losses were asymptomatic in the 4 and 8 kHz region, there were four patients who developed low or middle frequency losses. Previous aminoglycoside therapy or an abnormal audiogram prior to treatment were particularly potent factors in the genesis of hearing loss.

There are fewer prospective trials of the most recently introduced aminoglycosides – sisomicin and netilmicin. Feld *et al.* (1977) found a high frequency loss in five out of 41 patients treated with sisomicin. Two of the five had abnormal renal function, but no mention is made as to whether the hearing was normal before treatment.

The recent experience with netilmicin has shown lesser degrees of cochlear toxicity. Vesterhauge *et al.* (1980) carefully evaluated 30 patients and found no change in their pure tone or speech audiometry following treatment. They also noticed that 12 out of 30 had moderate symmetrical losses, usually in the high frequencies, prior to therapy. Tjernstrom (1980) in another prospective evaluation published similar findings. Eighteen of his 74 patients had abnormal hearing prior to treatment and there were no changes following treatment that could be ascribed to netilmicin.

However carefully all these prospective trials have been performed, they all suffer from the major criticism of being uncontrolled. Only one group comments on this failing:

> 'owing to our favourable experience of controlling infection with gentamicin, it was not justified to run a control group of similar patients from whom gentamicin had been withheld.' (Winkel *et al.*, 1978).

An important and well planned study of this problem has been performed by Davey *et al.* (1983). This group first assessed the validity of using portable audiometers on the ward, rather than in quiet surroundings, in a group of 24 healthy volunteers with no history of ear disease. They concluded 'that the low frequency thresholds obtained in the ward should not be compared with those recorded in an anechoic chamber and that changes in threshold of < 20 dB should not be regarded as significant when measured in a ward'. Subsequently 35 patients who were being treated with gentamicin were tested on the ward during treatment and at follow up at least 3 months later. This group was compared with a control group of 27 patients who had major surgery, infections treated with beta-lactam antibiotics or were receiving cytotoxics, and who were tested on admission to hospital, during treatment and again at long-term follow up. In a comparison of the controls on admission, and the gentamicin treated patients at follow up, members of both groups had hearing losses at 4, 6 and 8 kHz, but there was no significant difference in the numbers in each group. More interestingly, there were fluctuations in the hearing of the control patients while they were in hospital and were unwell, and two of the controls had a sustained hearing loss at 3 months. Because of the marked fluctuations in the hearing of the control group only sustained changes were described in the treatment group. An improvement in hearing was found in four gentamicin-treated patients coincidental with recovery from infection, while a sustained unilateral loss, accompanying clinical deterioration, occurred in two. One of these two died 2 weeks after the cessation of gentamicin and the other had undergone anaesthesia and major surgery.

The authors suggested that, had the control group received aminoglycosides, the hearing losses would probably have been labelled as having been caused by the drug, and wondered how, in patients, aminoglycoside hearing loss could ever be distinguished from other causes.

Basis of aminoglycoside ototoxicity

Aminoglycosides are positively charged molecules which would not normally be expected to cross the cell membrane. Their toxic side effects are also quite specific. Besides the inner ear, only the kidney and neural tissue are affected if the drug crosses the blood–brain barrier. In the inner ear itself it is the sensory cells, which are vulnerable. Any hypothesis which attempts to explain the ototoxic nature of these drugs must take these factors into account.

Although as pointed out above, there is variation between aminoglycosides in their reputed primary site of action and in their ototoxic potency, there is a general pattern to the effects produced (Lindeman, 1969; Hawkins and Johnsson, 1981; McDowell, 1982). Aminoglycosides cause loss of hair cells. In the cochlea, outer hair cells in the basal coil are preferentially affected. With increasing dosage or period of dosing, the damage spreads apically. This correlates with a loss of hearing sensitivity initially at high frequencies that may progress to involve successively lower frequencies. At any one location in the cochlea, damage spreads radially from the innermost to the outermost row of outer hair cells. Loss of outer hair cells is accompanied by expansion of adjacent supporting cells, which appear to remain undamaged by the drug and effect repair of the lesions (Forge, 1985) (Figure 20.3). Inner hair cells usually appear to survive until all the outer hair cells in their vicinity have been lost, although swelling of the afferent terminals beneath inner hair cells may occur as a quite early response and may be a reversible effect (Nicol *et al.*, 1992). In the vestibular system, hair cell loss is first apparent at the crest of the cristae and in the striolar region of the maculae and spreads outwards towards the peripheries with time. There is differential sensitivity between the different vestibular sensory regions, the crista showing proportionately greater hair cell loss than the utricular macula, and the utricular macula more than the saccular macula

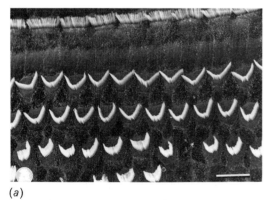
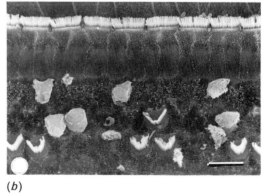

(a)   (b)

Figure 20.3 (*a*) Scanning electron micrograph of the apical surface of the normal organ of Corti. A single row of inner hair cells and three, or occasionally four, rows of outer hair cells are present. On inner hair cells, the stereocilia are organized in an almost straight line, whereas those on outer hair cells adopt a characteristic W-like configuration. The heads of pillar cells separate the row of inner hair cells from the outer hair cell rows, Deiters' cells intervene between outer hair cells, and Hensen's cells are present outside the outer hair cell. (*b*) Organ of Corti after gentamicin treatment. Outer hair cells are lost and undergoing degeneration; the first (innermost) row of hair cells is most affected but at this stage during the progress of aminoglycoside-induced damage, inner hair cells appear unaffected. The lost hair cells are replaced at the surface by expansion of adjacent supporting cells which produce characteristic scar patterns where they come together to occlude the lesion: Scale bar = 10 μm

(Lindeman, 1969). The regions where hair cell loss is first apparent in the vestibular epithelia are those where the type 1 hair cells predominate and these cells appear to be more sensitive than the type 2 cells. It is to be noted that the more sensitive sensory cell in the vestibular system, the type 1 cell, has an exclusively afferent innervation, whereas the cochlear hair cell which also has an exclusively afferent innervation, the inner hair cell, appears relatively resistant to aminoglycoside ototoxicity.

Studies of the pharmacokinetics of aminoglycosides have shown that the drugs enter perilymph relatively slowly. The peak concentration in perilymph is achieved at approximately 4 h after a single injection, but is always an order of magnitude lower than the peak concentration in serum (Tran Ba Huy *et al.*, 1981; Harpur and Gonda, 1982). The drug may persist in perilymph for some time, the half-life being approximately 15 h (Tran Ba Huy *et al.*, 1981; Harpur and Gonda, 1982). There is no correlation, however, between the levels different aminoglycosides reach in perilymph and their varying ototoxic potencies. Thus, so-called 'accumulation' in perilymph has been discounted as a factor involved in the specific ototoxic effects (Henley and Schacht, 1988). Entry of aminoglycoside to endolymph is very slow and it may persist there for some days (Tran Ba Huy, Bernard and Schacht, 1986). It has been suggested that this could be a factor in determining the delayed onset of toxic responses. This would imply that the action of the drug is dependent upon it reaching the apical surface of the hair cells, but this has not been demonstrated conclusively.

From early morphological studies of aminoglycoside ototoxicity it was concluded that one of the initial effects of the drug is to cause fusion of stereocilia (Wersall, 1981). Consequently, it was suggested that following entry of the drug into endolymph, stereocilia may be a primary site of drug action, the cationic aminoglycoside disrupting the negatively-charged cell coat over the stereociliary surface, enabling the membranes of adjacent stereocilia to come closely together so leading to their fusion. More recently, a loss of the stereociliary glycocalyx of cochlear hair cells soon after systemic administration of aminoglycoside has been reported (de Groot and Veldman, 1988). However, this effect was similar on both outer and inner hair cells whereas it is outer hair cells that are preferentially lost from the organ of Corti following aminoglycoside treatment. Furthermore, during aminoglycoside-induced hair cell degeneration, extensive alterations to the cell body may precede obvious morphological effects at the apical surface (Harpur and Bridges, 1979; Forge, 1985).

Nevertheless, acute effects of aminoglycosides at the apical surface of hair cells have been demonstrated directly in the lateral line systems of fish and reptiles (which contain hair cells phylogenetically related to those in the mammalian inner ears) (Kroese

and van den Bercken, 1982), and *in vitro* in the saccular maculae of frogs (Kroese, Das and Hudspeth, 1989) and cultured explants of the mammalian organ of Corti (Kossl, Richardson and Russell, 1990). Here, two separate effects of the direct application of aminoglycosides have been identified: an increase in stereociliary stiffness which is dependent upon the presence of calcium and may involve some interaction at the membrane surface; and a blocking of the transduction channels (which may be located at the tips of the stereocilia (Hudspeth, 1989)) that is inhibited by calcium. However, both these effects are reversible, their occurrence does not coincide with any obvious hair cell degeneration, and they do not appear to affect one hair cell type preferentially. Hair cell degeneration in the cultured explants occurs at much higher concentrations of the drug (approximately 1 mM) (Richardson and Russell, 1991) than those at which reversible effects on the stereocilia occur (approximately 50 μM), and is preceded, rapidly following the application of the drug at this higher concentration, by the formation of large membranous blisters at the cell apex suggesting some effect on lipid metabolism. Thus, while aminoglycosides potentially may act at the stereocilia and/or transduction channels, it is thought that these actions are probably independent of those which produce hair cell degeneration.

The pharmacokinetic studies also indicated there may be a two-stage process in the progression to ototoxicity, the drug entering a compartment from which it is released only very slowly (Tran Ba Huy, Barnard and Schacht, 1986). Examination of the levels of binding of the drugs to inner ear tissues has suggested that there is no difference between aminoglycosides with differing cochleotoxic or vestibulotoxic potentials and the concentration of each in inner ear tissues (Dulon *et al.*, 1986). However, studies using antibodies to aminoglycosides that enable immunocytochemical localization of the drugs in inner ear tissues have shown that they are selectively taken up by hair cells, soon after systemic administration (Hiel *et al.*, 1992). Furthermore, basal coil hair cells take up more than do apical coil hair cells (Hayashida *et al.*, 1989). In addition, greater amounts are taken up into the hair cells of animals maintained in a normal animal unit than in those of animals maintained in a sound-attenuated environment suggesting hair cell activity may be involved in the uptake. This increased uptake also corresponds with increased hair cell loss. Thus, there appears to be a selective uptake of the drug but this does not account for differing potencies of different aminoglycosides nor alone can it account for the cell death. After administration of 'non-ototoxic' doses of aminoglycosides the drug can be found within hair cells, sequestered inside what appear to be lysosomes, and it may persist there for up to at least a year without causing any apparent functional impairment or obvious injury to the hair cells (Dulon *et al.*, 1993).

The most complete hypothesis to date to account for the ototoxicity of the aminoglycosides envisages a specific, irreversible interaction of the drug with a particular cell membrane phospholipid, phosphatidy-linositol 4'5' bisphosphate (PhIP$_2$) (summarized in Schacht, 1986). This phospholipid is a 'second messenger' molecule that activates a cascade of intracellular biochemical pathways that control various aspects of cellular physiology including intracellular calcium levels. Although it is present in the membranes of most cells, neural tissue, including the ear, and the kidney show a much more active metabolism of phosphoinositides than do other tissues such as the liver or lung, and it has been demonstrated *in vivo* that neomycin inhibits the turnover of phospho-inositides in both the kidney and the inner ear. From *in vitro* studies of lipid bilayers and monolayers it has also been shown that the interaction of the aminogly-cosides with PhIP$_2$ is qualitatively different from their interaction with other anionic phospholipids and that they bind irreversibly. In addition, the extent to which different aminoglycosides alter the surface pressure of monomolecular films of PhIP$_2$, a measure of how well each one binds, correlates with the 'intrinsic' ototoxicity of each as determined by the concentration of drug perfused into the perilymph that is necessary to depress the cochlear microphonic; e.g. neomycin has the greatest effect on surface pressure and is the most effective in suppressing the cochlear microphonic, while amikacin is less 'ototoxic' and causes much less disturbance of the phospholipid monolayer (Lodhi *et al.*, 1980).

It has also been suggested that PhIP$_2$ is involved in the active motile responses of outer hair cells and that it is the second messenger system through which the direct efferent nerve supply to the outer hair cells acts. There may therefore be a much higher level of PhIP$_2$ metabolism in outer than inner hair cells. This could account for differential susceptibilities, but there is no direct evidence for this. PhIP$_2$ thus seems a likely candidate as a specific binding site for aminoglycosides in the inner ear, but as it is located on the inner leaflet of the plasma membrane the drug has to cross the membrane to reach it. A three-stage process to describe the interaction of aminogly-cosides with the hair cell has therefore been proposed (Schacht, 1986):

1 There is an initial reversible binding of the drug, possibly to anionic phospholipids exposed at the extracellular surface of the membrane. Changes in the cochlear microphonic following perfusion of aminoglycoside can be inhibited if calcium is perfused simultaneously or shortly after drug perfusion.
2 An active, selective uptake into hair cells.
3 A specific, irreversible binding to PhIP$_2$ with different aminoglycosides binding to greater or lesser degrees. Once the drug is bound, those reactions

dependent upon phosphoinositide turnover would be inhibited. In addition, the interaction with membrane phospholipids may also affect membrane permeability, enabling the subsequent direct entry of the drug into the cell. Competitive binding between calcium and neomycin, energy dependent uptake and binding to PhIP$_2$ have all been demonstrated in isolated outer hair cells (Williams, Zenner and Schacht, 1987). They have also been demonstrated in the vestibular sensory epithelia *in vitro* (Williams, Smith and Schacht, 1987).

On the other hand, it has also been found that when isolated hair cells are incubated with gentamicin, cell viability is unimpaired (Dulon *et al.*, 1989). This might be due to relative inactivity of isolated hair cells maintained in a non-physiological environment limiting the extent of uptake or metabolism, since hair cells *in vitro* in organotypic culture which show significant membrane-associated activity (Forge and Richardson, 1993) do show an obvious ototoxic response (Richardson and Russell, 1991). It might also imply that additional, as yet unidentified factors, are involved. It has been reported recently that isolated hair cells can be killed with gentamicin that has been exposed to a drug-metabolizing extract from liver cells suggesting that a product of aminoglycoside metabolism rather than the drug itself might in fact be the active agent (Huang and Schacht, 1990), but it is generally considered that aminoglycosides are excreted from the body without being metabolized and the putative metabolite has not been identified.

In addition to their effects on the organ of Corti, the aminoglycoside antibiotics also affect the stria vascularis. Originally, it was reported (Hawkins, 1973) that atrophy of the stria occurred several weeks after a course of aminoglycoside administration and it was suggested that the primary action of these drugs was in fact upon the stria with effects in the organ of Corti and the loss of hair cells occurring subsequently. Although it is now generally accepted that the hair cells are a primary site of aminoglycoside action, there is evidence that the stria also is affected in the initial stages of the response of the cochlea to these drugs; immediately following the end of a course of aminoglycoside treatment alterations to the stria can be seen at the same time as the earliest effects in the organ of Corti are apparent (Forge and Fradis, 1985). However, as both the organ of Corti and stria show drug-induced abnormalities at these earliest stages, it is not possible to determine the relative chronology of these events, nor whether effects in the stria and the organ of Corti are related or occur independently. The lateral wall of the cochlea has been shown to contain a high level of PhIP$_2$, higher in fact than that of the organ of Corti (Schacht, 1986), and thus, it is possible that the stria may be directly susceptible to the drugs if, as discussed above, this phospholipid serves as the target for aminoglycoside action. However, there is no direct evidence for an interaction between aminoglycosides and strial tissues.

Following the end of aminoglycoside treatment, over the period during which loss of outer hair cells from the organ of Corti progresses, the stria becomes thinner. This decrease in thickness is due to an atrophy almost exclusively of marginal cells (Forge, Wright and Davies, 1987). Some cells are lost by a process which shows morphological attributes of apoptosis, a process of controlled cell death, but the majority of marginal cells remain but with much reduced volume. Such alteration might be expected to affect the endocochlear potential and the ionic profile of endolymph, but the endocochlear potential at least is reported to be maintained at close to normal levels after the end of aminoglycoside treatment (Komune and Snow, 1982). Thus, the functional consequences of the affects of aminoglycoside ototoxicity on the stria are not clear. Obviously, the reorganization in the organ of Corti resulting from the loss of hair cells and their replacement by supporting cells that occurs following aminoglycoside treatment will have profound effects on cochlear physiology. This might be expected to influence the activity of the stria, but as yet there is no indication of whether and how there might be an interrelationship between effects in the stria and in the organ of Corti.

Nevertheless, it seems reasonable to suppose that the full expression of the ototoxic response to aminoglycoside involves effects not only on the organ of Corti but also in the stria vascularis.

Cisplatin

Cisplatin, a divalent platinum compound has been in clinical use as a chemotherapeutic agent since the late 1970s. It has been found to be effective in the treatment of cancer of the bladder, testes, ovaries, cervix, breast, prostate and some head and neck malignancies. Its antineoplastic action is thought to be mediated through its irreversible binding to DNA and inducing frameshift and base substitution mutations (Eastman, 1986).

Clinical manifestation of cisplatin ototoxicity is less pronounced than that of aminoglycoside ototoxicity, presumably because in the former case the drug administration is in single dose and the interval between administration of the drug is longer. Tinnitus is one of the earlier clinical features of cisplatin ototoxicity and it may be transient or permanent (Hayes, Cvitkovic and Golbey, 1977). The incidence of cisplatin-induced hearing loss ranges from 11% to 91% (Helson, Okonkwo and Anton, 1978; Peytral *et al.*, 1981). It is difficult to compare accurately the various clinical studies, as the number of patients in each study and the dose regimen differs significantly. With the high-dose regimen the hearing loss may be bilateral and permanent (Waters, Ahmad and Katsarkas, 1991). Cisplatin appears to be predominantly cochleotoxic, but there are a few reports confirming cisplatin-induced vestibulotoxicity (Schaefer, Wright and Post, 1981; Black, Myers and Schramm, 1982). Various chemoprotective agents, known as 'rescue' or blocking agents are currently being evaluated for their potential role in reducing or preventing the unwanted adverse systemic toxicity without altering the antitumour activity of cisplatin. These agents include acetazolamide, sulphur nucleophiles, free oxygen radical scavengers and phosphonic acid antibiotics. These compounds in the main reduce the nephrotoxicity and to a lesser extent the ototoxic effects (Litterst, 1981; Federspil, Tiesler and Schnatzle, 1983; Ozols, Deisroth and Jaradpour, 1983). A cisplatin analogue, known as carboplatin (*cis*-diammine-1, 1 cyclobutanedicarboxylate-platinum II) has been recently introduced as an equally effective chemotherapeutic agent. Morphological and physiological studies have shown carboplatin to be less ototoxic than its mother compound cisplatin (Schweitzer, Rarey and Dolan, 1986).

Basis of cisplatin ototoxicity

Cisplatin (*cis*-platinum; *cis*-dichlorodiammine platinum II or *cis*-DDP), like the aminoglycosides, is a highly charged molecule. It, too, is nephrotoxic as well as ototoxic. It induces a progressive loss of hair cells, the extent of which correlates with the dose of drug administered (Hoeve *et al.*, 1988). This occurs following repeated injections of relatively low drug doses (1 mg/kg daily) administered by intramuscular, intraperitoneal or subcutaneous routes, and after a single intravenous high dose (approximately 10–12.5 mg/kg) (Laurell and Engstrom, 1989a; Laurell and Bagger–Sjoback, 1991a, b). The pattern of hair cell damage in the cochlea also resembles that of the aminoglycosides, with outer hair cells in the basal turn preferentially affected.

As yet, however, there is no consistent idea of the basis of cisplatin's ototoxicity. It has been reported (McAlpine and Johnstone, 1990) that a rapid deterioration in the auditory nerve response threshold is produced when cisplatin is present in the scala media at concentrations of approximately 5 μM, but no effect is apparent with perilymphatic perfusion at drug concentrations of less than 3 mM. This suggests that one possible site of the drug action is at the apical end of the hair cells, and from other characteristics of the response to a single systemic administration it has been concluded that the drug blocks transduction channels. However, as with similar experiments with aminoglycosides, it is difficult from these results to explain differential effects on inner and outer hair cells. Nor is it known whether, and how, they might be related to hair cell degeneration. In recent studies (Saito, Moataz and Dulon, 1991), incubation of isolated hair cells with concentrations of cisplatin as high as 1 mM for up to 6 hours did not impair cell viability.

Cisplatin also causes a decline in the endocochlear potential indicating an action in the stria (Komune, Asakuma and Snow, 1981). It has been reported to cause strial atrophy but the effects appear to vary depending upon the dose of drug administered (Laurell and Engstrom, 1989b). Following a single intravenous high dose (10–12.5 mg/kg) the endocochlear potential begins to decline within 1 day and becomes permanently lost in parallel with the loss of hair cells that also ensues. However, with lower doses of the drug given repeatedly (e.g. daily injections of approximately 2 mg/kg for 10–14 days) by subcutaneous or intramuscular routes, although hair cell loss occurs, the endocochlear potential does not show any immediate alteration. Ultimately, strial atrophy develops several days or weeks after the end of the chronic treatment. The target for the drug action in the stria is unknown, but the differing responses to the different dosing regimens suggests that effects in the stria and in the organ of Corti are independent of each other and that the stria may be less susceptible to damage from cisplatin than are the outer hair cells.

Thus, at present neither the site of drug action nor the mechanisms that cause cell death are known. It seems likely that the mechanisms of cisplatin mediated ototoxicity are dependent upon actions at different sites. It is of interest to note, however, that there is some evidence that in the kidney, a cisplatin metabolite has been proposed as an active agent producing toxicity in renal tubule cells (Dedon and Borch, 1987).

Salicylates

Salicylate ototoxicity was first reported in 1877 by Muller. The effects that were described were due to high doses, but subsequently ototoxicity has been reported from even therapeutic doses of salicylates (Schwabach, 1884; Kapur, 1965; Jarvis, 1966).

Generally, the ototoxic effects of salicylates are thought to be reversible; however, some cases of permanent damage have been described (Kapur, 1965; Jarvis, 1966). The main ototoxic effects secondary to salicylates are hearing loss and tinnitus but vestibular effects, though rare, have been described (Bernstein and Weiss, 1967).

Salicylate-induced hearing loss is usually mild to moderate and symmetrical provided there is no pre-existing hearing loss. The hearing loss may be variable but 'flat' loss is commoner (McCabe and Dey, 1965; Myers and Bernstein, 1965; Bernstein and Weiss, 1967; Jardini, Findlay and Burgi, 1978) and recovery is usually seen 24 to 72 hours post-treatment. Some studies (Myers and Bernstein, 1965; Bernstein and Weiss, 1967) have shown that consumption of 6–8 g of aspirin per day is necessary

before symptoms of hearing loss (20–40 dB) and tinnitus are encountered. An interesting study by Day, Graham and Bieri (1989) revealed that in subjects in whom 1.95–5.85 g of aspirin/day was administered, hearing loss at 1 and 2 kHz increased approximately linearly with serum salicylate levels of 5–40 mg/dl. Other authors (Myers and Bernstein, 1965; Bernstein and Weiss, 1967) have also reported a high correlation between hearing loss and serum salicylate concentration provided the serum level was less than 40 mg/dl. The above studies did not suggest a minimum serum salicylate concentration required to detect a threshold shift. In addition to changes in hearing sensitivity, it has also been suggested that aspirin causes a decrease in temporal integration (McCabe and Dey, 1965), poorer temporal resolution (McFadden, Plattsmier and Pasanen, 1984) and impaired frequency selectivity (Bonding, 1979).

Salicylate-induced tinnitus has been characterized as tonal and high frequency, i.e. 7–9 kHz (McCabe and Dey, 1965). The onset of tinnitus is usually considered as the initial sign of salicylate ototoxicity. An interesting study conducted by Mongan, Kelly and Nies (1973) looked at the relationship between tinnitus and serum salicylate levels. They reported that the minimum salicylate serum level of 19.6 mg/dl was required for tinnitus to develop. In their study all patients with normal hearing developed tinnitus whereas only one-third of the patients with pre-existing hearing loss developed salicylate-induced tinnitus. In contrast to the above study, Day, Graham and Bieri (1989) found that tinnitus was present at serum salicylate concentration as low as 5 mg/dl.

Basis of salicylate ototoxicity

Early experimental studies indicated that one action of salicylates was upon the cochlear blood supply. Constriction of the vessels in the spiral ligament, stria vascularis and the vessels lying beneath the basilar membrane was observed after systemic administration (Hawkins, 1976). This may occur as a consequence of the effects of salicylate upon prostaglandin synthesis. It has, therefore been argued that the acute suppression of the compound action potential, also reported to occur after salicylate treatment, may be related to a salicylate-induced ischaemia. This could affect the inner hair cells which are highly sensitive to anoxia and thereby affect the compound action potential. An interference with the blood supply might also be expected to affect the stria leading to a diminution of the endocochlear potential; this declines rapidly during anoxia, but does not appear to be affected by salicylates. Effects on the vasculature should not be discounted, and may be a confounding factor (Didier, Miller and Nuttall, 1993), but there is compelling evidence that salicylates act directly upon the outer hair cells. Indeed, the studies from which this conclusion derives provide an excellent illustration of how the different techniques for examination of the cochlea can be used to delineate the site of drug action.

Salicylates are known to enter perilymph rapidly after administration. Potentially, therefore they might act on the bodies of inner or outer hair cells, the synapses, or the nerves, all of which are directly exposed to perilymph, but histological examination of the cochlea after systemic drug treatment has shown abnormalities to occur specifically in outer hair cells (Douek, Dodson and Bannister, 1983). In addition, otoacoustic emissions, which derive from the active responses of outer hair cells, are reversibly suppressed in humans after aspirin ingestion (Long, Tubis and Jones, 1986; Martin *et al.*, 1988), and acoustic distortion products have been shown to be depressed in experimental studies in animals (Stypulkowski, 1990). The cochlear microphonic is also affected although it has been variously reported to be depressed (Puel, Bobbin and Fallon, 1990) or to rise (Stypulkowski, 1990). Furthermore, following systemic administration (Stypulkowski, 1990) and with perilymphatic perfusion (Puel *et al.*, 1989; Puel, Bobbin and Fallon, 1990) the compound action potential responses to low intensity stimulation are suppressed but those to high intensity signals are unaffected. This, too, suggests an effect on the outer hair cell as the compound action potential response to signals of low intensity is thought to be elicited after amplification of the signal reaching the inner hair cells through the active processes associated with the outer hair cell (Kim, 1986). It has also been demonstrated *in vitro* that the fast motile responses of isolated outer hair cells that are normally elicited by electrical stimulation are reversibly inhibited by salicylate (Shehata, Brownell and Dieler, 1991).

This last observation suggests that *in vitro*, at least, salicylates affect the outer hair cells directly. This is probably also the case *in vivo*. As noted above, endocochlear potential is not affected after systemic administration (Stypulkowski, 1990) nor with perilymphatic perfusion (Puel, Bobbin and Fallon, 1990) of salicylate indicating that the observed depression of outer hair cell function is not an indirect effect of a reduction in the driving current to the hair cells. Furthermore, although it is well known that salicylates inhibit prostaglandin synthesis, the perilymphatic perfusion of agents which are more potent than salicylates in this regard do not affect cochlear function (Puel, Bobbin and Fallon, 1990).

It is therefore considered that salicylates may interact directly at the basolateral membrane of the outer hair cell leading to inhibition of the active mechanical response. Salicylates are known to affect membrane permeability, in particular causing an increase in K^+ and decrease in Cl^- conductance and it has been argued (Stypulkowski, 1990) that this occurs in the cochlea. Numerous K^+-channels have been localized to the basolateral membrane of the outer hair cell

(Ashmore and Meech, 1986). There is, however, no direct evidence that salicylates have any action upon these.

While an action of salicylates on the active processes of the outer hair cells would produce the observed loss in hearing sensitivity, it is not clear whether the tinnitus that also occurs is a separate or related phenomenon. Some clinical evidence suggests that tinnitus is the more prevalent effect and does not always coincide with hearing loss. It has been shown that following systemic salicylate administration there is an increase in the spontaneous firing rate of auditory neurons (Evans and Borerwe, 1982), i.e neural stimulation in the absence of an acoustic signal. As salicylate enters perilymph it has access to and could act directly upon the afferent nerve synapses, but in other systems salicylates usually decrease and eventually block neural excitation (Neto, 1980). Furthermore, it is neurons which respond normally to high frequencies that are affected whereas low frequency fibres do not show an increased spontaneous firing rate, and the perceived tinnitus in humans is reported to be of high frequency; it is difficult to see why only high frequency fibres should be affected by perilymphatic salicylate acting upon synapses. As an alternative there have been suggestions that the effects of salicylate upon the active processes of the hair cells are directly related to the production of tinnitus, or may affect the mechanical relationship of the outer and inner hair cells in such a manner so as to stimulate activity in the inner hair cells at the basal end of the cochlea (Stypulkowski, 1990). However, at present such explanations are entirely speculative and the mechanisms underlying the development of tinnitus after salicylate administration are still not understood.

Quinine

The quinine derivatives have long been used as antiprotozoal agents in the treatment of malaria and for other diseases such as rheumatoid arthritis. The toxicity is similar to that produced by salicylates, reversible tinnitus and sensorineural hearing loss being the principal symptoms. Some patients may also experience vertigo and permanent deafness if larger doses are administered (Toone, Hayden and Ellman, 1965).

Basis of quinine ototoxicity

The effects of quinine resemble those of salicylate. It produces a reversible hearing loss and tinnitus that disappears upon withdrawal of the drug, and the degree of threshold shift correlates closely with, and can be used as a predictor of, the concentration of the drug in blood plasma (Alvan *et al.*, 1991). It has been reported that quinine also causes constriction of cochlear capillaries (Hawkins, 1976) which was thought to be the basis of its ototoxicity and to indicate a similar mechanism of action to salicylate. More recently, it has been considered that quinine may act directly upon outer hair cells to affect cochlear mechanics, but its mechanism of action may be different from that of salicylate.

Electron microscopy of thin sections of the organ of Corti fixed at the time of maximal effect following systemic application of the drug has shown swelling of the lateral cisternae (Karlsson, Flock and Flock, 1991), an organized endoplasmic reticulum immediately inside the lateral plasma membrane, in the outer hair cells. Perilymphatic perfusion of quinine (Puel, Bobbin and Fallon, 1990) has been shown to produce a depression of the cochlear microphonic and of the compound action potential, but the effect is different from that of salicylate because quinine affects the compound action potential across all stimulus intensities as opposed to just the low intensity responses which salicylate suppresses. As the endocochlear potential is unaffected, these results indicate a direct effect on outer hair cells. Studies using isolated hair cells (Karlsson and Flock, 1990) have shown quinine to initiate slow changes in shape, (whereas salicylate inhibits fast motile responses) and direct examination of the organ of Corti in intact cochlea preparations has shown quinine to affect the micromechanics of the organ of Corti (Karlsson *et al.*, 1991).

Thus, the hearing loss due to quinine may result from a direct effect on the outer hair cells affecting their slow contractile properties and thereby the vibrational characteristics of the basilar membrane. It is known that quinine induces and enhances muscular contraction by affecting the availability of intracellular calcium released from the sarcoplasmic reticulum and it has been argued that quinine may act similarly on outer hair cells affecting intracellular calcium levels, possibly mediated by some event at the lateral cisternae that follows an initial action of the drug at the lateral plasma membrane.

Loop diuretics

Members of this group of drugs include ethacrynic acid, frusemide (furosemide), bumetanide and piretanide. The ototoxic effects of deafness and sometimes vertigo are usually encountered when the drug is give intravenously. Maher and Schreiner (1965) were the first to report immediate and reversible sensorineural hearing loss and vertigo following administration of ethacrynic acid to patients with renal failure. Transient cochleotoxic effects, occasionally with vertigo, have been observed after rapid infusion of high doses of frusemide by Schwartz *et al.* (1970). Permanent hearing losses with this drug have also been reported by Lloyd–Mostyn and Lord (1971) and Quick and Hoppe (1975).

An important synergic interaction between the loop diuretics and the aminoglycoside antibiotics is discussed below.

Basis of loop diuretic ototoxicity

All the so-called 'loop' diuretics including ethacrynic acid, frusemide (furosemide), bumetanide and piretanide, whose primary diuretic action is in the ascending limb of the loop of Henle, cause temporary hearing loss and decline in the compound action potential through an action upon the stria vascularis that inhibits maintenance of the endocochlear potential. They also affect the vestibular system in a similar manner through effects on the active ion transport mechanisms in the vestibular dark cells.

The stria vascularis and the dark cell regions are ion-transporting epithelia involved in the local production of endolymph. Any agent which injures these tissues will affect the transduction process and reduce hair cell responsiveness to stimuli. The dark cell regions consist of a single layer of cells directly overlying connective tissue. Their basolateral surfaces form extensive infoldings that enclose numerous mitochondria and contain high levels of Na^+/K^+ ATP-ase (Spicer, Schulte and Adams, 1990). The general morphology of dark cells is consistent with cells engaged in active ion transport and they are presumed to be directly involved in the production and maintenance of vestibular endolymph.

The stria vascularis is formed of three cell types: marginal, intermediate and basal cell. In addition, and unusually for an epithelium, it also contains a complex network of intraepithelial capillaries. The *marginal cells* resemble the vestibular dark cells with extensively infolded basolateral membranes to which Na^+/K^+ ATP-ase (Kerr, Ross and Ernst, 1982; Schulte and Adams, 1989) and adenyl cyclase (Zajic, Anniko and Schacht, 1983) are localized. They are ultimately responsible for the maintenance of endolymph. The *intermediate cells* are enclosed entirely within the corpus of the stria, reaching neither the apical surface nor the basal limit of the tissue. The *basal cells* separate the stria from the underlying spiral ligament which is freely permeable to perilymph. Numerous gap-junctions, regions of direct cell-to-cell coupling, are present between adjacent basal cells, between basal cells and cells in the spiral ligament, and between basal cells and each of the other two strial cell types (Forge, 1984). This suggests an important role for basal cells in the formation of intercellular communication in the stria.

The potassium that is transported into the scala media to produce the endocochlear potential does not derive from the blood supply. Studies with radioactive tracers have shown that systemically applied radioactive potassium (^{36}K) enters perilymph quite rapidly but enters endolymph only later (Sterkers *et al.*, 1982). Furthermore, the use of artificial oxygen carriers that enable perfusion of the blood supply with solutions of controlled composition has shown that the endocochlear potential is maintained when potassium-free solutions are used to perfuse the cochlear vasculature, but the endocochlear potential falls rapidly when the perilymphatic space is perfused with potassium-free solutions (Marcus, Marcus and Thalmann, 1981). These results show that potassium is circulated locally from endolymph to perilymph and back via the stria.

The loop diuretics interfere with the ion transport processes involved in endolymph homeostasis (Bosher, 1980a). The effects occur very rapidly following systemic administration. With frusemide administered by intravascular injection, the endocochlear potential begins to decline within seconds and reaches a nadir after about 2–3 minutes (Pike and Bosher, 1980); with ethacrynic acid the effect is somewhat slower and when this agent is administered by intraperitoneal injection the maximum decline in the endocochlear potential may not occur until 15–30 minutes post-injection (Forge, 1981). The effects are almost entirely reversible, the endocochlear potential being almost fully recovered within 4–6 hours. The maximum reduction in endocochlear potential (which can fall to -40 mV) and the time required for its recovery are directly proportional to the dose of drug administered (Rybak, Whitworth and Scott, 1991). The decline in the endocochlear potential coincides with the development of an extensive oedema in the stria vascularis (Bosher, 1980b; Forge, 1981; Forge and Brown, 1982) that can cause the tissue to swell to almost twice its normal thickness. This, too is reversible, the stria regaining a normal morphology approximately in parallel with the recovery of the endocochlear potential (Bosher, 1980b; Pike and Bosher, 1980; Forge, 1981) (Figures 20.4 and 20.5).

The development of oedema indicates that diuretics interfere with the normal ion transport processes in the stria, and the rapid onset of their effects suggests they gain direct access to their site of action through entry from the strial vasculature. This mode of entry would give direct access to the basolateral membranes of the marginal cells. Alterations to marginal cells are among the earliest detectable responses observed in structural studies and it has been demonstrated that loop diuretics inhibit Na/K ATPase and adenyl cyclase in the stria (Thalmann *et al.*, 1977); these enzymes are present predominantly in the basolateral membranes of the marginal cells. Consequently at one time it was considered that the ototoxic effect of the diuretics was due to a direct effect of the drug at the marginal cell basolateral membrane affecting active potassium influx into the scala media. However, diuretic-induced inhibition of the endocochlear potential follows a faster time course than that of the reduction of endolymphatic potassium that also occurs indicating that the generation of the potential is separate from the processes that maintain the ionic profile within the scala media (Bosher, 1980a; Pike and Bosher, 1980). Furthermore, it has also been shown that the concentration of diuretic that will completely abolish the positive component of the endocochlear potential is one to two orders of magnitude lower than that required for the inhibition of strial Na^+/K^+ ATP-ase or adenyl cyclase (Kusakari *et al.*, 1978). Thus, in the cochlea the primary action of the diuretics is not upon these enzymes.

In the kidney, a $Na^+/K^+/Cl$ co-transporter has been characterized as a site of diuretic action (Wangemann and Greger, 1990). A similar co-transporter is present in vestibular dark cells and the stria vascularis (Marcus, Marcus and Greger, 1987). It is thought

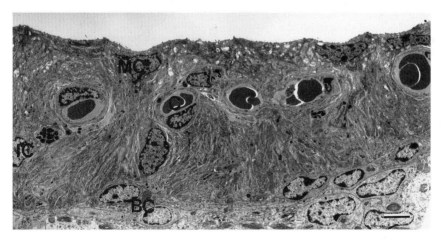

Figure 20.4 Normal stria vascularis. The stria vascularis consists of three cell types: the marginal cells (MC), intermediate cells (IC), and basal cells (BC), together with intraepithelial capillaries (C). The marginal cells line the endolymphatic space and the cell base is extensively infolded. Numerous large mitochondria are present within the infoldings. The intermediate cells reach neither the apical nor the normal basal aspect of the tissue. These cells possess melanin pigment granules. The basal cells are flattened and in one to three layers. They separate the stria from the underlying spiral ligament (the extracellular spaces of which contain perilymph). Scale bar $= 5 \mu m$

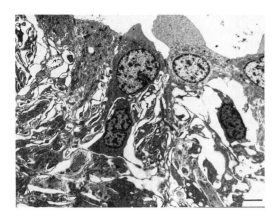

Figure 20.5 Human stria vascularis after diuretic administration (frusemide). An extensive oedema develops to create large extracellular spaces within the corpus of the tissue, and the marginal cells balloon outwards into the endolymphatic space. These responses indicate an effect of the diuretic on ion transport within the stria, but the effects are rapidly reversible. Scale bar = 2.5 μm

to play a crucial role in the homeostasis of endolymph. *In vitro* studies of isolated strips of dark cell epithelium and of the stria have also shown that diuretic acting from the serosal side inhibits its activity reversibly (Marcus, Marcus and Greger, 1987; Wangemann, Liu and Marcus, 1995). At present it seems reasonable to conclude that the ototoxic side effects of diuretics are due to interaction with this $Na^+/K^+/Cl^-$ co-transporter.

Erythromycin

Erythromycin, a macrolide antibiotic, has been in clinical use since the 1950s. Its ototoxic side effects were first reported by Mintz *et al.* in 1973. Ototoxic effects of erythromycin are rare and most reports state the adverse effects to be that of tinnitus and sensorineural hearing loss. Deafness in most cases is reversible, however, permanent deafness has been reported (Dylewski, 1988). Patients with poor renal and hepatic function are at increased risk as the drug elimination from the body in these patients is impaired. There is no experimental work to account for this transient loss.

Ototoxic synergism

Drugs

If several ototoxic drugs are administered concurrently, potentiation of the ototoxicity is likely to occur, even when the dose of either drug is within the recommended limits (Johnson and Hamilton,

1970). A classical example is that of aminoglycoside-loop diuretic interaction. The damage observed in the organ of Corti when an aminoglycoside is given followed by a loop diuretic is essentially the same as that produced when the aminoglycoside is used alone, but occurs at a lower overall dosage and usually much more rapidly (Nakai, 1977; Russell, Fox and Brummett, 1979). Brummett *et al.* (1974) demonstrated that the interaction did not occur with the non-loop-inhibiting diuretics and kanamycin. The ototoxic interaction appears to be specific to the loop-inhibiting diuretics but not specific to the aminoglycosides, since the interaction of ethacrynic acid with viomycin, capreomycin and polymixin B produces cochlear hair cell damage similar to that produced by aminoglycosides administered with ethacrynic acid (Davis *et al.*, 1982).

It has been shown that if the loop diuretic is given first and then an aminoglycoside, the cochleotoxic effect is no different to that caused by using either of the drugs alone. However, if the aminoglycoside is given first, followed by the loop diuretic then there is potentiation of cochleotoxicity (Brummett, 1980). This could be explained by the fact that aminoglycoside–inner ear cell membrane interaction increases cell membrane permeability thus facilitating a higher concentration of the loop diuretic to penetrate into the cells and resulting in more severe damage.

Noise exposure and ototoxicity

Noise exposure has been reported to increase susceptibilty to drug-induced cochleotoxicity (Darrouzet and De Lima Sobrinho, 1962; Hawkins, Marques and Clark, 1975), although Vernon and Brummett (1977) found no potentiation effect associated with exposure to environmental noise. The above studies looked at kanamycin and suggested that the effect of the noise and the drug were synergistic rather than additive.

Various studies have been conducted in order to study the combined effects of aspirin and noise but the results seem to be conflicting. McCabe and Dey (1965) and McFadden and Plattsmier (1983) have reported the combined effect of aspirin and noise as being additive when considering hearing loss. Carson *et al.* (1989) have also shown that combination of high dose aspirin and noise exposure will produce a potentiating effect in that there is a significantly greater hair cell loss in animals treated with both noise and aspirin than in those treated with noise or aspirin alone. In contrast, Woodford, Henderson and Hamernik (1978) found no significant difference in the hearing threshold in the combined noise and aspirin treated group. Some investigators (Durrant, 1978) have suggested that following noise-induced inner ear damage there is cochlear vasoconstriction, whereas others (Prazma *et al.*, 1987) have shown that there is a highly significant increase in blood flow after high intensity noise exposure. If the latter were true, then one might assume that the increase in cochlear blood flow would result in a larger amount of salicylate reaching the inner ear and thus causing a greater hearing loss.

Ototopical ototoxicity

There exists a great deal of concern among general practitioners about the potential ototoxicity of aminoglycoside antibiotic-containing ear drops. Bickerton, Roberts and Little (1988) found in their survey that 80% of the general practitioners were avoiding the use of antibiotic ear drops because of the potential damage the drops could cause to the inner ear. Solomons and Madden (1992) conducted a survey on the use of ear drops by consultant otolaryngologists in the UK. They reported that only 2% of the consultants did not use preparations containing antibiotics and only 2% had seen a patient who had developed sensorineural hearing loss following the use of antibiotic ear drops. In an American survey by Lundy and Graham (1992), 80% of the otolaryngologists believed that the risk of sensorineural hearing loss due to otitis media was greater than the risk of ototopical therapy, and less than 4% of the participants had claimed to have witnessed irreversible hearing loss secondary to the use of antibiotic ear drops. A study by Browning, Gatehouse and Calder (1988) on the medical management of active chronic otitis media found no evidence of ototoxic inner ear damage in patients using ear drops containing gentamicin over a 4–6 week period. In the British National Formulary, however, the Committee on Safety of Medicines has stated that there is an increased risk of drug-induced deafness secondary to antibiotic ear drops and that they should be used cautiously in patients with perforation of the tympanic membrane. Numerous animal studies have demonstrated inner ear damage following direct application of aminoglycoside to the middle ear cavity. Some animal studies have shown that alcohol-containing antiseptic solutions for cleaning the ear prior to surgery may cochleotoxic (Morizono and Sikora, 1981) as may chlorhexidine (Aursnes, 1981). The route of drug absorption is thought to be mainly through the round window membrane. In humans however, the round window membrane is much thicker (Wright and Meyerhoff, 1984) and is also partially protected by a bony niche, thus relatively reducing the amount of drug absorbed into the inner ear.

Management of ototoxicity

It is not always possible to monitor inner ear function in all patients receiving ototoxic drugs, as a large number of these patients are too unwell to cooperate with any form of audiovestibular investigations. Our aim, however, must be to prevent or diminish adverse effects secondary to ototoxic drugs. This can be achieved by avoiding or discontinuing the ototoxic drug if a satisfactory alternative is available. This may not always be possible as can be illustrated by the use of life-saving cisplatin therapy that may be offered in the treatment of certain malignant disorders. If possible, baseline audiometric and vestibular function tests should be performed. There is a group of high-risk patients that we must bear in mind. These include patients with impaired renal function, patients being treated with more than one ototoxic drug concurrently and patients with pre-existing sensorineural hearing loss. In the case of aminoglycosides, it is necessary to measure peak and trough serum levels of the drug and refer to the relevant drug company data sheets for the so-called, 'safe' levels so that the dose can be titrated to remain within the therapeutic range. In cases of permanent hearing loss, a hearing aid may be of help in the rehabilitation process. Patients with severe tinnitus may be helped by using a tinnitus masker. Prolonged dysequilibrium and bobbing oscillopsia may severely impair the patients' quality of life. These patients may benefit from performing Cooksey-Cawthorne vestibular rehabilitation exercises. As mentioned above, 'rescue' or blocking agents against the adverse effects of cisplatin are being developed and evaluated. It would indeed be interesting to see how effective these could be in preventing ototoxic damage.

Research methods for evaluation of ototoxicity
Physiology and function

Techniques for assessing the activity of the inner ear have largely been developed for the cochlea. Physiological investigation of the vestibular system is difficult to perform especially with experimental animals and there are no widely used sensitive tests of vestibular function. In the context of ototoxicity this is probably not a significant drawback. There are no agents known to affect only the vestibular system without also being potentially damaging to the cochlea, and chemical agents which are cochleotoxic also have effects in the vestibular system.

Cochlear function can be assessed at a number of different levels. Auditory cues detected by the cochlea evoke responses at higher brain centres which can be monitored through the specific reflexes which are elicited (the Preyer reflex) or by behavioural audiograms; the electrical activity associated with the passage of neural signals in the brain stem can be monitored; or the electrophysiological and biomechanical activity of the cochlea itself can be evaluated.

The Preyer reflex and behavioural response audiometry

The Preyer reflex is a twitching of the external pinna of the ear in response to sound. The test can be refined by presenting tones of different frequencies and different intensities (sound pressure levels expressed in decibels, dB SPL) but clearly there is a subjective element in determining whether there is a response and the twitching is elicited only at quite high sound pressure levels so that quite significant losses in hearing acuity can accrue before any effect on the reflex is noticeable. This test therefore is not generally recommended other than to derive some crude evaluation.

More sophisticated and sensitive estimation of the ability of an animal to 'hear' can be obtained through behavioural response audiometry to derive behavioural audiograms (Stebbins *et al.*, 1981). For these, an animal is trained to perform some task when sounds are presented. The threshold of the response, i.e. the lowest sound pressure level at which a response is elicited, can be determined for a number of different frequencies over the frequency range to which the animal is sensitive. Any change in the threshold concomitant with the administration of some ototoxic agent can then be evaluated. Such procedures have the advantage that repeated testing of the same animal is possible allowing pre- and post-administration thresholds to be compared and the progression of alteration to be followed. However, training is very time consuming and some animals which are in other ways useful for studies of the auditory system, such as the guinea pig, are very difficult to train at all, although some success in obtaining behavioural audiograms from guinea pigs has been achieved recently (Nicol *et al.*, 1992). In addition, the behaviourally determined response threshold does not come very close to the actual auditory threshold, and it is very difficult from a behavioural audiogram to determine the site of any lesion. Because of the limitations, therefore, these procedures are not used widely.

Brain stem auditory evoked potential

The stimulation of the auditory nerve following reception of a sound in the cochlea leads to successive stimulations of a number of centres along the auditory neural pathway in the brain stem to the auditory cortex. The electrical activity associated with such stimulations can be recorded with electrodes placed on the skull as a succession of waves of different amplitudes and latencies. The recording of these evoked responses is a non-invasive procedure that can potentially be used repeatedly in a single animal (Finitzo-Hieber, 1981) thereby allowing examination of the progression of a hearing impairment following an ototoxic insult. The signals are small and this creates problems in extracting the auditory response from background noise and from larger electrical signals evoked for example by muscular activity, but with the current ready availability of computer systems to perform signal analysis these problems can be overcome relatively simply. Consequently, brain stem auditory evoked potential recording is finding increasing use as a means to monitor the occurrence and progression of hearing loss after potentially ototraumatic insults, although it should be pointed out that it is difficult to determine the location of a lesion using this method and the level of sound necessary to produce a response may be somewhat higher than the actual auditory threshold so that initial stages of a progressive hearing loss, or a relatively small impairment of hearing may not be detectable. Nevertheless, the procedure has been used successfully in a number of studies. The threshold of the response, defined as the sound pressure level at which the wave chosen as a measure is no longer detectable, is determined over a range of frequencies prior to treatment and the change in threshold is monitored with time post-treatment, possibly for several months. It has been shown that permanent increases in brain stem auditory evoked potential thresholds at particular frequencies correlate with loss of hair cells at appropriate locations in the cochlea, and that it is possible to monitor transient, i.e. recoverable, changes in hearing acuity using this procedure (Schmidt, Anniko and Hellstrom, 1990).

Physiological and biomechanical activities of the cochlea

A number of different variables of cochlear functioning can be monitored; the resting endocochlear potential, or various sound-evoked responses that derive from the activity of particular parts of the transduction pathway. Assessment of changes to each of these can be used to make some kind of differentiation of the possible locations of lesions caused by injurious agents.

Endocochlear potential

A positive electrical potential of approximately 80 mV, the endocochlear potential, is present in the scala media. It is generated and maintained by active ion transport mechanisms in the stria vascularis. The endocochlear potential provides a driving force for current flow through the hair cells and, therefore, a decline in the level of the endocochlear potential decreases the sensitivity of the organ of Corti to sound stimuli resulting in deterioration of auditory threshold. The endocochlear potential can be monitored via a potassium-filled glass electrode inserted into the scala media either through the round window membrane and the basal coil of the organ of Corti, or through the lateral wall. Alterations of the endocochlear potential generally reflect an effect on the stria vascularis.

Cochlear microphonic potential

The modulation of current flow through the hair cells during transduction is associated with an alternating extracellular electrical potential that mimics exactly the orginal sound stimulus, i.e. the frequency and polarity of the cochlear microphonic potential follows precisely that of the stimulus (hence 'microphonic'). The cochlear microphonic potential predominantly derives from the activity of the outer hair cells. It can be recorded at particular locations within the cochlea with two electrodes, one either side of the organ of Corti, in the scala vestibuli and scala tympani. Alternatively, and more easily, it can be recorded from a more remote location by placing an electrode close to the round window. This can be used to assess the cochlear microphonic potential across all frequencies; by varying the frequency of the acoustic stimulus the cochlear microphonic potential originating from different regions of the cochlea can be assessed. The sound level at each frequency required to produce a constant cochlear microphonic potential output, or the amplitude of the cochlear microphonic potential in relation to sound intensity at each frequency can be measured.

Compound action potential

Neural excitation following sound stimulation results in the generation of action potentials in the auditory nerve. The gross activity of all the neural units responding to the particular sound stimulus can again be recorded remotely from electrodes placed close to the round window as the compound action potential. Nearly all the afferent nerves from the cochlea innervate inner hair cells and therefore the compound action potential reflects the activity of these cells. The procedures for measurement are essentially similar to those used for the cochlear microphonic potential; at different stimulus frequencies the sound intensity necessary to elicit a particular 'criterion' level of compound action potential response (usually 7–10 mV) is determined. The compound action potential is a measure of the actual ultimate output from the cochlea and consequently it has been argued it is the most meaningful measure for rapid assessement of the functional effects of potentially ototraumatic agents (Liberman, 1990).

The recording of the endocochlear, cochlear microphonic and compound action potentials are invasive techniques. Generally, these procedures are used acutely and the animal has to be sacrificed after the recording has been made. This means that in examination of ototoxic agents, pre- and post-administration levels of these potentials, or the progression of any alteration, cannot be made unless this occurs over a time period sufficiently short for the animal to be maintained under anaesthesia; this may be the case with some agents such as diuretics which produce acute effects on the endocochlear potential. It also means that determination of the abnormality must be made by comparison with untreated control subjects. However, these disadvantages can be overcome by permanently implanting a round window electrode for recording the cochlear microphonic and compound action potentials. With such a procedure long-term, continuous electrophysiological assessment of the effects of ototoxic agents in individual conscious animals has been successfully undertaken (Aran and Darrouzet, 1975).

Otoacoustic emissions

As well as electrical responses, sound stimuli also elicit active mechanical responses. These are thought to derive from stimulus-induced activity of the outer hair cells that influences the movement of the basilar membrane. The active mechanical response leads to the emission of sounds from the ear, a 'cochlear echo' or otoacoustic emission (Kemp, 1978) that is detected in the external auditory meatus some microseconds after the stimulating input signal. Otoacoustic emissions provide a non-invasive, yet very sensitive, objective means to assess cochlear function which merely involves the insertion of a small probe consisting of a microphone and loudspeaker assembly into the external auditory meatus. This procedure can be used repeatedly and reproducibly in individual subjects and is finding increasing clinical application, especially for testing cochlear function in newborn babies. There are a number of different types of otoacoustic emission signal depending upon the stimulus parameters used and for animals the most useful is the distortion product otoacoustic emission (Brown, McDowell and Forge, 1989; Norton, Bargones and Rubels, 1991). It has been shown that recording of distortion product otoacoustic emissions is a sensitive, reproducible method for assessment of ototoxic effects in the cochleae of animals (Brown, McDowell and Forge, 1989; Johnson and Canlon, 1994). As the technique is non-invasive, requires a minimum of animal preparation, and allows repetitive measurements from a single animal, it is likely that it will find increasing application.

Structural examinations

Examination of the inner ear structures by light or electron microscopy is widely used in assessing the effects of ototoxic agents. For the vestibular system, in the absence of reliable functional tests, such procedures may be the only ready means to evaluate ototoxic injury, and in the cochlea they allow assessment of the location and extent of lesions. Most, though not all, ototoxic agents affect the sensory hair cells and permanent functional impairment, i.e deafness or vestibular dysfunction, following ototoxic insult is due to the permanent loss of hair cells. Thus, at its simplest level, histological assessment of the inner ear involves an analysis of whether or not hair cells are present and, if loss has occurred, where the lesion is located and how extensive it is.

The most straightforward means for assessing the neuroepithelia of the inner ear is to examine the features at the surface in whole mounts of the tissue (Engstrom, Ades and Andersson, 1966). Following fixation, either by direct perfusion using the round and oval windows to gain access to the labyrinth, or after intra-vital perfusion of the whole animal, the bone enclosing the inner ear is picked away and the neuroepithelia dissected out. The organ of Corti is removed in segments, usually sequentially from apex to base, which can be examined by using phase-contrast (Figure 20.6), differential interference contrast (Figure 20.7), or, after additional processing, fluorescence microscopy (Figure 20.8). Hair cells are easily recognized by their distinctive hair bundles and it becomes possible to draw up a 'cytocochleogram', essentially a map depicting the position of each hair cell along the entire length of the organ of Corti. The location and number of damaged or missing hair cells can then be accurately determined and related to physiological data from the same cochlea if this is available. In general, light microscopy is best used to quantify and map the extent of missing hair cells once the damage caused by an ototoxic agent has stabilized, although by focusing beneath the surface to examine the larger cell organelles, some assessment of possible damage to hair cells which are still present in the organ of Corti can be made. It is also possible to examine details of the stereociliary bundles using light microscopy (Liberman, 1990) especially using fluorescence microscopy to visualize fluorescent markers for actin (Raphael and Altschuler, 1991). The fungal toxin, phalloidin, interacts specifically with filamentous actin and when conjugated with the fluorescent marker molecules fluorescein or rhodamine can be used to localize filamentous actin in cells. Actin is present in large amounts in the stereocilia and cuticular plates of the hair cells and is also associated with the intercellular junction between adjacent cells. Consequently these structures are intensely stained by labelled phalloidin. This enables the easy identification of hair cells and their borders and clearly shows individual stereocilia. (see Figure 20.8).

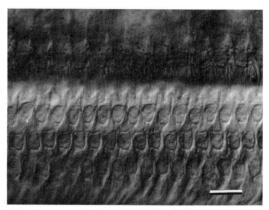

Figure 20.7 Nomarski differential interference contrast image of the apical surface of the organ of Corti. Again, the hair cells can be easily recognized and counted. Scale bar = 20 μm

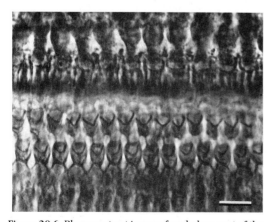

Figure 20.6 Phase-contrast image of a whole mount of the organ of Corti, focused at the apical surface. The hair cell stereocilia are easily distinguished and the number of hair cells can be easily counted. Scale bar = 20 μm

Examination of the surface features of the organ of Corti at higher resolution, though, is more easily achieved with scanning electron microscopy (Figure 20.9) which has found increasing use in studies of the inner ear (Davies and Forge, 1987; Forge *et al.*, 1992). With scanning electron microscopy it is not only possible to map the location of missing hair cells as with light microscopy, but it is also possible to assess more subtle alterations at the surface of the organ of Corti. Thus, some of the earliest events in the progression of damage to the hair cells can be identified or relatively minor alterations, especially to the stereociliary bundle, which would not be visible by light microscopy but may have quite significant functional implications, can be assessed. High resolution scanning electron microscopy has shown the presence of fine fibrils between stereocilia, 'tip-links', which are considered to be intimately involved in the transduction process (Pickles, Comis and Osborne, 1984; Hudspeth, 1989), and which may be damaged without there being any

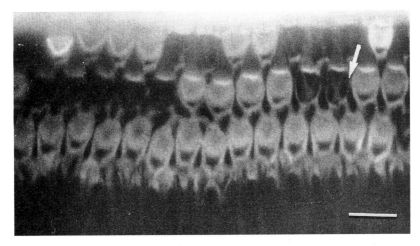

Figure 20.8 Fluorescence microscopy image of whole-mount organ of Corti stained with FITC-conjugated phalloidin. Phalloidin binds to f-actin which is present in the stereocilia, the cuticular plate of the hair cells, and in a ring around the apex of all the cells, associated with the intercellular junctions. These regions of the cells therefore show fluorescent staining. The hair cells are easily recognized by their stereocilia and cuticular plates, and the locations of missing hair cells can be identified. Where hair cells are lost, the lesion is occluded by expansion of the adjacent supporting cells which form junctions that seal the space and produce a characteristic x-or y-shaped 'scar' figure (arrow). Scale bar = 20 μm

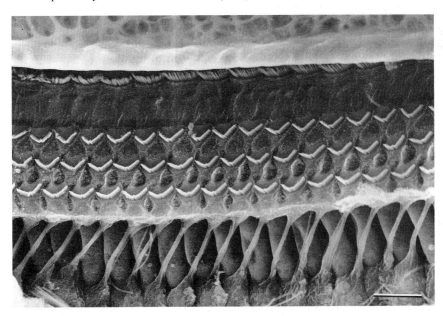

Figure 20.9 Scanning electron micrograph of the organ of Corti. The Hensen's cells towards the outside of the tissue have been removed to expose some of the internal structural organization of the tissue. The tectorial membrane at the top of the figure has shrunk away during processing of the tissue for scanning electron microscopy. The single row of inner hair cells and three rows of outer hair cells are evident. The cell bodies of the outer hair cells are cylindrical. The cell body of each Deiters' cell encloses the base of a single outer hair cell and the phalangeal process ascends diagonally to the apical surface where it expands to fill the space between adjacent hair cells. Scale bar = 20 μm

other significant alterations to the stereociliary bundle (Osborne and Comis, 1990). However, scanning electron microscopy only allows study of the cell surface and, in some situations, effects on the cell body may precede any detectable abnormalities at the apical surface (Harpur and Bridges, 1979; Forge, 1985).

These 'surface specimen techniques' can also be

applied to the vestibular neuroepithelium (Lindeman, 1969) but phase-contrast and differential interference contrast are more difficult to apply here because of the relative thickness of the tissue and because these tissues, particularly the cristae, are not flat. Furthermore, the sensory cells are not organized in a recognizable pattern as they are in the organ of Corti and it is almost impossible to distinguish between the two types of vestibular hair cell from their surface characteristics. Thus, maps of the vestibular neuroepithelia equivalent to a cochleogram cannot be drawn up. Only a rather more general assessment of hair cell loss is possible. For more accurate determination of the extent and location of hair cell loss it is necessary to cut serial sections for light microscopy (Aran *et al.*, 1982) where the two hair cell types can be identified from their morphology.

Sectioning is also an alternative method for examining cochlear tissues. For light microscopy, the intact cochlea is usually decalcified prior to embedding and sections of the whole cochlea in a plane parallel to the central core of the spiral (the modiolus) are obtained. For electron microscopy it is more usual to dissect out the tissues from the cochlea prior to embedding. Sectioning has the advantage that it allows examination of tissues other than the neuro-epithelium, in particular the stria vascularis, which may be sites of action for ototoxic agents or which are affected as damage following the initial ototoxic insult progresses. Furthermore, when sections of the entire cochlea are taken the tissues are retained in their original relationship. This allows assessment of more gross changes in tissue arrangement; e.g. swelling or collapse of Reissner's membrane occurring as a consequence of interference with the mechanisms that maintain the volume of cochlear fluids. It is also possible to obtain 'cytocochleograms' from cochlear sections by examining serial sections, reconstructing the length of the cochlear spiral and determining the absolute distance from the apex or base of any particular hair cell (Figure 20.10). This technique is far more laborious than surface examination of whole mounts but is favoured in some laboratories (Liberman, 1990) because damage to hair cells can be evaluated from effects other than those occurring at the surface, and it is possible to examine the non-sensory tissues at the precise locations where hair cells are affected and thereby obtain a more integrated view of the effects of damaging agents.

Methods to examine the direct effects of ototoxic agents

Many studies of the effects of ototoxic agents involve examination of structure and/or function after systemic application of the agent, a situation which mimics clinical conditions. However, such a regimen has many obvious disadvantages not least that it is

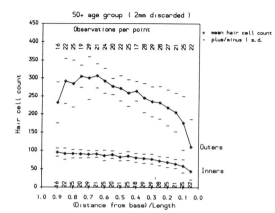

Figure 20.10 A composite cytocochleogram for humans aged 50 years and over. In this graph the x-axis represents the location of the hair cell count in the cochlea. By convention and to provide some concordance at least with the audiogram, the apex of the cochlea is to the left and corresponds with the low frequency end of the range of hearing. The base of the cochlea is at the right to correspond with high frequencies. Because of the wide range of lengths of the cochlear duct between individuals the cochlea was thought of as being of unit length and distances along the cochlea were presented as a proportion of the total length in the range 0.0 to 1.0. At each proportional site in the cochlea the average hair cell density from all the specimens collected was calculated and the standard deviation of the counts were computed and plotted. This proportional representation of the cochlea seems to give the appropriate description of many of the properties of the inner ear.

difficult to separate the initial interaction of the agent from the ensuing sequelae.

Perfusion of the fluid spaces of the inner ear with ototoxic substances provides one means of assessing direct effects (Nuttall, 1981; Bobbin and Ceasar, 1987). In an anaesthetized animal, the cochlea is exposed and two small holes are made in the bony wall over the perilymphatic scalae. A solution of salts of similar composition to perilymph and containing the substance under study is gently pumped into the cochlea through one hole and flows out from the other. The effects can be determined by simultaneous monitoring of the endocochlear, cochlear microphonic and compound action potentials and/or otoacoustic emissions and the reaction terminated at some specified point to examine the attendant structural correlates by perfusion of fixative.

Examination of the direct effects of ototoxic agents at a cellular level is also possible. Procedures have been developed for isolating hair cells from the cochlea or vestibular system and maintaining them in short-term culture (Brownell *et al.*, 1984; Zajic and Schacht, 1987), and for culturing explants of the developing organ of Corti (Richardson and Russell, 1991). These systems allow direct access to the hair cells and examination of the immediate effects of ototoxic agents using physiological, biochemical and cell biological methods. Increasingly such approaches are being adopted in efforts to understand the molecular basis of the interaction of ototoxic agents with the sensory cells of the inner ear.

In vitro studies

An alternative to using the whole animal as a test system, either for predicting ototoxicity or studying its mechanism, has been to use parts of the sensory epithelia maintained *in vitro* outside the animal. Several such systems have been developed each with their own advantages and disadvantages.

Isolated hair cell systems

Individual hair cells or clusters of hair cells can be dissected from segements of the organ of Corti removed from the cochlea after treatment with colla-

genase or repeated passage through a fine pipette (ticturition). The use of these isolated cells has been described in the sections above.

The major disadvantage of such systems is that they are non-physiological, although the cells survive with normal intracellular potentials for some hours and therefore are extremely useful in acute experiments.

Organotypic cultures

Organotypic cultures are blocks of tissue which are either the whole organ or which have the functional capacity resembling that of the intact whole organ.

Richardson and Russell (1991) have suggested that organotypic tissue cultures prepared from neonatal mouse cochlea may provide a useful model system for evaluating potentially ototoxic drugs. A comparative study (Kotecha and Richardson, 1994) was set up to look at the cochleotoxicity of five different aminoglycosides (Figure 20.11). The hair cells in

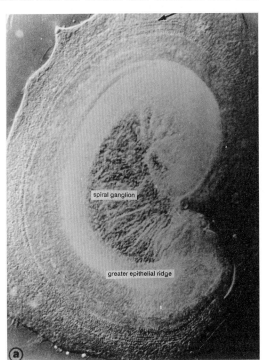
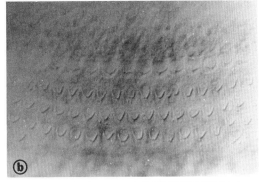
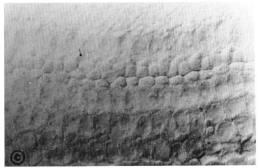

Figure 20.11 Whole organ tissue culture. Cultures were prepared from the inner ears of 1–2 day postnatal mice. The cochleae were dissected from the cartilaginous capsule in Hank's balanced salt solution buffered with an additional 10 mM Hepes pH 7.2 and, after removal of the lateral wall, divided into an apical and a basal coil. Apical coil explants consisted of the top one-and-a-quarter turn, of the cochlea and the basal coil explants consisted of the remainder of the spiral. After dissection the coils were explanted onto collagen coated round glass coverslips, fed with one drop of complete medium including heat inactivated horse serum, sealed into Maximow slides and maintined in the lying drop position at 37°C for 1 or 2 days before use. All cultures were routinely screened for viability and quality using Nomarski interference contrast optics before use in experiments. (*a*) Apical coil culture. The spiral ganglion is left in place during dissection and is marked. The arrow indicates the region of the organ of Corti which is shown in higher power in Nomarski optics in (*b*) and (*c*). (*b*) Nomarski micrograph focused at the level of the outer hair cell stereociliary bundles. The clusters of stereocilia are clearly seen and look 'healthy' by comparison with freshly mounted specimens. (*c*) Nomarski micrograph focused at the level of the nuclei of the bodies of the inner and outer hair cells. The nuclei can be seen as clearly rounded discrete masses and this is consistent with a 'healthy' cell

these tissue cultures are known to have normal physiological responses (Russell and Richardson, 1987).

Increase in ototoxic damage is seen as the drug concentration is increased (Figure 20.12). The basal coil explant was found to be more susceptible to ototoxic damage than the apical coil. This reflects the situation one would encounter clinically, namely that of patients

BASAL   APICAL

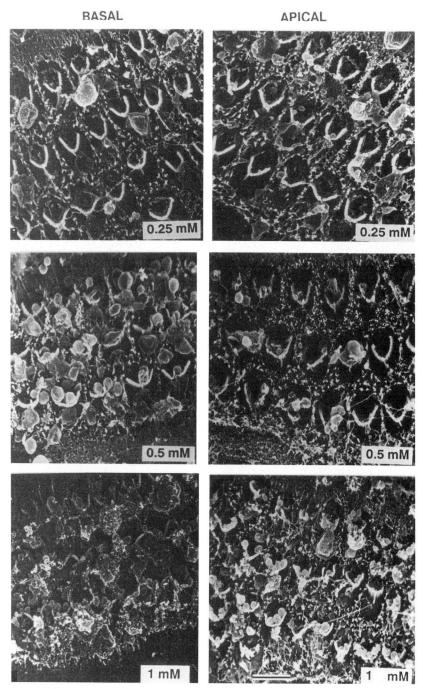

Figure 20.12 Basal and apical coil explants incubated with different concentrations of neomycin. As the concentration increases, the damage progressively worsens and is more marked in the basal than the apical coil explants. Scale bar = 10 μm

presenting with high frequency sensorineural hearing loss. The effects that different compounds have on the apical surface of the outer hair cells can be observed with the scanning and transmission electron microscope and are illustrated in Figure 20.13.

Most of the *in vitro* morphological studies reported

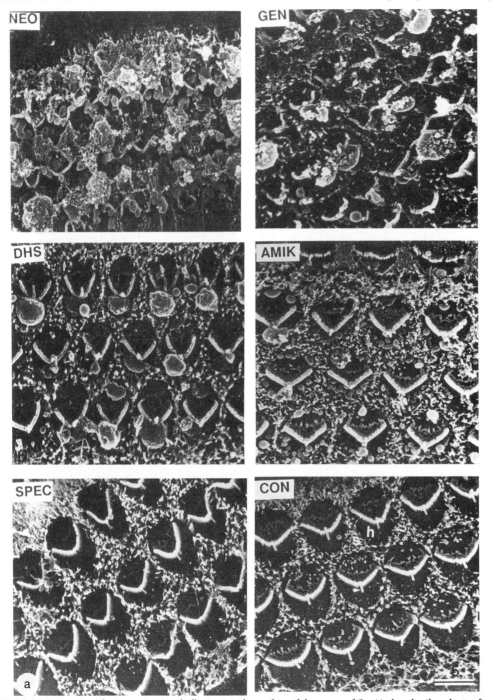

Figure 20.13 (*a*) A scanning electron micrograph illustrating the surface of the organ of Corti in basal coil explants after treatment for 1 h at room temperature in medium containing: 1 mM neomycin (NEO), 1 mM gentamicin (GEN), 1 mM dihydrostreptomycin (DHS), 1 mM amikacin (AMIK) and 1 mM spectinomycin (SPEC). A sample was incubated in the medium alone for 1 h as a control (CON). Scale bar = 5 μm and applies to all six micrographs

to date have been performed at room temperature. Kotecha (1993) conducted a study to illustrate some important morphological changes secondary to in-creasing the experimental temperature to a more physiological value of 37°C. In this study, various experiments were set up using the drug neomycin

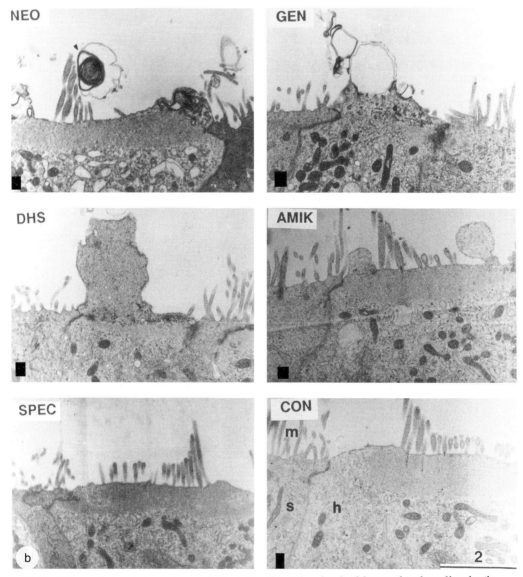

Figure 20.13 (*b*) Transmission electron micrograph illustrating the surface details of the apical surface of basal coil explant outer hair cell after treatment with the agents described above in (*a*). The apical whorls and blisters are a notable feature of changes in this system, h = outer hair cell, s = supporting cell, m = microvilli on supporting cell surface. Scale bar = 2 μm and applies to all six micrographs

sulphate at a concentration of 1 mM. Examining the damage caused after 1 and 4 hours at room temperature (Figure 20.14), it can be seen that the degree of damage at the two time points is essentially similar. It seems that a saturation point with regard to the degree of morphological damage has been achieved after 1 hour at room temperature. At 37°C (Figure 20.15), it is obvious that ototoxic damage progresses between 1 and 4 hours of treatment.

Some of the features seen in the degenerating cochlear hair cells following treatment at 37°C (e.g. nuclear condensation and cytoplasmic darkening) resemble the phenomenon of apoptosis (Kerr, Bishop and Searle, 1984). Similar hair cell degenerative changes have been observed *in vivo* following aminoglycoside treatment (Forge, 1985). However, not all hair cells appeared to undergo apoptosis, some appear necrotic, and whether aminoglycosides really

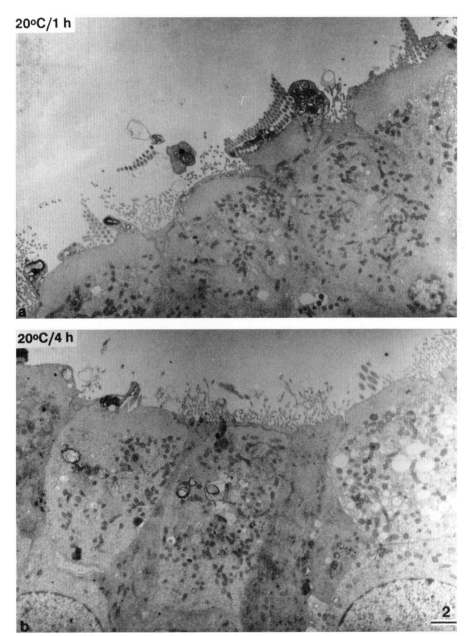

Figure 20.14 Transmission electron micrograph illustrating the surface details of basal coil explants treated with 1 mM neomycin. (*a*) Incubation for 1 h at 20°C; (*b*) incubation for 4 h at 20°C. Scale bar = 2 μm and applies to both micrographs

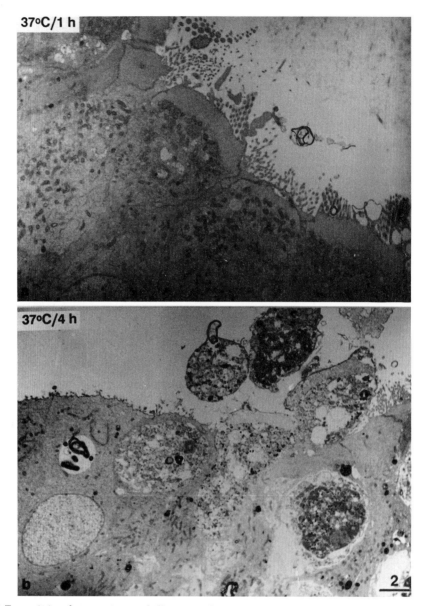

Figure 20.15 Transmission electron micrograph illustrating the surface details of basal coil explants treated with 1 mM neomycin. (*a*) Incubation for 1 h at 37°C; (*b*) incubation for 4 h at 37°C

trigger apoptosis requires further careful evaluation. Apoptosis or programmed cell death may be interrelated to cell-cycle control (Rubin, Philpott and Brooks, 1993). Active cell death by apoptosis results from a decision by the cell, based on information from its environment and its genome, and it is possible that the process of apoptosis is blocked at 20°C. It seems very probable that various factors may alter with the increase in the experimental temperature to 37°C. Recent studies (Huang and Schacht, 1990; Crann *et* *al.*, 1992) have shown that the cytotoxic metabolite produced from gentamicin is more cochleotoxic than the parent drug. At the higher temperature, aminoglycoside metabolite may be produced in the cultures which is more cochleotoxic than the parent drug. In the former studies (Huang and Schacht, 1990; Crann *et al.*, 1992), however, experiments on isolated hair cells were carried out at room temperature and sometimes in presence of drug-metabolizing hepatic enzymes. Takada, Bledsoe and Schacht (1985) have shown that a metabolic process is essential in the expression of gentamicin toxicity and also that the entry of gentamicin into hair cells is prevented by a reduction in their transmembrane electrical potential brought about by factors such as anoxia. It is possible that the changes in the experimental temperature may induce similar effects. The resting membrane potential has been shown to be maintained *in vitro* for several hours at room temperature (Russell and Richardson, 1987; Kros, Rusch and Richardson, 1992).

The *in vitro* organotypic model has advantages and disadvantages. It allows cochleotoxicity to be evaluated far more rapidly than the *in vivo* model. With the *in vitro* model the cochlear hair cells are directly exposed to the ototoxic drugs, and although this may not resemble the *in vivo* situation, it is interesting to note that the cochleotoxicity observed from this direct effect is essentially similar to that seen in many *in vivo* studies (Brown and Feldman, 1978). With *in vitro* models it is quite easy to alter experimental variables such as temperature. An obvious disadvantage of this *in vitro* model system is that it does not reflect the true situation as to what happens to a drug in the body, in terms of absorption, metabolism or excretion. It would be totally inappropriate solely to use an *in vitro* model system to evaluate a potentially ototoxic drug, but a model system as described above could well be used to screen potentially ototoxic drugs rapidly prior to performing time-consuming *in vivo* studies or formal clinical trials.

Vestibular organotypic cultures can also be established and one of their uses is described in the next section.

Hair cell regeneration

Until recently it was thought that in warm-blooded vertebrates, i.e. birds and mammals, hair cells are produced only during embryonic life and that the hair cells in the mature inner ear, once lost, cannot be replaced. Thus, the hair cell loss from noise trauma or ototoxic challenge results in permanent functional deficits. Over the last few years, however, this dogma has been revised. Evidence has accumulated to establish that in birds following noise- or aminoglycoside-induced hair cell loss, new hair cells appear in both the auditory (Cotanche, 1987; Cruz, Lambert and Rubel, 1987; Lippe, Westbrook and Ryals, 1991; Cotanche *et al.*, 1994) and vestibular (Weisleder and Rubel, 1993) portions of the inner ear. These new hair cells arise spontaneously through damage-induced stimulation of mitotic activity among undamaged supporting cells (Corwin and Cotanche, 1988; Ryals and Rubel, 1988; Lippe, Westbrook and Ryals, 1991; Cotanche *et al.*, 1994). This regeneration of hair cells leads to functional recovery (McFadden and Saunders, 1989; Tucci and Rubel, 1990; Cotanche *et al.*, 1994). Very recent observations also suggest that

a regenerative capacity may exist in the mammalian inner ear.

Examination of the vestibular sensory epithelia of guinea-pigs that had been given chronic systemic treatment with gentamicin (Forge, Corwin and Nevill, 1993) showed that, at 1–2 weeks post-treatment, hair cells were lost from the striolar regions of the utricle. By 4 weeks post-treatment, however, in the regions where hair cell loss had been extensive at earlier times, scanning electron microscopy showed cells with characteristics at their apical surfaces typical of those seen in immature hair cells at various stages of development (Figures 20.16, 20.17 and 20.18). Examination of thin sections showed that the type 1 hair cells usually present in the striolar regions of the utricle were degenerating or missing at 1 week post-treatment but at 4 weeks post-treatment had been replaced by cells with characteristics of type 2 hair cells, but also showing features typical of immaturity. Examination of utricles at 12 weeks post-treatment showed that many of these type 2 cells were now innervated and scanning electron microscopy revealed that the hair bundles had continued to develop towards a more mature form. Counts of hair cells, assessed from the number of hair bundles seen by scanning electron microscopy (Li Lin, personal communication), showed that a decrease in the number of hair cells across the striolar region to about one-third of normal at 1 week post-treatment, was followed by an increase to about two-thirds of normal numbers by 12 weeks. Counting of hair cells in thin sections of the utricle produced a similar result. In subsequent studies (Forge and Li, 1994), gentamicin was administered topically to the middle ear cavity in a single dose. This treatment protocol induced hair cell loss in the saccule as well as the utricle and there was a recovery in hair cell numbers by 12 weeks post-treatment in both the utricle and saccule to a similar extent to that found in the utricle after systemic treatment regimens.

These observation provided the first indication that hair cell recovery could occur spontaneously in the mature mammalian inner ear, but they do not of themselves demonstrate conclusively that regeneration is occurring. In a parallel study (Warchol *et al.*, 1993), organotypic cultures of mature utricles from guinea-pigs and from human patients who had undergone surgery for vestibular schwannomas were exposed to aminoglycosides to induce hair cell loss. The cultures were subsequently incubated in the presence of radioactive thymidine, an analogue of one of the bases in DNA that is incorporated into DNA when it is synthesized. Subsequent autoradiography of sections of the treated cultures showed radioactively-labelled nuclei in supporting cells at 1 week post-treatment and in putative hair cells at 4 weeks post-treatment. The presence of the label in these nuclei demonstrated that the cells possessing them had arisen following DNA synthesis and then

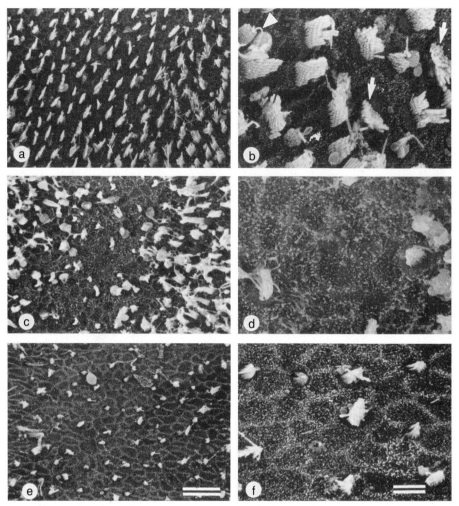

Figure 20.16 Scanning electron micrographs of the striola of the normal guinea-pig utricular macula (*a*, *b*); and 4 days (*c*, *d*) and 4 weeks (*e*, *f*) after gentamicin treatment. The utricular macula is normally evenly covered with hair cells, distinguishable by their hair bundles. Each bundle consists of stereocilia which increase in height in one direction towards the single kinocilium (arrowheads in *b*). In the striola, hair bundle orientation changes by 180°; in (*b*) arrows point to two bundles in opposite orientation to the others. By 4 days post-treatment, hair cells within the striola are lost (*c*) and replaced by expansion of adjacent supporting cells (*d*); but by 4 weeks, immature hair bundles are appearing (*e,f*) within the region where hair cell loss is pronounced at earlier times. Scale bars: *a,c,e* = 20 μm; *b,d,e,* = 5 μm

cell division subsequent to the drug-induced hair cell loss. This evidence together with the morphological observation showing recovery of hair cell numbers suggested that indeed hair cell regeneration may occur in the mature mammalian inner ear.

These studies showed a potential spontaneous re-generative capacity only in the mature mammalian vestibular system. There was no morphological evidence for regenerating hair cells in the damaged organs of Corti in the inner ears of those animals which showed recovery of vestibular hair. However,

other very recent work has suggested that it may be possible to stimulate hair cell regeneration at least in the immature mammalian cochlea (Lefebvre *et al.*, 1993, 1994). In organotypic cultures of the organ of Corti of neonatal rats, hair cell loss was induced by exposure of the cultures to aminoglycoside. After subsequent incubation of the cultures for a further 7 days in the presence of retinoic acid and fetal calf serum the tissue appeared to be re-populated by new hair cells. Both retinoic acid and fetal calf serum were necessary for this to occur (Lefebvre

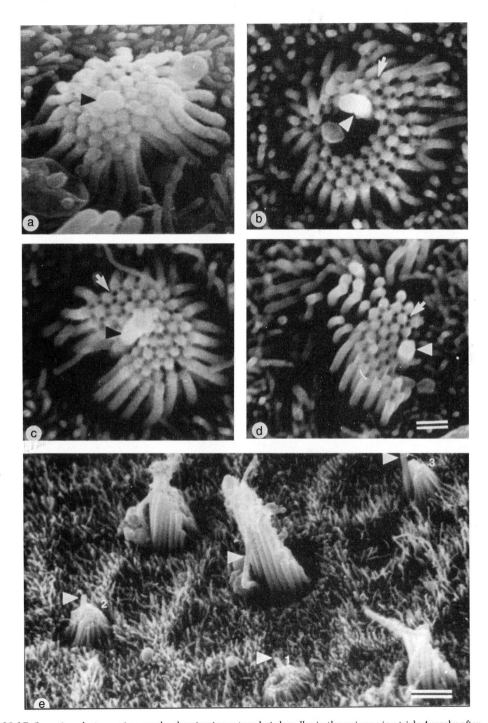

Figure 20.17 Scanning electron micrographs showing immature hair bundles in the guinea-pig utricle 4 weeks after gentamicin treatment. The bundles consist of immature stereocilia and a kinocilium (arrowhead). The stereocilia are of approximately equal height but regularly arranged with cross-links (arrows) between them. (*a–d*) show what appear to be successive stages in orientation of the bundle. In (*e*), it can be seen that as the stereocilia increase in height (bundles labelled 1–3), the bundles adopt the orientation of the mature hair bundle (centre of the field) in their vicinity (arrowheads indicate position of the kinocilium). Scale bars: (*a–d*) = 500 μm; (*e*) = 2 μm

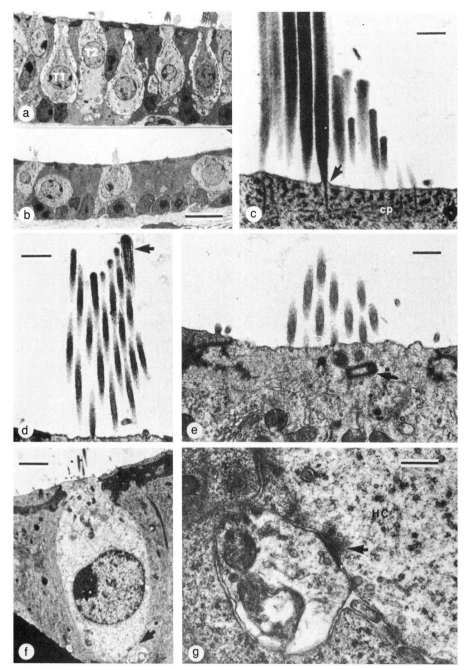

Figure 20.18 Thin sections of utricle in normal guinea-pig (*a,c*) and at 4 weeks after gentamicin treatment (*b,d–g*). The type 1 hair cells normally present across the striola (T1 in *a*) are lost after treatment (*b*) and replaced by cells with characteristics of immature type 2 hair cells (*b*). These cells show immature stereocilia and undeveloped cuticular plates (compare *d,e* with the normal mature hair cell apex in *c*). Some immature hair cells possess a small number of synaptic connections (*f,g*), suggesting the reappearing hair cells acquire innervation. Scale bars: (*a,b*) = 10 μm; (*c,d,e*) = 500 nm; (*g*) = 400 nm

et al., 1993) but further work has suggested that transforming growth factor alpha may substitute for the fetal calf serum (Lefevbre *et al.*, 1994).

While this work seems to offer the prospect that regeneration of cochlear hair cells could be induced, it should be pointed out that it was conducted *in vitro* using immature tissue in which the supporting cells have not fully differentiated. Furthermore, no evidence has yet been presented to demonstrate conclusively that what appear to be new hair cells have arisen through stimulation of renewed mitotic activity. At present the factors that control regeneration phenomena are unknown, but work in a number of centres is currently in progress and over the next few years it may become apparent whether a new dawn in therapies for treatment of the hearing and balance disorders caused by ototoxic drugs is a realistic possibility.

References

ALVAN, G., KARLSSON, K. K., HELLGREN, U. and VILLEN, T. (1991) Hearing impairment related to plasma quinine concentration in healthy volunteers. *British Journal of Clinical Pharmacology*, **31**, 409–412

ARAN, J. M. and DARROUZET, J. (1975) Observation of click-evoked compound VIII nerve responses before, during and over seven months after kanamycin treatment in the guinea pig. *Acta Otolaryngologica*, **79**, 24–32

ARAN, J. M., ERRE, J. P., GUILHAUME, A. and AUROUSSEAI, C. (1982) The comparative ototoxicities of gentamicin, tobramycin and dibekacin in the guinea pig. A functional and morphological cochlear and vestibular study. *Acta Otolaryngologica*, Supplement 300, 1–30

ASHMORE, J. F. and MEECH, R. W. (1986) Ionic basis of the resting potential in outer hair cells isolated from guinea pig cochlea. *Nature*, **322**, 368–371

AURSNES, J. (1981) Cochlear damage from chlorhexidene in guinea pigs. *Acta Otolaryngologica*, **92**, 259–271

BAMFORD, M. F. M. and JONES, L. F. (1978) Deafness and biochemical imbalance after burns treatment with topical antibiotics in young children – report of six cases. *Archives of Disease in Childhood*, **53**, 326–329

BERK, D. P. and CHALMERS, T. (1970) Deafness complicating antibiotic therapy of hepatic encephalopathy. *Annals of Internal Medicine*, **73**, 393–396

BERNSTEIN, J. M. and WEISS, A. D. (1967) Further observations on salicylate ototoxicity. *Journal of Laryngology and Otology*, **89**, 915–925

BICKERTON, R. C., ROBERTS, C. and LITTLE, J. T. (1988) Survey of general practitioners' treatment of the discharging ear. *British Medical Journal*, **296**, 1649–1650

BLACK, F., MYERS, E. and SCHRAMM, V. (1982) Cisplatin vestibular ototoxicity: preliminary report. *Laryngoscope*, **92**, 1363–1368

BOBBIN, R. P. and CEASAR, G. (1987) Kynurenic acid and gamma D-glutamyl-aminomethylsulfonic acid suppress the compound action potential of the auditory nerve. *Hearing Research*, **25**, 77–81

BONDING, P. (1979) Critical bandwidth in patients with a hearing loss induced by salicylates. *Audiology*, **18**, 133–144

BOSHER, S. K. (1980a) The nature of the ototoxic actions of ethacrynic acid upon the mammalian endolymph system. I. Functional aspects. *Acta Otolaryngologica*, **89**, 407–418

BOSHER, S. K. (1980b) The nature of the ototoxic actions of ethacrynic acid upon the mammalian endolymph system. II. Structural-functional correlates in the stria vascularis. *Acta Otolaryngologica*, **90**, 40–54

BROWN, A. M., MCDOWELL, B. and FORGE, A. (1989) Acoustic distortion products can be used to monitor the effects of chronic gentamicin treatment. *Hearing Research*, **42**, 143–156

BROWN, H. A. and HINSHAW, H. C. (1946) Toxic reactions of streptomycin on the eighth nerve apparatus. *Proceedings of Staff Meetings at Mayo Clinic*, **21**, 347

BROWN, R. D. and FELDMAN, A. M. (1978) Pharmacology of hearing and ototoxicity. *Annual Reviews of Pharmacology and Toxicology*, **18**, 233–252

BROWNELL, W. E., BADER, C. R., BERTRAND, D. and DE RIBEAUPIERRE, Y. (1984) Evoked mechanical responses of isolated cochlear outer hair cells. *Science*, **227**, 194–196

BROWNING, G. G. and DAVIS, A. C. (1983) Clinical characterisation of the hearing of the adult British population. *Advances in Oto-Rhino-Laryngology*, **31**, 217–223

BROWNING, G. G., GATEHOUSE, S. and CALDER, I. T. (1988) Medical management of active chronic otitis media: a controlled study. *Journal of Laryngology and Otology*, **102**, 491–495

BRUMMETT, R. E. (1980) Drug-induced ototoxicity. *Drugs*, **19**, 412–428

BRUMMETT, R. E., WEST, B. A., TRAYNOR, J. and MANOR, N. (1974) Ototoxic interaction between aminoglycoside antibiotics and diuretics. *Toxicology and Applied Pharmacology*, **29**, 97

CARSON, S. S., PRAZMA, J., PULVER, S. H. and ANDERSON, T. (1989) Combined effects of aspirin and noise in causing permanent hearing loss. *Archives of Otolaryngology – Head and Neck Surgery*, **115**, 1070–1075

CORWIN, J. T. and COTANCHE, D. A. (1988) Regeneration of sensory hair cells after acoustic trauma. *Science*, **240**, 1772–1774

COTANCHE, D. A. (1987) Regeneration of hair cell stereociliary bundles in the chick cochlea following severe acoustic trauma. *Hearing Research*, **30**, 181–196

COTANCHE, D. A., LEE, K. H., STONE, J. S. and PICARD, D. A. (1994) Hair cell regneration in the bird cochlea following noise damage or ototoxic drug damage. *Anatomy and Embryology*, **189**, 1–18

COX, C. E. (1976) Amikacin therapy of urinary tract infections. *Journal of Infectious Disease*, **134**, S362–S368

CRANN, S. A., HUANG, M. Y., MCLAREN, J. D. and SCHACHT, J. (1992) Formation of a toxic metabolite from gentamicin by a hepatic cytosolic fraction. *Biochemical Pharmacology*, **43**, 1835–1839

CRUZ, R. M., LAMBERT, P. R. and RUBEL, E. W. (1987) Light microscopic evidence of hair cell regeneration after gentamicin toxicity in chick cochlea. *Archives of Otolaryngology – Head and Neck Surgery*, **113**, 1058–1062

DARROUZET, J. and DE LIMA SOBRINHO, E. (1962) The internal ear, kanamycin, and acoustic trauma. Experimental study. *Revue de Laryngologie, Otologie et Rhinologie*, **83**, 781

DAVEY, P. G., JABEEN, F. J., HARPUR, E. S., SHENOI, P. M. and GEDDES, A. M. (1983) A controlled study of the reliability of pure tone audiometry for detection of gentamicin auditory toxicity. *Journal of Laryngology and Otology*, **97**, 27–36

DAVIES, S. and FORGE, A. (1987) Preparation of the mammalian organ of Corti for scanning electron microscopy. *Journal of Microscopy*, **147**, 89–101

DAVIS, R. R., BRUMMETT, R. E., BENDRICK, T. W. and HIMES, D. L. (1982) The ototoxic interaction of viomycin, capreomycin and polymixin B with ethacrynic acid. *Acta Otolaryngologica*, **93**, 211–217

DAY, R. O., GRAHAM, G. G. and BIERI, D. (1989) Concentration-response relationships for salicylate-induced ototoxicity in normal volunteers. *British Journal of Clinical Pharmacology*, **28**, 695–702

DEDON, P. C. and BORCH, R. F. (1987) Characterisation of the reactions of platinum antitumor agents with biologic and non-biologic sulfur-containing nucleophiles. *Biochemical Pharmacology*, **36**, 1955–1964

DE GROOT, J. C. M. J. and VELDMAN, J. E. (1988) Early effects of gentamicin on inner ear glycocalyx cytochemistry. *Hearing Research*, **35**, 39–46

DIDIER, A., MILLER, J. F. and NUTTALL, A. L. (1993) The vascular component of sodium salicylate ototoxicity in the guinea pig. *Hearing Research*, **69**, 199–206

DOBBS, S. M. and MAWER, G. E. (1976) Intravenous injection of gentamicin and tobramycin without impairment of hearing. *Journal of Infectious Disease*, **134**, S114–S117

DOUEK, E. E., DODSON, D. C. and BANNISTER, L. C. (1983) The effects of sodium salicylate on the cochlea of guinea pigs. *Journal of Laryngology and Otology*, **93**, 793–799

DULON, D., ARAN, J. M., ZAJIC, G. and SCHACHT, J. (1986) Comparative uptake of gentamicin, netilmicin and amikacin in the guinea pig cochlea and vestibule. *Antimicrobial Agents and Chemotherapy*, **30**, 96–100

DULON, D., HIEL, H., AUROUSSEAU, C., ERRE, J.-P. and ARAN, J.-M. (1993) Pharmacokinetics of gentamicin in the sensory hair cells of the organ of Corti: rapid uptake and long term persistence. *Comptes Rendus de Academie des Sciences. Sciences de la Vie (Paris)*, **316**, 682–687

DULON, D., ZAJIC, G., ARAN, J. M. and SCHACHT, J. (1989) Aminoglycoside antibiotics impair calcium entry but not viability and motility in isolated cochlear outer hair cells. *Journal of Neuroscience*, **24**, 338–346

DURRANT, J. D. (1978) Anatomic and physiologic correlates of the effects of noise on hearing. In: *Noise and Audiology*, edited by D. M. Lipscomb. Baltimore, MD: University Park Press

DYLEWSKI, J. (1988) Irreversible sensorineural hearing loss due to erythromycin. *Canadian Medical Association Journal*, **139**, 230–231

EASTMAN, A. (1986) Re-evaluation of interaction of cis-dichloro (ethylenediamine) platinum II with DNA. *Biochemistry*, **25**, 3912–3915

ENGSTROM, H., ADES, H. W. and ANDERSSON, A. (1966) *Structural Pattern of the Organ of Corti*. Stockholm: Almqvist and Wiksell

EVANS, E. F. and BORERWE, T. A. (1982) Ototoxic effects of salicylates on the responses of single cochlear nerve fibres and on cochlear potentials. *British Journal of Audiology*, **16**, 101–108

FARRINGTON, R. F., HULL–SMITH, H., BUNN, P. A. and MCDERMOTT, W. (1947) Streptomycin toxicity: reactions to highly purified drug on long continued administration to human subjects. *Journal of the American Medical Association*, **134**, 679–688

FEDERSPIL, P., TIESLER, E. and SCHNATZLE, W. (1983) Pharmakokinetics des Fosfomycin und otitis media. *Larungorhinootologie (Stuttgart)*, **61**, 591–594

FELD, R., VALDIVIESO, M., BODEY, G. P. and RODRIGUES, M. (1977) A comparative trial of sisomicin therapy by intermittent versus continuous infusion. *American Journal of Medical Science*, **274**, 178–188

FELDMAN, W. H. and HINSHAW, H. C. (1944) Effects of streptomycin in experimental tuberculosis in guinea pigs; a preliminary report. *Proceedings of Staff Meetings at Mayo Clinic*, **19**, 593–599

FINEGOLD, S. M. (1966) Toxicity of kanamycin in adults. *Annals of the New York Academy of Sciences*, **132**, 942–956

FINITZO–HIEBER, T. (1981) Auditory brainstem response in assessment of infants treated with amino-glycoside antibiotics. In: *Aminoglycoside Ototoxicity*, edited by S. A. Lerner, G. J. Matz and J. E. Hawkins Jr. Boston: Little Brown. pp. 269–280

FORGE, A. (1981) Ultrastructure in the stria vascularis of the guinea pig following intraperitoneal injection of ethacrynic acid. *Acta Otolaryngologica*, **92**, 439–457

FORGE, A. (1984) Gap junctions in the stria vascularis and effects of ethacrynic acid. *Hearing Research*, **13**, 189–200

FORGE, A. (1985) Outer hair cell loss and supporting cell expansion following chronic gentamicin treatment. *Hearing Research*, **19**, 171–182

FORGE, A. and BROWN, A. M. (1982) Ultrastructural and electrophysiological studies of acute ototoxic effects of furosemide. *British Journal of Audiology*, **16**, 109–116

FORGE, A. and FRADIS, M. (1985) Structural abnormalities in the stria vascularis following chronic gentamicin treatment. *Hearing Research*, **20**, 233–244

FORGE, A. and LI, L. (1994) Replacement of hair cells in guinea pig vestibular organs after losses induced by local application of gentamicin. *Abstracts, 17th Midwinter Meeting*, Academy for Research in Otolaryngology, pp. 131

FORGE, A. and RICHARDSON, G. P. (1993) Freeze-fracture analysis of apical membranes in cochlear cultures: differences between basal and apical-coil outer hair cells and effects of neomycin. *Journal of Neurocytology*, **22**, 854–867

FORGE, A., LI, L., CORWIN, J. T. and NEVILL, G. (1993) Ultrastructural evidence for hair cell regeneration in the mammalian inner ear. *Science*, **259**, 1616–1619

FORGE, A., WRIGHT, A. and DAVIES, S. J. (1987) Analysis of structural changes in the stria vascularis following chronic gentamicin treatment. *Hearing Research*, **31**, 253–266

FORGE, A., NEVILL, G., ZAJIC, G. and WRIGHT, A. (1992) Scanning electron microscopy of the mammalian organ of Corti: assessment of preparative procedures. *Scanning Microscopy*, **6**, 521–535

FOWLER, E. P. and SELIGMAN, E. (1947) Otic complications of streptomycin therapy. *Journal of the American Medical Association*, **133**, 87–91

GRIFFIN, J. P. (1988) Drug-induced ototoxicity. *British Journal of Audiology*, **22**, 195–210

HARPUR, E. S. and BRIDGES, J. B. (1979) An evaluation of the use of scanning and transmission electron-microscopy of the gentamicin-damaged guinea-pig organ of Corti. *Journal of Laryngology and Otology*, **93**, 7–23

HARPUR, E. S. and GONDA, I. (1982) Analysis of the pharmacokinetics of ribostamycin in serum and perilymph of guinea pigs after single and multiple doses. *British Journal of Audiology*, **16**, 95–99

HAWKINS, J. E. (1973), Ototoxic mechanisms. *Audiology*, **12**, 383–393

HAWKINS, J. E. (1976) Drbg ototoxicity. In: *Handbook of Sensory Physiology*, edited by W. D. Keidel and W. D. Neff, vol. 5. Berlin: Springer-Verlag. pp. 707–748

HAWKINS, J. E. and JOHNSSON, L. -G. (1981) Histopathology of cochlear and vestibular ototoxicity in laboratory animals. In: *Aminoglycoside Otoxicity*, edited by S. A. Lerner, G. J. Matz and J. E. Hawkins Jr. Boston: Little Brown. pp. 175–195

HAWKINS, J. E., MARQUES, D. M. and CLARK, C. S. (1975) Noise and kanamycin interaction in the guinea pig cochlea. *Journal of the Acoustical Society of America*, **58** (Supplement 1), 588

HAYASHIDA, T., HIEL, H., DULON, D., ERRE, J. -P., GUILHAUME, A. and ARAN, J.-M. (1989) Dynamic changes following combined treatment with gentamicin and ethacrynic acid with and without acoustic stimulation. Cellular uptake and functional correlates. *Acta Otolaryngologica*, **108**, 404–413

HAYES, D. M., CVITKOVIC, E. and GOLBEY, R. B. (1977) High dose cisplatinum diammine dichloride. *Cancer*, **39**, 1372–1381

HELSON, L., OKONKWO, E. and ANTON, L. (1978) Cisplatinum ototoxicity. *Clinical Toxicology*, **13**, 469–478

HENLEY, C. M. and SCHACHT, J. (1988) Pharmacokinetics of aminoglycoside antibiotics in blood, inner-ear fluids and tissues and their relationship to ototoxicity. *Audiology*, **27**, 137–146

HIEL, H., BENNANNI, H., ERRE, J. -P., AUROUSSEAU, C. and ARAN, J. -M. (1992) Kinetics of gentamicin in cochlear hair cells after chronic treatment. *Acta Otolaryngologica*, **112**, 272–277

HIGGINS, C. C. and KASTNERS, R. E. (1967) Nebramycin – a new broad spectrum antibiotic complex. II description of *Streptomyces tenebrarius*. *Antimicrobial Agents and Chemotherapy*, **7**, 324–331

HINCHCLIFFE, R. (1959) The threshold of hearing as a function of age. *Acoustica*, **9**, 304–308

HINSHAW, H. C. and FELDMAN, W. H. (1945) Streptomycin in the treatment of clinical tuberculosis: a preliminary report. *Proceedings of Staff Meetings at Mayo Clinic*, **20**, 313–318

HOEVE, L. J., MERTENS ZUR BORG, I. R., RODENBURG, M., BROCAAR, M. P. and GROEN, B. G. (1988) Correlations between cis-platinum dosage and toxicity in a guinea pig model. *Archives of Otorhinolaryngology*, **245**, 98–102

HUANG, M. Y. and SCHACHT, J. (1990) Formation of a cytotoxic metabolite from gentamicin by liver. *Biochemical Pharmacology*, **40**, R11–R14

HUDSPETH, A. J. (1989) How the ear's works work. *Nature*, **341**, 397–404

JARDINI, L., FINDLAY, R. and BURGI, E. (1978) Auditory changes associated with moderate blood salicylate levels. *Rheumatology and Rehabilitation*, **17**, 233–236

JARVIS, J. F. (1966) A case of unilateral permanent deafness following acetylsalicylic acid. *Journal of Laryngology and Otology*, **80**, 318–320

JOHNSON, A. -C. and CANLON, B., (1994) Toluene exposure affects the functional activity of the outer hair cells. *Hearing Research*, **72**, 189–196

JOHNSON, A. H. and HAMILTON, W. H. (1970) Kanamycin ototoxicity – possible potentiation by other drugs. *Southern Medical Journal*, **63**, 511–513

KAPUR, V. P. (1965) Ototoxicity of acetylsalicylic acid. *Archives of Otolaryngology*, **81**, 134–138

KARLSSON, K. K. and FLOCK, A. (1990) Quinine causes isolated outer hair cells to change length. *Neuroscience Letters*, **116**, 101–105

KARLSSON, K. K., FLOCK, B. and FLOCK, A. (1991) Ultrastructural changes in the outer hair cells of the guinea pig cochlea after exposure to quinine. *Acta Otolaryngologica*, **111**, 500–505

KARLSSON, K. K., ULFENDAHL, M., KHANNA, S. M. and FLOCK, A. (1991) The effects of quinine on the cochlear mechanics in the isolated temporal bone preparation. *Hearing Research*, **53**, 95–100

KAWAGUCHI, H., NAITO, T., NAKAGAWA, S. and FUJISAWA, K. (1972) BB-K8 a new semisynthetic aminoglycoside. *Journal of Antibiotics (Tokyo)*, **25**, 695–708

KEMP, D. T. (1978) Stimulated acoustic emission from within the human auditory system. *Journal of the Acoustical Society of America*, **64**, 1386–1391

KERR, J. F. R., BISHOP, C. J. and SEARLE, J. (1984) Apoptosis. *Recent Advances in Histopathology*, **12**, 1–15

KERR, T. P., ROSS, M. D. and ERNST, S. A. (1982) Cellular localisation of Na +, K + -ATPase in the mammalian cochlear duct: significance for cochlear fluid balance. *American Journal of Otolaryngology*, **3**, 332–338

KIM, D. O. (1986) Active and non-linear cochlear biomechanics and the role of outer-hair-cell sub-system in the mammalian auditory system. *Hearing Research*, **22**, 105–114

KOMUNE, S. and SNOW, J. B. (1982) Nature of the endocochlear DC potential in kanamycin poisoned guinea pigs. *Archives of Otolaryngology*, **108**, 334–338

KOMUNE, S., ASAKUMA, S. and SNOW, J. B. (1981) Pathophysiology of the ototoxicity of cis-diamminedichloroplatinum. *Otolaryngology – Head and Neck Surgery*, **89**, 275–282

KOSSL, M., RICHARDSON, G. P. and RUSSELL, I. J. (1990) Stereocilia bundle stiffness: effects of neomycin sulphate, A23187 and concanavalin A. *Hearing Research*, **44**, 217–230

KOTECHA, B. (1993) Aminoglycoside cochleotoxicity: An in vitro study. *M. Phil Thesis*, (University of Sussex)

KOTECHA, B. and RICHARDSON, G. P. (1994) Ototoxicity in vitro: effects of neomycin, gentamicin, dihydrostreptomycin, amikacin, spectinomycin, neamine, spermine and poly-L-lysine. *Hearing Research*, **73**, 173–184

KREIS, B. (1966) Kanamycin toxicity in adults. *Annals of the New York Academy of Sciences*, **132**, 957–967

KROESE, A. B. A. and VAN DEN BERCKEN, J. (1982) Effects of aminoglycosides on sensory hair cell functioning. *Hearing Research*, **6**, 183–197

KROESE, A. B. A., DAS, A. and HUDSPETH, A. J. (1989) Blockage of transduction channels of hair cells in the bullfrog's sacculus by aminoglycosides. *Hearing Research*, **37**, 203–218

KROS, C. J., RUSCH, A. and RICHARDSON, G. P. (1992) Mechano-electrical transducer currents in hair cells of the cultured mouse cochlea. *Proceedings of the Royal Society of London*, **B249**, 185–193

KUSAKARI, J., ISE, I., COMEGYS, T. H., THALMANN, I. and THALMANN, R. (1978) Effects of ethacrynic acid, furosemide and oubain upon the endolymphatic potential and upon high energy phosphates of the stria vascularis. *Laryngoscope*, **88**, 12–37

LAST, P. M. and SHERLOCK, S. (1960) Systemic absorption of orally administered neomycin in liver disease. *New England Journal of Medicine*, **262**, 385–389

LAURELL, G. and BAGGER–SJOBACK, D. (1991a) Degeneration of the organ of Corti following intravenous administration of cisplatin. *Acta Otolaryngologica*, **111**, 891–898

LAURELL, G. and BAGGER–SJOBACK, D. (1991b) Dose-dependent inner ear changes after i.v. administration of cisplatin. *Journal of Otolaryngology*, **20**, 158–167

LAURELL, G. and ENGSTROM, B. (1989a) The ototoxic effect of cisplatin on guinea pigs in relation to dosage. *Hearing Research*, **38**, 27–34

LAURELL, G. and ENGSTROM, B. (1989b) The combined effect of cisplatin and furosemide on hearing function in guinea pig. *Hearing Research*, **38**, 19–16

LEACH, W. (1962) Ototoxicity of neomycin and other antibiotics. *Journal of Laryngology and Otology*, **76**, 774–790

LEFEBVRE, P. P., MALGRANGE, B., STAEKER, H., MOONEN, G. and VAN DE WATER, T. R. (1993) Retinoic acid stimulates regeneration of mammalian auditory hair cells. *Science*, **260**, 692–695

LEFEBVRE, P. P., STAEKER, H., MALGRANGE, B., MOONEN, G. and VAN DE WATER, T. R. (1994) Transforming growth factor alpha (TGF) acts with retinoic acid to stimulate the regeneration of mammalian auditory hair cells. Abstracts, *17th Midwinter Meeting* Academy for Research in Otolaryngology, pp. 115

LIBERMAN, M. C. (1990) Quantitative assessment of inner ear pathology following ototoxic drugs or acoustic trauma. *Toxicologic Pathology*, **18**, 138–148

LINDEMAN, H. H. (1969) Regional differences in sensitivity of the vestibular sensory epithelia to ototoxic antibiotics. *Acta Otolaryngologica*, **67**, 177–189

LINDSAY, J. R., PROCTOR, L. R. and WORK, W. P. (1960) Histopathologic inner ear changes in deafness due to neomycin in a human. *Laryngoscope*, **70**, 382–392

LIPPE, W. R., WESTBROOK, E. W. and RYALS, B. M. (1991) Hair cell regeneration in the chicken cochlea following aminoglycoside ototoxicity. *Hearing Research*, **56**, 203–210

LITTERST, C. L. (1981) Alteration in the toxicity of cis-dichlorodiammine platinum II and in tissue localisation of platinum as a function of NaCl concentration in the vehicle of administration. *Toxicology and Applied Pharmacology*, **61**, 99–108

LITTLE, P. J. and LYNN, K. L. (1975) Neomycin toxicity. *New Zealand Medical Journal*, **81**, 445

LLOYD–MOSTYN, R. N. and LORD, I. J. (1971) Ototoxicity of intravenous frusemide. *Lancet*, ii, 1156–1157

LODHI, S., WEINER, N., MECHIGIAN, I. and SCHACHT, J. (1980) Ototoxicity of aminoglycosides correlated with their action on monomolecular films of polyphosphoinositides. *Biochemical Pharmacology*, **29**, 597–601

LONG, G. R., TUBIS, A. and JONES, K. (1986) Changes in spontaneous and evoked otoacoustic emissions and corresponding psychoacoustic threshold microstructures induced by aspirin consumption. In: *Peripheral Auditory Mechanisms*, edited by J. G. Allen, J. L. Hall, A. Hubbard S. T. Neely, and A. Tubis New York: Springer–Verlag. pp. 213–220

LOWRY, L. D., MAY, M. and PASTORE, P. (1973) Acute histopathologic inner ear changes in deafness due to neomycin; a case report. *Annals of Otology, Rhinology and Laryngology*, **82**, 876–880

LUNDY, L. B. and GRAHAM, M. D. (1992) Ototoxicity and ototopical medications: a survey of otolaryngologists. *American Journal of Otology*, **14**, 141–146

MCALPINE, D. and JOHNSTONE, B. M. (1990) The ototoxic mechanism of cisplatin. *Hearing Research*, **47**, 191–204

MCCABE, P. A. and DEY, D. (1965) The effect of aspirin upon auditory sensitivity. *Annals of Otology, Rhinology and Laryngology*, **74**, 312–325

MCDOWELL, A. (1982) Patterns of cochlear degeneration following gentamicin administration in both old and young guinea pigs. *British Journal of Audiology*, **16**, 123–129

MCFADDEN, D. and PLATTSMIER, H. S. (1983) Aspirin can potentiate the temporary hearing loss induced by intense sounds. *Hearing Research*, **9**, 295–316

MCFADDEN, D., PLATTSMIER, H. S. and PASANEN, E. G. (1984) Aspirin-induced hearing loss as a model of sensorineural hearing loss. *Hearing Research*, **16**, 251–260

MCFADDEN, E. A. and SAUNDERS, J. C. (1989) Recovery of auditory function following intense sound exposure in the chick. *Hearing Research*, **41**, 205–216

MAHER, J. F. and SCHREINER, G. E. (1965) Studies on ethacrynic acid in patients with refractory edema. *Annals of Internal Medicine*, **62**, 15–29

MARCUS, D. C., MARCUS, N. Y. and GREGER, R. (1987) Sidedness of action of loop diuretics and oubain on nonsensory cells of utricle: a micro-Ussing chamber for inner ear tissues. *Hearing Research*, **30**, 55–64

MARCUS, D. C., MARCUS, N. Y. and THALMANN, R. (1981) Changes in cation contents of stria vascularis with ouabain and potassium-free perfusion. *Hearing Research*, **4**, 149–160

MARTIN, G. K., LONSBURY–MARTIN, B. L., PROBST, R. and COATS, A. C. (1988) Spontaneous otoacoustic emissions in a nonhuman primate. 1. Basic features and relations to other emissions. *Hearing Research*, **33**, 49–68

MASUR, H., WHELTON, P. K. and WHELTON, A. (1976) Neomycin toxicity revisited. *Archives of Surgery* (Chicago), **111**, 822–825

MEYERS, R. M. (1972) Ototoxic effects of gentamicin. *Archives of Otolaryngology*, **92**, 160–162

MINTZ, U., AMIR, J., PINKHAS, J. and DE VRIES, A. (1973) Transient perceptive deafness due to erythromycin lactobionate. *Journal of the American Medical Association*, **225**, 1122–1123

MONGAN, E., KELLY, P. and NIES, K. (1973) Tinnitus as an indication of therapeutic serum salicylate levels. *Journal of the American Medical Association*, **226**, 142–145

MORIZONO, T. and SIKORA, M. A. (1981) Ototoxicity of ethanol in the tympanic cleft in animals. *Acta Otolaryngologica*, **92**, 33

MULLER, G. (1877) Beitrag zur wirking der salicylasuren natrons beim dibetes melleus. *Berlin klinik Wochenshrift*, **14**, 29–31

MYERS, E. N. and BERNSTEIN, J. M. (1965) Salicylate ototoxicity. *Archives of Otolaryngology*, **82**, 483–493

NAGABUSHAN, T., MILLER, G. H. and WEINSTEIN, M. J. (1982) Structure-activity relationships in the aminoglycoside aminocyclitol antibiotics. In: *The Aminoglycosides; Microbiology, Clinical Use and Toxicology*, edited by A. Whelton and H. C. Neu. New York: Marcel Dekker

NAKAI, Y. (1977) Combined effect of 3′, 4′-di-deoxy kanamycin B and potent diuretics on the cochlea. *Laryngoscope*, **87**, 1548–1558

NETO, F. R. (1980) Further studies on the actions of salicylates on nerve membranes. *European Journal of Pharmacology*, **68**, 155–162

NEU, H. C. and BENDUSH, C. L. (1976) Ototoxicity of tobramycin: a clinical overview. *Journal of Infectious Disease*, **134**, (suppl.), S206–S218

NICOL, K. M., HACKNEY, C. M., EVANS, E. F. and PRATT, S. R. (1992) Behavioural evidence for recovery of auditory function in guinea pigs following kanamycin administration. *Hearing Research*, **61**, 117–131

NORTON, S. J., BARGONES, J. Y. and RUBEL, E. W. (1991) Development of otoacoustic emissions in gerbil: evidence for micromechanical changes underlying development of the place code. *Hearing Research*, **51**, 73–92

NUTTALL, A. L. (1981) Perfusion of aminoglycosides in perilymph. In: *Aminoglycoside Ototoxicity*, edited by S. A. Lerner, G. J. Matz and J. E. Hawkins Jr. Boston: Little Brown. pp. 51–61

OSBORNE, M. P. and COMIS, S. D. (1990) High resolution

scanning electron microscopy of stereocilia in the cochlea of normal, postmortem, and drug-treated guinea pigs. *Journal of Electron Microscopy*, **15**, 254–260

OZOLS, R. G., DEISROTH, N. and JARADPOUR, A. B. (1983) Treatment of poor prognosis non-seminomatous tubular cancer with a 'high-dose' platinum combination chemotherapy regimen. *Cancer*, **51**, 1803–1807

PEYTRAL, C., HENIN, J. M., VACHER, S. and ISRAEL, V. (1981) Ototoxicite du cisplatinum (CDDP). *Annales d'Otolaryngologie et de Chirurgie Cervicofaciale*, **98**, 85–88

PICKLES, J. O., COMIS, S. D. and OSBORNE, M. P. (1984) Cross-links between stereocilia in the guinea pig organ of Corti, and their possible relation to sensory transduction. *Hearing Research*, **15**, 103–112

PIKE, D. A. and BOSHER, S. K. (1980) The time course of the strial changes produced by intravenous furosemide. *Hearing Research*, **3**, 79–89

PRAZMA, J., VANCE, S. G., BOLSTER, D. E., PILLSBURY, H. C. and POSTMA, D. S. (1987) Cochlear bloodflow: the effect of noise at 60 minutes exposure. *Archives of Otolaryngology – Head and Neck Surgery*, **113**, 36–39

PUEL, J-L., BOBBIN, R. P. and FALLON, M. (1990) Salicylate, mefenamate, meclofenamate, and quinine on cochlear potentials. *Otolaryngology – Head and Neck Surgery* **102**, 66–73

PUEL, J-L., BLEDSOE, S. C. JR, BOBBIN, R. P., CEASAR, G. and FALLON, M. (1989) Comparative actions of salicylate on the amphibian lateral line and guinea pig cochlea. *Comparative Biochemistry and Physiology*, **93C**, 73–80

QUICK, C. A. and HOPPE, W. (1975) Permanent deafness associated with furosemide administration. *Annals of Otology, Rhinology and Laryngology*, **84**, 94–101

RAPHAEL, Y. and ALTSCHULER, R. A. (1991) Scar formation after drug-induced cochlear insult. *Hearing Research*, **51**, 173–184

RICHARDSON, G. P. and RUSSELL, I. J. (1991) Cochlear cultures as a model system for studying aminoglycoside induced ototoxicity. *Hearing Research*, **53**, 293–311

ROCKSTROH, B., ELBERT, T., LUTZENBERGER, W., ALTENMULLER, E., DIENER, H-C., BIRBAUMER, N. *et al.* (1988) Effects of the anticonvulsant carbamazepine on event related brain potentials in humans. In: *Evoked Potentials III, The third evoked potentials symposium*, edited by C. Barber and T. Blum. London: Butterworths

ROWEN, M. J., O'CONNOR, J. J. and ANWYL, R. (1988) Changes in auditory evoked responses in the inhibitory action of 5-hydroxytryptophan following chronic treatment with imipramine in the rat. *Psychopharmacology*, **96**, 408–413

RUBIN, L. L., PHILPOTT, K. L. and BROOKS, S. F. (1993) The cell cycle and cell death. *Current Biology*, **3**, 391–393

RUSSELL, I. J. and RICHARDSON, G. P. (1987). The morphology and physiology of hair cells in organotypic cultures of the mouse cochlea. *Hearing Research*, **31**, 9–24

RUSSELL, W. J., FOX, K. E. and BRUMMETT, R. E. (1979) Ototoxic effects of the interaction between kanamycin and ethacrynic acid. *Acta Otolaryngologica*, **88**, 369–381

RYALS, B. M. and RUBEL, E. W. (1988) Hair cell regeneration after acoustic trauma in adult Coturnix quail. *Science*, **240**, 1774–1776

RYBEK, L. P., WHITWORTH, C. and SCOTT, V. (1991) Comparative acute ototoxicity of loop diuretic compounds. *European Archives of Otorhinolaryngology*, **248**, 353–357

SAITO, T., MOATAZ, R. and DULON, D. (1991) Cisplatin blocks depolarization-induced calcium entry in isolated cochlear outer hair cells. *Hearing Research*, **56**, 143–147

SCHACHT, J. (1986) Molecular mechanisms of drug-induced hearing loss. *Hearing Research*, **22**, 297–304

SCHAEFER, S. D., WRIGHT, C. G. and POST, J. D. (1981) Cisplatinum vestibular therapy toxicity. *Cancer*, **47**, 857–859

SCHATZ, A., BUGIE, E. and WAKSMAN, S. A. (1944) Streptomycin, a substance exhibiting antibiotic activity against Gram positive and Gram negative bacteria. *Proceedings of the Society for Experimental Biology and Medicine*, **55**, 66–69

SCHMIDT, S-H., ANNIKO, M. and HELLSTRON, S. (1990) Electrophysiological effects of the clinically used local anasthetics lidocaine, lidocaine-prilocaine and phenol on the rat's inner ear. *European Archives of Otorhinolaryngology*, **248**, 87–94

SCHULTE, B. A. and ADAMS, J. C. (1989) Distribution of immunoreactive Na + , K + -ATPase in gerbil cochlea. *Journal of Histochemistry and Cytochemistry*, **37**, 127–134

SCHWABACH, D. (1884) Ueber Bleibende storungen im gehororgan nach chinin-und salicylsauregebrauch. *Deutsche Medizinische Wochenschrift (Stuttgart)*, **10**, 163–166

SCHWARTZ, G. A., DAVID, D. S., RIGGIO, R. R., STENZEL, K. H. and RUBIN, A. L. (1970) Ototoxicity induced by furosemide. *New England Journal of Medicine*, **282**, 1413–1414

SCHWEITZER, V. G., RAREY, K. E. and DOLAN, D. F. (1986) Ototoxicity of cisplatin vs. platinum analogs CBDCA (JM-8) and CHIP (JM-9). *Otolaryngology – Head and Neck Surgery*, **94**, 458–470

SHEHATA, W. E., BROWNELL, W. E. and DIELER, R. (1991) Effects of salicylate on shape, electromotility and membrane characteristics of isolated outer hair cells from the guinea pig cochlea. *Acta Otolaryngologica*, **111**, 707–718

SMITH, C. R., BAUGHAN, K. L., EDWARDS, C. Q., ROGERS, J. F. and LEITMAN, P. S. (1977) Controlled comparison of amikacin and gentamicin. *New England Journal of Medicine*, **296**, 349–353

SOLOMONS, N. and MADDEN, G. (1992) Are antibiotic-containing ear drops ototoxic when applied to the middle ear? *Health Trends*, **24**, 64–65

SPICER, S. S., SCHULTE, B. A. and ADAMS, J. C. (1990) Immunolocalisation of Na + , K + -ATPase and carbonic anhydrase in the gerbil's vestibular system. *Hearing Research*, **43**, 205–218

STEBBINS, W. C., MCGINN, C. S., FEITOSA, M. A. G., MOODY, D. B., PROSEN, C. A. and SERAFIN, J. V. (1981) Animal models in the study of ototoxic hearing loss. In: *Aminoglycoside Ototoxicity*, edited by S. A. Lerner, G. J. Matz and J. E. Hawkins Jr. Boston: Little Brown. pp. 5–25

STEPHENS, S. D. G. (1982) Some historical aspect of ototoxicity. *British Journal of Audiology*, **16**, 76–80

STERKERS, O., SAUMON, G., TRAN BA HUY, P. and AMIEL, C. (1982) K, Cl, and H$_2$0 entry in perilymph, endolymph and cerebrospinal fluid of the rat. *American Journal of Physiology*, **243**, F173–F180

STYPULKOWSKI, P. H. (1990) Mechanisms of salicylate ototoxicity. *Hearing Research*, **46**, 113–145

SUGARBAKER, P. H., SABATH, L. D. and MORGAN, A. P. (1974) Neomycin toxicity from porcine skin xenografts. *Annals of Surgery*, **179**, 183–185

TAKADA, A., BLEDSOE, S. and SCHACHT, J. (1985) An energy-dependent step in aminoglycoside ototoxicity; prevention of gentamicin ototoxicity during reduced endolymph potential. *Hearing Research*, **19**, 245–251

THALMANN, R., ISE, I., BOHNE, B. A. and THALMANN, I. (1977) Actions of 'loop' diuretics and mercurials upon the cochlea. *Acta Otolaryngologica*, **83**, 221–232

TJERNSTROM, O. (1980) Prospective evaluation of vestibular and auditory function in 76 patients treated with netilmicin. *Scandinavian Journal of Infectious Disease*, Supplement 23, 122–125

TJERNSTROM, O., BANCK, G., BELFRAGE, S., JUHLIN, I., NORDSTROM, L. and TORREMALM, N. G. (1973) The ototoxicity of gentamicin. *Acta Pathologica Microbiologica Scandinavica*, Supplement 241, 73–78

TOONE, E. C. Jr, HAYDEN, G. D. and ELLMAN, H. M. (1965) Ototoxicity of chloroquine. *Arthritis and Rheumatism*, **8**, 475–476

TRAN BA HUY, P., BERNARD, P. and SCHACHT, J. (1986) Kinetics of gentamicin uptake and release in the rat: comparison of inner ear tissues and fluids with other organs. *Journal of Clinical Investigation*, **77**, 1492–1500

TRAN BA HUY, P., MANUEL, C., MEULEMANS, A., STERKERS, O. and AMIEL, C. (1981) Pharmacokinetics of gentamicin in perilymph and endolymph of the rat as determined by radioimmunoassay. *Journal of Infectious Disease*, **143**, 476–486

TUCCI, D. L. and RUBEL, E. W. (1990) Physiological status of regenerated hair cells in the avian inner ear following aminoglycoside ototoxicity. *Otolaryngology – Head and Neck Surgery*, **103**, 443–450

VERNON, J. and BRUMMETT, R. E. (1977) Noise trauma induced in presence of loop-inhibiting diuretics. *Transactions of the American Academy of Ophthalmology and Otolaryngology*, **84**, 407–413

VESTERHAUGE, S., JOHNSEN, N. J., THOMSEN, J. and SVARE, J. (1980) Netilmicin treatment followed by monitoring of vestibular and auditory function using highly sensitive methods. *Scandinavian Journal of Infectious Disease*, Supplement 23, 117–121

WAKSMAN, S. A., BUGIE, E. and SCHATZ, A. (1944) Isolation of antibiotic substances from soil microorganisms with special reference to streptothricin and streptomycin. *Proceedings of Staff Meetings at Mayo Clinic*, **19**, 537–548

WALBY, A. P. and KERR, A. G. (1982) Streptomycin sulphate and deafness: a review of the literature. *Clinical Otolaryngology*, **7**, 63–68

WANGEMANN, P. and GREGER, R. (1990) Piretanide inhibits the $Na + 2Cl - K +$ carrier in the thick ascending limb of the loop of Henle and reduces the metabolic fuel requirement of this nephron segment. In: *Diuretics III: Chemistry, Pharmacology and Clinical Applications*, edited by J. B. Puschett and Greenberg. Amsterdam: Elsevier. pp. 220–224

WANGEMANN, P., LIU, J. and MARCUS, D. C. (1995) Ion transport mechanisms responsible for K^+ secretion and the transepithelial voltage across marginal cells of the stria vascularis in vitro. *Hearing Research*, **84**, 19–29

WARCHOL, M. E., LAMBERT, P. R., GOLDSTEIN, B. J., FORGE, A. and CORWIN, J. T. (1993) Regenerative proliferation in inner ear sensory epithelia from adult guinea pigs and humans. *Science*, **259**, 1619–1622

WARD, K. M. and ROUTHWAITE, F. J. (1978) Neomycin ototoxicity. *Annals of Otology, Rhinology and Laryngology*, **87**, 211–215

WARD, P. R., TUCKER, A. M., TUDOR, C. A. and MORGAN, D. C. (1977) Self assessment of hearing impairment. *British Journal of Audiology*, **11**, 33–39

WATERS, E. S., AHMAD, M. and KATSARKAS, A. (1991) Ototoxicity due to cis-diamminedichloroplatinum in the treatment of ovarian cancer: influence of dosage and schedule of administration. *Ear and Hearing*, **12**, 91–102

WEINSTEIN, M. L., LEUDEMANN, G. M., ODEN, E. M. and WAGMAN, G. H. (1963) Gentamicin a new broad spectrum antibiotic complex. *Antimicrobial Agents and Chemotherapy*, **3**, 1–7

WEINSTEIN, M. L., MARQUEZ, J. A., TESTA, R. T., WAGMAN, G. H., ODEN, E. M. and WAITZ, J. A. (1970) Antibiotic 66–40: a new micromonospora produced aminoglycoside antibiotic. *Journal of Antibiotics (Tokyo)*, **23**, 551–554

WEISLEDER, P. and RUBEL, E. W. (1993) Hair cell regeneration after streptomycin toxicity in the avian vestibular epithelium. *Journal of Comparative Neurology*, **331**, 97–110

WERSALL, J. (1981) Structural damage to the organ of Corti and the vestibular epithelia caused by amino-glycoside antibiotics in the guinea pig. In: *Aminoglycoside Ototoxicity*, edited by S. A. Lerner, G. J. Matz and J. E. Hawkins Jr. Boston: Little Brown. pp. 197–214

WILLIAMS, S. E., SMITH, D. E. and SCHACHT, J. (1987) Characteristics of gentamicin uptake in the isolated crista ampullaris of the inner ear of the guinea pig. *Biochemical Pharmacology*, **36**, 89–95

WILLIAMS, S. E., ZENNER, H.-P. and SCHACHT, J. (1987) Three molecular steps of aminoglycoside ototoxicity demonstrated in outer hair cells. *Hearing Research*, **30**, 11–18

WINKEL, O., HANSEN, M. M., KAABER, K. and ROZARTH, Z. (1978) A prospective study of gentamicin ototoxicity. *Acta Otolaryngologica*, **86**, 212–216

WOODFORD, C. M., HENDERSON, D. and HAMERNIK, R. P. (1978) Effects of combinations of sodium salicylate and noise on the auditory threshold. *Annals of Otology, Rhinology and Laryngology*, **87**, 117–127

WRIGHT, C. and MEYERHOFF, W. (1984) Ototoxicity of otic drops applied to the middle ear in the chinchilla. *American Journal of Otolaryngology*, **5**, 166–176

WRIGHT, J. J. (1976) Synthesis of 1-N ethyl sisomycin: a broad spectrum, semi-synthetic aminoglycoside antibiotic. *Chemical Communication*, 206–208

ZAJIC, G. and SCHACHT, J. (1987) Comparison of isolated outer hair cells from five mammalian species. *Hearing Research*, **26**, 249–256

ZAJIC, G., ANNIKO, M. and SCHACHT, J. (1983) Cellular localization of adenylate-cyclase in the developing and mature inner ear of the mouse. *Hearing Research*, **10**, 249–261

21

Vestibular schwannoma

Richard T. Ramsden

History

Vestibular schwannomas (acoustic neuromas) have always held a great fascination for otolaryngologists. There are a number of reasons for this. The great majority of tumours present with deafness and tinnitus, so the initial responsibility for diagnosis lies with the otologist. Microsurgical skills, which are so important in the removal of these tumours, were first used by otologists whose familiarity with temporal bone anatomy has had a significant effect on surgical results. It is probably also fair to state that otologists have traditionally regarded the physical and psychological effects of facial paralysis with more gravity than was the custom of the earlier neurosurgeons, many of whom felt that the loss of the facial nerve was a small and acceptable price to pay for the removal of an intracranial tumour. Up until the postwar period the surgery of vestibular schwannomas was almost exclusively performed by neurosurgeons who regarded occasional sorties by otologists into their territories with some disdain. It has, however, become increasingly apparent during the past 30 years that it is only by close cooperation between the otologists and neurosurgeons that the high ideals of early diagnosis, total removal, low mortality and morbidity, preservation of the facial nerve and on occasion the hearing can be achieved. The internal auditory meatus instead of being a boundary between otologists and neurosurgeons has become a zone of mutual activity neatly though unintentionally implied in its classical source (*meatus*, 'a coming together').

Pirsig, Ziemann-Becker and Teschler-Nicola (1992) described the temporal bone findings in two Early Bronze Age children excavated from the prehistoric burial site at Franzhausen, Austria. These skulls date from around 2000–2300 BC and are thus approxi-

mately 4000 years old. Both children exhibited marked widening of one internal auditory meatus and in one there appears to be expansion into the vestibule and cochlea. The changes are particularly elegantly and hauntingly demonstrated on CT images of the cadaver temporal bones. The authors suggested that these two children suffered from neurofibromatosis type 2 (NF2).

It would appear, however, that the first case of acoustic neuroma or vestibular schwannoma, to be fully documented was that of Sandifort of Leiden, in 1777, in an article entitled 'De duro quodam corpusculo, nervo auditorio adhaerente', in which he described the post-mortem finding of a small firm tumour of the auditory nerve, emerging from the internal auditory meatus and compressing the medulla in a patient who had complained of deafness. Sandifort declared that because of its position the tumour was accessible 'neither to medicines nor the hand'. Sir Charles Bell, in 1830, provided one of the earliest clinicopathological correlations in a patient who was referred to him as a case of tic douloureux, and went on to develop deafness, dizziness and facial paralysis before dying of apparent brain stem compression and raised intracranial pressure. At post mortem, a semicystic tumour the size of a pigeon's egg was found in the cerebellopontine angle, indenting the pons, extending into the internal meatus and involving the Vth and VIIth cranial nerves.

Throughout the nineteenth century there appeared an increasing number of clinicopathological descriptions of what, despite somewhat ambiguous histopathological reports, were certainly vestibular schwannomas (e.g. Cruveilhier, 1835; Toynbee, 1853; Stevens, 1879; Oppenheim, 1890), and the reader is referred to the review by Harvey Cushing (1917) for further details of this fascinating period. Ballance (1907) is usually credited with the first successful removal of an acoustic neuroma in 1892, but Cushing felt that his case was more likely to have been a meningioma and attributes the honour to Thomas Annandale of Edinburgh in 1895 – 'a brilliant surgical result, the first recorded'. Generally, however, the mortality and morbidity of early surgical series were dauntingly high, due to late presentation, poor anaesthesia and instrumentation, haemorrhage, and above all to the feeling that these tumours could be enucleated rapidly with the finger, a manoeuvre that inevitably resulted in serious bleeding from the anterior inferior cerebellar artery, the importance of which was not appreciated. Indeed, it is significant that Ballance, in 1907, expressed the view that the surgical results might be improved if that artery could be ligated prior to removal of the tumour.

The first attempts at surgical removal were by way of the unilateral suboccipital approach favoured by Krause (1903), that particular writer reporting an operative mortality of 83.8%. In a visionary article in 1904, Panse proposed that an approach through the labyrinth might allow removal of an acoustic neuroma as large as a hen's egg. He defined the anatomical limits of that exposure, the lateral sinus, the jugular bulb, the carotid artery and the temporal lobe but felt that the facial nerve must inevitably be sacrificed. However, he suggested that in certain tumours of this region the facial nerve should be rerouted after being mobilized from the geniculate ganglion to the stylomastoid foramen, thus anticipating Fisch by three-quarters of a century. The translabyrinthine approach appears to have been first employed, in 1911, by Kummel in Heidelberg (Marx, 1913) and Quix (1912), in Utrecht, but failed to find widespread acceptance, Ballance dismissing it as 'objectionable for obvious reasons'. In 1917, Harvey Cushing, in his monograph 'Tumours of the Nervus Acusticus and the Syndrome of the Cerebellopontile Angle', described his bilateral suboccipital approach to the posterior fossa which allowed not only a wide decompression, but also the possibility of exploring both sides in cases in which there was doubt as to the side of the lesion. He recommended a subtotal intracapsular removal, and was able to reduce the operative mortality by 1931 to 4%, this despite the fact that the tumours were almost always very large with hydrocephalus, brain stem compression and failing vision. Dandy (1925), however, was strongly in favour of a total removal via a unilateral suboccipital approach.

The surgical results of these two great American neurosurgeons were certainly an encouraging improvement on those of their predecessors, but despite that and the invaluable contribution of Atkinson (1949) in clarifying the importance of the anterior inferior cerebellar artery, there remained a certain reluctance on the part of neurosurgeons to embark on this type of surgery unless the tumour was so large as to be causing pressure effects on the brain stem, or raised intracranial pressure. Many patients were in effect told that their tumours were too small for surgery and to return when they had grown larger!

It was to this unique surgical anomaly that William House directed his attention in the early 1960s, developing first the middle fossa, and shortly afterwards the translabyrinthine approach to the internal auditory meatus (House, 1961, 1964). The great improvement in results achieved by his group, in terms both of mortality and morbidity, particularly to the facial nerve, is largely the consequence of the policy of early diagnosis and surgery and owes much to advances in diagnostic techniques in the fields of both radiology and audiology and the evolution of microsurgery as an essential skill for both otologist and neurosurgeon. Rand and Kurze (1965) were among the first neurosurgeons to apply microsurgical techniques to acoustic neuroma removal via the suboccipital transmeatal route. The middle fossa approach has been shown by a number of workers, particularly Wigand, Haid and Berg (1989) to be less restrictive than previously thought, with good access to the posterior fossa for all but the very largest tumours. In recent years, there have been rapid changes in the audiological and radiological assessment of patients suspected of having an acoustic neuroma. Audiological localization in cases of unilateral sensorineural deafness developed in the postwar period, and culminated in the use of the auditory brain stem response (ABR). In the past decade the role of traditional audiological testing has lessened with the advent of sensitive imaging techniques, initially the CT scan and, in the last 5 years with magnetic resonance imaging (MRI). The latter provides the surgeon with the ability to demonstrate even the smallest of lesions, always assuming he is prepared to use it. Surgery remains the preferred treatment for most tumours, despite claims from the proponents of stereotactic radiosurgery (the gamma knife). Preservation of the facial nerve has become the norm rather than the exception, and conservation of useful hearing is possible in a small number of selected patients. The detection of tumour growth factors, markers which can accurately predict patterns of growth in individual tumours may allow surgeons to identify patients for whom surgery is unnecessary. Perhaps the most exciting recent developments have been in the field of molecular biology which has revealed the fundamental chromosomal abnormality in vestibular schwannoma and in neurofibromatosis type 2. The possibilty in the future of treating these tumours by chromosomal manipulation is one which should not be discounted.

Anatomy

The cerebellopontine angle is a triangular area bounded laterally by the medial portion of the posterior surface of the temporal bone, medially by the edge of the pons and posteriorly by the anterior surface of the cerebellar hemisphere and the flocculus, and is part of the lateral medullary cistern. Superiorly it is limited by the trigeminal nerve as it crosses the petrous apex and by the edge of the tentorium. Its inferior limit is formed by the lower cranial nerves (IX, X, XI) as they enter the jugular foramen, and by the hypoglossal nerve. It contains one important artery, the anterior inferior cerebellar artery, and two cranial nerves, the facial and vestibulocochlear, as they pass from their points of origin at the pontomedullary junction towards the internal auditory meatus.

The internal meatus is a passage through the petrous bone leading from the posterior surface of the temporal bone to the medial wall of the vestibule. It has a porus, or inlet, medially with a sharply defined crescentic posterior lip and a rather poorly demarcated anterior edge, a canal proper which is roughly cylindrical and a fundus laterally which is separated from the vestibule by a thin plate of bone. The lateral wall of the meatus presents several features of great surgical importance (see Plate 3/21/I). It is divided into superior and inferior halves by the falciform crest. The upper compartment is further separated into an anterior area for the facial nerve and a posterior area for the superior vestibular nerve by a sharp vertical ridge of bone known as 'Bill's bar' after William House. The lower half also comprises two areas: anteriorly, the tractus spiralis foraminosus or cribrose area through which the spiralling fibres of the cochlear nerve pass, and posteriorly the rather smaller area for the inferior vestibular nerve supplying the saccule. The singular nerve, a branch of the inferior vestibular nerve supplying the ampulla of the posterior semicircular canal, passes through a small canal on the floor of the meatus, about 1 mm from the fundus.

The VIIth and VIIIth nerves leave the brain stem at the region of the pontomedullary junction, at which point they are closely related to each other and here it is impossible to make out the individual components of the vestibulocochlear nerve. As they pass laterally separation between them becomes more apparent, and at the level of the porus, four individual nerves can be identified, the facial and nervus intermedius anterosuperiorly, the superior vestibular posterosuperiorly, the cochlear anteroinferiorly, and the inferior vestibular posteroinferiorly (see Figure 21.3).

The anterior inferior cerebellar artery usually arises from the basilar artery as a single trunk, and in the cerebellopontine angle forms a loop which has an intimate, but somewhat variable, relationship with the facial and vestibulocochlear nerves and with the internal auditory meatus; on occasion the artery may in fact loop right into the meatus (see Figure 2.13*b*). The main branches of the anterior inferior cerebellar artery are the internal auditory and subarcuate arteries, and these tend to tether the anterior inferior cerebellar artery to the posterior surface of the temporal bone. It is important to realize that this is a region of considerable anatomical variation, and for further details the reader is referred to the excellent post-mortem studies of Mazzoni and Hansen (1970) and of Rhoton *et al.* (1982).

The most important venous structures in this region are the lateral sinus and the jugular bulb which sweeps up below the internal meatus, but which may, if high, be a posterior relation of the meatus, and may interfere with surgical access to the meatus. On rare occasions a diverticulum of the jugular bulb may extend up as far as the middle fossa dura. The superior petrosal sinus runs in the line of attachment of the tentorium to the petrous ridge, from the cavernous sinus anteriorly to the lateral sinus posteriorly. The petrosal vein drains into it anteriorly, and is commonly encountered in the surgical field during tumour removal.

The relationship of the meninges to the internal meatus and its contents is of considerable surgical importance. The dura of the posterior surface of the temporal bone is firmly adherent round the porus where it merges with the periosteal lining of the meatus. The pia-arachnoid, on the other hand, continues into the meatus investing the VIIth and VIIIth nerves in individual or common sheaths, and blending with the neurilemma. The subarachnoid space, therefore, extends laterally to the fundus of the meatus, and may even follow the labyrinthine portion of the facial nerve as far as the middle ear.

Pathology

Site of origin

The term 'acoustic neuroma' though hallowed by long usage is doubly inaccurate and should be replaced in scientific communications by 'vestibular schwannoma', although such is its place in history that it will doubtless persist for years in the demotic patois of otology. As Schuknecht (1974) has pointed out, over the years there have been a number of terms that have been used to describe these tumours, neuromas, neurofibromas, neurolemmomas, perineural fibroblastomas, none of which accurately reflects the tissue of origin. It would seem that they arise from the Schwann cells which envelope the distal portion of the VIIIth nerve from the point at which the neuroglial elements cease. This area, the glial neurilemmal junction is thought to be a zone of cellular instability and is considered by some authorities to be the site of origin of these tumours. Schuknecht (1974) disagreed with this view and stated that a tumour can arise from any point on the VIIIth nerve between the glial neurolemmal junction and the cribrose area. It is, however, clear that, because this junctional area is usually situated within the internal auditory meatus, most tumours originate within that canal, an observation that was first made by Henschen in 1912. It also apparent that the majority of tumours arise on one or other branch of the vestibular nerve rather than the cochlear nerve (Nager, 1969), hence the desire for semantic purity. A small but important percentage of tumours arises more medially, in the cerebellopontine angle itself rather than the meatus, presumably because of variation in the location of the glial neurolemmal junction. In fact Schuknecht (1974) observed that the glial neurolemmal junction of the cochlear nerve is situated more medially than that of the vestibular nerve. The importance of this group of tumours lies in the fact that they can expand silently in the cerebellopontine angle without the early audiovestibular symptoms associated with an intrameatal mass, and may thus reach a considerable size by the time they present (Moffat *et al.*, 1993a). A recent study by Tallan, Harner and Beatty (1993), however, casts some doubt on these orthodox views about tumour origin. Using digital morphological analysis of the facial and vestibulocochlear nerves as well as light microscopy and immunohistochemical techniques, they were unable to explain the observed distribution of schwannomas by the distribution of Schwann cells and could find no disordered arrangement of Schwann cells in the region of the glial Schwann cell junction.

Little was known about the aetiogical factors that might render a subject liable to develop a vestibular schwannoma until the recent advances in molecular biology made it clear that a defect of chromosome 22q is responsible for the development of both sporadic unilateral vestibular schwannomas and of the bilateral lesions of neurofibromatosis type 2, a topic which will be examined later in this chapter. An important paper which has been largely ignored in the literature is that of Shore–Freedman *et al.* (1983). They located 2311 subjects who had had childhood irradiation treatment for enlarged tonsils and adenoids at the Michael Reece Hospital in Chicago; the mean follow up was 35 years. The authors found 29 'neurolemmomas', two neurofibromas and one ganglioneuroma, and 10 of the total presented as vestibular schwannomas (compare this with the usually quoted annual incidence of 1:100 000). As an aside it is interesting to record that there were, in addition, 54 salivary gland tumours in the group.

Pattern of growth

As the tumour grows within the internal auditory meatus, it causes progressive but slow destruction of the vestibular nerve from which it arises and produces pressure effects on the adjacent cochlear and facial nerves as well as changes in the meatal blood vessels. Because the tumour arises in the nerve

sheath it tends in the early stages to compress rather than invade nerve fibres, so that there appears to be a good plane of surgical dissection between tumour and nerve. Several studies have suggested that this plane may be more apparent than real and that microscopic invasion of the cochlear and facial nerves may occur (Neely, 1981; Luetje *et al.*, 1983; Marquet *et al.*, 1990). These observations are of great relevance to the hearing preservation debate and will be discussed in more detail later. The tumour is invested in a layer of arachnoid, and as it expands in a medial direction it invaginates the arachnoid and creates a double layer which covers the whole tumour and separates it from adjacent structures (Di Tullio, Malkasian and Rand, 1978) (Figure 21.1).

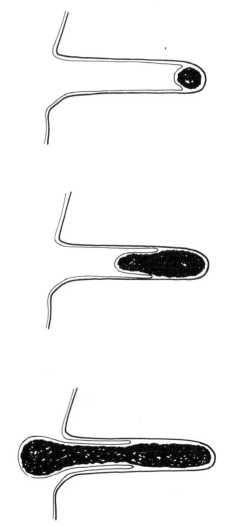

Figure 21.1 The expanding tumour grows medially and invaginates the arachnoid, producing a double layer plane of dissection

This is an important surgical plane, adherence to which minimizes trauma to the facial nerve, the brain stem and the major vessels in the posterior fossa during tumour removal. At an early stage of growth the tumour causes a rise in cerebrospinal fluid protein, which in turn may cause an arachnoiditis, often leading to development of an arachnoid cyst in relation to the tumour. The tumour may be small and the cyst large or vice versa. Erosion of the walls of the internal meatus occurs, particularly at the porus; occasionally in a well pneumatized temporal bone, the tumour may break through into a supralabyrinthine air cell system, and continue to grow within the petrous bone. The relationship of such an extension to the facial nerve may be complex and the situation demands extra vigilance on the part of the surgeon. Extensive intrapetrous spread is rare but Woolford, Birzgalis and Ramsden (1994) described a very large vestibular schwannoma which caused widespread destruction of the petrous bone and presented with a mass in the external ear canal and neck (in addition to the 4 cm intracranial component!).

Within the meatus, the facial nerve is usually to be found on the anterior surface of the tumour, between the tumour and the anterior wall of the meatus. A tumour arising on the cochlear division of the VIIIth nerve may however displace the facial nerve upwards and backwards, and the surgeon has to be aware of this variation, because the facial nerve will then be the first neural structure he will encounter on opening the posterosuperior aspect of the meatus in the translabyrinthine operation. As expansion continues in a medial direction, the cerebellopontine angle is entered, and because this is a relatively large empty space, growth may proceed quite silently. The facial nerve becomes progressively more attenuated usually over the anterior surface of the expanding tumour. The tumour also displaces the anterior inferior cerebellar artery and develops a blood supply from it, although Perneczky (1981) maintains that most of the tumour blood supply is from meningeal vessels. Lye, Elstow and Weiss (1986) described an endothelial cell stimulating angiogenic factor (ESAF) which is responsible for new vessel formation in a number of intracranial neoplasms including vestibular schwannoma. The anterior inferior cerebellar artery and the facial nerve, though often considerably displaced by the tumour, remain separated from it by the double arachnoid layer referred to previously. Rarely, a loop of anterior inferior cerebellar artery may become compressed within the meatus, between the tumour and the bony meatal wall with resultant ischaemic effects on the cerebellum.

When the tumour reaches about 2 cm intracranial diameter, its upper pole makes contact with the trigeminal nerve as it crosses the petrous apex to enter Meckel's cave, and compresses it against the pons and midbrain. At this stage sensory changes on the face and in particular depressed corneal sensation may be apparent to the examiner. The lower pole of the tumour displaces the IXth, Xth and XIth cranial nerves but these seem relatively resistant to pressure and stretching. Brain stem and cerebellar involvement follow and quite marked degrees of brain stem shift may occur (Figure 21.2) to the extent that ultimately contralateral false localizing signs may be seen. (Cushing's bilateral suboccipital approach was developed partly because of the problems of false lateralization.) In addition, the tumour may pass ventral to the brain stem and may ultimately reach almost to the opposite temporal bone. The VIth cranial nerve may become stretched over the surface. Because of the size of the cerebellopontine angle, the slow rate of growth of the tumour, and the capacity of the brain to accomodate to quite a striking degree of shift, if slowly applied, the posterior fossa can accommodate a surprisingly large mass before serious changes in CSF hydrodynamics occur. A stage is, however, eventually reached when there is no more slack in the system. Hydrocephalus with papilloedema and brain stem embarrassment may rapidly ensue, especially if, as may often happen, there is spontaneous haemorrage into the tumour. Hydrocephalus may be obstructive or communicating. In the former, the distortion of the brain stem from the tumour causes obstruction of the aqueduct with

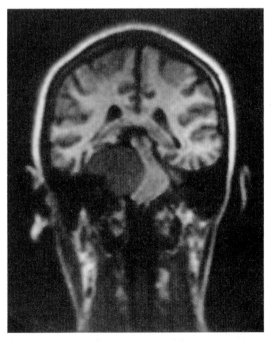

Figure 21.2 MRI of large cerebellopontine angle lesion (meningioma) to demonstrate marked degree of brain stem distortion (but no hydrocephalus)

dilation of the third and lateral ventricles, but compression of the fourth ventricle. Communicating hydrocephalus is seen as a result of high protein levels in the CSF and in this situation, typically there is dilation of the fourth ventricle.

Tumour growth factors

Most vestibular schwannomas grow slowly, on average approximately 2 mm per year (Valvassori and Guzman, 1989). It is clear, however, that there may be considerable variation in growth rate and in clinical progression. Some patients harbour small tumours for decades, without any perceivable change in clinical findings; indeed, it is well known that small asymptomatic tumours are often found by chance at post-mortem examination. On the other hand, it is not uncommon to encounter instances of rapid tumour growth of up to, or exceeding, 10 mm per year (Nedzelski *et al.*, 1992; Sterkers *et al.*, 1992). Much effort has recently been directed towards identifying methods of evaluating tumour growth, as well as factors that may account for the great variations seen. The ability to predict the future growth pattern of an individual tumour would be of great value in planning treatment, and might allow the identification of a group of patients for whom surgery is unnecessary. One of the most obvious ways to monitor tumour growth is by the use of CT or MR imaging; the latter is much more useful because of its higher resolution and ability to demonstrate tumour within the bony internal meatus. Most recent studies have measured linear growth either in a true lateral to medial axis, or in a plane parallel to the posterior surface of the petrous bone. Better information, however, may in future be gained from three-dimensional volumetric studies, and a recent study by Arriaga, Long and Nelson (1993) did show that facial nerve outcome at surgery was significantly related to tumour volume and was best predicted as a nonlinear function of diameter. In other words even small changes in tumour diameter may be associated with significant volume changes that can adversely affect the facial nerve result.

Sterkers *et al.* (1992) in a CT/MR study found an average annual growth rate of 1.4 mm in 21 unoperated elderly patients (range 0– > 5 mm). In patients with tumour recurrence or regrowth following surgery, they found the rate to be higher (3 mm per year). These authors also suggested that the rate of growth might be higher in younger patients than in the elderly. In a similar study, Nedzelski *et al.* (1992) analysed the growth rate in 50 unoperated patients most of whom were over 65 years of age. They quoted an annual growth rate of 1.1 mm, ranging from an actual reduction in size of 5 mm to an increase of 9.8 mm. The majority of tumours (78%) showed little or no growth. These two studies cer-

tainly suggest that in old patients tumour growth may be slow, and could justify a 'wait and rescan' policy. Comparative data for younger patients would be of interest, but because younger patients are usually advised to have their tumours removed early, this information is not available. Nedzelski *et al.* (1992) also stated that tumour growth is linear (i.e. a slowly growing tumour is always a slowly growing tumour). There is some evidence from Charabi *et al.* (1995) that this is not always the case. There are of course factors other than mitotic activity that may cause sudden rapid tumour expansion, such as arachnoid cyst formation and haemorrhage into the tumour.

At the present time there are no simple laboratory tests that will allow one to predict the biological behaviour of a vestibular schwannoma. Several teams of workers have employed a number of different techniques to look at certain aspects of cellular function. In a number of studies flow cytometry has been used to examine the DNA content of vestibular schwannoma cells and to examine the number of cells in S phase (the S phase percentage); S phase is that part of the cell cycle during which DNA replication occurs. The study of Rasmussen *et al.* (1984) failed to reveal a relationship between the S phase percentage and growth rate. Wennerberg and Merke (1989) in a similar study could find no correlation between the S phase percentage and the volume of tumour assessed at surgery. Studies using Ki 67 monoclonal antibody to label proliferating cells have been reported by Lesser *et al.* (1991) and by Pasquier *et al.* (1992). In the former study, the authors identified two groups of tumours, one with a proliferation rate five times that of the other and felt that this test could be used to differentiate between aggressive and non-aggressive tumours. Pasquier *et al.* (1992), on other hand, were unable to gain useful information regarding tumour growth using this technique. These authors did, however, report a weak correlation between between tumour size and the number of nuclear organizer regions (NOR) in the cell nucleus. The nuclear organizer regions are made up of ribosomal RNA and their numbers are related to the transcription rate. Wiet, Ruby and Bauer (1994) looked at proliferating cell nuclear antigen (PCNA), which is formed during S phase and is essential for DNA synthesis. They found a statistically significant relationship between proliferating cell nuclear antigen levels and tumour size, but only comparing tumours greater or smaller than 3 cm. With a 2 cm cut off no correlation was seen.

It has frequently been stated that there is a female to male preponderance in the incidence of vestibular schwannoma, and this has led to a number of studies to try to identify sex hormone receptors associated with these tumours. Martuza, MacLaughlin and Ojemann (1981) reported demonstrating receptors, but the studies of Curley *et al.* (1990), Klinken *et al.*

(1990) and Martin, Prades and Cuelikh (1992) all failed to confirm these findings. Analysis of the sex incidence in the present author's series of over 400 vestibular schwannomas has been carried out with a statistical correction for the known extra longevity of women, and the conclusions suggested that the previously reported female preponderance may have been more apparent than real (Evans *et al.*, 1995). The other factor which affects the biological behaviour of vestibular schwannomas is the presence of neurofibromatosis type 2. Most sporadic unilateral tumours present in the fifth and sixth decades, whereas in neurofibromatosis type 2 most cases are clinically apparent by the age of 20–30 years. The genetics of neurofibromatosis type 2 will be discussed later in this chapter.

If a reliable cytological marker could be identified, then one could imagine a therapeutic regimen based on analysis of biopsy material obtained at a minimally invasive procedure, such as cerebellopontine angle endoscopy, a technique which is being used by some for examination of the posterior fossa and for vestibular nerve section (Magnan *et al.*, 1994). The search to identify an immunological marker in the bloodstream has, as yet, met with little success, although Rasmussen, Thomsen and Tos (1981) were able to demonstrate cell-mediated immunity against vestibular schwannoma in four patients out of 11 before surgery, as well as in one normal control (out of 16), using the leucocyte inhibition capillary tube technique. The identification of a reliable marker in the bloodstream might possibly allow one to predict tumour growth by means of a simple blood test. Anniko, Arndt and Noren (1981) were able to grow vestibular schwannoma cells in organ culture and demonstrated that they were highly radioresistant.

Effects on the inner ear

Degenerative changes in the cellular structures of the inner ear, and biochemical alterations in the inner ear fluids secondary to the presence of a vestibular schwannoma in the internal auditory meatus have been frequently described (De Moura, Hayden and Conner, 1969; Schuknecht, 1974), and may account for the fact that in many cases of vestibular schwannoma the audiological picture may appear to be cochlear, or exhibit mixed cochlear and retrocochlear features. Suga and Lindsay (1976) postulated that cochlear changes may result from interference with the arterial blood supply of the inner ear from pressure of the tumour on branches of the internal auditory artery. They pointed out, however, that the venous drainage of the inner ear is mainly by way of the canals for the cochlear and vestibular aqueducts, rather than via the internal meatus, and that venous backpressure on the cochlea from meatal obstruction is unlikely to be responsible for the inner ear changes

suggested by Brunner (1925) and Watkyn-Thomas (1939). Degeneration is more commonly seen in the cochlea than in the otolith organs or in the semicircular canals. There may be atrophy of the organ of Corti, most frequently seen in the basal turn, but occasionally widespread or complete. Vacuolization of the stria vascularis has been frequently reported, notably by Suga and Lindsay (1976), who observed that quite extensive strial damage could be associated with surprisingly good preservation of the organ of Corti, and of the endolymphatic spaces of the cochlea and vestibule, leading them to conclude that only a small amount of normal stria is necessary for the maintenance of the normal volume of endolymph in the inner ear. The other notable change reported has been in the spiral ganglion, the cells of which may be extensively or totally lost. Jahnke and Neuman (1992) described the fine structural changes in the vestibular end organ seen on transmission electron microscopy: high amounts of fibrous long-spacing collagen, marked thickening and doubling of the capillary basement membrane, mucoid degeneration in the subepithelial space and severe degeneration of sensory and non-sensory epithelia. They considered these changes to be the result of high protein levels in the perilymph.

Protein elevation in the inner ear fluids was first described by Dix and Hallpike (1950) and has been the subject of many subsequent studies (Silverstein and Schuknecht, 1966). An exudate may even be seen in the perilymphatic spaces of the cochlea (Figure 21.3). Several attempts have been made to identify the protein electrophoretically, in samples of perilymph taken at the time of translabyrinthine surgery, but the main problem appears to be in obtaining a sample free from contamination with blood. O'Connor *et al.* (1982) were unable to identify a protein pattern specific to vestibular schwannoma. Palva and Raunio (1982) carried out immunodiffusion tests using anticerebrospinal fluid, antitumour antiserum pooled from five patients with vestibular schwannomas and were able to demonstrate cerebrospinal fluid and tumour specific proteins in the perilymph. They suggested that cerebrospinal fluid proteins could enter through the cochlear aqueduct, and tumour protein through small channels in the cribrose area.

The occurrence of tiny schwannomas confined to the cochlea or vestibule was considered to be uncommon, but with precise MR imaging has been shown to less of a rarity than was previously thought. Johnsson and Kingsley (1981) described their chance post-mortem findings of a small tumour of 1.5 mm diameter within the scala tympani seeming to have originated in the distal process of the cochlear neuron. Such a tumour could well have given rise to a Menière-like syndrome. Thomsen and Jorgensen (1973) reported a case of an intracochlear schwannoma which was seen to originate in the spiral ganglion. Storrs (1974) presented two cases in which a vestibular schwannoma presented as a middle ear tumour. More recently, Birzgalis, Curley and Ramsden (1991) and Saeed, Birzgalis and Ramsden (1994) described two further cases one of which was predicted preoperatively on MR imaging which demonstrated a high signal in the labyrinth of a shape which conformed to the vestibule and the lateral and posterior canals. Intracochlear neurofibromatosis is a well recognized feature of neurofibromatosis type 2 (Linthicum, 1972), in which an intralabyrinthine lesion may be independent of, separate from or in continuity with a meatal tumour (Figure 21.4).

Gross appearance

The typical vestibular schwannoma is a firm, well encapsulated tumour with a somewhat nodular surface which, as the tumour enlarges tends to mould itself to the contours of the cerebellopontine angle.

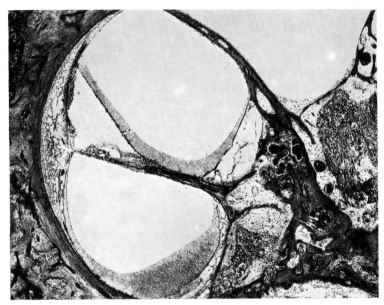

Figure 21.3 Inner ear changes – exudate in cochlea

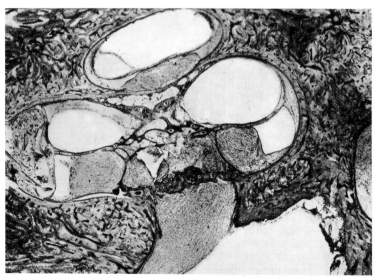

Figure 21.4 Inner ear changes – intracochlear extension of tumour

There is a relatively well-defined plane of separation between the tumour and the arachnoid, but in places it may be rather firmly adherent to its surroundings, particularly in the proximity of branches of the anterior inferior cerebellar artery, making safe removal at times difficult or occasionally impossible. The medial pole of the tumour usually displaces the brain stem before it, but on occasion may almost appear to infiltrate into the brain stem, and may enter the fourth ventricle through the foramen of Luschka. The interior of the tumour is usually rather softer than the capsule and, although there is considerable variation from one tumour to another and in different parts of the same tumour; generally the consistency resembles that of a grape. The cut surface is rather variegated, with grey, yellow and purplish areas. Cyst formation within the substance of the tumour is common, and in some instances these cysts may constitute the main bulk of the tumour (Hitselberger and House, 1968). They contain serous yellow or haemorrhagic fluid which may be cerebrospinal fluid. Surgical removal of the cystic vestibular schwannoma is more difficult than that for a solid tumour with a less favourable outcome for the facial nerve (Charabi *et al.*, 1994). Spontaneous haemorrhage into the tumour is not uncommon and in a large tumour may cause a sudden dangerous increase in intracranial pressure. Calcification is seen occasionally, usually in quite small patches, but Thomsen, Klinken and Tos (1984) described an acoustic neuroma which was almost totally calcified.

Histological appearance

Microscopically the neoplastic cells show two characteristic patterns, the Antoni types A and B, thoroughly described by Antoni in 1920. In the Antoni A (Figure 21.5*a*) or fasciculated type, there is an orderly arrangement of parallel cells with dark staining fusiform nuclei arranged in bundles or whorls separated from each other by areas of relatively acellular fibrous tissue. The term 'palisading' is applied to describe this appearance. In the more common Antoni type B (Figure 21.5*b*) or reticular pattern, there is a looser reticular arrangement with fewer cellular elements and a more disorderly arrangement of nuclei. Areas of degeneration may be seen, the result, according to Hitselberger and House (1968), of the tumour outgrowing its blood supply. There are also pale tumour cells containing lipid, giving a generally rather foamy appearance, and responsible for the yellow colour of the tumour. This picture has been referred to by Nager (1969) as Antoni B, subgroup 1. His subgroup 2 describes an appearance in which there is a relative paucity of cells with transformation of tumour tissue into a hyaline substance. All of these histological variants may coexist in the same tumour. Malignant change

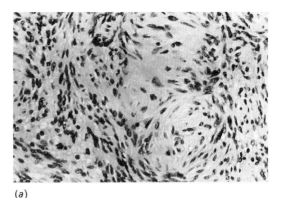

(*a*)

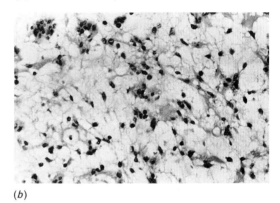

(*b*)

Figure 21.5 Photomicrographs of a vestibular schwannoma. (*a*) Antoni type A showing whorl formation and palisading; (*b*) Antoni type B showing reticular appearance

in a vestibular schwannoma is rare, but Schuknecht (1974) described and illustrated a case of a 9-year-old girl in whom this did occur.

Clinical presentation

Vestibular schwannomas are uncommon, but their true incidence is difficult to ascertain with any degree of accuracy. All of the frequently reported early estimates were based on post-mortem studies, usually of unsuspected cases, and these are fallacious for two important reasons. First, such a study will inevitably select an aged population, and furthermore, they are usually not consecutive. The estimate of 2.4% by Hardy and Crowe (1936) is based on a non-consecutive series of post-mortem studies, and is therefore likely to be too high, and the famous Witmaak collection of 1720 temporal bones was collected over no less a period than 37 years (Tos and Thomsen, 1984). Perhaps the most realistic epidemiological estimate comes from Tos and Thomsen (1984), who calculated a diagnosis rate for symptomatic tumours of 1 per 100 000 of the population per year, although these authors emphasized that this figure understates the true incidence of the condition, because of missed diagnoses. Sporadic unilateral tumours have their greatest incidence in the fourth, fifth and sixth decades, whereas in neurofibromatosis type 2 presentation is earlier, usually in the second and third decades.

The evolution of the usual clinicopathological picture in patients with VIIIth nerve tumours may be considered in five stages:

1 The 'otological' stage in which the changes are confined to the vestibulocochlear, and to a limited extent facial, nerves. This stage includes all intrameatal lesions, and extrameatal tumours up to about 2 cm
2 Stage of trigeminal nerve involvement, suggesting a diameter of 2 cm or greater
3 Stage of brain-stem and cerebellar compression, e.g. ataxia, direction changing nystagmus and long tract signs, and of involvement of the lower cranial nerves
4 Stage of rising intracranial pressure, with failing vision, headache and vomiting
5 Terminal stage, with severe disturbance of the vital brain stem centres, and tonsillar herniation.

There may also be another group of patients, in long-term institutional care, because of behavioural or personality changes who, if examined with CT scanning, would be found to be harbouring large posterior fossa lesions, and who could be transformed and rehabilitated following successful surgery.

Otological stage (stage 1)

Deafness and tinnitus

The commonest symptoms are unilateral hearing loss and tinnitus, which occur in over 90% of patients. The deafness is usually gradual in onset and slowly progressive over a period varying from as little as a few months to 20 years or more, but averaging about 2 years (King, Gibson and Morrison, 1976). The patient may volunteer the information that his ability to discriminate speech seems disproportionately poor, especially when conversing on the telephone. In perhaps 10% of cases the hearing loss is sudden and may be profound, due presumably to a vascular accident to the cochlea. Nedzelski and Dufour (1975) estimated that 3% of sudden 'idiopathic' deafness cases turn out to be due to vestibular schwannoma. The presence of a clinically silent tumour may render the cochlea more sensitive to other damaging influences, particularly barotrauma and noise, and a unilateral 4 kHz dip, appearing suddenly and perhaps only transiently after a relatively brief period of noise exposure may be the first indication of the presence of a vestibular schwannoma. At times there may be a fluctuating hearing loss both for pure tones and more especially for speech which, if accompanied by attacks of vertigo

may lead one to suspect a diagnosis of Ménière's disease. The tinnitus has no particular diagnostic features, except that it is non-pulsatile, and usually commences at about the same time as, or precedes, the deafness. Occasionally one will encounter the patient with no measurable hearing loss and with no tinnitus who, nevertheless, insists that there is 'something the matter with the hearing' in one ear. It is worth remembering that there are more subtle aspects of hearing than those which are measurable on hearing tests, and to take such a complaint seriously.

Imbalance

The slowly growing tumour destroys the vestibular nerve from which it arises so gradually that the central nervous system is able to compensate for the unilateral loss of peripheral input. Severe disturbances of equilibrium are therefore the exception. Many patients may suffer a total loss of caloric response on the affected side without ever experiencing any dysequilibrium, and others may complain of no more than slight imbalance or light-headedness on change of head or body position, especially in the dark. A minority of patients, 30% in the series of Hitselberger and House (1968), suffer from true rotatory vertigo. Many of that group experience a prolonged episode of acute labyrinthine failure, lasting for a few days or more, to which a diagnosis of labyrinthitis or vestibular neuronitis may be attached, and which probably has a vascular cause similar to the sudden loss of cochlear function alluded to previously. A small number of patients have recurrent attacks which seem identical to those of Ménière's disease, but a carefully taken history, particularly with respect to the duration, temporal pattern and associated features of the attacks would allow this diagnosis to be excluded with confidence in most instances. The author has encountered a small number of patients whose only vestibular symptom was a Tullio phenomenon brought about by the noise of traffic.

Facial nerve involvement

Although the facial nerve is compressed and may be considerably attenuated by the expanding tumour, obvious facial weakness is uncommon. This is because motor neurons, as elsewhere in the body, are more resistant to pressure than sensory fibres. Minor degrees of weakness not apparent to the patient may be detectable on close examination, and myographic and blink reflex abnormalities may be apparent on electrophysiological testing but, if a severe facial weakness occurs in association with other features of a cerebellopontine angle syndrome, the cause is more likely to be a facial neuroma, meningioma or primary cholesteatoma than a vestibular schwannoma. Facial tic is surprisingly rare, but may occur. Pain in or behind the ear is seen in about 25% of patients although is rarely a presenting complaint (Moffat *et al.*, 1989a). It may be due to involvement of the sensory branch of the facial nerve, or to stretching of the richly innervated dura at the porus. Nervus intermedius involvement is frequently manifested by altered lacrimation, the patient complaining of either a dry irritating eye, or of excessive tearing, and less commonly by alterations in the sensation of taste, with cachoguesia at times. Thomsen and Zilstorff (1975), employing a simple test of the nasolacrimal reflex, found evidence of nervus intermedius involvement in 85% of 125 patients with a vestibular schwannoma, an incidence higher than that of trigeminal nerve symptoms, and concluded that apart from audiovestibular findings, a defective nasolacrimal reflex was the most significant clinical evidence of cerebellopontine angle pathology.

Trigeminal nerve involvement (stage 2)

The earliest sensory change, occurring when the tumour has reached 2–2.5 cm is nearly always in the cornea, and may result in a feeling of irritation in the eye especially if there is coexisting alteration in tear production. With further growth of the tumour, pain, tingling or numbness may be felt in any or all of the three divisions of the nerve, and occasionally typical trigeminal neuralgia may occur as in the beautiful description of Bell's case (1830). There may also be altered thermal sensation with a feeling of cold on the face or on the edge of the tongue. There is usually an interval of about 2 years between the first audiovestibular presentation and the appearance of trigeminal signs and symptoms (King, Gibson and Morrison, 1976), but with medially arising tumours facial numbness or pain may be the presenting complaint (Moffat *et al.*, 1993a).

Brain stem and cerebellar compression (stage 3)

As the tumour enlarges still further, more evidence of neurological involvement appears. Ataxia of the ipsilateral upper and lower limbs is manifested as clumsiness due to dysmetria, dyssynergia and dysdiadochokinesia, and with disturbances of gait, the patient tending to lean or stagger to the side of the lesion. Intention tremor may develop and it is important to differentiate it from that of Parkinson's disease which decreases during voluntary movement. Direction changing horizontal nystagmus, vertical nystagmus and rotatory nystagmus are all evidence of involvement of the central vestibular pathways, and although often violent, this is not usually associated with severe imbalance. Clinical involvement of the

lower cranial nerves is infrequent, but if present implies the presence of a large tumour. Sterkers has recorded unilateral pharyngeal pain in one case and recurrent laryngeal nerve palsy in another (Portmann *et al.*, 1975).

Increasing intracranial pressure (stage 4)

As the intracranial pressure starts to increase, headache becomes more severe and although generalized, is usually worst in the suboccipital region and in the upper neck, and is often associated with nausea and vomiting. The patient may adopt a peculiar head posture, with the neck flexed, a manoeuvre which increases the volume of the cisterna magna by 5–10 ml. There may also be titubation, a rhythmic side-to-side or nodding movement of the head caused by extreme cerebellar distortion. Failing vision due to papilloedema may, even today, be the mode of initial presentation, the earlier otological and neurological symptoms having been ignored by the patient, or worse, by his doctor. Occasionally, however, a cerebellopontine angle lesion can reach this stage with a minimum of symptoms (Figure 21.6a, b). A patient may present with raised intracranial pressure, no localizing signs, dementia from hydrocephalus and a tremor attributed to Parkinson's disease. Alternatively, vomiting from raised intracranial pressure may be regarded as being of gastrointestinal origin (King, Gibson and Morrison, 1976).

Terminal stage (stage 5)

The terminal events in the history are related to failure of the vital centres in the brain stem.

Examination

General examination may reveal the presence of cutaneous lesions suggestive of neurofibromatosis type 2, cutaneous neurofibromas and café-au-lait blemishes. Minor manifestations may not be apparent in the fully clad outpatient, but he should be questioned about the presence of such lesions and if necessary treated to a full examination.

Ears

The tympanic membranes will be normal in most cases, but they must nevertheless be examined. Chronic middle ear disease can coexist with a vestibular schwannoma and even if it is inactive, may present problems to the surgeon by limiting his access

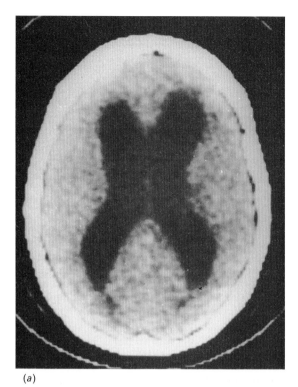

(a)

(b)

Figure 21.6 CT image from patient presenting with dementia, tremor wrongly attributed to Parkinson's disease, and nausea caused by (*a*) hydrocephalus secondary to (*b*) an unsuspected vestibular schwannoma

to the internal auditory meatus through a sclerotic and acellular petrous bone. Furthermore, there are other causes of cerebellopontine angle syndrome apart from a vestibular schwannoma, and evidence of primary cholesteatoma or glomus jugulare tumour may be apparent on otoscopy. Tuning fork tests will usually confirm a unilateral sensorineural hearing loss.

Cranial nerves

These merit the closest scrutiny, in particular the Vth and VIIth nerves.

Trigeminal nerve

All three sensory divisions of the trigeminal nerve should be tested for pin-prick and fine touch, not forgetting to include the tongue, and bearing in mind the fact that the cutaneous branches of the cervical plexus extend up over the angle of the mandible. The most important area for sensory loss is the cornea, which is usually the first to be involved by an expanding lesion in the cerebellopontine angle. The reflex is elicited by stroking the cornea lightly with a wisp of cotton wool, remembering first to remove any contact lenses. Motor function is only rarely impaired, but can be checked by asking the patient to clench the teeth.

Facial nerve

Testing of the facial nerve requires some care. Severe facial weakness is uncommon even with large tumours. All that may be apparent is a slight impairment in the patient's ability to bury the eyelashes on the affected side when screwing the eyes up tightly. Minor degrees of weakness are more likely to be seen during involuntary movement of the face. Throughout the interview, the examiner should be observing the patient's face and may notice the occasional slight delay in the blink on one side. This may be confirmed by testing the blink reflex by means of a well-regulated tap on the forehead with the finger.

The cutaneous branch of the facial nerve may be tested by touching the skin of the posterosuperior aspect of the external auditory meatus with the tip of a needle. Loss of sensation (Hitselberger's sign) may occur while the tumour is still confined within the internal meatus, but not all clinicians find this a very reliable test (Portmann *et al.*, 1975).

Function of the nervus intermedius is evaluated by testing for lacrimation and taste on the anterior two-thirds of the tongue. Lacrimation may be assessed by carrying out Schirmer's test, in which short strips of filter paper are hooked over the lower eyelid for half a minute. This is a useful test, but there may be a slight theoretical criticism in those patients who have reduce corneal sensation and thus an unequal stimulus to tear production. A more accurate, though more time consuming, test may be that of the nasolacrimal reflex as described by Thomsen and Zilstorff (1975). This involves blowing a stream of saturated benzene fumes, 500 ml/minute, in the nostril for 30 seconds directed towards the olfactory area, with Schirmer's paper in the eye. The paper is left in place for a further 30 seconds, before removal, and the lacrimation measured in millimetres. Unfortunately both sides cannot be tested at the same time, and an interval of 10 minutes is recommended between tests. A difference of 20% between the two sides is considered significant. An elevation in the taste threshold on the anterior two-thirds of the tongue is best measured on electrogustometry, a difference of more than 20 μA between the two sides being considered significant (Pulec and House, 1964). The other general visceral function served by the nervus intermedius is saliva production in the submandibular gland. There is a submandibular salivary flow test (Magielski and Blatt, 1958), but it is rarely used.

Examination of palatal and pharyngeal sensation and mobility is important, and abnormalities of either may indicate pressure on the glossopharyngeal or vagus nerves by the lower pole of a large tumour, although clinical involvement of the lower nerves is rare.

Eyes

The eye is a most fruitful source of information to the neuro-otologist who should be as conversant with the use of the ophthalmoscope as with the otoscope. As stated previously, there is still a surprising number of patients who first present to hospital at the stage of increasing intracranial pressure, and failing vision, and the otologist should be able to recognize not only florid papilloedema, but also the earlier changes of venous congestion and loss of venous pulsation. Posterior lens opacities and retinal hamartomas are commonly seen in neurofibromatosis type 2, as are Lisch nodules in neurofibromatosis type 1. Nystagmus is a very common and important sign, its pattern changing at different stages in the growth of the tumour, thus providing useful information about its size. When the tumour is small, fine first degree vestibular nystagmus to the contralateral side may be observed, particularly if optical fixation is abolished using Frenzel's glasses. As the mass enlarges it comes into contact with the brain stem, producing rather complex changes in the central vestibular connections. Dix and Hallpike (1966) suggested that as the mass made contact with the ipsilateral vestibular nucleus, there was an increase in this fine contralateral nystagmus. Later as the cerebellar connections are involved,

the nystagmus becomes direction changing, that is beating to the right on rightward gaze and beating to the left on leftward gaze. The nystagmus to the contralateral side remains fine, rapid and of low amplitude, whereas the nystagmus to the side of the lesion is more coarse and of higher amplitude. The former remains enhanceable when visual fixation is inhibited, whereas this is not true of the latter. The term Brun's nystagmus is often applied to this pattern of direction changing nystagmus (Croxson, Moffat and Baguley, 1988). When cerebellar involvement is even more marked, other patterns such as vertical nystagmus, rotatory nystagmus and rebound nystagmus may be seen (Hood, Kayan and Leech, 1973).

The other reflex eye movement that may be disturbed by a large mass in the posterior fossa is the smooth pursuit reflex (Nedzelski, 1983). This is a low velocity tracking movement that allows the eyes to follow accurately an oscillating target such as a finger at frequencies up to about 1–1.5 Hz. At greater frequencies, the eyes cannot follow the target smoothly and the previously clean sinusoidal movement becomes contaminated with small rapid saccadic jumps. 'Saccadic pursuit' is also seen at normal frequencies if there is interruption of the brain stem pathways that subserve it. The reflex can be rapidly assessed by asking the patient to follow with his eyes the examiner's finger as it moves slowly from side to side, or it can be recorded graphically using electronystagmography (Figure 21.7).

Coordination, gait and posture

The finger-nose test performed with the eyes shut is a very sensitive indicator of cerebellar function. The inability to execute it accurately is known as dysmetria. The inability accurately to carry out rapidly altering changes in the direction of hand movements is dysdiadokokinesia and is also a sign of cerebellar dysfunction. Romberg's test performed with the eyes closed was primarily a test of proprioceptive function, but may be deranged in cerebellar, brain stem and uncompensated vestibular disorders. The larger the tumour the more likely is Romberg's test to be positive. Unterberger's test, which involves marking time on the spot with the eyes closed, is a more sensitive test of vestibular function and is more likely to be abnormal with smaller tumours, and may indeed be the only discernable abnormality on physical examination (Moffat et al., 1989b). Usually, but not invariably, deviation is towards the side of the tumour, i.e. in the direction of the slow phase of nystagmus.

Investigation and diagnosis

For many years surgeons have realized that the results of vestibular schwannoma surgery are better

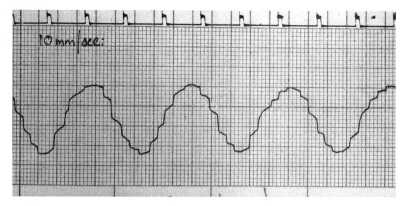

Figure 21.7 Smooth pursuit reflex. The normal smooth pursuit is broken up by a series of saccadic jumps. From a patient with a large tumour with brain stem compression

with small than with large tumours, in terms of perioperative mortality, major neurological sequelae and facial nerve preservation and function. As the majority of tumours present with symptoms which lead the patient to an otolaryngological clinic, it is essential that the otologist has a strategy based on the best currently available technology that minimizes his chances of missing a tumour. The whole approach to this problem has been revolutionized in the past decade with the widespread availability of MR imaging, and the holy grail of early diagnosis is now within our grasp in the majority of cases. There will often be patient delay in seeking advice, there will sadly often be delay at the level of the general practitioner/primary care physician, but at specialist level it should now be exceptional to miss the diagnosis of a vestibular schwannoma.

Audiovestibular investigation

In the last edition of this volume in 1987, much space was devoted to descriptions of tests of audiological function which had evolved in the 1940s, 1950s and 1960s, and which it was hoped would allow differentiation of cochlear from neural deafness. These included tests of speech discrimination (Schuknecht and Woellner, 1955; Hood and Poole, 1971), of loudness recruitment (Dix, Hallpike and Hood, 1948) and of abnormal adaptation (Carhart, 1957). Ramsden *et al.* (1992) in a series of 105 proven tumours reported a definite neural pattern in 68% on recruitment testing (loudness balance), 47% on speech audiometry, and only 24% in adaptation testing (tone decay). These tests are thus seen to be highly unreliable and now have no place in the vestibular schwannoma diagnostic protocol, although speech audiometry is a test which should still be available for a functional evaluation of hearing especially if hearing preservation surgery is contemplated. Stapedial reflex testing has been shown to be more reliable

than those tests already mentioned. Hirsch and Anderson (1980) reported abnormalities of the reflex threshold and/or adaptation of the response in 98% of a series of proven tumours. In the series reported by Ramsden *et al.* (1992) the figure was only 84%. When one considers that the response cannot be elicited with a hearing loss greater than 60–75 dB (Flood *et al.*, 1984), and that as many as 30% of patients with vestibular schwannoma have that degree of deafness or worse at presentation, it will be realized that with better options now available stapedial reflex testing has a very small contribution to make. It may, however, have a role in clinics where expensive imaging facilities are not readily available. For details of the test the reader is referred to Volume 2, Chapter 12.

Electric response audiometry

Electric response audiometry (ERA) remains the most reliable audiological tool in the investigation of the vestibular schwannoma suspect. Two techniques are in common use in the evaluation of the individual with a unilateral sensorineural deafness: electrocochleography (ECochG) and brain stem electric response audiometry (BERA, BSER). The main role of the former seems to be in the identification of endolymphatic hydrops, particularly in Menière's disease (Gibson, Moffat, and Ramsden, 1977). Brain stem electric response audiometry records the electric events which occur in the VIIIth nerve and the brain stem in the first 7 milliseconds following acoustic stimulation. The response is referred to as the auditory brain stem response (ABR). The full details of the test technique are described elsewhere (Volume 2). In brief, a sound wave entering the cochlea is transduced into an electric potential in the organ of Corti. Electrical events of very low voltage then occur in rapid succession in the auditory nerve and in a series of brain stem stuctures, as activation of the auditory pathways occurs. At a simple level one can imagine each 'relay station' being associated with its own electric event of precise latency, and rather less precise amplitude. The overall response (auditory brain stem response) can be recorded from scalp electrodes, amplified using the technique of 'time domain averaging', displayed, analysed and stored for future reference. The response comprises a series of five negative deflections, JI–JV (Figure 21.8) after Jewett who was one of the first to describe them (Jewett, Romano and Williston, 1970). Their sites of origin have traditionally been thought to be as follows:

JI   cochlear nerve
JII   cochlear nucleus
JIII superior olivary complex
JIV   lateral lemniscus
JV   inferior colliculus.

However, as Abramovich (1990) pointed out, this is amost certainly an oversimplification. For example, JII may well contain a contribution from the proximal cochlear nerve as well as the cochlear nucleus. To imagine that the sequence of waves corresponds to a

straightforward rostral propagation of the response is also unlikely to be accurate, and the individual components of the auditory brain stem response probably represent the resultants of a number of electrical vectors arising from a number of different generators within the brain stem.

While the exact sources of these phenomena remain to be clarified, their clinical value is established. In normal subjects, the latency of these responses is very predictable, not only from person to person, but also from test to test in the same individual. The early identification of these potentials was largely the result of the work of Jewett, Romano and Williston (1970). Selters and Brackmann (1977) were the first to explore the possible applications of the technique to the detection of lesions of the VIIIth nerve. They argued that any delay in electrical transmission in the nerve caused for example by a tumour would be passed on to all subsequent points in the auditory pathway, and would be detectable as a delay in the latency of JV which is the largest and therefore the most convenient component of the auditory brain stem response for study. They found the interaural latency difference of JV to be superior to the absolute latency of JV for the detection of vestibular schwannomas. They used the term 'TV' to identify the latency of JV and 'ITV' for the interaural difference, and regarded the upper limit of normal for ITV to be 0.2 ms. They correctly identified 91% of tumours using this criterion. Terkildsen and Thomsen (1983) regarded an ITV of 0.3 ms as significant. Of perhaps more value is the JI–JV interpeak interval (IPI) which is normally approximately 4 ms. Its measurement demands a precise JI response and if this not clear on brain stem electrical response audiometry, it may be measured by electrocochleography. Any delay in the JI–JV IPI is usually the result of delay between JI and JIII, rather than between JIII and JV, although the converse is possible (Abramovich, 1990).

Apart from delay in JV latency, two other abnormalities of the auditory brain stem response may be seen in patients with vestibular schwannoma. In some patients there may be no recognizable waveform despite adequate hearing levels, and this is thought to result from loss of the synchrony of neural firing necessary to produce an identifiable wave-form. The other common observation with large tumours causing brain stem distortion is delay in the contralateral auditory brain stem response; this frequently returns to normal after tumour removal.

Many studies have attested to the high reliability of auditory brain stem response in detecting vestibular schwannoma with a sensitivity approaching 100% (Ramsden *et al.*, 1992; Walstead *et al.*, 1992). However most of these studies were retrospective reviews of surgical series and may have failed to identify those individuals with probably small, tumours who were not diagnosed because their investigations ceased when the auditory brain stem response

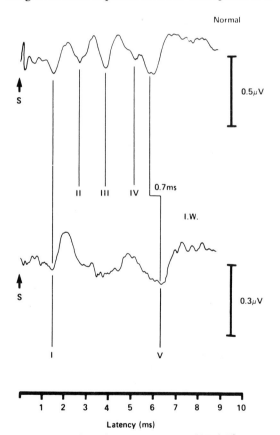

Figure 21.8 Auditory brain stem response (ABR). The upper trace is from the normal ear and the lower from the tumour ear. The latencies of JI are equal but there is a highly significant 0.7 ms delay in JV on the side of the vestibular schwannoma

was seen to be normal. Because the majority of tumours arise on the vestibular nerve, a small lesion is capable of existing for a period of time without causing any changes in the auditory nerve. A number of recent studies suggest that the sensitivity of the auditory brain stem response might not be as high as hitherto suggested. Lai, Gibson and Scrivener (1991) quoted an incidence of 24% normal or equivocal auditory brain stem response in their series of proven tumours. Hashimoto *et al.* (1992) found normal auditory brain stem response in 22% of a series of 20 small vestibular schwannomas (intracranial diameter ≤ 1.5 cm).

The lack of specificity of brain stem electric response audiometry is a major disadvantage. It can only be relied upon to produce clear wave-forms from ears with a hearing level of 75 dB or better. At higher threshold levels the absence of a response may simply be a reflection of the severity of the hearing loss regardless of cause, rather than the presence of a vestibular schwannoma. If therefore the absence of a response is construed as an abnormal auditory brain stem response, there will be a very high number of 'false-positive' results. It should also be remembered that as high a figure as 30% of patients with vestibular schwannoma present with a hearing loss of that magnitude, so the absence of a wave-form is meaningless. Despite these caveats brain stem electric response audiometry remains the single most useful audiological test currently available, and still has a key role in diagnosis, especially in centres where access to MR is impossible or restricted.

Gibson and Beagley (1976) and Morrison, Gibson and Beagley (1976) have reported on the electrocochleographic abnormalities in cases of vestibular schwannoma, and described three typical findings – broadening of the compound VIIIth nerve action potential (CAP), good preservation of the cochlear microphonic (CM), and preservation of the compound nerve action potential at stimulus intensities that are inaudible to the patient. Unfortunately, as these authors point out, broadening of the compound auditory potential is not pathognomonic of retrocochlear disease, and a very similar wave-form is also seen in Ménière's disease and other hydropic disorders. In addition, cochlear microphonic measurements are notoriously variable and hard to standardize. For these reasons electrocochleography has not gained widespread acceptance in the diagnosis of retrocochlear pathology.

Caloric testing

Because the majority of tumours arise on one or other division of the vestibular nerve, it is hardly surprising that the bithermal caloric test of Fitzgerald and Hallpike (1942) frequently reveals a canal paresis. The frequency of a significant difference between the two sides depends upon tumour size. Whereas with large tumours it may approach 100%, King, Gibson and Morrison (1976) reported that 20% of patients with tumours of 2 cm or less had normal caloric responses. Welling and Glasscock (1992) reported a significant canal paresis in only 66% of tumours. It does appear that in the quest for diagnosis of small tumours the caloric test has been largely superseded by more sensitive techniques. One should remember that the caloric test produces a maximum stimulus in the horizontal semicircular canal which is innervated by the superior vestibular nerve. A small tumour arising on the inferior vestibular nerve may not cause any reduction in the caloric response. Some surgeons regard this finding as a good prognostic indication for hearing preservation, but there is not universal agreement on this point. The most suggestive finding on caloric testing is a significant reduction in the response in the absence of a history of dizziness. This should alert one to the presence of slowly progessive vestibular pathology of which vestibular schwannoma is the commonest example.

Radiological investigation

Temporal bone radiology

For many years the mainstay of radiological screening for vestibular schwannoma was plain radiology supplemented by tomography. Valvassori (1969) established well known criteria for diagnosis of abnormality of the internal auditory meatus on tomography. Using them, definite abnormalities were detectable in approximately 80% of a series of proven tumours (Ramsden *et al.*, 1992), and this figure seems close to the best achievable with this investigation. It has now been largely superseded by better techniques.

CT scanning

The development of computerized tomography of the brain was a very great step forward in the diagnosis of VIIIth nerve tumours. From its introduction in the 1970s it progressed through a series of new generations of hardware and software programs to a high level of sophistication, and will demonstrate most intracranial lesions. CT does have a number of disadvantages. It requires the administration of an intravenous contrast agent to which some patients are allergic. It cannot demonstrate the smallest of tumours, in particular the intrameatal lesions, without the introduction of intrathecal contrast such as air (Figure 21.9). It delivers a dose of ionizing radiation (see also Figures 2.52 and 2.53).

Magnetic resonance imaging

With the advent of MRI, we have attained the gold standard in imaging of vestibular schwannomas

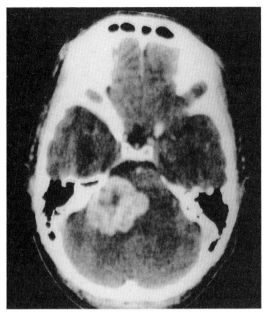

(a)

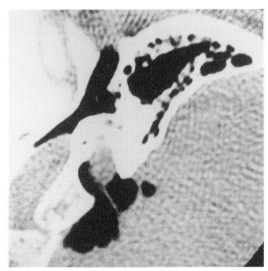

(b)

Figure 21.9 (*a*) CT scan of a large irregular tumour with a cystic area in the centre. Note the absence of detail of the internal meatus. (*b*) An intrameatal schwannoma demonstrated by the use of intrathecal air. The adjacent neural bundle is easily seen

(Figure 21.10). The theoretical aspects of the technique are reviewed in Volume 1. Its advantages over conventional techniques are a high intrinsic contrast between tissues, an absence of bone artefacts, an ability to image directly in the coronal, sagittal and axial planes, as well as an absence of ionizing radiation. On T1-weighted images, a vestibular schwan-

noma has a similar signal intensity to brain; on T2 images the tumour is hyperintense compared with brain (see Figure 2.55). Large tumours can be more readily demonstrated than with contrast enhanced CT, and details of brain stem distortion are more easily visible. Intracanalicular tumours and the intracanalicular component of large tumours are readily demonstrated. The use of the paramagnetic enhancing agent gadolinium diethylene triaminpenta acetic acid (Gd DTPA) (see Figure 2.54) clarifies the images (Curati *et al.*, 1986) but new software programs promise to make that unnecessary. Lesions as small as 2 mm can be imaged quite clearly. Telischi *et al.* (1993) investigated the reliability of MR in predicting the lateral extent of tumour in the meatus and found a positive predictive value of 98.5%. This is of value in decisions regarding attempted hearing preservation surgery, as hearing is less likely to be preserved in tumours which extend to the fundus. One of the criticisms levelled at MRI as a primary investigation is expense, but a number of recent studies have indicated that the cost of MR need not be any greater than a protocol based on conventional audiovestibular testing and auditory brain stem response (Moffat and Hardy, 1989: Robson *et al.*, 1993; Saeed *et al.*, 1995). It is the author's contention that any case of unilateral audiovestibular failure in which the diagnosis is not readily apparent should have MR studies as an initial procedure. It is the acid test which neuro-otologists have been seeking for decades and it seems wrong, now that it is available, to avoid it on the fallacious grounds that it is too complicated, invasive or expensive.

In parts of the world where access to MR is limited a protocol based on the following three tests is recommended:

1 Auditory brain stem response
2 Radiological studies of the temporal bone, employing CT scanning with i.v. contrast, or even plain tomography using the criteria of Valvassori
3 Bithermal caloric testing.

Differential diagnosis

The vestibular schwannoma is by far the commonest lesion of the cerebellopontine angle and in the series of Moffat *et al.* (1993b) constituted 80% of all cerebellopontine angle pathologies. The next most frequently encountered tumour is the meningioma which usually arises from a broad base on the posterior surface of the temporal bone (see Figure 2.56) or from the petrous ridge but is not usually centred over the internal auditory meatus (see Figure 2.57). Radiologically there may be hyperostosis or erosion of the temporal bone but expansion of the internal auditory meatus is uncommon. Patchy calcification may be seen within the tumour itself. On CT, dense homogeneous enhancement is seen. On MR, meningiomas

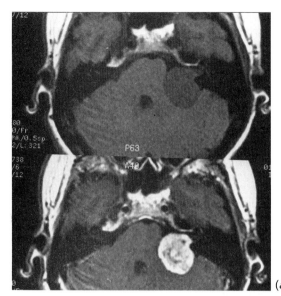

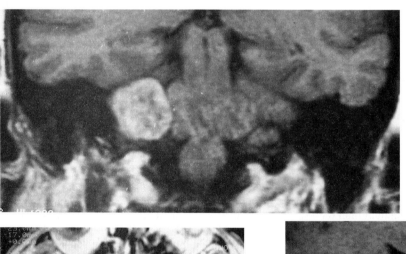

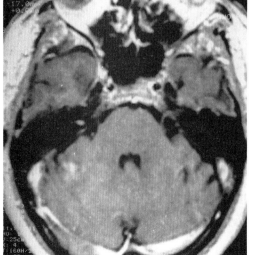

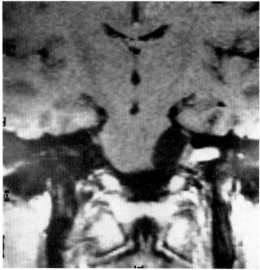

Figure 21.10 MR images. (*a*) Typical vestibular schwannoma with tumour in the cerebellopontine angle and medial half of internal meatus (pre- and post-gadolinium axial views). (*b*) Large intracranial tumour with no meatal involvement (coronal view). (*c*) Tiny intrameatal schwannoma (axial view). (*d*) Intrameatal schwannoma with cystic intracranial component (coronal view)

(*a*)

(*b*)

(*c*)

(*d*)

have a heterogeneous appearance. They are isodense with brain on T1 images; on T2-weighted images they may be seen either as areas of decreased signal intensity or of high intensity (Valvassori *et al.*, 1988). Their enhancement with gadolinium tends to be rather less intense than with vestibular schwannomas. Meningiomas may be seen, either single or multiple in association with vestibular schwannoma in neurofibromatosis type 2 (see Figure 2.58).

Next most common are primary cholesteatomas which arise from congenital epithelial rests in the temporal bone or posterior cranial fossa. These typically present with a progressive facial paralysis or hemifacial spasm. Radiologically there is often characteristic widespread destruction of the temporal bone with scalloping of the bony edge (Fisch, 1978). On CT, there is typically no enhancement with contrast because of the avascular nature of the lesion. On MR, the image is hypointense on T1, but hyperintense on T2 images. As Moffat *et al.* (1993b) pointed out it is possible and indeed important to differentiate between a cholesteatoma and a cholesterol cyst of the petrous apex; the latter is hyperintense on both T1- and T2-weighted images. Arachnoid cysts of the posterior fossa may occur in the cerebellopontine angle. The hypotheses that have been suggested to explain their development include congenital malformation, infection with adhesive arachnoiditis, trauma, increased intraventricular pressure and embryonic rests (Little, Gomez and MacCarty, 1973). They are thin walled and seem to develop between the layers of the arachnoid. They contain CSF and are therefore hypointense on T1-weighted MR images and hyperintense on T2-weighted images. Arachnoid cysts are not uncommonly seen in association with a vestibular schwannoma and are probably a response to high CSF protein levels (chemical arachnoiditis). Schwannomas of other cranial nerves are less common than the VIIIth. Lesions of cranial nerves IX, X, XI and XII do not usually present with hearing loss, but with symptoms appropriate to the individual nerve in question. On radiological imaging they are seen to be situated low in the posterior fossa and may be associated with expansion of the jugular foramen (see Figure 2.58). Facial neuromas usually present with facial nerve symptoms and signs. It is worth bearing in mind that in neurofibromatosis type 2 the trigeminal nerve is the most frequently involved after the audiovestibular (see Figure 2.59). Other less common space-occupying lesions in the cerebellopontine angle include lipoma which is often difficult to remove totally (Rosenbloom *et al.*, 1985; Pensak *et al.*, 1986), choroid plexus papilloma which may occur in isolation (Panizza, Jackson and Ramsden, 1992) or as part of the von Hippel Lindau disease (Moffat *et al.*, 1993b), haemangioma and haemangiopericytoma of the temporal bone, which carries a very gloomy prognosis (Birzgalis *et al.*, 1990). Other skull base tumours may extend into the cerebellopontine angle, notably the

glomus jugulare tumour (Fisch type IV), but also on occasion carcinoma of the middle or external ears or of the postnasal space. Vascular causes of a cerebellopontine angle syndrome include basilar artery ectasia (Gibson and Wallace, 1975), aneurysm and compression of the VIIIth nerve by a vascular loop of the anterior inferior cerebellar artery (Figure 21.11) (see also Figure 2.13b).

Menière's disease is often said to be the condition that most frequently has to be differentiated from vestibular schwannoma. As mentioned above the clinical features of Menière's disease, and in particular the characteristics of the vertigo are rarely found with vestibular schwannoma. Nevertheless, it is important to be aware of the possibility and to subject all apparent Menière's patients to rigorous investigation including MR imaging (see Chapter 19).

Treatment

Surgery

The results of surgical removal of vestibular schwannomas have improved immensely in the last 30 years, for a number of reasons. There has been a healthy collaboration between otologists and neurosurgeons, with the emergence of the otoneurologist or neuro-otologist as a superspecialist and the establishment of units with a special interest in the surgery of the inner ear, the cerebellopontine angle and the skull base. Advances in other fields of knowledge have contributed. Radiologists have at their disposal more and more sophisticated imaging techniques which have allowed diagnosis at an ever earlier stage. With MR lesions as small as 2–3 mm can be accurately imaged. Advances in neuroanaesthesia allow surgeons to indulge their time-consuming passions, and intraoperative monitoring both of vital functions and of the facial nerve are routine. The most significant single advance was the introduction of the operating microscope initially to otology and more belatedly to neurosurgery (Rand and Kurze, 1965) and with it the evolution of microsurgical technique. The other advance was the realization, remarkable for its very belatedness (Atkinson, 1949), that the anterior inferior cerebellar artery was essential for life and well-being and had to be treated with the greatest of respect.

Perioperative mortality has dropped from 16% in 1950 (Pennybacker and Cairns, 1950) to 1% or less, and is related to the size of the tumour. Morrison and King (1982) reported no mortality for small tumours, rising to 2% when the tumour was large. A similar incidence of serious neurological sequelae may be expected. Anatomical preservation of the facial nerve is achieved in well over 90% of cases regardless of size, although functional results are better in small tumours (under 2.5 cm intracranial diameter) (Dutton *et al.*, 1992). Facial nerve function is usually

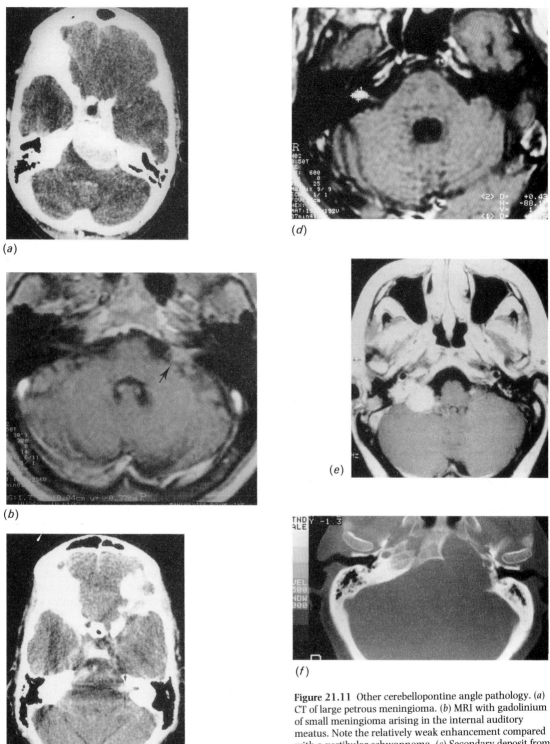

(a)

(b)

(c)

(d)

(e)

(f)

Figure 21.11 Other cerebellopontine angle pathology. (a) CT of large petrous meningioma. (b) MRI with gadolinium of small meningioma arising in the internal auditory meatus. Note the relatively weak enhancement compared with a vestibular schwannoma. (c) Secondary deposit from pinealoma (CT). (d) Lipoma. (e) Glomus jugulare with intrapetrous and intracranial components. (f) Petrosal cholesteatoma (CT)

assessed on the House Brackmann six point scale (I is normal, VI is total paralysis; see Chapter 24). Grade I or II results can be seen in approximately 75% of cases regardless of size. Peroperative facial nerve monitoring by recording the EMG from the facial muscles is a useful adjunct to surgery and may speed up surgery but it is no substitute for precise anatomical knowledge. One of the roles it may have is as a predictor of functional outcome (Babighian *et al.*, 1992). By recording stimulus response measurements at the end of the operation the surgeon may eventually be able to identify those patients who, despite having a facial nerve in anatomical continuity, are unlikely to achieve a good funtional grade, and should therefore have an immediate grafting procedure.

In the light of these results the majority of patients will be advised to have surgery in the anticipation that total tumour removal will be achieved with preservation of a facial nerve that will probably function well. There are, of course, certain exceptions to this generalization. A small tumour in an elderly or infirm patient should be monitored with annual MR imaging. A similar course of action might be advised in a younger patient with a small tumour if the hearing is good and if binaural hearing is essential in his work, bearing in mind that the statistics all show that the best hearing preservation procedure is no procedure. The increasing numbers of small tumours being revealed by MRI has prompted some authors to state that all intracanalicular tumours should be managed conservatively (Cox, 1993). The case for early removal has been put by Ramsden and Moffat (1994) who listed a number of factors which have to be weighed up in arriving at a decision in an individual case, namely: age, tumour growth characteristics, general health, the hearing level in the tumour ear, the hearing level in the opposite ear, the risks of death or morbidity from surgery and the costs both human and financial in prolonged follow up.

Broadly speaking there are three approaches to the cerebellopontine angle, from above, from the side or from behind. The superior approach or middle fossa technique has the advantage of allowing the possibility of preserving hearing, but the disadvantages of a slightly increased risk to the facial nerve, and cramped access, although the greatest proponents of the technique can remove tumours of up to 4 cm intracranial diameter through it (Haid and Wigand, 1992). It also carries a slight risk of epilepsy from retraction of the temporal lobe. The posterior approach or retrosigmoid technique also has the advantage of being applicable in hearing preservation operations, but carries the risk of cerebellar retraction. Early facial nerve identification is less secure than with the translabyrinthine procedure. The lateral approach or the translabyrinthine operation has two great advantages, early identification of the facial nerve and avoidance of cerebellar retraction but almost inevitably is associated with the total loss of hearing (but see 'Hearing preservation', below). The transotic approach of Jenkins and Fisch (1980) is an extension of the translabyrinthine operation in which the cochlea is also drilled out and the internal auditory meatus skeletonized through 360°. In the view of these authors, this approach gives better control over the whole length of the facial nerve. A blind sac closure of the ear canal is fashioned to deal with the problem of the large cavity.

Apart from considerations of hearing preservation one can as a general rule state that in the best hands the choice of approach has little effect on the outcome, the two most important determinants of which are tumour size and the experience of the surgical team.

Stereotactic radiosurgery

Stereotactic radiosurgery, the so-called gamma knife, was introduced in 1951 at the Karolinska Institute in Stockholm by Leksell, but has yet to find an accepted place in the treatment of vestibular schwannomas. Nevertheless, it does have its protagonists and because it is being represented as a serious alternative to surgery, the available facts merit earnest scrutiny. The technique involves the delivery of a highly focused high dose of ionizing radiation from a 201 cobalt-60 source in one 20-minute session to the tumour, the location of which has been precisely identified stereotactically. The dose gradient is extremely steep and as a result the lesions produced are said to be very circumscribed, with apparently little irradiation of adjacent normal structures. The dose delivered to the centre of the tumour is 15–25 Gy and to the periphery 10–15 Gy. It differs from more conventional techniques which rely for their effectiveness on the difference in the radiosensitivity of tumour tissue and normal structures. The main aim in treatment with the gamma knife is not total destruction of the tumour but the long-term arrest of growth (Norén *et al.*, 1992). To this has been added the claims of enhanced facial nerve and hearing preservation compared with surgery.

A number of centres have recently published results of cobalt-60 gamma knife therapy for vestibular schwannoma (Lunsford, Linskey and Flickinger, 1992; Myrseth *et al.*, 1992; Norén *et al.*, 1992). Norén *et al.* (1992) and Hirsch and Norén (1992) described the Karolinska results of treatment in 254 patients with a minimum follow up of 1 year (mean $4\frac{1}{2}$ years) and quoted arrest of growth or decrease in size in 85% of cases with increase in size in 15%, the results being worse for bilateral tumours of which 24% continued to grow. The authors claimed 17% facial weakness after treatment, always temporary and with a final grading of III or better, and a 19% incidence of trigeminal dysaesthesia, the majority of which were mild and transient. Of 29 patients with 'useful hearing' (PTA < 50 dB SDS > 80%), seven (24%) retained their pretreatment levels for 2 years. Cerebellar oedema occurred in 8% of cases, and hydrocephalus requiring shunting in 1.5%. These authors concluded that the technique should be offered to all patients with a vestibular schwannoma as an alternative to microsurgery.

The Pittsburgh study described by Lunsford, Linskey and Flickinger (1992) presents broadly similar figures for tumour response. The authors drew attention to a loss of central tumour enhancement on CT in 78% of patients after treatment although in 17% this enhancement subsequently returned. They were as optimistic as Norén on facial nerve results and presented similar though not directly comparable results for hearing preservation (35% with PTA $\leq$ 50 dB SDS > 50% at 1 year). Communicating hydrocephalus without change in tumour size was seen in 5% and all these patients required shunting. These authors were more circumspect in their indications for radiosurgery, advocating its use in the elderly, the infirm, bilateral tumours or a tumour in the only hearing ear, or on tumour recurrence after surgery.

The advantages to the patient of the gamma knife are obvious: a single outpatient treatment with no operation or anaesthetic and no need for prolonged rehabilitation or convalescence. Surgeons, however, have expressed a number of anxieties about stereotactic radiosurgery. Perhaps the most important concerns the long-term uncertainty about the biological behaviour of the tumour remnant. Tumour growth may continue after treatment in 15–24% of tumours. In the remainder growth is arrested, or shrinkage occurs but total eradication is exceptional. Little is known about the long-term growth potential of these remnants so it is clear that every patient treated with the gamma knife will require a life-long follow up with repeated radiological examinations. This fact alone would seem to render the treatment inappropriate for the patient with a small tumour who, if treated surgically, can expect total removal with little risk to the facial nerve, and a finite period of follow up of perhaps 2 years. Thomsen, Tos and Børgesen (1990) also pointed out that stereotactic radiosurgery is unsuitable for tumours greater than 2.5 cm intracranial diameter. Myrseth *et al.* (1992) were clearly of the same mind when they stated that they would only use the gamma knife for tumours between 1.5 and 2.5 cm intracranial diameter. Thomsen, Tos and Børgesen (1990) drew attention to the fact that surgery on vestibular schwannomas that have been irradiated carries an increased risk to the facial nerve over unirradiated tumours of similar size. In view of the numbers that continue to grow after irradiation, this is an important consideration. The hearing preservation issue is unconvincing, because it still relates to such a small percentage of diagnosed vestibular schwannomas, and because the best results are still no better than those achieved by surgery. Sterkers and Hocsman (1992) described their experience of four patients referred for gamma knife treatment all of whom lost the hearing in their only hearing ears after treatment and all of whose tumours continued to grow. Finally, the incidence of hydrocephalus is not negligible after irradiation. Hydrocephalus requiring shunting occurred in the patient described by Thomsen, Tos and Børgesen (1990) irradiated for a small tumour in the vain hope of preserving hearing. By way of contrast, these authors have not seen hydrocephalus in 500 cases of vestibular schwannoma removed via the translabyrinthine route.

At the present time, stereotactic irradiation is not favoured by the majority of surgeons but it is clearly very important that all those involved in the management of patients with vestibular schwannomas remain informed about the published results from the centres that are using the technique, and about technical developments in the field.

Surgical techniques

Middle fossa approach (see Plate 3/21/II)

The incision begins in front of the ear at the level of the zygomatic arch and curves gently upwards and backwards to the superior temporal line. The temporalis muscle may be divided in a linear manner to expose the squamous temporal bone, and a 4 cm square craniectomy cut, the lower edge of which is on a level with the upper surface of the petrous bone. Approximately two-thirds of the bone flap should be in front of the external meatus and one-third behind it. Alternatively, the flap may be left attached to a pedicle of temporalis muscle and turned inferiorly. The dura is then gently elevated first to the arcuate eminence, and then anteriorly and medially until the superior petrosal sinus is reached and the middle meningeal artery is exposed as it enters the skull through the foramen spinosum.

The greater superficial petrosal nerve is found about 1 cm behind and slightly lateral to the artery and, using a diamond burr, is followed to the geniculate ganglion which may, in fact, be immediately under the dura without any bony covering. The facial nerve is then traced backwards and medially to the meatus, passing deeply between the cochlea and the superior semicircular canal, neither of which should be opened. As it leaves the meatus, the facial nerve is separated from the superior vestibular nerve by a very obvious vertical crest of bone – 'Bill's bar'. The meatus is exposed from its lateral to medial ends through as wide a bony trough as possible and the dura is incised along the posterior wall of the meatus, i.e. away from the facial nerve. After positive identification, the tumour is carefully dissected off the facial nerve, taking care to minimize the manipulation of both it and the cochlear nerve which is to some extent protected by the facial nerve. Both superior and inferior vestibular nerves must be totally ablated as the tumour is removed otherwise there is a risk of postoperative imbalance.

If hearing is to be conserved, care must be taken to avoid damage to the internal auditory artery. Division of the superior petrosal sinus may be necessary to facilitate removal of a tumour extending into the posterior fossa. After careful haemostasis, the internal auditory meatus is sealed using fascia or muscle, the middle fossa dura is allowed to sink back over the defect, and the wounds is closed in layers, replacing the bone.

Translabyrinthine approach (Figures 21.12–21.16; see Plates 3/21/III and 3/21/IV)

The incision is an extension of the standard post-auricular wound, the upper end reaching as far as the line of the anterior wall of the external meatus, and the lower limit being a point about 2 cm behind the tip of the mastoid. A superiorly-based periosteal flap is preserved in continuity with the lower edge of the temporalis muscle for use in eventual wound closure. An extended mastoidectomy is carried out paying particular attention to creating as wide an access as possible. The bone over the middle fossa must shelve upwards and the posterior canal wall must be thinned. Bone should be removed over and behind the lateral sinus, so that the sinus can later be compressed posteriorly. The facial nerve is identified at the second genu and the retrofacial air cells removed. A total labyrinthectomy is then performed taking particular care to avoid trauma to the facial nerve as the inferior crus of the posterior canal is followed into the vestibule, a point at which the drill is immediately medial to the second genu. The endolymphatic duct will be seen leaving the vestibule in the line of the common crus before turning through 90° and running downwards and backwards into the endolymphatic sac on the posterior fossa dura. The subarcuate artery is encountered under the superior semicircular canal and after the labyrinthectomy is the only feature in a dense triangular wall of bone separating the surgeon from the internal auditory meatus. The meatus is now skeletonized superiorly, posteriorly and inferiorly through at least 180°. Dissection is easier if there is a well developed air cell system.

The anatomical limit above the meatus is the middle fossa dura with the superior petrosal sinus. With a larger tumour one should be prepared to remove bone quite extensively over the middle fossa to allow access to the upper pole of the tumour. Posteriorly, bone is removed from a wedge-shaped

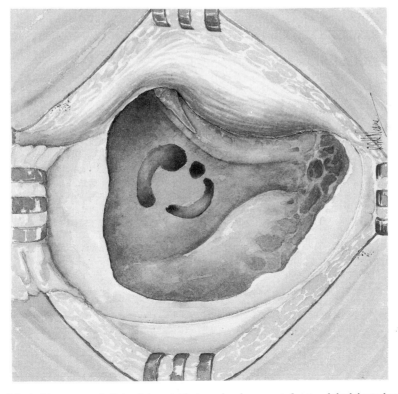

Figure 21.12 Translabyrinthine approach. Extended mastoidectomy has been carried out and the labyrinthectomy begun (right ear)

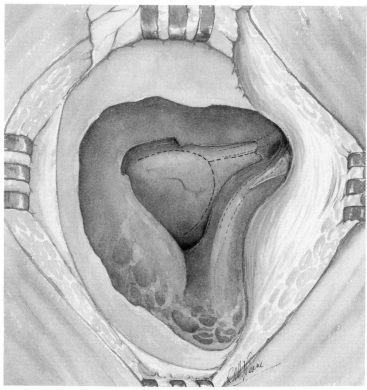

Figure 21.13 Translabyrinthine approach. Total labyrinthectomy has been carried out. Bone has been removed to expose the posterior fossa dura and the dura of the internal auditory meatus. The dotted line represents the dural incision (right ear)

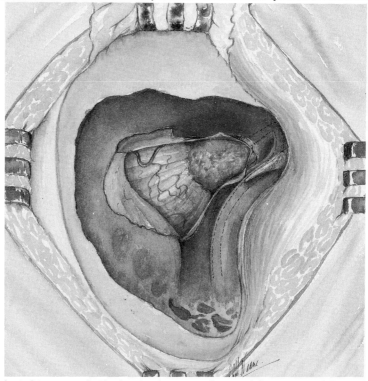

Figure 21.14 Translabyrinthine approach. The dura has been opened to reveal the tumour and the cerebellum (right ear)

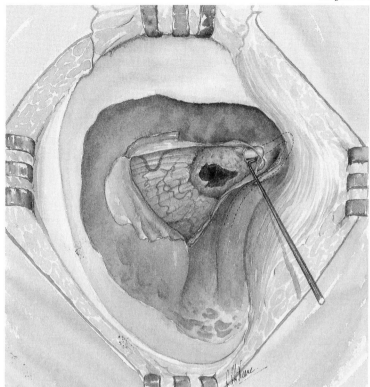

Figure 21.15 Translabyrinthine approach. Much of the interior of the tumour has been removed and the facial nerve has been identified at Bill's bar (right ear)

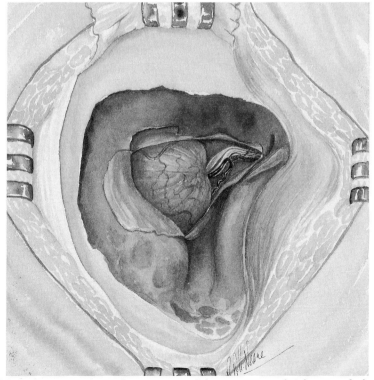

Figure 21.16 Translabyrinthine approach. Total tumour removal showing an intact facial nerve and a loop of anterior inferior cerebellar artery (right ear)

area between the internal meatus and the posterior fossa and, eventually, when the porus is reached, continuity between the meatus and the posterior fossa can be demonstrated. Inferior to the meatus the limiting factor for bone removal is the jugular bulb. If this is high or there is a jugular diverticulum, it must be skeletonized and packed inferiorly with bone wax to allow access. As one passes medial to the jugular bulb beneath the meatus, the cochlear aqueduct is encountered and CSF may escape. This has the effect of slackening off the intracranial contents and allows the tumour and cerebellum to fall away from the posterior fossa dura, facilitating eventual opening of the posterior fossa. The cochlear aqueduct is very closely related to the lower cranial nerves. In order to avoid damage to them in further anterior dissection one must keep above the aqueduct, close to the inferior wall of the meatus. Bone is finally picked off the dura of the posterior and middle fossae, and the internal auditory meatus. The thin bone over the lateral sinus may be retained as an island (Bill's island), or removed. Either way the sinus can be compressed posteriorly, to allow greatly increased access into the posterior fossa.

The transverse crest is readily identified and above it the superior vestibular nerve which can be traced to the ampulla for the superior semicircular canal. The facial nerve may now be identified at the lateral end of the meatus separated by 'Bill's bar' from the superior vestibular fibres as they enter the vestibule. The dura of the internal auditory meatus is then incised and, after division of the superior vestibular nerve, the intrameatal portion of the tumour can be separated from the facial nerve, and dissected medially. The posterior fossa is then opened by cutting a laterally based U-shaped dural flap, a manoeuvre which has to carefully performed in order to avoid damage to cerebellar vessels which may be very close to the dura especially if CSF has not already been run off. The main bulk of the tumour is exposed, and the plane between the tumour and the cerebellum defined. An intracapsular removal is performed, using the House Urban rotary dissector, or the Cavitron Ultrasonic Surgical Aspirator (CUSA). The remaining capsule is then removed by careful dissection in the plane between the tumour and the arachnoid taking particular care to avoid damage to the branches of the anterior inferior cerebellar artery and the lower cranial nerves which are in the arachnoid layer and to the brain stem and trigeminal nerve. The previously identified facial nerve is traced medially. At the porus, it turns sharply forwards and may become very thin and hard to follow but, by careful adherence to the arachnoid plane, it is usually possible to preserve it. Often it is possible to identify the facial nerve at the brain stem, just medial to the root of the vestibulocochlear nerve, in which position it is usually seen to run upwards for several millimetres rather than laterally. A combination of medial and lateral dissection often leaves one with a firm fragment at the porus which can prove stubborn. If the facial nerve is known to have been lost, an immediate repair should be effected preferably by re-routing the intrapetrous portion from just above stylomastoid foramen into the posterior fossa and carrying out an end-to-end anastomosis with the proximal stump at the brain stem, using fibrin glue and a cuff of connective tissue. If this does not reach, a cable graft may be employed using a segment of cervical plexus or sural nerve (Barrs, Brackmann and Hitselberger, 1984; Samii, 1984). After tumour removal is complete, and haemostasis ensured, meticulous closure is important in order to minimize the risk of CSF leakage. The middle ear and attic should be packed with muscle, the dural defect lined with fascia, and the cavity filled with 1 cm strips of abdominal fat, held in place with the periosteal flap. A pressure dressing should be retained in place for a week.

Retrosigmoid approach (Figures 21.17–21.20; see Plate 3/21/III)

The retrosigmoid approach has evolved from the more extensive suboccipital operation. The patient is positioned in the 'park bench' position and an S-shaped retromastoid incision is made from the level of the upper edge of the pinna to the spine of C2, taking care to avoid the vertebral artery. After separation of the muscular attachments, the craniectomy is carried out. In the classic suboccipital approach the limits were the transverse sinus superiorly, the foramen magnum inferiorly and the sigmoid sinus laterally, but this can be reduced to an opening approximately 5 cm by 3 cm. In siting the craniotomy it is important that the surgeon's line of vision should be along the posterior surface of the petrous bone, thus minimizing the amount of cerebellar retraction necessary. The dura is opened through a triradiate incision and cerebellar retractors gently introduced protecting the underlying cerebellum with patties. The intracranial segment of the tumour is debulked intracapsularly, as described above, taking care to identify and protect the lower nerves, and the trigeminal nerve, as well as the anterior inferior cerebellar artery. A laterally based dural flap is raised over the internal auditory meatus, and the posterior wall of the meatus carefully drilled off, exposing the intrameatal portion of tumour which protects the facial and cochlear nerves in the anterior half of the meatus. If hearing preservation is intended, the labyrinth must not be entered, but if this is unimportant there is no doubt that extending the bone removal as far laterally as possible increases the chances of total tumour removal and allows one to identify the transverse crest and 'Bill's bar'. The tumour is gently separated from the facial nerve. If hearing preservation is the goal, dissection should be in a medial to lateral direction to

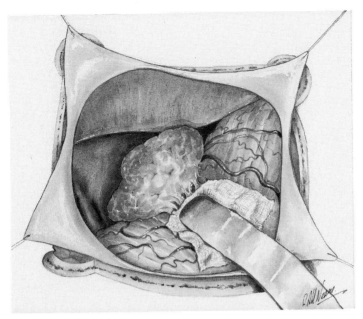

Figure 21.17 Retrosigmoid approach. The cerebellum is retracted to reveal tumour in the cerebellopontine angle (left ear)

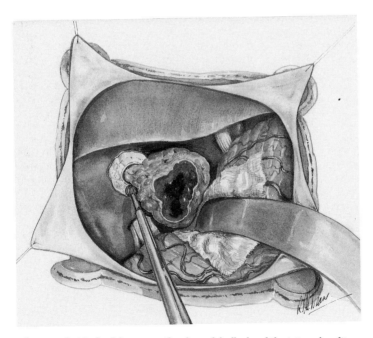

Figure 21.18 Retrosigmoid approach. Much of the tumour has been debulked and the internal auditory meatus is being opened to reveal the intrameatal portion of the tumour (left ear)

avoid avulsion of auditory neurons from the cribrose area. The operation is completed by removing tumour capsule from the adjacent structures in the manner outlined above, and before closing the wound the internal auditory meatus should be sealed with a muscle plug, and any mastoid air cells that have been opened should be sealed with bone wax to prevent a CSF leak. The craniectomy may be filled using the bone fragment removed in order to prevent adhesions between the dura and the overlying

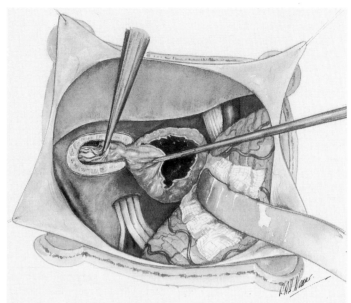

Figure 21.19 Retrosigmoid approach. Dissection of the intrameatal portion of the tumour with identification of the facial nerve (left ear)

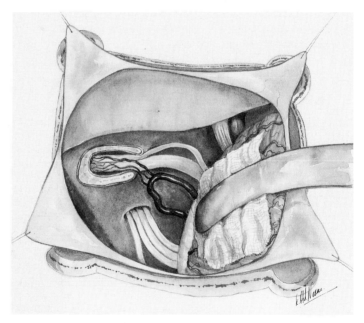

Figure 21.20 Retrosigmoid approach. Total tumour removal. The facial and cochlear nerves have been preserved and may be seen entering the brain stem. A loop of the anterior inferior cerebellar artery is seen (left ear)

muscles, which may be the cause of the occipital headache that many patients complain of after this surgery. Facial nerve repair is much more difficult through the retrosigmoid approach because of the inaccesibility of the intrapetrous portion of the nerve, but cable grafting is possible.

Postoperative care

The patient is returned from theatre to an intensive care unit for regular neurological observations and cardiac monitoring. Ventilation should be avoided as it masks neurological changes. A nasogastric tube is unnecessary unless there is genuine fear that there has been damage to the lower cranial nerves which should be an uncommon occurrence. Similarly tracheostomy is exceptionally rarely indicated unless there has been vagal nerve damage. The patient will be catheterized and on intravenous fluids, but over-hydration must be avoided. Many surgeons will pre-scribe intravenous broad-spectrum antibiotics, and possibly steroids if there has been any threat of brain swelling. Steroids do not seem to have any beneficial effect on facial nerve function after tumour surgery. The cornea should be protected until it is obvious that facial function is satisfactory. As a temporary meas-ure the upper lid may be taped on to the cheek but an eye pad should be avoided in case of corneal abrasion. If the weakness is marked, and the Bell's phenomenon poor, and particularly if there is coexisting corneal anaesthesia, a formal lateral tarsorrhaphy should be performed. The eye should be kept moist with artifi-cial tears. Cerebrospinal fluid fistula is a dangerous condition which cannot be allowed to persist. It may settle spontaneously, with repeated lumbar punctures or with a lumbar drain but, if in doubt, it is advisable to return the patient to theatre for repair.

As recovery proceeds, the patient is mobilized quickly, and is usually ready to go home by about the tenth postoperative day. Very rarely, in the case of a large tumour, postoperative hydrocephalus may be seen and this may require treatment by daily lumbar puncture or possibly ventriculoperitoneal shunting. Imbalance from loss of vestibular function is not usually a major problem because, in most instances, vestibular function has already been consid-erably reduced prior to surgery. The great majority of patients are fully rehabilitated to their previous levels of activity, and should for example be able to play golf, jog, and cycle, although some may experience imbalance in the dark. Tinnitus is a surprisingly rare long-term complaint. One of the least appreciated problem areas is the eye in patients who have suffered partial or total facial weakness. Not only may the loss of the protective blink reflex expose the eye to the risk of foreign bodies, but there may be subtle changes in the physical properties of the tear film with resultant pain, grittiness, blurring, dryness or watering. If there is coexisting loss of corneal sensa-tion, neurotrophic changes may occur with the risk of corneal ulceration. It is a clinical problem which demands close ophthalmological attention and poss-ible tarsorrhaphy.

One of the most difficult problems concerns the non-recovering facial nerve. If the nerve is known to have been severed, immediate repair is indicated if possible. If that is not possible, an immediate hypoglosso-facial anastomosis should be carried out. The problem arises when the nerve is thought to be partially preserved but no recovery ensues over a long period of observation. Recovery from a degener-ated nerve will usually be apparent by 1 year after surgery. If no recovery is visible at 2 years, a hypoglosso-facial anastomosis should be carried out, but by then much valuable time will have been lost, and the final outcome of the delayed grafting pro-cedure may have suffered. The answer may lie in identifying an electrophysiological indicator which could determine which patients should be offered an early nerve graft.

Hearing preservation

The issue of hearing preservation in vestibular schwannoma surgery remains one of the most contro-versial among surgeons who treat large numbers of these tumours. On the face of it any attempt to preserve hearing might seem entirely laudable, but the problems are not as clear cut as they might at first appear. Several questions have to be asked. Is the hearing that one is attempting to save worth preserving? Does the effort of attempting hearing preservation expose the patient to any risks in other areas? For example is there any increased risk of incomplete tumour removal and thus tumour recur-rence? Is there any increased risk of damage to the facial nerve? What are the chances of a successful outcome? Let us consider these factors.

Otologists are becoming increasingly aware of the criteria which determine a successful outcome in tympanoplasty surgery. Until recently closure of the air bone gap was regarded as the main index of success. The work of Smyth and Patterson (1985), and of Browning, Gatehouse and Swann (1991), however, has led us to regard the postoperative inter-aural difference as a more important measure of a good result. In general, however technically success-ful the tympanoplasty might have been in closing the air bone gap, if the postoperative difference in thresh-old between the two ears is greater than a certain level (usually defined as 30 dB or better across the speech frequencies), the patient will not be aware of the benefits of the operation. These studies suggest that there may be a difference between a result which satisfies the surgeon (i.e. closure of the air bone gap) and that which is appreciated by the patient (i.e. improvement to within 30 dB or less of the opposite ear). The tympanoplasty argument can be applied to the hearing preservation operation for vestibular schwannoma. If the hearing in the oper-ated ear cannot be retained at a level of within 30 dB of the opposite (and usually normal) ear, it is unlikely that the patient will appreciate the residual hearing, although some authorities will settle for 50 dB. Fur-thermore, in contrast to the majority of patients undergoing tympanoplasty surgery, patients with ves-tibular schwannoma are likely to have superadded distortion factors related to neural damage, particu-larly debased speech discrimination. Fifty per cent speech discrimination has been regarded by some as the minimum acceptable level, and the 50/50 criterion is one which many take as their cut-off for attempting a hearing preservation operation (50 dB interaural difference, 50% maximum SDS). The present writer however employs the stricter 30/70 criterion (30 dB interaural difference, 70% maximum SDS). The application of these figures immediately reduces the number of patients with vestibular schwannoma suitable for attempted hearing preservation. Tumour size is another factor which has to be taken into account. Hearing preservation is rarely possible with tumours greater than 2 cm intracranial diameter. As tumour size and preoperative hearing level are independent variables, the pool is further decreased if one excludes patients with tumours greater than 2 cm in diameter. Hinton *et al.* (1992) for example found that using a 30/50 criterion (30 dB interaural difference, 50% or better SDS) and eliminating all tumours larger than 2 cm, only 8% of a large series were suitable candidates for hearing preservation surgery.

Is there any disadvantage to the patient from attempted hearing preservation? The translabyrinthine approach is clearly not appropriate for most hearing preservation operations although the novel work of McElveen *et al.* (1991) suggested that hearing can be saved in some instances using this approach. Most neuro-otologists agree that the translabyrinthine operation has distinct advantages in terms of facial nerve preservation and avoidance of cerebellar retraction, and many feel that the increased certainty of facial nerve identification is a more important consideration than the benefits of binaural hearing, especially if the criteria of useful hearing are not met.

Hearing preservation can usually only be achieved via the middle fossa or retrosigmoid approaches. The main disadvantage of the former approach, apart from temporal lobe retraction, is the increased risk of damage to the facial nerve, because the surgeon has to work past the nerve in order to remove the tumour. Furthermore, the access is quite cramped for all but the smallest tumours, although Wigand, Haid and Berg (1989) who are the main proponents of the technique were able through their extended middle fossa approach to remove tumours of up to 3–4 cm in intracranial diameter. The advantage is that one can visualize the lateral end of the internal auditory meatus quite clearly and be sure of total tumour removal even when tumour extends into the labyrinthine portion of the facial canal.

The retrosigmoid approach requires some degree of cerebellar retraction, which in addition to the recognized risk to the cerebellum itself and brain stem may also put the auditory nerve and the internal auditory artery on the stretch. In addition, the view of the lateral end of the internal meatus is restricted, and there is the danger that the surgeon will open the posterior semicircular canal in the attempt to gain access to the fundus of the meatus, or alternatively, in an attempt to avoid that complication will inadvertantly leave tumour in the fundus. The cases which do best with hearing preservation surgery are those in which there is very little tumour in the meatus; little or no drilling is needed and tumour can therefore be dissected off the VIIIth nerve with minimal trauma. Accurate preoperative MR imaging can indicate the lateral extent of the tumour in the meatus; those that extend to the fundus are regarded by many surgeons as being unsuitable for a hearing preservation operation. Neely (1981) and more recently Marquet *et al.* (1990) pointed to another possible danger in cochlear nerve preservation. These authors have studied the interface between tumour and cochlear nerve in a series of vestibular schwannoma cases and using immunohistochemical techniques, have shown that there is no clear cleavage plane between tumour and nerve and that there is invasion of the cochlear nerve by tumour cells. The latter authors go so far as to state that, as a result of their findings, they reject the principle of hearing preservation surgery in favour of total tumour removal. As if to underline this fear, Tucci *et al.* (1994) reported a 9% recurrence on MRI following 'total' tumour removal in hearing preservation operations. On the other hand, Schessel *et al.* (1992) found no recurrences in a series of 28 hearing preservation cases followed up for between 5 and 13 years although CT rather than MR was used for imaging. Lye *et al.* (1992) have demonstrated that small tumour fragments of 2–3 mm knowingly left behind at the end of surgery may undergo involution and may cease to be visible on MR imaging.

What sort of results can be obtained from hearing preservation operations? Here the literature is full of haphazard and incomplete reports and is bedevilled by a lack of agreement as to the criteria for success. Terms such as 'useful', 'serviceable' and 'measurable' hearing are frequently encountered but unless supported by audiometric data, are meaningless. From the well documented reports that are available it seems that the 30/70 criterion can be met in 10–30% of attempted hearing preservation operations (Sanna *et al.*, 1992). Failure may occur even in the presence of an apparently well preserved nerve because of vascular changes especially in the cochlea. Dissection of the tumour from the VIIIth nerve may avulse cochlear nerve fibres from the modiolus. The success of these operations may be improved by refinements in intraoperative VIIIth nerve monitoring. At present, the most commonly employed technique is peroperative auditory brain stem response measurement, but the responses may take several minutes to acquire and that may not be immediate enough to provide a real warning of impending damage. It may in effect tell the surgeon that he has just irrevocably damaged the hearing, rather than warn him that he is about to do so. Direct VIIIth nerve recording would be more useful but the technique is still in the process of evolution.

Another issue to be considered concerns the stability of the postoperative hearing assuming the operation to have been successful. There is evidence from Shelton *et al.* (1992) of progressive subsequent deterioration over a period of years, due presmably to long-term vascular changes or scarring in the VIIIth nerve. Tucci *et al.* (1994) on the other hand described stable long-term results.

It will be seen that the issues regarding hearing preservation surgery for unilateral vestibular schwannomas are far from resolved, and in considering them it is worth remembering that many patients report an improvement in their subjective overall hearing ability after the removal of a debased or distorted input from the tumour side after a 'hearing destroying' operation. Each case has to be treated on its merits and the pros and cons discussed fully with the patient. The possibility, as suggested by Fisch (1994) of withholding surgery as long as good hearing exists should be offered assuming there is no neurosurgical necessity for surgery, and that regular follow up is available.

The situation in neurofibromatosis type 2 with bilateral tumours is of course entirely different. Any aidable hearing that can be preserved may prove of immense value to the patient.

Neurofibromatosis types 1 and 2

In the past 5 years the problems of the definition, classification, diagnosis and treatment of the neuro-fibromatoses have, to a very considerable extent, been clarified thanks to advances in the fields of molecular biology, diagnostic imaging and microelectronics. In 1882, von Recklinghausen described an entity characterized by multiple skin tumours, axillary freckling, and skin pigmentation and this condition became known as von Recklinghausen's disease. In his original description there is no mention of hearing loss and no suggestion of the presence of VIIIth nerve tumours. The occurrence of bilateral auditory nerve tumours was first described by Wishart in 1822. In his case there were a number of coexisting intracranial and spinal tumours but no suggestion of cutaneous lesions. With the passage of time, however, differentiation between the two conditions became so vague that for almost all of the twentieth century it was generally held that the presence of multiple cutaneous neurofibromas and café-au-lait skin spots was associated with bilateral acoustic neuromas and that the term 'von Recklinghausen's disease' described the entire syndrome. Advances in the fields of molecular biology and of human genetics now enable us to define two nosologically separate entities – neurofibromatosis type 1 (NF1: von Recklinghausen's disease) and neurofibromatosis type 2 (NF2: bilateral vestibular schwannoma syndrome) (Kanter *et al.*, 1980). The different features of these two conditions have been defined and reviewed by the National Institutes of Health (NIH) Consensus Development Conference on Neurofibromatosis (1990). Neurofibromatosis type 1, or peripheral neurofibromatosis, is true von Recklinghausen's disease and has recently been identified as being the result of a defect on chromosome 17q. It is an autosomal dominant disorder with a birth incidence of 1 in 2500, approximately 50% of which represent new mutations. It is characterized *inter alia* by the occurrence of multiple skin neurofibromas, numerous café-au-lait lesions and by iris hamartomas (Lisch nodules). The NIH criteria are listed in Table 21.1. There is no predisposition to vestibular schwannoma in neurofibromatosis type 1. The incidence of VIIIth nerve tumours is the same as in the general population.

Table 21.1 Criteria for diagnosis of neurofibromatosis types 1 and 2

Neurofibromatosis type 1 may be diagnosed in Caucasians when two or more of the following are present:

Six or more café-au-lait macules whose greatest diameter is more than 5 mm in prepubescent patients and more than 15 mm in postpubescent patients

Two or more neurofibromas of any type *or* one plexiform neurofibroma

Freckling in the axillary *or* inguinal region

A distinctive osseous lesion as sphenoid dysplasia *or* thinning of long-bone cortex, with or without pseudoarthrosis

Optic glioma

Two or more Lisch nodules (iris hamartomas)

A parent, sibling, *or* child with neurofibromatosis type 1 on the basis of the previous criteria

Neurofibromatosis type 2 may be diagnosed when one of the following is present:

Bilateral VIIIth nerve masses seen by MRI with gadolinium

A parent, sibling, *or* child with neurofibromatosis type 2 and either unilateral VIIIth nerve mass or any one of the following:

    neurofibroma
    meningioma
    glioma
    schwannoma
    posterior capsular cataract or opacity at a young age

Neurofibromatosis type 2, sometimes referred to as central neurofibromatosis, is an autosomal dominant disorder predisposing to tumours of neurogenic origin, the most common of which are bilateral vestibular schwannomas. It has a birth incidence of approximately 1 in 35 000, and a very high degree of penetrance so that nearly all carriers of the gene express it by the age of 50 years. It has been shown to be due to loss of a tumour suppressor gene which has recently been cloned on chromosome 22q (Troffater *et al.*, 1993). Fifty per cent of an affected individual's offspring are likely to inherit the disorder but it is also clear that there is a high spontaneous mutation rate and that as many as 50% of sufferers have not inherited the condition. Neurofibromatosis type 2 is an example of the so-called 'two hit' hypothesis which states that both copies of the gene need to be affected in a single cell before an individual develops a tumour. With a sporadic vestibular schwannoma both tumour suppressor genes have to be knocked out by the noxious influence whatever that may be. In neurofibromatosis type 2, because every cell already contains one inherited faulty copy, only one further noxious event is necessary before tumour suppression is inhibited. For this reason, vestibular schwannoma formation in neurofibromatosis type 2 occurs at a much younger age than with sporadic tumours. Typically bilateral vestibular schwannomas develop in teenage, with schwannomas also occurring in other cranial nerves, on spinal nerve roots and in the skin. There are two clinical phenotypes. In the milder type described by Gardner and Frazier (1930), bilateral VIIIth nerve lesions occur in isolation, but in the more aggressive Wishart pattern there may be multiple lesions on other cranial nerves particularly the trigeminal, and in the spinal cord. Meningioma is another common feature of the disease, as indeed Wishart himself pointed out. Other intracranial tumours such as gliomas and ependymomas are also seen. Café-au-lait lesions are few in number compared with type 1. As in type 1 the occurrence of eye abnormalities is common. In neurofibromatosis type 2, the typical abnormality is the posterior lens opacity, which is entirely different from the Lisch nodule of type 1 (Kaiser-Kupfer *et al.*, 1989). The lens abnormality of type 2 may occur very early in life; one should always suspect that a patient with an apparently sporadic unilateral vestibular schwannoma who had a 'cataract' removed in childhood may be suffering from neurofibromatosis type 2.

The diagnostic criteria for neurofibromatosis type 2 are under constant review by the NIH. Table 21.1 lists the currently accepted guidelines.

The cloning of the neurofibromatosis type 2 gene was a great milestone in the rapidly changing field of molecular biology. The possibility of presymptomatic and even prenatal diagnosis is now highly feasible with an accuracy of 95–99%. The great hope for the future is that manipulation of and correction of the faulty gene will eventually become a real possibility and will prevent the evolution of these tumours and cause regression of those already present.

With MR imaging (Figure 21.21) we now have at our disposal an accurate method of evaluating not only the status of the vestibular schwannomas but also any other intracranial and spinal tumours that may coexist, allowing classification of individuals into either Wishart or Gardner Frazier phenotypes. By having a comprehensive picture of the whole central nervous system the surgical team can rank the sequence of surgery. A patient with two vestibular schwannomas may be at greater immediate risk from a high thoracic or cervical tumour. Therapy can thus be tailored to individual requirements. All patients known to have neurofibromatosis type 2 and all relatives thought to be at risk should have MRI of the brain and spinal cord performed promptly to allow accurate staging of the disease.

Surgical dilemmas

It is essential that these difficult clinical problems are managed by a multidisciplinary team comprising a neuro-otologist, neurosurgeon, geneticist, ophthalmologist, neuroradiologist and psychosocial worker. Ideally treatment should be on a regional or supraregional basis (Evans *et al.*, 1993). The team faced with a subject with neurofibromatosis type 2 and bilateral vestibular schwannomas has a number of factors to consider in deciding how to advise the patient. Reduced to its simplest distillate, the most important factors are tumour size and hearing level. The ideal situation would be the patient with two small vestibular schwannomas and good hearing. A successful hearing preservation operation via the middle or posterior fossa on one side is followed some months later by a similarly successful procedure on the opposite side, leaving the patient with two tumour free and normally hearing ears. This is an uncommon not to say exceptional situation. Another presentation might be the patient with a large tumour and poor hearing on one side and a small tumour with good hearing on the opposite side. Here the obvious treatment option would be to remove the large tumour and to watch the contralateral small tumour until such times as it became so large as to demand removal, or until hearing was lost in which case there would be no point in not removing the tumour. Unfortunately nature is not always so obliging and it is not uncommon to see a patient with a large tumour with good hearing on one side, and a small tumour with a dead ear on the other. What are the options in this situation? Neurosurgical considerations may dictate that the large tumour must be removed with total deafness as an inevitable consequence. The advent of implantable electrical auditory prostheses offers the surgeon a possible means of alleviating the burden of total deafness. There are two possible situations in which an implantable prosthesis might be indicated. It is not uncomon during an attempted hearing preservation operation to preserve a healthy cochlear nerve but to lose the hearing from vascular damage to the cochlea. Such an ear would respond to promontory stimulation or round window testing and would be amenable to subsequent intracochlear implantation with a multichannel cochlear implant (Hoffman, Kohan and Cohen, 1992).

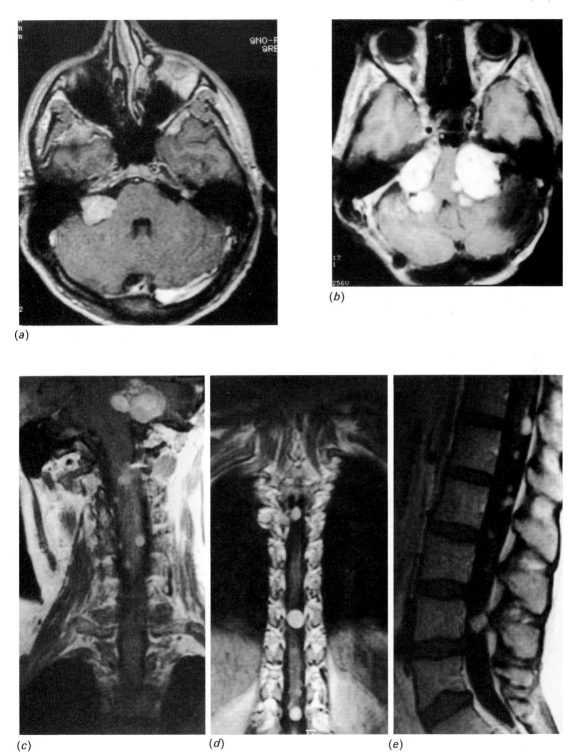

Figure 21.21 Neurofibromatosis type 2 (NF2). (*a*) Bilateral vestibular schwannomas but no other tumours (Gardiner Frazier type). (*b*) Multiple posterior fossa tumours. (*c, d, e*) Composite view from patient with Wishart type NF2. At least one posterior fossa tumour is seen, and there are multiple spinal tumours in the cervical, thoracic and lumbar regions

Alternatively, there is now the real possibility of stimulating the auditory pathways through the cochlear nucleus by means of the auditory brain stem implant (ABI). This device (Figure 21.22) which has evolved from cochlear implant technology is inserted into the lateral recess of the fourth ventricle through the foramen of Luschka at the time of tumour removal. It has a multichannel electrode array which is positioned on the surface of the dorsal cochlear nucleus and is connected to a receiver stimulator under the skin. The stimulus is delivered by an external component comprising a microphone, a signal processor and a transmitter coil similar to a cochlear implant system. Although this surgery is still at an experimental stage, early results from North America and Europe indicate that such patients are capable of pitch discrimination and some degree of open set speech discrimination (Laszig *et al.*, 1995).

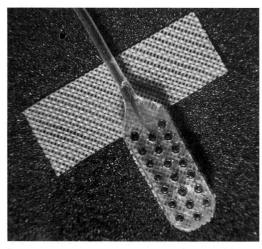

Figure 21.22 The current European design auditory brain stem implant (ABI) showing the 21 electrode array which is positioned on the dorsal cochlear nucleus. The dacron mesh is for support. (Reproduced by courtesy of Cochlear AG, Basel)

References

ABRAMOVICH, S. (1990) *Electric Response Audiometry in Clinical Practice*. Edinburgh: Churchill Livingstone

ANNIKO, M., ARNDT, J. and NOREN, G. (1981) The human acoustic neuroma in organ culture. II. Tissue changes after gamma irradiation. *Acta Otolaryngologica*, **91**, 223–235

ANTONI, N. (1920) *Ueber Ruckensmarkstumoren und Neurofibrome; Studien zur pathologischen Anatomie und Embryologie; mit einem kinischen Anhang*. Munich: J. F. Bergmann

ARRIAGA, M. A., LONG, S. and NELSON, R. (1993) Clinical correlates of acoustic neuroma volume. *American Journal of Otology*, **14**, 465–468

ATKINSON, W. J. (1949) The anterior inferior cerebellar artery: its variations, pontine distribution, and significance in the surgery of cerebello-pontine angle tumours. *Journal of Neurology, Neurosurgery and Psychiatry*, **12**, 137–151

BABIGHIAN, G., DE MIN, G., AMADORI, M. and GALAVERNI, D. (1992) Intraoperative monitoring of the facial nerve during acoustic neuroma surgery. In: *Acoustic Neuroma* (*Proceedings of First International Conference on Acoustic Neuroma, Copenhagen 1991*) edited by M. Tos, and J. Thomsen. Amsterdam: Kugler Publications. pp. 593–598

BALLANCE, C. (1907) *Some Points in the Surgery of the Brain and its Membranes*. London: Macmillan and Co. p. 276

BARRS, D. M., BRACKMANN, D. E. and HITSELBERGER, W. E. (1984) Facial nerve anastomosis in the cerebellopontine angle: a review of 24 cases. *American Journal of Otology*, **5**, 268–272

BELL, C. (1830) *The Nervous System of the Human Body*, embracing the papers delivered to the Royal Society on the subject of nerves. London: Longman, Rees, Orme, Brown and Green. pp. 112–114

BIRZGALIS, A. R., CURLEY, J. W. A. and RAMSDEN, R. T. (1991) Intralabyrinthine schwannoma. *Journal of Laryngology and Otology*, **105**, 659–661

BIRZGALIS, A. R., RAMSDEN, R. T., LYE, R. H. and RICHARDSON, P. L. (1990) Haemangiopericytoma of the temporal bone. *Journal of Laryngology and Otology*, **104**, 998–1004

BROWNING, G. G., GATEHOUSE, S. and SWANN, I. R. C. (1991) The Glasgow Benefit Plot: a new method of reporting benefits from middle ear surgery. *Laryngoscope*, **101**, 180–185

BRUNNER, H. (1925) Pathologie und Klinik der Erkrankung des Innenohres nach stumpfen Schadeltraumen. *Monatsschrift für Ohrenheilkunde und Laryngo-Rhinologie*, **59**, 697–709

CARHART, R. (1957) Clinical determination of abnormal auditory adaptation. *Archives of Otolaryngology*, **65**, 32–39

CHARABI, S., MANTONI, M., TOS, M. and THOMSEN, J. (1994) Cystic vestibular schwannomas: neuroimaging and growth. *Journal of Laryngology and Otology*, **108**, 375–379

CHARABI, S., THOMSEN, J., MANTONI, M., CHARABI, B., JORGENSEN, B., BORGENSEN, S. E. *et al.* (1995) Acoustic neuroma (vestibular schwannoma); growth, surgical and non-surgical consequences of wait and see policy. *Otolaryngology – Head and Neck Surgery* (in press)

COX, G. J. (1993) Intracanalicular acoustic neuromas: a conservative approach. *Clinical Otolaryngology*, **18**, 153–154

CROXSON, G. R., MOFFAT, D. A. and BAGULEY, D. (1988) Brun's bidirectional nystagmus in cerebello positive angle tumours. *Clinical Otolaryngology*, **13**, 153–157

CRUVEILHIER, J. (1935) quoted by Cushing, H. (1917) *Tumors of the Nervus Acusticus and the Syndrome of the Cerebellopontile Angle*, ch. 1, reprinted 1963. New York: Haffner Publishing Company. p. 4

CURATI, W. L., GRAIF, M., KINGSLEY, D. P. E., NEINDORF, H. P. and YOUNG, I. R. (1986) Acoustic neuromas. Gd - DTPA enhancement in MR imaging. *Radiology*, **158**, 447–451

CURLEY, J. W. A., RAMSDEN, R. T., HOWELL, A., HEALEY, K. and LYE, R. H. (1990) Oestrogen and progesterone receptors in acoustic neuroma. *Journal of Laryngology and Otology*, **104**, 865–867

CUSHING, H. (1917) *Tumors of the Nervus Acusticus and the Syndrome of the Cerebellopontile Angle*, reprinted 1963, New York: Haffner Publishing Company

DANDY, W. E. (1925) An operation for the total removal of

cerebellopontine (acoustic) tumors. *Surgery, Gynecology and Obstetrics*, **41**, 129–148

DE MOURA, L. F. P., HAYDEN, R. C. and CONNER, G. H. (1969) Bilateral acoustic neuroma and neurofibromatosis *Archives of Otolaryngology*, **90**, 28–34

DI TULLIO, M. V. JR, MALKASIAN, D. and RAND, R. W. (1978) A critical comparison of neurosurgical and otolaryngological approaches to acoustic neuromas. *Journal of Neurosurgery*, **48**, 1–12

DIX, M. R. and HALLPIKE, C. S. (1950) Observations on the pathological mechanism of conductive deafness in certain cases of neuroma of the VIIIth nerve. *Journal of Laryngology and Otology*, **64**, 658–666

DIX, M. R. and HALLPIKE, C. S. (1966) Observations on the clinical features and neurological mechanism of spontaneous nystagmus resulting from unilateral acoustic neurofibroma. *Acta Otolaryngologica*, **61**, 1–22

DIX, M. R., HALLPIKE, C. S. and HOOD, J. D. (1948). Observations on the loudness recruitment phenomenon, with especial reference to the differential diagnosis of the inner ear and VIII nerve. *Proceedings of the Royal Society of Medicine*, **41**, 516–526

DUTTON, J. E. M., RAMSDEN, R. T., LYE, R. H., MORRIS, K., PAGE, R. D., KEITH, A. O. et al. (1992) The neuro-otological team approach to the surgical management of acoustic neuroma: the Manchester experience In: *Acoustic Neuroma (Proceedings of First International Conference on Acoustic Neuroma, Copenhagen 1991)* edited by M. Tos and J. Thomsen. Amsterdam: Kugler Publications. pp. 503–507

EVANS, D. G. R., BLAIR, V., STRACHAN, T., LYE, R. H. and RAMSDEN, R. T. (1995) Variation in expression of the gene for type II neurofibromatosis: absence of a gender effect on vestibular schwannoma. *Journal of Laryngology and Otology*, **109**, 830

EVANS, D. G. R., RAMSDEN, R., HUSON, S., HARRIS, R., LYE, R. and KING, T. T. (1993) Type 2 neurofibromatosis: the need for supraregional care. *Journal of Laryngology and Otology*, **107**, 401–406

FISCH, U. (1978) 'Congenital' cholesteatomas of the supralabyrinthine region. *Clinical Otolaryngology*, **3**, 369–376

FISCH, U. (1994) In panel discussion Hearing preservation in acoustic neuroma surgery. *4th International Symposium & Workshops. Inner Ear Medicine and Surgery* – July 16–23 1994: Snowmass, Colorado: Prosper Meniere Society

FITZGERALD, E. and HALLPIKE, C. S. (1942) Studies in human vestibular function; observations on the directional preponderance of caloric nystagmus resulting from cerebellar lesions. *Brain*, **65**, 115–137

FLOOD, L. M., BRAMMER, R. E., GRAHAM, M. O. and KEMINK, J. L. (1984) Pitfalls in the diagnosis of acoustic neuroma. *Clinical Otolaryngology*, **9**, 165–170

GARDNER, W. J. and FRAZIER, C. H. (1930) Bilateral acoustic neurofibromas: a clinical study and field survey of a family of five generations with bilateral deafness in thirty eight members. *Archives of Neurology and Psychiatry*, **23**, 266–302

GIBSON, W. P. R and BEAGLEY, H. A. (1976) Electrocochleography in the diagnosis of acoustic neuroma. *Journal of Laryngology and Otology*, **90**, 127–139

GIBSON, W. P. R. and WALLACE, D. (1975) Basilar artery ectasia (an unusual cause of a cerebello-pontine lesion and hemifacial spasm). *Journal of Laryngology and Otology*, **89**, 721–731

GIBSON, W. P. R., MOFFAT, D. A. and RAMSDEN, R. T. (1977)

Clinical electrocochleography in the diagnosis and management of Meniere's disorder. *Audiology*, **16**, 389–401

HAID, C. T. and WIGAND M. E. (1992) Surgery of acoustic neuromas through the enlarged middle cranial fossa approach. In: *Acoustic Neuroma (Proceedings of First International Conference on Acoustic Neuroma, Copenhagen 1991)* edited by M. Tos and J. Thomsen. Amsterdam: New York Kugler Publications. pp. 483–488

HARDY, M. and CROWE, S. J. (1936) Early asymptomatic acoustic tumour. Report of 6 cases. *Archives of Surgery*, **32**, 292–301

HASHIMOTO, S., TOSHIMA, M., SAKURADA, T., ISHIGAKI, M., KOIKE, S., INAMURA, N. et al. (1992) Strategy for the early diagnosis of acoustic neuromas. In: *Acoustic Neuroma (Proceedings of First International Conference on Acoustic Neuroma, Copenhagen 1991)* edited by M. Tos and J. Thomsen. Amsterdam: Kugler Publications. pp. 83–86

HENSCHEN, F. (1912) Die Akustikustumoren, eine neue Gruppe radiologisch darstellbarer Hirntumoren *Fortschritte auf dem Gebiet der Roentgenstrahlen*, **18**, 207–218

HINTON, A. E., RAMSDEN, R. T., LYE, R. H. and DUTTON, J. E. M. (1992) Criteria for hearing preservation in acoustic schwannoma surgery: the concept of useful hearing. *Journal of Laryngology and Otology*, **106**, 500–503

HIRSCH, A. and ANDERSON, H. (1980) Elevated stapedius reflex threshold and pathologic reflex decay. Clinical occurrence and significance. *Acta Otolaryngologica Supplementum*, **368**

HIRSCH, A. and NORÉN, G. (1992) Audiological evaluation after stereotactic radiosurgery in acoustic neurinomas. In: *Acoustic Neuroma (Proceedings of First International Conference on Acoustic Neuroma, Copenhagen 1991)* edited by M. Tos and J. Thomsen. Amsterdam: Kugler Publications. pp. 293–295

HITSELBERGER, W. E. and HOUSE, W. F. (1968) *Otolaryngology*, ch 24. Maryland: Harper and Row

HOFFMAN, R. A., KOHAN, D. and COHEN N. L. (1992) Cochlear implants in the management of acoustic neuromas. *American Journal of Otology*, **13**, 525–528

HOOD, J. D. and POOLE, J. P. (1971) Speech audiometry in conductive and sensorineural hearing loss. *Sound*, **5**, 30–38

HOOD, J. D., KAYAN, A. and LEECH, J. (1973) Rebound nystagmus. *Brain*, **96**, 507–526

HOUSE, W. F. (1961) Surgical exposure of the internal auditory canal and its contents through the middle cranial fossa. *Laryngoscope*, **71**, 1363–1385

HOUSE, W. F. (1964) Evolution of transtemporal bone removal of acoustic tumours. *Archives of Otolaryngology*, **80**, 731–741

JAHNKE, K. and NEUMAN, T. A. (1992) The fine structure of vestibular end organs in acoustic schwannoma patients In: *Acoustic Neuroma (Proceedings of First International Conference on Acoustic Neuroma, Copenhagen 1991)*, edited by M. Tos and J. Thomsen. Amsterdam: Kugler Publications. pp. 203–207

JENKINS, H. A. and FISCH, U. (1980) The transotic approach to resection of difficult acoustic neuromas of the cerebellopontine angle. *American Journal of Otology*, **2**, 70–76

JEWETT, D. L., ROMANO, M. N. and WILLISTON, J. S. (1970) Human auditory evoked potentials: possible brain stem components detected on the scalp. *Science*, **167**, 1517–1518

JOHNSSON, L. G. and KINGSLEY, T. C. (1981) Asymptomatic acoustic neuroma. A temporal bone report. *Archives of Otolaryngology*, **107**, 377–381

KAISER-KUPFER, M. I., FRIEDLIN, V., DATILES, M. B. and EL-DRIDGE, R. (1989). The association of posterior capsular lens opacities with bilateral acoustic neuromas in patients with neurofibromatosis type 2. *Archives of Ophthalmology*, **107**, 541–544

KANTER, W. R., ELDRIDGE, R., FABRICANT, R., ALLEN, J. C. and KOERBER, T. (1980). Central neurofibromatosis with bilateral acoustic neuroma. genetic, clinical and biochemical distinctions from peripheral neurofibromatosis. *Neurology*, **30**, 851–859

KING, T. T., GIBSON, W. P. R. and MORRISON, A. W. (1976) Tumours of the eighth cranial nerve. *British Journal of Hospital Medicine*, **16**, 259–272

KLINKEN, L., THOMSEN, J., RASMUSSEN, B. B., WIET, R. J. and TOS, M. (1990) Estrogen and progesterone receptors in acoustic neuromas. *Archives of Otolaryngology – Head and Neck Surgery*, **116**, 202–203

KRAUSE, F. (1903) Zur Freilegung der hinteren Felsenbein-flache und des Kleinhirns. *Beitrage zur klinischen Chirurgie*, **37**, 728–764

LAI, D., GIBSON, W. and SCRIVENER, B. (1991). Prognostic factors for facial nerve function after acoustic neuroma surgery. *Journal of the Otolaryngological Society of Australia*, **5**, 414–418

LASZIG, R., SOLLMANN, W. P., MARANGOS, N. and RAMSDEN, R. T. (1995) The European ABI: Early results. *Proceedings of International Cochlear Implant, Speech and Hearing Symposium, Melbourne, 1994* (in press)

LEKSELL, L. (1951) The stereotaxic method and radiosurgery of the brain. *Acta Chirurgica Scandinavica*, **102**, 316–319

LESSER, T. H. J., JANZER, R. C., KLEIHUIS, P. and FISCH, U. (1991) Clinical growth rate of acoustic schwannomas: correlation with the growth factor as defined by the monoclonal antibody Ki67. *Skull Base Surgery*, **1**, 11–15

LINTHICUM, F. H. Jr (1972) Unusual audiometric and histological findings in bilateral acoustic neurinomas. *Annals of Otology, Rhinology and Laryngology*, **81**, 433–437

LITTLE, J. R., GOMEZ, M. R. and MACCARTY, C. S. (1973) Infratentorial arachnoid cysts. *Journal of Neurosurgery*, **39**, 380–386

LUETJE, C. M., WHITTAKER, C. K., CALLAWAY, L. A. and VERAGA, G. (1983) Histological acoustic tumor involvement of the VIIth nerve and multicentric origin in the VIIIth nerve. *Laryngoscope*, **93**, 1133–1139

LUNSFORD, L. D., LINKSEY, M. E. and FLICKINGER, J. C. (1992) Stereotactic radiosurgery for acoustic nerve sheath tumours. In: *Acoustic Neuroma (Proceedings of First International Conference on Acoustic Neuroma, Copenhagen 1991)*, edited by M. Tos M and J. Thomsen. Amsterdam: Kugler Publications. pp. 279–287

LYE, R. H., ELSTOW, S. F. and WEISS, J. B. (1986) Neovascularisation of intracranial tumours In: *Biology of Brain Tumours*, edited by M. D. Walker and D. G. T. Thomas. Boston: Martinus Nijhoff. pp. 61–66

LYE R. H., PACE-BALZAN, A., RAMSDEN, R. T., GILLESPIE, J. E. and DUTTON, J. M. (1992) The fate of tumour rests following removal of acoustic neuromas: an MRI-DTPA study. *British Journal of Neurosurgery*, **6**, 195–202

MCELVEEN, J. T., WILKINS, R. H., ERWIN, A. C. and WOLFORD, R. D. (1991) Modifying the translabyrinthine approach to preserve hearing during acoustic tumour surgery. *Journal of Laryngology and Otology*, **105**, 34–37

MAGIELSKI, J. E. and BLATT, I. M. (1958) Submaxillary salivary flow: a test of chorda tympani nerve funtion as an aid in diagnosis and prognosis of facial paralysis. *Laryngoscope*, **68**, 1770–1789

MAGNAN, J., CHAYS, A., LEPETRE, C., PENCROFFI, E. and LOCATELLI, P. (1994) Surgical perspectives of endoscopy of the cerebellopontine angle. *American Journal of Otology*, **15**, 366–370

MARQUET, J. F. E., FORTON, G. E. J., OFFECIERS, F. E. and MOENECLAEY, L. L. M. (1990) The solitary schwannoma of the eighth cranial nerve. *Archives of Otolaryngolgy – Head and Neck Surgery*, **116**, 1023–1025

MARTIN, C., PRADES, J. M. and CUELIKH, L. (1992) Growth rate of acoustic neuromas. In: *Acoustic Neuroma (Proceedings of First International Conference on Acoustic Neuroma, Copenhagen 1991)* edited by M. Tos and J. Thomsen. Amsterdam: Kugler Publications. pp. 177–182

MARTUZA, R. L., MACLAUGHLIN, D. T. and OJEMANN, R. G. (1981) Specific estradiol binding in schwannomas, meningiomas and neurofibromas. *Neurosurgery*, **9**, 665–670

MARX, H. (1913) Zur Chirurgie der Kleinhirnbrückenwinkeltumoren. *Mitteilungen an den Grenzgebieten der Medizin und Chirurgie*, **26**, 117–134

MAZZONI, A. and HANSEN, C. C. (1970) Surgical anatomy of the arteries of the internal auditory canal. *Archives of Otolaryngology*, **91**, 128–135

MOFFAT, D. A., and HARDY, D. G. (1989) Early diagnosis and surgical management of acoustic neuromas: is it cost effective? *Journal of the Royal Society of Medicine*, **82**, 329–332

MOFFAT, D. A., BAGULEY, D. M., EVANS, R. A., and HARDY, D. G. (1989a) Mastoid ache in acoustic neuroma. *Journal of Laryngology and Otology*, **103**, 1043–1044

MOFFAT, D. A., GOLLEDGE, J., BAGULEY, D. M., and HARDY, D. G. (1993a). Clinical correlates of acoustic neuroma morphology. *Journal of Laryngology and Otology*, **107**, 290–294

MOFFAT, D. A., HARRIES, M. L. L., BAGULEY, D. M. and HARDY, D. G. (1989b) Unterberger's stepping test in acoustic neuroma. *Journal of Laryngology and Otology*, **103**, 839–841

MOFFAT, D. A., SAUNDERS, J. E., MCELVEEN, J. T., MCFERRAN, D. J. and HARDY, D. G. (1993b) Unusual cerebello-pontine angle tumours. *Journal of Laryngology and Otology*, **107**, 1087–1098

MORRISON, A. W. and KING, T. T. (1982) Translabyrinthine removal of acoustic neuromas. In: *Neurological Surgery of the Ear and Skull Base*, edited by D. E. Brackmann. New York: Raven Press. pp. 227–233

MORRISON, A. W., GIBSON, W. P. R. and BEAGLEY, H. A. (1976). Transtympanic electrocochleography in the diagnosis of retrocochlear tumours. *Clinical Otolaryngology*, **1**, 153–167

MYRSETH, E., MØLLER, P., GANZ, J. C., JENSEN, Ø., KRÅKENES, J., LARSEN, J. L. et al. (1992) Acoustic neuroma: some principles for the selection of method of treatment, with particular reference to suboccipital surgery and stereotactic radiosurgery. In: *Acoustic Neuroma (Proceedings of First International Conference on Acoustic Neuroma, Copenhagen 1991)* edited by M. Tos and J. Thomsen. Amsterdam: Kugler Publications. pp. 297–299

NAGER, G. T. (1969) Acoustic neurinomas. Pathology and differential diagnosis. *Archives of Otolaryngology*, **89**, 252–279

NATIONAL INSTITUTES OF HEALTH CONSENSUS DEVELOPMENT CONFERENCE (1990) Neurofibromatosis 1 (von Recklinghausen disease) and neurofibromatosis 2 (bilateral acoustic neurofibromatosis). *Annals of Internal Medicine*, **113**, 39–52

NEDZELSKI, J. M. (1983) Cerebellopontine angle tumours: bilateral flocculus compression as cause of associated oculomotor abnormalities. *Laryngoscope*, **93**, 1251–1260

NEDZELSKI, J. M. and DUFOUR, J. J. (1975) Acoustic neurinomas presenting as sudden deafness. *Otorhinolaryngology and its Borderlands*, **37**, 271–279

NEDZELSKI, J. M., SCHESSEL, D. A., PLEIDERER, A., KASSEL, E. E. and ROWED, D. W. (1992) The natural history of the growth of acoustic neuromas and its role in nonoperative management. In: *Acoustic Neuroma (Proceedings of First International Conference on Acoustic Neuroma, Copenhagen 1991)* edited by M. Tos and J. Thomsen. Amsterdam: Kugler Publications. pp. 149–158

NEELY, J. G. (1981) Gross and microscopic anatomy of the eighth cranial nerve in relation to the solitary schwannoma. *Laryngoscope*, **91**, 1512–1531

NORÉN, G., GREITZ, D., HIRSCH, A. and LAX, I. (1992) Gamma knife radiosurgery in acoustic neurinomas In: *Acoustic Neuroma (Proceedings of First International Conference on Acoustic Neuroma, Copenhagen 1991)*, edited by M. Tos and J. Thomsen. Amsterdam: Kugler Publications. pp. 289–292

O'CONNOR, A. F., LUXON, L. M., SHORTMAN, R. C., THOMPSON, E. T. and MORRISON, A. W. (1982) Electrophoretic separation and identification of perilymph proteins in a case of acoustic neuroma. *Acta Otolaryngologica*, **93**, 195–200

OPPENHEIM, H. (1890) Ueber mehrere Fälle von endocraniellem Tumor in welchem es gelang eine genaue Localdiagnose zu stellen. *Berliner klinische Wochenschrift*, **27**, 38–40

PALVA, T. and RAUNIO, V. (1982) Cerebrospinal fluid and acoustic neurinoma specific proteins in perilymph. *Acta Otolaryngologica*, **93**, 201–203

PANIZZA, B. J., JACKSON, A. and RAMSDEN, R. T. (1992) Choroid plexus papilloma of the cerebellopontine angle. *Skull Base Surgery*, **2**, 155–159

PANSE, R. (1904) Klinische und pathologische Mitteilungen. IV. Ein Gliom des Akustikus. *Archiv für Ohrenheilkunde*, **61**, 251–255

PASQUIER, B., WOZNIAK, Z. M., MOURET, P., GRATACAP, B. and CHARACHON, R. (1992) Evaluation of acoustic neuroma growth rates by immunochemical techniques. In: *Acoustic Neuroma (Proceedings of First International Conference on Acoustic Neuroma, Copenhagen 1991)*, edited by M. Tos and J. Thomsen. Amsterdam: Kugler Publications. pp. 173–176

PENNYBACKER, J. B. and CAIRNS, H. (1950) Results in 130 cases of acoustic neurinoma. *Journal of Neurology, Neurosurgery and Psychiatry*, **13**, 272–277

PENSAK, M. L., GLASSCOCK, M. E., GULYA, A. J., HAYS, J. W., SMITH, H. P. and DICKENS, J. R. E. (1986) Cerebellopontine lipomas. *Archives of Otolaryngology–Head and Neck Surgery*, **112**, 99–101

PERNECZKY, A. (1981) Die arteria cerebelli inferior anterior. *Fortschritte der Medezin*, **99**, 511–514

PIRSIG, W., ZIEMANN–BECKER, B. and TESCHLER–NICOLA, M. (1992) Acoustic neuroma: four thousand years ago. In: *Acoustic Neuroma (Proceedings of First International Conference on Acoustic Neuroma, Copenhagen 1991)*, edited by M. Tos and J. Thomsen. Amsterdam: Kugler Publications. pp. 7–12

PORTMANN, M., STERKERS, J.-M., CHARACHON, R. and CHOUARD, C. H. (1975) *The Internal Auditory Meatus. Anatomy, Pathology and Surgery*. Edinburgh: Churchill Livingstone. pp. 75–76

PULEC, J. L. and HOUSE, W. F. (1964) Trigeminal nerve testing in acoustic tumours. *Archives of Otolaryngology*, **80**, 681–684

QUIX, F. H. (1912) Ein Fall von translabyrinthisch operiertem Tumor Acusticus. *Verhandlung der deutschen Otologischen Gesellschaft*, **21**, 245–255

RAMSDEN, R. T., DUTTON, J. E. M., LYE, R. H. and KEITH, A. O. (1992) The value of traditional audiological tests in the diagnosis of acoustic neuroma. In: *Acoustic Neuroma (Proceedings of First International Conference on Acoustic Neuroma, Copenhagen 1991)* edited by M. Tos and J. Thomsen. Amsterdam: Kugler Publications. pp. 73–76

RAMSDEN, R. T. and MOFFAT, D. A. (1994) Intracanalicular acoustic neuromas: the case for early surgery. *Clinical Otolaryngology*, **19**, 1–2

RAND, R. W. and KURZE, T. (1965) Micro-neurosurgical resection of acoustic tumors by a transmeatal posterior fossa approach. *Bulletin of the Los Angeles Neurological, Society*, **30**, 17–20

RASMUSSEN, N., THOMSEN, J. and TOS, M. (1981) Possible cellular immunity against acoustic neuroma. *Acta Otolaryngologica*, **92**, 337–341

RASMUSSEN, N., TRIBUKAIT, B., THOMSEN, J., HOLM, L. E. and TOS, M. (1984) Implications of DNA characteristics of human acoustic neuromas. *Acta Otolaryngologica*, Supplement 406, 278–281

RHOTON, A. L. JR, MARTIN, R. G., GRANT, J. L. and PEACE, D. (1982) Microsurgical relationships of the anterior inferior cerebellar artery and the facial-vestibulocochlear nerve complex. In: *Neurological Surgery of the Ear and Skull Base*, edited by D. E., Brackmann. New York: Raven Press. pp. 23–27

ROBSON, A. K., LEIGHTON, S. E. J., ANSLOW, P. and MILFORD, C. A. (1993) MRI as a single screening procedure for acoustic neuroma: a cost effective protocol. *Journal of the Royal Society of Medicine*, **86**, 455–457

ROSENBLOOM, S. B., CARSON, B. S., WANG, H., ROSENBAUM, A. E. and UDVARHELYI, G. B. (1985) Cerebellopontine angle lipoma. *Surgical Neurology*, **23**, 134–138

SAEED, S. R., BIRZGALIS, A. R. and RAMSDEN, R. T. (1994) Intravestibular schwannoma shown by magnetic resonance imaging. *Neuroradiology*, **36**, 63–64

SAEED, S. R., RAMSDEN, R. T., WOOLFORD, T. J. and LYE, R. H. (1995) Magnetic resonance imaging: a cost effective first line investigation in the detection of acoustic neuromas. *Journal of Neurosurgery*. (in press)

SAMII, M. (1984) Facial nerve grafting in acoustic neurinoma. *Clinics in Plastic Surgery*, **11**, 221–225

SANDIFORT, E. (1777) *De duro quodam corpusculo, nervo auditorio adhaerente; observationes anatomico-pathologicae.* P v.d. Eyk & D Vygh. Book 1, 116–120

SANNA, M., GAMOLETTI, R., TOS, M. and THOMSEN, J. (1992) Synopsis on hearing preservation following acoustic neuroma surgery. In: *Acoustic Neuroma (Proceedings of First International Conference on Acoustic Neuroma, Copenhagen 1991)* edited by M. Tos and J. Thomsen. Amsterdam: Kugler Publications. pp. 985–987

SCHESSEL, D. A., NEDZELSKI, J. M., KASSEL, E. E. and ROWED, D. W. (1992) Recurrence rates of acoustic neuroma in hearing preservation surgery. *American Journal of Otology*, **13**, 233–235

SCHUKNECHT, H. F. (1974) Neoplastic growth. In *Pathology of the Ear*, ch. 11. Cambridge, Massachusetts: Harvard University Press. pp. 415–451

SCHUKNECHT, H. F. and WOELLNER, R. C. (1955) An experimental and clinical study of deafness from lesions of the cochlear nerve. *Journal of Laryngology and Otology*, **69**, 75–97

SELTERS, W. A. and BRACKMANN, D. E. (1977) Acoustic tumour detection with brain stem electric response audiometry. *Archives of Otolaryngology* **103**, 181–187

SHELTON, C., HILZELBERGER, W. E., HOUSE, W. F. and BRACKMANN, D. E. (1992) Long term results of hearing preservation after acoustic tumor removal. In: *Acoustic Neuroma (Proceedings of First International Conference on Acoustic Neuroma, Copenhagen 1991)* edited by M. Tos and J. Thomsen. Amsterdam: Kugler Publications. pp. 661–664

SHORE – FREEDMAN, E., ABRAHAMS, C., RECANT, W. and SCHNEIDER, A. B. (1983) Neurilemomas and salivary gland tumours of the head and neck following childhood irradiation. *Cancer*, **51**, 2159–2163

SILVERSTEIN, H. and SCHUKNECHT H. F. (1966) Biochemical studies of inner ear fluid in man. *Archives of Otolaryngology*, **84**, 395–402

SMYTH, G. D. L. and PATTERSON, C. C. (1985) Results of middle ear reconstruction: do patients and surgeons agree? *American Journal of Otology*, **6**, 276–279

STERKERS, J.-M. and HOCSMAN, E. (1992) Results in four consecutive cases of acoustic neuroma treated with the gamma knife. In: *Acoustic Neuroma (Proceedings of First International Conference on Acoustic Neuroma, Copenhagen 1991)* edited by M. Tos and J. Thomsen. Amsterdam: Kugler Publications. p. 309

STERKERS, O., EL DINE, M. B., MARTIN, N., VIALA, P. and STERKERS, J. M. (1992) Slow versus rapid growing acoustic neuromas. In: *Acoustic Neuroma (Proceedings of First International Conference on Acoustic Neuroma, Copenhagen 1991)* edited by M. Tos and J. Thomsen. Amsterdam: Kugler Publications. pp. 145–147

STEVENS, G. T. (1879) A case of tumor of the auditory nerve occupying the fossa for the cerebellum. *Archives of Otology*, **8**, 171–176

STORRS, L. A. (1974) Acoustic neurinomas presenting as middle ear tumors. *Laryngoscope*, **84**, 1175–1180

SUGA, F. and LINDSAY, J. R. (1976) Inner ear degeneration in acoustic neuroma. *Annals of Otology, Rhinology and Laryngology*, **85**, 343–358

TALLAN, E. M., HARNER, S. G. and BEATTY, C. W. (1993) Does the distribution of Schwann cells correlate with the observed occurrence of acoustic neuromas? *American Journal of Otology*, **14**, 131–134

TELISCHI, F. F., LO, W. W. M., ARRIAGA, M. A. and DE LA CRUZ, A. (1993) Lateral extent of internal auditory canal involvement by acoustic neuromas: a surgical- radiological correlation. *American Journal of Otology*, **14**, 446–450

TERKILDSEN, K. and THOMSEN, J. (1983) Diagnostic screening for acoustic neuromas. *Clinical Otolaryngology*, **8**, 295–296

THOMSEN, J. and JORGENSEN, M. B. (1973) Undiagnosed acoustic neurinomas. A presentation of 4 cases. *Archiv für klinische und experimentelle Ohren Nasen und Kehlkopfheilkunde*, **204**, 175–182

THOMSEN, J. and ZILSTORFF, K. (1975) Intermedius nerve involvement and testing in acoustic neuromas. *Acta Otolaryngologica*, **80**, 276–282

THOMSEN, J., KLINKEN, L. and TOS, M. (1984). Calcified acoustic neuroma. *Journal of Laryngology and Otology*, **98**, 727–732

THOMSEN, J., TOS, M. and BORGESEN, S. E. (1990) Gamma knife: hydrocephalus as a complication of stereotactic radiosurgical treatment of an acoustic neuroma. *American Journal of Otology*, **11**, 330–333

TOS, M. and THOMSEN, J. (1984) Epidemiology of acoustic neuromas. *Journal of Laryngology and Otology*, **98**, 685–692

TOYNBEE, J. (1853) Neuroma of the auditory nerve. *Transactions of the Pathological Society of London*, **4**, 259–260

TROFFATER, J. A., MACCOLLIN, M. M., RUTTER, J. L., MURRELL, J. L., DUYAO, M. P., PARRY, D. M. *et al.* (1993) A novel Moesin-Ezrin-Radixin like gene is a candidate for the neurofibromatosis type 2 tumor suppressor. *Cell*, **72**, 791–800

TUCCI, D. L., TELIAN, S. A., KILENY, P. R., HOFF, J. T. and KEMICK, J. L. (1994) Stability of hearing after acoustic neuroma surgery. *American Journal of Otology*, **15**, 183–188

VALVASSORI, G. E. (1969) The diagnosis of acoustic neuromas. *Seminars in Roentgenology*, **4**, 171–177

VALVASSORI, G. E. and GUZMAN, M. (1989) Growth rate of acoustic neuromas. *American Journal of Otology*, **10**, 174–176

VALVASSORI, G. E., BUCKINGHAM, R. A., CARTER, B. L., HANAFEE, W. N. and MAFEE, M. F. (1988) *Head and Neck Imaging.* New York: Thieme Medical Publications. pp. 124–126

VON RECKLINGHAUSEN, F. D. (1882) *Ueber die multiplen Fibrome und ihre Beziehung zu den multiplen Neuromen.* Berlin: Hirschwald

WALSTED, A., NIELSEN, K. B., SALOMON, G., THOMSEN, J. and TOS, M. (1992) Auditory brainstem response in the diagnosis of acoustic neuroma. In: *Acoustic Neuroma (Proceedings of First International Conference on Acoustic Neuroma, Copenhagen 1991)* edited by M. Tos and J. Thomsen. Amsterdam: Kugler Publications. pp. 87–90

WATKYN–THOMAS, F. W. (1939) Discussion on internal ear deafness. *Proceedings of the Royal Society of Medicine*, **32**, 487–491

WELLING, D. B. and GLASSCOCK, M. E. (1992) The diagnostic work-up of acoustic neuromas. In: *Acoustic Neuroma (Proceedings of First International Conference on Acoustic Neuroma, Copenhagen 1991)* edited by M. Tos and J. Thomsen. Amsterdam: Kugler Publications. pp. 101–105

WENNERBERG, J. and MERKE, U. (1989) Growth potential of acoustic neuromas. *American Journal of Otology*, **10**, 293–296

WIET, R. J., RUBY, S. G. and BAUER, G. P. (1994) Proliferating nuclear cell antigen in the determination of growth rates in acoustic neuromas. *American Journal of Otology*, **15**, 294–298

WIGAND, M. E., HAID, C. T. and BERG, M. (1989) The enlarged middle cranial fossa approach for surgery of the temporal bone and cerebello-pontine angle. *Archives of Otorhinolaryngology*, **246**, 299

WISHART, J. H. (1822) Case of tumours in the skull, dura mater and brain. *Edinburgh Medical and Surgical Journal*, **18**, 393–397

WOOLFORD, T. J., BIRZGALIS, A. R. and RAMSDEN, R. T. (1994) An extensive vestibular schwannoma with both intracranial spread and lateral extension to the external auditory canal. *Journal of Laryngology and Otology*, **108**, 149–151

22

Epithelial tumours of the external auditory meatus and middle ear

O. H. Shaheen

Historical perspective

Claims that Schwartze and Wilde published the earliest reports on middle ear cancer in 1775 are seriously open to question (Peele and Hauser, 1941; Lewis, 1960), because as Stell (1984b) pointed out neither of these distinguished clinicians was living in that era and histopathology had not as yet evolved. Quite clearly the date mentioned was incorrect and if Schwartze and Wilde were to be credited with descriptions of aural tumours, their publications would have appeared some 100 years later.

Although it is entirely possible that they may have written on this subject, it was Politzer (1883) who published the first authoritative account of the disease, and this was followed by reports from Kretschmann (1886) and Zeroni (1899).

Newhart (1917) reviewed 34 cases of carcinoma of the middle ear which had been reported in the literature between 1899 and 1917, and Broders (1921) studied 63 cases of epithelioma of the pinna, external meatus and middle ear in some detail.

There have been many reports on the subjects since then, with major contributions from Peele and Hauser (1941), Parsons and Lewis (1954), Lederman (1965), Tucker (1965) and Lewis (1973, 1975, 1983).

Pathogenesis

Nearly every report refers to the possible link between long-standing chronic suppurative otitis media and squamous carcinoma of the middle ear cleft and external auditory meatus. The incidence of chronic otitis in cases of cancer is put at 38% (Conley and Novack, 1960) and 85% (Newhart, 1917), and strongly suggests a relationship between the inflammatory complaint and the development of carcinoma. The fact that some cancers also arise in old mastoid cavities would tend to support the existence of a causal link, but clearly factors other than chronic otitis must be invoked, since malignant tumours are not invariably seen in the presence of suppuration. Squamous cell carcinoma of the external auditory meatus arising separately and independently from a middle ear neoplasm and epithelial tumours of glandular origin would generally appear not to exhibit a prior history of long-standing discharge.

Whereas actinic rays, trauma, frostbite, psoriasis and xeroderma pigmentosa (Towson and Shofstall, 1950; Fredericks, 1956–1957) are possible aetiological factors, it is doubtful that they would apply to more deep-seated tumours. Chronic otitis externa however, would appear to be a plausible predisposing factor in the pathogenesis of external meatus tumours. The view has also been put forward that the evolution of carcinoma of the middle ear and external meatus can be likened to a Marjolin's ulcer, which by virtue of its site, indolence, and the presence of irritation ultimately turns to cancer.

Causes other than chronic suppuration include exposure to radiotherapy and possibly the carcinogen aflatoxin B which is produced by *Aspergillus flavus* and known to be hepatocarcinogenic (Johns and Headington, 1974); the evidence in support of the latter is, however, somewhat speculative.

On an experimental level, it is known that one dose of azoxymethane injected into rats induces squamous carcinoma in 15% of animals (Ward, 1975) and, doubtless, other known carcinogens painted onto the skin of the external auditory meatus of conditioned animals could also ultimately induce carcinoma.

Incidence

Tumours of the external auditory meatus and middle ear as a group are extremely uncommon and the neoplasm most likely to be encountered in this group is a squamous cell carcinoma, usually in a patient who has suffered from chronic suppurative otitis media.

Various authors have attempted to quantify the incidence of aural tumours by noting the frequencies of neoplasms in a given number of otological or general otolaryngological attendances over a given period. Figures such as 1:4000 or 1:20 000 are quoted, but are not really helpful since the spectrum of disease, sex, age and race of any given sample may vary considerably from one centre to another (Robinson, 1931; Schall, 1934; Towson and Shofstall, 1950).

Stell (1984b) has reported that the official age adjusted incidence or rate of registration of new cases has remained steady at approximately 1 per million for women and 0.8 per million for men over a 10-year period ending in 1977. It would also seem that the incidence rises with age in men, but is proportionately less after 75 years of age in women. This contrasts with a decreasing mortality rate after 70–75 years in men, while that for women continues to rise with advancing age (Morton, Stell, and Derrick, 1984).

Pathology

The majority of tumours arising in the external auditory meatus and the middle ear are squamous cell carcinomas. Uncommonly, other epithelial tumours which are mainly glandular in origin, may be encountered in either area, of which a small minority are adenomas.

External auditory meatus

Hidradenoma (hidradenocarcinoma, ceruminoma)

The term ceruminoma still in current usage, should be discarded in favour of hidradenoma or hidradenocarcinoma, since the ceruminous glands of the external canal are sweat glands and do not secrete cerumen. In fact wax is produced not by these glands but by the sebaceous glands of the external auditory meatus (Johnstone, Lennox and Watson, 1957). Tumours derived from the ceruminous glands (hidradenomas) are more often malignant than benign, the former evolving as differing histological entities including adenoid cystic carcinoma, mucoepidermoid tumour and adenocarcinoma.

Adenomas derived from ceruminous glands are histologically identical to benign sweat gland tumours seen elsewhere in the body; it should be pointed out that some authorities employ the term hidradenoma loosely in the context of the ear to cover both benign and malignant variants arising from the ceruminous glands (Moss, 1987; Peters, 1988; Batsakis, 1989; Benecke, 1990).

Basal cell carcinoma, sebaceous tumours and malignant melanoma

All three tumours are exceedingly rare, but basal cell carcinoma is the type most likely to be encountered in the UK. Basal cell tumours usually arise on the pinna and subsequently invade the external auditory meatus, but can in fact develop within the canal itself. Once bony invasion has taken place its behaviour is similar to that of squamous carcinoma, but with the difference that it rarely metastasizes (Stell, 1984a). According to Paparella and Meyerhoff (1980), the prognosis is better if the disease occurs on the pinna, rather than the external auditory meatus, possibly because of late detection and bone erosion in the case of the latter. Jesse, Healey and Wiley (1967) considered basal cell cancers to be slow growing and to remain within the confines of the meatus for a considerable period of time before eventually growing mediolaterally to involve the middle ear and pinna. In Stell's series (1984a), local excision was sufficient to cure most tumours arising from within the meatus in contradiction to the view put forward by Paparella and Meyerhoff (1980). Sebaceous tumours which are exceedingly rare are noted for their local invasiveness, whereas malignant melanomas are characterized more by their tendency to metastasize.

Middle ear

Apart from squamous cell carcinoma, the occasional adenoma, adenocarcinoma, basal cell carcinoma and choristoma may be seen in the middle ear. A choristoma is a collection of normal tissue observed at a location other than its normal site of origin and those found in the middle ear are usually collections of salivary tissue (Joachims, 1988; Batsakis, 1989; Bottrill, 1992).

The temporal bone is not infrequently the site of metastasis from tumours arising elsewhere, but may also be the seat of an exceedingly rare primary tumour, namely a papillary neoplasm of the endolymphatic sac, otherwise known as Heffner's tumour (Batsakis and El-Naggar, 1993).

Behaviour of squamous carcinoma of the external auditory meatus and middle ear

Many cases diagnosed as carcinoma of the middle ear or external meatus are found at the first visit to be straddling both areas, so that it may be very difficult to determine the site of origin. Often the designation is based more on the history and the observed extent of involvement of the areas in question, rather than any certain knowledge of the exact site of origin. Clearly if carcinoma of the meatus arises adjacent to the tympanic membrane, it can quite easily and quickly spread beneath the fibrous annulus of the drum to invade the middle ear, or alternatively destroy the tympanic membrane in its passage medially.

The opposite situation of a tumour arising in the middle ear invading the meatus is just as likely to occur and perhaps more so, since the majority of cases of squamous cell carcinoma are associated with chronic otitis media and a perforation. The existence of such a defect would accelerate the spread of tumour from middle ear to meatus, or vice versa. This has led many to regard carcinoma of the middle ear and deep meatus as one and the same disease.

There are instances, however, in which the carcinoma is sharply localized to the external auditory meatus some distance away from an intact drum, when it would be quite wrong to implicate the middle ear in the disease process.

Carcinoma of the meatus tracks outwards towards the concha, but at the junction of cartilaginous and bony meatus, the disease may escape anteriorly into the parotid gland and temporomandibular joint and posteriorly into the retroauricular sulcus (see Plate 3/22/I).

Cervical lymphadenopathy from meatal carcinoma is not uncommon; by contrast, cancer within the middle ear rarely metastasizes. The sites most often involved in metastasis are the pre- and postauricular nodes, and those lying along the anterior border of the trapezius in the posterior triangle of the neck.

Escape from the middle ear and mastoid occurs in several directions and along different routes. The thin wall of the tegmen is quickly penetrated, allowing cancer to become attached to the middle fossa dura. Spread posteriorly through the mastoid antrum and the mastoid process leads to exposure and infiltration of the posterior fossa dura and sigmoid sinus (Figures 22.1 and 22.2).

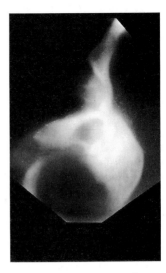

Figure 22.2 Lateral tomogram showing destruction of the mastoid and adjacent posterior tympanic plate of bone by cancer

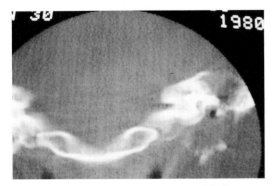

Figure 22.1 Axial CT showing destruction of the bony interface between the mastoid and posterior cranial fossa

Inferiorly, the jugular bulb may become involved by extension from the hypotympanum and, in time, the last four cranial nerves become paralysed. Disease may then extend quite far medially beneath the petrous bone and anterior to the vertebral column, there being no barrier to restrict spread in this direction.

Not uncommonly carcinoma will spread down the eustachian tube with invasion of the adjacent peritubal cells and destruction of the bony septum between tube and carotid canal (Phelps and Lloyd, 1981). Escape into the infratemporal fossa may occur via this route, but equally may spread directly through the petrotympanic fissure or circuitously via the parotid gland and temporomandibular joint.

Destruction of the fallopian canal is common, especially the thin horizontal segment, but surprisingly the cochlea, which one would expect to be resistant, is not immune to invasion (Michaels and Wells, 1980; Hiraide, Inouye and Ishii, 1983).

Involvement of the posterior and middle cranial fossa dura is often extensive, the disease presenting as a sheet of cancer covering a large surface. Penetration due to active infiltration as opposed to surface spread is slow to take place and at operation the deep surface of excised dura is not infrequently free of disease.

Certain parts of the petromastoid seem to be resistant to spread, namely those composed of thick sclerotic bone; typically the inferomedial part of the mastoid lying posterolateral to the jugular bulb is just such an area.

Symptoms and signs

Invasion of both bone and dura is characteristically painful and this would explain the deep-seated, boring, severe and unrelenting pain of middle ear and external meatal cancer.

Discharge is a common symptom in patients with a pre-existing history of chronic suppurative otitis media, but with the onset of carcinoma the discharge usually becomes blood-stained.

Involvement of the middle ear cleft is associated with deteriorating hearing, and in the event of inner ear invasion, unsteadiness and total loss of hearing.

Facial paralysis is generally due to invasion of the fallopian canal, especially when disease is confined mainly to the middle ear, but may also occur when meatal carcinoma escapes into the parotid gland via the osseocartilaginous junction of the external auditory meatus.

Escape from the middle ear into the infratemporal fossa leads to infiltration of the pterygoid muscles and trismus, while subpetrosal spread in a medial direction causes paralysis of the last four cranial nerves (see Plate 3/22/II).

Cancers of the external meatus will metastasize to the regional lymph nodes in 20% of cases.

Investigations

The most useful investigations at present are CT and MRI. The former serves to demonstrate areas of bony destruction and the latter soft tissue invasion. CT scans in the coronal plane will reveal the extent of bony destruction in the external auditory meatus, loss of the spur forming the outer attic wall, and destruction of the tegmen tympani. Axial films are helpful in detecting posterior and medial invasion of the petrous pyramid, and erosion into the carotid canal (Phelps and Lloyd, 1981) (Figure 22.3).

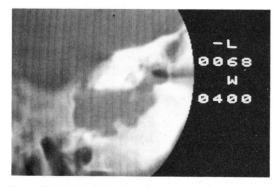

Figure 22.3 Axial CT showing destruction of the petrous pyramid and floor of the middle cranial fossa

MRI will complement the information obtained by CT in respect of soft tissue involvement and ideally, therefore, both types of imaging should be used. The frequency of dural involvement is such that, before embarking on surgery, it is advisable to ascertain whether the dura is thickened or penetrated by using MRI. In many instances penetration of the dura is incomplete, although spread within its substance will occur over a wide area. MRI will provide a useful indication of the resectability or otherwise of the disease.

Both CT and MRI are of some benefit in delineating smaller non-palpable lymph node metastasis of 1 cm or greater, and also spread in the prevertebral region which would not otherwise be detected clinically.

Angiography may be helpful when major vessel involvement is suspected.

Treatment

Most authorities agree that a combination of surgery and radiotherapy, in that order, as opposed to single modality treatment is likely to yield the best results (Dalley, 1965; Lederman, 1965; Tucker, 1965; Lewis, 1983).

The rationale behind this choice is well-founded. Primary surgery has the merit of allowing the surgeon to confirm the findings of the radiological investigations, to exenterate most if not all of the disease, and to impart useful information to the radiotherapist about those areas which are considered to contain residual disease. Furthermore, the removal of a large block of sclerotic bone facilitates access for the radiotherapist, and pre-empts infection and necrosis of bone, which would otherwise engender complications during and after radiotherapy. Having a mastoid bowl also serves as a useful observation port and an avenue for aural toilet.

Selection of patients for combined treatment

Clearly the selection must be based on the premise that treatment should have a reasonable prospect of success, and it is therefore essential to appreciate the deterrents to and limitations of surgery.

Dural involvement *per se* does not constitute a contraindication to surgery now that resection of large areas of dura with replacement by fascia lata can be undertaken with a much reduced morbidity. However, widespread dural involvement, perhaps even more than its penetration, should deter the surgeon from operating, since it is rarely possible to encompass the area of disease and a significant volume of tumour will then be left behind. Equally, major invasion of the brain must be viewed as a bad prognostic sign, with little prospect for cure.

Escape outwards along the external auditory meatus and thence into the pinna, retroauricular sulcus and parotid gland does not preclude a satisfactory result, provided it is recognized at the outset, and surgery tailored to encompass the extent of the disease.

Invasion of the infratemporal fossa, reflected clinically by the existence of trismus, or radiologically by erosion of the skull base and the presence of a mass, is unlikely to be controlled by radical surgery and should cause one to reconsider the advisability of surgery.

Facial palsy, on the other hand, does not invariably carry the bad prognosis associated with primary cancers of the parotid gland which have infiltrated the facial nerve, particularly adenocystic carcinoma, with its propensity for perineural spread. This is especially true when involvement of the facial nerve is strictly confined to the middle ear, but less so when the disease has escaped medially towards the petrous apex and laterally out of the canal into the parotid gland.

The decision whether or not to operate when disease has been identified as escaping from the meatus and middle ear may be difficult. It should be remembered that the findings at operation are nearly always in excess of those anticipated preoperatively, and this should restrain the surgeon when selecting the more advanced cases for operation.

To this end, some have tried to devise a staging system for the exclusion of those cases which are patently incurable, while at the same time defining the group of patients in whom limited escape has occurred and for whom surgery might be beneficial. Stell (1984a,b) suggested the following staging system, in the absence of any official staging either by the UICC or the AJCC.

T1: tumour limited to the site of origin without facial nerve paralysis or bone destruction
T2: tumour extending beyond the site of origin indicated by facial paralysis or radiological evidence of bone destruction, but no extension beyond the organ of origin
T3: clinical or radiological evidence of extension to surrounding structures such as the dura, base of skull, parotid gland and temporomandibular joint
TX: patients with insufficient data for classification, including patients previously seen and treated elsewhere.

Clark *et al.* (1991), on the other hand, questioned the usefulness of a preoperative staging system on the basis that at operation they frequently found that the disease was much more advanced than they had anticipated. They did, however, consider that the staging system would allow them to select patients for palliative surgery while sparing those patients who had very advanced disease from any type of operation.

Surgery

Until quite recently, surgery in the UK took the form almost exclusively of a radical mastoidectomy, whereas surgical thinking in the USA from the middle 1950s to the 1970s was dominated by the concept of monobloc petrosectomy as propounded by Parsons and Lewis (1954). This procedure, which was designed to widen the limits of excision and to conform to the ideals of a proper cancer operation, was applied in general to the more extensive cancers but, in time, it was recognized that the technique as originally advocated was flawed. Its major drawback was its reliance on the placement of osteotomy cuts in certain critical positions such as the jugular foramen and the bone adjacent to the carotid canal, in order to prise away the temporal bone. Damage to the last four cranial nerves and major haemorrhage were common sequelae, and the postoperative morbidity was consequently high (Mladick *et al.*, 1974; Wilson *et al.*, 1974).

With the growing realization that the monobloc concept was not an imperative when dealing with the petrous bone and that drilling would achieve an even better clearance, the operation as devised by Parsons and Lewis (1954) gave way to the more pragmatic modern approach of drilling under the microscope (Lewis, 1975) (see Plate 3/22/III). This is not to say however, that every case of middle ear and external meatus cancer should be treated in this way.

If disease is confined to the middle ear, mastoid and éxternal meatus, a radical mastoidectomy will generally suffice.

Small tumours confined to the external meatus can be treated by a core excision with removal by drilling of the underlying bone and skin grafting of the defect.

In instances where escape of disease is known to have occurred on a relatively limited scale, a larger operation is required, and subtotal petrosectomy using the drill and the microscope is the logical option. This procedure will usually entail ablation of the facial nerve, and may also require excision of segments of dura. A hypoglossal–facial nerve anastomosis will serve to reanimate the facial musculature and thereby lessen the cosmetic deformity, and repair of dural defects is accomplished by the use of fascia lata, taken from the thigh and either stitched or glued in position. The dural patch should be covered by a large free muscle graft or a bulky flap to prevent any further escape of CSF.

In cases where the disease has infiltrated the hypotympanum and involved the jugular bulb, excision of the tympanomastoid complex together with the jugular bulb, as practised for glomus tumours, should be carried out in order to maximize tumour clearance.

Disease that has reached the infratemporal fossa in bulk is unlikely to be encompassed by surgery and therefore should be considered inoperable.

Tumours of the middle ear and external meatus which have extended laterally to involve the pinna and adjacent areas require pinnectomy, parotidectomy, and excision of the pre- and postaural skin. There may, in consequence, be a significant soft tissue defect at the conclusion of the operation which will need closure by a transposition flap. Large bulky myocutaneous flaps are ideal for providing surface cover, deep padding, and a seal for a potential CSF leak. On a technically more difficult and laborious plane, a free revascularized myocutaneous graft is an attractive, albeit riskier, alternative.

Radical neck dissection would seem to have no place as an elective procedure in the management of squamous carcinoma of the ear, but clearly is required in cases of overt metastasis. The operation may be effective when involved nodes are high up in the neck and limited in number, but even when cure is not achieved, may help to minimize the tendency to local recurrence.

With any form of surgery, postoperative radiotherapy should be considered as a vital and an integral part of treatment aimed at eliminating any microscopical or macroscopical residues of cancer. The surgeon having observed the extent and location of the disease at operation must impart his findings to the radiotherapist so as to maximize the effectiveness of treatment.

Complications of surgery

Cerebrospinal fluid leak and meningitis are major complications. Prevention of the former depends on the effectiveness of the seal used to plug a dural defect and the latter on appropriate broad-spectrum intravenous antibiotic cover during the operation and postoperatively.

Damage to the last four cranial nerves is characterized by hoarseness, dysphagia, and aspiration during swallowing, and may require restitution by cricopharyngeal myotomy and thyroplasty. The problem of sacrificing the facial nerve can be addressed at the time of the definitive operation by performing a hypoglossal–facial anastomosis.

Petrosectomy in a patient with a functioning labyrinth will leave him with a dead ear and imbalance for several months after surgery.

Radiotherapy

There are certain recognized sequelae following radiotherapy to the ear. The skin in the meatus becomes dry and the wax hard and crusty. Patients with an intact labyrinth who are irradiated frequently complain at a much later stage of diminished hearing and disordered balance. The most distressing complication is osteoradionecrosis, manifesting as severe pain, discharge and sequestration of bone over a prolonged period (see Plate 3/22/IV).

Results

It is difficult to be certain about the results of treatment for squamous carcinoma of the middle ear and external meatus since reports in the literature rarely compare like with like. Goodwin and Jesse (1980) reported 56% cures for the osseous meatus and 23% for the middle ear, whereas Lewis (1975) gave an overall cure rate of 27%.

The numbers of the rarer glandular epithelial tumours are so small that percentages relating to prognosis are of little value.

References

BATSAKIS, J. G. (1989) Adenomatous tumours of the middle ear. *Annals of Otology, Rhinology and Laryngology*, **98**, 749–752

BATSAKIS, J. G. and EL-NAGGAR, A. K. (1993) Papillary neoplams (Heffner's tumors) of the endolymphatic sac. *Annals of Otology, Rhinology and Laryngology*, **102**, 648–651

BENECKE, J. L. (1990) Adenomatous tumours of the middle ear and mastoid. *American Journal of Otology*, **11**, 20–26

BOTTRILL, I. D. (1992) Salivary gland choristoma of the middle ear. *Journal of Laryngology and Otology*, **106**, 630–632

BRODERS, A. C. (1921) Epithelioma of the ear: a study of 63 cases. *Surgical Clinics of North America*, **1**, 1401–1410

CLARK, L. J., NARULA, A. A., MORGAN, D. A. L. and BRADLEY, P. J. (1991) Squamous carcinoma of the temporal bone: a revised staging. *Journal of Laryngology and Otology*, **105**, 346–348

CONLEY, J. J. and NOVACK, A. J. (1960) The surgical treatment of malignant tumours of the ear and temporal bone. *Archives of Otolaryngology*, **71**, 635–652

DALLEY, V. M. (1965) Radiation therapy in relation to malignant tumours of the temporal bone. In: *Progress in Radiation Therapy*, vol 3. New York: Grune and Stratton

FREDERICKS, S. (1956–57) External ear malignancy. *British Journal of Plastic Surgery*, **9**, 136–160

GOODWIN, W. J. and JESSE, R. H. (1980) Malignant neoplasms of the external auditory canal and temporal bone. *Archives of Otolaryngology*, **106**, 675–679

HIRAIDE, F., INOUYE, T. and ISHII, T. (1983) Primary squamous cell carcinoma of the middle ear invading the cochlea. A histopathological case report. *Annals of Otology, Rhinology and Laryngology*, **92**, 290–294

JESSE, R. H., HEALEY, J. E. and WILEY, D. B. (1967) External auditory canal, middle ear and mastoid. In: *Cancer of the Head and Neck*. Baltimore: Williams and Wilkins

JOACHIMS, H. Z. (1988) Basal cell carcinoma of the middle ear – a natural history. *Journal of Laryngology and Otology*, **102**, 932–934

JOHNS, M. E. and HEADINGTON, J. T. (1974) Squamous cell carcinoma of the external auditory canal: a clinicopathologic study. *Archives of Otolaryngology*, **100**, 45–49

JOHNSTONE, J. M., LENNOX, B. and WATSON, A. J. (1957) Five

cases of hidradenoma of the external auditory meatus. *Journal of Pathology and Bacteriology*, **73**, 421–427

KRETSCHMANN, F. (1886) Uber carcinoma das schlafenbeines. *Archives für Ohrenheilkunde*, **24**, 231–262

LEDERMAN, M. (1965) Malignant tumours of the ear. *Journal of Laryngology and Otology*, **79**, 85–119

LEWIS, J. S. (1960) Cancer of the ear. A report of 150 cases. *Laryngoscope*, **70**, 3–31

LEWIS, J. S. (1973) Squamous carcinoma of the ear. *Archives of Otolaryngology*, **97**, 41–42

LEWIS, J. S. (1975) Temporal bone resection. Review of 100 cases. *Archives of Otolaryngology*, **101**, 23–25

LEWIS, J. S. (1983) Surgical management of tumors of the middle ear and mastoid. *Journal of Laryngology and Otology*, **97**, 299–311

MICHAELS, L. and WELLS, M. (1980) Squamous cell carcinoma of the middle ear. *Clinical Otolaryngology*, **5**, 235–248

MLADICK, R. A., HORTON, C. E., ADAMSON, J. E. and CARRAWAY, J. H. (1974) The core resection for malignant tumors of the auricular area and subjacent bones. *Plastic and Reconstructive Surgery*, **53**, 281–287

MORTON, R. P., STELL, P. M. and DERRICK, P. P. (1984) Epidemiology of cancer of the middle ear cleft. *Cancer*, **53**, 1612–1617

MOSS, R. (1987) Ceruminoma revisited. *American Journal of Otology*, **8**, 485–488

NEWHART, H. (1917) Primary carcinoma of the middle ear: report of a case. *Laryngoscope*, **27**, 543–555

PAPARELLA, M. M. and MEYERHOFF, W. L. (1980) In: *Otolaryngology*, 2nd edn. Philadelphia: W. B. Saunders. p. 1366

PARSONS, H. and LEWIS, J. S. (1954) Subtotal resection of the temporal bone for cancer of the ear. *Cancer*, **7**, 995–1001

PEELE, J. C. and HAUSER, C. H. (1941) Primary carcinoma of the external auditory canal and middle ear. *Archives of Otolaryngology*, **34**, 254–266

PETERS, B. R. (1988) Pleomorphic adenoma of the middle ear and mastoid. *Archives of Otolaryngology*, **114**, 676–678

PHELPS, P. D. and LLOYD, G. A. S. (1981) The radiology of carcinoma of the ear. *British Journal of Radiology*, **54**, 103–109

POLITZER, A. (1883) *Textbook of Diseases of the Ear*. Translated by J. P Cassells. London: Baillière Tindall and Cox. pp. 650–655

ROBINSON, G. A. (1931) Malignant tumours of the ear. *Laryngoscope*, **41**, 467–473

SCHALL, L. A. (1934) Neoplasms involving the middle ear. *Archives of Otolaryngology*, **32**, 548–553

STELL, P. M. (1984a) Basal cell carcinoma of the external auditory meatus. *Clinical Otolaryngology*, **9**, 187–190

STELL, P. M. (1984b) Carcinoma of the external auditory meatus and middle ear. *Clinical Otolaryngology*, **9**, 281–299

TOWSON, C. E. and SHOFSTALL, W. H. (1950) Carcinoma of the ear. *Archives of Otolaryngology*, **51**, 724–738

TUCKER, W. N. (1965) Cancer of the middle ear. A review of 89 cases. *Cancer*, **18**, 642–650

WARD, J. M. (1975) Dose response of azoxymethane in rats. *Veterinary Pathology*, **12**, 165–177

WILSON, J. S. P., BLAKE, G. B., RICHARDSON, A. E. and WESTBURY, G. (1974) Malignant tumours of the ear and their treatment. II tumours of the external auditory meatus, middle ear cleft and temporal bone. *British Journal of Plastic Surgery*, **27**, 77–91

ZERONI (1899) Ueber das carcinom des gehoerorganes. *Archivs für Ohrenheilkunde*, **8**, 141–190

23

Glomus and other tumours of the ear

A. D. Cheesman

Glomus jugulare

The glomus jugulare is a collection of ganglionic tissue within the temporal bone in close relation with the jugular bulb. The first descriptions of this tissue were probably by Valentin (1840), who described his 'ganglia tympanica', and Krause (1878), his 'glandula tympanica'. Both writers described ganglionic-like tissue, but the credit for recognizing the histological relationship to the carotid body goes to Guild in 1941. He originally called the structure the glomus jugularis, but in a later report (Guild, 1953) he accepted the terminology glomus jugulare accorded by Lattes and Waltner (1949). They also suggested that the generic term for these structures in the body should be non-chromaffin paraganglia (any associated tumour being called a non-chromaffin paraganglioma).

The paraganglia are cells derived from the neural crest and are found widely distributed in the autonomic nervous system, the usual sites being the carotid, ciliary and vagal bodies, along the aorta and its main branches, the glomus jugulare complex, in the bladder, in the para-adrenal area, and most notably the adrenal medulla. The paraganglia of the adrenal medulla secrete adrenalin and noradrenalin. Histologically they stain chromaffin positive, hence the term 'chromaffin paraganglia'. Paraganglia having a negative chromaffin reaction are termed 'non-chromaffin'; they do not normally secrete hormones. The nerve supply of the latter is mainly sensory and, although the carotid body has been shown physiologically to be a chemoreceptor, responding to changes in blood pH and oxygen tension, the glomus jugulare has never been shown to be a physiologically active chemoreceptor.

Guild's (1953) anatomical studies were based on 88 temporal bones, in which he found an average of three glomus bodies in each bone. They were usually found in close relationship with either the tympanic branch of the glossopharyngeal nerve or the auricular branch of the vagus nerve; both nerves had an equal distribution of glomus bodies. The bodies were supplied with non-medulated sensory fibres from the adjacent nerve and, in most cases, the blood supply was from the ascending pharyngeal artery. Apart from their close relationship with the two nerves, their anatomical position was very variable, but 50% could be found in the adventitia of the jugular bulb and 25% in the mucosa of the promontory. Histologically, they were similar to the carotid body with epithelioid cells interspersed in a highly vascular stroma of capillary and precapillary vessels. The proportion of cells to vessels was variable and Guild recognized two groups, the cellular glomus bodies and the vascular glomus bodies, with a slight preponderance of the former. Their size was variable, but they tended to be ovoid in shape with a long diameter of 0.5 mm, equally distributed between the two ears in both sexes and found more commonly in the middle age group.

Glomus jugulare tumours

There are several reports of vascular tumours in the ear over the latter part of the eighteenth and early part of the nineteenth century (Simpson and Dallachy, 1958). In particular, Lubbers (1937) reported a case of metastatic carotid body tumour in the ear, with a contralateral carotid body tumour.

Rosenwasser (1945) was the first surgeon to recognize the relationship between these tumours and the normal glomus jugulare. In 1942, he removed a vascular tumour from the middle ear and mastoid and, on histological examination, found it to be very similar to the carotid body, but he could find no other primary tumours in the neck, and called it a carotid-body-like tumour. In his 1945 paper, Rosenwasser proposed that the tumour arose from the glomus jugularis described by Guild. Since that time there have been a variety of names attached to the tumour in an attempt to indicate its pathological origin.

Winship, Klopp and Jenkins (1948) first used the term 'glomus jugulare', and Lattes and Waltner (1949) proposed that the tumours were called non-chromaffin paragangliomas. Mulligan (1950) introduced the general term 'chemodectoma' for the carotid body and glomus jugulare tumours, based on their common histological appearances and probable origin from chemoreceptor tissue. Boyd, Lever and Griffith (1959) objected to this term as the glomus jugulare has no demonstrable chemoreceptor function.

Current usage suggests that these tumours should be considered as non-chromaffin paragangliomas. The most common term used is 'glomus tumours', and the terms 'glomus tympanicus' and 'glomus jugulare tumours' are used primarily for the clinical description of a particular tumour.

Pathology

Histological examination of the glomus jugulare tumour shows a similar appearance to the normal glomus jugulare; cytologically they are not very active with only rare mitotic figures, and they usually have a well-defined thin fibrous capsule. Clinically, however, they can be locally invasive and destructive of bone and facial nerve. In the author's series, they have shown a great propensity to infiltrate through the mastoid air-cell system, as well as invading the cancellous bone of the skull base. Makek *et al.* (1990) have demonstrated a high degree of neural infiltration in jugulotympanic paragangliomas; some 66 cases out of the 83 studied had neural infiltration. They described four grades of neural invasion with clinical correlation.

Sex, age and familial incidence

The glomus tumour, in contradistinction to the glomus body, shows a predominance in females of 6:1. Glomus tumours tend to be more common in the middle age groups. Although most glomus tumours occur as sporadic events there are increasing reports of familial glomus tumours. The hereditary pattern appears to be autosomal dominant with variable penetrance. One such series had 16 documented glomus tumours in 95 members over five generations (Heutink *et al.*, 1992).

Endocrine activity

They are usually considered to be non-chromaffin paragangliomas with no endocrine function, but there has been an increasing number of reports of vasoactive tumours (Duke *et al.*, 1964; Matishak, Symon and Cheesman, 1987), and clinically it is important to look for evidence of endocrine activity by urinary assay of the metabolites dopamine and 3-methoxy-4-hydroxymandelic acid (vanillylmandelic acid).

Multicentricity

Glomus tumours are sometimes multicentric presenting in both ears (Winship and Louzan, 1951), or in conjunction with other paragangliomas, the carotid body commonly being the second site (Spector *et al.*, 1975).

Metastases

The glomus jugulare tumour is generally considered to be of low malignancy, mainly causing problems because of its site in the complex anatomy of the skull base. However, there are well documented cases of malignant glomus jugulare tumours, with both nodal and distant metastases; fortunately the incidence is very rare (Brown, 1967; Johnston and Symon, 1992).

Natural history of presentation

The slow growth of these tumours means that the diagnosis is often missed until the tumour is very extensive. Alford and Guilford (1962) found the average delay to diagnosis was 6 years from the original symptoms, the extremes being 42 years and 2 weeks. The first symptoms noted generally follow middle ear involvement, and are often ignored. Pulsatile tinnitus and conductive deafness are, equally, the commonest presenting symptoms. A red mass (the rising sun behind the drum) on routine examination is not uncommon, but quite a high proportion do not present until cranial nerve palsies occur. Some 30% of cases, in most series, present with facial palsy. The pareses resulting from involvement of the nerves of the jugular foramen, often do not cause sufficient symptoms in most cases to warrant presentation. Table 23.1 shows the clinical findings in the author's series of 61 cases (Watkins *et al.*, 1994) and is similar to most other reports. Otalgia and aural bleeding are other fairly common symptoms.

Classification

There have been many attempts at classification. Lundgren (1949) used a basic division into glomus

Table 23.1 Presenting features in glomus tumours of temporal bone (%)

Deafness	69
Middle ear mass	75
Pulsatile tinnitus	55
Imbalance	8
Otorrhoea	5
Facial palsy	8
Endocrine syndrome	3
Cranial nerve deficits	
hoarseness	16
dysphagia	16
Headache	15
Visual disturbance	6

tympanicus tumours arising from the promontory, and glomus jugulare tumours arising from the jugular bulb. This had clinical value in planning the surgical approach for small tumours. Bickerstaff and Howell (1953) used a symptomatic classification,

but this had little value, either for management or prognosis. Alford and Guilford (1962) reviewed the world's literature and proposed a staging system for their own cases. The staging was determined by the degree of spread shown radiologically and symptomatically; they then used the staging to indicate various combinations of surgery and radiotherapy.

The most widely used classification was devised by Oldring and Fisch (1979). They proposed four types, A, B, C, D based on site and size (Figure 23.1):

Type A: tumours localized to the middle ear cleft (glomus tympanicus tumours)

Type B: tympanomastoid tumours with no destruction of bone in the infralabyrinthine compartment of the temporal bone

Type C: tumours invading the infralabyrinthine region and extending towards the petrous apex with destruction of infralabyrinthine compartment of temporal bone

Type D: tumours with intracranial extension.

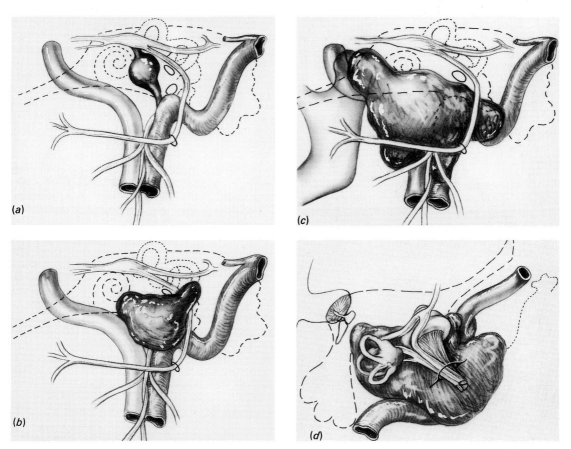

Figure 23.1 Classification after Oldring and Fisch (1979) with permission. (*a*) Type A tumour; (*b*) type B tumour; (*c*) type C tumour showing erosion of infralabyrinthine bone; (*d*) type D tumour viewed from above, showing intracranial spread (from Cheesman and Symon (1987) *Operative Surgery*, 4th edn, Neurosurgery, edited by L. Symon, D. G. Thomas and K. Clarke. London: Butterworths)

The classification, although anatomically based, was primarily differentiated by the surgical approaches used. In 1982, Fisch further subdivided types C and D to cope with the different surgical problems encountered. While the original classification into four types has considerable clinical value, Fisch's further subdivision is of limited value unless one follows his surgical approach exactly.

Investigation

Those cases presenting to the otologist usually have a red mass behind the tympanic membrane and this should indicate the probable diagnosis. Two other conditions mimic this appearance – a high jugular bulb or an aberrant carotid artery. The red drum of otitis media should be obvious from the history. More extensive spread involving the external auditory meatus may appear to be a squamous cell carcinoma, which can often bleed profusely. Those cases presenting to the neurologist often cause considerable diagnostic problems, as neuromas of the last four cranial nerves have a common symptomatology.

The first step in investigation entails a careful clinical examination. Observation of the drum under the microscope will frequently show a pulsation of the mass, which will be soft and often blanch on palpation. The hearing loss is generally conductive. Neurological assessment of the cranial nerves is very important, and often gives considerable information regarding the extent of the tumour.

Radiology

The main investigation must be radiological and, with the advances in imaging over the last decade, a very detailed assessment of the tumour can be made.

CT scanning remains the most valuable method of imaging giving information about bone erosion but more importantly, relates the extent of the tumour to the bony anatomy of the ear which is vital in operative planning. MR imaging with gadolinium enhancement gives a better indication of soft tissue involvement but is more difficult to correlate with the anatomy (Phelps and Cheesman, 1990) (see Figures 2.45–2.48). Finally, angiography indicates the blood supply of the tumour and with preoperative embolization allows a significant reduction in operative bleeding.

Mention should be made of the more traditional methods of imaging. With Type A and B tumours, plain mastoid X-rays will show only clouding of the middle ear and mastoid air cells, although special views of the jugular foramen may show unilateral enlargement. Type C tumours may show bone erosion on plain films, but the jagged erosion of the normally well corticated jugular bulb is best seen on polytomography. The absence of the normal crest of bone between the carotid canal and jugular fossa on lateral tomography is virtually diagnostic of a glomus jugulare tumour (Phelps' sign).

Retrograde venography by catheterization of the internal jugular vein was popular to differentiate between a glomus tympanicus and glomus jugulare, the latter showed as a filling defect. However, with modern CT scanning this invasive technique is no longer necessary.

High resolution CT scanning is the technique of choice for establishing the diagnosis in those cases presenting with a red mass behind the drum (the rising sun sign). Figure 23.2 shows the diagnostic pathway using high resolution CT scans. The first step is a conventional axial scan; this will show whether the jugular bulb is enlarged and, if there is any erosion of the cortex, a glomus jugulare tumour

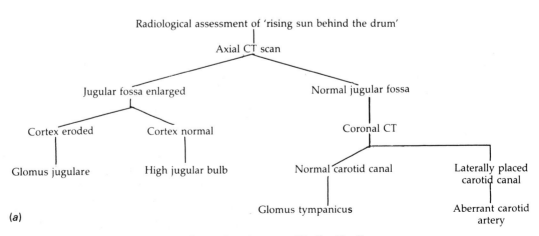

(a)

Figure 23.2 (a) Flow diagram for radiological assessment (courtesy of Dr Glyn Lloyd)

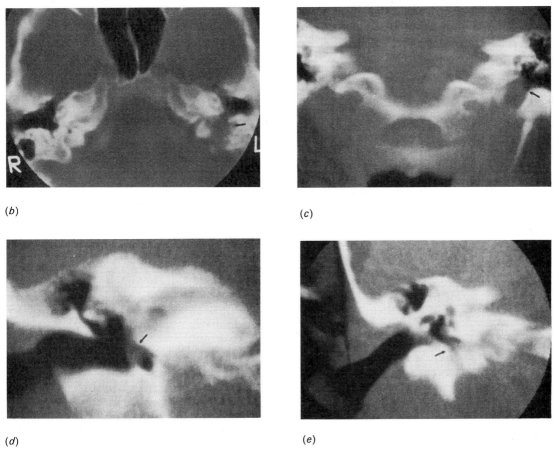

(b)   *(c)*

(d)   *(e)*

Figure 23.2 (*b*) axial CT scan of left glomus jugulare showing enlarged jugular fossa with eroded cortex; (*c*) coronal CT scan showing high jugular bulb with well corticated fossa, but absent bone in the hypotympanum; (*d*) coronal CT scan showing a small glomus tympanicus tumour; (*e*) coronal CT scan showing an aberrant carotid artery with a laterally placed carotid canal, again with absent bone in the hypotympanum, a more anterior cut than (*c*)

is likely (see Figure 2.44). Smooth well-corticated enlargement is generally due to the abnormally high jugular bulb. If the jugular fossa has normal dimensions, coronal CT scanning is necessary (the coronal cuts obtained by scanning with the patient's head in the submentovertical position are necessary as the coronal computer reconstructions do not give adequate detail) (see Figure 2.46*a*). If on coronal cuts the carotid canal is normal, the mass must be a glomus tympanicus. An aberrant carotid artery is demonstrated by a more laterally placed carotid canal often with a deficient bony wall. With the more extensive glomus tumours, the erosion of the infralabyrinthine part of the temporal

bone and intracranial spread are clearly demonstrated.

In the unlikely event of doubts as to the correct diagnosis still existing after CT scanning, angiography will demonstrate virtually all glomus tumours apart from the very early glomus tympanicus tumour which may not be obvious even with selective angiography of the ascending pharyngeal artery. If the requirement is to establish the diagnosis, digital subtraction angiography using intravenous contrast injection will often confirm it (Figure 23.3). More recently MR angiography has also demonstrated its value in diagnosis. Arteriography is best reserved for the preoperative detailed assessment of the extent of

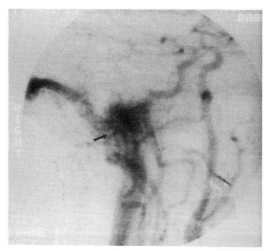

Figure 23.3 Digital subtraction angiogram showing a right glomus jugulare tumour

the tumour and indication of the arterial blood supply (see Figure 2.49). If the arteriography is accompanied by preoperative embolization, it should not be performed more than 8 days prior to the planned surgery, otherwise collateral vessels may open, thereby restoring the tumour's vascularity.

Extension of the tumour along the carotid artery towards the cavernous sinus remains a difficult area to image. Extension towards the petrous apex is not easily demonstrated on MR as the signal enhancement of tumour and fat is similar in T1-weighted sequences. More recently subtraction MR (Lloyd *et al.*, 1992) has given better tissue characterization in this area. CT may also suggest extent by showing erosion of the carotid canal.

Follow-up imaging by MR is also complicated by the difficulty in differentiating between the fat used to obliterate the operative cavity and recurrent tumour. Unless subtraction MR is used it is probable that recurrence rates will be understated.

Endocrine

Prior to any surgery, it is important to exclude the secretion of any vasoactive hormones by the tumour, particularly in those cases with an elevated blood pressure. A 24-hour urine collection will demonstrate any raised vanillylmandelic acid levels (normal level up to 7 mg/24 hours). Direct biopsy of the tumour should not be necessary if the suggested radiological assessment is used.

Biopsy of an obvious tumour presenting in the external auditory meatus is occasionally performed to exclude a squamous cell carcinoma; in such cases

bleeding will occur, but it is rarely severe and always stops with a bismuth iodoform and paraffin paste (BIPP) pack.

Management

After many years of controversy, it is now possible to propose a series of reasonable therapeutic options in the management of glomus jugulare tumours. In the past, the main arguments have been over the value and place of radiotherapy. Initially it was used when surgical resection was deemed impossible or, more often, when the operation had to be curtailed because of unpredicted technical problems in the hands of a surgeon unfamiliar with this particular tumour. Subsequently, it was used as the sole form of treatment in many centres, and presently tends to be used mainly as an adjunct to surgery.

The main types of surgical procedure described over the years have often reflected the interests of general otology. In the 1940s and 1950s, open techniques were usually performed. In the 1960s the intact canal wall procedures were popular, and since 1970 increasingly more sophisticated skull base procedures have been described.

The use of other modalities of treatment have been suggested, but none have found wide acceptance. Tumour reduction by diathermy was initially popular and, with the evolution of cryotherapy, the cryoprobe was suggested, but in both cases it was found impossible to treat any tumours apart from the smallest glomus tympanicus. Intra-arterial embolization under radiological control is useful for intracranial vascular malformations, but when used for glomus tumours the duration of tumour reduction is very limited. It has no place as a permanent treatment, but is excellent as a preoperative adjunct to surgical resection.

The current treatment options for glomus tumours may be summarized as follows:

1 No active treatment and continuous observation
2 Primary radiotherapy
3 Surgical resection
4 Surgical resection with planned adjunctive radiotherapy

No treatment

Glomus tumours are extremely slow growing and may have a long natural history. They usually present in the middle age groups and, where general health is good, treatment is definitely indicated in view of the patient's expected life span. Some patients do not present until the latter part of the sixth or seventh decades and, providing that repeat CT scans do not show very extensive spread or rapid growth, and the patient's symptoms are minimal, no treatment is indicated apart from explanation and reassurance.

Radiotherapy

There have been several detailed studies on the effects of radiotherapy monitored clinically and radiologically, and several workers have also looked at the histopathological changes in irradiated tumours (Capps, 1952; Silverstone, 1973; Spector, Maisel and Ogura, 1974). Unfortunately, there is too much variation in both method and dose of radiation to draw definite conclusions. Most clinicians agree that radiotherapy is rarely curative, but it does have some effect on slowing tumour growth. Rosenwasser (1968) made the profound generalization, 'that the inherent tendency of the glomus jugulare tumours to slow growth may be more important in determining its radiocurability than is its actual responsiveness to irradiation'. Clinically, following irradiation, visible tumour often shrinks and bleeding generally ceases, and although tinnitus and vertigo may improve, the deafness and other cranial nerve palsies persist. Repeat angiography shows little changes in either vascularity or in the extent of the tumour, apart from intracranial extensions which often regress.

Histopathological examination of irradiated tumour shortly after radiotherapy may not give the true picture, as radiation fibrosis generally develops 6–12 months later. Most advocates of radiotherapy stress that improvement may take several years to become obvious. Cytologically, the epithelioid or chief cells show very little change apart from being broken up into nests of tumour surrounded by sheets of fibrous tissue. Most of the radiation effects appear to involve the stroma with changes typical of endarteritis obliterans, and this in some cases causes thrombosis of some areas of the tumour.

Many of the documented complications of radiation, such as cerebral necrosis and radionecrosis of the temporal bone, can probably be attributed to the use of older methods of radiation such as orthovoltage (Jackson and Koshiba, 1974). Today, 3-D imaging gives better tumour localization and with megavoltage irradiation should result in fewer complications (Cole and Beiler, 1994). The usual practice is to deliver 4000–5000 cGy (rads) over a 3–4 week period.

Most clinicians agree that an elderly or infirm patient with a symptomatic, growing tumour should be treated solely with radiotherapy. In the absence of an experienced surgical team, radiotherapy will probably cause less problems than surgery with types C and D tumours, but it must be remembered that 40% of tumours may continue to grow after initial radiation control (Spector, Maisel and Ogura, 1974). Rosenwasser, reviewing the results of treatment in 1969, came to the conclusion that surgery, if possible, was the method of choice in the management of glomus jugulare tumours. Despite the advances in skull base surgery over the last decade, it is extremely difficult to eradicate those extensive tumours that invade the cancellous bone or cells of the petrous apex around the internal carotid artery. If such cases have limited neurological deficit on presentation, surgery may well increase the neurological deficit, and in such cases subtotal resection with postoperative radiotherapy is probably the method of choice. In this respect, the use of the newer interstitial radioactive implants, such as iodine-125 with its long half-life, may well be the ideal form of treatment in future (Glaser *et al.*, 1995).

Surgery

The objectives of surgery are total resection of the tumour where possible, and this should ideally be achieved without increasing the patient's neurological deficit. In certain cases improvement of the hearing may also be achieved.

Most of the frightening complications described in the past have resulted from inadequate appreciation of the extent of the tumour preoperatively, and from inadequate exposure of the tumour at the time of surgery.

Type A tumours, or glomus tympanicus tumours, can usually be approached via the external auditory meatus.

Type B tumours can often be encompassed by a combined approach (intact canal wall) procedure.

Type C tumours need some form of skull base approach utilizing an upper cervical dissection and transmastoid approach.

Type D tumours require a skull base approach and posterior fossa craniotomy, some surgeons preferring to perform the resection in two stages.

Surgical technique

The various techniques available are well described in the textbooks of operative surgery, but considerable experience is also required for the surgery to be performed safely.

Various methods of reducing the tumour's vascularity have been suggested. Spector, Maisel and Ogura (1974) favoured preoperative irradiation which reduced vascularity and, by inducing stromal fibrosis, permitted easier tumour dissection. Other surgeons including the author have favoured the use of preoperative embolization. This requires the help of an experienced neuroradiologist as there is about a 1% chance of inadvertent embolization of the internal carotid artery system leading to a stroke. Selective angiography of the individual vessels supplying the tumour is performed and embolization achieved either with gelfoam or polyvinyl alcohol sponge (Ivalon). The procedure should be performed some 4–8 days prior to planned resection, and a light general anaesthetic is used (Figure 23.4).

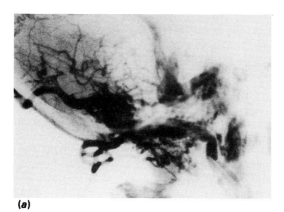

(a)

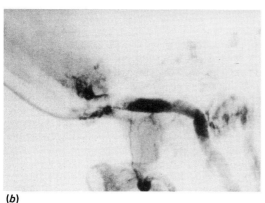

(b)

Figure 23.4 Preoperative embolization of a right glomus jugulare tumour; (*a*) occipital circulation to tumour prior to embolization; (*b*) occipital circulation after intra-arterial embolization with Ivalon

The highest quality of anaesthetic help is required for this type of surgery. Careful work-up should have excluded any production of vasoactive hormones by the tumour. Profound hypotension controlled by intra-arterial monitoring reduces bleeding to an acceptable level, and dissection with gauze soaked in 1:1000 adrenalin is also useful.

Transmeatal approach (Figure 23.5)

The very small glomus tympanicus tumours can be removed by simple tympanotomy if all their borders can be visualized and additional exposure can be obtained by dissecting the malleus handle free of the drum.

Additional exposure can also be obtained by lowering the inferior annulus in the hypotympanic approach described by Shambaugh (1955); in 1967, Farrior described further extension of this approach by removing the mastoid tip and mobilizing the vertical portion of the facial nerve.

Extended facial recess approach (Figure 23.6)

With the advent of combined approach mastoidectomy for cholesteatoma, it became clear that large type A and moderate-sized type B glomus tumours could be removed with an intact canal wall procedure instead of by the traditional radical cavity. House (1968) combined the intact canal wall procedure with a neck approach to the jugular bulb, but did not transpose the facial nerve. Glasscock, Harris and Newsome (1974) further developed this technique.

By extending the facial recess inferiorly, reasonably good access is obtained to the hypotympanum, particularly if the chorda tympani is sacrificed. Even

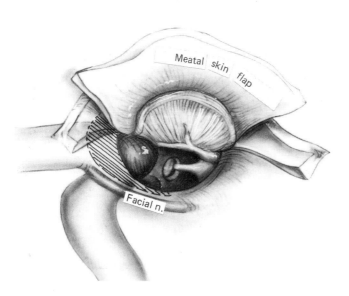

Figure 23.5 Transmeatal approach showing extended tympanotomy. Access to hypotympanum is obtained by removal of shaded area of tympanic bone anterior to facial nerve (from Cheesman and Symon (1987) *Operative Surgery*, 4th edn, Neurosurgery, edited by L. Symon, D. G. Thomas and K. Clarke. London: Butterworths)

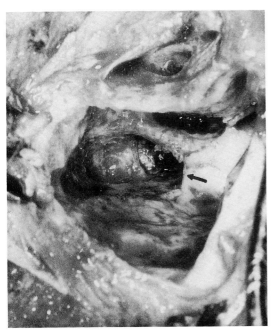

Figure 23.6 Extended facial recess approach showing tumour in the hypotympanum exposed by removing bone of the tympanic recess posteromedial to the fallopian canal

better exposure is obtained by skeletonizing in turn, the vertical portion of the facial nerve, the sigmoid sinus, and the posterior semicircular canal. With these structures clearly identified, the tympanic recess can be opened widely medial to the vertical portion of the facial nerve and this gives adequate exposure for type B tumours. In such cases, total tumour removal can be accomplished with preservation of normal ossicular function.

Infratemporal fossa approach (lateral approach) (Figure 23.7)

The essential features of this approach are: the resection of the jugular bulb after ligating the internal jugular vein in the neck, and packing off the sigmoid sinus superiorly, and the anterior transposition of the facial nerve to allow direct access to the jugular bulb region. Such an approach was attempted by Capps in 1955, but the stormy postoperative period caused him to recommend radiotherapy for such extensive tumours. The approach was successfully used by Shapiro and Neues (1964) and Gejrot (1965). Gejrot, in particular, emphasized the importance of preserving the

medial wall of the sinus if possible, thus protecting the neural compartment of the jugular bulb and maintaining intact the dura of the posterior fossa. Since that time, many surgeons have utilized this basic approach but especial credit must be given to Fisch (Fisch, Fagan and Valvanis, 1984) who extended the approach for a variety of lesions in the lateral skull base.

The basic steps of Fisch's infratemporal fossa approach are as follows: a postaural incision is extended both superiorly and inferiorly into the neck. The facial flap and pinna are raised and reflected anteriorly. The cartilaginous meatus is transected and closed off as a blind-ending sac. The parotid region is dissected to mobilize the peripheral branches of the facial nerve, and the nerves and vessels of the upper neck are carefully mobilized up to the skull base. Control ligatures are placed around the internal jugular vein and internal carotid artery, but not tied at this stage. A complete mastoidectomy (subtotal petrosectomy) is performed removing all the air cells, the posterior meatal wall, the drum, malleus and incus. The outer wall of the hypotympanum is drilled away and the facial nerve skeletonized along both its horizontal and vertical portions. It is dissected free from the canal and permanently transposed anteriorly.

If, during mobilization of the facial nerve, it becomes apparent that it has been invaded by the tumour, removal of the nerve sheaths becomes necessary or resection of the involved section of nerve and a cable-graft using sural nerve is placed between the cut ends (see Figures 24.15 and 24.16).

The sigmoid sinus is ligated in the region of the sinodural angle and the internal jugular vein is ligated in the neck. The tumour is then mobilized, first peripherally then centrally. If possible the medial wall of the sinus is preserved, but if infiltrated with tumour it is resected along with the nerves of the medial compartment. At this stage bleeding occurs from the inferior petrosal sinus where it enters the jugular bulb medially. It is controlled by packing the lumen with Surgicel gauze. A plane of cleavage can often be found between the tumour and the internal carotid artery, otherwise the tumour on the wall of the carotid is controlled with judicious bipolar diathermy. At the completion of the procedure, any dural defect is repaired with fascia, the eustachian tube is closed off with bone wax, and the whole cavity filled with a free fat graft.

The anterior transposition of the facial nerve may occasionally be achieved without immediate loss of function. It is more usual to develop a temporary paresis which recovers in 2–3 months with a satisfactory final result in 85% of cases.

Intracranial extensions of greater than 2 cm are best managed, according to Fisch, by a second-stage procedure to reduce the chances of cerebrospinal fluid leak and meningitis.

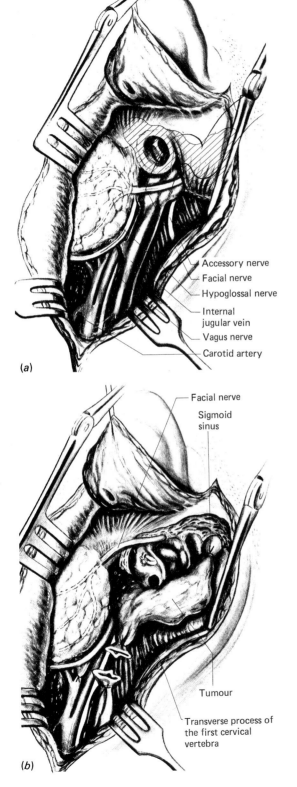

(a)

Accessory nerve
Facial nerve
Hypoglossal nerve
Internal jugular vein
Vagus nerve
Carotid artery

Facial nerve
Sigmoid sinus

Tumour

Transverse process of the first cervical vertebra

(b)

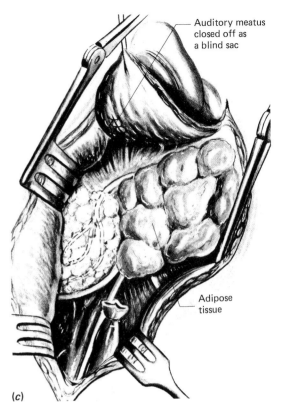

Auditory meatus closed off as a blind sac

Adipose tissue

(c)

Figure 23.7 Infratemporal fossa approach after Fisch. (*a*) Exposure of jugular foramen from upper neck dissection; (*b*) anterior transposition of facial nerve, subtotal petrosectomy and ligaton above and below the tumour; (*c*) closure of external auditory meatus and obliteration of cavity with fat free graft (from Cheesman and Symon (1987) *Operative Surgery*, 4th edn, Neurosurgery, edited by L. Symon, D. G. Thomas and K. Clarke. London: Butterworths)

Posterolateral approach (Figure 23.8)

Cheesman and Symon (1987) have described a modification to the infratemporal fossa (or lateral) approach of Fisch. They have termed it the 'posterolateral approach' and with it have been able to achieve total resection of many type C and D tumours without transposition of the facial nerve. They originally managed type D tumours by combining a posterior fossa craniotomy with a 'Fisch-type' infratemporal fossa approach at the same operation, and were fortunate not to suffer the same complications as seen by Fisch. Their wide posterolateral exposure allows preservation of the posterior meatal wall and does not require transposition of the facial nerve in most cases. Radical mastoidectomy and transposition of the facial nerve was only necessary in those cases with extensive tumour around the internal carotid artery. In such

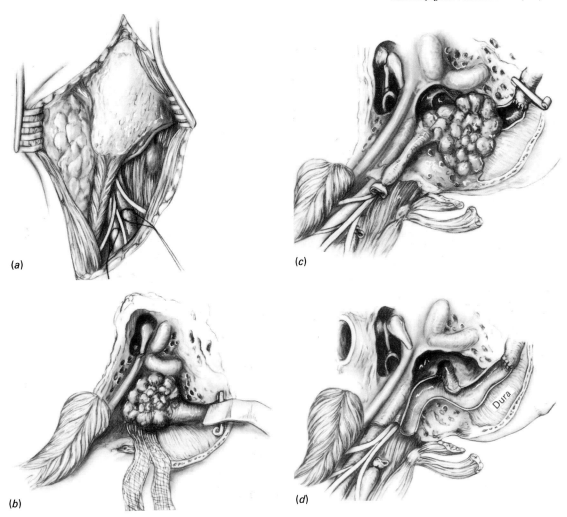

(a)

(b)

(c)

(d)

Figure 23.8 Posterolateral approach. (*a*) Upper neck dissection and posterior reflection of sternomastoid muscle to show lateral process of atlas; (*b*) cortical mastoidectomy and exposure for suboccipital approach; (*c*) ligation above and below tumour and mobilization of tumour from medial wall of jugular bulb; (*d*) completed resection showing preserved neural compartment with packing in inferior petrosal sinus (from Cheesman and Symon (1987) *Operative Surgery*, 4th edn, Neurosurgery, edited by L. Symon, D. G. Thomas and K. Clarke. London: Butterworths)

cases the necessary medial dissection of the skull base often resulted in increased neurological deficit, particularly when the intracranial extension reached anterior to the internal auditory meatus, and they currently feel postoperative irradiation is a useful adjunct in such cases, enabling a more conservative resection. However, long-term follow up will be necessary to validate their views.

Management of secretory glomus jugulare tumours

There has been an increasing number of functionally active paragangliomas reported (Matishak, Symon and Cheesman, 1987), of which nine have been functional glomus jugulare tumours. Many of these cases present as phaeochromocytomas and their localization often creates diagnostic problems. The management of the blood pressure, however, creates even greater problems for the anaesthetist. The initial hypertension often requires both alpha and beta blockade and, following embolization and surgical resection, the loss of vasoconstrictor tone may result in circulatory collapse, needing correction with massive intravenous infusions, and the use of an antigravity suit to the lower body to increase venous return.

To anticipate these potential problems, it is prudent to perform a routine vanillylmandelic acid estimation of a 24-hour urine collection preoperatively.

Postoperative neurological complications

The slow development of nerve palsies preoperatively generally allows adequate compensation, and few patients on presentation have any aspiration or swallowing problems. However, if the vagus and glossopharyngeal nerves are further damaged at surgery there is often an acute swallowing problem postoperatively. Fortunately, most patients rapidly adapt to the unilateral paresis and generally return to normal function after 1–2 weeks. In a few patients persistent problems require the use of nasogastric feeding or even temporary PEG-type (per-cutaneous endoscopic gastrostomy) gastrostomy and occasionally a temporary tracheostomy is necessary. Hoarseness also generally improves with time, but if it persists for more than 6 months the unilateral paralysed cord can be corrected with a thyroplasty which corrects the prolapsed cord more effectively than a Teflon injection. The temporary facial palsy following anterior transposition has already been discussed. When the patient has a facial palsy on presentation, nerve grafting is invariably needed and the results depend on the duration of the preoperative facial palsy. Palsies of greater than one year's duration often achieve poor results, and adjunctive facial rehabilitation is often necessary.

Other tumours of the petrous apex

Tumours and cysts of the petrous apex are rare and are described in both the otological and neurosurgical literature indicating how they have traditionally presented. They usually present by erosion of either the internal auditory meatus or the inner ear and mimic tumours of the cerebellopontine angle. Diagnosis is generally made by comparing the results of both CT and MR scanning. The MRI characteristics of such lesions including enhancement with gadolinium are summarized in Table 23.2.

Chordoma

Chordomas are rare tumours that are derived from notochordal remnants and are predominantly found in relation to the axial skeleton, more specifically 40% are in the region of the clivus and petrous apex. They are locally malignant, but can metastasize following surgical interference. They produce symptoms by pressure on the inner ear or cranial nerves and pain is a prominent feature. Radiologically they are well demonstrated on CT by irregular bone erosion and often central areas of calcification; they generally enhance with contrast. MR scanning shows a non-homogeneous appearance on T1-weighted protocols and heterogeneous enhancement with gadolinium. Careful histological study with immunocytochemistry is vital to differentiate them from chondrosarcoma and to identify the chondroid chordoma which forms 30% of skull base chordomas. Treatment is by wide surgical resection and, by the nature of the anatomy, often more than one approach is necessary in each patient. Even in very experienced hands complete removal is often impossible and should be supplemented by postoperative radiotherapy either by brachytherapy using I^{125} implants or stereotactic radiation. Primary irradiation has little effect.

Prognosis depends on histological type, the average survival of patients with chondroid chordoma is some 16 years but with the ordinary chordoma survival is only 4 years. However, with the concentration of cases in skull-base centres using multiple procedures and radiation, we are beginning to see better survival figures.

Chondrosarcoma

Chondrosarcomas of the petrous apex are probably derived from cartilaginous rests in the foramen lacerum and they are rarer than those found in relation to the nasal cavities. They are locally malignant and cause symptoms by bone erosion exerting

Table 23.2 MRI characteristics of rare lesions of the internal auditory meatus and cerebellopontine angle

Tumours	T1	T1 gado	T2
Epidermoid	Hypo, hetero	Isointense	Hyperintense
Lipoma	Hyperintense	No change	Hypointense
Facial neuroma	Hypointense	Hyperintense	Variable
Arachnoid cyst	Hypointense	Hypointense	Hyperintense
Choroid plexus pap	Variable	Hyper, hetero	Hyper, hetero
Metastatic adenocarcinoma	Hypointense	Hyperintense	Hyper-variable
Lymphoma	Iso, hetero	Hyperintense	Hyper, hetero
Cholesterol cyst	Hyperintense	Hyperintense	Hyperintense
Cavernous angioma	Hyperintense	Hyperintense	Hyperintense

IAM = internal auditory meatus; CPA = cerebellopontine angle; Hypo = hypointense; Hyper = hyperintense; Iso = isointense; Hetero = heterogeneous

Reproduced by kind permission of Dr Darius Kohan. Presented at the 31st Annual Scientific Meeting of American Neurotology Society, Orlando, Florida 4th May 1996

pressure on the inner ear or cranial nerves. Radiologically they appear very similar to the chordomas (see above) but tend to enhance to a greater degree. Histological differentiation from the chordomas is important because of the considerably better prognosis. Treatment is similar, aiming for wide local resection supplemented by postoperative irradiation. The 5-year survival is at least 70%.

Meningioma

Meningiomas are the commonest benign intracranial tumour and are thought to arise from arachnoid villi. They also arise extracranially within the middle cleft (Nager, 1963) although personal experience suggests that some of these middle ear tumours actually arise from outside the temporal bone and merely secondarily invade the middle ear cleft from an enplaque meningioma of the middle or posterior fossae. Nager reported a poor prognosis for these tumours but this probably reflects the limited surgical procedures available at that time. With the advances in neuro-otological surgery, otologists are showing a greater interest in meningiomas of the cerebellopontine angle and petroclival region which constitute some 5–10% of all meningiomas. They present with the well described symptoms of the cerebellopontine angle tumour and are diagnosed radiologically by their wide based dural attachment, smooth outline, focal calcium deposits and dense homogeneous enhancement (see Figures 2.56 and 2.57). There is often hyperostosis of the underlying petrous ridge. Primary radiotherapy is not indicated, but postoperative irradiation has been shown to slow recurrence following subtotal resection. The myriad of surgical approaches described for petroclival meningiomas indicates the problems in approach and ability to resect these tumours and with the development of the various transpetrous approaches adding to the accessibility, neurosurgeons are increasingly utilizing the assistance of their neuro-otological colleagues for this challenging tumour.

Surgical approaches to the petrous apex and adjacent clivus

The traditional neurosurgical approaches have been generally unsuccessful because of the narrow exposure and, increasingly, skull base approaches are being adopted for tumours in this region. However, the complex anatomy of the skull base forms a significant barrier to the wide exposure of the petroclival region and a variety of anterior and lateral skull base approaches have been described depending on the relationship of the petrosal portion of the internal carotid artery to the tumour.

Fisch, Fagan and Valvanis (1984) have tended to favour the lateral approach whereas Crockard has described a transmaxillary approach (James and Crockard, 1991). While both techniques have their virtues, in practice the author has found that often both approaches in staged operations are necessary, in particular with the chordoma. Such procedures are best carried out as a combined otoneurosurgical procedure as both intra- and extradural techniques are often utilized. With radical debulking of these tumours, postoperative radiotherapy either with implants or by stereotactic means has been shown to be valuable in extending survival.

Infratemporal fossa route to lateral skull base and petroclival region

Fisch (1982), in particular, has developed the infratemporal fossa approach as a route to the lateral skull base. He has described a type B approach to the region of the clivus, and a type C approach to the posterior aspect of the maxillary antrum, parasellar region, nasopharynx and sphenoid sinus.

He uses the type B approach primarily for a chordoma of the clivus, cholesteatoma of the petrous apex, and meningiomas. The operation is an anterior extension of his glomus approach (type A) and he gains further access by removing bone of the posterior zygomatic arch and occasionally the head of the mandible. He then works forward along the eustachian tube, dividing the mandibular branch of the trigeminal nerve and middle meningeal artery to gain access to the clivus anterior to the carotid artery. His type C approach is basically the same, except that the zygoma is divided more anteriorly and he continues the dissection more medially by removing the pterygoid plates, and also divides the nerves of the pterygopalatine fossa to enter the nasopharynx and sphenoid region. He uses this latter approach for the removal of some large juvenile angiofibromas, adenoid cystic carcinoma and squamous cell carcinoma of the nasopharynx, which extend laterally into the infratemporal fossa. Both the type B and C approaches are anterior to the facial nerve which is left in the fallopian canal but the facial nerve is potentially at danger from stretching where it enters the parotid gland and it should be mobilized within the parotid to give better mobility.

Anterior approaches to the petroclival region

Archer, Young and Uttley (1987) used a Le Fort I osteotomy to approach tumours of the clival region and this approach was subsequently extended by James and Crockard (1991) who, in addition to the horizontal Le Fort I osteotomy, used a midline sagittal split to separate the two maxillae giving further access to the clivus. The upper jaw is reconstructed at the end of the procedure using mini-plates to restore the occlusion. The author has used these techniques for tumours of the clivus and supplements the surgical resection with an intraoperative implant of radioactive gold (Au^{198}) or iodine (I^{125}) and finds that the need for the extended maxillotomy depends on the degree of oral opening that the patient has preoperatively. However, in surgery, the description of any particular technique merely increases the number of possible approaches to solve any particular problem. The way forward in skull base surgery is to consider all the possibilities for each case, and to provide an individual solution for each. This often entails the combined approach by both otolaryngologist and neurosurgeon; if they can work well together the patient benefits.

Neuronavigation systems

Now the problems of access to the central skull base have been rationalized, we are left with the need to determine accurately our anatomical location and relationship to both the tumour and vital structures during the procedure. This can now be achieved by using neuronavigational systems which have been extensively developed over the last few years (Carney *et al.*, 1996; Carran *et al.*, 1996). Preoperative images, both MRI and CT, are fed into a computer to relate soft tissue tumour extent to bony anatomical landmarks. At the time of surgery the surgical field can also be related to the computer images using a probe or wand mounted on a robotic arm. The 3-D location of its tip is continually fed into the computer and related to the preoperative images in all planes giving the surgeon a real time indication of his precise location to a few millimetres. The ISG Wand system is already in use (Figure 23.9) and further significant advances are expected over the next few years.

Epithelial tumours

The only benign epithelial tumour found in the middle ear is the rare adenoma and this can usually be excised by the standard combined approach mastoidectomy with preservation of hearing.

The common malignant tumour is the squamous cell carcinoma and this is dealt with in Chapter 22, the essence of treatment being a combination of

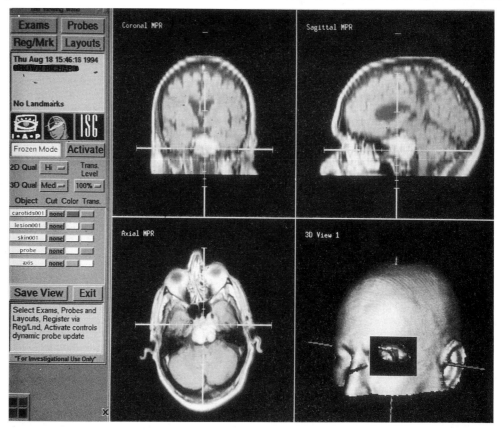

Figure 23.9 Chordoma prior to Wand-guided removal. (Reproduced by kind permission of Professor H. B. Coakham, Frenchay Hospital, Bristol)

radiotherapy and radical surgery. The other malignant epithelial tumours are adenocarcinoma and adenoid cystic carcinoma, both being relatively radioresistant, and initial radical surgery offers the best chance of cure. Radiotherapy postoperatively may have some effect on residual disease.

Mesenchymal tumours

The paragangliomas have already been discussed in detail.

Schwannomas

Schwannomas of the jugular foramen are being increasingly encountered as a result of better radiological imaging in cases of the various jugular foramen syndromes. They arise from the Antoni A and Antoni B cells of the nerve sheaths, are benign and cause symptoms from pressure on the associated nerve and subsequently the adjacent otolabyrinth. It is generally impossible to identify from which particular nerve sheath the tumour arises and at surgery the tumour often envelops all the nerves of the neural compartment even though they may have normal function when tested clinically.

Radiologically it is necessary to distinguish them from the glomus tumours. This is easily done as the bone expansion is smooth with preservation of the cortex; there is also less intense enhancement with contrast, and angiography (especially MR angiography) demonstrates its avascular nature.

These tumours are readily excised completely and the ensuing neurological deficit is amenable to rehabilitation. Many surgical approaches originally described for glomus tumours have been recommended but their associated morbidity, while acceptable for glomus tumours, is unacceptable for the simpler problem of the schwannoma. The posterolateral approach of Cheesman and Symon allows easy removal, even of the hypoglossal schwannoma, with minimal morbidity (Tan *et al.*, 1990).

Facial schwannoma

A schwannoma may occur on the facial nerve. Providing the facial palsy has been of short duration, simple resection and repair by cable-graft can produce excellent results. However, if the facial palsy has been present for more than 1 year, the results of grafting are less than satisfactory, and a hypoglossofacial anastomosis for rehabilitation is often more beneficial (Symon *et al.*, 1993).

Rhabdomyosarcoma

Primary sarcomas of the temporal bone are rare, the most common type being the embryonal rhabdomyo-

sarcoma. This is the most common childhood malignancy; unfortunately it is sometimes initially missed, being reported on pathologically as a granulation tissue, but the rapid growth and extensive destruction should make the diagnosis obvious. The more recent use of combination chemotherapy and radiotherapy has produced spectacular improvements in prognosis and, although these must remain the main modalities, primary surgical debulking if it can be achieved without increased morbidity can be beneficial (Wiatrak and Pensak, 1989).

Secondary tumours

The temporal bone may occasionally be the site of metastatic tumour, usually the hypernephroma. More commonly, it is involved by direct spread from tumours of the parotid and nasopharynx. In most cases, palliative radiotherapy is indicated, unless the primary tumour can be controlled, in which case, the metastasis can occasionally be encompassed by radical surgery.

Granulomas of the temporal bone

Wegener's granulomatosis may occasionally present in the middle ear and, if the general condition of the patient is good, may present a diagnostic problem with histological reports of granulation tissue only (see Figures 4.35a and b). Management is discussed in Volume 4, but see also Chapters 15 and 17.

Eosinophilic granuloma or histiocytosis X is a rare condition of unknown aetiology, typified by single or multiple osteolytic lesions with granulomatous replacement. The granulomas are composed of histiocytes and eosinophils. Three distinct clinical variants are recognized: eosinophilic granuloma, Hand-Schüller-Christian disease and Letterer-Siwe disease.

Eosinophilic granuloma is a disease of young adults with a male predominance. The granulomas present in the middle ear and meatus often complicated with secondary infection. The osteolytic lesions seen on X-ray are generally assumed to be cholesteatoma preoperatively, but at surgery the granulomatous replacement of bone is obvious, and confirmed by histological examination. Local resection followed by low dose radiotherapy is generally curative.

Hand-Schüller-Christian disease was originally described as a triad of skull base granulation, exophthalmos and diabetes insipidus. It is a more severe form of the disease with multifocal granulomas. It is usually a disease of childhood and there is accompanying systemic upset with recurrent respiratory infection, hepatosplenomegaly, lymphadenopathy and frequently, diabetes insipidus if the sella is involved. Low dose chemotherapy has been used to control the condition, but it tends to be a chronic disease with a mortality of 10–20%. Letterer-Siwe disease is a fulminating condition in children under 3 years old. The diffuse granulomatous deposits replace the bone marrow, and skin deposits are frequent. Death generally follows intercurrent infection and bleeding diathesis (see also Chapter 15).

References

ALFORD, B. R. and GUILFORD, F. R. (1962) A comprehensive study of tumours of the glomus jugulare. *Laryngoscope*, **72**, 765–787

ARCHER, D. J., YOUNG, S. and UTTLEY, D. (1987) Basilar aneurysms: a new trans-clival approach via maxillotomy. *Journal of Neurosurgery*, **67**, 54–58

BICKERSTAFF, E. R. and HOWELL, J. S. (1953) The neurological importance of tumours of the glomus jugalare. *Brain*, **76**, 576–593

BOYD, J. D., LEVER, J. D. and GRIFFITH, A. N. (1959) Electron microscopic observations on a glomus jugulare tumour. *Annals of Otology, Rhinology and Laryngology*, **68**, 273–277

BROWN, J. S. (1967) Glomus jugulare tumours: methods and difficulties of diagnosis and surgical treatment. *Laryngoscope*, **77**, 26–67

CAPPS, F. W. (1952) Glomus jugulare tumours of the middle ear. *Journal of Laryngology and Otology*, **66**, 302–314

CAPPS, F. W. (1955) Tumours of the glomus jugulare or tympanic body. *Journal of the Faculty of Radiologists*, **8**, 312–324

CARNEY, A. S., PATEL, N., BALDWIN, D. L., COAKHAM, H. B. and SANDEMAN, D.R. (1996) Intra-operative image guidance in otolaryngology – the use of the ISG viewing wand. *Journal of Laryngology and Otology*, **110**, 322–327

CARRAU, R. L., SNYDERMAN, C. H., CURTIN, H. D., JANECKA, I. P., STECHISON, M. and WEISSMAN, J. L. (1996) Computer-assisted intraoperative navigation during skull base surgery. *American Journal of Otolaryngology*, **17**, 95–101

CHEESMAN, A. D. and SYMON, L. (1987) Surgery of glomus jugulare tumours. In: *Operative Surgery*, Neurosurgery volume, edited by L. Symon, D. G. Thomas and K. Clarke. London: Butterworths. pp. 365–380

COLE, J. M. and BEILER, D. (1994) Long-term results of treatment for glomus jugulare and glomus vagale tumours with radiotherapy. *Laryngoscope*, **104**, 1461–1465

DUKE, W. W., BOSHELL, B. R., SOTERES, P. and CARR, J. H. (1964) A norepinephrine-secreting glomus jugulare tumour presenting as a phaeochromocytoma. *Annals of Internal Medicine*, **60**, 1040–1047

FARRIOR, J. B. (1967) Glomus tumours; postauricular hypotympanotomy and hypotympanoplasty. *Archives of Otolaryngology*, **86**, 367–373

FISCH, U. (1982) Infratemporal fossa approach for glomus tumours of the temporal bone. *Annals of Otology, Rhinology and Laryngology*, **91**, 474–479

FISCH, U., FAGAN, P. and VALVANIS, A. (1984) The infratemporal fossa approach for the lateral skull base. *Otolaryngologic Clinics of North America*, **17**, 513–552

GEJROT, T. (1965) Surgical treatment of glomus jugulare tumours. With special reference to the diagnostic value of retrograde jugularography. *Acta Otolaryngologica*, **60**, 150–168

GLASER, M. G., LESLIE, M. D., COLES, I. and CHEESMAN, A. D. (1995) Iodine seeds in the treatment of slowly proliferating tumours in the head and neck region. *Clinical Oncology*, **7**, 105–108

GLASSCOCK, M. E., HARRIS, P. F. and NEWSOME, G. (1974) Glomus tumors. Diagnosis and treatment. *Laryngoscope*, **84**, 2006–2032

GUILD, S.R. (1941) A hitherto unrecognized structure, the glomus jugularis, in man. *Anatomical Record*, **79**, 28

GUILD, S. R. (1953) The glomus jugulare: a nonchromaffin paraganglion in man. *Annals of Otology, Rhinology and Laryngology*, **62**, 1045–1071

HEUTINK, P., VAN DER MAY, A. G., SANDKUIJI, L. A., VAN GILS, A. P., BARDOEL, A., BREEDVELD, G. J. *et al.* (1992) A gene subject to genomic imprinting and responsible for hereditary paragangliomas maps to chromosome 11q23-qter. *Human Molecular Genetics*, **1**, 7–10

HOUSE, W. (1968) Panel discussion: management of glomus tumours. *Archives of Otolaryngology*, **89**, 170–178

JACKSON, A. W. and KOSHIBA, R. (1974) Treatment of glomus jugulare tumours by radiotherapy. *Proceedings of the Royal Society of Medicine*, **67**, 267–270

JAMES, D. and CROCKARD, H. A. (1991) Surgical access to the base of skull and upper cervical spine by extended maxillotomy. *Neurosurgery*, **29**, 411–416

JOHNSTON, F. and SYMON, L. (1992) Malignant paragangliomas of the glomus jugulare; a case report. *British Journal of Neurosurgery*, **6**, 255–260

KRAUSE, W. (1878) Die glandula tympanica des menschen. *Zentralblatt für Medizin Wissenesch*, **16**, 737–739

LATTES, R. and WALTNER, J. G. (1949) Nonchromaffin paraganglioma of the middle ear. *Cancer*, **2**, 447–468

LLOYD, G. A., CHEESMAN, A. D., PHELPS, P. D. and KING, C. M. (1992) The demonstration of glomus tumours by subtraction MRI. *Neuroradiology*, **34**, 470–474

LUBBERS, J. (1937) Gezwel van het os petrosum net gecombineerde hersenzenuwverlamming (syndroom foramen jugulare, BURGER) en gelijktijdig gezwel van caroticum aan de andere zijde. *Nederlands Tijdschrift voor Geneeskunde*, **81**, 2566–2567

LUNDGREN, N. (1949) Tympanic body tumours in the middle ear: tumours of the carotid body type. *Acta Otolaryngologica*, **37**, 366–379

MAKEK, M., FRANKLIN, D. J., JIN-CHENG, Z. and FISCH, U. (1990) Neural infiltration of glomus temporale tumours. *American Journal of Otology*, **11**, 1–5

MATISHAK, M., SYMON, L., CHEESMAN, A. D. and PAMPHLETT, R. (1987) Catecholamine secreting paragangliomas of the base of the skull. Report of two cases. *Journal of Neurosurgery*, **66**, 604–608

MULLIGAN, R. M. (1950) Chemodectoma in the dog. *American Journal of Pathology*, **28**, 680–681

NAGER, G. T. (1963) *Meningiomas involving the Temporal Bone*. Springfield: Charles C. Thomas. pp. 365–380

OLDRING, D. and FISCH, U. (1979) Glomus tumors of the temporal region: surgical therapy. *American Journal of Otolaryngology*, **1**, 7–18

PHELPS, P. D. and CHEESMAN, A. D. (1990) Imaging jugulotympanic glomus tumours. *Archives of Otolaryngology – Head and Neck Surgery*, **116**, 940–945

ROSENWASSER, H. (1945) Carotid body tumor of the middle ear and mastoid. *Archives of Otolaryngology*, **41**, 64–67

ROSENWASSER, H. (1968) Glomus jugulare tumors. Newer diagnostic procedures in therapy. *Archives of Otolarnygology*, **88**, 53–60

ROSENWASSER, H. (1969) Glomus jugulare tumors. Long term results. *Archives of Otolaryngology*, **89**, 160–166

SHAMBAUGH, G. E. (1955) Surgical approach for so-called glomus jugulare tumors of the middle ear. *Laryngoscope*, **65**, 185–198

SHAPIRO, M. J. and NEUES, D. K. (1964) Technique for the removal of glomus jugulare tumors. *Archives of Otolaryngology*, **79**, 219–224

SILVERSTONE, S. (1973) Radiation therapy of glomus tumors. *Archives of Otolaryngology*, **97**, 43–48

SIMPSON, L. C. and DALLACHY, R. (1958) A review of tumours of the glomus jugulare with reports of three further cases. *Journal of Otology and Laryngology*, **72**, 194–226

SPECTOR, G. J., CIRALSKY, R., MAISEL, R. H. and OGURA, J. H. (1975) Multiple glomus tumors in the head and neck. *Laryngoscope*, **85**, 1066–1075

SPECTOR, G. J., MAISEL, R. H. and OGURA, J. H. (1974) Glomus jugulare tumours. A clinico-pathological analysis of the effects of radiotherapy. *Annals of Otology, Rhinology and Laryngology*, **83**, 26–32

SYMON, L., CHEESMAN, A. D., KAWAUCHI, M. and BORDI, L. (1993) Neuromas of the facial nerve. A report of 12 cases. *British Journal of Neurosurgery*, **7**, 13–22

TAN, L. C., BORDI, L., SYMON, L. and CHEESMAN, A. D. (1990) Jugular foramen neuromas. *Surgical Neurology*, **34**, 205–211

VALENTIN, G. (1840) Ueber eine gangliöse Anschwellung in der Jacobsonchen anastomose des Menschen. *Archiv für Anatomie, Physiologie und Wissenschaftliche Medicin Novorno*, Leipzig, 287–290

WATKINS, L. D., MENDOZA, N., CHEESMAN, A. D. and SYMON, L. (1994) Glomus jugulare tumours: a review of 61 cases. *Acta Neurochirurgica*, **130**, 66–70

WIATRAK, G. E. and PENSAK, M. L. (1989) Rhabdomyosarcoma of the ear and temporal bone. *Laryngoscope*, **99**, 1188–1192

WINSHIP, T., KLOPP, C. T. and JENKINS, W. H. (1948) Glomus jugularis tumors. *Cancer*, **1**, 441–448

WINSHIP, T. and LOUZAN, J. (1951) Tumours of the glomus jugulare not associated with jugular vein. *Archives of Otolaryngology*, **54**, 378–383

24

Disorders of the facial nerve

Barry Schaitkin and Mark May

The material presented is based on the authors' experience in managing more than 3000 patients over a period of 25 years. The emphasis is on management in terms of diagnosis, prognosis, and treatment. The presentation begins with applied basic science and progresses to clinical evaluation, stressing pathophysiology, differential diagnosis, special tests, natural history, and the treatment of specific disorders.

Embryology

Normal and abnormal presentations of the facial nerve can best be understood through an awareness of its embryonic development (Gasser, 1967a, b). The main pattern of the nerve's complex course, branching pattern, and relationships is established during the first 3 months of prenatal life. During this period the muscles of expression also differentiate, become functional, and actively contract. Important steps in facial nerve development occur throughout gestation and the nerve is not fully developed until approximately 4 years after birth (Table 24.1).

Congenital anomalies can be understood by relating them to embryological development. The facial nerve develops within the second pharyngeal arch during the time that closely adjacent derivatives of the first arch and first external groove and internal pouch are forming the external and middle ear regions. Anomalies of the facial nerve within the temporal bone should therefore be anticipated whenever there is an associated malformation of the external or middle ear. If the stapes or incus is deformed the surgeon should be on guard for a possible misplaced and exposed facial nerve; a soft tissue mound over the footplate of the stapes or the promontory may actually be the facial nerve (Jahrsdoerfer, 1981).

A great variety of facial nerve arrangements has been encountered within the temporal bone (Proctor and Nager, 1982). The nerve may course with the chorda tympani nerve, bifurcate, trifurcate, or take innumerable other aberrant pathways within the temporal bone. When a large chorda tympani nerve is encountered it may be carrying motor fibres to the face. In such instances, the vertical segment of the

Table 24.1 Time during gestation that anatomical structures appear

Week of gestation	Structures noted
Week 3	Collection of neural crest cells to become VIIth cranial nerve identifiable
Week 5	Chorda tympani, greater petrosal, VIIth motor nucleus
Week 6	External genu, postauricular branch, branch to posterior belly of digastric
Week 7	Geniculate ganglion, nervus intermedius
Week 7–8	Myoblasts that will form the facial muscles are noted
Week 8	Stapedius nerve, temporofacial and cervicofacial part of extracranial facial nerve becomes apparent
End of week 8	Rest of terminal branches of VII form
Week 12	All facial muscles are identifiable

facial nerve just distal to the point where the chorda tympani nerve branches off may dwindle to a fibrous strand and lie in a narrowed fallopian canal. This condition has been encountered in children born with facial paralysis. The nerve may be dehiscent and it may herniate into the middle ear cavity (Johnson and Kingsley, 1970). This unusual presentation of the facial nerve, when encountered during otological surgery, must not be confused with a facial nerve schwannoma. Excision or biopsy of such a structure would cause iatrogenic facial paralysis that would have to be repaired by surgery.

Anatomy

A general knowledge of the anatomy of the VIIth cranial nerve is essential for diagnosis and treatment of facial nerve disorders. For example, specific differential diagnostic possibilities can be derived by localizing the site of the lesion (Table 24.2 and Figure 24.1) and, in the event that surgical treatment is appropriate, defining the level of facial nerve involvement is critical.

Table 24.2 Signs indicating probable diagnosis of lesions of the facial nerve at various levels*

Level	Signs	Probable diagnosis
I Supranuclear		
Cortex and internal capsule	Tone and upper face intact, loss of volitional movement with intact spontaneous expression, slurred speech (tongue weakness), hemiparesis (arm greater than leg) on side of facial involvement Paresis of upper extremity begins with involvement of thumb, finger and hand movement	Lesion of motor cortex or internal capsule on opposite side of facial involvement Paresis upper extremity usually middle cerebral artery Paresis lower extremity usually anterior cerebral artery
Opercular syndrome	Voluntary facial and lingual movements impaired, emotional and automatic movements preserved or exaggerated Speech is dysarthric; laryngeal, sternocleidomastoid, and trapezius muscles involved Weakness of the tongue, pharynx, jaws, neck muscles, and upper extremity may occur EEG may not be abnormal because of depth of lesion in operculum (insula or island of Reil complex) Upper face usually not spared as with other motor cortex lesions	Vascular, neoplastic, encephalitic or traumatic lesion
Extrapyramidal	Increased salivary flow, spontaneous facial movement impaired, volitional facial movement intact Masked face of parkinsonism or dystonia, progressive hemifacial spasm Grimacing and choreiform movements	Tumour or vascular lesion of basal ganglia Parkinsonism Meige's syndrome (cervical facial dystonia)
Midbrain	Involvement of face and oculomotor roots; loss of pupillary reflexes, external strabismus, and oculomotor paresis on opposite side of facial paresis	Unilateral Weber's syndrome (vascular lesion)
	Bilateral facial paresis with other cranial nerve deficits, emotional lability, hyperactive gag reflex, marked hyperflexia associated with hypertension	Pseudobulbar palsy associated with multiple infarcts
Pontine nucleus	Involvement of cranial nerves VII and VI on side of lesion with gaze palsy on side of facial paresis Contralateral hemiparesis, ataxia, cerebellovestibular signs	Involvement of pons at level of VII and VI nuclei by pontine glioma, multiple sclerosis, encephalitis, infection, or polio
	Contralateral hemiplegia with ipsilateral facial palsy Internal strabismus may be present on side of facial palsy	Possible lesion just above pontine facial nucleus, below decussation of corticobulbar tract Millard–Gubler syndrome, Foville's syndrome
	Deficits of cranial nerves VII and VI noted from time of birth with or without other congenital anomalies Facial motor involvement usually incomplete sparing of corner of mouth or lower lip common Another type of presentation is involvement of the lower lip with complete or partial sparing of upper face Anomalies of the pinna, canal or mandible associated with facial palsy indicate developmental defect of facial nerve	Developmental facial palsy (noted at birth) Oculofacial syndrome or Moebius' syndrome Thalidomide toxicity Non-developmental facial palsy due to facial or abducens nerve anomalies are most often due to infranuclear lesions
II Infranuclear intracranial		
Cerebellopontine angle (CPA)	Impairment of hearing, especially discrimination out of proportion to pure tone scores Possible ataxia, abnormalities of tearing or taste, staples reflex decay, decreased corneal sensation	Vestibular schwannoma

Table 24.2 *(Continued)*

Level	Signs	Probable diagnosis
	Facial motor deficit (late sign) Prolongation of the latency of waves III–V of auditory brain stem response (ABR) Anomalies on CT scan (usually not enhanced with contrast)	
	Abnormalities in trigeminal, acoustic-vestibular and facial nerve function, starting with facial pain or numbness Lesion noted on CT (enhancement with contrast)	Meningioma
	Abnormalities of facial and acoustic-vestibular nerve function May start with facial twitchings Erosion or lytic area evident on plain radiographs of temporal bone	Cholesteatoma or facial schwannoma arising in temporal bone
	Abnormalities of cranial nerves VII, VIII, IX, X, XI, and XII Pulsatile tinnitus and purple-red pulsating mass bulging through the tympanic membrane	Glomus jugulare tumour
	Abnormalities of abducens nerve in addition to above	Glomus jugulare tumour extending to petrous apex to involve middle fossa
Skull base	Conductive or sensorineural hearing loss, acute or recurrent facial palsy Positive family history, abnormalities of bone density on skull radiograph	Osteopetrosis
	Multiple cranial nerve involvement in rapid succession	Carcinomatous meningitis, leukaemia, Landry–Guillain–Barré syndrome, mononucleosis, diphtheria, tuberculosis, sarcoidosis, malignant otitis externa
III *Transtemporal bone*		
Internal auditory meatus and labyrinthine segment of facial nerve	Ecchymosis around pinna and mastoid prominence (Battle's sign) Haemotympanum with sensorineural hearing loss (tuning fork lateralizes to normal side), vertigo, nystagmus (fast component away from involved side) Sudden complete facial paralysis following head trauma Usually associated with basilar skull fracture, loss of consciousness and CSF leak Transection of facial nerve more likely with this injury compared to longitudinal fracture	Temporal bone fracture (transverse, longitudinal or combination)
Geniculate ganglion	Dry eye, decreased taste and salivation. Erosion of geniculate ganglion area or middle fossa demonstrated by pluridirectional tomography and CT scan of temporal bone	Schwannoma, meningioma, cholesteatoma, haemangioma, arteriovenous malformation
	Ear pain, vesicles in pinna, dry eye, decreased taste and salivary flow Sensorineural hearing loss, nystagmus, vertigo, red chorda tympani nerve Facial palsy may be complete, incomplete, or progress to complete over 14 days	Herpes zoster cephalicus (Ramsay Hunt syndrome)
	Same as above without vesicles, no other cause evident Facial palsy may be complete, incomplete, or progress to complete over 10 days	Idiopathic (Bell's) palsy, (viral inflammatory immune disorder)
	Same as above but no recovery in 6 months	Tumour

Table 24.2 *(Continued)*

Level	Signs	Probable diagnosis
	Ecchymosis around pinna and mastoid (Battle's sign), haemotympanum Conductive hearing loss (tuning fork lateralizes to involved ear) No vestibular involvement unless stapes subluxed into vestibule (causes fluctuant sensorineural hearing loss and vertigo with nystagmus)	Longitudinal fracture of temporal bone May be proximal or at geniculate ganglion (dry eye), or distal to geniculate ganglion (tearing symmetrical) (Tear test valid only in acute injury)
Tympanomastoid	Decreased taste and salivation, loss of stapes reflex and symmetrical tearing Sudden onset facial palsy which may be complete or incomplete or may progress to complete	
	Pain, vesicles, red chorda tympani	Herpes zoster cephalicus
	Pain without vesicles, red chorda tympani	Bell's palsy
	Red, bulging tympanic membrane, conductive hearing loss Usually history of upper respiratory tract infection Lower face may be involved more than upper	Acute suppurative otitis media
	Foul drainage through perforated tympanic membrane History of recurrent ear infection, drainage, and hearing loss	Chronic suppurative otitis media, most likely associated with cholesteatoma
	Pulsatile tinnitus, purple-red pulsatile mass noted through tympanic membrane	Glomus tympanicum or jugulare
	Recurrent facial paralysis, positive family history, facial oedema, fissured tongue May present with simultaneous bilateral facial paralysis	Melkersson–Rosenthal syndrome
IV *Extracranial*	Incomplete facial nerve paresis Hearing, balance, tearing, stapedial reflex, taste, salivary flow spared	Penetrating wound of face; sequelae of parotid surgery; malignancy of parotid, tonsil or oronasopharynx; rarely, with benign lesion of parotid gland compressing facial nerve
	Uveitis, salivary gland enlargement, fever	Sarcoidosis (Heerfordt's syndrome), lymphoma
V *Sites variable*	Bilateral facial paralysis from birth	Moebius' syndrome
	Bilateral facial paralysis, acquired	Landry–Guillain–Barré syndrome, sarcoidosis, mononucleosis, leukaemia, idiophatic (Bell's) palsy
	Facial paralysis, especially simultaneous bilateral facial paralysis with symmetrical ascending paralysis, decreased deep tendon reflexes, minimal sensory changes Abnormal spinal fluid (protein and few cells, albumino-cytological dissociation)	Landry–Guillain–Barré syndrome
	Deficits of cranial nerves VI and VII or VII, VI, and III, possibly in association with other neurological signs	Carcinoma of nasopharynx, metastatic carcinoma from breast, ovary, prostate; meningitis, leukaemia, diabetes mellitus
VI *Pseudobulbar palsy*	Inappropriate or exaggerated laughing or crying May be associated with marked increase in jaw jerk, or gag reflex	Polyneuritis Toxic, viral or vascular lesion involving bilateral corticobulbar pathways

*From May (1986)

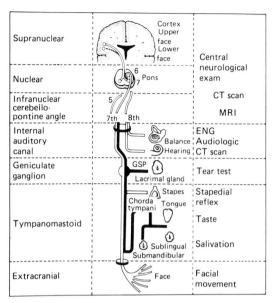

Figure 24.1 Topographical anatomy of the facial nerve

Cortex and internal capsule

Anatomy of the pyramidal system from the cortex to the pontine nucleus is illustrated in Figure 24.2. Facial motor nerves are represented with the forehead uppermost and the eyelids, midface, and lips located sequentially below the representation of the forehead. Note that the tracts to the lower face are crossed, whereas innervation to the forehead is both crossed and uncrossed. Sparing of forehead movement is considered to be characteristic of a cortical lesion. However, it is also possible to have forehead sparing with a lesion of the pontine facial nucleus, with selective lesions within the temporal bone, or even in association with an injury to the nerve in its distribution in the face. Since preservation of forehead function is insufficient to make a diagnosis of a central lesion, other neurological signs must be sought (Table 24.3).

Extrapyramidal system

The extrapyramidal system consists of the basal ganglia and the descending motor projections other than the fibres of the pyramidal or corticospinal tracts. This system provides for automatic associated movements and spontaneous, emotional, mimetic human facial language which accompanies the more precise voluntary responses. The interplay between the pyramidal and extrapyramidal system accounts for tonus and stabilizes the motor responses. The affect of parkinsonism is known to be the result of extrapyramidal pathway destruction, and the facial dystonia

of Meige's syndrome, a rare clinical entity, is thought to be due to basal ganglion disease. The severe progressive hemifacial spasm that accompanies Meige's syndrome will be discussed further under central nervous system facial nerve disorders.

Emotion is another function of the extrapyramidal cortical system and is mediated by discharges passing through the cingulate, orbital, and other frontal cortical areas and the basolateral portion of the amygdala.

Upper midbrain

A lesion in the upper midbrain will involve the oculomotor pathways and result in ipsilateral loss of direct and consensual pupillary light reflexes, ipsilateral external strabismus, and oculomotor paresis. In addition, paresis of contralateral muscles of the head and body will be noted. This symptom complex is referred to as unilateral Weber's syndrome.

Lower midbrain

A lesion in the lower midbrain that is central to the facial nerve nucleus involves the tracts of the abducens nerve and may cause contralateral paresis of the face and muscles of the extremities, ipsilateral abducens paresis, and internal strabismus. A lesion that extends far enough laterally to include the emerging facial nerve fibres may present as peripheral ipsilateral facial paralysis associated with loss of taste papillae on the anterior two-thirds of the tongue, and a dry eye on the same side. In addition, salivary flow from the submaxillary gland on the side of the lesion may be greatly diminished or absent.

It is important to emphasize that the peripheral topognostic tests for tearing, taste, and lacrimal flow can be altered by supranuclear lesions. However, a lesion in this region of the brain stem would involve other neural functions as well, and would be highly unlikely to involve only facial function.

Pontine nucleus

The facial motor nucleus contains approximately 7000 neurons and is seated in the lower third of the pons, beneath the fourth ventricle. The neuronal processes that leave the nucleus pass around the abducens nucleus (VIth cranial nerve) before emerging from the brain stem. A peripheral VIIth nerve paralysis, an internal strabismus on the same side, and inability to turn the non-paralysed eye towards the nose when asked to look towards the paralysed side of the face all suggest a single lesion near the

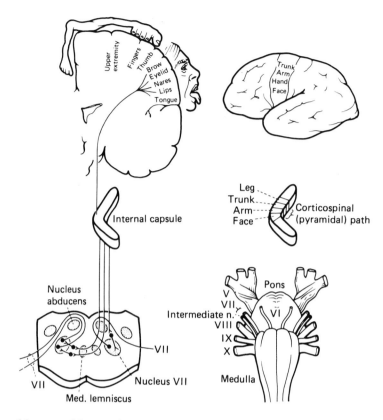

Figure 24.2 Anatomy of the pyramidal system from cortex to pontine nucleus

floor of the fourth ventricle involving the VIth and VIIth cranial nerves. A lesion near the ventricle at the level of the superior salivary nucleus causes peripheral facial paralysis, a dry eye, paralysis of voluntary muscles, loss of following gaze toward the side of the facial paralysis, and often vertical or rotatory nystagmus.

Cerebellopontine angle

The facial nerve emerges from the brain stem with a more slender nerve, the nerve of Wrisberg or nervus intermedius. Because of the association of the facial nerve with the nervus intermedius and the vestibulocochlear nerve at the level of the cerebellopontine angle and in the internal auditory meatus, tearing, taste, submandibular salivary flow, and hearing and balance may be disturbed with a facial nerve lesion at this level. Large lesions filling the cerebellopontine angle may compress other cranial nerves and cause deficits of the Vth cranial nerve and later the IXth, Xth, and XIth cranial nerves. Lesions that may

occur in the area include temporal bone fractures, vestibular schwannomas (neuromas), meningiomas, primary cholesteatomas, and perhaps hyper- or hypokinetic disorders from vascular cross-compression of cranial nerves (see Figure 5.33).

Transtemporal bone portion of the facial nerve

An understanding of the gross and microscopic anatomical relationships between the facial, auditory, and vestibular nerves, described by Silverstein and Norrell (1980), is essential for performing a retrolabyrinthine vestibular neurectomy (Figure 24.3). The intracranial segment of the facial nerve from the brain stem to the fundus of the internal auditory meatus is covered only by a thin layer of glia, which makes it quite vulnerable to any type of surgical manipulation but also quite resistant to a slow process of stretching or compression. Thus, the facial nerve in this region can become quite elongated and spread out over the surface of a sizeable but slow-

Table 24.3 Signs differentiating supranuclear from infranuclear lesions*

Supranuclear	Infranuclear
Forehead intact bilaterally	Total facial palsy (usually unilateral)

Emotion intact
    If patient has volitional but not spontaneous smile, a deeper basal ganglion lesion should be suspected
    If patient coughs and cries appropriately but has marked increase in jaw jerk and gag reflex in response to minor stimulus involvement of both corticobulbar tracts (pseudobulbar palsy) should be suspected
	Emotion impaired

Deficit of tongue, thumb, fingers, hand	No deficit
Hemiplegia on side of facial palsy Ipsilateral facial palsy with contralateral hemiplegia suggests pontine lesion near facial nucleus	No hemiplegia
Ataxia	No ataxia
Reflexes intact (can be decreased with acute lesion)	No reflexes
Tone maintained	Flaccid
Drooping corner of mouth	Not an isolated finding
Slight flattening of nasolabial fold	Not an isolated finding
No muscle atrophy No muscle fasciculations	Muscle atrophy Muscle fasciculations
Electrical tests† MST responses equal bilaterally	MST responses decreased or absent
EEMG responses normal	EEMG responses decreased or absent
EEMG responses normal	EEMG fibrillations
MUAP present	MUAP decreased or absent

*From May (1986)

†MST, Maximal stimulation test; EEMG, evoked electromyography; EMG, needle electromyography; MUAP, motor unit action potential. Presence or absence of signs listed depend upon level and completeness of injury. The following alterations in function can occur with supranuclear as well as infranuclear lesions: autonomic-tearing, salivary flow; special sensory-taste; motor function-stapes reflex (stapes nucleus separate from pontine facial motor nucleus)

growing vestibular nerve schwannoma without any gross evidence of facial weakness (see Figure 2.17 and Plate 3/21/IV).

Fallopian canal

The course of the facial nerve through the fallopian canal is unique. No other nerve in the body covers such a long distance through a bony canal. The nerve is also remarkable for the Z shape of its intratemporal portion, in that it has a ganglion, and that the length of its course is 28–30 mm. The nerve in the fallopian canal can be divided into three segments:

labyrinthine, tympanic; and mastoid (Figure 24.4). The labyrinthine segment is the thinnest part of the facial nerve within the fallopian canal. The narrowest part is at its entrance, where it averages 0.68 mm in diameter (Fisch and Esslen, 1972, a,b). Fisch (1977) feels that this bottleneck at the entrance of the fallopian canal predisposes the nerve to strangulation in cases of oedematous swelling. The observation is supported by post-mortem findings reported by Fowler (1963) and by Proctor, Corgill and Proud (1976). The blood supply to the nerve in this region is unique; this is the only segment of the facial nerve in which there are no anastomosing arterial arcades.

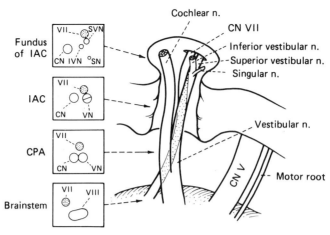

Figure 24.3 Anatomical relationships of the facial, auditory, and vestibular nerves viewed through a left postauricular approach. IAC, internal auditory canal (meatus); CPA, cerebellopontine angle

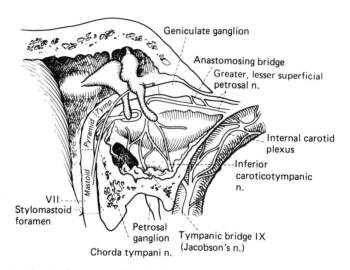

Figure 24.4 The tympanic and vertical segments of the facial nerve as viewed through the middle ear

The labyrinthine segment of the facial nerve includes the geniculate ganglion. The somatosensory (pain), and special sensory (taste) fibres are afferent fibres that synapse in the geniculate ganglion, while the autonomic secretomotor fibres to the lacrimal gland pass through the geniculate ganglion and form the first branch of the facial nerve, the greater superficial petrosal nerve (Figure 24.5). The secretory fibres to the parotid gland are carried with the IXth cranial nerve. They travel through the tympanic plexus and form the lesser superficial petrosal nerve (see Figure 24.4). There are communications with the nervus intermedius, which provides an alternative route for the parasympathetic fibres to reach the parotid, thus bypassing the tympanic plexus and the IXth cranial nerve branch of Jacobson.

This might explain why sectioning Jacobson's nerve, in many cases, may have little effect on parotid salivary flow.

In the region of the geniculate ganglion there are ample alternative pathways and connections for parasympathetic fibres to reach their terminations (see Figure 24.5). Such alternative pathways explain how lacrimal flow may be unaffected by slow-growing lesions at or proximal to the geniculate ganglion, and the spontaneous recovery of tearing following resection of the geniculate ganglion or nervus intermedius, such as might occur with posterior fossa surgery. The geniculate ganglion lacks a bony covering in approximately 15% of temporal bones, an arrangement that makes the facial nerve quite vulnerable to injury during surgery involving the middle cranial

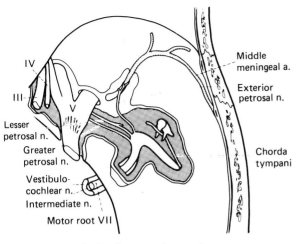

Figure 24.5 The facial nerve and some of its connections as seen through a dissection of the right middle cranial fossa

fossa, especially in children. Further, the bone of the tegmen tympani and middle fossa plate over this region may be quite thin.

In the authors' experience with temporal bone fractures, this is the area of the facial nerve most often compressed by crushed, thin, bony fragments. The change in direction taken by the facial nerve at the genu is another reason why this site is the most common focus of injury when severe traction is applied to the nerve along the axis of its tympanic segment, as may occur in longitudinal fracture of the petrous pyramid. The fact that the arachnoid pia mater extends to the geniculate ganglion, as well as the complex embryological development of this portion of the nerve, may explain why this area of the facial nerve is so often the site of primary cholesteatomas, vascular malformations, meningiomas, and schwannomas (Fisch, 1977).

The geniculate ganglion marks the proximal end of the tympanic portion, and from this point the nerve courses 3–5 mm, before passing just behind the cochleariform process and the tensor tympani tendon. The cochleariform process is a useful landmark to find the facial nerve when other landmarks are obscured by granulation tissue, cholesteatoma, or in cases of trauma. The entire tympanic segment is approximately 8–11 mm long and the tympanic wall of this part of the fallopian canal is thin and easily fractured. In addition, dehiscences occur frequently, allowing the uncovered nerve to prolapse into the oval window niche, partly or completely concealing the footplate of the stapes; this makes the nerve subject to trauma during stapes surgery. The tympanic segment is divided from the mastoid portion by the pyramidal eminence (see Figure 2.11*b*).

At this point the fallopian aqueduct makes another turn downward, forming the second genu. The latter

is another area where the facial nerve is vulnerable to injury during mastoid surgery. The distal aspect of the tympanic segment is found by the surgeon through the mastoid approach by entering the suprapyramidal recess (retrofacial recess) as illustrated in Figure 24.6. Here, the facial nerve is lateral and distal to the pyramidal process. In the presence of chronic infection, care must be taken not to confuse a pathological dehiscence of the facial nerve in this region with a mound of granulation tissue. The best way to avoid this is to identify the nerve proximal and distal to the area that looks suspicious. The second genu, which marks the beginning of the mastoid segment, is lateral and posterior to the pyramidal process, which houses the stapedius muscle that lies on the deep side of the facial nerve; this explains the fact that the facial nerve lies lateral to the pyramidal process. The nerve continues vertically down the anterior wall of the mastoid process to the stylomastoid foramen (see Figure 2.17). The distance from the beginning of the second genu to the stylomastoid foramen varies between 10 and 14 mm. This segment of the facial nerve has three branches:

1 The nerve to the stapedius muscle
2 The chorda tympani nerve
3 The nerve from the auricular branch of the vagus.

The nerve to the stapedius muscle arises from small neurons within the pons, located outside the main facial nerve nucleus, which interface with the rostral end of the facial nucleus and the caudal end of the lateral superior salivatory nucleus (Lyon, 1978; Joseph *et al.*, 1985). Although Lyon (1978) studied

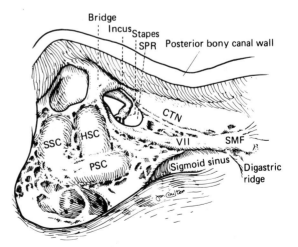

Figure 24.6 Anatomical landmarks for the surgeon to identify the mastoid segment of the facial nerve. SSC, superior semicircular canal; HSC, horizontal semicircular canal; PSC, posterior semicircular canal; CTN, chorda tympani nerve; SMF, stylomastoid foramen; SPR, suprapyramidal recess

cats and Joseph *et al.* (1985) studied rabbits to determine the location of the motor neurons relative to the stapedius muscle, it is quite likely that these neurons lie in a similar location in humans. If so, this may help to explain why alterations in the middle ear reflex occur when a brain stem lesion is present. Further, the separate nucleus for the stapedius muscle innervation provides the anatomical basis for sparing of the stapedius muscle in patients with congenital facial palsy such as Moebius' syndrome.

Surgical landmarks to identify the facial nerve

The facial nerve (see Figure 24.6) will usually be found just deep to the short process of the incus, in a line between the short process of the incus and the anterior extent of the digastric ridge. The facial nerve is thus posterior to the chorda tympani nerve and just lateral to the ampullary end of the posterior semicircular canal. Skeletonizing the posterior canal is helpful in order to avoid fenestrating this part of the labyrinth. The tympanomastoid suture line is another useful landmark, because it lies just anterior to the facial nerve and close to the course of the chorda tympani nerve. The chorda tympani nerve and facial nerve are deep to this suture. The facial nerve lies anterior to the sigmoid sinus and leaves the temporal bone through the stylomastoid foramen just anterior and lateral to the sigmoid sinus, where the digastric ridge turns and runs in the direction of the stylomastoid foramen.

Facial nerve sheath

The sheath that surrounds the facial nerve through its course in the fallopian canal consists of periosteum, epineurium, and perineurium (Figure 24.7). Although surgical decompression and opening the perineurium of the facial nerve are controversial in the management of Bell's palsy and herpes zoster cephalicus, opening the sheath is imperative in cases of suspected tumour or trauma. A tumour of the facial nerve may be discovered when the sheath is opened, or a traumatic haematoma may be found compressing the nerve deep to the sheath. Finally, when the nerve has been disrupted, it is necessary to open the sheath to find the proximal and distal ends for repair.

Spatial orientation

Agreement is lacking, despite investigations into the matter as to whether the facial nerve is spatially oriented in its extra-axial course from the brain stem to the periphery, as it is in the cortex and pontine nucleus. Evidence against topographical organization of these facial nerve fibres has come from several investigators who have found that the fibres destined for each peripheral branch are diffusely located in the facial nerve trunk (Sunderland and Cossar, 1953; Harris, 1968; Sade, 1975; Thomander, Aldskogius and Grant, 1982).

Thomander, Aldskogius and Grant (1982) exposed the individual peripheral facial nerve branches to horseradish peroxidase, permitting retrograde trans-

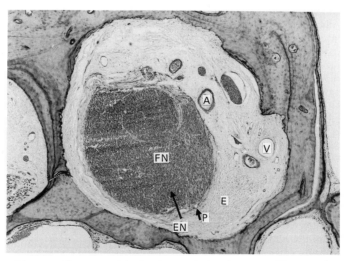

Figure 24.7 Cross-section of the mastoid segment of the facial nerve (FN) in the temporal bone. In this section also it is monofunicular and covered by the perineurium (P), endoneurium (EN) and epineurium (E); arteriole (A); venule (V). (From May (1986) with permission of the Publishers, Thieme-Stratton Inc.)

port of the tracer to demonstrate the location of these fibres in the cat facial nerve trunk. The study indicated that the fibres to each peripheral branch were diffusely arranged in the facial nerve trunk at least as far proximally as the tympanic segment.

Gacek and Radpour (1982) studied the cross-sectional anatomy of the facial nerve through its course in the temporal bone by making discrete lesions in the facial nerve of the cat proximal to the geniculate ganglion and documenting anterograde wallerian degeneration. They discovered degenerated myelin sheaths in all three of the peripheral branches studied, regardless of whether the lesion involved the rostral, caudal, or middle fascicles of the facial nerve. From this, they concluded that small fascicles of the facial nerve at the level of the internal auditory meatus carry motor fibres to all peripheral branches, and that motor axons of the facial nerve in the cat are not topographically arranged in the facial nerve trunk, as had previously been proposed. Jannetta (1975) described 31 patients with hemifacial spasm treated by removing a vessel compressing the facial nerve in the cerebellopontine angle. In those cases where the compressing vessel was found on the cephalic aspect of the nerve, the spasm was more severe in the upper part of the face. In cases where the vessel compressed the caudal aspect of the nerve, the spasm began in the lower face in an atypical fashion. This observation lends support to the existence of spatial orientation of the nerve in its most proximal intracranial portion.

Considering all the evidence, it is likely that there is some degree of spatial organization of facial nerve fibres, especially at the level at which the axon processes leave the brain-stem nucleus and course toward the periphery. Accepting the fact that the peripheral facial nerve is at best only partially topographically oriented, with some axons carried with the upper division terminating in muscle groups of the lower face and vice versa, it is understandable that regeneration following facial nerve injuries usually results in some degree of mass movement and synkinesis.

Blood supply

The nerve receives its nourishment from the anterior inferior cerebellar artery, which enters the internal auditory meatus in close association with the VIIth and VIIIth cranial nerves, the petrosal branch of the middle meningeal artery which runs along with the greater petrosal nerve, and the stylomastoid branch of the postauricular artery, which enters the facial canal at the stylomastoid foramen. The territories supplied by the three arteries tend to overlap at any given level. As mentioned previously, the anastomosis between the arterial systems is immediately proximal to the geniculate ganglion, making this segment of the facial nerve vulnerable to ischaemia from oedema.

This might have bearing on the pathogenesis of facial paralysis following embolization of the middle meningeal artery (Metson and Hanson, 1983).

Extracranial segment of the facial nerve

The facial nerve leaves the fallopian canal at the stylomastoid foramen. In newborns and in children up to 2 years of age, the facial nerve as it exits the skull is just deep to the subcutaneous tissue underlying the skin. After 2 years of age, as the mastoid tip and tympanic ring form, the facial nerve takes a deeper position and, in an adult, it may be up to 5 cm below the level of the skin. Beyond the age of 2 years, the facial nerve is protected by the tympanic bone, the mastoid tip, the ascending ramus of the mandible, and the fascia between the parotid and cartilaginous external canal.

The position of the facial nerve in the young child must be kept in mind by the otologist and head and neck surgeon. To avoid unintentional injury to the facial nerve, a postauricular incision should be modified to avoid coursing near the junction of the tympanic ring and mastoid tip, and this area should be protected by placing a finger over the area at the time the incision is made. The surgeon is cautioned not to depend upon a nerve stimulator to find the facial nerve in the region of the stylomastoid foramen. A muscle response may be noted in spite of the fact that the stimulator is not directly on the facial nerve, or the stimulator may give no response when on the facial nerve, if a thin layer of connective tissue is insulating the nerve. The nerve must therefore be identified by its anatomical location and appearance.

The main trunk may be identified entering the substance of the parotid and then bifurcating into an upper and a lower division. The facial nerve passes through the parotid gland and emerges over the fascia of the masseter muscle. There are communications between the upper and lower divisions in the majority of patients, and these form a variety of patterns. The rich plexus of nerve filaments that forms in the peripheral zone, just before entering the undersurface of the facial muscles, provides for free intermingling between branches carried by the upper and lower divisions, which may explain the diffuse distribution of axons within the main trunk of the facial nerve throughout its course from the brain stem.

Communications of the facial nerve

There are diffuse intra-axial connections within the central nervous system and, in addition, the facial nerve communicates with the vestibulocochlear nerve within the internal auditory meatus, with the otic ganglion and sympathetic fibres in the area of the geniculate ganglion and, just before it leaves the stylomastoid foramen, with the auricular branch of the vagus nerve. Outside the stylomastoid foramen the facial nerve communicates with the glossopharyngeal nerve, the vagus nerve, the great auricular nerve, and the auriculotemporal nerve. The peripheral branches communicate behind the ear with the lesser occipital, on the face with branches of the trigeminal, and in the neck with the cervical cutaneous nerve. These relationships have been documented by the meticulous dissections of Bischoff (1977). The fact that myriads of strands of the facial nerve interconnect with the Vth, VIIth, VIIIth, IXth, Xth, XIth and XIIth cranial nerves, and with the cervical cutaneous nerves, may help to explain the symptoms of many syndromes; head and face pain, and ear, throat, eustachian tube, and neck pain. These syndromes are extremely hard to treat when the cause is malignant disease or a functional imbalance such as that which causes cluster headaches or atypical facial neuralgia. These interconnections also explain mastoid, ear, face or neck pain associated with Bell's palsy and herpes zoster cephalicus, the presence of residual facial sensation after the trigeminal nerve has been cut, preservation of taste and tearing after facial nerve severance, and the occurrence of pain with skull base cancer after resection of the Vth, VIIth, IXth, and Xth cranial nerves, the 1st or 2nd cervical nerves or the nervus intermedius.

Spontaneous recovery of facial nerve function

This free intermingling of fibres of the facial nerve with fibres of other neural structures (particularly the Vth cranial nerve) has been proposed as the mechanism of spontaneous return of facial nerve function after peripheral injury to the nerve. Although spontaneous recovery of facial function was noted in approximately 25% of patients studied by Martin and Helsper (1957), this potential should not be relied upon for spontaneous reanimation of the face following resection of the facial nerve. There is no question that appropriate nerve repair at the earliest possible time following injury yields the best results. Nevertheless, spontaneous recovery does occur and may play a part in some of the cases in which the results of surgical reanimation are superior.

One other mechanism for the spontaneous recovery of facial function should be discussed. The plasticity hypothesis was first proposed by Cajal (1894), and was discussed in detail by Kandel (1977). This hypothesis offers the most plausible explanation, not only for spontaneous recovery of facial function following facial nerve sectioning, but also for repair after interruption of infranuclear pathways. The

plasticity hypothesis, according to Cajal, proposes that connections exist between groups of cells and that these are reinforced by multiplication of terminal branches of protoplasmic appendices and nerve collaterals, thus bringing about functional transformations in particular systems of neurons as the result of appropriate stimuli or combinations of stimuli combinations.

Neuropathophysiology

Nerve injury

The facial nerve carries approximately 10 000 fibres, of which 7000 are myelinated motor axons that reach the facial muscles (Van Buskirk, 1945). It must be understood that none of the various injuries and disorders involving the facial nerve causes an all-or-nothing lesion, but rather each of the fibres is capable of being spared or injured to a different degree at any one time.

Classification of injury and recovery

Sunderland (1978) described five possible degrees of injury that a peripheral nerve fibre might undergo. This classification system is depicted diagrammatically in Figure 24.8, and is more comprehensive than the classification system of Seddon (1943), which described only neuropraxia, axonotmesis, and neurotmesis. Figure 24.8 and Table 24.4 show the pathological changes that occur in the nerve and the anticipated responses of the nerve to electrical testing, as well as the type of recovery that might be expected with the various types of injuries. The span of possibilities in terms of electrical responses, as well as recovery, reflects the possible mixtures of degree of injury that might occur. The five suggested by Sunderland describe very nicely the pathophysiological events associated with all types of disorders that afflict the facial nerve. The first three degrees of injury can occur with the viral inflammatory immune disorders, such as Bell's palsy and herpes zoster cephalicus. The fourth and fifth degrees occur when there is disruption of the nerve, as in transection, which might occur during surgery, as a result of a severe temporal bone fracture, or from a rapidly growing benign or malignant tumour.

Fortunately, the pathological processes causing facial paralysis in patients with Bell's palsy and herpes zoster cephalicus usually do not progress past the first or second degree of injury, which accounts for the fact that most individuals recover satisfactorily. A similar process causes facial paralysis due to acute suppurative otitis media, chronic otitis media associ-

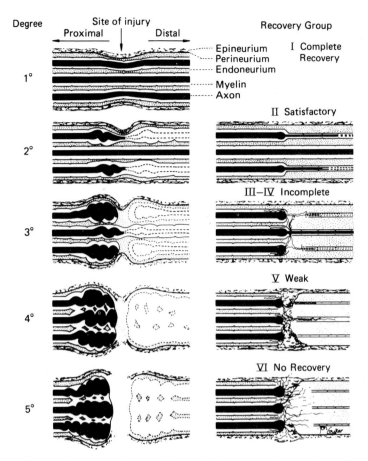

Figure 24.8 Correlation of degree of injury, morphological changes in the nerve, and expected type of recovery. First degree: compression. Second degree: interruption of axoplasm and myelin. Third degree: disruption of endoneurium. Fourth degree: disruption of endoneurium and perineurium. Fifth degree: transection of nerve. Regeneration: as the degree of injury becomes more severe the quantity and quality of recovery become worse. (From May (1986) with permission of the Publishers, Thieme-Stratton Inc.)

ated with a cholesteatoma, slow-growing benign neoplasms, and temporal bone fractures. In each of these disorders, the nerve is usually not transected, but rather compressed. In acute otitis media and trauma, compression may be sudden or slowly progressive, evolving over 5–10 days, just as is noted with Bell's palsy and herpes zoster cephalicus. However, unlike the process that occurs with Bell's palsy or herpes zoster cephalicus, in these other disorders pressure is exerted on the nerve from without rather than from within the intraneural space; nevertheless, the results of compression of the nerve are the same. Eventually, axoplasm is dammed up, compression of venous drainage leads to further compression of the nerve and loss of axons, and eventually loss of endoneurial tubes occurs, leading to third-degree injury. In fourth- or fifth-degree injury, since most or all of the endoneurial tubes have been disrupted,

as well as the perineurium in the fourth-degree injuries and the perineurium and epineurium in the fifth-degree injuries, recovery even under ideal conditions is never as good as with the first three degrees.

Altered function of the facial nerve following injury

Three major changes that occur in the axon following regeneration may contribute to a combination of hypo- and hyperkinesis:

1 The distance between the nodes of Ranvier is altered
2 The newly formed axons are covered with myelin that is much thinner than the normal axon
3 There is a splitting and crossing of axons that

Table 24.4 Neuropathology and spontaneous recovery correlated with degree of facial nerve injury*

Degree of injury	Pathology of injury	EEMG†, MST response	Neurobiology of recovery	Clinical recovery begins	Spontaneous recovery – result one year postinjury
1	Compression Damming of axoplasm No morphological changes (Neuropraxia)	Normal	No morphological changes noted	1–4 weeks	Grade I Complete: without evidence of faulty regeneration
2	Compression persists Increased intraneural pressure Loss of axons but endoneurial tubes remain intact (Axonotmesis)	0–10% of normal	Axons grow into intact empty myelin tubes at a rate of 1 mm/day which accounts for longer period for recovery in 2° injuries compared to 1° Less than complete recovery is due to some fibres with 3° injury	1–2 months	Grade II Fair: some noticeable difference with volitional or spontaneous movement, minimal evidence of faulty regeneration
3	Intraneural pressure increases Loss of myelin tubes (Neurotmesis)	No response	With loss of myelin tubes the new axons have an opportunity to get mixed up and split causing mouth movement with eye closure referred to as synkinesis	2–4 months	Grades III–IV Moderate to poor: obvious incomplete recovery to crippling deformity with moderate to marked complications of faulty regeneration
4	Above plus disruption of perineurium (Partial transection)	No response	In addition to problems caused by 2° and 3° injuries, now the axons are blocked by scarring which impairs regeneration	4–18 months	Grade V Motion barely perceptible
5	Above plus disruption of epineurium (Complete transection)	No response	Complete disruption with a scar-filled gap presents an insurmountable barrier to the regrowth of axons and neuromuscular reanastomosis	Never	Grade VI None

*From May (1986)
† EEMG = evoked electromyography; MST = maximal stimulation test
Classification by groups I–VI modified from House and Brackmann (1985)

reinnervate denervated muscle groups without necessarily corresponding to the cell body-motor unit arrangement that was present prior to degeneration.

As a result of these factors a tic or involuntary twitching occurs. In addition, inappropriate movement may be noted, such as movement of the mouth with blinking, or closing of the eye with smiling. Another cause of abnormal facial movements following regeneration may be changes that occur at the myoneural junction. In addition to these factors, it is quite likely that there are changes within and around the facial nerve nucleus in the brain stem, as well as alterations in central connections to the cell body. The combination of these factors may lead to spasms that occur on the involved side of the face, causing the eye to close and the corner of the mouth to pull. These spasms may be quite painful.

Facial hyperkinesis may be due to another mechanism referred to as ephaptic transmission. This term describes facial hyperkinesis or a hemifacial spasm that seems to occur spontaneously, without any discoverable cause. It is theorized that depolarization at the site of injury acts as a stimulus to the intact portion of the fibre, and that the action potential in one fibre is capable of exciting adjacent fibres in the area of injury. Granit, Leksell and Skoglund (1944) demonstrated ephaptic transmission at the site of compression in a nerve that was still capable of transmitting impulses across the site, and Kugelberg and Cobb (1951) demonstrated an acute, reversible phenomenon in the peripheral nerve of humans.

After producing ischaemia by means of pneumatic cuffs, Kugelberg demonstrated the development of foci of spontaneous, repetitive, and synchronized discharges, both during the ischaemia and after release of the cuff.

Four types of altered function are described next: synkinesis, crocodile tears, stapedius tendon contraction and facial myokymia.

Synkinesis

Synkinesis is an abnormal synchronization of movement, occurring with voluntary and reflex activity of muscles that normally do not contract together. It may be grossly deforming and debilitating. In its worst form, mass movement of all parts of the involved side of the face occurs; the patient is unable to move each part of the face separately. In its subtlest form it may consist of no more than a tiny twitch of the chin accompanying blinking on the side of the involvement. This may be the only sign of previous facial paralysis, and to detect it requires very close observation.

Crocodile tears

Increased unilateral lacrimation on the involved side associated with eating may occur with a severe denervating lesion when it involves the facial nerve at or above the site of the geniculate ganglion or along the greater petrosal nerve. This phenomenon is probably the result of faulty regeneration of parasympathetic fibres, which innervate the lacrimal gland instead of the salivary glands.

Stapedius tendon contraction

Stapedius tendon contraction is a hyperkinetic syndrome that occurs with faulty facial nerve regeneration and causes fullness or roaring in the ear. The complaint is noted with facial movements and often coincides with facial spasm. The diagnosis can be confirmed by tympanometric recordings with an electroacoustic bridge; sectioning the stapedius tendon through a tympanotomy approach has been effective in relieving the spasm.

Facial myokymia

A continuous, fine, fibrillary or undulating movement of the facial muscles gives the face an appearance suggesting a 'bag of worms'. This condition has been associated with multiple sclerosis and intrinsic tumours of the brain stem.

Approach to the patient with facial paralysis

Peripheral facial paralysis is a diagnostic challenge (Schaitkin and May, 1993). Every effort must be made to determine the aetiology, because Bell's palsy is a diagnosis of exclusion. The differential diagnosis is quite broad (Table 24.5); however, a careful history, physical examination, and the use of special tests will quickly narrow the possibilities (Tables 24.6 and 24.7). The causes in our practice's patients are shown in Table 24.8.

History

Although suggestive, the history of palsy onset − whether incomplete, complete, sudden, or delayed − is not diagnostic. All of these patterns have been noted with idiopathic (Bell's) palsy as well as with infection or neoplastic aetiologies. The exception is the patient whose paralysis progresses over a period longer than 3 weeks or who does not begin to recover after 6 months of paralysis. These patients should undergo thorough evaluation for a neoplasm affecting the facial nerve.

Recurrent facial paralysis occurs with idiopathic (Bell's) palsy, Melkersson–Rosenthal syndrome, and tumours. The incidence of recurrence in the authors' experience is 12%. One-third of these occur on the same side and two-thirds on the opposite side of the initial facial weakness. Of all patients with an ipsilateral recurrence of facial paralysis, 17% were found to have tumours on further evaluation; thus, *ipsilateral* recurrence also necessitates evaluation for a neoplasm. Suspicion should be increased if there is a history of previous malignancy. This is especially true in patients who have had breast, lung, thyroid, kidney, ovary, or prostate cancer and then present with a facial paralysis.

In contrast to recurrent facial palsy on the same side, recurrence on the opposite side is almost always idiopathic (Bell's) palsy, because alternating recurrent facial palsy has been noted only rarely with other disorders. Melkersson–Rosenthal syndrome (Figure 24.9) is characterized by two or more of the following: recurrent alternating facial paralysis; recurrent oedema of the lips, face, or eyelids; cheilitis; fissured tongue; or family history. A bilateral simultaneous paresis may be a medical emergency and presents special diagnostic and therapeutic challenges. Early diagnosis and appropriate treatment of potentially progressive and life-threatening disorders must be initiated. The most common cause in the authors' experience has been Guillain–Barré syndrome. Other causes included idiopathic (Bell's) palsy, leukaemia, sarcoidosis, skull fracture, Moebius' syndrome, rabies, Lyme disease, and infectious mononucleosis.

Table 24.5 Causes of facial palsy identified in a review of medical literature (1900–1983)*

Birth
Moulding
Forceps delivery
Dystrophia myotonica
Moebius' syndrome (facial diplegia associated with other
   cranial nerve deficits)

Trauma
Basal skull fracture
Facial injuries
Penetrating injury to middle ear
Altitude paralysis (barotrauma)
Scuba diving (barotrauma)
Lightning

Neurological
Opercular syndrome (cortical lesion in facial motor area)
Millard–Gubler syndrome (abducens palsy with
   contralateral hemiplegia due to lesion in base of pons
   involving corticospinal tract)

Infection
Otitis externa
Otitis media
Mastoiditis
Chicken pox
Herpes zoster cephalicus (Ramsay Hunt syndrome)
Encephalitis
Poliomyelitis (type I)
Mumps
Infectious mononucleosis (glandular fever)
Leprosy
Coxsackievirus
Malaria
Syphilis
Scleroma
Tuberculosis
Botulism
Acute haemorrhagic conjunctivitis (enterovirus 70)
Gnathostomiasis
Mucormycosis
Lyme disease

Metabolic
Diabetes mellitus
Hyperthyroidism
Pregnancy
Hypertension
Acute porphyria

Neoplastic
Cholesteatoma
VIIth nerve tumour
Glomus jugulare tumour
Leukaemia
Meningioma
Haemangioblastoma
Sarcoma
Carcinoma (invading or metastatic)
Anomalous sigmoid sinus
Haemangioma of tympanum
Hydradenoma (external auditory meatus)
Facial nerve tumour
Schwannoma
Teratoma
Hand–Schüller–Christian disease
Fibrous dysplasia
von Recklinghausen's disease

Toxic
Thalidomide (Miehlke syndrome, cranial nerves VI, VII with
   congenital malformed external ears and deafness)
Tetanus
Diphtheria
Carbon monoxide

Iatrogenic
Mandibular block anaesthesia
Antitetanus serum
Vaccine treatment for rabies
Postimmunization
Parotid surgery
Mastoid surgery
Post-tonsillectomy and adenoidectomy
Iontophoresis (local anaesthesia)
Embolization
Dental

Idiopathic
Bell's, familial
Melkersson–Rosenthal syndrome (recurrent alternating
   facial palsy, furrowed tongue, faciolabial oedema)
Hereditary hypertrophic neuropathy (Charcot–Marie–Tooth
   disease, Déjérine-Sottas disease)
Autoimmune syndrome
Temporal arteritis
Thrombotic thrombocytopenic purpura
Polyarteritis nodosa
Landry–Guillain–Barré syndrome (ascending paralysis)
Multiple sclerosis
Myasthenia gravis
Sarcoidosis (Heerfordt syndrome – uveoparotid fever)
Osteopetrosis

*From May (1986)

Even though idiopathic paralysis accounts for the vast majority of facial nerve dysfunctions seen by the practitioner, it behoves one to entertain other possibilities when confronted by:

1 Signs of tumour
2 Bilateral simultaneous palsy
3 Vesicles
4 Involvement of multiple cranial nerves
5 History and findings of trauma
6 Signs of ear infection
7 Signs of central nervous system lesions
8 Facial palsy noted at birth.

Table 24.6 Differential diagnosis of aetiology of facial palsy by history and physical findings*

Bell's palsy
1 Acute onset of unilateral facial palsy
2 Numbness or pain of ear, face, neck, or tongue (50%)
3 Viral prodrome (60%)
4 Recurrent facial palsy (12%)
    (ipsilateral 36%, alternating 64%)
5 Positive family history (14%)
6 Loss of ipsilateral tearing and/or submandibular salivary flow (10%)
7 Decrease in or loss of ipsilateral stapedial reflex (90%)
8 Red chorda tympani nerve (noted in 40% of patients evaluated in first 10 days in whom the chorda typmani could be seen; also noted with herpes zoster cephalicus and Guillain–Barré syndrome)
9 Self-limiting and spontaneously remitting

Herpes zoster cephalicus
1 Same as for Bell's, except pain more common and severe
2 Vesicles on pinna, face, neck, or oral cavity (100%)
3 Sensorineural hearing loss and/or vertigo (40%)

Tumour
1 Sudden complete onset similar to Bell's; EEMG results abnormal (10% within 5 days)
2 Recurrent same side (17%)
3 Slowly progressive weakness beyond 3 weeks (59%)
4 No recovery after 6 months
5 Twitching with paresis
6 Mass in parotid, submandibular gland, or neck
7 Mass between ascending ramus and mastoid tip
8 Progression of other motor cranial nerve deficits
9 Some of branches of facial nerve spared
10 History of cancer

Bilateral simultaneous facial palsy
1 Guillain–Barré syndrome
2 Moebius' syndrome
3 Sarcoidosis
4 Myotonic dystrophy
5 Skull trauma
6 Infectious mononucleosis
7 Cytomegalovirus
8 Acute porphyria
9 Botulism
10 Lyme disease
11 Bell's–*Herpes simplex*

Birth
1 Congenital diplegia (Moebius' syndrome, thalidomide toxicity)
2 Lower lip palsy (developmental)
3 Trauma
4 Tumour

Trauma
    Skull fracture (acute or delayed)

Infection
1 Bulbar palsy (viral meningitis, encephalitis, or immune reaction)
2 Postinfluenza, rabies, or poliomyelitis immunization
3 Infectious mononucleosis
4 Botulism
5 Tetanus
6 Syphilis
7 Malaria
8 Lyme disease
9 Herpes zoster cephalicus
10 Otitis media (acute or chronic, with or without cholesteatoma)
11 Leprosy

Metabolic
    Acute porphyria

Neoplastic
    Acute leukaemia

Iatrogenic
    Bilateral arterial embolization

Idiopathic
1 Guillain–Barré syndrome
2 Sarcoidosis (Heerfordt syndrome – uveoparotid fever)
3 Polyarteritis nodosa
4 Bell's palsy

Melkersson–Rosenthal syndrome
1 Recurrent alternating facial palsy
2 Fissured tongue
3 Labial-periorbital facial oedema
4 Non-specific labial granuloma
5 Positive family history

* from May (1986)
EEMG, evoked electromyography

Physical examination

A thorough head and neck examination is a minimum for evaluating facial nerve dysfunction. This examination must be expanded as indicated by the individual patient's history.

On otoscopy, a red chorda tympani nerve or vascular flaring in the posterior superior aspect of the tympanomeatal area is an important sign of idiopathic (Bell's) palsy. Other signs are mastoid or preauricular pain, numbness, hyperacusis, dizziness, loss of tearing, and altered taste. Otoscopy may also reveal signs of acute or chronic otitis media or of blunt or penetrating trauma.

More than 50% of patients in our series had pain, generally located over the mastoid region. Severe pain should prompt a thorough evaluation for the vesicles seen with Herpes zoster cephalicus (Ramsay Hunt syndrome). These vesicles are most commonly found in the ear canal and on the pinna, face, or

Table 24.7 Special diagnostic tests to evaluate patients with facial palsy*

Topognostic tests
    Hearing† and balance tests
    Schirmer test†
    Stapes reflex†
    Submandibular flow test
    Taste test†

Electrical tests
    Maximal stimulation test (MST)
    Evoked electromyography (EEMG)†
    Electromyography (EMG)

Radiographic studies
    Plain views of mastoid and internal auditory meatus
    Pluridirectional tomography of temporal bone
    Computerized tomography of brain stem, cerebellopontine angle, temporal bone, skull base; contrast sialography of parotid
    Magnetic resonance imaging
    Chest radiographic survey to detect sarcoidosis, lymphoma, carcinoma

Surgical exploration
Special laboratory tests
    Lumbar puncture (cerebrospinal fluid) to detect meningitis, encephalitis
    Guillain–Barré syndrome, multiple sclerosis, meningeal carcinomatosis
    Complete white blood cell count and differential to detect infectious mononucleosis, leukaemia
    Monospot test to detect infectious mononucleosis
    Heterophil titre to detect infectious mononucleosis
    Fluorescent treponemal antibody titre to detect syphilis
    Erythrocyte sedimentation rate to detect sarcoidosis, collagen vascular disorders

Urine and faecal examinations
    Acute porphyria–elevated porphyrins and urinary porphobilinogen
    Botulism—*Clostridium botulinum* toxin in stool specimen
    Sarcoidosis–urinary calcium

Serum cryoglobulins and immune complexes to detect Lyme disease

Serum globulin level to detect sarcoidosis

Serum and urine calcium determinations to detect sarcoidosis

Serum angiotensin-converting enzyme (ACE) level to detect sarcoidosis

Serum antinuclear antibody test (ANA), and rheumatoid factor (RF) to detect collagen vascular disorders (polyarteritis nodosa)

Bone marrow examination to detect leukaemia, lymphoma

Glucose tolerance test to detect diabetes mellitus

* From May (1986)
† Performed routinely; the rest of the studies are ordered based on suspicion raised by history and physical examination or abnormalities noted in the routine tests

Table 24.8 Facial paralysis – diagnoses in 3454 patients seen in one practice 1963–1994

Diagnosis	Number (%) of patients with this diagnosis
Bell's palsy	1762 (51)
Atypical Bell's palsy	18 (0.5)
Trauma	806 (23)
Tumour	185 (5)
Suspected tumour	11 (0.3)
Herpes zoster oticus	237 (7)
Infection	123 (4)
Present at birth	124 (4)
Hemifacial spasm	91 (3)
Central nervous system	26 (0.8)
Other	71 (2)
Totals	3454 (101)*

* Percentages add to more than 100 because of rounding.

neck extending down to the shoulder, as in Figure 24.10, but they can affect the sensory distributions of cranial nerves V, VII, X, and XI and the cervical plexus by way of extension from the facial nerve.

The intraoral examination should document a fissured tongue or regional oedema. A pharyngeal lesion or a mass in the parotid gland, submandibular region, or neck warrants further study.

During the ocular examination, the physician should assess the integrity of the IInd to VIth cranial nerves, the presence of uveitis, and the equality of tearing in the two eyes according to the results of Schirmer's test. The presence of an intranuclear ophthalmoplegia suggests multiple sclerosis, whereas ptosis and weakness of the muscles coupled with laryngeal or facial weakness suggest myasthenia gravis.

Special tests

Trying to locate the site of lesion using the results of tests for tearing (Zilstorff–Pedersen, 1965), taste (Kvarup, 1958), and salivary flow (Blatt, 1965) as popularized by Tschiassny (1953) has been found to be of limited value when the lesion is acute and of little or no value when facial paralysis is long-standing. Likewise, the prognostic value of these tests is limited, contrary to a previous report (May, Blumenthal and Taylor, 1981). The lack of correlation between test results and the location of the lesion is related to a number of variables:

1 The anatomy of the facial nerve and its branches is quite variable, so that axons may follow a variety of alternative pathways

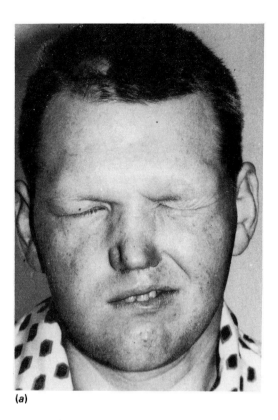

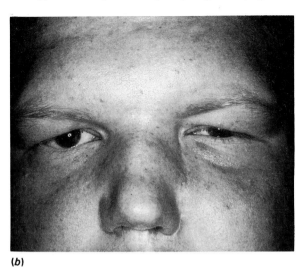

(b)

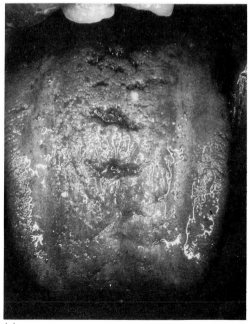

(a)

Figure 24.9 Melkersson–Rosenthal syndrome. History of recurrent *alternating* facial paralysis on 10 occasions occurring every 6 to 24 months over a total of 14 years. (*a*) Facial weakness, right side; (*b*) oedema of eyelids, especially on the left side; (*c*) fissured tongue; (*d*) fissured tongue in another patient was an isolated finding since there was no history of facial paralysis. The presence of a fissured tongue has no clinical significance when it occurs in the absence of other manifestations of Melkersson–Rosenthal syndrome. (From May (1986) with permission of the Publishers, Thieme-Stratton Inc.)

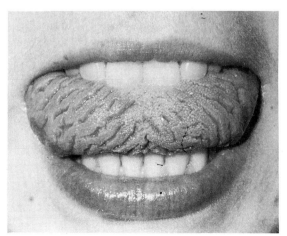

(c)

(d)

2 The lesion responsible for the paralysis may be diffuse rather than focal, so that the nerve is affected at various levels and with different degrees of severity

3 Recovery of the various components may occur at different times

4 The techniques used to measure the various facial nerve functions may not be completely reliable.

Electrical testing

Whereas tearing, salivary flow, and taste tests have not been useful for diagnosis or prognosis, the prognosis for acute facial palsy can be accurately determined by serial electrical testing. Most patients who have undergone serial testing have had idiopathic (Bell's) palsy, and the tests have been used to follow the clinical course from complete paralysis to spontaneous recovery or to the decision to intervene surgically.

Maximal stimulation test (MST)

Using the MST is an excellent way to evaluate facial nerve degeneration soon after its onset. The test can be performed with any stimulator for which strength and duration of stimulus can be varied. Stimulation is begun with a 1 mA current, which does not cause pain. The examiner increases the current slowly up to 5 mA, or until the patient begins to note discomfort, recording the amount of muscle twitching at each level of stimulation applied. The response on the involved side is compared to that on the normal side for each area tested and recorded as absent, markedly decreased, minimally decreased, or equal.

In our series of patients, when the response remained equal bilaterally up to 10 days after onset of Bell's palsy, 92% of the patients had complete return of function. However, when the response was lost within 10 days the test was 100% reliable in predicting an incomplete return of facial function. When the response was markedly decreased, 73% of the patients had incomplete return of facial function (May, Blumenthal and Klein, 1983). Other authors used a five-point grading system to report results of MST, and they found the test to be 94% accurate in prognosis for Bell's palsy (Ruboyianes *et al.*, 1994).

Evoked electromyography (EEMG)

Fisch and Esslen (1972a, b) popularized the study of evoked compound action potentials, which they called electroneurography (ENOG). However, the term *evoked electromyography* (*EEMG*) is more accurate for this test, because the action potentials are recorded for muscle, not nerve. EEMG is similar to MST except that EEMG responses are recorded and

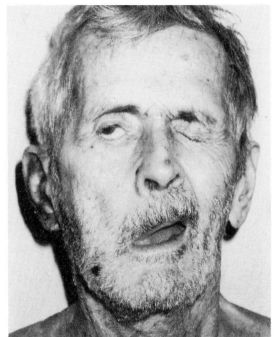

(*a*)

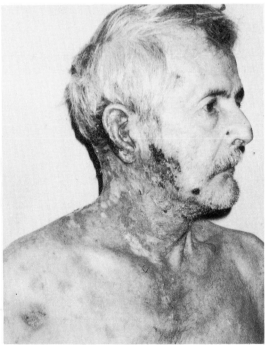

(*b*)

Figure 24.10 Patient with chronic lymphocytic leukaemia with an acute Herpes zoster cephalicus eruption along the distribution of C2, C3, and C4. (*a*) Total facial paralysis on the right side; (*b*) herpetic eruption extending from the angle of the jaw (region of the parotid) to lower half of the lateral pinna and external canal and down to the neck

measured electrically rather than by visual observation.

As Figure 24.11 shows, the more steeply the EEMG response decreases within the first 10 days, the worse the prognosis for recovery of facial nerve function. This was shown by Fisch (1984) and in a study by May, Klein and Taylor (1985) in which, if a response to MST or EEMG of 25% of normal or greater was maintained up to the tenth day after onset, the patient had a 98% chance of having a satisfactory recovery. If the response was between 11% and 24% within the first 10 days, the patient had an 84% chance of having a satisfactory recovery, but had only a 21% chance of satisfactory recovery when the response to MST or EEMG dropped to below 10% within the first 10 days.

A review of our patients' responses to EEMG 14 days after onset of facial paralysis (Table 24.9, House–Brackmann classification for 387 patients), showed that those with an EEMG at least 25% of normal or more had a 97% chance of satisfactory recovery. If the response remained between 11% and 24% of normal within the first 14 days, there was a 63% chance of satisfactory recovery, but there was only a 30% chance of satisfactory recovery when the response to MST or EEMG dropped below 10% of normal within the first 10 days.

Electromyography (EMG)

EMG is an indispensable test of nerve function when significant nerve degeneration has occurred and the response to MST and to EEMG are lost. A denervated muscle produces spontaneous electrical potentials (fibrillations) that are diagnostic of denervation. Generally fibrillation potentials do not appear until 10–21 days after injury.

Voluntary motor unit action potentials may be detected by EMG in the first few days after onset of facial palsy. The persistence of voluntary motor unit action potentials indicates that the lesion is incomplete, which is particularly important to know in patients whose facial paralysis is of traumatic aetiology because it obviates the need for surgical exploration in most cases.

Table 24.9 Prognostic value of EEMG results within first 14 days of onset of facial paralysis in 387 patients*

Outcome	EEMG results (% of normal)		
	>25% (n = 304)	11–24% (n = 49)	<10% (n = 34)
Satisfactory	97%	63%	30%
Unsatisfactory	3%	37%	70%

* Satisfactory results are House-Brackmann class I or II; unsatisfactory results are House–Brackmann class III or IV (House and Brackmann, 1985).

Even though EMG has limitations, it is still the most reliable test available to follow the course of severe

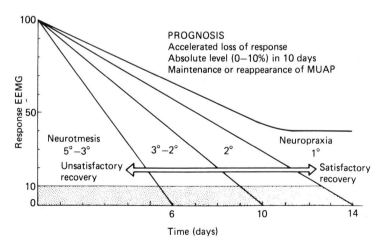

Figure 24.11 The prognosis for recovery is related to the response to evoked electromyography (EEMG) noted within the first 10 days of onset of facial paralysis. Prognosis is poor if the response to evoked electromyography is lost within the first 5 days, but is favourable if the response is maintained beyond 10 days, and especially beyond 14 days, after onset. Early return of voluntary motor unit action potentials noted by electromyography within the first 14 days indicates that the nerve is recovering. MUAP = motor unit action potential. (From May (1986) with permission of the Publishers, Thieme-Stratton Inc.)

denervation. Furthermore, EMG results offer the earliest evidence of recovery of facial nerve function, as indicated by decrease in fibrillations followed by the appearance of prolonged polyphasic voluntary motor unit action potentials (Blumenthal and May, 1986).

The prognostic value of EMG was shown by Sillman *et al.* (1992), who corroborated the results of May, Blumenthal and Klein (1983) and Fisch (1984) in finding that patients who had greater than 90% degeneration on EEMG, but who demonstrated the early presence of voluntary motor unit action potentials, had a better clinical outcome and thus did not require surgical decompression of the nerve.

Magnetic stimulation of the facial nerve

One of the major disadvantages of all of the evoked electrical tests is that they rely on extratemporal stimulation. Several clinicians have reported on proximal stimulation of the facial nerve by a magnetic coil placed over the scalp (Kartush *et al.*, 1989; Metson *et al.*, 1991; Rimpilainen *et al.*, 1992). Current techniques for magnetic stimulation cause the patient a degree of discomfort similar to that felt with EEMG, but latency studies suggest that placing the coil properly to stimulate the nerve at the route exit zone of the brain stem and using a smaller coil to decrease the zone of stimulation may reduce this.

The main advantage of magnetic stimulation over other nerve stimulation techniques is its potential for intracranial stimulation. All of the electrical tests just described are used to stimulate the extratemporal facial nerve and can only register changes after notable nerve degeneration has occurred. With magnetic stimulation, the nerve proximal to the zone of injury can be evaluated, and because this can be performed early in the course of idiopathic (Bell's) palsy, such stimulation may permit an earlier prognosis (Rimpilainen *et al.*, 1992). To date, however, magnetic stimulation has not been used to arrive at decisions for or against surgical decompression of the facial nerve.

Radiology

Imaging of the facial nerve frequently requires a combination of modalities, depending on the site of the lesion and the pathological process involved. Computerized tomography (CT) is an excellent way to document changes within the temporal bone. Magnetic resonance imaging (MRI) with gadolinium enhancement highlights lesions both proximally and distally, and often shows abnormalities associated with idiopathic (Bell's) palsy. For example, Murphy and Teller (1991) found increased signal intensity in 18 out of 25 patients with Bell's palsy. The most common sites for enhancement were the labyrinthine segment, geniculate ganglion, and proximal tympanic segments, with some correlation being noted between lack of enhancement and a better outcome.

Enhancement on MRI is also seen in patients with Ramsay Hunt syndrome (Weber and McKenna, 1992).

The most common neoplasm affecting the facial nerve is a neuroma. The appearance of these lesions on imaging studies depends on their location, and those in the cerebellopontine angle portion of the facial nerve can be indistinguishable from a vestibular schwannoma. Erosion and expansion in the labyrinthine segment and geniculate ganglion are classic for these tumours. Neuromas in the parotid gland will appear brightly enhanced by gadolinium, which helps to differentiate them from pleomorphic adenomas (Weber and McKenna, 1992).

Reporting results – facial function recovery

In 1983, House proposed a six-point classification system for reporting the results of facial nerve surgery; this system was modified and named the House–Brackmann system (House and Brackmann, 1985) (Table 24.10). The House–Brackmann system is still widely used, although it relies on subjective assessment of surgical results. As an alternative, Burres and Fisch (1986) proposed an objective grading system. We studied 41 patients with facial weakness using both systems and compared the results; the correlation was very high (Croxson, May and Mester, 1990). A recently reported classification system, the Nottingham system, has both objective and subjective components; it appears easier to use than the Burres–Fisch system and correlates well with results using the House–Brackmann system (Murty *et al.*, 1994).

These systems are the clinical correlates of the five degrees of nerve injury described by Sunderland (1978) (see Figure 24.8), and one can see how injuries from neuropraxia to complete transection in Sunderland's classification result in clinical symptoms ranging from minimal to severe impairment in facial nerve function.

Diagnosis of acute facial paralysis

Patients and their families were satisfied during their consultation if answers could be provided to three questions: what is the cause of the facial weakness (diagnosis)?; when can recovery be expected (prognosis)?; what can be done to promote recovery (treatment)?

For most patients who present with an acute facial palsy, these three questions can be answered after a thorough evaluation at the initial consultation. When

Table 24.10 Classification system for reporting results of recovery from facial paralysis*

Degree of injury	Grade	Definition
Normal (1°)	I	Normal symmetrical function in all areas
Mild dysfunction (barely noticeable) (1°–2°)	II	*Slight weakness noticeable* only on close inspection Complete eye closure with minimal effort Slight asymmetry of smile with maximal effort Synkinesis barely noticeable, contracture, or spasm absent
Moderate dysfunction (obvious difference) (2°–3°)	III	*Obvious weakness*, but not disfiguring May not be able to lift eyebrow Complete eye closure and strong but asymmetrical mouth movement with maximal effort Obvious, but not disfiguring synkinesis, mass movement or spasm
Moderately severe dysfunction (3°)	IV	*Obvious disfiguring weakness* *Inability to lift brow* Incomplete eye closure and asymmetry of mouth with maximal effort *Severe synkinesis, mass movement, spasm*
Severe dysfunction (3°–4°)	V	*Motion barely perceptible* Incomplete eye closure, slight movement corner mouth *Synkinesis, contracture, and spasm usually absent*
Total paralysis	VI	*No movement*, loss of tone, no synkinesis, contracture, or spasm

* System proposed by House and Brackmann (1985), and adopted by the Facial Nerve Disorders Commitee of the American Academy of Otolaryngology–Head and Neck Surgery, September 16, 1984
Recovery results noted one year or longer after onset

no specific cause such as trauma, infection, or tumour can be identified and the patient's symptoms fit the picture of idiopathic (Bell's) palsy, as described previously (see Table 24.6), the patient is told that facial nerve weakness is most probably due to a viral inflammatory immune disorder often referred to as Bell's palsy. The prospects for recovery from this disorder are excellent, and the patient should be reassured that he has not had a stroke and will not be permanently deformed.

The probable timing and final degree of recovery are predicted at the initial and later consultations on the basis of:

1 The completeness of the palsy
2 The patient's responses to MST or EEMG
3 The time recovery first begins.

Almost every patient with idiopathic (Bell's) palsy or acute facial palsy due to trauma or infection who retains some facial movement beyond 14 days after onset will have a satisfactory recovery from this disorder (House–Brackmann Grade I or II recovery). Nevertheless, patients must be followed carefully, both to document recovery and to watch for signs of paresis progression that indicate a worse prognosis.

Bell's palsy

The term *Bell's palsy* is used to designate acute peripheral facial palsy that occurs due to a viral inflammatory immune mechanism. The disorder is self-limiting, non-progressive, not life-threatening, spontaneously remitting, and currently is neither preventable nor curable. The incidence of Bell's palsy has been reported to be between 15 and 40 per 100 000 population (Hauser *et al.*, 1971; Adour *et al.*, 1978; Peitersen, 1982).

Bell's palsy is characterized by a viral prodrome in the majority of patients (60%), often accompanied by pain around the ear (50%), facial numbness (40%), changes in taste (50%), and numbness of the tongue (20%) (May and Hardin, 1977). In that series, a positive family history was obtained in 14% of patients, and the syndrome recurred in 12%.

Peitersen (1982) studied the natural history of Bell's palsy occurring in more than 1000 patients seen over a 15-year period. He found that in 84% recovery was satisfactory, 71% recovered without sequelae, and 13% had deficits that were barely noticeable. The other 16% of patients had obvious incomplete recovery of facial function, but sequelae were crippling in only 4% and there was not a single patient who did not have some recovery. Peitersen noted that 85% of the patients in his study began to recover facial function within 3 weeks of the onset of the palsy, which was incomplete in 31%. Peitersen concluded that there is a relationship between the degree of injury and ultimate recovery and the time that recovery is first noted; the earlier recovery is noted, the better the prognosis for a satisfactory and rapid recovery.

So long as the palsy is first evaluated within 14 days of onset and is incomplete, patients can be given an appointment to return in 3 weeks for further evaluation. However, they should be told to check daily for progression and to return sooner if the palsy worsens. Daily home evaluation of facial movement should be performed by the patient standing in front of a mirror or having a family member observe the effects of the patient raising the eyebrows, squeezing the eyes closed, wrinkling the nose, attempting to whistle, blowing out the cheeks, and grinning so as to show the teeth. The patient with an incomplete palsy should begin to recover in 6 weeks; if not, or the paresis worsens, a tumour should be suspected.

To determine prognosis and develop a management plan for the patient with complete facial motor deficit, the physician must rely on the patient's response to MST or EEMG and the time after onset that recovery of facial nerve function first appears. If return of facial function starts within the first 3 weeks after onset of paralysis and the response to EEMG remains more than 11% of normal up to day 14 after onset, satisfactory recovery of facial function is likely. On the other hand, if the response to EEMG drops below 11% of normal or is lost completely within the first 14 days, then the prognosis for satisfactory recovery drops to 30%.

Facial function is re-evaluated 3 months, 6 months, 1 year, and 2 years after onset of paralysis. Medical treatment is provided as needed to manage the sequelae of facial nerve paralysis and to prevent complications.

Medical treatment

There are three main types of treatment for acute facial palsy: physical, pharmacological, and psychophysical.

Physical therapy includes application of heat, massage, and exercises performed twice a day. Patients are advised to follow these steps:

1 Wet a cotton towel with hot water, wring it out, and keep the hot towel on the face until the towel cools
2 Massage facial cream into the skin around the eyes and mouth and over the mid-face for a few minutes
3 Stand in front of a mirror and watch your face while performing a series of facial exercises. Even though no facial movement may be noted, intact nerve fibres will be activated, and the exercises may help to maintain muscle tone.

Several types of medication, including steroids, have been used to treat facial paralysis, but none has been shown to be effective (DeVriess, 1977; Stankiewicz, 1987).

Psychophysical modalities such as motor-sensory re-education have been useful for patients with facial palsy (Balliet, 1984; Schram and Burres, 1984). In the acute phase, integrated EMG tracings of motor strength can often be displayed on an oscilloscope, offering the patient significant encouragement at a time when no visible movement can be seen. The course of actual nerve recovery is related to the response, recorded on the oscilloscope, to voluntary effort. During the post-acute phase, when recovery has begun, the patient can benefit from a number of self-help activities, including biofeedback techniques such as looking in a mirror and touching the face while trying to contract the facial muscles. These strategies are particularly useful when facial recovery has reached a plateau.

Depression

Patients who suddenly suffer complete facial paralysis initially fear that they have suffered a stroke and that the loss of function will be permanent. Even when patients have been reassured that facial function might return, they often become depressed by the facial deformity. If the prognosis is favourable for early recovery of facial function, the patient should be encouraged to adopt a positive outlook, but if recovery is not expected for 2 to 4 months, the patient should be informed of this openly and offered counselling. Group therapy has been effective in helping patients deal with this deformity, especially when group members are selected to be of the same sex and similar age and the patient counsellor has had a satisfactory recovery or learned to adapt to permanent deformity in a positive way.

Physical pain

Approximately one-half of patients with acute idiopathic (Bell's) palsy and almost all with Herpes zoster cephalicus have pain. In most cases the pain can be controlled with a non-narcotic analgesic, and although prednisone has not been shown to improve the function of the facial nerve, it has been effective for decreasing the pain associated with Bell's palsy (Adour, 1980). In rare instances a narcotic may be required for pain control.

Eye care

Patients with facial palsy will need to take steps to keep the affected ocular globe moist, to prevent keratitis and corneal breakdown. The patient should voluntarily close the eyelids on the involved side whenever the eye feels irritated or dry, about two to four times a minute, and drops should be used during the day and ointment at night. In addition, a moisture chamber should be worn over the involved eye whenever the patient is out of doors or the eye becomes irritated.

Surgery to reanimate the paralysed eyelids should be considered if medical treatment is ineffective, in particular when patients lack Bell's phenomenon, have corneal *a*naesthesia, and lack tears or have a *d*ry eye – the BAD syndrome (Figure 24.12). A tarsorrhaphy should be a last resort – it produces a cosmetic blight, limits vision, and often does not protect the exposed cornea (Figure 24.13). Furthermore, even when the tarsorrhaphy can be reversed, sequelae often result, including notching of the lid margin and trichiasis. Implantation of a gold weight or eyelid spring for the upper eyelid and lower eyelid tightening procedures or implantation of cartilage have been so effective that a tarsorrhaphy is rarely indicated. If a patient has undergone tarsorrhaphy, it should be reversed and one of the eye reanimation procedures performed as soon as possible.

Other viral causes of acute facial palsy

A number of viruses can cause facial paralysis that is similar to Bell's palsy.

Herpes zoster cephalicus (Ramsay Hunt syndrome)

Hunt (1907, 1908) first described the syndrome – now called Herpes zoster cephalicus or Herpes zoster oticus – of viral prodrome, severe pain in and around the ear, and vesicles involving the pinna. In its mildest form, Herpes zoster oticus may not be associated with any neurological signs, but in its severe form it may be accompanied by sensorineural hearing loss, disturbance of vestibular function, and even viral encephalitis.

The natural history of Herpes zoster cephalicus differs from that of Bell's palsy in several ways:

1 Bell's palsy recurs in 12% of cases, but Herpes zoster rarely recurs
2 With Bell's palsy the decrease in response to electrical testing peaks in 5–10 days, but in Herpes zoster the peak is later (10–14 days)
3 84% of individuals suffering from Bell's palsy have satisfactory recovery, but only 60% of those with Herpes zoster oticus recover to a satisfactory degree.

Treatment of herpes zoster is similar to that of Bell's palsy. However, the pain that patients with Herpes zoster oticus suffer from the vesicular eruption often requires narcotics to control. Acyclovir proved effective in ameliorating the symptoms of patients with Herpes zoster oticus in a small study (Dickins, Smith and Graham, 1988).

Other viruses

Other herpes viruses can cause facial nerve disorders similar to Bell's palsy. The Epstein-Barr virus is known to be the cause of infectious mononucleosis, and it has been isolated in cases of the Guillain–Barré syndrome. The fact that cytomegalovirus has also been isolated in patients with Guillain–Barré syndrome suggests that multiple viral agents are capable of producing this disorder.

Melkersson–Rosenthal syndrome is yet another

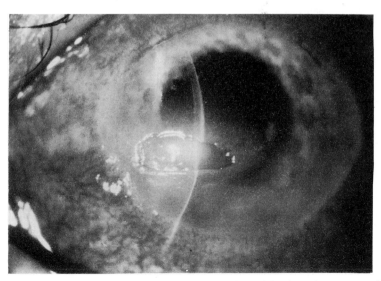

Figure 24.12 Keratitis and corneal ulceration 10 days after acoustic surgery and facial paralysis. BAD syndrome present: lack of *B*ell's phenomenon, *A*naesthetic cornea, and *D*ry eye due to absence of tearing

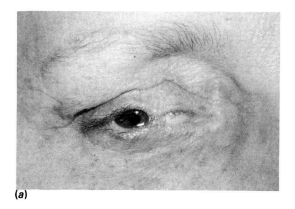

(a)

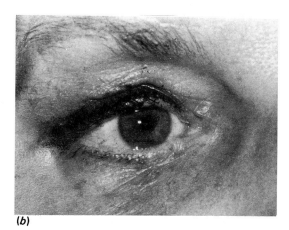

(b)

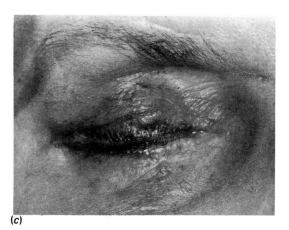

(c)

Figure 24.13 (*a*) Medial and lateral tarsorrhaphy after acoustic surgery and facial nerve sacrifice. Note cosmetic blight and limitation of vision. In spite of tarsorrhaphy cornea still exposed. (*b*) Tarsorrhaphy lysed and eyelid spring in place; eyelids opened. (*c*) Eyelids closed

clinical entity that may masquerade as Bell's palsy. However, although it is possible that a viral agent may play a role in Melkersson–Rosenthal syndrome, there is strong evidence that it is actually an inherited autoimmune disorder.

Lyme disease

Lyme disease, first reported in 1975 as an outbreak near Lyme, Connecticut (Clark *et al.*, 1985), is now known to be caused by a spirochaete transmitted primarily by tick bite. Although initially limited in its scope of occurrence, Lyme disease is now found essentially world-wide. The disease is characterized by erythema at the site of the tick bite, 1–4 weeks after the bite, often accompanied by fever, malaise, stiff neck, headache, fatigue, depression, myalgias, arthralgias, pharyngitis, and lymphadenopathy.

Within weeks to months of these initial signs, 10% of patients develop neurological abnormalities such as meningitis, encephalitis, and cranial neuritis, including unilateral and bilateral facial palsy. In a series of patients with Lyme disease reported upon by Clark *et al.* (1985), more than 10% evidenced facial palsy and one-quarter of these patients had bilateral paralysis. Their prognosis for recovery was excellent. Only one of the 124 patients in this series had significant sequelae. A 3-week course of tetracycline is the treatment of choice, although amoxycillin, cephalosporins, and penicillin have all been reported to be effective. The antibiotic therapy is directed at concurrent symptoms and to prevent complications; antibiotic medication does not appear to alter the course of the paralysis itself.

Surgical management of facial nerve paralysis

Surgical management may be appropriate for facial paralysis resulting from certain causes.

Indications for surgery

The benefit of facial nerve surgical decompression through the transmastoid or middle fossa route has not been clearly established for idiopathic (Bell's) palsy or Herpes zoster cephalicus. Furthermore, surgical decompression of the nerve to treat acute suppurative otitis media, necrotizing otitis external, or facial paralysis occurring after iatrogenic or externa temporal bone trauma is indicated only in selected cases (Maiman *et al.*, 1985). However, facial paralysis due to an ongoing process such as chronic suppurative otitis media, with or without cholesteatoma, can only be relieved by eradicating the primary disease. Surgery should be performed prior to electrical denervation to give the most satisfactory facial function recovery, and must not be delayed if the palsy has progressed from incomplete to complete over a period of hours or days and if the response to evoked EEMG is less than 25% of normal or dropping precipitously after the third day following onset.

There are two other situations in which surgical exploration of the facial nerve is absolutely indicated: facial nerve transection and tumour infiltration. The presence and extent of these conditions may be suspected by reviewing CT and MRI images, which play very important roles in the preoperative evaluation of suspected temporal bone fracture or tumour involving the facial nerve.

Peitersen's (1982) landmark study of the natural history of Bell's palsy found that 84% of patients with this disorder recover satisfactorily without intervention. Treatment for Bell's palsy must therefore be directed at identifying the remaining 16% early in the course of disease and intervening effectively to improve their prognosis. Marsh and Coker (1991) noted that anatomical, electrophysiological, radiological, pathological, and clinical factors point to the meatal segment of the facial nerve as a frequent site for entrapment.

Patients who are being prospectively entered into surgical trials to assess the role of decompression for an idiopathic palsy or Herpes zoster oticus should meet the criteria for surgery listed by Marsh and Coker (1991):

1 Acceptable anaesthetic risk
2 Age less than 60 years
3 EEMG results greater than 90% of normal
4 No evidence of neuropraxia deblocking on EMG
5 Paralysis of less than 21 days' duration
6 Provision of informed consent.

Approach and exposure

Although the majority of surgeons performing surgical decompression use a middle fossa approach, we prefer the transmastoid sublabyrinthine approach to explore the facial nerve from its labyrinthine segment to the stylomastoid foramen. The technique for exposure and decompression is outlined in Figure 24.14.

The transmastoid approach to the facial nerve begins with mastoidectomy. Air cells are removed from the antrum downward to the mastoid tip and the ridge of the digastric groove is defined. Cells are also removed from the antrum forward to the root of the zygoma until the upper edge of the incus and the prominence of the bony horizontal canal are identified. Care is taken not to disturb the ossicles. The bony meatal wall, although thinned, is left intact.

The landmark for the vertical mastoid portion of the facial nerve is the posterior tip of the incus above and the anterior end of the digastric groove below. Under the operating microscope, the periosteum of the digastric groove is exposed and followed forward and upward until the stylomastoid foramen is reached. Then the bone between the foramen and the horizontal semicircular canal is thinned with a diamond burr, used parallel to the course of the nerve, under continuous irrigation with Ringer's solution or Tis-U-Sol to remove bone dust and blood and prevent overheating. As the nerve is approached, it begins to appear through the paper-thin bone as a pink streak.

Brisk bleeding may be encountered from the artery that enters the fallopian canal at the pyramidal bend.

Finally, the surgeon uses the diamond burr gently to thin bone over the fallopian canal from its tympanic portion to the stylomastoid foramen, taking care not to disturb the incus or to open the horizontal semicircular canal. Right and left dental curettes are used to lift off the thinned bone covering the facial epineurium, thus exposing the contents of the fallopian canal. With magnification provided by the operating microscope, this can be accomplished without injuring the nerve.

Decompression

When the horizontal segment of the facial nerve is involved, decompression is carried out through a triangle bounded by the facial nerve medially, the chorda tympani nerve and tympanic annulus laterally, and the short process of the incus superiorly. In constructing this triangular window into the facial recess, it is advisable to leave a small pillar of bone over the fossa incudis to prevent accidental brushing of the incus by the burr, which could result in serious, irreversible acoustic trauma.

When the patient's hearing is normal and the entire horizontal segment of the facial nerve must be decompressed, it may be necessary to disarticulate the incus. In most cases this manoeuvre can be performed quite safely through the facial recess by gently separating the capsules of the incudostapedial and malleoincudal joint, leaving the short process of the incus attached to the fossa incudis. Then the incus can be rotated toward the middle ear to facilitate dissection over the proximal tympanic, geniculate, and distal labyrinthine segments of the facial nerve. When this dissection is complete, the incus is rotated towards the mastoid so that the midtympanic portion of the facial nerve can be dissected without concern for transmitting vibrations from the incus to the stapes and thus into the inner ear. After decompression, the incus is restored to its natural anatomical position, where it will remain providing the fossa incudis has been preserved.

Decompression of the facial nerve is completed by slitting the nerve sheath vertically on its posterior aspect with a disposable Beaver knife. If bleeding is troublesome it should be controlled with Surgicel. Use of electric cautery is discouraged, because even a wet-field bipolar cautery can cause injury if inadvertently applied to the nerve. If the use of cautery cannot be avoided, a bipolar wet-field cautery may be applied while the area is being irrigated.

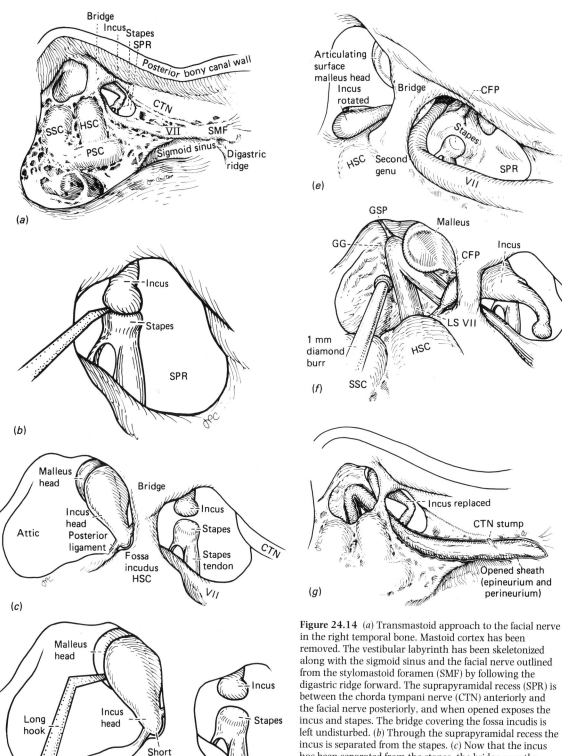

Figure 24.14 (*a*) Transmastoid approach to the facial nerve in the right temporal bone. Mastoid cortex has been removed. The vestibular labyrinth has been skeletonized along with the sigmoid sinus and the facial nerve outlined from the stylomastoid foramen (SMF) by following the digastric ridge forward. The suprapyramidal recess (SPR) is between the chorda tympani nerve (CTN) anteriorly and the facial nerve posteriorly, and when opened exposes the incus and stapes. The bridge covering the fossa incudis is left undisturbed. (*b*) Through the suprapyramidal recess the incus is separated from the stapes. (*c*) Now that the incus has been separated from the stapes, the bridge over the fossa incudis is shaved so that the entire head of the incus with its posterior suspensory ligaments is exposed and preserved. (*d*) The incus is separated from the malleus, but

Traumatic facial nerve injury

Trauma is the second most common cause of facial paralysis. The choice of approach to the treatment of these patients is based on the cause of injury to the facial nerve, location of the lesion, status of hearing, and length of time since paralysis was first noted.

Temporal bone fractures

Incomplete or delayed onset of facial paralysis following a temporal bone fracture calls for conservative management, because in these cases the nerve has almost certainly not been transected. Thus, complete or satisfactory recovery of facial nerve function without surgical intervention can be expected if some facial movement persists beyond 10 days. Even when facial movement is present initially and then lost, some recovery can be expected despite loss of responses to electrical tests (EEMG, MST, or voluntary motor unit action potentials on electromyography).

Facial nerve disruption is most likely in patients who experience a sudden onset of complete facial paralysis, loss of consciousness, cerebrospinal fluid (CSF) leak, loss of response to electrical stimulation by the fifth day, and marked disruption of temporal bone fragments on CT scan. Such patients should undergo exploratory surgery at the earliest possible moment.

These patients are best treated by submiddle fossa exploration via a transmastoid extralabyrinthine approach (see Figure 24.14) – from the stylomastoid foramen to the labyrinthine segment – to rule out multiple fracture sites. This approach permits adequate exposure of the geniculate ganglion and labyrinthine segment of the facial nerve, an area found by the authors to be involved in 18 (47%) of 38

patients who underwent exploration for temporal bone fracture. In the past, the geniculate ganglion and distal labyrinthine segment could only be reached by a middle fossa procedure, necessitating craniotomy. Most authors still choose this middle fossa approach, first proposed by Fisch (1974) and Glasscock *et al.* (1979).

Once the disrupted segment of nerve has been exposed, by whatever approach the surgeon chooses, treatment consists of freshening the proximal and distal ends of the nerve and placing an interposition graft without sutures. The results with this approach have been uniformly successful when it was employed within 30 days after the injury, before fibrosis and distortion of structures begins. When patients are first evaluated 4 years or longer after injury, anastomosis gives less than satisfactory results, and regional reanimation techniques should be considered.

Injury during surgery

It has been said that the facial nerve should be re-explored 'before the sun sets' when facial paralysis occurs following otological surgery. We have found, however, that in most cases it is best to wait a day or longer before re-exploration. This wait allows time for discussion with the patient and family and for the surgeon to regain his composure. Most importantly, it allows time for assessment of the circumstances of injury, which may preclude the need for re-operation.

Otological surgery

If, at the completion of an otological surgical procedure, the surgeon noted that the facial nerve was intact and the face moved with proximal nerve stimulation, the nerve can be expected to recover spontaneously; re-exploration is unnecessary. If the surgeon is unsure about the status of the nerve at the completion of surgery, serial electrical tests can be performed. If the nerve's electrical response is lost by the fifth postoperative day, re-exploration is appropriate. However, what appeared to be total paralysis immediately after surgery may prove to be incomplete paralysis when the effects of local and general anaesthesia dissipate fully, thus eliminating the need to consider re-operation.

Finally, the prognosis is favourable for satisfactory spontaneous recovery when:

1 Response to electrical stimulation is maintained beyond 10 days
2 Voluntary motor unit action potentials on EMG persist or return within 14 days

---

left attached to the fossa incudis by its ligaments. (*e*) With the incus rotated towards the mastoid the facial nerve can be followed proximal to the cochleariform process (CFP). (*f*) The incus is next rotated into the middle ear so that the facial nerve can be exposed as it courses past the malleus head to form the geniculate ganglion (GG) and bends acutely back towards the horizontal semicircular canal (HSC) as the labyrinthine segment (LS). The bone is shaved away from the nerve using a 1 mm diamond burr, working from the geniculate ganglion towards the ampullated end of the horizontal semicircular canal (HSC). The superior semicircular canal (SSC) has been skeletonized. (*g*) Once the facial nerve has been skeletonized from the stylomastoid foramen to the labyrinthine segment the sheath is opened and the chorda tympani nerve is divided. The incus is then replaced in its anatomical position and the wound is closed. PSC, posterior semicircular canal. (From May (1986) with permission of the Publishers, Thieme-Stratton Inc.)

3 Visible facial movement is maintained or begins to appear within 3 weeks.

To help avoid nerve injury during surgery, the otological surgeon must remember that the nerve can be in an anomalous location or be dehiscent. One of these conditions occurs in the majority (up to 60%) of cases (Welling, Glasscock and Gantz, 1992).

Parotid gland surgery

When performing surgery on the parotid gland, the surgeon should inspect and stimulate the main trunk of the facial nerve before closing the incision. If the patient's facial muscles jump briskly, the surgeon can be sure that the nerve has not been disrupted and, even if the patient awakes with a facial paralysis, nothing more needs to be done. Recovery can be expected within 4–6 months and, although the nerve may not recover completely, recovery will be adequate. On the other hand, if the nerve does not respond to direct stimulation prior to closure, the surgeon should inspect the nerve carefully for an area of disruption.

Repair of severed facial nerve by approximation

Theoretically, it might seem that regeneration of the facial nerve would be more satisfactory across a single junction than across two junctions at either end of a free graft. For this reason it is tempting to reapproximate the facial nerve when there are just a few millimetres between the two ends. Additional length can be obtained for end-to-end approximation if the injury to the facial nerve is proximal to the geniculate ganglion and hearing and balance function have been destroyed. In this case the facial nerve can be freed from its first genu, separating the nerve from the geniculate ganglion and mobilizing the vertical and horizontal segments posteriorly towards the internal auditory meatus. It is also possible to gain length for end-to-end anastomosis to repair injuries of the facial nerve in the region of the parotid gland.

However, re-routing the facial nerve to gain length for end-to-end approximation in the horizontal and vertical segments by mobilizing the proximal and distal ends is not the procedure of choice. Often, the more the nerve is freed up, the more it seems to shorten and the more the blood supply to the nerve is jeopardized. In the authors' experience, results were as good or better when a free graft was introduced as when a nerve was re-routed. Furthermore, if the ends cannot be brought together without tension, then a free graft must be inserted: lack of tension at the site of approximation is the best guarantee that the repair will be a success.

Repair of a severed facial nerve by graft

When there is a gap between the cleanly cut ends of a severed facial nerve, so that the distal segment of the nerve cannot be brought up to establish contact with the proximal end without tension, a nerve graft should be inserted. The cervical cutaneous and sural cutaneous nerves are most suitable for facial nerve grafting. The cervical cutaneous nerve is ideal for grafts up to 10 cm in length and the sural cutaneous for longer grafts (Figure 24.15).

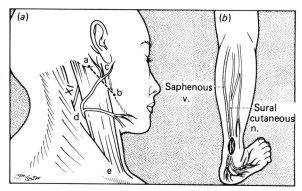

Figure 24.15 Donor nerves for grafting facial nerve. (*a*) Landmarks for finding the great auricular nerve to be used as a graft. A line is drawn between (a) the mastoid tip and (b) the angle of the jaw. That line is bisected at right angles by the great auricular nerve as it passes from behind the posterior border of the sternocleidomastoid at a point halfway (d) between the mastoid tip (a) and the clavicle (e) and courses obliquely towards the parotid gland (d–c). Just above the great auricular nerve, emerging from the posterior border of the sternocleidomastoid muscle, is the XIth cranial nerve. Care must be taken not to injure this nerve when removing the great auricular nerve. (*b*) Sural cutaneous nerve is preferred for grafts greater than 10 cm; 30–40 cm in length can be obtained with the sural nerve. It can be found between the lateral malleolus and the Achilles tendon. It runs just deep to the saphenous vein. (From May (1986) with permission of the Publishers, Thieme-Stratton Inc.)

A segment of nerve, measured so as to be slightly longer than the gap to be bridged, is removed, and its ends are cut sharply at right angles with a safety razor blade against a wooden tongue depressor. The nerve graft is handled carefully to avoid pinching or other trauma. Under a microscope, the nerve graft is carefully approximated to the distal and proximal stumps using 10–0 monofilament suture and the technique illustrated in Figure 24.16. By accomplishing a fascicular anastomosis, the graft need not be protected by covering it with a vein graft or Silastic tubing. As long as the two ends of the graft lie within

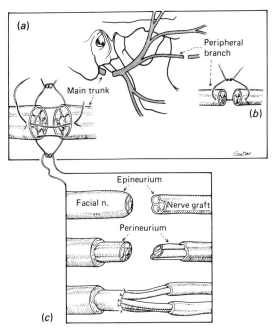

Figure 24.16 Techniques for nerve grafting. (*a*) Several epineurial sutures in a main trunk; (*b*) a single suture in the peripheral branch; (*c*) Millesi technique of interfascicular repair. Theoretically it should enhance return and minimize mass movement, but this has not been demonstrated clinically. (From May (1986) with permission of the Publishers, Thieme-Stratton Inc.)

the temporal bone and do not extend outside the stylomastoid foramen or into the internal auditory meatus, suturing is unnecessary.

Recently, the idea of nerve repair using autogenous axially aligned freeze-thawed skeletal muscle has been proposed (Glasby, Hitchcock and Huang, 1986). Early work with this technique suggests it to be an alternative to the sacrifice of a sensory nerve, and it may be less difficult technically to perform (Glasby and Sharp, 1992).

Facial reanimation

When at all possible, the best results for facial reanimation come from immediate restoration of nerve continuity. This includes the use of immediate facial nerve grafting at the time of vestibular schwannoma resection if the nerve has been sacrificed. When nerve continuity cannot be restored we prefer a XII–VII cranial nerve jump graft to restore tone and function without causing tongue paralysis (May, 1991).

This works best within 6 months of onset of paralysis and should not be employed after 2 years. The eye is reanimated independently using a gold weight if possible. If an adequate weight to achieve closure causes excessive ptosis, an eyelid spring is placed. Lower

eyelid position is restored with a combination of a lower eyelid tightening procedure and a cartilage implant.

For facial paralysis greater than 2 years in duration, the patient should undergo temporalis muscle transposition in combination with eye reanimation.

Tumours involving the facial nerve

Tumours of the head and neck may lie in close proximity to, envelop, or invade the facial nerve as it courses from the brain stem through the temporal bone and parotid gland to reach the facial muscles.

Tumour types

The benign lesion most frequently seen to involve the facial nerve is a schwannoma. Half of these tumours are vestibular schwannomas (neuromas) and are located in the cerebellopontine angle or internal auditory meatus and, in the authors' experience, half were found to involve the facial nerve or chorda tympani nerve within the temporal bone.

Vascular lesions such as meningiomas, angiomas, intraosseous haemangiomas, and arteriovenous malformations were the next most common types of benign tumours causing facial palsy and, with few exceptions, involved the facial nerve extraneurally at, or proximal to the geniculate ganglion. Unlike a schwannoma, these lesions often could be separated from the facial nerve with preservation of residual function.

Malignant tumours may also involve the facial nerve. The most common types of malignancy affecting the nerve in the authors' series of patients have been adenoid cystic and mucoepidermoid carcinomas, and the most common site of origin of these lesions has been the parotid gland.

Facial nerve and acoustic tumours

Excision of a vestibular schwannoma with anatomical preservation of the facial nerve is possible in more than 90% of patients (Nadol *et al.*, 1992; Arriaga *et al.*, 1993). Similar to that which may be seen with traumatic injury of other types, iatrogenic nerve trauma has a predictable progression. Patients with good facial function postoperatively on discharge from the hospital have a 98% probability of regaining acceptable facial function, compared with 77% of patients with poor function on discharge (Arriaga *et al.*, 1993).

In the patient whose facial nerve is disrupted during tumour resection, performing a direct VII–VII (facial nerve-to-facial nerve) anastomosis provides results superior to those of any other type of nerve anastomosis used in this context. The length of graft has not been shown to be important to the long-term outcome. However, in patients who had preoperative facial paralysis, the results of nerve interposition are not reliable (Luetje and Whittaker, 1991; Stephanian *et al.*, 1992).

Intraoperative nerve monitoring

Many surgeons monitor facial nerve function intraoperatively. Clearly, monitoring has been advantageous in vestibular schwannoma surgery (Delgardo, Buchheit and Rosenholta, 1979; Harner *et al.*, 1987), and many physicians now use monitors routinely in otological and extratemporal facial nerve surgery. We follow more closely the practice of Roland and Meyerhoff (1993) and do not use monitors except in unusual cases with greatly distorted anatomy or in vestibular schwannoma surgery.

Facial nerve disorders in newborns and children

Facial disorders in children can be due to a variety of causes and should not be assumed to be of the Bell's type. Further, the type of treatment and ultimate outcome depend on early, accurate diagnosis of the cause of the palsy. The principles of managing facial paralysis in children are the same as those for adults with a few exceptions, and these will be noted. The information presented is based on the diagnosis and management of facial paralysis in 559 patients, from newborn to 18 years, seen between 1963 and 1994. The causes of facial palsy in these children were similar to those in adults, with the exception of paralysis noted at birth and the number of cases due to acute otitis media (Table 24.11).

Facial paralysis noted at birth

The differential diagnosis and treatment of facial paralysis in the newborn has been reviewed by May, Blumenthal and Taylor (1981) and Harris *et al.* (1983). The two main differential diagnostic possibilities are developmental and traumatic; the factors that aid in differentiating between them are listed in Table 24.12.

The most common finding associated with congenital facial paralysis was the presence of one or more other anomalies. Weakness of the lower lip has particular significance in that it may be associated with multiple congenital anomalies (Pape and Pickering, 1972). Developmental bilateral facial palsy is frequently incomplete, with the lower portion of the face usually less affected than the upper part. This

Table 24.11 Causes of facial palsy in 559 children (0–18 years)

Diagnosis	Number (%) children with this diagnosis
Bell's palsy	203 (36)
Atypical Bell's palsy	6 (1)
Trauma	120 (22)
Tumour	26 (5)
Suspected tumour	1 (0.2)
Herpes zoster oticus	15 (3)
Infection	52 (9)
Present at birth	123 (22)
Hemifacial spasm	1 (0.2)
Central nervous system	2 (0.4)
Other	10 (2)
Totals	559 (101)*

* Percentages add to more than 100 because of rounding

distinguishes it from facial palsy due to trauma, which is rarely bilateral and in which the upper and lower parts of the face are equally involved. Bilateral immobility of the face may not be apparent at birth and may be manifested by incomplete eyelid closure when asleep, an open mouth, and/or inability to suck.

Syndromes associated with congenital facial paralysis

A number of syndromes evidence facial paralysis at birth.

Moebius' syndrome

Moebius' syndrome is a rare congenital disorder that is usually marked by bilateral facial palsy, unilateral or bilateral abducens palsy, anomalies of the extremities, absence of various muscles, particularly the pectoral group, and involvement of other cranial nerves, particularly the last four and especially the hypoglossal (Figure 24.17).

Dystrophia myotonica

Dystrophia myotonica is a steadily progressive familial distal myopathy with associated weakness of the muscles of the face, jaw, neck, and levators of the eyelids. Children with muscular dystrophy usually present at birth with congenital facial diplegia, although without abducens nerve paralysis; only later does the progressive nature of the myopathy become evident (Hanson and Rowland, 1971).

Table 24.12 Facial palsy at birth: differential diagnosis*

Developmental		Traumatic
	History	
No recovery of facial function after birth		Total paralysis at birth with some recovery noted subsequently
Family history of facial and other anomalies		
	Physical	
Other anomalies, bilateral palsy, lower lip or upper face palsy		Haemotympanum, ecchymosis, tics, synkinesis
Other cranial nerve deficits		
	Radiograph of temporal bone	
Anomalous external, middle, or inner ear; mandible; or vertical segment of facial nerve		Fracture
	Maximal stimulation/ evoked electromyography	
Response decreased or absent and without change on repeat testing		Normal at birth, then decreasing to possible loss of response
	Electromyography	
Reduced or absent response, no evidence of degeneration		Normal at birth, then loss of spontaneous motor units and 10–21 days later appearance of fibrillations and giant motor unit potentials
	Auditory brain stem response	
Abnormality in waves III–V		Normal, providing hearing is normal

*From May (1966)

Congenital facial diplegia associated with dystrophia myotonica that appears at birth is the earliest manifestation of the disease in its severest form. Unlike Moebius' syndrome, there is muscle wasting, particularly of the sternocleidomastoid, temporal, and facial muscles, creating an expressionless face that is so characteristic it is referred to as the myopathic facies.

Extramuscular dystrophies such as cataract, premature frontal baldness, and testicular atrophy are also present, and the neck is usually described as swan-like (Figure 24.18). This latter defect is due to wasting of the muscles of mastication and the sternocleidomastoid muscle.

Thalidomide embryopathy

Phocomelia (seal-like limbs) has apparently been known since Babylonian times, and was described by Ballantyne (1904), but the sudden increased incidence of this rare deformity between 1958 and 1962 focused attention on the disorder. Investigations discovered that the sedative thalidomide taken by the mother between days 28 and 42 of pregnancy led to thalidomide embryopathy with associated arrested development of the ear and abducens paralysis (Miehlke, 1965).

Osteopetrosis (malignant variant)

Malignant osteopetrosis is a rare cause of facial paralysis at birth, although it may be present later in childhood (see Table 15.2).

Management of developmental facial paralysis

At present, with the exception of free muscle neurovascular transplantation, which we are working on, there is no effective way to restore facial function in the newborn or young child with facial paralysis due to a congenital anomaly. It is in the child's best interest to delay reanimation surgical procedures until the patient reaches adolescent years. Therefore, management of the newborn or young child with a congenital facial paralysis should be directed towards preventing complications and performing reanimation techniques that have very low morbidity.

The main area of concern for reanimation is the eye. Children with facial paralysis from birth usually do not have problems with keratitis and corneal scarring. However, this may occur, particularly if the

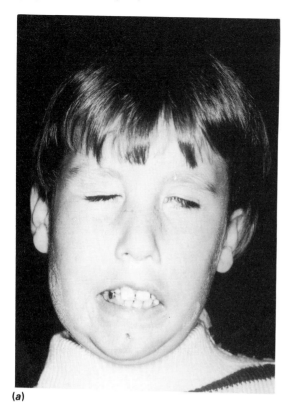

(a)

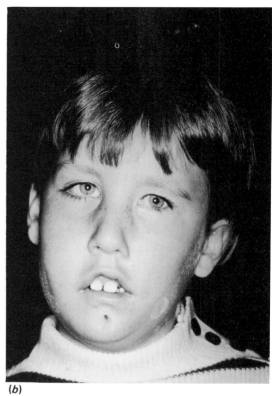

(b)

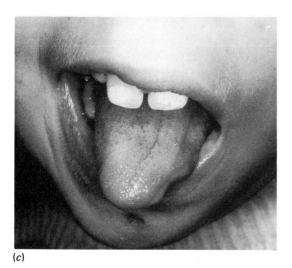

(c)

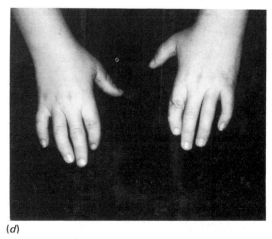

(d)

Figure 24.17 (*a*) Child born with bilateral facial paralysis due to Moebius' syndrome. Note asymmetric involvement with left eye more involved than right and normal lower face. (*b*) Attempting to look right or left. No eye movement indicates involvement of the VIth cranial nerve. Head tilt to left is the result of efforts to compensate for eye muscle imbalance. (*c*) Partial atrophy of left side of tongue indicates involvement of XIIth cranial nerve. (*d*) Anomalous fingers. (From May (1986) with permission of the Publishers, Thieme-Stratton Inc.)

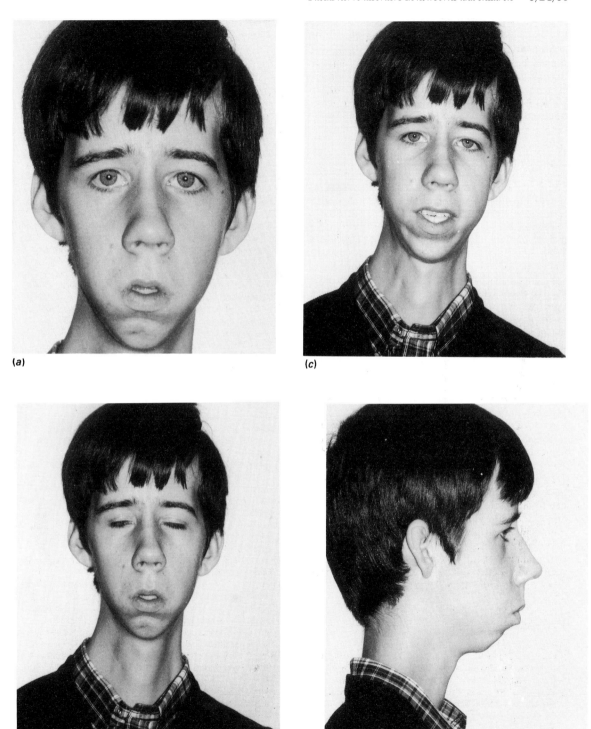

Figure 24.18 An expressionless face and swan-like neck due to atrophy of the masticatory, facial, and sternocleidomastoid muscles as part of the syndrome of myotonia dystrophica. (*a*) In repose; (*b*) eyes closed tightly; (*c*) smiling; (*d*) lateral view showing the atrophy of the neck muscles. (From May (1986) with permission of the Publishers, Thieme-Stratton Inc.)

child has poor Bell's phenomenon, decreased tearing, or entropion with irritation of the globe from eyelashes rubbing against the cornea. The child should be evaluated periodically by an ophthalmologist and, if there is any evidence of irritation or corneal keratitis, medical and perhaps surgical measures should be considered to correct the deformities.

Hyperkinetic disorders

The three most common hyperkinetic disorders are essential hemifacial spasm, blepharospasm, and aberrant regeneration.

Primary hemifacial spasm is most effectively treated by retromastoid vascular decompression of the nerve. When this procedure fails to correct the problem sufficiently or the patient is not a candidate for an intracranial procedure, selective peripheral neurolysis may be tried. This procedure causes weakness, however. Another alternative is injection of botulinum A toxin, which lasts from 6 weeks to 6 months. The injections relieve the spasm by interfering with release of acetylcholine at the terminal ends of the motor neuron.

Blepharospasm does not respond to retromastoid vascular decompression but has been effectively relieved by peripheral selective neurolysis, or selective resection of muscles in or around the eyelids (Anderson, 1982; Guerrissi, 1991). A more conservative approach is botulinum A toxin injections, which can offer significant relief (Biglan, May and Walden, 1986).

In the vast majority of patients in our practice who have a hyperkinetic disorder, the problem is secondary to faulty regeneration after a neuronal insult – any type of injury, from Bell's palsy to tumour resection. Ninety-two per cent of our patients with aberrant regeneration after idiopathic facial paralysis experience improvement in synkinesis and hyperkinesis with the injection of botulinum toxin (oculinum) (May, Croxson and Klein, 1989).

References

ADOUR, K. (1980) Corticosteroid therapy for acute facial paralysis. In: *Controversies in Otolaryngology*, edited by J. Snow. Philadelphia; W. B. Saunders. pp. 395–400

ADOUR, K. K., BYL, F. M., HILSINGER, R. L. JR, KAHN, Z. M. and SHELDON, M. (1978) The true nature of Bell's palsy: analysis of 1000 consecutive patients. *Laryngoscope*, **88**, 787–801

ANDERSON, R. L. (1982) A periorbital approach to blepharospasm. In: *New Orleans Academy of Ophthalmology: Symposium on Diseases and Surgery of the Lids, Lacrimal Apparatus, and Orbit.* St Louis: C. V. Mosby Co. pp. 336–351

ARRIAGA, M. A., LUXFORD, W. M. ATKINS, J. S., and KWARTLER,

J. A. (1993) Predicting long-term facial nerve outcome after acoustic neuroma surgery. *Otolaryngology – Head and Neck Surgery*, **108**, 220–224

BALLANTYNE, J. W. (1904) *Manual of Antenatal Pathology and Hygiene. The Embryo.* London: Green

BALLIET, R. (1984) Motor control strategies in the retraining of facial paralysis. In: *Proceedings of the Fifth International Symposium on the Facial Nerve*, edited by M. Portmann. New York: Masson Publishing. pp. 465–469

BIGLAN, A. W., MAY, M. and WALDEN, P. C. (1986) Treatment of facial spasm with oculinum (*Clostridium botulinum* toxin): a preliminary report. *American Journal of Otology*, **7**, 65–70

BISCHOFF, E. P. E. (1977) *Microscopic Analysis of the Anastomosis between the Cranial Nerves*, translated – edited by E. Sacks Jr. and E. W. Valtin. Hanover, New Hampshire: University Press of New England

BLATT, I. M. (1965) Bell's palsy. I. Diagnosis and prognosis of idiopathic peripheral facial paralysis by submaxillary salivary flow-chorda tympani nerve testing. A study of 102 patients. *Laryngoscope*, **75**, 1081–1091

BLUMENTHAL, F. and MAY, M. (1986) Electrodiagnosis. In: *The Facial Nerve*, edited by M. May. New York: Thieme-Stratton. pp. 241–265

BURRES, S. and FISCH, U. (1986) The comparison of facial grading systems. *Archives of Otolaryngology*, **112**, 755–758

CAJAL, S. R. Y. (1894) La fine structure des centres nerveux. *Proceedings of the Royal Society*, Series 55, 444–468

CLARK, J. R., CARLSON, R. D., SASAKI, C. T., PACHNER, A. R. and STEERE, A. C. (1985) Facial paralysis in Lyme disease. *Laryngoscope*, **95**, 1341–1344

CROXSON, G., MAY, M. and MESTER, S. J. (1990) Grading facial nerve function: House–Brackmann versus Burres–Fisch methods. *American Journal of Otolaryngology*, **11**, 240–246

DELGARDO, T. E., BUCHHEIT, W. A. and ROSENHOLTA, H. R. (1979) Intraoperative monitoring of facial muscle evoked responses obtained by intracranial stimulation of the facial nerve: a more accurate technique for facial nerve dissection. *Neurosurgery*, **4**, 418–421

DEVRIESS, P. P. (1977) Prednisone in idiopathic facial paralysis (Bell's palsy). *ORL Journal of Otorhinolaryngology and Related Specialties*, **39**, 257–271

DICKINS, J. R., SMITH, J. T. and GRAHAM, S. S. (1988) Herpes zoster oticus: treatment with intravenous acyclovir. *Laryngoscope*, **98**, 776–779

FISCH, U. (1974) Facial paralysis in fractures of the petrous bone. *Laryngoscope*, **84**, 2141–2154

FISCH, U. (1977) Total facial nerve decompression and electroneuronography. In: *Neurological Surgery of the Ear*, edited by H. Silverstein and H. Norrell. Birmingham, Alabama: Aesculapius Publishing Co. pp. 21–33.

FISCH, U. (1984) Prognostic value of electrical tests in acute facial paralysis. *American Journal of Otology*, **5**, 494–498

FISCH, U. and ESSLEN, E. (1972a) The surgical treatment of facial hyperkinesia. *Archives of Otolaryngology*, **95**, 400–404

FISCH, U. and ESSLEN, E. (1972b) Total intratemporal exposure of the facial nerve: pathologic findings in Bell's palsy. *Archives of Otolaryngology*, **95**, 335–341

FOWLER, A. P. JR (1963) The pathological findings in a case of facial paralysis. *Transactions of the American Academy of Ophthalmology and Otolaryngology*, **67**, 187–197

GACEK, R. R. and RADPOUR, S. (1982) Fibre orientation of the facial nerve: an experimental study in the cat. *Laryngoscope*, **92**, 547–556

GASSER, R. F. (1967a) The development of the facial nerve in man. *Annals of Otology, Rhinology, and Laryngology*, **76**, 37–56

GASSER, R. F. (1967b) The development of the facial muscles in man. *American Journal of Anatomy*, **120**, 357–376

GLASBY, M. A., HITCHCOCK, R. J. and HUANG, C. L. (1986) Effect of muscle basement membrane on regeneration of rat sciatic nerve. *Journal of Bone and Joint Surgery*, **68**, 829–833

GLASBY, M. A. and SHARP, J. R. (1992) New possibilities for facial nerve repair. *Facial Plastic Surgery*, **8**, 100–108

GLASSCOCK, M. E., WIET, R. J., JACKSON, C. G. and DICKENS, J. R.. (1979) Rehabilitation of the face following traumatic injury of the facial nerve. *Laryngoscope*, **89**, 1389–1404

GRANIT, R., LEKSELL, L. and SKOGLUND, C. R. (1944) Fibre interaction in injured or compressed region of nerve. *Brain*, **67**, 125–140

GUERRISSI, J. O. (1991) Selective myectomy for postparetic facial synkinesis. *Plastic and Reconstructive Surgery*, **87**, 459–466

HANSON, P. A. and ROWLAND, L. P. (1971) Moebius' syndrome and fascioscapulohumeral muscular dystrophy. *Archives of Neurology*, **24**, 31–39

HARNER, S. G., DAUBE, J. R., ABERSOLD, M. J. and BEATTY, C. W. (1987) Improved preservation of facial nerve function with use of electrical monitoring during removal of acoustic neuromas. *Mayo Clinic Proceedings*, **62**, 92–102

HARRIS, J. P., DAVIDSON, T. M., MAY, M. and FRIA, T. (1983) Evaluation and treatment of congenital facial paralysis. *Archives of Otolaryngology*, **109**, 145–151

HARRIS, W. D. (1968) Topography of the facial nerve. *Archives of Otolaryngology*, **88**, 264–267

HAUSER, W. A., KARNES, W. E., ANNIS, J. and KARLAND, L. T. (1971) Incidence and prognosis of Bell's palsy in the population of Rochester, Minnesota. *Mayo Clinic Proceedings*, **46**, 258–264

HOUSE, J. W. (1983) Facial nerve grading systems. *Laryngoscope*, **93**, 1056–1068

HOUSE, J. W., and BRACKMANN, D. E. (1985) Facial nerve grading system. *Otolaryngology – Head and Neck Surgery*, **93**, 146–147

HUNT, J. R. (1907) On herpetic inflammations of the geniculate ganglion. A new syndrome and its complications. *Journal of Nervous and Mental Diseases*, **34**, 73–96

HUNT, J. R. (1908) A further contribution to herpetic inflammations of the geniculate ganglion. *American Journal of Medical Sciences*, **136**, 226–241

JAHRSDOERFER, R. A. (1981) The facial nerve in congenital middle ear malformations. *Laryngoscope*, **91**, 1217–1224

JANNETTA, P. J. (1975) The cause of hemifacial spasm: definitive microsurgical treatment at the brainstem in 31 patients. *Transactions of the American Academy of Ophthalmology and Otolaryngology*, **30**, 319–322

JOHNSON, L. G. and KINGSLEY, T. C. (1970) Herniation of the facial nerve in the middle ear. *Archives of Otolaryngology*, **91**, 598–602

JOSEPH, M. P., GUINAN, J. J. JR., FULLERTON, B. C., NORRIS, B. E. and KIANG, N. Y. S. (1985) Number and distribution of stapedius motoneurons in cats. *Journal of Comparative Neurology*, **232**, 43–54

KANDEL, E. R. (1977) Neuronal plasticity and the modification of behaviour. In; *Handbook of Physiology*, edited by American Physiological Society, Section 1, vol. 1, part 2, ch 29. Baltimore: Williams & Wilkins Co. pp. 1139–1140

KARTUSH, J. M., BOUCHARD, K. R., GRAHAM, M. D. and LINSTROM, C. L. (1989) Magnetic stimulation of the facial nerve. *American Journal of Otology*, **10**, 14–19

KUGELBERG, E. and COBB, W. (1951) Repetitive discharges in the human motor nerve fibres during the postischemic state. *Journal of Neurology, Neurosurgery and Psychiatry*, **14**, 88–94

KVARUP, V. (1958) Electro-gustometry: a method for clinical taste examinations. *Acta Otolaryngologica*, **49**, 294–305

LUETJE, C. and WHITTAKER, C. K. (1991) The benefits of VII–VII neuroanastomosis in acoustic tumor surgery. *Laryngoscope*, **101**, 1273–1275

LYON, M. J. (1978) The central location of the motor neurons to the stapedius muscle in the cat. *Brain Research*, **143**, 437–444

MAIMAN, D. J., CUSICK, J. F., ANDERSON, A. J. and LARSON, S. J. (1985) Nonoperative management of traumatic facial nerve palsy. *Journal of Trauma*, **25**, 644–648

MARSH, M. A. and COKER, N. J. (1991) Surgical decompression of idiopathic facial palsy. *Otolaryngologic Clinics of North America*, **24**, 675–689

MARTIN, H. and HELSPER, J. T. (1957) Spontaneous return of function following surgical section or excision of the seventh cranial nerve in surgery of parotid tumors. *Annals of Surgery*, **146**, 715–727

MAY, M. (ed.) (1986) *The Facial Nerve*. New York: Thieme-Stratton

MAY, M. (1991) Jump graft hypoglossal facial nerve. *Otolaryngology – Head and Neck Surgery*, **106**, 818–825

MAY, M. and HARDIN, W. B. (1977) Facial palsy: interpretation of neurologic findings. *Transactions of the American Academy of Ophthalmology and Otolaryngology*, **84**, 710–722

MAY, M., BLUMENTHAL, F. and KLEIN, S. R. (1983) Acute Bell's palsy: prognostic value of evoked electromyography, maximal stimulation, and other electrical tests. *American Journal of Otology*, **1**, 1–7

MAY, M., BLUMENTHAL, F. and TAYLOR, R. H. (1981) Bell's palsy: surgery based upon prognostic indicators and results. *Laryngoscope*, **91**, 2092–2103

MAY, M., CROXSON, G. R., and KLEIN, S. R. (1989) Bell's palsy: management of sequelae using EMG rehabilitation, botulinum toxin, and surgery. *American Journal of Otolaryngology*, **10**, 220–229

MAY, M., KLEIN, S. R. and TAYLOR, F. H. (1985) Idiopathic (Bell's) facial palsy: natural history defies steroid or surgical treatment. *Laryngoscope*, **95**, 406–409

METSON, R. and HANSON, D. G. (1983) Bilateral facial nerve paralysis following arterial embolization for epistaxis. *Otolaryngology – Head and Neck Surgery*, **91**, 299–303

METSON, R., REBEIZ, E., WEST, C. and THORNTON, A. (1991) Magnetic stimulation of the facial nerve. *Laryngoscope*, **101**, 25–30

MIEHLKE, A. (1965) Anatomy and clinical aspects of the facial nerve. *Archives of Otolaryngology*, **81**, 444–445

MURPHY, T. P. and TELLER, D. C. (1991) Magnetic resonance imaging of the facial nerve during Bell's palsy. *Otolaryngology – Head and Neck Surgery*, **105**, 667–674

MURTY, G. E., DIVER, J. P., KELLY, P. J., O'DONOGHUE, G. M. and BRADLEY, P. J. (1994) The Nottingham system: objective assessment of facial nerve function in the clinic. *Otolaryngology – Head and Neck Surgery*, **110**, 156–161

NADOL, J. B., CHIONG, C. M., OJEMAN, R. G., MCKENNA, M. J., MARTUZA, R. L., MONTGOMERY, W. W. *et al.* (1992) Preservation of hearing and facial nerve function in resection of acoustic neuroma. *Laryngoscope*, **102**, 1153–1158

PAPE, K. E. and PICKERING, B. (1972) Asymmetric crying facies: an index of other congenital anomalies. *Journal of Pediatrics*, **81**, 21–30

PEITERSEN, E. (1982) The natural history of Bell's palsy. *American Journal of Otology*, **4**, 107–111

PROCTOR, B., CORGILL, D. A. and PROUD, G. (1976) The pathology of Bell's palsy. *Transactions of the American Academy of Ophthalmology and Otolaryngology*, **82**, 70–80

PROCTOR, B. and NAGER, G. T. (1982) The facial canal: normal anatomy, variations and anomalies. *Annals of Otology, Rhinology and Laryngology*, **91** (suppl. 93), 33–61

RIMPILAINEN, I., KARMA, P., LARANNE, J., ESKOLA, H. and HAKKINEN, V. (1992) Magnetic facial nerve stimulation in Bell's palsy. *Acta Otolaryngologica*, **112**, 311–316

ROLAND, P. S. and MEYERHOFF, W. L. (1993). Intraoperative facial nerve monitoring: what is its appropriate role? Editorial. *American Journal of Otology*, **14**, 1

RUBOYIANES, J. M., ADOUR, K. K., SANTOS, D. Q. and DOERSTEN P. G. VON (1994) The maximal stimulation and facial nerve conduction latency tests: predicitng the outcome of Bell's palsy. *Laryngoscope*, **104**, 1–6

SADE, J. (1975) Facial nerve reconstruction and its prognosis. *Annals of Otology, Rhinology and Laryngology*, **84**, 695–703

SCHAITKIN, B. and MAY, M. (1993) Evaluation and management of facial nerve disorders. *Current Opinion in Otolaryngology & Head and Neck Surgery*, **1**, 79–83

SCHRAM G. H. and BURRES, S. (1984) Non-surgical rehabilitation after facial paralysis. In: *Proceedings of the Fifth International Symposium on the Facial Nerve*, edited by M. Portmann. New York: Masson Publishing. pp. 461–464

SEDDON, H. J. (1943) Three types of nerve injury. *Brain*, **66**, 237–288

SILLMAN, J. S., NIPARKO, J. K., LEE, S. S. and KILENY, P. R.

(1992) Prognostic value of evoked and standard electromyography in acute facial paralysis. *Otolaryngology – Head and Neck Surgery*, **107**, 377–381

SILVERSTEIN, H. and NORRELL, H. (1980) Retrolabyrinthine vestibular neurectomy. *Otolaryngology – Head and Neck Surgery*, **90**, 778–782

STANKIEWICZ, J. A. (1987) A review of the published data on steroids and idiopathic facial paralysis. *Otolaryngology – Head and Neck Surgery*, **97**, 481–486

STEPHANIAN, E., SEKHAR, L. N., JANECKA, I. P. and HIRSCH, B. (1992) Facial nerve repair by interposition nerve graft: results in 22 patients. *Neurosurgery*, **31**, 73–77

SUNDERLAND, S. (1978) *Nerve and Nerve Injuries*, 2nd edn. London: Churchill Livingstone. pp. 88–89, 96–97, 133

SUNDERLAND, S. and COSSAR, D. F. (1953) The structure of the facial nerve. *Anatomical Record*, **116**, 147–166

THOMANDER, L., ALDSKOGIUS, H. and GRANT, G. (1982) Motor fibre organization in the intratemporal portion of a cat and rat facial nerve studied with the horseradish peroxidase technique. *Acta Otolaryngologica*, **93**, 397–405

TSCHIASSNY, K. (1953) Eight syndromes of facial paralysis and their significance in locating lesions. *Annals of Otology, Rhinology and Laryngology*, **62**, 677–691

VAN BUSKIRK, C. (1945) The seventh nerve complex. *Journal of Comparative Neurology*, **82**, 303–333

WEBER, A. L. and MCKENNA, M. J. (1992) Radiological evaluation of the facial nerve. *Israeli Journal of Medical Science*, **28**, 186–192

WELLING, D. B., GLASSCOCK, M. E. and GANTZ, B. J. (1992) Avulsion of the anomalous facial nerve at stapedectomy. *Laryngoscope*, **102**, 729–733

ZILSTORFF–PEDERSEN, K. (1965) Quantitative measurements of the nasolacrimal reflex in normal and in peripheral facial paralysis. *Archives of Otolaryngology*, **81**, 457–462

25

Cochlear implants

W. P. R. Gibson

The purpose of this chapter is to describe the otologist's role in a cochlear implant programme. The otologist is primarily involved with the medical assessment, surgical techniques, and postoperative care. It is common for the otologist to act also as the initial point of referral and to be the director of the programme. The otologist should have an understanding of candidate selection, the importance of neural plasticity and the broad categories of results that can be obtained. Specific audiological and speech test methods, language assessments and techniques for teaching the child to listen and speak will not be covered in this chapter.

In the past, there was little anyone could offer to alleviate profound sensory hearing loss and the deaf person had to learn to cope as normally as possible in the absence of hearing. For the adult deafened later in life, deafness entailed learning lip-reading and practising maintaining speech without any feedback of sound. For the child, born deaf or deafened before learning speech, lip-reading and clear speech could only be obtained with intensive, individual tuition. It was accepted by most otologists, audiologists, teachers and other professionals that the most practical means of educating deaf children was to teach them primarily using 'sign', utilizing the visual system. Speech was either taught simultaneously or later as the secondary language. Generations of deaf people have evolved who can only communicate freely using sign, and these people form the basis of a deaf culture. They feel it is normal for deaf people to communicate using sign and seek acceptance from the hearing community for their special culture and language.

The cochlear implant has radically changed the outlook for profoundly deaf adults and children. The cochlear implant can provide sufficient hearing sensations to enable most deafened persons to continue communicating using speech (see Table 25.5); and can provide the opportunity for children born deaf or deafened early in life to use speech as their primary means of communication (see Table 25.6).

To most hearing people, it appears that the cochlear implant provides a miraculous escape from a terrible disability. To deaf 'signing' people, the cochlear implant is a denial of the success they have achieved in living effectively as deaf people and the community that they have established. The otologist must be aware of the sensitivities involved.

Development of cochlear implants

The first suggestion that electricity could be used to help the deaf to hear has been attributed to Benjamin Franklin, the inventor of the lightning conductor. During the 1930s some work was undertaken stimulating the VIIIth nerve electrically during surgical procedures (Andreev, Gersuni and Volokhov, 1934). In 1957, Djourno and coworkers (Djourno and Eyriès 1957; Djourno, Eyriès and Vallancien, 1957a, b) published the first description of cochlear implants inserted into two totally deaf patients. This stimulated much interest especially in the USA.

In 1961, House et al. (1976) implanted a single electrode into the cochlea and soon afterwards Simmons et al. (1964) inserted six stainless steel electrodes directly into the auditory nerve. Both devices were initially successful but met a howl of criticism as the scientific community did not feel sufficient basic research had been accomplished to justify human implantation. Several workers began some careful animal experimentation (Michelson, 1968; Clark, 1969).

It was William House who recommended human

implantation in 1969 (House *et al.*, 1976) despite criticism that further animal work was needed. Three subjects were implanted in 1969 and 1970, and studied intensively. In 1972, the single wire intra-cochlear device designed by House and Urban (1973), which was later commercially developed by the 3M company, was made available and many patients received the device in Los Angeles. Other devices were developed over the next 10 years in many countries. Loeb (1990) provides an overview of the myriad of devices that have been developed.

Clark and coworkers developed a multielectrode, intracochlear implant (Clark *et al.*, 1984, 1987) at The University of Melbourne. This device was developed further as a 22 electrode array by a commercial company called Nucleus Ltd. The Melbourne/Nucleus device was the first commercially available cochlear implant which was capable of providing recognition of speech without any contextual clues ('open set') by listening alone. The device is now being produced commercially by Cochlear Ltd and since 1994 several improvements to the speech processing strategies have occurred. The Cochlear™ device has obtained FDA approval for use in both adults and children and it has been the most widely used worldwide. There are now several other commercial companies producing effective multielectrode cochlear implants. This chapter describes the Cochlear implant™ device but the conclusions apply equally to the other devices.

Basics of a cochlear implant

The cochlear implant prosthesis consists of two main parts (Figure 25.1). The implant is the internal part which is placed surgically beneath the scalp, with an array of electrodes placed inside the cochlea. The body of the implant contains a receiver/stimulator that decodes the signals from the external prosthesis and sends the electrical charges to the individual electrodes. The external part consists of a microphone, speech processor and the transmitting coil.

The microphone receives sound and transduces it to an electrical wave-form which is sent to the speech processor. The latter alters the electrical signal to emphasize the speech signals and divides the signal into components for each of the electrodes. There are two main strategies used in the most popular commercially available cochlear implants at present: continuous interleaved sampling (CIS) which uses high electrode stimulation rates; and the spectral peak processing (SPEAK). The Med-el™ and Clarion™ devices currently use CIS which has replaced the older method of compressed analogue processing (CA). More detail is available in Volume 2, Chapter 15.

The Cochlear™ implant now uses SPEAK which has replaced the older MSP (mini speech processor) strategy. The MSP digitizes the signal and extracts the early formats of speech (F0, F1, F2) and some high frequency bands. The SPEAK strategy uses a filterbank (20 filters) to cover a frequency range from 150 Hz to 10 kHz. After the analysis of the incoming sound signals, each electrode is allocated a specific filter with the most apical electrode being assigned to the lowest filter. The incoming speech is analysed and frequency ranges containing the highest amplitudes (maxima) are presented to the corresponding electrodes. The older versions of SPEAK presented six maxima while the newer versions can present up to 10 maxima. The rate of stimulation on each electrode varies from 180–300 Hz but clusters of closely spaced electrodes can be stimulated within a region of the cochlea providing a close spectral representation of the neural patterns obtained in a normal cochlea.

Trials comparing the MSP and SPEAK processors demonstrate an overall improvement using the SPEAK processor especially in the open set recognition of speech in the presence of background noise (McKay and McDermott, 1993).

The Combi-40 device produced by Med-el™ uses only eight electrodes but each electrode is capable of firing at rates of up to 12,000 per second. The Clarion device™ can use either CIS with fast stimulation rates or be programmed using CA. All these devices have been shown to provide open set speech recognition and the studies comparing the different devices are awaited.

Selection of candidates

Apart from their lack of hearing, deaf people are usually completely healthy (Fritsch and Sommer, 1991). Some deaf people feel they have overcome the disability aspect of deafness by becoming fluent in sign language and joining deaf groups. The term 'patient' is best avoided except for that period when the person is in hospital and recovering from surgery. During the assessment period, the term 'candidate' is used and after surgery, the term 'implantee' is used.

Importance of neural plasticity

The main factor which influences candidacy is neural plasticity. Neural plasticity is the ability of the central nervous system to be programmed to learn a task. For example, soon after birth a foal learns to walk within a few hours beside the mare. If the foal is restricted at birth by a plaster cast, after 3 weeks, when the cast is removed, it is no longer possible to teach the foal to walk. The brain no longer has the ability to learn this task as those neurons, normally available for the task of walking, have lost the 'plasticity' to adapt.

In humans, the physiology of neural plasticity associated with many motor or sensory tasks must be appreciated (Buchwald, 1990). The clinician recognizes the need to correct strabismus (ocular squint)

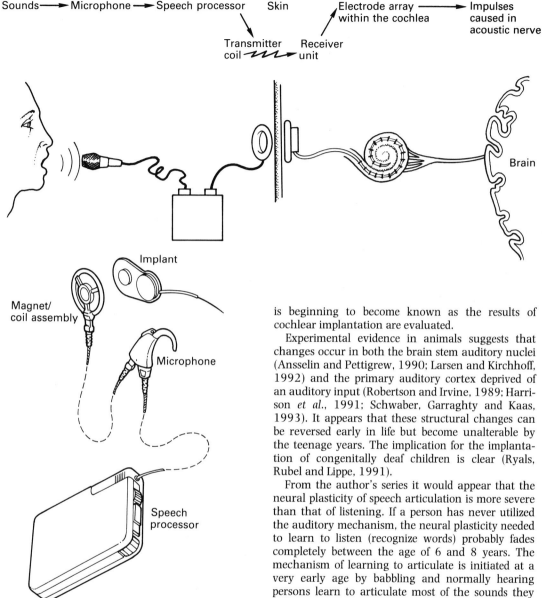

Sounds ⟶ Microphone ⟶ Speech processor   Skin   Electrode array ⟶ Impulses
                                                                  within the cochlea   caused in
                                                                                          acoustic nerve

                                        Transmitter   Receiver
                                        coil   unit

Brain

Implant

Magnet/
coil assembly

Microphone

Speech
processor

Figure 25.1 (*a*) and (*b*) A diagrammatic representation of the components of a cochlear implant (Cochlear™ device)

within the first 2 years of life as after this age the brain cannot adapt to the change in the eye position and anopia occurs. If vision is restored after the first 5 years of life, the child suffers 'cortical blindness' and can see the shapes and colours but is unable to recognize objects. The neural plasticity associated with listening and with speech articulation is less well understood (Clopton and Silverman, 1978), but

is beginning to become known as the results of cochlear implantation are evaluated.

Experimental evidence in animals suggests that changes occur in both the brain stem auditory nuclei (Ansselin and Pettigrew, 1990; Larsen and Kirchhoff, 1992) and the primary auditory cortex deprived of an auditory input (Robertson and Irvine, 1989; Harrison *et al.*, 1991; Schwaber, Garraghty and Kaas, 1993). It appears that these structural changes can be reversed early in life but become unalterable by the teenage years. The implication for the implantation of congenitally deaf children is clear (Ryals, Rubel and Lippe, 1991).

From the author's series it would appear that the neural plasticity of speech articulation is more severe than that of listening. If a person has never utilized the auditory mechanism, the neural plasticity needed to learn to listen (recognize words) probably fades completely between the age of 6 and 8 years. The mechanism of learning to articulate is initiated at a very early age by babbling and normally hearing persons learn to articulate most of the sounds they will require before uttering any meaningful words.

From the author's series, it seems that excellent speech articulation can only be accomplished if the speech sounds are learnt before the age of 2–3 years.

Sadly many families seek a cochlear implant for their older deaf child believing that if the child can hear, articulation of speech can improve naturally. Unfortunately, neural plasticity studies would suggest that, even with intensive speech therapy, only limited gains are possible.

It is possible that in the future positron electron transmission (PET) scanning will be available to show if the auditory areas of the brain can still respond to auditory input or whether these areas have been allocated during development to other sensory inputs.

Candidacy categories (Table 25.1)

The main factor that influences candidacy for a cochlear implant is whether the person has already acquired speech before becoming completely deaf (postlingual), or became deaf before learning speech (prelingual). Sometimes, people who lost their hearing at the time of beginning to utter speech are known as 'perilingual', but these people can be categorized as prelingual for all clinical purposes.

Candidates who seek an implant are categorized into four main groups:

Table 25.1 Categorization of candidates

Postlingual	Onset of deafness has occurred after completion of speech development
Perilingual	Onset of deafness has occurred while speech development was occurring
Prelingual	Onset of deafness occurred prior to any development of speech
	a Primary candidates: have not acquired language by any other means of communication
	b Secondary candidates: have used another mode of communication (usually sign) to develop language
	c Change-over candidates: have developed auditory skills using a hearing aid

Postlingual candidates

This category can be divided into prepubertal and postpubertal groups.

The postpubertal group are adults and teenagers who become deaf after experiencing normal hearing during their childhood; they are excellent candidates providing they have realistic expectations of the hearing they are likely to regain. Speech appears to lose all plasticity by puberty, so that after this time, there are no gross articulation changes even over prolonged periods of deafness. There may be errors such as inappropriate loudness, pitch changes and loss of intonation. These errors may be improved after implantation.

The duration of deafness in postpubertal candidates is also a factor. In general, those who have been unable to use a hearing aid for over 13 years do less well than those completely deafened for a shorter period (Clark *et al.*, 1987).

The prepubertal group are children aged 2–12 years of age. If all useable hearing is lost before puberty, plasticity is still present. If articulation errors occur, these may not be correctable after puberty.

The younger the child, the more likely speech will be lost. The older the child, the less speech is lost. Intensive oral teaching can preserve useable speech but articulation errors may be hard to avoid. Even after a successful cochlear implant, speech errors are difficult to correct.

The term 'perilingual' is sometime used to describe the children who become deaf between 2 and 4 years of age who lose all memory of speech within a few months of total deafness. Once speech has been lost, the child has to be taught to listen and to speak again exactly as if born deaf.

Prelingual candidates

Prelingually deaf candidates are those who were born deaf or who became deaf within the first 2 years of their life. They can be considered in three groups:

Prelingual primary candidates

Those who have no other means of communication and seek to learn speech as the primary method of acquiring language. Usually these candidates are young children.

Neural plasticity is all important. The key to success appears to the ability to establish an effective cochlear implant at as early an age as possible and then teaching the child to hear and speak ('habilitation'). All groups agree that an oral approach to habilitation must be undertaken and auditory-verbal techniques appear to give optimal results.

It is rare to have candidates other than very young children, as some alternative form of communication has usually been established in older children in order to provide some means of teaching language (education).

Prelingual secondary candidates

These are prelingually deaf people who have developed language, or who are developing language, using an alternative means of communication to speech. They seek an implant to improve their oral skills. Sometimes these oral skills may be minimal.

Lack of neural plasticity may hamper progress, especially after 5 years of age. In general, older secondary subjects perform poorly with a cochlear implant and may not meet the expectations of their family. As they are unable to distinguish speech or to improve their vocalization, some will become 'non-users'.

Preoperative counselling is vital. Both the candidate and the family must be aware of the limitations imposed by lack of auditory and articulation neural plasticity. Older subjects can only expect to hear prosodic rhythms that will help existing lip-reading skills and are unlikely to get any significant improvement in speech intelligibility.

Younger children who still have some remaining plasticity are most likely to gain benefit but only if this can be combined with effective habilitation. Learning to listen and to speak at an older age appears to be a full-time effort. It seems unlikely that 1 or 2 hours of oral therapy mingled with predominantly manual communication can succeed. If signing continues after implantation, then a truly 'total' communication is needed with extended periods of oral training.

Prelingual 'change-over' candidates

These are people who have learnt to communicate orally using a hearing aid. They may have succeeded by intensive tutorage in using tiny amounts of residual hearing, or they may have lost residual hearing so that their hearing aid is no longer effective.

These 'change-over' candidates make excellent implantees. It seems that the auditory system has been primed for distinguishing minimal sounds. As most 'change-over' implantees achieve excellent 'open set listening', the audiological guidelines for candidacy may have to be relaxed in these cases. If a child is using a hearing aid effectively, loss of auditory neural plasticity does not occur, although loss of neural plasticity for articulation still remains.

Older candidates who have been deaf since childhood will not get any marked changes in their speech production but they may gain better volume control and intonation. There probably is an advantage in performing the change-over at an earlier age while some plasticity for articulation still remains.

Medical selection of candidates (Table 25.2)

The otologist is often the first person to see a prospective candidate. Much depends on the age of the candidate. Most cochlear implant groups have separate teams (Table 25.3) and inclusion protocols for children and for adults.

After deciding which category the prospective candidate represents, there is usually enough background information to decide whether or not that person will be best helped by an implant. If it appears that an implant is indicated some preliminary counselling is usually undertaken and referrals are made to other members of the implant team.

Medical history

It is important to try to determine the cause of the deafness, the status of the cochlea, the extent of spiral ganglion survival and the viability of the auditory nerve and CNS pathway. It is useful to reveal otic capsule abnormalities, internal auditory meatal abnormalities and intralabyrinthine ossification so that surgery can be planned accordingly.

Table 25.2 Medical history, examination and investigations

History
- Extent, timing and cause of the hearing loss
- Whether a hearing aid has been useful
- How the patient communicates
- Is there any usable speech?
- Language level
- Any major health problems
- Any evidence of developmental delay
- Past otological history: ear infections, ear surgery, otitis media with effusion
- Family history: how does the family communicate?
- Social history: does the patient understand and want the implant?

Examination
- Appearance including congenital stigmata
- Any abnormal behaviour
- Status of the meatus, tympanic membrane and middle ear, presence of a mastoid cavity or atticotomy
- Nose and throat, and general examination
- Preoperative investigations
- Audiology: adults, pure tone audiogram, impedance and CID speech testing
  - children, aided pure tone audiogram, special speech tests to measure discrimination
- Electrophysiological testing
- Electrocochleography, steady state potential testing, brain stem auditory potential testing
- Promontory stimulation testing/electrically evoked brain stem auditory potentials
- Vestibular tests: caloric testing in adults
- Radiological tests: high quality CT scans (MRI, PET) chest X-ray

Referrals
- Audiologist
- Speech therapist
- Teacher of the deaf
- Language assessment
- Developmental paediatrician
- Ophthalmologist
- Physician

Present otological history

The extent and timing of the hearing loss and the likely cause should be determined. Whether or not a hearing aid has been useful, is a crucial question.

Usually there is a pure tone audiogram available and obviously only people who have a severe to profound loss in both ears are considered. A sudden total loss of hearing needs urgent consideration, especially in young children, as deterioration in speech can occur very quickly. A gradual deterioration of hearing can occur in adults and children so that careful audiological testing has to be undertaken to discover whether or not a cochlear implant would be more effective than a hearing aid. The deterioration can be caused by otosclerosis and sometimes a stapedectomy is undertaken prior to implant surgery.

Table 25.3 Cochlear implant teams

Adults	Director
	Otologists (medical and surgical care)
	Audiologists
	Speech therapists
	(Psychologist)
	Patient support group
	Electrical engineer
	(Research staff)
	Radiologist and staff
	Medical staff
	Nursing staff
	Administration
	Secretarial staff
Children	As for adults, plus the following:
	audiologists need paediatric experience
	Teachers of the deaf ('habilitationists')
	Family counsellor

A fluctuant hearing loss, especially in children, is a concern. The differential diagnosis includes auto-immune disease, perilymph fistula and vestibular aqueduct syndrome.

If there is a long-standing profound hearing loss, then the usefulness of a hearing aid must be determined. If a hearing aid has been abandoned, neural plasticity becomes important as that person may have lost the ability to discriminate sounds; usually such people are no longer candidates. If the person manages to use a hearing aid effectively despite a profound hearing loss, the probability is that he will be an excellent implantee.

The author only considers adults and teenagers as candidates if they can communicate using speech. The exact criteria vary but candidates should have speech tracking scores using lip-reading and residual audition of over 10 words per minute. Most groups have found that children in oral classes (auditory verbal or auditory oral) benefit more from a cochlear implant than those who also use sign to communicate. Unless the school is supportive, it is unwise to consider a cochlear implant.

It was thought that if a child had developed a high language level using sign, he would be able to grasp listening and speech skills more effectively. Unfortunately this philosophy is incorrect as loss of neural plasticity overrides any advantage gained by better language.

Non-otological history

It is important to discover if there are any other health problems before undertaking lengthy elective surgery. Elderly patients may have cardiovascular or diabetic problems. Congenitally deaf children may have cardiac, visual or developmental problems. It is useful to have medical specialists in these areas associated with the implant team so that appropriate referrals can be made.

Past otological history

Past ear infections may have caused labyrinthitis which can be associated with ossification. If there is a perforation present, then this must be closed before undertaking implant surgery. Otosclerosis can be associated with abnormal bone which is less dense than normal bone and may result in facial nerve stimulation when some adjacent electrodes are stimulated.

A mastoid cavity is not a contraindication as the cavity can be obliterated with a blind sac closure of the ear canal. Usually this is performed as a staged procedure to ensure that there is no infection or cholesteatoma formation at the time of the implant surgery.

In children, recurrent otitis media needs to be controlled before surgery, usually by using prolonged courses of antibiotics. The immunological status of the child may have to checked to exclude immunoglobulin deficiency syndromes.

Otitis media with effusion ('glue ear') without any recurrent infections is not usually a problem. At surgery, the implant array can be packed off from the middle ear cavity with muscle and fibrous tissue.

Past non-otological history

In particular, the otologist should discover if there has ever been any problem associated with a previous general anaesthetic. Allergies to drugs and bleeding disorders should be noted.

Family history

It is rare to get a positive family history when a recessive congenital hearing loss is present. Dominant genetic conditions, such as Usher's syndrome more commonly affect close family relatives.

It is important to discover how the family communicates. Only a few hearing parents of deaf children can sign fluently and siblings can rarely sign. Although the parents may want a signing child to have an implant to learn speech, in reality if the child is older, it is better that the family are encouraged to learn signing.

Social history

It is very important that the candidate and his family understand exactly what gain is likely after receiving a cochlear implant. The most effective method of providing this information is for the candidate and family to meet someone who is using a cochlear implant. In Sydney, this service is provided by a support group called CICADA (Cochlear Implant Club and Advisory Association). Similar support groups exist in most countries. It is important that the meeting is not only with 'star' implant performers but with an implantee who matches the age and type of hearing loss of the candidate. The author does not undertake any surgery until such a meeting has been completed.

If a child is being considered, then the family should meet the family of an implanted child. If possible they should also visit the school. A meeting with the family counsellor on the implant team also is arranged.

It is vital to ensure that the adult or teenager wants the cochlear implant himself and it is not the family who is pushing him into surgery with unrealistic expectations. For children, it is important that the family realize that there will be little or no natural acquisition of listening and speech skills and that these can only be gained by intensive tutorage over a prolonged period.

Medical examination

If the person was born deaf, the otologist should look for any congenital stigmata and it is often worthwhile asking the parents if there were any unusual features. For example, the white forelock suggestive of Waardenberg's syndrome may have been hidden. Unusual behaviour suggestive of autism may need further referral.

The ears are checked to ensure the ear canal is healthy, the tympanic membranes intact and there is no middle ear effusion. If there was previous surgery, check for previous mastoid surgery or even a cavity or atticotomy. Children who rely on hearing aids often have a constant mild otitis externa. Soft debris may have to be removed before a view of the tympanic membrane can be obtained and before impedance testing can be performed.

A nose and throat examination should be performed and a general examination if indicated.

Preoperative investigations

Audiological tests

Preoperative testing is needed to ensure that the candidate will benefit more from a cochlear implant than a hearing aid, and to provide baseline measurements so that the effect of the cochlear implant can be assessed postoperatively. The preoperative testing is summarized below.

The pure tone audiogram is useful as it shows the severity of the loss. It is unusual to recommend an implant if hearing thresholds better than 100 dBHL exist at 2 kHz or higher frequencies.

The speech audiogram is helpful. Usually maximum discrimination scores of over 10% on Central

Institute for the Deaf (CID) testing exclude the use of a cochlear implant.

As cochlear implants continue to improve, the decision as to whether to continue with a hearing aid, or to proceed to a cochlear implant becomes more difficult. Recently, some groups have been considering candidates who still have some usable hearing in one ear (Shallop, Arndt and Turnacliff, 1992).

Congenitally deaf children are more difficult to assess as speech discrimination testing is often impossible except in experienced hearing aid users (change-over candidates). These change-over children tend to do very well with a cochlear implant and 'open set' scores of up to 40% on testing such as the Bamford-Kowal-Bench (BKB) sentences or phonetically balanced kindergarten (PBK) lists does not necessarily exclude the use of an implant.

Other congenitally deaf children who have little concept of speech are more difficult to assess. The aided audiogram is helpful. If the aided thresholds reach the 'speech zone' at frequencies above 2 kHz, then the child is unlikely to be a candidate. Such a result would suggest that a hearing aid will provide as much audition as the implant and if there are difficulties it is due to loss of neural plasticity or lack of auditory training, or both!

A more detailed account of the range of audiological tests available is given in Volume 2, Chapter 14.

Electrophysiological tests

Electrophysiological tests are an important adjunct to behavioural testing, especially for young children. The purpose is to verify the degree of the hearing loss and to ensure that the acoustic nerve and brain stem auditory pathway are sufficiently preserved to support a cochlear implant.

The most commonly used electrophysiological testing involves brain stem auditory evoked potentials (BAEP). This test is not affected by sedation or natural sleep and gives an accurate estimate of the hearing especially in the higher audiometric frequencies. There are some disadvantages: the waveform is minute and requires prolonged averaging; it is not often feasible to obtain an accurate estimate of frequencies below 2 kHz, and it is difficult to be certain that no residual cochlear function remains in profound hearing loss.

Electrocochleography (ECochG) provides a very certain measure of residual cochlear function, especially if a round window electrode is used (Gibson, 1994). The drawback is that testing in young children must be performed under general anaesthesia. Steady state potentials (evoked SSEP) (Rickards and Clark, 1984) provide an alternative, non-invasive, method for the lightly sedated child.

Promontory stimulation testing involves placing a transtympanic electrode onto the promontory of the ear close to the round window membrane, and exciting the cochlea with small bursts of electricity. Postlingually deafened subjects usually report a hearing sensation but prelingual subjects may be confused by the resulting sensations. Promontory testing has proved disappointing as it does not correlate with postoperative results (Gantz, 1989). It does, however, provide a gross response which shows that the ear does respond to electrical stimulation and it is useful in revealing which congenitally deaf candidates are likely to be able to recognize hearing sensations if they receive a cochlear implant. As a general rule, it is unwise surgically to implant an ear which does not provide clear hearing sensations preoperatively.

Preoperative electrically evoked brain stem potentials should provide the opportunity to check the intactness of the auditory pathway without the need for a subject response. Unfortunately, it is difficult to obtain the electrically evoked brain stem auditory potentials because of the initial artefact caused by the electrical stimulation. Transtympanic electrodes and electrodes placed on the round window membrane tend only to provide gross responses. Some groups have resorted to intracochlear testing (Montandon, Kasper and Pelizzone, 1992).

Vestibular testing

Commonly all labyrinthine function is lost when hearing is lost due to meningitis. The children remain unsteady for some months but eventually cope well. Adults are less able to cope without vestibular function and may develop bothersome oscillopsia or be unable to walk freely in the dark.

Vestibular function testing is required for adults preoperatively to ensure that the cochlear implant is not inserted into the ear with the only functioning labyrinth. A simple caloric test, using iced water if necessary, suffices.

If the deafness was caused by labyrinthitis, then it is usual for the better hearing ear to have the better vestibular function. If the better ear is to be implanted, then the possibility of postoperative vestibular problems have to be discussed with the prospective patient.

Radiological tests

A high quality CT scan is essential before surgery. The scan is especially useful for the detection of bony obliteration within the cochlea (labyrinthitis ossificans), to detect demineralization of the cochlea in severe otosclerosis, and to detect any congenital abnormalities of the otic capsule or internal auditory meatus (Phelps, Annis and Robinson, 1990; Weit et al., 1990).

Labyrinthitis ossificans can occur after labyrinthitis (see Figures 2.68 and 17.1). Labyrinthitis can occur as a result of meningitis especially in young children in whom the cochlear aqueduct is patent. This usually results in localized ossification near the round window. If the infection spreads via the internal auditory meatus, then total ossification of the cochlea may result (see Figure 2.31). Meningitis in children, aged under 10 years, invariably results in some limited ossification near the round window. In 20% of these children there is extensive ossification preventing the complete insertion of the electrode array (author's figures). The otologist faces a dilemma: if surgery is undertaken too soon, the possibility of spontaneous recovery is lost. If surgery is delayed unduly, the cochlea may ossify denying the child the opportunity of an effective cochlear implant. Brookhauser, Auslander and Meskan (1988) followed a series of 87 children deafened by meningitis and showed that the hearing altered in 7% of the children. About 4% of the ears showed some recovery but these ears appeared to have had some residual remaining hearing. McCormick et al. (1993) have published the case of a child with near total hearing loss who showed recovery in both the implanted and non-implanted ear. This child is using both the implant and a hearing aid successfully, and it is probable that the implant has been worthwhile as it provides high frequencies not available through the hearing aid.

The guidelines for cochlear implantation in post-meningitic children in Sydney are as follows: if total or near total hearing loss has occurred and if there is any evidence of ossification, then cochlear implant surgery is offered 3 months after the meningitis. For ears with some residual hearing, an observation period of at least 9 months is recommended. Serial radiology to check for evidence of progressive ossification after six months is advisable. The final decisions are made by the parents who are fully informed of all possibilities.

Severe congenital abnormalities, such as a Michel deformity or a severe Mondini abnormality, can provide a contraindication to implantation. Absence of the internal auditory meatus or a very narrow meatus may indicate the absence of the VIIth nerve.

Magnetic resonance imaging is not used so commonly at present, partly because of the costs involved. MRI can confirm the presence of the acoustic nerve and reveal any degeneration by the brightness of the T2-weighted image (Laszig et al., 1988). In the future, MRI may be capable of showing if the cochlear coils contain fluid or fibrous tissue (see Figure 2.70).

Positive electron transmission (PET) scanning may become available to show if the auditory areas of the brain can still respond to auditory input (LeScao et al., 1993). Awareness of certain abnormalities may encourage the surgeon to offer a cochlear implant. For example, the vestibular aqueduct syndrome may be associated with deterioration of hearing especially after head trauma. When hearing aid use becomes very limited, these candidates tend to do well with a cochlear implant.

A simple chest radiograph is usually carried out before surgery on all patients.

Blood investigations

Blood tests are usually requested after hospital admission. All patients have a full blood count preoperatively. Other tests of liver or kidney function are only undertaken when suggested by the patient's history. Serology and HIV testing are only undertaken at present with the patient's consent. Blood grouping and the saving of serum is only recommended for very small children or those at special risk.

Electrocardiography

This is undertaken on admission for patients with a history of cardiovascular problems.

Referrals

A multidisciplinary approach has to be followed especially when considering children for cochlear implantation. The otologist is often responsible for organizing these referrals.

Audiology

All candidates have to undergo extensive audiological testing. The audiologist's approach to cochlear implants is described in Volume 2, Chapter 14.

Speech therapy

A preoperative visit to the speech pathologist is useful to document the level of speech intelligibility and to note any voicing errors.

Teacher of the deaf (auditory habilitator)

A specially trained teacher of the deaf should work with the prelingually deaf children for a period of 10 weeks prior to implantation. During this time, the child is familiarized with the tasks which will be needed postoperatively. The teacher will report subjectively on the progress of the child during this period and the oral capabilities of the child.

Language assessor

The spoken and non-spoken language levels of the child are assessed according to age appropriate measures. Tests such as The Peabody Picture Vocabulary Tests and The Expressive One-word Picture Vocabulary Tests are used. The language assessment may be undertaken by a teacher of the deaf or by a specially trained person.

Psychologist

A psychologist or family counsellor should see the family of a prospective child implantee to work out any problems that may occur postoperatively. Children who become deaf due to meningitis at ages between 3 and 8 years often become emotionally disturbed and difficult to manage. Although this behaviour improves dramatically in most cases as soon as they can hear effectively again, the disturbances can cause some concern during the initial postoperative period.

The parents of congenitally deaf children may not understand the limitations imposed by loss of neural plasticity and can have inappropriate expectations. Success involves an intensive effort on behalf of the parents and specialized teachers, and the parents have to understand that their role is crucial.

In Sydney, the parents' attitude is monitored carefully during the 10 week pre-implant trial period.

Child development paediatrician

Before considering an implant on a young child it is useful to have a developmental assessment. The paediatrician may also give useful advice on the genetics and may detect syndromes. At present most teams are cautious about implanting children with developmental problems although in the future these children may be considered important candidates.

Implant support groups

All postlingual adult and teenage candidates in Sydney are required to visit an implantee. This is arranged by the support group. The parents of prospective children also visit the parents of children who have received an implant, but this visit is usually arranged by the staff to ensure an appropriate choice.

Other professionals

Visits to other professionals, if there is a specific need, are arranged. An ophthalmologist can often detect retinitis pigmentosa, or detect eye signs associated with Cogan's syndrome. For elderly candidates, a specialist physician may be required.

The final assessment meeting

After the completion of all preoperative testing and visits, a final assessment meeting is held.

Postlingually deaf adults or teenagers usually visit the otologist who has all the relevant reports compiled; often the audiologist will attend. The results are explained and the likely benefits of the implant outlined. The candidate will decide usually whether or not to have surgery; most candidates are eager to proceed, insisting on a date for operation.

The otologist now has a surgical patient. The possible complications of surgery have to be explained. The otologist should mention postoperative discomfort, the dangers of postoperative infection, the rare possibility of a facial palsy, and the probability that the device may break down or become outmoded in the future. Many hospitals now use an informed consent form.

The final assessment meeting for a child is more complex. Usually all the professional staff involved with the 10 week assessment of the child gather with the parents. If possible a representative of the school or the itinerant teacher will also attend. Each professional tables a written report of their assessment which is explained to the parents. Then each professional states whether or not they feel an implant would or would not benefit the child. Finally, the parents are asked to decide; usually after 10 weeks' assessment they have a clear idea and many are enthusiastic to continue. The otologist then outlines the surgical procedure and the possible complications in front of all the team. The parents sign an informed consent form and a form expressing a commitment to the habilitation programme.

The choice of the ear to be implanted is made at the final assessment meeting. If one ear has sufficient hearing for speech recognition using a hearing aid, then this ear is preserved. If neither ear can be used with a hearing aid, then most surgeons prefer to implant the most recently deafened ear or the ear with better audiometric thresholds. Other factors such as the radiological appearance and the results of promontory electrical stimulation should also be considered.

Surgery

The surgery basically involves a cortical mastoidectomy, a limited posterior tympanotomy and the insertion of an array of electrodes through the basal coil of the cochlea. General anaesthesia is needed for children and is usual for adults. The body of the implant is inserted into a niche drilled in the skull behind the ear.

Incision

There are many different incisions used for implant surgery. In general, C-shaped postaural incisions are avoided as there is a risk of poor healing especially in young children and elderly patients.

The following general principles apply: the width of the incision should be at least $2\frac{1}{2}$ times the depth of the incision. Transverse incisions may cause long-term numbness and discomfort in the scalp. The external meatus should be avoided, especially in hear-

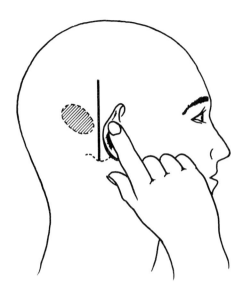

Figure 25.2 The simplest incision for cochlear implant surgery. This incision is suitable for children

ing aid users, as this is a source of infection. The incision should not be within 1 cm of the body of the implant body as it may become painful if the transmitter coil presses into the scar.

The author uses two different incisions. The choice depends on the thickness of the scalp. The simplest is a vertical incision (Gibson, Harrison and Prowse, 1995) which is chosen when it is not necessary to thin the scalp and is suitable for children, most women and some men (Figure 25.2). The vertical incision is placed close behind the attachment of the pinna so that it crosses the mastoid cavity anteriorly where the electrode array should be medially placed. The upper end of the incision extends at least 3 cm above the pinna so that the scalp can be 'bowstringed' backwards to provide adequate exposure of the scalp for the drilling and securing of the receiver/ stimulator package. A step incision of the periosteum is performed about 1 cm posterior to the skin incision to provide greater security against a possible postoperative fistula. The incision is similar to that suggested by Graham, East and Fraser (1989) except that the author does not curve the incision and cuts slightly behind the postauricular crease. The author has used this incision for over 60 children and over 30 adults with no complications to date. The major advantages are the rapid postoperative healing and the lack of any scalp numbness. A minor advantage is the minimal need to shave off any of the hair.

The second incision (Figure 25.3) is required when there is a thicker scalp and there are concerns that the transmitter coil magnet will have difficulty maintaining contact with the buried receiver/stimulator. For this incision, a posteriorly placed limb allows the scalp to be hinged backwards to allow the scalp to be thinned over the position of the receiver/stimulator. Attempts to thin the scalp using a vertical incision often resulted in button-holing the skin. This incision has been used extensively by Cohen (1995, personal communication). The only disadvantage is that adults may complain of scalp numbness above the incision but the complaint is rarely persistently bothersome. It is necessary to shave the hair from a wider area of the scalp than for the vertical incision.

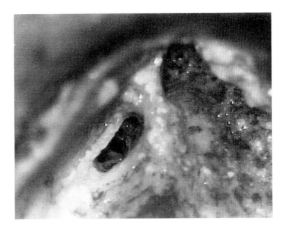

Figure 25.4 The surgeon's view of the posterior tympanotomy. The bone covering the facial nerve and the chorda tympani should be kept intact

The site of exposure should be carefully documented, preferably with photography.

It is usually possible to preserve the chorda tympani nerve. The author routinely exposes this nerve as a guide to the position of the facial nerve.

Exposure of the round window niche usually requires the drilling of a ledge of bone on the medial rim of the posterior tympanotomy which is anterior and medial to the facial nerve. If exposure of the round window niche is still difficult, the angle of viewing can be improved by removing some of the external end of the posterior meatal wall ('a mouse nibble'). It is unnecessary to visualize the entire round window niche as drilling of the anterior lip of the round window niche usually brings the round window membrane nicely into view. In very difficult cases, after locating the position of the round window blindly, using a curved needle, an opening can be made through the promontory into the basal coil.

The cochlea should not be opened until all drilling has finished to prevent fluid and bone chips entering the duct.

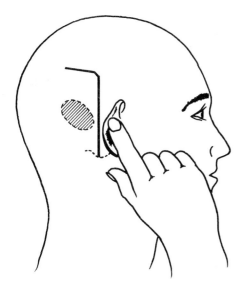

Figure 25.3 The extended incision for cochlear implant surgery allows the scalp to be thinned over the stimulator/receiver

Approach to the middle ear

The cortical mastoidectomy should be fashioned leaving overhanging edges as these are useful for containing the electrode array after insertion. The usual surgical technique of rounding the edges should be avoided.

Most surgeons create a limited posterior tympanotomy through the facial recess leaving the incus and a superior bridge of bone intact (Figure 25.4). The facial nerve should not be exposed and a thin layer of bone should be left covering it. It is extremely hazardous re-operating when previous surgery has exposed the facial nerve. Since change-overs will be needed in the future, as better implants become available, protection of the facial nerve is important.

If the surgeon uncovers the facial nerve sheath, care should be taken to prevent any part of the electrode array becoming adherent to the facial nerve.

Drilling the site of the cochlear implant package

The current Cochlear™ implant is 6 mm in width; it is necessary therefore to expose the dura to get sufficient depth in children to avoid undue pressure on the overlying skin. Future implants will probably be thin enough to make this step unnecessary.

In Sydney, the bone is removed back to the dura at the edge of the device at a right angle but leaving a thin, mobile island of bone covering over the dura in the centre (Scriv's oasis). On revision surgery, it appears that this allows bone to regenerate under the device.

There are several methods of securing the body of the implant in the bony niche. It is very important that the implant lies naturally in position with no tendency to extrude. The author takes some time fashioning the niche to exact proportions so that the implant fits snugly.

Insertion of the electrode array

The round window anatomy must be understood by the surgeon and the basal coil must be identified with certainty (Clifford and Gibson, 1987). The window often lies superiorly in the niche and there is an inferior ridge of bone called the 'crista semilunaris' around which the cochlear duct almost hooks. It is always best to identify the round window, and to even test for the round window reflex by manipulating the stapes.

The main trap which can fool the inexperienced surgeon is when the mastoid is extensively pneumatized and a chain of large air cells lies parallel to the basal coil (the hypotympanic cells). The surgeon should always drill the crista semilunaris and gain a direct view down the basal turn of the cochlea. A micro-drill is essential. The Xomed microdrill, or 'Skeeter drill', is highly recommended. Some surgeons prefer to fashion a cochleostomy through the promontory immediately in front of the round window feeling that this gives a more direct line of access for the electrode array (Gantz, McCabe and Tyler, 1988).

After inserting the electrodes, the monopolar diathermy cannot be used for fear of damaging the implant. Immediately before electrode insertion, the surgeon should check for bleeding vessels and that the skin thickness over the expected implant site is no thicker than 5 mm. If the scalp is thicker it must be thinned to provide adequate stability of the transmitter coil which is attracted magnetically to the receiver/stimulator package. The monopolar is then removed and replaced with bipolar diathermy.

The implant is then given to the surgeon who checks that the body will fit snugly into the drilled out site. The implant array is inserted gently to prevent buckling. After 10–15 electrodes are inserted, the body of the device can be rotated to encourage the passage of the tip around the bend of the cochlea. All active electrodes should be inserted plus a few of the stiffening rings (Figure 25.5). The surgeon should not try to force the electrodes into the cochlea if some active electrodes remain outside. There is no known advantage in inserting extra stiffening rings, but most surgeons will do so should the opportunity arise.

After the implant is positioned, the rest of the electrode lead has to be gently manipulated into the mastoid cavity without the electrodes falling out of the cochlea. It helps considerably if a bony rim has been left behind around the mastoid cavity under which the lead can be placed. The lead should lie naturally with no tendency to extrude. Some surgeons place a special tie, others use an adhesive, to prevent the electrode array extruding from the coch-

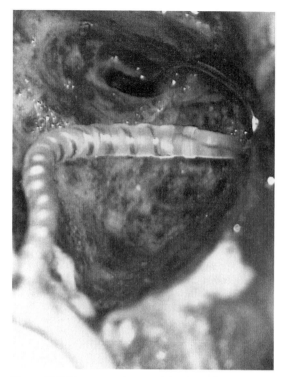

Figure 25.5 The surgeon's view of the electrode array inserted correctly inside the basal turn of the cochlea

lea. The author bends the electrode array so that a stiffening ring rests behind the medial margin of the tympanotomy. Some technique to prevent extrusion is particularly important in very young children because of the anticipated skull growth.

The electrode insertion is then rechecked and the number of stiffening rings outside the cochlea is noted. Usually a photograph is taken for the record, to aid any future surgeon if a revision is needed.

Next, the round window is sealed with copious amounts of muscle, covering the entire electrode array in the middle ear. The posterior tympanotomy and attic also are obliterated with muscle. This should lessen the risk of infection reaching the cochlear implant if the middle ear becomes infected. The electrode lead is kept away from any site where the facial nerve sheath has been exposed.

The wound is closed with clips or removable sutures. Absorbable sutures are not used in children as they can provide a focus for infection. Continuous sutures are also unwise as these may encourage the formation of a haematoma. Surgical drains should *never* be used.

Prophylactic antibiotics are used by most surgeons, even though there is no scientific evidence of benefit (Robinson and Chopra, 1989). The author uses amoxycillin for 7–10 days and erythromycin for patients with a penicillin allergy. The patient usually remains in hospital for 12–24 hours after surgery as it takes a while to recover from the long anaesthetic. Postoperatively the pain is usually related to any surgical trauma to the top of the sternomastoid and this should be kept to a minimum whenever possible. Surprisingly few patients experience any vertigo even when there has been good vestibular function in the implanted ear preoperatively.

Tinnitus is less of a problem than expected. All patients are warned that tinnitus could increase after surgery but this only occurs in 2% of patients. In 76% of patients, tinnitus is either relieved or improved (Gibson, 1992).

Special considerations for very young children

In children under the age of 2 years, special care has to be taken to avoid damaging the facial nerve which may arise quite superficially from the anterior surface of the mastoid bone. The author finds the anterior incision is satisfactory (see Figure 25.2). The skull can be very thin and monopolar diathermy should be used cautiously for fear of burning the intracranial contents. The mastoid can be very small and may still contain marrow cells which bleed. There should be no tendency for the implant body or array to spring laterally as over time this is certain to result in scalp breakdown and device extrusion. As a future update may be required, special care should be taken not to expose the facial nerve. The middle ear should be packed off with muscle or fibrous tissue to isolate the implant from infection should otitis media occur.

Osteogenesis

In most cases this can be predicted from the preoperative CT scan. Total osteogenesis is not a contraindication to using a multiple channel electrode array but the patient should be counselled carefully as a less than optimal result may occur which may preclude the possibility of 'open set' listening. Ears with labyrinthitis ossificans have a higher risk of ganglion cell depletion (Gantz, 1989) and there is a probability that less than 15 functioning electrodes will be available.

If the surgeon finds osteogenesis obstructing the round window niche, he should take careful note of the anatomy and probable course of the basal turn. He should attempt to drill out the new bone without straying outside the cochlea. Drilling too medially may open into the internal auditory meatus. Anteriorly beneath the opening of the eustachian tube is the carotid artery which has a tough sheath making it unlikely to be damaged. Providing the osteogenesis is restricted to the basal coil, it is usually possible eventually to drill out the obstructing bone and insert all or most of the electrode array. The problem arises when the osteogenesis extends around the bend of the basal turn as it is impossible to continue the drilling.

The surgeon may then attempt to insert the electrode through the scala vestibuli by removing the stapes superstructure and drilling into the cochlea anterior and slightly inferior to the anterior crus of the stapes (Steenerson, Gary and Wynens, 1990). On two occasions, the author has found it possible to insert 22 and 17 electrodes through this route.

If both the scala tympani and the scala vestibuli are obstructed, the surgeon can join the two openings together and then develop a cleft in the promontory along the site of the basal coil and under the facial nerve. Usually 15 electrodes can be inserted into this cleft (Aso and Gibson, 1995). The results after partial insertion can be surprisingly good (Cohen and Waltzman, 1993).

Surgery on the discharging ear

It is unwise to attempt cochlear implant surgery on a discharging or infected ear as the infection may spread to the implant package necessitating explantation. Most patients are treated vigorously with aural toilet and antibiotics until the ear is completely clear of infection and stable. If a perforation is present this must be closed preoperatively.

At the time of surgery, many surgeons now advocate blind sac closure of the external meatus to lessen any risk of breakdown at a future date. This is done by removing the tympanic membrane and the medial half of the external meatus. Great care has to be taken to remove all epithelial tissue and the bony margins are usually polished with a burr. The external half of the meatus is then raised and delivered out through the meatus. The middle ear and external meatus are filled with abdominal fat and the meatus is closed by careful suturing.

Surgery on a mastoid cavity

Most surgeons undertake a two-stage procedure. First, the cavity is rendered as free from infection as possible by vigorous preoperative aural toilet and antibiotics. At the first operation, the mastoid cavity is obliterated with fat and a blind sac closure of the external meatus is undertaken. Great care has to be taken to remove all epithelial tissue from the mastoid cavity. The second operation occurs about 4–6 months later. The ear is re-opened and a careful inspection is made for any skin pockets or infection. If the ear is free from any such problems, the surgeon proceeds to insert the cochlear implant in the usual fashion.

Postoperative complications and care

Immediate complications (Table 25.4)

Facial palsy is often the main concern of the patient or the parents. Permanent facial palsy seems to be very rare as the author has discovered no such case on asking many colleagues. Temporary facial palsy can occur either immediately or a few days after

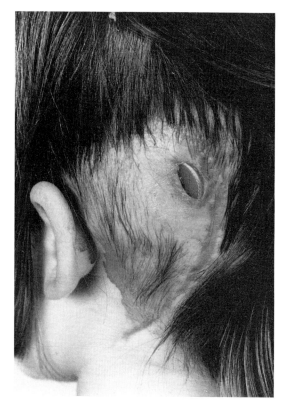

Figure 25.6 Extrusion of a cochlear implant in a young child

surgery in approximately 2% of operations (Cohen, Hoffman and Strascheim, 1988). It appears that a temporary palsy is more likely if the facial sheath has been exposed, especially in the elderly. Temporary facial palsy in children appears to be very rare.

The most serious immediate complications are infection, necrosis of the skin flap, and misplacement of the electrode array. As with any surgical implant, infection must be avoided by meticulous observance of sterility. If infection does occur, intravenous antibiotic therapy will usually rescue the situation. If infection persists, the overlying scalp will breakdown and the implant will extrude (Figure 25.6). If this event is threatened, the implant has to be removed and the tissues rested before re-implantation can be undertaken. The electrode array cannot be removed from the cochlear duct for longer than a few hours without fibrous obliteration resulting. The usual technique is to cut the array as close to the round window as feasible leaving the portion within the cochlea. The intracochlear portion is removed only immediately prior to insertion of the new cochlear implant.

Scalp flap breakdown and necrosis were associated with poorly shaped incisions. Usually these were C-shaped postaural incision and inverted U-shaped flaps with a narrow neck or extended pedicles. Scalp break-

down is more likely to occur in very young children and in the elderly.

Misplacement of the electrode array can occur in ears with extended pneumatization and in ears in which extensive drilling has been required because of labyrinthitis ossificans. If the surgeon has any doubts a simple mastoid X-ray can be performed (Marsh *et al.*, 1993).

The incidence of immediate postoperative complications becomes less as the surgical team becomes more experienced (Gibson, Lam and Scrivener, 1991).

Immediate postoperative care

The following postoperative care is recommended:

The patient receives intravenous antibiotic therapy during surgery and in the immediate postoperative period. The antibiotics are continued orally for 1 week. The wound is inspected for any haematoma formation 12 hours postoperatively and the tight bandaging removed and replaced with a looser dressing. Most patients are discharged the day after surgery. Simple analgesia is offered but rarely needed. The sutures or clips are removed 7 days after surgery and the external auditory meatus checked and cleaned if necessary. Children are usually quarantined for 14 days after surgery. They are kept away from play groups or school and have limited visitors. The initial programming of the implant usually commences 14–28 days after surgery when all swelling over the device has subsided.

Long-term complications (see Table 25.4)

A major concern voiced when cochlear implants were introduced was that long-term electrical stimulation might cause damage to the surviving nerve cells and preclude the use of a more sophisticated device in the future. Animal studies have been quite favourable showing little or no loss of spiral ganglion cells after long periods of electrical stimulation (Hartshorn, Miller and Altschuler, 1991). Human studies over the years have also reduced fears (House and Urban, 1973) and most surgeons now feel that the advantages of early implantation while the child has the necessary remaining plasticity to learn speech and listening, outweigh the concerns.

Some cases of apparent hearing deterioration have been reported after more than 5 years of implant use (Staller *et al.*, 1991). The author has two such cases in over 200 patients, but both patients continue to use the implant successfully.

Some fluctuations in hearing using the device can occur with illness – especially with viral 'flu'. The reason for these fluctuations is unclear, perhaps a neuritis occurs. In some patients, a perilymph fistula has been suspected and the ears may recover after resealing the round window niche. An alternative cause of fluctuation can be related to an abnormal

Table 25.4 Commonest complications of cochlear implant surgery

			Author's series (%) (n = 200)
Immediate	Facial paralysis	permanent	0
		temporary	1.5
	Wound infection	requiring explantation	1.5
		treated without explantation	6.0
	Skin necrosis	using C incision	1
		using other incisions	0
	Misplacement of electrode array		0.5
	Short-term increase in tinnitus		3
Long term	Gradual hearing deterioration		1
	Device failure		1.5
	Extrusion of electrode array		0.5
	Extrusion of implant through scalp		0.5
	Facial nerve twitching on stimulation		3.5
	Progressive partial facial nerve paralysis		0.5
	Long-term balance disturbance		0
	Long-term increased tinnitus		0
	Troublesome numbness of scalp		4
	Troublesome taste disturbance		2
	Non-users: prelingual adults and teenagers ($n = 10$)		50
	postlingual adults ($n = 88$)		1.2

vestibular aqueduct with probable back flow of debris from the endolymphatic sac to the cochlea. In all cases, bedrest is helpful and the use of steroids is yet to be evaluated.

Device breakdown occurs in approximately 1% of the Cochlear™ implant users. Device failure is usually reported by the patient and verified by an integrity test (the electrical output of each of the electrodes is recorded from surface electrodes and displayed using an oscilloscope). If a device fails, it is surgically simple to replace the device providing the facial nerve was not widely exposed at the initial surgery.

Extrusion of the electrode array from the cochlea has been reported but only encountered once by the author in over 200 operations. If the device extrudes it can be difficult to reinsert the array as fibrosis may occur within the cochlea. Under these circumstances it is usually possible to reinsert the device through the scala vestibuli approach.

Extrusion of the body of the implant through the scalp is also very rare (see Figure 25.6). When the implant is placed initially, there should be no tendency for the implant to lift up from the surface of the skull. Using the newer, vertical incision (Figure 25.2), the package is placed into a subperiosteal pocket which is firmly attached at the edges to the underlying scalp.

Facial nerve problems can occur in the long term. The commonest long-term facial nerve problem is twitching of the facial nerve when certain electrodes are activated. This can occur in ears affected by cochlear otosclerosis and some congenitally abnormal otic capsules. The solution is to switch off the offending channels. The author has had one patient gradually develop a partial facial palsy some 4 years after implantation in a congenitally abnormal ear which was found to be due to the tip of the electrode array entering the internal auditory meatus (Birman and Croxson, 1993). Radiological studies should be obtained from any patient who develops any facial twitching or weakness.

Balance problems due to cochlear implant surgery have not been reported which persist long term (Cohen, Hoffman and Strascheim, 1988). The caloric response is rarely lost completely after cochlear implantation. Adults who lose hearing and balance due to infections such as meningitis may suffer some chronic instability but this is not altered by implant surgery. Children compensate well to total bilateral labyrinthine failure.

Numbness or even neuralgia over the scalp can occur if a transverse incision is made above the ear as this will divide the cutaneous nerves. Although it only causes a minor amount of discomfort, the inverted U incision is not recommended because it is particularly likely to cause the problem. Persistent neuralgia may also be experienced in the region of the insertion of the sternomastoid muscle.

Loss of taste can occur if the chorda tympani nerve is divided when the posterior tympanotomy is fashioned. With experience, most implant surgeons can avoid the nerve.

Middle ear infections occur commonly in young children and may occur at any time after implant surgery, immediately postoperatively or much later. The danger of the infection spreading into the tissues around the implant should be recognized. Acute otitis media in the implanted ear requires effective antibiotic therapy without any delay and the antibiotics must be continued for 2 weeks. The situation is analogous to any surgical implant which is threatened by spread of adjacent infection. If the site of the body of the implant becomes tender or fluctuant, the child should be admitted to hospital for intravenous therapy. In Sydney, the parents of implanted children have a specially written information sheet which they can give to their family physician.

A head injury which has caused damage to the implant has been uncommon although the author has one such adult patient. Sports which could damage the implant have to be curtailed. A reasonable approach is to restrict sports activities to those which can be undertaken wearing a wrist-watch.

Non-use of the device should be considered a tragedy in view of all the effort expended by the cochlear implant team, the implantee and his family. Very few if any postlingually deafened people become non-users unless they have had totally unrealistic expectations and have been deaf for many years. The main group of non-users are secondary prelingual candidates who find they are unable to distinguish speech using the device and grow frustrated at their inability to fulfil unrealistic expectations from their family. At present prelingually deaf people over the age of 8 years should only be considered after extensive counselling.

Problems at the 'switch on' of the device

The initial 'switch on' of the cochlear implant is an exciting time for the implantee and all the cochlear implant team. The procedure is usually performed by an audiologist. If there are problems, the otologist is often contacted. The simplest problem is that there is still too much postoperative swelling over the site of the transmitter coil. If the implantee can hear nothing despite lack of any swelling, the following possibilities have to be considered:

1 The electrode array is misplaced. A simple mastoid X-ray should be obtained (Marsh *et al.*, 1993)
2 There is no spiral ganglion cell survival. An implant evoked brain stem potential is extremely helpful
3 In young children, some difficulty may occur in

recognizing the response of the child to hearing sensations.
4 The device is not functioning. An electrode integrity test can be performed

Older prelingually deaf people may complain of a sensation of dizziness or even pain initially and it can take some days before the sensations are accepted as auditory. A delay in perception of cochlear implant stimulation in children with postmeningitic ossified cochleae has been reported (Geier *et al.*, 1993). Often, after a few months, the situation improves.

After the initial 'switch on', the implantee has to return several times to have the 'map'. The map is the stimulation threshold and maximum comfort levels of each of the electrodes. It can take several months before a stable map is achieved which is a problem if the implantee lives far away from the implant centre.

Implant evoked brain stem auditory potentials (IMPEBAP)

Brain stem auditory potentials which have been evoked by stimulating the cochlea electrically through the implant can be very helpful especially in very young children. In Sydney, all the children under the age of 8 years have this test performed under general anaesthesia prior to the behavioural 'switch on' (Brown, Antognelli and Gibson, 1993). The threshold of the implant evoked brain stem auditory potential response appears to correlate reasonably with the behavioural maximum comfort levels.

Electrically elicited stapedius reflex

The stapedius muscle can be observed during surgery. It visibly contracts when the electrode array is stimulated at levels above the comfort settings (Battmer, Laszig and Lehnhardt, 1990). The Hannover cochlear implant group perform testing during surgery and test up to seven electrodes.

Results

The results of cochlear implantation require complex analysis depending on the age and category of the implantee. The otologist should find the following simplified method of reporting results helpful when considering candidates for cochlear implant surgery.

Results in adults

The results for listening are shown in Table 25.5. 'Open set' listening relates to being able to distinguish speech without any contextual clues. There are various methods of testing for 'open set' listening. Table 25.5 is simply based on the Central Institute for the

Table 25.5 Results of implants in adults (%) **(aged 15 years and over)**

	Listening results without lipreading		
	Good open set	*Some open set*	*Closed set only*
Postlingually deaf for less than 15 years (*n* = 64)	29	47	24
Postlingually deaf for over 15 years (*n* = 22)	0	32	68
Prelingually deaf (*n* = 10)	0	0	100

Good open set Central Institute for the Deaf (CID) single word scores over 10%
Some open set CID single word scores 0–10%
Closed set CID score 0%

Deaf (CID) word scores. Good 'open set' listening was when the implantee detected over 10% of single words. Some 'open set' was for scores between 0–10% and 'closed set' relates to detection of sound without any word recognition unless there was a contextual clue. The minimum follow-up period was 4 months.

Adults do continue to improve over time but usually it is clear whether or not they will achieve 'open set' listening after 4 months of implant use. The quality of speech is not mentioned but generally some features improve such as intensity and pitch. Overall speech intelligibility does not alter dramatically. There is one non-user in the author's series who had been totally deaf for over 40 years and became psychoneurotic about the presence of an implant inside her head.

Postlingually deafened adults can be very pleased with 'closed set' listening as it can make lip-reading much easier for them. Prelingually deaf adults do not find 'closed set' listening much help and may be annoyed by everyday sounds. There are five non-users in this group.

Results in children

The results in 54 children are shown in Table 25.6. The minimum follow up for all children is 1 year but many have been followed up for several years.

All the children, especially the primary prelingually deaf group, tend to improve over time and to move to a higher category. Primary prelingual children may take 2–3 years to reach their final category.

The classification is done on the basis of speech intelligibility and listening skills. Language levels are not included as the author finds that this measure is of little help in choosing a candidate.

Category A children are those who achieve listening 'open set' scores of 10% or more on BKB sentences and have a speech phonological deviancy score of 20 points or less on Assessment of Phonological Processes – Revised (APP-R) testing. Some of these children have 'open set' listening scores of over 90%. Category B children have similar 'open set' listening scores but their speech is less intelligible with scores of over 80% on all the subsets of the CID phonetic inventory test. Both category A and category B are able to attend regular schooling.

Category C children have less than 10% 'open set' listening scores. On 'closed set' testing they achieve scores of over 75% (NUCHIPS, MTSP or WIPI (see Appendix 25.1) testing). The speech can be quite variable in this group with a few children achieving quite intelligible speech.

Category D children are the least successful and it is doubtful if they gain any real help from their implants. They have listening scores between chance and 75% on 'closed set' testing and their speech is

Table 25.6 Results of cochlear implants in children using Cochlear MSP processor (%) **(All children with over 15 usable electrodes – aged 1–14 years inclusive at time of implant)**

	A *Open set listening* *Good speech*	*B* *Open set listening* *Average speech*	*C* *Good closed set* *Variable speech*	*D* *Limited closed set* *Limited speech*
Postlingually deafened (6)	83 (5)	0	17 (1)	0
Prelingual: primary (23)	30 (7)	22 (5)	30 (7)	18 (4)
Prelingual: secondary (11)	0	0	27 (3)	73 (8)
Prelingual: change-over (14)	43 (6)	43 (6)	14 (2)	0

Open set and listening criteria explained in text

unintelligible (less than 80% on CID phonetic inventory test). Often their speech is merely single word utterances. With intensive tuition, three secondary prelingual children have now reached category C after 2–3 years of implant use. There are unfortunately three non-users in this group and it is likely that the number of non-users will increase as the children grow older, more independent of their family, and become associated with signing deaf groups.

Conclusions

The cochlear implant will change the outlook for totally deaf and profoundly deaf people. Most postlingually deafened people can return to the hearing world after a cochlear implant. Prelingually deaf children can benefit greatly if they receive a cochlear implant but the neural plasticity of auditory development effectively precludes benefit from older prelingually deaf children who have not been able to utilize audition in their communication. The younger the congenitally deaf child receives audition, the more effective that device becomes in providing usable listening and speech skills.

Although this chapter has concentrated on specific medical and surgical roles, the otologist is advised to read the other chapters on cochlear implants in this book. The cochlear implant will improve greatly over the next decade and will be available even for severely deaf people. It is an important ingredient of the future for otology.

Appendix 25.1

Simple explanation of some specialized tests used to assess children. There are a great number of different tests. The following are the tests used in The Sydney Children's Cochlear Implant programme.

Speech perception tests

The Discrimination After Training test (DAT) (Thielemeir, 1984). This is a closed-set recognition test which primarily tests a child's ability to discriminate the non-segmental aspects (pitch, loudness and duration) of speech. There are 12 levels in the test and for the first 10 levels the child is required to select the stimulus item from a choice of two pictures. At level 11, the choice is one out of three items. At level 12, the choice is one out of four items.

The Monosyllable, Trochee, Spondee, Polysyllable test (MTSP). This test is subtest 3 from the NAL PLOTT test regimen (NAL is the National Acoustic Laboratory, an Australian organization). The MTS test was designed in 1976 by Erber and Alencewicz. The MTSP is a modification of this test (Plant, 1984) which adds the polysyllable testing.

The MTSP test measures a child's ability to:

1 categorize words according to their syllable number and type
2 Identify individual words with syllable categories.

There are three items in each syllable category. The child points to the pictured word pattern perceived.

Word Intelligibility by Picture Identification (WIPI) (Lerman, Ross and McLauchlin, 1965). This is a closed set task which provides a forced choice of between six pictures for each word presented. There are four lists of 25 suitable words. In Sydney, a modification of this test for Australian children was used.

The Northwestern University Children's Perception of Speech test (NUCHIPS) (Elliot and Katz, 1980). This is a closed set task in which the child must select one out of a choice of four pictures depicting single syllable words.

Bamford-Kowal-Bench Sentence test (BKB sentences) (Bench and Bamford, 1979). This is an open set task which measures word perception in sentences. There are 50 key words in 16 sentences. The children are required to repeat, or where possible, write down their responses.

Phonetically Balanced Kindergarten Word List (PBK) (Haskins, 1949). This is an open set test of a child's ability to recognize words of one syllable. The test is scored on words correctly identified and the number of phonemes correctly identified. The child is required to repeat or write down the responses.

Speech production assessment

Assessment of Phonological Processes – Revised (APP-R) (Hodgson, 1986). Although originally designed for the pre-school child, this test is now widely used for older children. It consists of 50 stimulus items and assesses all English consonants at least twice. Thirty one consonant clusters are also assessed, four with three elements. A percentage incorrect score is obtained by totalling the number of errors and dividing by the number of presentations.

CID Phonetic Inventory (Moog, 1988). This assessment provides a quantitative measure of suprasegmental and phonetic aspects of a child's vocalizations/speech. All responses are in imitation of a model presented with live voice by the examiner. The percentage of correctly pronounced vowels, consonants, and other word features is scored.

References

ANDREEV, A. M., GERSUNI, S. V. and VOLOKHOV, A. A. (1934) Electrical stimulation of the hearing organ. *Journal of Physiology*, 17, 546–559

ANSSELIN, A. D. and PETTIGREW, A. G. (1990) Patterns of

functional innervation in the auditory nuclei of the chick brainstem following early unilateral removal of the otocysts. *Developmental Brain Research*, **54**, 177–186

ASO, S. and GIBSON, W. P. R. (1995) Surgical techniques for the insertion of a multi-electrode implant into a postmeningitic ossified cochlea. *American Journal of Otology*, **16**, 210–214

BATTMER, R. D., LASZIG, R. and LEHNHARDT, E. (1990) Electrically elicited stapedius reflex in cochlear implant patients. *Ear and Hearing*, **5**, 370–374

BENCH, R. J. and BAMFORD, J. (1979) *Speech-Hearing Test and Spoken Language of Hearing-Impaired Children*. London: Academic Press

BIRMAN, C. and CROXSON, G. (1993) Delayed palsy, a complication of cochlear implant. *Australian Journal of Otolaryngology*, **1**, 252–254

BROOKHAUSER, P. E., AUSLANDER, M. C. and MESKAN, M. E. (1988) The pattern and stability of postmeningitic hearing loss in children. *Laryngoscope*, **98**, 940–945

BROWN, C., ANTOGNELLI, T. and GIBSON, W. P. R. (1993) Auditory brainstem response evoked by electrical stimulation with a cochlear implant. *Advances in Oto-Rhino-Laryngology*, **48**, 125–129

BUCHWALD, J. S. (1990) Comparison of plasticity in sensory and cognitive processing systems. *Clinical Perinatology*, **17**, 57–66

CLARK, G. M. (1969) Responses of cells in the superior olivary complex of the cat to electrical stimulation of the auditory nerve. *Experimental Neurology*, **24**, 124–136

CLARK, G. M., TONG, Y. C., PATRICK, J. F., SELIGMAN, P. M., CROSBY, P. A., KUZMA, J. A. *et al.* (1984) A multichannel hearing prothesis for profound-to-total hearing loss. *Journal of Medical Engineering and Technology*, **8**, 3–8

CLARK, G. M., BLAMEY, P. J., BROWN, A. M., BUSBY, P. A., DOWELL, R. C. *et al.* (1987) The University of Melbourne/Nucleus multiple electrode cochlear prosthesis. In: *Advances in Oto-Rhino-Laryngology*, edited by C. R. Pfaltz. Basel: Karger. p. 38

CLIFFORD, A. and GIBSON, W. P. R. (1987) The anatomy of the round window with respect to cochlear implant insertion. *Annals of Otology, Rhinology and Laryngology*, Suppl. 128, 17–19

CLOPTON, B. M. and SILVERMAN, M. S. (1978) Changes in latency and duration of neural responding following developmental auditory deprivation. *Experimental Brain Research*, **32**, 39–47

COHEN, N. L. and WALTZMAN, S. B. (1993) Partial insertion of the Nucleus multichannel cochlear implant: technique and results. *American Journal of Otology*, **14**, 357–361

COHEN, N. L., HOFFMAN, R. A. and STRASCHEIM, M. (1988) Medical and surgical complications related to the Nucleus multichannel cochlear implant. *Annals of Otology, Rhinology and Laryngology*, **97**, 8–13

DJOURNO, A. and EYRIÈS, C. (1957) Prosthese auditive par excitation electrique a distance du nerf sensoriel a l'aide d'un bobinage inclus a demeure. *Presse Medicale*, **35**, 14–17

DJOURNO, A., EYRIÈS, C. and VALLANCIEN, B. (1957a) De l'excitation electrique du nerf cochleaire chez l'homme, par induction a distance, a l'aidi d'un micro-bobinage inclus a demeure. *Compte Rendu Societé Biologie (Paris)*, **151**, 423–425

DJOURNO, A., EYRIÈS, C. and VALLANCIEN, B. (1957b) Premiers essais d'excitation electric du nerf auditif chez l'homme, par microappareils inclus a demure. *Bulletin Nationale d'Academie Medicale (Paris)*, **141**, 481–483

ELLIOT, L. L. and KATZ, D. R. (1980) *Northwestrn University Children's Perception of Speech (NUCHIPS)*. St Louis: Auditec

ERBER, N. P. and ALENCEWICZ, C. M. (1976) Audiologic evaluation of deaf children. *Journal of Speech and Hearing Disorders*, **41**, 256–267

FRITSCH, M. H. and SOMMER, A. (1991) *Handbook of Congenital and Early Onset Hearing Loss*. New York and Tokyo: Igaku-Shoin. Ch. 1

GANTZ, M. D. (1989) Issues of candidate selection for a cochlear implant. *Otolaryngologic Clinics of North America*, **22**, 239–247

GANTZ, M. D., MCCABE, B. F. and TYLER, R. S. (1988) Use of multichannel cochlear implants in obstructed and obliterated cochleas. *Otolaryngology, Head and Neck Surgery*, **98**, 72–81

GEIER, L., GILDEN, J., LUETJE, C. M. and MADDOX, H. E. (1993) Delayed perception of cochlear implant stimulation in children with postmeningitic ossified cochleae. *American Journal of Otology*, **14**, 556–561

GIBSON, W. P. R. (1992) The effect of electrical stimulation and cochlear implantation on tinnitus. In: *Tinnitus 91*, edited by J–M. Aran and R. Dauman. Amsterdam and New York: Kugler Publications. pp. 403–408

GIBSON, W. P. R. (1994) The role of electrocochleography in a children's cochlear implant program. In: *Proceedings of the First International Conference on ECoG, OAE and Intraoperative Monitoring*, edited by D. Hoehmann. Amsterdam and New York: I. K. Kugler & Ghedini.

GIBSON, W. P. R., LAM, P. and SCRIVENER, B. (1991) The postoperative complications encountered in 100 cochlear implant surgeries–The Sydney experience. *Journal of the Otolaryngological Society of Australia*, **6**, 399–404

GIBSON, W. P. R., HARRISON, H. C. and PROWSE, C. (1995) A new incision for placement of the 'cochlear' multichannel cochlear implant. *Journal of Laryngology and Otology*, **109**, 821–825

GRAHAM J. M., EAST, C. A. and FRASER, J. G. (1989) UCH/RNID single channel cochlear implant: surgical technique. *Journal of Laryngology and Otology*, Supplement 18, 14–19

HARRISON, R., NAGASAWA, A., SMITH, D. W., STANTON, S. and MOUNT, R. J. (1991) Reorganisation of the auditory cortex after neonatal high frequency cochlear hearing loss. *Hearing Research*, **54**, 11–19

HARTSHORN, D. O., MILLER, J. F. and ALTSCHULER, R. A. (1991) Protective effect of electrical stimulation in the deafened guinea pig cochlea. *Otolaryngology – Head and Neck Surgery*, **104**, 311–319

HASKINS, J. (1949) *Kindergarten Phonetically Balanced Word Lists (PBK)*. St Louis: Auditec

HODGSON, B. W. (1986) *The Assessment of Phonological Processes – Revised*. Austin, Texas: Pro-ed, Inc

HOUSE, W. F. and URBAN, J. (1973) Long term results of electrode implantation and electronic stimulation of the cochlea in man. *Annals of Otology, Rhinology and Laryngology*, **82**, 504–517

HOUSE, W. F., BERLINER, K., CRARY, W., GRAHAM. M., LUCKEY, R., NORTON, N. *et al.* (1976) Cochlear implants. *Annals of Otology, Rhinology and Laryngology*, Supplement 27, 1–93

LARSEN, S. A. and KIRCHHOFF, T. M. (1992) Anatomical evidence of synaptic plasticity in the cochlear nuclei of deaf white cats. *Experimental Neurology*, **115**, 151–157

LASZIG, R., TERWEY, B., BATTMER, R. D. and HESSE, G. (1988) Magnetic resonance imaging (MRI) and high resolution computer tomography (HRCT) in cochlear implant candidates. *Scandanavian Audiology*, Supplement 30, 197–200

LERMAN, J., ROSS, M. and MCLAUCHLIN, R. (1965) A picture-identification test for hearing-impaired children. *Journal of Audiological Research*, 5, 273–278

LESCAO, Y., ROBIER, A., BAULIEU, J. L., BEUTTER, P. and POURCELOT, L. (1993) Perfusion response during electrical stimulation of the auditory nerve in profoundly deaf patients: study with single photon emmision computed tomography. *American Journal of Otology*, 14, 70–73

LOEB, G. E. (1990) Cochlear prosthetics. *Annual Review of Neurosciences*, 13, 357–371

MCCORMICK, B., GIBBIN, K. P., LUTMAN, M. E. and O'DONOGHUE, G. M. (1993) Late partial recovery from meningitic deafness after cochlear implantation: a case study. *American Journal of Otology*, 14, 610–612

MCKAY, C. M. and MCDERMOTT, H. J. (1993) Perceptual performance of subjects with cochlear implants using the spectral maxima sound processor (SMSP) and the Mini Speech Processor (MSP). *Ear and Hearing*, 14, 350–367

MARSH, M. A., XU, J., BLAMEY, P. J., WHITFORD, L. A., XU, S. A., SILVERMAN, J. M. *et al.* (1993) Radiologic evaluation of multichannel intracochlear implant insertion depth. *American Journal of Otology*, 14, 386–391

MICHELSON, R. P. (1968) The crossed cochlea effect. *Transactions of the American Laryngology, Rhinology and Otology Society*, 1, 626–644

MOOG, J. S. (1988) *CID Phonetic Inventory: a Speech Rating for Hearing Impaired Children*. St Louis: Central Institute for the Deaf

MONTANDON, P., KASPER, A. and PELIZZONE, M. (1992) Exploratory cochleotomy: assessment of auditory nerve excitability and anatomical conditions in cochlear implant candidates. *Oto-rhino-laryngology*, 54, 295–298

PHELPS, P. D., ANNIS, A. D. and ROBINSON, P. J. (1990) Imaging for cochlear implants. *British Journal of Radiology*, 63, 512–516

PLANT, G. (1984) A diagnostic speech test for severely and profoundly hearing-impaired children. *Australian Journal of Audiology*, 6, 1–9

RICKARDS, F. W. and CLARK, G. M. (1984) Steady-state evoked potentials to amplitude-modulated tones. In: *Evoked Potentials II*, edited by R. H. Nodar and C. Barber. Boston: Butterworths. pp. 163–168

ROBERTSON, D. and IRVINE, D. R. F. (1989) Plasticity of frequency organization in auditory cortex of guinea pigs with partial unilateral deafness. *Journal of Comparative Neurology*, 282, 456–471

ROBINSON, P. J. and CHOPRA, S. (1989) Antibiotic prophylaxis in cochlear implantation: current practice. *Journal of Laryngology and Otology*, Supplement 18, 20–21

RYALS, B. M., RUBEL, E. W. and LIPPE, W. (1991) Issues in neural plasticity as related to cochlear implants in children. *American Journal of Otology*, Supplement 12, 22–27

SCHWABER, M. K., GARRAGHTY, P. E. and KAAS, J. H. (1993) Neuroplasticity of the adult primate auditory cortex following cochlear hearing loss. *American Journal of Otology*, 14, 252–258

SHALLOP, J. K., ARNDT, P. L. and TURNACLIFF, K. A. (1992) Expanded indications for cochlear implantation: perceptual results in seven adults with residual hearing. *Journal of the Speech and Language Association*, 16, 141-147

SIMMONS, F. B., MONGEON, C. J., LEWIS, W. R. and HUNTINGTON, D. A. (1964) Electrical stimulation of the acoustical nerve and inferior colliculus. *Archives of Otolaryngology*, 79, 559–567

STALLER, S., GIBSON, W. P. R., BEITER, A., CHUTE, P., GOIN, D., PORTMANN, M. *et al.* (1991) Cochlear implants in children: results and complication. In: *Surgery of the Inner Ear*, edited by I. K. Arenberg. Amsterdam and New York: Kugler Publications. pp. 533–536

STEENERSON, R. L., GARY, L. B. and WYNENS, M. S. (1990) Scala vestibuli cochlear implantation for labyrinthine ossification. *American Journal of Otology*, 13, 117–123

THIELEMEIR, M. (1984) *Discrimination After Training Test (DAT) – version 2*. Los Angeles: House Ear Institute.

WEIT, R., PYLE, M., O'CONNOR, A., RUSSEL, E. and SCHRAMM, D. (1990) Computer tomography: how accurate a predictor for cochlear implantation? *Laryngoscope*, 100, 687–692

Volume index